AIRWAY MANAGEMENT
Principles and Practice

AIRWAY MANAGEMENT
Principles and Practice

Edited by

JONATHAN L. BENUMOF, M.D.

Professor of Anesthesiology
University of California at San Diego Medical Center
San Diego, California

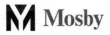 Mosby

St. Louis Baltimore Boston Carlsbad Chicago Naples New York Philadelphia Portland
London Madrid Mexico City Singapore Sydney Tokyo Toronto Wiesbaden

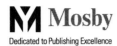

Mosby
Dedicated to Publishing Excellence

A Times Mirror
Company

Acquisition Editor: Susan Gay
Managing Editor: Kathryn H. Falk
Project Manager: Trish Tannian
Editing and Production: Graphic World Publishing Services
Book Design Manager: Gail Morey Hudson
Manufacturing Supervisor: Dave Graybill
Cover Design: Teresa Breckwoldt

Printed in the United States of America
Composition by Graphic World Inc.
Printing/binding by Maple-Vail Book Mfg. Group

Mosby–Year Book, Inc.
11830 Westline Industrial Drive
St. Louis, Missouri 63146

Library of Congress Cataloging in Publication Data

Airway management : principles and practice / edited by Jonathan L. Benumof.
    p.   cm.
    Includes bibliographical references and index.
    ISBN 0-8151-0625-4
    1. Airway (Medicine) 2. Respiratory therapy. 3. Anesthesia.
  4. Trachea—Intubation. I. Benumof, Jonathan, 1942-
    [DNLM: 1. Intubation, Intratracheal. 2. Anesthesia—methods.
  3. Airway Obstruction—etiology. WO 280 A298 1995]
RC735.I5A396 1995
616.2—dc20
DNLM/DLC
for Library of Congress   95-31859
                                          CIP

95 96 97 98 99 / 9 8 7 6 5 4 3 2 1

CONTRIBUTORS

CEDRIC R. BAINTON, M.D.

Professor of Anesthesia
Vice Chairman, Department of Anesthesia
University of California–San Francisco
Chief of Anesthesia, San Francisco General Hospital
San Francisco, California

ANIS BARAKA, M.D, F.R.C. Anaesth (Hon)

Professor and Chairman
Department of Anesthesiology
American University of Beirut
Beirut, Lebanon

ROBERT F. BEDFORD, M.D.

Clinical Professor, Department of Anesthesiology
University of Virginia School of Medicine
Charlottesville, Virginia

JONATHAN L. BENUMOF, M.D.

Professor of Anesthesiology, Department of Anesthesiology
University of California–San Diego
San Diego, California

MICHAEL J. BISHOP, M.D.

Profesor, Department of Anesthesiology
University of Washington School of Medicine
Chief, Anesthesiology/OR Services
Veterans Affairs Medical Center
Seattle, Washington

SUSAN BLASER, M.D., F.R.C.P.C.

Assistant Professor, University of Toronto
Staff Neuroradiologist, Department of Diagnostic Imaging
The Hospital for Sick Children
Toronto, Ontario, Canada

THOMAS F. BOERNER, M.D.

Assistant Professor
Department of Anesthesiology and Critical Care Medicine
University of Pittsburgh School of Medicine
Pittsburgh, Pennsylvania

ROY D. CANE, M.B.B.Ch.

Professor, Department of Anesthesiology
Director, Department of Critical Care Medicine
University of South Florida College of Medicine
Tampa, Florida

ROBERT A. CAPLAN, M.D.

Staff Anesthesiologist, Virginia Mason Medical Center
Clinical Professor, Department of Anesthesia
University of Washington
Seattle, Washington

ROGER S. CICALA, M.D.

Associate Professor, Department of Anesthesiology
Director, Department of Trauma Anesthesia
Presley Trauma Center, University of Tennessee
Memphis, Tennessee

MARY V. CLEMENCY, M.D.

Associate Chief of Anesthesiology
Grady Memorial Hospital
Assistant Professor, Department of Anesthesiology
Emory University School of Medicine
Atlanta, Georgia

NEAL H. COHEN, M.D., M.P.H., M.S., F.C.C.M.

Professor, Department of Anesthesia and Medicine
Vice Chairman, Department of Anesthesia
Director, Department of Critical Care Medicine
President, Medical Staff
University of California–San Francisco
San Francisco, California

RICHARD M. COOPER, B.Sc., M.Sc., M.D., F.R.C.P.C.

Assistant Professor, Department of Anesthesia
The Toronto Hospital
Toronto, Ontario, Canada

SHEILA D. COOPER, M.D.

Assistant Clinical Professor, Department of Anesthesia
University of California at San Diego Medical Center
San Diego, California

EDWARD T. CROSBY, B.Sc., M.D., F.R.C.P.C.

Director, Department of Obstetrical Anaesthesia
Ottawa General Hospital
Associate Professor, Department of Anesthesia
University of Ottawa
Ottawa General Hospital
Ottawa, Ontario, Canada

TERENCE M. DAVIDSON, M.D., F.A.C.S.

Professor, Department of Surgery/Head & Neck Surgery
Associate Dean, Department of Continuing Medical
    Education
University of California
San Diego School of Medicine
Veterans Administration Hospital
San Diego, California

STEPHEN F. DIERDORF, M.D.

Professor, Department of Anesthesia
Indiana University School of Medicine
Indianapolis, Indiana

JOHN V. DONLON, Jr., M.D.

Associate Clinical Professor, Department of Anesthesia
Harvard Medical School
Chief, Department of Anesthesia
Massachusetts Eye and Ear Infirmary
Boston, Massachusetts

THOMAS B. DOUGHERTY, M.D., Ph.D.

Associate Professor, Director of Clinical Research
Department of Anesthesiology and Critical Care
The University of Texas, M.D. Anderson Cancer Center
Houston, Texas

D. JOHN DOYLE, M.D., Ph.D., F.R.C.P.C.

Staff Anaesthetist, Department of Anaesthesia
The Toronto Hospital
Assistant Professor, Department of Anaesthesia
University of Toronto
Toronto, Ontario, Canada

JOYCE DRAKE, M.A.

Director of Health Care Programs
Medic Alert Foundation
Turlock, California

ORLANDO G. FLORETE, Jr., M.D.

Clinical Assistant Professor, Department of Anesthesiology
University of Florida Health Science Center
Jacksonville, Florida

MICHAEL FRASS, M.D.

Professor of Medicine, Head, Intensive Care Unit
Department of Internal Medicine I
University of Vienna
Vienna, Austria

GORDON GIBBY, M.D.

Associate Professor, Department of Anesthesiology and
    Cardiology
University of Florida College of Medicine
Gainesville, Florida

MEDHAT S. HANNALLAH, M.D., F.F.A.R.C.S.

Associate Professor, Department of Anesthesia
Georgetown University Medical Center
Washington, DC

STEPHEN J. HERMAN, M.D., F.R.C.P.C.

Associate Professor, Department of Medical Imaging
The University of Toronto
Associate Professor, Department of Radiology
The Toronto Hospital
Toronto, Ontario, Canada

ORLANDO RICARDO HUNG, B.Sc. (Pharm), M.D., F.R.C.P.(C)

Associate Professor, Department of Anesthesia
Assistant Professor, Department of Pharmacology
Dalhousie University
Halifax, Nova Scotia, Canada

GIRISH P. JOSHI, M.B.B.S., M.D., F.F.A.R.C.S.I.

Assistant Professor, Department of Anesthesiology and Pain
    Management
The University of Texas Southwestern Medical School
Dallas, Texas

M. ANNE KELLER, M.D., F.R.C.P.C.

Assistant Professor, Department of Medical Imaging
The University of Toronto
Assistant Professor, Department of Radiology
The Toronto Hospital
Toronto, Ontario, Canada

HAE K. KIL, M.D., M.S.

Assistant Professor, Department of Anesthesiology
Yonsei University College of Medicine
Seoul, Korea

LETTY M.P. LIU, M.D.

Associate Profesor, Department of Anesthesia
Harvard Medical School
Anesthetist, Department of Anesthesia
Massachusetts General Hospital
Boston, Massachusetts

PHIL LIU, M.D.

Associate Professor, Department of Anesthesiology
University of California, Irvine
Orange, California

ANTHONY E. MAGIT, M.D., F.A.A.P.

Assistant Professor/Head and Neck Surgery
Department of Surgery, University of California
San Diego School of Medicine
San Diego, California

S. RAO MALLAMPATI, M.D.

Assistant Professor, Department of Anesthesiology
Harvard Medical School
Brigham and Women's Hospital
Boston, Massachusetts

LYNETTE MARK, M.D.

Assistant Professor, Department of Anesthesiology and
    Critical Care Medicine
Department of Otolaryngology-Head and Neck Surgery
The Johns Hopkins Medical Institutions
Baltimore, Maryland

JOHN P. McGEE II, M.S., M.D.

Assistant Professor of Clinical Anesthesia
Northwestern University Medical School
Chicago, Illinois
Senior Attending, Department of Anesthesia
Evanston Hospital
Evanston, Illinois

RICHARD J. MELKER, M.S., M.D., Ph.D.

Associate Professor
Department of Anesthesiology and Pediatrics
University of Florida College of Medicine
Gainesville, Florida

DEBRA E. MORRISON, M.D.

Assistant Clinical Professor
Department of Anesthesiology
University of California, Irvine
Orange, California

**MICHAEL F. MURPHY, M.D., F.R.C.P.C. (Anes),
F.R.C.P.C. (Em)**

Clinical Chief, Department of Emergency Medicine
Chedoke McMaster Hospitals
McMaster University Hospital
Hamilton, Ontario, Canada

JOHN F. NOLAN. M.D.

Fellow, Department of Anesthesiology/Critical Care
University of South Florida College of Medicine
Tampa, Florida

KEVIN O'GRADY, B.A.Sc., M.H.Sc.

Institute of Biomedical Engineering
University of Toronto
Toronto, Ontario, Canada

ANDRANIK OVASSAPIAN, M.D.

Professor, Department of Anesthesia
Northwestern University
Chief, Department of Anesthesia Service
V.A. Lakeside Medical Center
Chicago, Illinois

VINCENTE PALLARES, M.D.

Professor of Anesthesia
Department of Anesthesiology
University of Miami Medical School
Miami, Florida

KAREN L. POSNER, Ph.D.

Research Assistant Professor
Department of Anesthesiology
Adjunct Research Assistant Professor
Department of Anthropology
University of Washington
Seattle, Washington

MARC DECKER POSNER, M.D.

Resident
Department of Medicine
Louis A. Weiss Memorial Hospital
University of Chicago
Chicago, Illinois

SIVAM RAMANATHAN, M.D.

Chief, Department of Anesthesiology
Magee-Women's Hospital
Professor, Department of Anesthesiology
University of Pittsburgh School of Medicine
Pittsburgh, Pennsylvania

JALIL RIAZI, M.D.

Associate Clinical Professor and Vice Chair
Director of Pediatric Anesthesia
Department of Anesthesiology
UCI Medical Center
Orange, California

M. RAMEZ SALEM, M.D.

Chairman, Department of Anesthesiology
Illinois Masonic Medical Center
Clinical Professor, Department of Anesthesiology
University of Illinois College of Medicine
Chicago, Illinois

ANTONIO SANCHEZ, M.D.

Associate Clinical Professor, Department of Anesthesiology
University of California, Irvine
Orange, California

ALAN N. SANDLER, M.B., Ch.B., F.R.C.P.C.

Associate Professor, Department of Anaesthesia
University of Toronto
Anaesthetist-in-Chief, Department of Anaesthesia
The Toronto Hospital
Toronto, Ontario, Canada

JAMES SCHAUBLE, M.D.

Associate Professor
Department of Anesthesiology and Critical Care Medicine
Johns Hopkins Hospital
Baltimore, Maryland

DAVID E. SCHWARTZ, M.D., F.C.C.M.

Associate Professor, Department of Anesthesiology
University of Illinois
Chicago, Illinois

GEORGE J. SHEPLOCK, M.D.

Assistant Clinical Professor
Department of Anesthesia
Indiana University School of Medicine
Indianapolis, Indiana
Center Associate
Center for Excellence in Education
Indiana University
Bloomington, Indiana

IAN SMITH, B.Sc., M.B., B.S., F.R.C.A.

Senior Lecturer in Anaesthesia
Keele University
North Staffordshire Hospitals
Stoke on Trent, United Kingdom

MITCHEL B. SOSIS, M.D., Ph.D.

Assistant Professor, Department of Anesthesiology
Rush Medical College
Chicago, Illinois

RONALD D. STEWART, O.C., M.D., F.A.C.E.P., F.R.C.P.C., D.Sc. (Hon)

Professor of Anaesthesia, Department of Emergency
    Medicine
Dalhousie University
Minister of Health
Province of Nova Scotia
Halifax, Nova Scotia, Canada

ROBERT K. STOELTING, M.D.

Professor and Chair, Department of Anesthesia
Indiana University School of Medicine
Indianapolis, Indiana

JOHAN P. SUYDERHOUD, M.D.

Assistant Professor, Department of Anesthesia
Georgetown University Medical Center
Washington, DC

MARK D. TASCH, M.D.

Associate Professor, Department of Anesthesia
Indiana University School of Medicine
Indianapolis, Indiana

NARENDRA S. TRIVEDI, M.D.

Associate Clinical Professor
Department of Anesthesiology
University of California, Irvine
Orange, California

SUSAN TURLEY, M.A. (Educ.), R.N.

Independent Consultant
Words Plus
Ellicott City, Maryland

JEFFREY S. VENDER, M.D., F.C.C.M.

Professor, Department of Anesthesiology
Northwestern University Medical School
Chief, Department of Anesthesia
Director, Medical-Surgical ICU
Evanston Hospital
Evanston, Illinois

DAVID O. WARNER, M.D.

Associate Professor, Department of Anesthesiology
Mayo Medical School
Consultant, Department of Anesthesiology, Mayo Clinic
Mayo Clinic and Foundation
Rochester, Minnesota

CHARLES B. WATSON, M.D., F.C.C.M.

Chairman, Department of Anesthesia
Co-Director, SICU
Clinical Associate Professor, Department of Anesthesiology
Bridgeport Hospital
University of Connecticut
Bridgeport, Connecticut

MELISSA WHEELER

Assistant Professor, Department of Anesthesia
Children's Memorial Hospital
Chicago, Illinois

PAUL F. WHITE, Ph.D., M.D.

Professor, Holder of Margaret Milam McDermott Chair
Department of Anesthesiology and Pain Management
University of Texas Southwestern Medical Center
Dallas, Texas

TO ALL THOSE WHO HAVE
STRUGGLED WITH A PATIENT'S AIRWAY
AND
TO MY FAMILY WHO HAVE
GREATLY HELPED ME WIN ALL MY STRUGGLES

PREFACE

Complications related to airway management are frequent and very often severe; taking the area under-the-curve approach (frequency times severity) it is widely accepted that for the last two decades, and at the present time, airway complications were and are the most serious and significant negative medical outcome facing the anesthesia community. It is also widely accepted that if one could give enough forethought and planning to the management of the airway of any given patient, then the vast majority of airway complications/problems could be avoided/solved. The goal and purpose of this book is to encompass and clearly present the knowledge and forethought that will allow the clinician to avoid airway complications and solve airway problems.

The body of knowledge that allows one to think well about airway management has several components. First, one needs to have a good clinical science knowledge base (Part I: Basic Clinical Science Considerations). Second, one must be able to recognize an airway problem and have a good conceptual framework (i.e., the American Society of Anesthesiologists Difficult Airway Algorithm) in which to place the problem (Part II). Third, one must be adept with a broad armamentarium of airway techniques in order to effectively administer the plan (Part III). Fourth, one must fully understand all the clinical situations in which airway problems are particularly likely to occur in order to choose the best techniques to solve the problem (Part IV). Finally, we must effectively teach those that follow us not to repeat our past mistakes but rather to profit from the best knowledge and forethought of today and to establish educational mechanisms that will ensure continuing growth and success in the broad, across-many-disciplines, specialty of airway management.

Jonathan L. Benumof

CONTENTS

PART I

BASIC CLINICAL SCIENCE CONSIDERATIONS

Chapter 1

FUNCTIONAL ANATOMY OF THE AIRWAY

Thomas F. Boerner
Sivam Ramanathan

I. INTRODUCTION

The air passages starting from the nose and ending at the bronchioles are vital to the delivery of respiratory gas to and from the alveoli. During clinical anesthesia, the anesthesiologist uses these air passages to deliver the anesthetic gases to the alveoli while, at the same time, maintaining vital respiratory gas transport. To accomplish proper airway management, the anesthesiologists often gain access to the airways by means of an endotracheal tube or other devices that are directly introduced into the patient's upper or lower air passages. In addition, the anesthesiologists are called upon to establish access to the airways in certain cases of dire emergencies. For the purpose of description, the airway is divided into the upper airway, which extends from the nose to the glottis, and the lower airway, which includes the trachea, the bronchi, and the subdivisions of the bronchi. The airways also serve other important functions such as olfaction, deglutition, and phonation. A detailed anatomic description of these structures is beyond the scope of this chapter. Structural details as they relate to function in health and disease will be described.

II. THE UPPER AIRWAY

A. THE NOSE

The airway functionally begins at the nares and the mouth where air first enters the body. Phylogenetically, breathing was intended to occur through the nose. This arrangement enables the animal not only to smell danger but permits uninterrupted conditioning of the inspired air while feeding. However, during exercise or respiratory distress, mouth breathing occurs to facili-

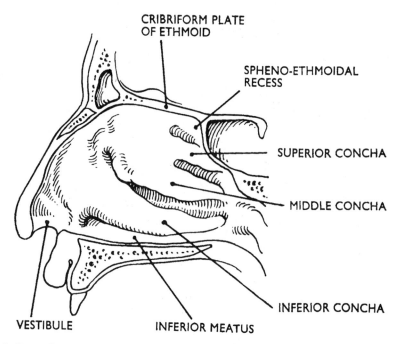

Fig. 1-1. Lateral wall of right nasal cavity. Conchae are also known as turbinate bones. Sphenoid sinus opens into the sphenoethmoidal recess. Frontal, maxillary, and ethmoidal sinuses open into meatuses of the nose. (From Ellis H, Feldman S: *Anatomy for anaesthetists,* ed 6, Oxford, 1993, Blackwell Scientific.)

tate decreased airway resistance and increased airflow.

The nose serves two functions: respiratory and olfactory. In the adult human, the two nasal fossae extend 10 to 14 cm from the nostrils to the nasopharynx. The two fossae are divided mainly by a midline quadrilateral cartilaginous septum together with the two extreme medial portions of the lateral cartilages. Each fossa is convoluted and provides approximately 60 cm^2 surface area per side for warming and humidifying the inspired air.[1] The nasal fossa is bounded laterally by inferior, middle, and superior turbinate bones (conchae),[2] which divide the fossa into scroll-like spaces called the inferior, middle, and superior meatuses (Fig. 1-1).[1,3,4] The inferior turbinate usually limits the size of the nasotracheal tube that can be passed through the nose. The vascular mucous membrane overlying the turbinates can be damaged easily, leading to profuse hemorrhage. The paranasal sinuses, which comprise the sphenoid, ethmoid, maxillary and frontal sinuses open into the lateral wall of the nose.

The olfactory portion of the nasal fossa consists of the middle and upper septum and the superior turbinate bone; the respiratory portion consists of the rest of the nasal fossa.[3] The respiratory mucous membrane consists of ciliated columnar cells and the goblet cells. The olfactory mucous membrane contains the nonciliated supporting cells and the olfactory cells. The olfactory cells have specialized hairlike processes, called the olfactory hair, innervated by the olfactory nerve.[3] The nonolfactory sensory nerve supply to the nasal mucosa is derived from the first two divisions of the trigeminal nerve. The parasympathetic autonomic nerves reach the mucosa from the facial nerve after relay through the sphenopalatine ganglion, and sympathetic fibers are derived from the plexus surrounding the internal carotid artery via the vidian nerve.[5]

Approximately 10,000 L of ambient air passes through the nasal airway per day, and 1 L of moisture is added to this air in the process.[6] The moisture is derived partly from transudation of fluid through the mucosal epithelium and from secretions produced by glands and goblet cells. These secretions have significant bacteriocidal properties. Foreign body invasion is further minimized by the stiff hairs (vibrissae), the ciliated epithelium, and the extensive lymphatic drainage of the area.

A series of complex autonomic reflexes controls the blood supply to the nasal mucosa and allows it to shrink and swell quickly. Reflex arcs also connect this area with other parts of the body. For example, the Kratschmer reflex leads to bronchiolar constriction upon stimulation of the anterior nasal septum in animals. A demonstration of this reflex may be seen in the postoperative period when a patient becomes agitated when the nasal passage is packed.[5]

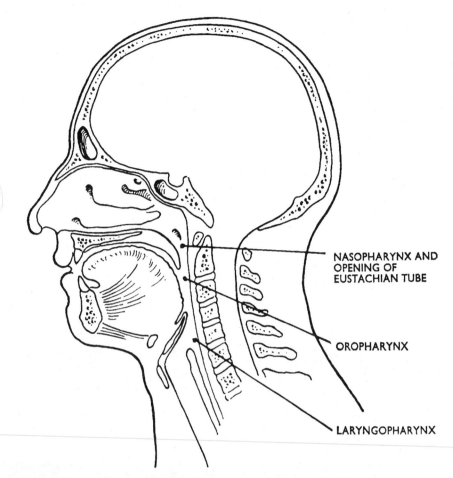

NASOPHARYNX AND
OPENING OF
EUSTACHIAN TUBE

OROPHARYNX

LARYNGOPHARYNX

Fig. 1-2. Diagrammatic representation of a sagittal section through head and neck to show divisions of the pharynx. Laryngopharynx is also known as the hypopharynx. (From Ellis H, Feldman S: *Anatomy for anaesthetists,* ed 6, Oxford, 1993, Blackwell Scientific.)

B. THE PHARYNX

The nasopharynx lies posterior to the termination of the turbinates and nasal septum and extends to the soft palate.[1] The eustachian tubes open into the lateral walls of the nasopharynx. The oropharynx starts below the soft palate and extends to the hyoid bone. In the lateral walls of the oropharynx are situated the tonsillar pillars of the fauces. The anterior pillar contains the glossopharyngeus muscle and the posterior pillar, the palatoglossus muscle.[7] The hypopharynx lies behind the larynx and is also called the laryngopharynx (Fig. 1-2). The pharynx is surrounded by two layers of muscles, an external and an internal. The stylopharyngeus, the salpingopharyngeus, and the palatopharyngeus form the internal layer. They elevate the pharynx during deglutition. The superior, middle, and inferior constrictors form the external layer, and they advance the food into the esophagus.

The constrictors are innervated by filaments arising out of the pharyngeal plexus (formed by motor and sensory branches from the vagus and the glossopharyngeal nerves). The inferior constrictor is additionally innervated by branches from recurrent laryngeal and external laryngeal nerves. The internal layer is innervated by the glossopharyngeal nerve.

1. The pharynx and defense against pathogens

Inhaled particles of size greater than 10 μ are removed by inertial impaction upon the posterior nasopharynx. In addition, the inhaled airstream changes direction sharply at 90 degrees at the nasopharynx, thus causing some loss of momentum of the suspended particles. Being unable to remain suspended, the particles are trapped by the pharyngeal walls. The impacted particles are trapped by the circularly arrayed lymphoid tissue known as the ring of Waldeyer (Fig. 1-3). The ring includes the two large palatine tonsils, the lingular tonsils, the eustachian tonsil, and the nasopharyngeal tonsil (adenoids, Fig. 1-3).[8,9] These structures occasionally impede the passage of endotracheal tubes, especially

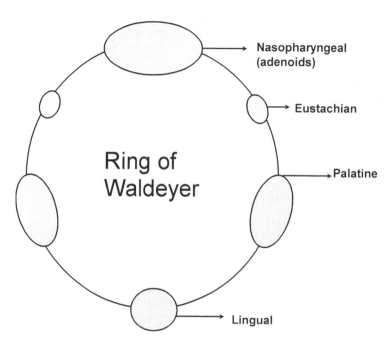

Fig. 1-3. Ring of Waldeyer, a collection of lymphoid tissue that guards against pathogen invasion. (From Hodder Headline PLC, London.)

if they are infected and enlarged. In addition, sepsis originating from one of the numerous lymphoid aggregates may lead to a retropharyngeal or peritonsillar abscess, which indeed poses anesthetic challenges.[5]

2. The pharynx and upper airway obstruction

a. SEDATION AND ANESTHESIA

The pharynx is the common pathway for food and the respiratory gases. Patency of pharynx is vital to the patency of the airway and a proper gas exchange. Decrease in the size of the pharynx can lead to airway obstruction. It is usually believed that upper airway obstruction occurs in sedated or anesthetized patients (without an endotracheal tube) as a result of the tongue falling back onto the posterior pharyngeal wall. With the aid of magnetic resonance imaging (MRI), Shorten et al.[10] have shown that, during general anesthesia or intravenous sedation, airway obstruction occurs as a result of decrease in the anteroposterior diameter of the pharynx at the level of the soft palate and epiglottis and not as a result of the dorsum of the tongue coming into contact with the posterior pharyngeal wall (Fig. 1-4).

b. OBSTRUCTIVE SLEEP APNEA

The reduction in the size of the pharynx is also a factor in the development of respiratory obstruction in patients with obstructive sleep apnea (OSA).[11] This problem has recently been studied using MRI. Nasal continuous positive airway pressure (nasal CPAP) has been found to be effective in treating airway obstruction in these patients. The major defect appears to be

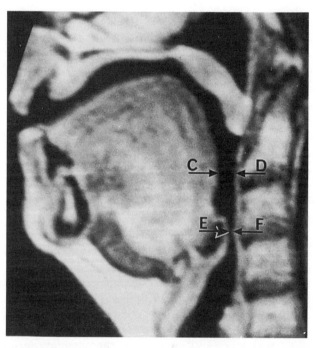

Fig. 1-4. Medial sagittal view of upper airway showing site of airway obstruction in sedated patients. Soft palate is in contact with the posterior pharyngeal wall. *CD,* Minimum anteroposterior diameter at level of tongue; *EF,* minimum anteroposterior diameter at level of epiglottis. (From Shorten GD, Opie NJ, Graziotti P: *Anaesth Intensive Care* 22:165, 1994.)

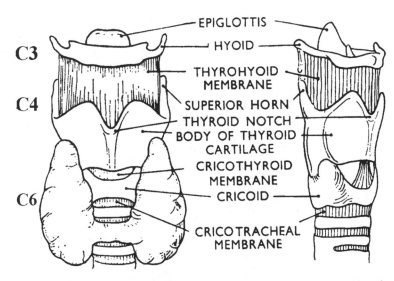

Fig. 1-5. External frontal *(left)* and anterolateral *(right)* views of the larynx. Note location of cricothyroid membrane and thyroid gland in relation to thyroid and cricoid cartilage in the frontal view. Horn of the thyroid cartilage is also known as the cornu. In the anterolateral lateral view, the shape of the cricoid cartilage and its relation to thyroid cartilage is shown. (From Ellis H, Feldman S: *Anatomy for anaesthetists,* ed 6, Oxford, 1993, Blackwell Scientific.)

reduced size of the oropharynx.[12] The loss of activity in the pharyngeal dilator, the genioglossus (GG) muscle appears to bring about this pharyngeal collapse during sleep.[13] Patients prone to OSA appear to have increased activity in the basal GG activity in the electromyogram. Any loss of tone in this muscle during sleep is likely to cause a pharyngeal collapse. The application of nasal CPAP appears to increase the volume and also the cross-sectional area of the oropharynx by reducing the water content of the pharyngeal tissues.[12]

It must be stressed, however, that decrease in pharyngeal size as a predisposing factor to the development of OSA is not universally supported.[11] Measurements of differential pressures across the palate and the hypopharynx show that the site of airway obstruction occurs either at the level of the palate or at the level of the hypopharynx,[11] and the site of obstruction is specific in a given subject.[11] It must be noted, however, that, although the obstruction occurs at a specific site, it might extend downwards, as the inspiratory suction pressure further extends the collapse.[11]

C. THE LARYNX

The larynx, which lies in the adult neck opposite the third through sixth cervical vertebrae,[7] is situated at the crossroads between the food and air passages (or conduits). It acts as a "watchdog," allowing passage only to air and preventing secretions and food from entering the trachea. In addition, it functions as the organ of phonation. The larynx may be somewhat higher in females and children. Until puberty, no differences in the laryngeal sizes exist between males and females. At

puberty, the male larynx develops more rapidly than that of the female. The female larynx is smaller and more cephalad.[7] Most larynges develop somewhat assymetrically.[14] The inlet to the larynx is bounded anteriorly by the upper edge of the epiglottis, posteriorly by a fold of mucous membrane stretched between the two arytenoid cartilages, and laterally by the aryepiglottic folds.[5]

1. The bone of the larynx

The hyoid bone suspends and anchors the larynx during respiratory and phonatory movement. This sesamoid bone is horseshoe shaped. It is attached to the temporal bone by the stylohyoid ligament and to the thyroid cartilage by the thyrohyoid membrane and muscle. Intrinsic tongue muscles originate on the hyoid, and the pharyngeal constrictors are attached here as well.[1,7,15]

2. The cartilages of the larynx

Cartilages provide the framework of the larynx (Figs. 1-5 and 1-6). The laryngeal cartilages are the unpaired epiglottis, thyroid and cricoid, and the paired arytenoids, corniculates and cuneiforms. They are connected and supported by membranes, synovial joints, and ligaments. The ligaments, when covered by mucous membranes, are called the folds.

a. THE THYROID CARTILAGE

The thyroid cartilage, the largest structure in the larynx, acquires its shieldlike shape from the embryological midline fusion of the two distinct quadrilateral laminae.[16] In females, the sides join at approximately 120 degrees, and in males it is closer to 90 degrees. This

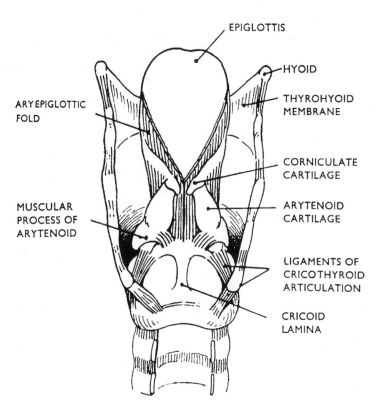

Fig. 1-6. Cartilages and ligaments of the larynx seen posteriorly. Note location of the corniculate cartilage within the aryepiglottic fold. (From Ellis H, Feldman S: *Anatomy for anaesthetists*, ed 6, Oxford, 1993, Blackwell Scientific.)

smaller thyroid angle explains the greater laryngeal prominence in males (the "Adam's apple"), the longer vocal cords, and the lower-pitched voice.[17] The thyroid notch lies in the midline at the top of the fusion site of the two laminae.[18] On the inner side of this fusion line are attached the vestibular ligaments and, below them, the vocal ligaments (Fig. 1-7). The superior (greater) and inferior (lesser) cornu of the thyroid are the slender, posteriorly directed extensions of the edges of the lamina. The lateral thyrohyoid ligament is attached to the superior cornu, and the cricoid cartilage articulates with the inferior cornu.

b. THE CRICOID CARTILAGE

The cricoid cartilage represents the anatomic lower limit of the larynx and helps support it.[16] The cricoid is shaped like a signet ring, with the signet part, or lamina, rising posteriorly.[19] The cricoid is the only complete cartilaginous ring in the upper airway.[16] The tracheal rings connect to the cricoid by ligaments and muscles. The cricoid lamina has ball and socket synovial articulations, with the arytenoids posterosuperiorly and the thyroid cartilage more inferolaterally and anteriorly.[16] It also attaches to the thyroid cartilage by the cricothyroid membrane, a relatively avascular and easily palpated landmark in most adults. The cricothyroid membrane can provide surgical access to the airway via transtracheal jet ventilation or surgical cricothyroidotomy.

c. THE ARYTENOIDS

The two light arytenoid cartilages are shaped like three-sided pyramids, and they lie in the posterior aspect of the larynx.[20] The arytenoid's medial surface is flat and covered with only a firm, tight layer of mucoperichondrium.[21] The base of the arytenoid is concave and articulates by a true synovial ball and socket joint with the posterosuperior lamina of the cricoid cartilage.

The lateral extension of the arytenoid base is called the muscular process. Important intrinsic laryngeal muscles originate here. The medial extension of the arytenoid base is called the vocal process. Vocal ligaments, the bases of the true vocal folds, extend from the vocal process to the midline of the inner surface of the thyroid lamina (Fig. 1-7). The fibrous membrane that connects the vocal ligament to the thyroid cartilage actually penetrates the body of the thyroid. This membrane is called the Broyles' ligament.[16] This ligament contains lymphatics and blood vessels and therefore can act as an avenue for extension of laryngeal cancer outside the larynx.[21,22] The relationship between the anterior commissure of the larynx and the inner aspect of the thyroid cartilage is important to laryngeal surgeons, for they perform thyroplasties and supraglottic laryngectomies based on its location. A study on cadavers reported that the anterior commissure of the larynx can usually be found above the midpoint of the

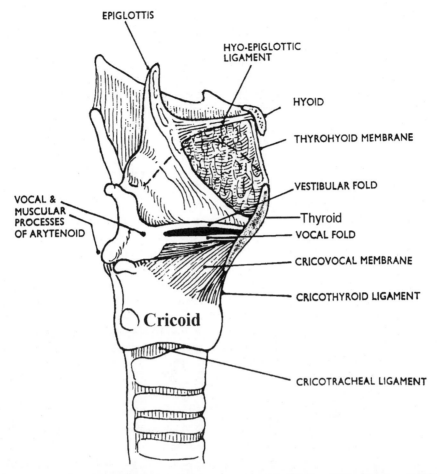

EPIGLOTTIS

HYO-EPIGLOTTIC
LIGAMENT

HYOID

THYROHYOID MEMBRANE

VESTIBULAR FOLD

VOCAL &
MUSCULAR
PROCESSES
OF ARYTENOID

Thyroid

VOCAL FOLD

CRICOVOCAL MEMBRANE

CRICOTHYROID LIGAMENT

Cricoid

CRICOTRACHEAL LIGAMENT

Fig. 1-7. Sagittal *(lateral)* view of the larynx. Vocal and vestibular folds and thyroepiglottic ligament attach to midline of inner surface of the thyroid cartilage. Also note relationship between cricovocal membrane to vocal folds. (Modified from Ellis H, Feldman S: *Anatomy for anaesthetists,* ed 6, Oxford, 1993, Blackwell Scientific.)

vertical midline fusion of the thyroid cartilage ala.[21,23]

d. THE EPIGLOTTIS

The epiglottis is considered to be vestigial by many authorities.[24] Composed primarily of fibroelastic cartilage, the epiglottis does not ossify and maintains some flexibility throughout life.[16,20,25] It is shaped like a leaf or a tear and is found between the larynx and the base of the tongue (Fig. 1-6).[15,21] The upper border of the epiglottis is attached by its narrow tip, or petiolus, to the midline of the thyroid cartilage by the thyroepiglottic ligament (Figs. 1-7 and 1-8). The hyoepiglottic ligament connects the epiglottis to the back of the body of the hyoid bone.[17,26] The mucous membrane that covers the anterior aspect of the epiglottis sweeps forward to the tongue as the median glossoepiglottic fold and to the pharynx as the paired lateral pharyngoepiglottic folds.[16] The pouchlike areas found between the median and lateral folds are the valleculae. The tip of a properly placed Macintosh laryngoscope blade rests in this area. The vallecula is a common site of impaction of foreign bodies, such as fish bones, in the upper airway.

e. THE CUNEIFORM AND THE CORNICULATE CARTILAGES

The epiglottis is connected to the arytenoid cartilages via the laterally placed aryepiglottic ligaments and folds (Fig. 1-6). Two sets of paired fibroelastic cartilages are embedded in each aryepiglottic fold.[20] The sesamoid cuneiform cartilage is roughly cylindrical and lies anterosuperior to the corniculate in the fold. The cuneiform may be seen laryngoscopically as a whitish elevation through the mucosa. The corniculate is a small triangular object visible directly over the arytenoid cartilage (Fig. 1-8). The cuneiform and corniculate cartilage reinforce and support the aryepiglottic folds[16,21] and may help the arytenoids to move.[7,25]

f. THE FALSE AND TRUE VOCAL CORDS

The thyrohyoid membrane (Figs. 1-6 to 1-8), attaching the superior edge of the thyroid cartilage to the hyoid bone, provides cranial support and suspension.[7] It is separated from the hyoid body by a bursa that facilitates movement of the larynx during deglutition.[21] The thicker median section of the thyrohyoid membrane is the thyrohyoid ligament, and its thinner lateral edges are pierced by the internal branches of the superior laryngeal nerves.

Beneath the laryngeal mucosa is a fibrous sheet containing many elastic fibers, the fibroelastic membrane of the larynx. Its upper area, the quadrangular membrane, extends in the aryepiglottic fold between the arytenoids and the epiglottis. The lower, free border of the membrane is called the vestibular ligament and forms the vestibular folds, or false cords (Figs. 1-7 and 1-8).[15,17,20]

The cricothyroid membrane joins the cricoid and thyroid cartilages. The thickened median area of this fibrous tissue, the "conus elasticus," extends up inside the thyroid lamina to the anterior commissure and continues and blends with the vocal ligament. The cricothyroid ligament thus connects the cricoid, thyroid, and arytenoid cartilages.[17,20] The thickened inner edges of the cricothyroid ligament, called the vocal ligament, forms the basis of the true vocal folds (Fig. 1-7).[7,21]

g. THE LARYNGEAL CAVITY

The laryngeal cavity (Fig. 1-9) extends from the laryngeal inlet to the lower border of the cricoid cartilage. Viewed laryngoscopically from above, two paired inward projections of tissue are visible in the laryngeal cavity (Fig. 1-8): the superiorly placed vestibular folds, or false cords, and the more inferiorly placed vocal folds, or true vocal cords (Figs. 1-7 to 1-9). The

space between the true cords is called the rima glottidis, or the glottis (Fig. 1-8). The glottis is divided into two parts. The anterior, intermembranous section is situated between the two vocal folds. The two vocal folds meet at the anterior commissure of the larynx (Fig. 1-8). The posterior intercartilaginous part passes between the two arytenoid cartilages and the mucosa stretching between them in the midline posteriorly, forming the posterior commissure of the larynx (Fig. 1-8).[17]

The area extending from the laryngeal inlet to the vestibular folds is known as the vestibule or supraglottic larynx (Fig. 1-9). The laryngeal space from the free border of the cords to the inferior border of the cricoid is called the subglottic, or infraglottic, larynx. The region between the vestibular folds and the vocal cords is termed the ventricle, or the sinus. The ventricle may expand anterolaterally to a pouchlike area with many lubricating mucous glands called the laryngeal saccule (Fig. 1-9).[16] The saccule is believed to help in voice resonance in apes.[21,24] The pyriform sinus lies laterally to the aryepiglottic fold within the inner surface of the thyroid cartilage (Fig. 1-8).[21]

The epithelium of the vestibular folds is the ciliated, pseudostratified variety (respiratory type), whereas the epithelium of the vocal folds is the nonkeratinized squamous type.[21] Thus, the entire interior of the larynx is covered with respiratory epithelium except the vocal folds.[5]

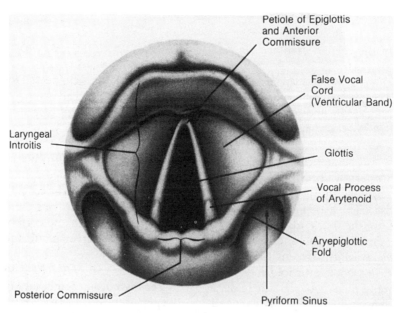

Fig. 1-8. Larynx viewed from above with a laryngeal mirror. Note location of the anterior and posterior commissures of the larynx and the aryepiglottic fold. Elevations in the aryepiglottic folds are the cuneiform cartilages. (From Tucker HM, Harvey M: Anatomy of the larynx. In Tucker HM, editor: *The larynx,* ed 2, New York, 1993, Thieme Medical Publishers.)

Airway protection is enhanced by the orientation of the cords. The false cords are directed inferiorly at their free border. This position can help to stop egress of air during Valsalva's maneuver. The true cords are oriented slightly superiorly. This prevents air or matter from entering the lungs. Great pressure is needed to separate adducted true cords.[25] Air trapped in the ventricle during closure pushes each false cord and true cord more tightly together.[18]

3. The muscles of the larynx

The complex and delicate functions of the larynx are made possible by an intricate group of small muscles. These muscles can be divided into the extrinsic and the intrinsic groups.[24,26] The extrinsic group connects the

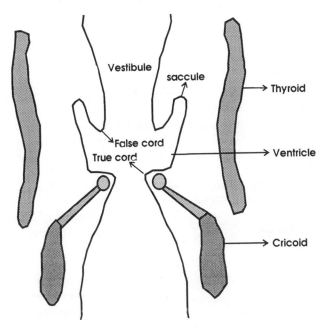

Fig. 1-9. Diagrammatic representation of the laryngeal cavity. Note location of false and true cords and laryngeal saccule. (Modified from Tucker HM, Harvey M: Anatomy of the larynx. In Tucker HM, editor: *The larynx*, ed 2, New York, 1993, Thieme Medical Publishers.)

larynx with its anatomic neighbors, such as the hyoid bone, and modifies the position and movement of the larynx. The intrinsic group facilitates the movements of the laryngeal cartilages against one another and directly affects glottic movement.[21,25]

a. THE EXTRINSIC MUSCLES OF THE LARYNX

The suprahyoid muscles attach the larynx to the hyoid bone and elevate the larynx. These muscles are the stylohyoid, geniohyoid, mylohyoid, thyrohyoid, digastric, and stylopharyngeus muscles. In the infrahyoid muscle group are the omohyoid, sternothyroid, thyrohyoid, and sternohyoid muscles. These "strap" muscles, in addition to lowering the larynx, can modify the internal relationship of laryngeal cartilages and folds to one another. The inferior constrictor of the pharynx primarily assists in deglutition (Table 1-1).[7,16-18]

b. THE INTRINSIC MUSCLES OF THE LARYNX

Some authors consider the cricothyroid muscle to be both an extrinsic and intrinsic muscle of the larynx, since its actions affect both laryngeal movements and the glottic structures.[21] The paired cricothyroid muscles join the cricoid cartilage and the thyroid cartilage (Fig. 1-10). The muscle has two parts. A larger, ventral section runs vertically between the cricoid and the inferior thyroid border. The smaller, oblique segment attaches the anteromedial cricoid to the posterior inner thyroid border and the lesser cornu of the thyroid. When the muscle contracts, the ventral head draws the anterior part of the cricoid cartilage towards the relatively fixed lower border of the thyroid cartilage. The oblique head of the muscle rocks the cricoid lamina posteriorly. Since the arytenoids do not move, the vocal ligaments are tensed, and the glottic length is increased 30%.[21,27]

The function of the intrinsic musculature is threefold: (1) they open the vocal cords during inspiration; (2) they close the cords and the laryngeal inlet during deglutition, and (3) they alter the tension of the cords during phonation.[7,16,21] The larynx can close at three levels: (1) the aryepiglottic folds close by the contraction of the aryepiglottic and oblique arytenoid muscles; (2) the false

Table 1-1. Extrinsic muscles of the larynx

Muscle	Function	Innervation
Sternohyoid	Indirect depressor of the larynx	Cervical plexus Ansa hypoglossi C1, C2, C3
Sternothyroid	Depresses the larynx Modifies the thyrohyoid and aryepiglottic folds	Same as above
Thyrohyoid	Same as above	Cervical plexus Hypoglossal nerve C1, C2
Thyroepiglottic	Mucosal inversion of aryepiglottic fold	Recurrent laryngeal nerve
Stylopharyngeus	Assists folding of thyroid cartilage	Glossopharyngeal
Inferior pharyngeal constrictor	Assists in swallowing	Vagus, pharyngeal plexus

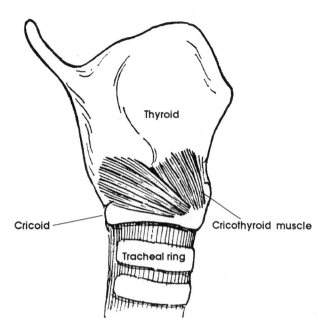

Fig. 1-10. Cricothyroid muscle and its attachments. (Modified from Ellis H, Feldman S: *Anatomy for anaesthetists,* ed 6, Oxford, 1993, Blackwell Scientific.)

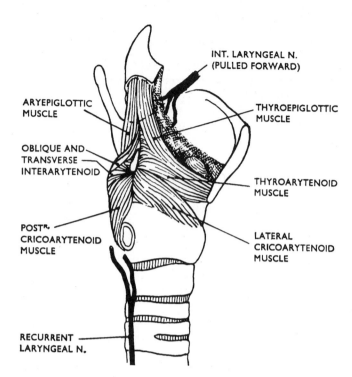

Fig. 1-11. Intrinsic muscles of the larynx and their nerve supply. (Modified from Ellis H, Feldman S: *Anatomy for anaesthetists,* ed 6, Oxford, 1993, Blackwell Scientific.)

vocal cords close by the action of the lateral thyroarytenoids; and (3) the true vocal cords close by the contraction of interarytenoids, lateral cricoarytenoids, and the cricothyroid.[7] The intrinsic muscles include the aryepiglottic, thyroarytenoid, oblique and transverse arytenoids, and lateral and posterior cricoarytenoids (Fig. 1-11). All but the transverse arytenoids are paired.

The thick posterior cricoarytenoid muscle originates near the entire posterior midline of the cricoid cartilage. Muscle fibers run superiorly and laterally to the posterior area of the muscular process of the arytenoid cartilage.[16] Upon contraction, the posterior cricoarytenoid rotates the arytenoids and moves the vocal folds laterally. The posterior cricoarytenoid is the only true abductor of the vocal folds.[17,20,21,25]

The lateral cricoarytenoid muscle joins the superior border of the lateral cricoid cartilage and the muscular process of the arytenoid. This muscle rotates the arytenoids medially, adducting the true vocal folds.[16] The unpaired transverse arytenoid muscle joins the posterolateral aspects of the arytenoids. The muscle, covered anteriorly by a mucous membrane, forms the posterior commissure of the larynx. Contraction of this muscle brings the arytenoids together and ensures posterior adduction of the glottis.[16,17,20]

The oblique arytenoids (Fig. 1-11) ascend diagonally from the muscular processes posteriorly across the cartilage to the opposite superior arytenoid and help close the glottis. Fibers of the oblique arytenoid may continue from the apex through the aryepiglottic fold as the aryepiglottic muscle that attaches itself to the lateral aspect of the epiglottis. The aryepiglottic muscle and the oblique arytenoid act as a "purse-string" sphincter during deglutition.[21]

The thyroarytenoid muscle (Fig. 1-11) is broad and sometimes divided into three parts. It is among the fastest contracting striated muscles.[25] The muscle arises along the entire lower border of the thyroid cartilage. It passes posteriorly, superiorly, and laterally to attach to the anterolateral surface and the vocal process of the arytenoid.

The segment of thyroarytenoid muscle that lies adjacent to the vocal ligament (and frequently surrounds it) is called the vocalis muscle. The vocalis is the major tensor of the vocal fold and can "thin" the fold to achieve a high pitch. Beneath the mucosa of the fold, extending from the anterior commissure back to the vocal process, is a potential space called Reinke's space. This area can become edematous if traumatized. The more laterally attached fibers of the thyroarytenoid function as the prime adductor of the vocal folds.[21]

The most lateral section of the muscle, sometimes called the thyroepiglottic muscle, attaches to the lateral aspects of the arytenoids, the aryepiglottic fold, and even the epiglottis. When it contracts, the arytenoids are pulled medially, down, and forward.[16,21] This shortens and relaxes the vocal ligament. The function and innervation of the extrinsic muscles are summarized in

Table 1-2. Intrinsic musculature of the larynx

Muscle	Function	Innervation
Posterior cricoarytenoid	Abductor of vocal cords	Recurrent laryngeal
Lateral cricoarytenoid	Adducts arytenoids closing glottis	Recurrent laryngeal
Transverse arytenoid	Adducts arytenoids	Recurrent laryngeal
Oblique arytenoid	Closes glottis	Recurrent laryngeal
Aryepiglottic	Closes glottis	Recurrent laryngeal
Vocalis	Relaxes the cords	Recurrent laryngeal
Thyroarytenoid	Relaxes tension cords	Recurrent laryngeal
Cricothyroid	Tensor of the cords	Superior laryngeal (external branch)

Table 1-1. Table 1-2 describes the intrinsic musculature of the larynx.

c. THE INNERVATION OF THE LARYNX

The external branch of the superior laryngeal nerve supplies motor innervation to the cricothyroid muscle. All other motor supply to laryngeal musculature is provided by the recurrent laryngeal nerves (Fig. 1-11). Both the superior and the recurrent laryngeal nerves are derivatives of the vagus nerve.

The superior laryngeal nerve generally separates from the main trunk just outside the jugular foramen. At approximately the level of the hyoid bone, the external branch comes off and travels below the superior thyroid artery to the cricothyroid muscle. The internal branch of the superior laryngeal nerve and the superior laryngeal artery pass through the thyrohyoid membrane laterally between the greater cornua of the thyroid and hyoid. The nerve divides almost immediately into a series of sensory branches and provides sensory innervation as far down as the vocal cords.[16,21] Sensory innervation of the epiglottis is dense, and the true vocal folds are more heavily innervated posteriorly than anteriorly.[25]

The left recurrent laryngeal nerve branches from the vagus in the thorax and courses cephalad after hooking around the arch of the aorta in close relation to the ligamentum arteriosum. On the right side, the nerve loops posteriorly beneath the subclavian artery before following a cephalad course to the larynx. Both nerves ascend the neck in the groove between the trachea and the esophagus before they reach the larynx. The nerves enter the larynx just posterior, or sometimes anterior, to the cricothyroid articulation. The recurrent laryngeal nerve supplies all the intrinsic muscles of the larynx except the cricothyroid. The recurrent laryngeal nerve also provides sensory innervation to the larynx below the vocal cords. Parasympathetic fibers to the larynx travel along the laryngeal nerves, and the sympathetics from the superior cervical ganglion travel to the larynx with blood vessels. Tables 1-1 and 1-2 summarize the innervation of the laryngeal musculature.

i. Glottic closure and laryngeal spasm. Stimulation of the superior laryngeal nerve endings in the supraglottic region can induce protective closure of the glottis. This short-lived phenomenon is a polysynaptic involuntary reflex.[25] Triggering of other nerves, notably cranial nerves such as the trigeminal and glossopharyngeal, can, to a lesser degree, also produce reflex glottic closure.[28,29] The nerve endings in the mammalian supraglottic area are highly sensitive to touch, heat, and chemical stimuli.[30] This sensitivity is especially intense in the posterior commissure of the larynx, close to where the pyriform recesses blend with the hypopharynx.[31] Complex sensory receptors, similar in structure to lingual taste buds, have been demonstrated here.[32] Instillation of water, saline, bases, and acids have been demonstrated to cause glottic closure in vitro and in vivo.[33] Infants also respond to stimulation with prolonged apnea, although this response disappears later in life.[25]

Laryngospasm occurs when glottic closure persists long after the removal of the stimulus.[28,31] This has led to speculation that laryngospasm represents a focal seizure of the adductors subtended by the recurrent laryngeal nerve.[34] This state is only initiated by repeated superior laryngeal nerve stimulation.[28] Symptoms abate, perhaps due to a central mechanism, as hypoxia and hypercarbia worsen.[35]

ii. Vocal cord palsies. The recurrent laryngeal nerve may be traumatized during surgery on the thyroid gland. Malignancy of the neck or trauma may affect the nerve.[5,26] The left recurrent nerve may be compressed by neoplasms in the thorax, aneurysm of the aortic arch, or an enlarged left atrium (mitral stenosis).[26] It may be occasionally injured during ligation of a patent ductus arteriosus. The left nerve is likely to be paralyzed twice as frequently as the right nerve because of its close relationship to many intrathoracic structures. The superior laryngeal (or the external laryngeal nerve) may also be damaged during thyroidectomy.

Under normal circumstances, the vocal cords meet in the midline during phonation (Fig. 1-12). On inspiration they move away from each other. They return towards midline on expiration, leaving a small opening between them. When laryngeal spasm occurs, both true and false vocal cords lie tightly in midline opposite each other. To

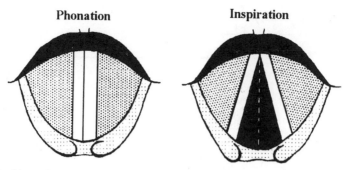

Fig. 1-12. Position of vocal cords during phonation and inspiration. Abbreviation used: *recur,* recurrent. (From Hodder Headline PLC, London.)

arrive at a clinical diagnosis of laryngeal nerve-muscle abnormality, the position of the cords must be examined laryngoscopically during phonation and inspiration (Figs. 1-12 and 1-13).

The recurrent laryngeal nerve carries both abductor and adductor fibers to the vocal cords. The abductor fibers are more vulnerable, and moderate trauma causes a pure abductor paralysis. Severe trauma will cause both abductor and adductor fibers to be affected.[5] Pure adductor paralysis does not occur as a clinical entity. In the case of pure unilateral abductor palsy, both cords will meet in the midline on phonation (because adduction is still possible on the affected side) (Fig. 1-13). However, only the normal cord will abduct during inspiration (Fig. 1-13). In the case of the complete unilateral palsy of the recurrent laryngeal nerve, both abductors and adductors will be affected. On phonation, the unaffected cord will cross the midline to meet its paralyzed counterpart, appearing to lie in front of the affected cord[5] (Fig. 1-13). On inspiration, the unaffected cord will move to full abduction. When abductor fibers are damaged bilaterally (incomplete bilateral damage to the recurrent laryngeal nerve), the adductor fibers will draw the cords towards each other, and the glottic opening will be reduced to a slit, resulting in severe respiratory distress[24,26] (Fig. 1-13). However, with a complete palsy, each vocal cord will lie midway between abduction and adduction. A reasonable glottic opening will exist. Thus, bilateral incomplete palsy is more dangerous than the complete variety (Fig. 1-13).

Damage to the external branch of the superior laryngeal nerve or to the superior laryngeal nerve trunk causes paralysis of the cricothyroid (the tuning fork of the larynx) and causes hoarseness that improves with time due to increased compensatory action of the opposite muscle. The glottic chink appears oblique during phonation. The aryepiglottic fold on the affected side appears shortened, and the one on the normal side is lengthened. The cords may appear wavy. The symptoms include frequent throat clearing and difficulty in

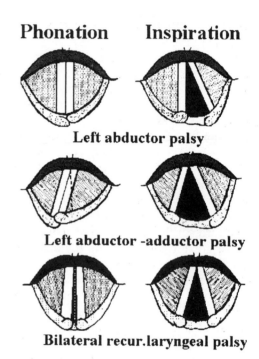

Fig. 1-13. Diagrammatic representation of different types of vocal cord palsies. Note that in complete bilateral recurrent laryngeal palsy *(bottom panel),* vocal cords remain in the abducted position and the glottic opening is preserved. Abbreviation used: *recur*, recurrent. For details see text. (From Hodder Headline PLC, London.)

raising the vocal pitch.[27] A total bilateral paralysis of vagus nerves will affect the recurrent laryngeal nerves and the superior laryngeal nerves. In this condition, the cords assume the abducted, cadaveric position.[5] The vocal cords are relaxed and appear wavy[5,27] (Fig. 1-14). A similar picture may be seen following the use of muscle relaxants.

Topical anesthesia of the larynx may affect the fibers of the external branch of the superior laryngeal nerve and paralyze the cricothyroid muscle, signified by a

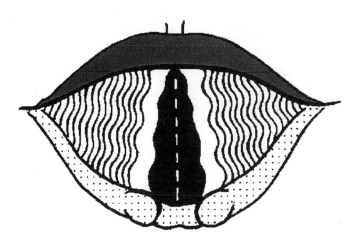

Fig. 1-14. Cadaveric position of vocal cords. For details see text. (From Hodder Headline PLC, London.)

"gruff voice." Similarly, superior laryngeal nerve block may affect the cricothyroid muscle in the same manner as surgical trauma does. These factors must be taken into consideration while evaluating postthyroidectomy vocal cord dysfunction following surgery.

d. BLOOD SUPPLY OF THE LARYNX

Blood supply to the larynx is derived from the external carotid and the subclavian arteries. The external carotid gives rise to the superior thyroid artery, which bifurcates forming the superior laryngeal artery. This artery courses with the superior laryngeal nerve through the thyrohyoid membrane to supply the supraglottic region. The inferior thyroid artery, derived from the thyrocervical trunk, terminates as the inferior laryngeal artery. This vessel travels in the tracheoesophageal groove with the recurrent laryngeal nerve and supplies the infraglottic larynx. There are extensive connections with the ipsilateral superior laryngeal artery and across the midline. A small cricothyroid artery may branch from the superior thyroid and cross the cricothyroid membrane. It most commonly travels near the inferior border of the thyroid cartilage.[21]

III. THE LOWER AIRWAY

A. GROSS STRUCTURE OF THE TRACHEA AND BRONCHI

The adult trachea begins at the cricoid cartilage, opposite the sixth cervical vertebra (Figs. 1-10 and 1-11). It is 10 to 20 cm long and 12 mm in diameter. It is flattened posteriorly and contains 16 to 20 horseshoe-shaped cartilaginous rings. At the sixth ring, the trachea becomes intrathoracic. The first and the last rings are broader than the rest. The lower borders of the last ring split and curve interiorly between the two bronchi to form the carina at the T-5 level (angle of Louis, second intercostal space). The posterior part of the trachea, void of cartilage, consists of a membrane of smooth muscle and fibroelastic tissue joining the ends of the cartilages. The muscle of the trachea is stratified in an inner circular and an outer longitudinal layer. The longitudinal

bundles predominate in children but are virtually absent in adults.[36,37]

In the adult, the right main bronchus is wider and shorter and takes off at a steeper angle than does the left mainstem bronchus. Thus, endotracheal tubes, suction catheters, or foreign bodies more readily enter the right bronchial lumen. However, the angulation of the two bronchi are nearly equal in children less than 3 years old. The right mainstem bronchus gives rise to three lobar bronchi and the left, two. Both main bronchi and the lower lobe bronchi are situated outside the lung substance (large bronchi, 7 to 12 mm in diameter). Main bronchi divide into 20 bronchopulmonary divisions supplying each respective lobule's medium bronchi (4 to 7 mm) that lead into small bronchi (0.8 to 4 mm). Bronchioles are bronchi that are less than 0.8 mm in size. Bronchioles do not have any cartilage in their walls.[38]

Bronchioles are of two types, terminal and respiratory. The terminal bronchioles do not bear any alveoli and lead into the alveoli-bearing respiratory bronchioles. Each terminal bronchiole leads to three respiratory bronchioles, and each respiratory bronchiole leads to four generations of alveolar ducts[38] (Fig. 1-15).

Although the diameter of each new generation of airway decreases progressively, the aggregate cross-sectional area increases. This is especially true beyond airways 2 mm in diameter or smaller, where further branching is not accompanied by concomitant decreases in caliber. The failure of the airway diameter to decrease with subsequent divisions produces the inverted thumbtack appearance on a graph depicting increasing surface area as a function of distance from mouth[5] (Fig. 1-16).

The bronchi are surrounded by irregular, cartilaginous rings similar in structure to the trachea except that the attachment of the posterior membrane is more anterior[39] (Fig. 1-17). Rings give way to discrete, cartilaginous plates as the bronchi become intrapulmonary at the lung roots (Fig. 1-18). Eventually, even these plates disappear, usually at airway diameters of about 0.6 mm.[39]

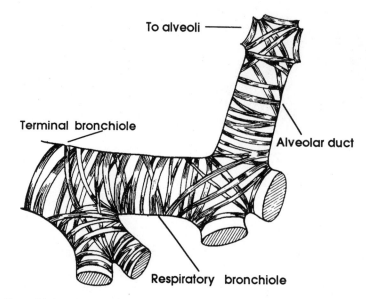

Fig. 1-15. Bronchiolar division and geodesic network of muscle layer surrounding the airway. (From Hodder Headline PLC, London.)

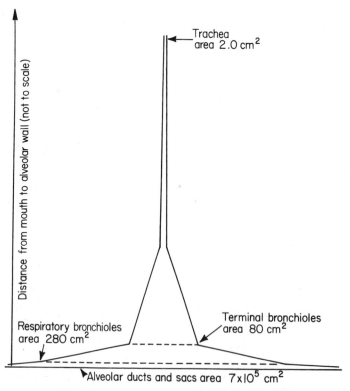

Fig. 1-16. Relationship between cross-sectional area and generation of the airway. Note abrupt increase in cross-section when the respiratory bronchiole is reached (inverted thumbtack arrangement). For details see text. (From Hodder Headline PLC, London.)

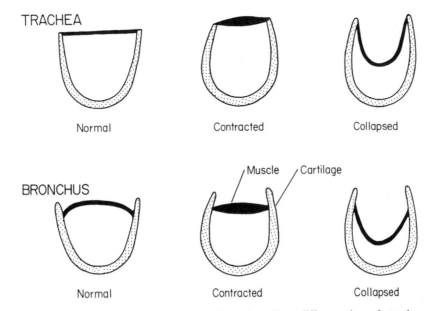

Fig. 1-17. Cross-sectional view of trachea and bronchus. Note different sites of attachment of posterior membrane in the tracheal and bronchial sections. Also note invagination of posterior membrane into the lumen in the collapsed state. (From Horsfield K: *Br J Dis Chest* 68:145, 1974.)

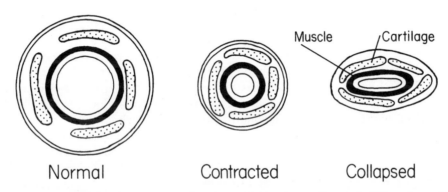

Fig. 1-18. Cross-sectional views of medium bronchi (4 to 8 mm diameter) with peribronchial space. (From Horsfield K: *Br J Dis Chest* 68:145, 1974.)

The rings or the plates of the bronchi are interconnected by a strong fibroelastic sheath within which a myoelastic layer consisting of smooth muscle and elastic tissue is arrayed.[5] The myoelastic band is arranged in a special pattern called the geodesic network representing the shortest distance between two points on a curved surface (Fig. 1-15). This architectural design serves as the strongest and most effective mechanism for withstanding or generating pressures within a tube without fiber slippage along the length of the outer surface of the tube. The primary function of the muscular component is to change the size of the airway according to the respiratory phase. The smooth muscle tone (bronchomotor tone) is predominently under the influence of the vagus nerve. The elastic layer runs longitudinally but encircles the bronchus at the points of division.[5]

The muscular layer becomes progressively thinner distally, but its thickness relative to the bronchial wall increases. Therefore, the terminal bronchiole with the narrowest lumen has perhaps the thickest muscle, nearly 20% of the total thickness of the wall that lacks cartilaginous support.[38,39] Thus, smaller bronchioles may be readily closed off by action of the musculature during prolonged bronchial spasm. Such an arrangement may facilitate closure of unperfused portions of the lung when a ventilation-perfusion mismatch occurs (pulmonary embolism). The smooth muscles and the glands of the cartilaginous airways are innervated by the autonomic nervous system. They are stimulated by the vagus and inhibited by sympathetic impulses derived from the upper thoracic ganglia.

B. AIRWAY EPITHELIUM AND AIRWAY DEFENSE MECHANISMS

The cartilaginous airways are lined by a tall, columnar, pseudostratified epithelium containing at least 13 cell types.[24] An important function of this lining is the production of mucus, a part of the respiratory defense mechanism. The mucus is steadily propelled to the outside by a conveyer belt mechanism. The large airways have a mucous secretory apparatus that consists of serous and goblet cells and submucous glands. The submucous glands empty into secretory tubules, which, in turn, connect with the larger connecting ducts. Several connecting ducts unite and form the ciliated duct that opens into the airway lumen. No mucous glands are seen in the bronchioles.[6,40]

The most populous cell of the large airways is the ciliated epithelial cell, bearing 250 cilia per cell.[6,24] The length of the cilia decreases progressively in the smaller airways. On the surface of the cell are found small claws and microvilli. The microvilli probably regulate the volume of secretions through resorption, a function that may be shared with the brush cell scattered along the airways. The basal cell, more numerous in the large airways, imparts the epithelium's pseudostratified appearance. The other cell types, except the K cell, develop from the basal cell *via* the intermediate cell. This cell lies in the layer above the basal cell and differentiates into cells with secretory or ciliary function.[6,24,40] The K cell, or Kulchitsky-like cell, resembles the Kulchitsky's cells of the gastrointestinal tract. These cells uptake, decarboxylate, and store amine precursors, such as levodopa (L-dopa), and are thus known as amine precursor uptake and decarboxylation (APUD) cells. The functions of the K cells are not definitely known, but proposed roles include mechanoreception or chemoreception (stretch, carbon dioxide [CO_2]). Globule leukocytes are derived from subepithelial mast cells and interact with them to transfer IgE to the secretions and to alter membrane permeability to locally produced or circulating antibodies. The ubiquitous lymphocytes and plasma cells defend against pathogens. Table 1-3 lists important cell types that constitute the airway epithelium.

The nonciliated bronchiolar epithelial cell, or Clara cell, largely composes the cuboidal epithelium of the bronchioles. The Clara cells assume the role of basal cells as a stem cell in the bronchiole. Only six cell types have been recorded in the human bronchiole: the ciliated, brush, basal, K, Clara, and the globular leukocyte. These cells form a single-layered simple cuboidal epithelium.

C. BLOOD SUPPLY

Bronchial arteries supply the bronchi and the bronchioles. Arterial supply extends into the respiratory

Table 1-3. Types of tracheobronchial cell

Cell	Probable function
Epithelial	
Goblet	Mucous secretion
Serous	Mucous secretion
Ciliated	Mucous propulsion-resorption, supportive
Brush	Mucous resorption
Basal	Supportive, parent
Intermediate	Parent
Clara	Supportive, parent
Kulchitsky	Neuroendocrine possible mechanoreceptor, chemoreceptor
Mesenchymal	
"Globule" leukocyte	Immunological defense
Lymphocyte	Defense

Modified from Jeffrey PK, Reid L: New features of the rat airway epithelium: a quantitative and electron microscopic study, *J Anat* 120:295, 1975.

bronchiole. Arterial anastomoses occur in the adventitia of the bronchiole. The branches enter the submucosa after piercing the muscle layer to form the submucosal capillary plexus. The venous radices arising from the capillary plexus reach the venous plexus in the adventitia by penetrating the muscle layer. When the muscle layer contracts, the arteries can maintain forward flow to the capillary plexus. However, the capillaries cannot force the blood back into the venous plexus. Thus, prolonged bronchial spasm can lead to mucous membrane swelling in the small airways.[5] The venous drainage of the bronchi occurs via the bronchial, azygous, hemiazygous, and intercostal veins. There is some communication between the pulmonary artery and the bronchiolar capillary plexus leading to normally occurring "anatomic shunting."

D. FUNCTION OF THE LOWER AIRWAY

1. Forces acting on the airway

Different forces act upon the airway to alter its morphology continuously. These forces are modified by (1) the location of a given airway segment (intrathoracic or extrathoracic), (2) the phases of respiration, (3) lung volume, (4) gravity, (5) age, and (6) disease.[39,40]

Intrathoracic, intrapulmonary airways such as the distal bronchi and bronchioles are surrounded by a potential space, the peribronchial space (Fig. 1-19). The bronchi are untethered and, therefore, move longitudinally within this sheath. However, the bronchiolar adventitia is attached by an elastic tissue matrix to the adjoining elastic framework of the surrounding alveoli and parenchyma. Consequently, the bronchioles are subject to transmitted tissue forces.[36,39]

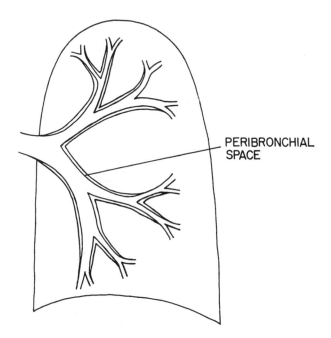

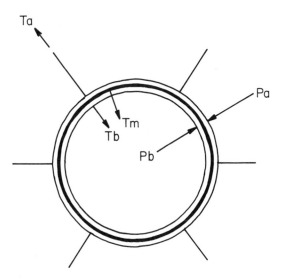

Fig. 1-19. Diagram showing formation of peribronchial space by invagination of the visceral pleura. (From Horsfield K: *Br J Dis Chest* 68:145, 1974.)

Fig. 1-20. Vector diagram showing transmural forces influencing airway caliber. *Ta,* alveolar elastic forces; *Tb,* bronchial elastic forces; *Tm,* bronchial muscular forces; *Pb,* barometric pressure; *Pa,* -alveolar gas pressure. Arrow direction indicates direction of the force. Algebraic sum of these forces determine size of airway lumen at any given time. (From Horsfield K: *Br J Dis Chest* 68:145, 1974.)

Many forces act in concert to modify the airway lumen (Fig. 1-20). The forces that tend to expand the lumen include pressure of the gas in the bronchi-bronchiole and the elastic tissue forces of the alveoli. Forces that tend to close the airway include the elasticity of the bronchial wall, which increases as the lumen expands; the forces due to bronchial muscle contraction; and the pressure of the gas in the surrounding alveoli. The algebraic sum of these forces at any given time determines the diameter of the airway.[38,39]

The lower part of the trachea and proximal bronchi are intrathoracic but extrapulmonary. Consequently, they are subject to the regular intrathoracic pressures (intrapleural pressure) but not to the tissue elastic recoil forces. The upper trachea is both extrathoracic and extrapulmonary. While it is unaffected by the elastic recoil of the lung, it is subject to the effects of ambient pressure and cervical tissue forces.[36,39]

During spontaneous inspiration, the lung expands, lowering the alveolar pressure more than it does the bronchial pressure, to create a pressure gradient that induces airflow. This increases the elastic retractive forces of the connective tissue and opens the intrathoracic airways. However, extrathoracic intraluminal pressure decreases relative to atmospheric pressure, with the result that the diameter of the upper trachea decreases. During expiration, alveolar pressure rises and exceeds the tissue retractive forces, thus decreasing intrathoracic airway diameter. In this case, the extrathoracic intraluminal pressure rises above the atmospheric pressure, and the upper trachea expands. On forced expiration alveolar pressure is greatly elevated, further reducing the diameter of the smaller airways.

The dynamic forces are altered by gravity such that those forces tending to expand the lung are greater at the top than at the bottom whether the patient is prone, supine, or erect.[41] The diameter and length of the airways of all sizes vary directly as the cube root of the lung volume varies when the lung expands.[42] On expiration below functional residual capacity (FRC), the retractive forces gradually decrease the airway size toward the point of closing volume. Because of the effect of gravity, the basal airways close first. The retractive forces of the elastic tissues decrease with aging, which explains why closing volume increases with age. This effect is exaggerated in diseases with elastic tissue damage (pulmonary emphysema).

2. The relationship between structure and function

The extent to which the retractive forces affect the airway morphology is related to the specific structure of the airway segment in question. When the fibromuscular membrane of the trachea contracts, the ends of the cartilages are approximated, and the lumen narrows in both the intrathoracic and extrathoracic trachea. When the radial forces decrease airway diameter, the posterior membrane invaginates into the lumen (Fig. 1-17). However, the rigid cartilaginous hoops prevent luminal occlusion. Extrapulmonary bronchi behave in a similar fashion.

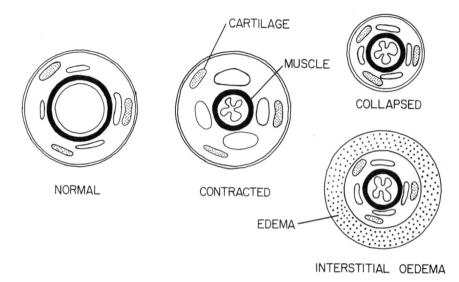

Fig. 1-21. Structure of small bronchi (0.8 to 4 mm in diameter). Note how the mucous membrane is thrown into folds in contracted and collapsed states, reducing the airway lumen. (From Horsfield K: *Br J Dis Chest* 68:145, 1974.)

The medium intrapulmonary bronchi within the peribronchial sheath are surrounded by cartilaginous plates. While these plates add some rigidity to the wall, they do not prevent collapse, and so these airways are dependent on the elastic retractive forces of the surrounding tissue (Fig. 1-20).[39] Therefore, forced expiration can collapse many bronchioles in emphysema.

The miniature carinas at small airway bifurcations maintain airway lumens. Intrinsic bronchial muscles reduce the lumen and increase the mean velocity of the airflow during forced expiratory maneuvers, particularly in the peripheral airways with small flow rates. Here, two additional anatomic adaptations contribute to increasing flow rates: (1) as the muscular ring contracts, the mucous lining is thrown into accordion-type folds that project into the lumen, further narrowing the lumen[39] (Fig. 1-21); (2) the venous plexus situated between the muscle and the cartilage fills and invaginates into the lumen during muscle contraction. These mechanisms permit bronchoconstriction without distorting the surrounding tissues and minimize the muscular effort required to reduce airway lumen. The drawback of such an arrangement is that even a small amount of fluid or sputum can result in complete occlusion of the small airways.[39] Thus, it is not at all surprising that the airway resistance is increased tremendously during an asthmatic attack that is characterized by both bronchospasm and increased secretions.[43-45] The small airways can also be affected by interstitial pulmonary edema, a condition in which the peribronchial space can accumulate fluid and isolate the bronchus from the surrounding retractive forces (see Fig. 1-21).

IV. CONCLUSION

In this chapter we described certain salient features of the human respiratory passages as they relate to their functional anatomy in health and disease from the anesthesiologist's point of view. It is necessary for students of anesthesia to possess some knowledge of the structures that they will most frequently use as a passageway to patient care in their professional career.

REFERENCES

1. Reznik GK: Comparative anatomy, physiology and function of the upper respiratory tract, *Environ Health Perspect* 85:171, 1990.
2. Roberts JT, Pino R: Functional anatomy of the upper airway. In Roberts JT, editor: *Clinical management of the airway*, Philadelphia, 1994, WB Saunders.
3. Williams P, Warwick R, Dyson M, et al: *Gray's anatomy*, ed 37, New York, 1989, Churchill Livingstone, p. 1171.
4. Williams P, Warwick R, Dyson M, et al: *Gray's anatomy*, ed 37, New York, 1989, Churchill Livingstone, p. 365.
5. Linton RF: Structure and function of the respiratory tract in relation to anaesthesia. In Churchill-Davidson HC, editor: *A practice of anaesthesia*, ed 5, Chicago, 1984, Year Book Medical Publishers.
6. Grande CM, Ramanathan S, Turndorf H: The structural correlates of airway function, *Problems in Anesthesia* 2:175, 1988.
7. Roberts J: *Fundamentals of tracheal intubation*, New York, 1983, Grune & Stratton.
8. Green GM: Lung defense mechanisms. Symposium on chronic respiratory disease, *Med Clin North Am* 57:547, 1973.
9. Newhouse M, Sanchis J, Bienstock J et al: Lung defense mechanisms, part I, *N Engl J Med* 295:990, 1976.
10. Shorten GD, Opie NJ, Graziotti P et al: Assessment of upper airway anatomy in awake, sedated and anaesthetised patients using magnetic resonance imaging, *Anaesth Intensive Care* 22:165, 1994.
11. Hudgel DW: The role of upper airway anatomy and physiology in obstructive sleep apnea, *Clin Chest Med* 13:383, 1992 (review).

12. Ryan CF, Lowe AA, Li D et al: Magnetic resonance imaging of the upper airway in obstructive sleep apnea before and after chronic nasal continuous positive airway pressure therapy, *Am Rev Respir Dis* 144:939, 1991.

13. Mezzanotte WS, Tangel DJ, White DP: Waking genioglossal electromyogram in sleep apnea patients versus normal controls (a neuromuscular compensatory mechanism), *J Clin Invest* 89:1571, 1992.

14. Hirano M, Kurita S, Yukizane K et al: Asymmetry of the laryngeal framework: a morphologic study of cadaver larynges, *Ann Otol Rhinol Laryngol* 98:135, 1989.

15. Roberts J: Functional anatomy of the larynx, *Int Anesthesiol Clin* 28:101, 1990 (review).

16. Hanafee WN, Ward PH: Anatomy and Physiology. In Hanafee WN, Ward PH, editors: *The larynx: radiology, surgery, pathology,* New York, 1990, Thieme Medical Publishers.

17. Fink RF: Anatomy of the Larynx. In *The human larynx: a functional study,* New York, 1975, Raven Press.

18. Tucker HM: Physiology of the larynx. In Tucker HM, editor: *The larynx,* ed 2, New York, 1993, Thieme Medical Publishers.

19. Finucane B, Santora AH: Anatomy of the airway. In *Principles of airway management,* Philadelphia, 1988, FA Davis.

20. Fried MP, Meller SM: Adult laryngeal anatomy. In Fried MP, editor: *The larynx: a multidisciplinary approach,* Boston, 1988, Little, Brown.

21. Tucker HM, Harvey M: Anatomy of the larynx. In Tucker HM, editor: *The larynx,* ed 2, New York, 1993, Thieme Medical Publishers.

22. Broyles EN: The anterior commissure tendon, *Ann Otol Rhinol Laryngol* 52:341, 1943.

23. Meitelles LZ, Lin P, Wenk EJ: An anatomic study of the external laryngeal framework with surgical implications, *Otolaryngol Head Neck Surg* 106:235, 1992.

24. Williams P, Warwick R, Dyson M et al: *Gray's anatomy,* ed 37, New York, 1989, Churchill Livingstone pp. 1248-86.

25. Pectu LP, Sasaki CT: Laryngeal anatomy and physiology, *Clin Chest Med* 12:415, 1991.

26. Ellis H, Feldman S: *Anatomy for the anaesthetists,* ed 6, Oxford, 1993, Blackwell Scientific.

27. Abelson TI, Tucker HM: Laryngeal findings in superior laryngeal nerve paralysis: a controversy, *Otolaryngol Head Neck Surg* 89:463, 1981.

28. Suzuki M, Sasaki CT: Laryngeal spasm: a neuroradiologic redefinition, *Ann Otol Rhinol Laryngol* 86:150, 1977.

29. Kirchner J: Laryngeal reflex system. In Baer T, Sasaki C, editors: *Laryngeal function in phonation and respiration,* Boston, 1987, Little, Brown.

30. Rex MAE: The production of laryngospasm in the cat by volatile anesthetic agents, *Br J Anaesth* 42:941, 1970.

31. Thach BT: Neuromuscular control of upper airway patency, *Clin Perinatol* 19:773, 1992.

32. Ide C: The cytologic composition of laryngeal chemosensory corpuscles, *Amer J Anat* 158:193, 1980.

33. Storey AT, Johnson P: Laryngeal water receptors initiating apnea in the lamb, *Exp Neurol* 47:42, 1975.

34. Sasaki CT: Physiology of the larynx. In English GM, editor: *Otolaryngology,* Philadelphia, 1984, Harper & Row.

35. Nishino T, Yonezawa T, Honda Y: Modification of laryngospasm in response to changes in $PaCO_2$ and PaO_2 in the cat, *Anesthesiology* 55:286, 1981.

36. Proctor DF: The upper airways. II. The larynx and trachea, *Am Rev Respir Dis* 137:296, 1977.

37. Richardson JB, Ferguson CC: *Morphology of the airways.* In Nadel JA, editor: *Physiology and pharmacology of the airways,* New York, 1980, Dekker.

38. Ranga V, Kleinerman J: Structure and function of the airways in health and disease, *Arch Pathol Lab Med* 102:609, 1978.

39. Horsfield K: The relation between structure and function of the airways of the lung, *Br J Dis Chest* 68:145, 1974.

40. Breeze R, Turk M: Cellular structure, function and organization in the lower respiratory tract, *Environ Health Perspect* 55:3, 1984.

41. West JB, Matthews FL: Stresses, strain and surface pressures in the lungs caused by weight, *J Appl Physiol* 32:332, 1972.

42. Hughes JM, Hoppin FG, Mead J: Effect of lung inflation on bronchial length and diameter in excised lungs, *J Appl Physiol* 32:25, 1972.

43. Salem MR, Baraka A: Bronchospasm: an early manifestation of pulmonary embolism during and after anesthesia, *Anesth Analg* 47:103, 1968.

44. Cropp G: The role of the parasympathetic nervous system in the maintenance of chronic airway obstruction in asthmatic children, *Am Rev Respir Dis* 112:599, 1975.

45. Wanner A: The role of mucociliary dysfunction in bronchial asthma, *Am J Med* 67:477, 1979.

Chapter 2

RADIOLOGY OF THE AIRWAY

M. Anne Keller
Susan Blaser
Stephen J. Herman

I. INTRODUCTION

The need for preoperative radiologic evaluation of the airway is dictated by basic principles of airway management: (1) safety for intubation; (2) mechanical ability to open the mouth; and (3) airway obstruction and/or displacement.

A safe intubation requires knowledge of an intact or stabilized cervical spine. In cases of clinical concern, such as trauma, tumor (Fig. 2-1), rheumatoid arthritis, or congenital anomalies, radiographs of the cervical spine will usually suffice to adequately clear the spine for alignment, stability, and integrity of bony architecture. It is essential that the entire cervical spine to the level of T1 be visualized, barring which a computerized tomographic (CT) scan in 1.5 mm increments with sagittal reformations must be done to adequately define the anatomy.

A safe intubation is also dependent on an intact skull base. A history of cerebrospinal fluid (CSF) rhinorrhea,

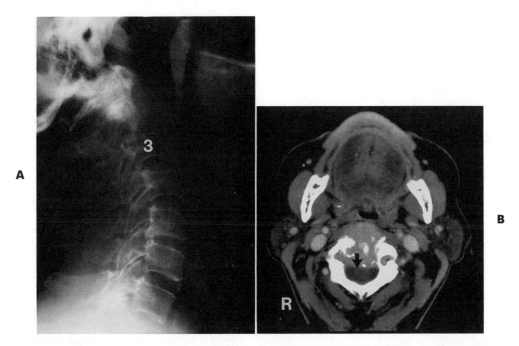

Fig. 2-1. A, *Metastatic thyroid carcinoma.* A 67-year-old woman was being evaluated for biopsy-positive thyroid carcinoma. Lateral radiograph of cervical spine demonstrates complete destruction of the body of C2 with a large anterior tissue mass encroaching on the airway. It is impossible to appreciate any posterior soft tissue and subsequent effect on the cervical spinal cord. **B,** Contrast-enhanced axial CT scan of neck showed metastatic destruction of the body of C2 resulting in an unstable spine. Note posterior epidural tumor *(arrow)* producing early spinal cord compression.

skull base fracture, or a known sinus, skull base, or nasopharyngeal tumor should trigger concerns as to the integrity of the bony skull base. A misdirected nasoendotracheal or nasogastric tube can very easily extend through a deficient skull base, with catastrophic positioning intracranially. These patients, by history, will be identified preoperatively, and the appropriate workup with CT and/or magnetic resonance imaging (MRI) will identify those areas of greatest danger for the anesthesiologist. In the pediatric population, blind placement of nasal airways should be avoided due to the potential complications of CSF leak and meningitis from unsuspected nasal cavity encephaloceles.[1]

The mechanical inability to open the mouth occurs in predictable circumstances. Severe degenerative arthritis, traumatic arthritis (Fig. 2-2), and juvenile rheumatoid arthritis result in destruction of the mandibular head and the joint space, resulting in varying degrees of limitations of mouth opening. Radiographs or panographic mandibular views may identify those patients at greatest risk for problems. If in doubt, CT provides the most helpful imaging for bony architecture and position of the mandibular heads. Limited mouth opening is also characteristically present with myositis ossificans progressiva. Fibrositis with progressive ossification of the muscles of mastication produces trismus. Eventual bony

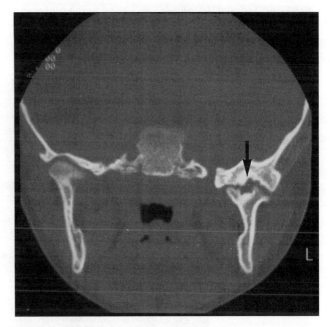

Fig. 2-2. *Posttraumatic degenerative temporomandibular arthritis.* Unenhanced coronal CT of temporomandibular joint demonstrates destruction of the left condylar head and the glenoid fossa *(arrow)*. Note also shortening of left mandibular ramus due to destruction of the growth center.

ankylosis of muscles to the mandible and skull base occur over time. This disease is best appreciated radiologically by CT.

Isolated fracture-dislocation of the mandible is identified by routine radiographs or a panograph. Complex trauma with multiple facial bone and mandibular fractures requires CT for adequate assessment. However, mandibular head dislocations are most frequently identified in the postoperative patient requiring a CT brain scan for evaluation of neurologic symptoms. The dislocations may be due to the recent intubation.

II. ANATOMY

Familiarity with the compartments of the head and neck and with the fascial planes of the neck is essential for an understanding of the extent to which the airway can be affected by both tumors and infections. While tumors of respiratory epithelial origin will have an obvious effect on the airway, the ability of more deeply located tumors to cause airway deformity or obstruction may be less readily appreciated.

The compartments of the head (Fig. 2-3) include: (1) the nasopharynx, which consists of respiratory mucosa and lymphoid tissue; (2) the parapharyngeal space, which consists predominantly of fat with a few small blood vessels and nerves and, occasionally, minor salivary gland tissue; (3) the infratemporal fossa (also known as the masticator space), which consists of the deep lobe of the parotid gland, the ramus of the mandible, the medial and lateral pterygoid muscles, the head of the temporalis muscle, cranial nerve V_3, the internal maxillary artery branches, fat, lymphatics, and occasionally minor sali-

vary gland tissue; (4) the neurovascular bundle (also known as the carotid space), which contains the internal carotid artery, internal jugular vein, cranial nerves IX, X, XII, and the sympathetic chain.[2]

The relationship of the compartments of the head to the oral cavity and its compartments must also be noted. The oral cavity is subdivided into (1) anterior tongue and floor of the mouth; (2) base of the tongue; (3) oropharynx, including the lateral oropharyngeal mucosal surface; (4) tonsil; (5) retromolar trigone; and (6) submandibular space. Those compartments of the head and oral cavity that are of special significance to each other are the parapharyngeal space, the neurovascular bundle, and the submandibular space. The parapharyngeal space extends from the skull base to the fascia covering the submandibular gland. Therefore, it is in direct continuity with the submandibular space, which is of paramount importance for the spread of infections. Since the parapharyngeal space also lies deep to the tonsillar pillars, it allows peritonsillar infections to spread to the submandibular space. Similarly, a deep lobe parotid abscess, lying in the infratemporal fossa and abutting the parapharyngeal space, can spread extensively. It is also obvious how carotid artery erosion and internal jugular vein thrombosis occur as complications of both tumors and infection, since both lie in intimate relationship to the parapharyngeal space and the infratemporal fossa.

The compartments of the head and oral cavity also have an extremely important relationship to the potential fascial planes of the neck, accounting for the other serious complications of peritonsillar and orodontal

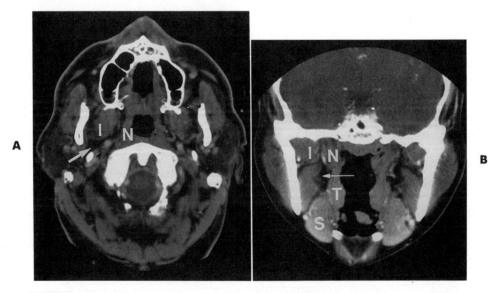

Fig. 2-3. A, *Compartments of the head. Axial CT scan. I,* Infratemporal fossa; *N,* nasopharynx; *black arrowhead,* neurovascular bundle; *long white arrowhead,* parapharyngeal space. **B,** *Coronal CT scan. I,* Infratemporal fossa; *N,* nasopharynx; *long white arrow,* parapharyngeal space; *S,* submandibular gland; *T,* tonsil.

infections, namely, tracking down the major vessels of the neck to the superior mediastinum, and down either the retropharyngeal space or danger space of the deep cervical fascia to the posterior mediastinum.[3]

The fascial compartments of the head and neck all interconnect with each other and can be divided into (1) localized compartments above the level of the hyoid, which include the submandibular space and parapharyngeal space; (2) localized compartments below the level of the hyoid, which include the anterior visceral (pretracheal) space. It extends from the hyoid bone to the anterior mediastinum and surrounds the trachea to lie along the anterior margin of the esophagus. It is contiguous with the retropharyngeal space and becomes involved following tracheal and esophageal perforations and hypopharyngeal trauma. The attachment of the pretracheal fascia to the pericardium and parietal pleura explains the occurrence of pericarditis and empyema with mediastinitis; and (3) spaces which involve the length of the neck. These include (a) the retropharyngeal space, which extends from the skull base to the superior mediastinum and is the commonest route by which oropharyngeal infections involve the mediastinum. The retropharyngeal space is limited anteriorly by the deep cervical fascia and posteriorly by the alar fascia (the deep layer of the deep cervical fascia) and lies posterior to the oral cavity, hypopharynx, and esophagus. The retropharyngeal space extends to the level of T6, at which point it is closed off by connective tissue at the carina, (b) the danger space, between the alar and prevertebral layers of the deep cervical fascia, extending from the skull base to the level of the diaphragm in the posterior mediastinum. This space becomes involved by infection in the retropharyngeal and parapharyngeal spaces, and (c) the vascular space along the neurovascular bundle, the fascia of which is connected to the three layers of the deep cervical fascia. Although involvement of this space by infection tends to remain localized, it can be a route for extension to the mediastinum.

With this compartmental approach in mind, an understanding of the tumors and infections encountered in the head and neck can be more readily understood. The most common reason for imaging the airway is a history of airway obstruction. Following the clinical history and endoscopic evaluation, imaging is nearly always required to adequately assess the airway. These studies are complementary in that the endoscopist can best evaluate the mucosa and the radiologist can best evaluate the submucosal anatomy. The role of imaging is to: (1) assess the deep extent of a lesion; (2) determine the length of the airway involved; (3) demonstrate lymphadenopathy that may not be palpable; and (4) determine the proximity of masses to the carotid artery and skull base, both of which may affect the operability

of the lesion. The single most useful imaging modality to assess the airway is CT. MRI has a varying contribution, and its use will be touched upon in the specific circumstances for which it is most suited.

III. PATHOLOGY

A. THE PEDIATRIC NASAL AIRWAY

1. Congenital atresias and stenoses

Nasal agenesis, as an isolated anomaly, is extremely uncommon. Variable presence of the premaxilla, and the symptoms related to airway obstruction, has been described.[4,5] CT is useful in defining the absence of nasal bones and the presence and thickness of bony atresia plates, while MR in the coronal plane confirms the presence or absence of olfactory nerves.

Bony atresias and stenoses of the nasal cavity are more common, with posterior choanal stenosis-atresia being the most frequent (Fig. 2-4). Unilateral or bilateral, these stenoses are predominantly bony and are due to defective development of the oronasal membrane at the level of the posterior choanae. Rare atresias posterior to this are membranous and are caused by a persistent buccopharyngeal membrane.[6] Infants with bilateral disease present at birth or during their first feed with respiratory distress, although they are able to breathe with crying. Unilateral atresia-stenosis presents later in life with unilateral nasal obstruction and a chronic nasal discharge. Patients with suspected choanal

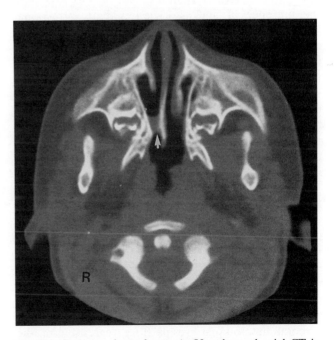

Fig. 2-4. *Posterior choanal stenosis.* Unenhanced axial CT in 7-month-old female demonstrates right posterior choanal obstruction by bony stenosis. Medial deviation of medial wall of the maxillary sinus and lateral deviation of the vomer form a cone-shaped nasal cavity, while soft tissue density bar obstructs the residual choanal opening *(arrow).*

atresia require a CT scan following the instillation of vasoconstrictive nasal drops. The most common CT features of posterior choanal atresia-stenosis include medial deviation of the medial maxillary wall, lateral deviation and thickening or splitting of the vomer, fusion or bridging of the vomer to the perpendicular plate of the palatine bone, elevation of the ipsilateral hard palate, hypoplastic inferior turbinates, and narrowing of the entire posterior nasal cavity.[7] Associated anomalies, more frequent with bilateral involvement,[8] are present in approximately 50% of patients and include defects of the anterior skull base with congenital absence of the cribriform plate and crista galli,[9] Treacher Collins syndrome, Pierre Robin anomaly, and the CHARGE association (coloboma, heart defects, atresia choanae, genital hypoplasia, retarded growth-development, ear anomalies). Due to the more contracted nasopharynx and narrowed posterior choanal region, there is a higher prevalence of both preoperative obstruction and surgical failures.[10]

Diffuse nasal cavity narrowing or stenosis may be associated with premature underdevelopment or midface hypoplasia, as in Crouzon's disease (craniofacial dysostosis), Treacher Collins syndrome (mandibulofacial dysostosis), kleeblattschädel syndrome, and Apert's syndrome (acrocephalosyndactyly).[8] CT evaluation in patients with midface hypoplasia is frequently performed to provide three-dimensional (3D) reconstructions prior to calvarial vault reshaping and to determine the presence of any associated midline intracranial anomalies. Any child with a midface hypoplasia syndrome and with a history of airway obstruction should be referred for anesthetic management of the airway during imaging. Multiple foci of airway stenosis or obstruction should be considered. Tracheal stenosis due to a completely cartilaginous trachea which lacks rings has been reported in a patient with Crouzon's disease,[11] and mandibular anomalies may make emergent airway access difficult in children with bronchial arch anomaly syndrome.

2. Congenital nasal masses

Nasal encephaloceles, dermoids, and gliomas are anomalies of nasofrontal development that result from incomplete regression of a transient projection of dura known to traverse the prenasal space during the end of the second gestational month. Herniation of brain parenchyma into this dural projection leads to nasal encephalocele, while nasal gliomas, also known as nasal cerebral heterotopias, result from regression of the craniad portion of the projection, sequestering herniated glial tissue either within the nasal cavity or in the subcutaneous preglabellar tissue. If the projection of dura remains adherent to the skin, a dermal sinus tract is formed that may terminate anywhere along the path of

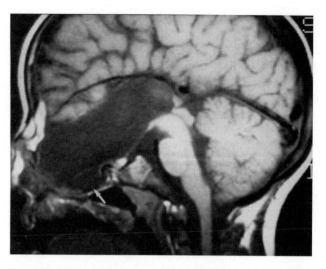

Fig. 2-5. *Sphenoidal-ethmoidal encephalocele.* T1-weighted (TR 600, TE 20) sagittal MRI in a 6-year-old child with frontonasal dysplasia reveals flattened nose, absence of corpus callosum, and dilated third ventricle that is herniating through a sphenoethmoidal defect to obstruct the nasal cavity. Note that anterior cerebral artery *(arrow)* is displaced into the nasal cavity by the encephalocele.

the dural projection. Desquamation of lining cells results in the formation of dermoid-epidermoid tumors along the tract.[12] These lesions commonly cause widening of the nasal bridge and palpable masses over the dorsum of the nose. Basal encephalocele (transethmoidal, sphenoethmoidal (Fig. 2-5), and nasoethmoidal) herniate into the nasal cavity and may cause significant obstruction.[13] CT and MRI are both able to detect these masses and define the extent of nasal cavity involvement and intracranial connections. Coronal CT best defines the bony defect in the crista galli, while MRI clearly differentiates the soft tissue components from CSF.[12]

Congenital nasolacrimal mucocele is an uncommon medial canthal mass with intranasal extension. CT is diagnostic, demonstrating the intranasal cystic mass and dilatation of both the lacrimal sac and nasolacrimal duct. These lesions may be unilateral or bilateral (Fig. 2-6).

3. Inflammatory lesions

Inflammatory polyps are associated with allergy, asthma, chronic infection, aspirin and nonsteroidal antiinflammatory drugs, along with cystic fibrosis and ciliary dyskinesia. Nasal obstruction in children with cystic fibrosis may be compounded by bony obstruction of the nasal cavity by medial bowing of the maxillary walls. Plain films or CT is usually adequate for evaluation. Sphenochoanal and antrochoanal polyps arise from the sphenoid and maxillary antra respectively, dilate their respective sinus ostia, and extend into the nasal cavity.[14] CT may demonstrate bone remodeling and, much less frequently, bone destruction

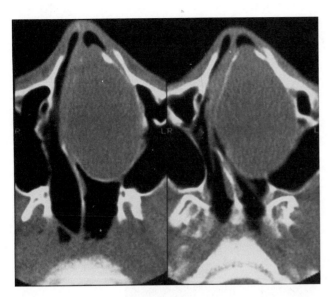

Fig. 2-6. *Nasal cavity epithelial cyst.* Unenhanced axial CT reveals a large, low attenuation nasal mass with a faintly calcified rim. The mass obstructs left nasal cavity, deviates the nasal septum to compromise the contralateral nasal cavity, distorts the nasal process of the maxillary bone, and deforms the medial wall of the left maxillary sinus.

that may simulate aggressive tumor erosion.[15]

Septal hematomas occur more frequently in childhood than in adulthood due to the more elastic mucoperichondrium in children. Intermittent bleeding and obstruction are suggestive of these lesions, which can develop immediately following birth, with later severe nasal trauma, or with occult trauma, such as that associated with an intranasal foreign body. Children with nasal foreign bodies may present with unilateral nasal obstruction and purulent nasal discharge. These may be associated with pyogenic granulomas or necrosis if the object has been present a short time and rarely may calcify or become a rhinolith if the object has been present for a long time.[16] Plain films may be all that is required in acutely impacted foreign bodies, while enhanced CT helps to define the extent of the associated vascular granulation tissue. Direct coronal CT is obviously required if any of the above is associated with CSF leakage.

4. Neoplasms

Malignant tumors of the nose are rare in children, the most common of these being rhabdomyosarcoma. Other lesions, such as lymphoma, chloroma, malignant teratoma, esthesioneuroblastoma, and histiocytosis, also occur. CT is used to define the degree of obstruction, associated bone destruction, and metastatic spread, while MRI provides information on intracranial invasion and potential subarachnoid spread.

Benign nasal tumors include squamous papilloma, teratoma, and proliferating hemangioma. Nasal papil-

lomas are extremely common small pedunculated, cauliflower-like growths arising from the septum or from the mucosa of the vestibule.[13] Imaging is rarely called for. Proliferating hemangiomas and venous malformations that are causing nasal obstruction and epistaxis, on the other hand, may require complex imaging with CT, MR, and angiography and endovascular or percutaneous embolization. Capillary hemangiomas, which are proliferating masses of endothelioid cells, need to be differentiated from venous malformations of the nasal vault due to their differing course and therapy. Proliferating hemangiomas exhibit dense, early enhancement of lobular masses with distinct margins on CT following the administration of intravenous contrast material. Intense staining with glandlike architecture is seen on arteriography. These lesions involute to fibrofatty tissue over time and may respond to steroid or interferon therapy. If obstructive or life threatening, endovascular embolization may be used to speed the process of involution. Venous malformations are vascular malformations present at birth, may contain phleboliths, and are composed of round or tubular structures that densely enhance following contrast material. Angiography may demonstrate an avascular mass or a faint blush without arteriovenous shunting. Venous malformations do not involute over time, nor do they respond to steroid or interferon therapy.

Nasal obstruction by fibroosseous lesions of the maxilla and midface, such as fibrous dysplasia, aggressive fibromatosis, ossifying fibroma, and extramedullary hematopoiesis (Fig. 2-7), may involve both soft tissue and bone. Nasal obstruction in fibrous dysplasia may be due to direct involvement of the turbinates and bony expansion by fibrous lesions.[17]

B. THE ADULT NASAL AIRWAY

1. Inflammatory lesions

The most common intrinsic pathology to encroach on the adult nasal airway is benign polyposis. Often, imaging is not done preoperatively. However, benign inflammatory disease of the paranasal sinuses and granulomatous disease such as Wegener's granulomatosis or midline lethal granuloma can aggressively destroy the bony margins of the sinuses and the skull base, usually at the cribriform plate, and behave in a malignant fashion. When required, CT will clearly demonstrate the presence of nasal polyps and the extent of secondary sinus and nasal obstruction and also will exclude other pathology such as benign or malignant tumors.

2. Neoplasms

Benign tumors arising at the nasoethmoid junction include angiofibroma and inverting papilloma (Fig. 2-8), both of which can behave aggressively and erode the skull base and/or the orbit. Although angiofibromas (Fig.

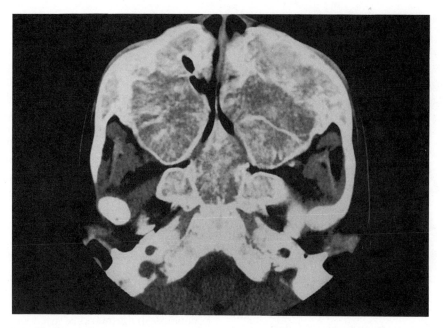

Fig. 2-7. *Thalassemia.* Unenhanced axial CT in 21-year-old female demonstrates severe nasal cavity obstruction secondary to marked bone marrow expansion in all facial bones.

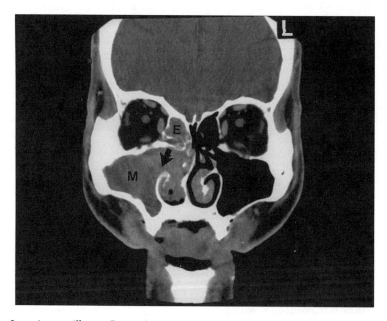

Fig. 2-8. *Inverting papilloma.* Coronal contrast-enhanced CT scan shows complete right nasal obstruction secondary to a mass in the nose, with extension through widened maxillary sinus ostium *(arrow)*. Note secondary obstruction of the right maxillary *(M)* and ethmoid sinuses *(E)*.

2-9) are most common in teenage males, they occasionally present between 18 and 30 years. Symptoms of nasal obstruction and epistaxis will ensure that a CT or MRI scan is done to assess the airway. Squamous cell carcinoma, the commonest malignancy of the paranasal sinuses, tends to destroy the bony margins of its sinus of origin and produce nasal or nasopharyngeal obstruction. The ethmoid and maxillary sinuses are most frequently involved. Of greatest concern for the surgeon and the anesthesiologist is the integrity of the skull base. Frequently, the cribriform plate and medial or inferior orbital walls are destroyed by the tumor, making biopsy-intubation more hazardous. Adenocarcinoma, lymphoma, adenoid cystic carcinoma, and esthesioneuroblastoma also behave in a similar manner. If any of these tumors erode bone at the skull base, either at the

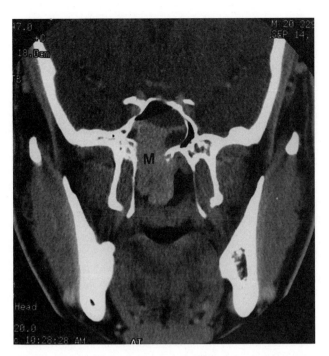

Fig. 2-9. *Juvenile angiofibroma.* Coronal contrast-enhanced CT scan shows vascular mass *(M)* in right side of the nasopharynx with extension into the sphenoid sinus.

cribriform plate, clivus, or orbit, an MRI with gadolinium enhancement is essential to assess for dural and/or brain invasion. Gadolinium is an intravenous contrast agent analogous to that used for CT enhancement, allowing better differentiation of pathology from normal structures.

C. THE PEDIATRIC NASOPHARYNGEAL AIRWAY

1. Congenital lesions

Teratomas are the most common symptomatic congenital nasopharyngeal mass. They tend to be in the midline and may have intracranial or mediastinal extension. These lesions may be solid or cystic, with distinct or infiltrative margins. Demonstration of calcification, ossification, and fat on CT or MR scans are highly suggestive of the diagnosis.[8] Intermittent airway obstruction has been described with congenital pedunculated nasopharyngeal lesions such as dermoid or lipoma. Brain heterotopia is an extremely rare cause of nasopharyngeal obstruction. The pathology is similar to nasal glioma, but there is no intracranial extension or apparent bony defect.[8]

Mucopolysaccharide storage (MPS) in the soft tissues of the upper airway is progressive, with nasopharyngeal infiltration leading to respiratory compromise. Submucosal thickening sequentially involves the upper, mid, and lower airway, leading to gradual deformity and collapse of the trachea.[18] At the same time, MPS deposition within the tectorial membrane at the craniocervical junction leads to severe cord compression in the region of the foramen magnum, and potential cervical spine instability renders airway management even more difficult.

2. Inflammatory lesions

Nasal obstruction from adenoidal hyperplasia can result in hypoventilation and eventual cor pulmonale. Obstruction can occur from hyperplasia of adenoidal tissue in a normal nasopharyngeal cavity[19] or superimposed on an abnormally small airway, seen in midfacial hypoplasia syndromes. A lateral plain film of the neck is all that is required to evaluate adenoidal hypertrophy, while CT is necessary to evaluate an underlying stenotic airway. Acute marked enlargement of the tonsillar-adenoidal tissue occurs in association with prevertebral soft tissue swelling in infectious mononucleosis.

Retropharyngeal abscesses comprise approximately 10% of peritonsillar and neck abscesses in children.[20] These lesions may occur secondary to penetrating trauma or infection of the nasopharynx or mastoid air cells. Neck stiffness in association with bulging of the prevertebral space on a well-positioned lateral plain film are suggestive. Contrast-enhanced CT scans demonstrate a low density mass with a thick enhancing rind if an abscess has evolved, but differentiation from adenitis or the presuppurative stage may be difficult in the absence of fluid-debris levels or gas within the collection.

Extension into the mediastinum is now a rare but potentially lethal complication, as are atlantoaxial subluxation and spinal epidural extension. Signs of these complications should be sought on all imaging studies evaluating retropharyngeal abscesses.[21]

3. Neoplasms

Juvenile angiofibromas are the most common benign nasopharyngeal tumors. Prepubescent males with juvenile nasopharyngeal angiofibromas present with nasal obstruction and recurrent epistaxis. CT demonstrates a densely enhancing nasopharyngeal mass that fills the nasopharynx and extends into the posterior nasal cavity, infratemporal fossa, and occasionally into the middle cranial fossa. Coronal CT is necessary to search for intracranial and subtle intraorbital extension. MRI, with gadolinium enhancement and fat suppression technique, further defines the extent of the tumor, particularly if CT determination of intracranial invasion is equivocal. Preoperative angiography defines any internal carotid arterial supply for the surgeon, while preoperative embolization of external carotid arterial supply to the tumor lessens intraoperative blood loss.[13]

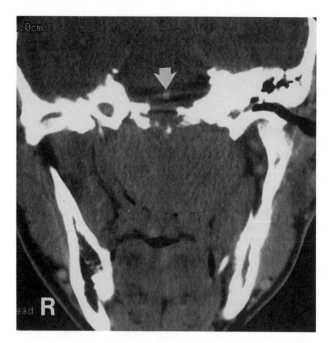

Fig. 2-10. *Squamous cell carcinoma of nasopharynx.* Contrast-enhanced coronal CT scan shows very large soft tissue mass in the nasopharynx involving both sides of the midline. Note destruction of the clivus with tumor in the prepontine cistern, displacing the basilar artery posteriorly *(arrow).*

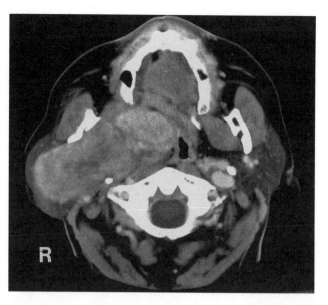

Fig. 2-11. *Pleomorphic adenoma of the parotid.* Axial contrast-enhanced CT image shows large pleomorphic adenoma arising in the deep lobe of right parotid gland (in infratemporal fossa). Note complete obliteration of the parapharyngeal fat and deformity of the nasopharyngeal airway.

Nasopharyngeal malignancies are uncommon in childhood but include rhabdomyosarcoma, lymphoma, and carcinoma.

D. THE ADULT NASOPHARYNGEAL AIRWAY

1. Neoplasms

The nasopharynx, while intrinsically affected by malignancy, also frequently is affected by tumors originating in the parapharyngeal space, neurovascular bundle, and infratemporal fossa. The major intrinsic tumors of the nasopharynx arise from the squamous epithelium or lymphoid tissue, with the occasional occurrence of adenocarcinoma or minor salivary gland tumor.

The clivus is frequently destroyed by squamous cell carcinoma (Fig. 2-10), even though only a small soft tissue tumor may be seen endoscopically in the nasopharynx. This abnormal bone is exceedingly soft and allows endotracheal-nasogastric tubes or biopsy needles to readily traverse the pathologic bone, allowing inadvertent intracranial access. Involvement of the cavernous sinus and perineural spread along cranial nerve V_2 or V_3 usually requires coronal MR imaging with gadolinium enhancement.

Non-Hodgkin's lymphoma in the nasopharynx presents with a considerable soft tissue mass, more often bilateral than unilateral, and most often spares the underlying bone. Extension down the tonsil is common.

Imaging characteristics are nonspecific and diagnosis is dependent on biopsy.

The parapharyngeal space is more often compressed by an adjacent tumor in the infratemporal fossa or nasopharynx than the primary site of origin of a tumor. Since the parapharyngeal space contains predominantly fat and a few small blood vessels and nerves, it infrequently gives rise to primary tumors. Minor salivary gland tissue, located everywhere in the head and neck, can occasionally give rise to a tumor in the parapharyngeal space. Similarly, infratemporal fossa pathology, most often arising in the deep lobe of the parotid (Fig. 2-11), can become sufficiently large to produce significant anatomic airway deformity rather than physiologic compromise. Neurogenic tumors, arising from branches of V_3, originate in the infratemporal fossa.

More unusual histologic malignancies include lymphoma, rhabdomyosarcoma, malignant fibrous histiocytoma, and metastases. Infratemporal fossa tumors often present late, having attained a large size before presenting with clinical symptoms. Since this area is neither visible intraorally nor palpable superficially, tumors rarely present before they have become large enough to produce trismus (by interference with the function of the muscles of mastication) or sensory dysfunction of V_2 or V_3. CT or MR imaging is essential to define the location and extent of the lesion.

Neurovascular bundle (carotid space) masses include paragangliomas, neurogenic tumors of cranial nerves IX, X, and XII and the sympathetic chain, pseudoaneurysms of the internal carotid artery, and thrombosis of the jugular vein. The first two categories of tumors may be sufficiently large to deform the airway.

E. THE PEDIATRIC ORAL CAVITY

1. Congenital lesions

Airway obstruction by the tongue occurs secondary to its size or its position. Glossoptosis or posterior displacement of the tongue is seen in many congenital syndromes associated with mandibular hypoplasia or micrognathia. Mandibular catch-up growth over the first year of life usually alleviates the obstruction. A partial list of the more common syndromes in which micrognathia and resultant glossoptosis occur would include Pierre Robin, Treacher Collins, Goldenhar's, Freeman-Sheldon, Hallermann-Streiff, and trisomy 18.

Macroglossia may be an isolated entity or a feature of a congenital disorder such as Down syndrome or Beckwith-Wiedemann syndrome. Systemic disorders that lead to macroglossia include congenital hypothyroidism and MPS diseases.[8] Macroglossia is also seen in association with intrinsic congenital tongue masses, such as choristomas, dermoids, teratomas, vallecular cysts, and vascular malformations. Radiographic appearance of these mass lesions is extremely variable, dependent on the tissues of origin.

Lingual thyroid is suggested in a child with congenital hypothyroidism and stridor. The presence of lingual thyroid may be confirmed by uptake of Tc-99m sodium pertechnetate on thyroid scintigraphy, contrast-enhanced CT which demonstrates a homogeneously enhancing mass, ultrasound, or MRI, which reveals a midline mass posterior to the foramen cecum. Sagittal MRI is ideally suited to demonstrate the intravallecular thyroid displacing the epiglottis posteriorly into the airway. The entire airway should be imaged to exclude multiple lesions and intratracheal thyroid tissue. Thyroglossal duct cysts, described in the adult section to follow, occur as well in the pediatric population.

Vascular malformations, common oral lesions, are particularly frequent in the tongue. Diffuse lymphangiomatosis and venous malformations may cause macroglossia from hemorrhage into focally dilated lymphatic channels or acute obstruction of venous drainage. Both may acutely and massively enlarge following trauma or infection. Rim enhancement or complete lack of augmentation and fluid-fluid levels are seen with lymphatic malformations, while pools of contrast material are seen with venous malformations on both CT and MRI.

2. Neoplasms

Rapidly enlarging neoplastic tongue lesions include proliferating hemangioma of infancy and rhabdomyosarcoma. Proliferating hemangiomas are the most common head and neck tumors seen in the pediatric population, with the lip, cheek, and tongue being the most common locations. Dense enhancement of gland-like lesions is frequently associated with enlarged feeding arteries. Lack of involvement of adjacent bony structures is usual. Rapid enlargement during the first year of life and slow involution over several years is typical. Airway obstruction is one of the few indications for aggressive therapy in these lesions. The head and neck region is the most common primary site for rhabdomyosarcoma during childhood, with the tongue, palate, or cheek commonly involved. Rhabdomyosarcomas are less densely enhancing than proliferating hemangiomas and are more likely to involve adjacent bone. In the absence of cutaneous involvement, angiography and/or biopsy may be needed to differentiate these two rapidly expanding oral masses. Other rare causes of macroglossia include plexiform neurofibroma in association with neurofibromatosis, lipoma, and lingual carcinoma.

F. THE ADULT ORAL CAVITY

1. Neoplasms

The oral cavity lesions that are of sufficient size to produce airway symptoms are usually malignant, 90% of which are squamous cell carcinoma.[22] The tonsil is the commonest site, followed by tongue, floor of mouth, and retromolar trigone. Five percent of oral cavity malignancies are non-Hodgkin's lymphoma, predominantly involving the palatine and lingual lymphoid tissue. These may also become extremely large and cause respiratory and swallowing difficulties. The spread of both these tumors is submucosally, along deep musculofascial planes, along nerves (XII and V_3), and along perivascular spaces into bone. The mucosal involvement is readily apparent by endoscopy or direct visualization, but the deep extent of tumors can often not be readily appreciated by clinical examination. CT is the preferred method of imaging when tumor is contiguous to bone. However, perineural spread is more readily identified by MRI with gadolinium, keeping in mind the necessity to follow the entire course of these nerves both extracranially and intracranially. Perineural tumor spread is most commonly encountered in adenoid cystic carcinoma (arising in minor salivary gland tissue), recurrent squamous cell carcinoma, lymphoma, and sarcomas.

Squamous cell carcinoma accounts for 90% of all tongue malignancies, the remainder being non-Hodgkin's lymphoma (Fig. 2-12) and minor salivary gland neoplasms.[22] Twenty-five percent of these tumors involve the base of the tongue. This location, because of frequent inferior extension to the preepiglottic space, has greater likelihood of airway problems. Surgical management may also be rejected as total glossectomy and laryngectomy required for control of disease are often considered untenable for a particular patient.

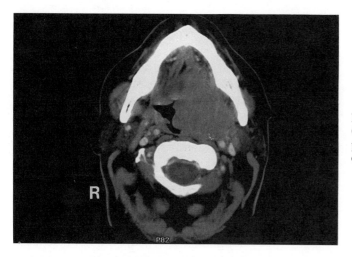

Fig. 2-12. *Lymphoma of the tongue.* Axial contrast-enhanced CT images demonstrate large hypodense mass arising from the posterior aspect of left side of the tongue. Note marked airway obstruction.

Partial glossectomy, common for anterior tongue and floor of mouth cancers, frequently cause swallowing difficulties, at least in the immediate perioperative period, resulting in aspiration problems. MR scanning is usually the only imaging examination required to define the lesion. Sagittal images are ideally suited to demonstrating extension of tumor from the tongue base into the preepiglotic space. While floor of the mouth carcinoma may invade the adjacent mandible, squamous cell carcinoma arising in the retromolar trigone does so more frequently and is more difficult to detect clinically. CT is indicated to assess this area adequately. Since mandibular invasion necessitates a much longer and more radical surgical procedure, it is essential to determine invasion preoperatively.

2. Inflammatory lesions

Infections of the oral cavity are potentially life threatening. Therefore, their early recognition is mandatory so that optimal treatment can be initiated. These patients frequently deteriorate extremely rapidly with acute respiratory obstruction; hence, an appreciation of the underlying abnormality and the extent of the infection is of paramount importance. An acute submandibular space cellulitis, Ludwig's angina, is usually secondary to an abscess arising in a periapical location around the second or third mandibular molar.[23] The marked swelling in the floor of the mouth causes elevation of the tongue and airway compromise. These patients often cannot tolerate lying flat, making early evaluation by CT impossible. A lateral soft tissue radiograph of the neck will demonstrate the marked submandibular swelling, allowing early diagnosis. If the patient fails to improve following 24 hours of intravenous antibiotics, and following the establishment of a safe airway, a CT scan should be done to define fully the extent of the infection, keeping in mind the need to assess the submandibular space, the parapharyngeal

space, the anterior visceral space, and the retropharyngeal and deep cervical fascial spaces into the mediastinum (Fig. 2-13). Ludwig's angina usually remains a diffuse cellulitis, without a well-defined abscess. As expected given its dental origin, the infection is usually of mixed flora, with both aerobic and anaerobic microorganisms.

Tonsillitis, pharyngitis, and peritonsillar abscesses (Fig. 2-14) are also potentially dangerous. These infections spread laterally into the parapharyngeal space, which allows inferior extension to the submandibular space. The retropharyngeal space and deep cervical fascial planes are at risk for extension to the mediastinum.[24] Similarly, the immediate proximity of the neurovascular bundle places the carotid artery at risk for erosion and the internal jugular vein at risk for thrombosis.

Uncommonly, an infection occurs in the infratemporal fossa from an infected maxillary molar.[25] Entry into this space is via alveolar canals in the posterior maxillary sinus wall through which run the posterior superior alveolar nerves and vessels. The dangerous structure within the infratemporal fossa is the pterygoid venous plexus, through which infection has direct access to the cavernous sinus and the orbit.

The radiologic evaluation of infection in the peritonsillar region, parapharyngeal space, and infratemporal fossa requires CT or MR scanning, following the establishment of a safe airway. CT will establish the extent of disease unless cavernous sinus thrombosis is suspected, in which case MR is the imaging technique of choice. Often these patients, because of respiratory compromise or increased secretions necessitating frequent swallowing, cannot cooperate fully for the length of time required for a diagnostic quality MRI. CT therefore is the imaging modality of choice.

By either CT or MRI, the earliest pathologic change in infection is haziness of the fat planes with loss of the

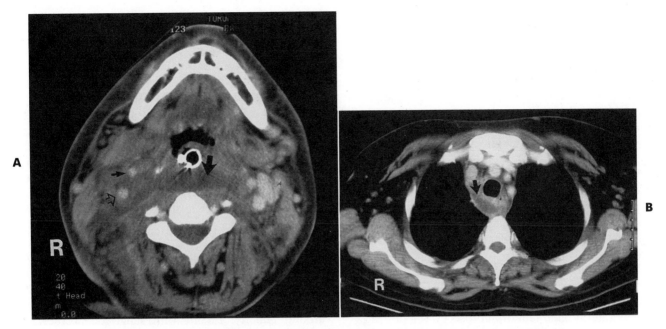

Fig. 2-13. A, *Retropharyngeal and mediastinal abscesses.* A 41-year-old woman presented with pharyngeal swelling resulting in acute airway obstruction requiring intubation for airway maintenance. Contrast-enhanced axial CT scans show extensive retropharyngeal low-density mass *(large arrow)* indicative of early abscess formation. Note extension to involve the neurovascular bundle, with inflammatory change separating the internal carotid artery *(small closed arrow)* from the internal jugular vein (small open arrow). **B,** The infection has tracked down the retropharyngeal space into the mediastinum, with a loculated collection seen in a paraesophageal location *(arrow).*

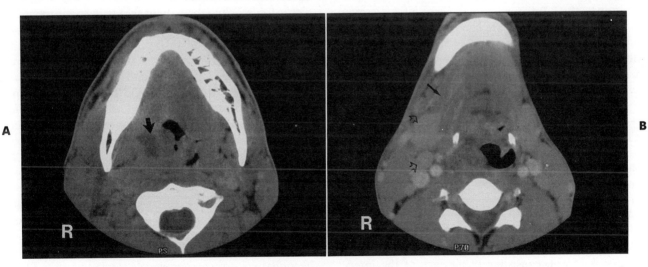

Fig. 2-14. A, *Peritonsillar abscess extending to submandibular space.* Contrast-enhanced axial CT scans show right peritonsillar abscess (arrow) extending to the parapharyngeal space. **B,** The infection descends to right submandibular space where early abscess formation is also evident *(closed arrow).* Note enlargement of submandibular and internal jugular lymph nodes *(open arrows).*

sharp margins of adjacent muscles and/or the neurovascular bundle. As the infection becomes localized, more focal pockets of inflammatory debris and pus become defined. The ability of imaging to define the location and extent of infection, to determine if abscess formation has occurred within the area of cellulitis, to suggest a possible source of infection, and to reveal vascular complications is essential information for the management of neck and orodontal infections.[26]

G. THE PEDIATRIC LARYNX

1. Congenital lesions

Laryngomalacia, or inspiratory laryngeal collapse, is the most common form of congenital laryngeal obstruction. This self-limiting disorder is thought to be due to immaturity of cartilaginous development and usually resolves by 18 months of age without the need for airway intervention. Rare severe cases may, however, require resection of redundant tissue, epiglottiplasty, or tracheostomy. Lateral plain film or fluoroscopy demonstrates anteroinferior displacement of the "floppy" aryepiglottic folds during respiration.

Vocal cord paralysis may be congenital or acquired, unilateral or bilateral. Unilateral lesions are more likely to involve the peripheral motor nerves, particularly the longer left recurrent laryngeal nerve that is easily damaged during birth or thoracotomy. Central nervous system lesions, such as Arnold-Chiari malformation or hydrocephalus, are more likely to result in bilateral paralysis due to stretching of the vagus nerve over the lip of the jugular foramen.[27,28]

Laryngeal webs are usually located in the region of the anterior commissure. These webs may be thin membranes, thick webs, or partial fusion of the cords. While identifiable on lateral plain films, thin slice, high resolution axial CT scans provide more detailed information about the thickness and position of the webs and the frequently encountered associated airway anomalies, such as congenital subglottic stenosis.[29] Rarely, laryngeal atresia, or complete cord fusion, occurs due to failure of laryngeal cannulation.[28] Several types of laryngeal atresia have been described. Supraglottic obstruction with absent vestibule and subglottic stenosis or supraglottic obstruction that separates a shallow primitive vestibule from a normal subglottis are both usually accompanied by other defects.

Arrest of the dorsal advance of the cricoid results in laryngotracheoesophageal cleft, or a variable failure of separation of larynx from esophagus.[30] The malformation may be focal, consisting of absence of the interarytenoid muscle, or diffuse, with the presence of a single tube representing the larynx, trachea, and esophagus.[28] Barium esophagram and CT are useful in the diagnosis of this lesion, although barium studies may misdiagnose clefts as high tracheoesophageal fistulae.

Maldevelopment of the cricoid cartilage or the subglottic submucosa results in congenital subglottic stenosis.[30] Diagnosis of congenital subglottic stenosis is made by failure to pass a 3.5 mm endoscope past the region of the cricoid.[27] Evaluation with plain films or CT demonstrates the extent of stenosis distal to the reach of the endoscope. Children with congenital subglottic stenosis, seen in Down syndrome, are at increased risk of developing obstruction with upper airway infection and may have frequent and recurrent episodes of laryngotracheobronchitis. While congenital stenosis tends to resolve with growth, obstruction may be severe enough to necessitate early tracheostomy.

2. Neoplasms

Laryngeal papillomatosis is the most common pediatric laryngeal tumor. Primarily affecting the glottis with multiple masses, these lesions can seed the distal respiratory tract. Spontaneous involution may occur around puberty. Infants with subglottic proliferating hemangioma develop progressive obstruction prior to 6 months of age, while maintaining a normal cry. Classically, a small, irregular soft tissue mass is seen below the true cords on plain films. Up to 50%, however, may demonstrate symmetric narrowing on frontal films due to a posterior or circumferential lesion.

3. Inflammatory lesions

Laryngotracheobronchitis, or croup, is a diffuse viral inflammation. Tapering of the subglottis or the "steeple sign," is seen on frontal plain films. Acute bacterial epiglottitis, usually due to *Haemophilus influenzae*, produces acute inflammation of the epiglottis and aryepiglottic folds. While the patient should never be moved to a radiology department for films, a portable lateral film may be requested when symptoms are atypical. In addition to swelling of the epiglottis and aryepiglottic folds, pharyngeal distension and cervical kyphosis are commonly seen.[29] Angioneurotic edema and Stevens-Johnson syndrome may cause a similar radiographic appearance. Aryepiglottic cysts and epiglottic cysts are seen as soft tissue masses in the region of the aryepiglottic folds or epiglottis.

H. THE ADULT LARYNGEAL AIRWAY

1. Neoplasms

The majority of patients with laryngeal airway obstruction who are sent for imaging have a malignancy. Ninety-nine percent of malignancies of the larynx and hypopharynx are squamous cell carcinoma.[31,32] T1 tumors frequently are not imaged, since the endoscopist can confidently stage these tumors. However, as larger tumors extend more deeply submucosally, imaging becomes extremely important. CT is the most accurate way to stage T3 and T4 tumors. Tumors of this size almost

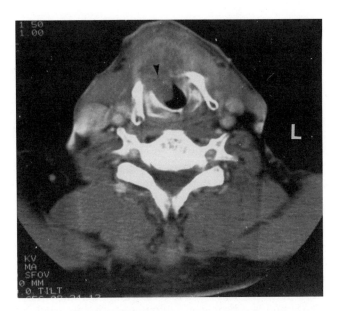

Fig. 2-15. *Transglottic squamous cell carcinoma.* Contrast-enhanced axial CT scan shows soft tissue tumor in the anterior aspect of the subglottis. This component and the airway narrowing are visible to the endoscopist. Extensive thyroid cartilage destruction *(arrow)* can only be clearly revealed by imaging, CT being the preferred modality.

always have a significant element of airway obstruction, making it impossible for the patient to remain still for the block of time required for each sequence of an MRI scan (3 to 10 minutes). As CT acquires images individually rather than as a block, the scanning time is 1 to 2 seconds per image. Even so, a severely obstructed patient will have difficulty lying flat and maintaining quiet respirations for CT. CT of the larynx very adequately evaluates the degree of airway compromise and the erosion of laryngeal cartilages and demonstrates the superior and inferior extent of pathology (Fig. 2-15). However, it can not reliably differentiate tumor edema from tumor, and the surgeon must rely on histologic results of biopsies for this information. MRI also fails to provide this differentiation.

The site of origin of carcinoma within the larynx is well identified by CT, as the supraglottic, glottic, and subglottic airways are clearly defined. Carcinoma most often remains within the larynx, rather than extending posteriorly into the hypopharynx or laterally into the neck. In the supraglottic larynx, tumor frequently involves the fat of the preepiglottic space, allowing inferior extension to the anterior commissure and the vocal cords. At the level of the glottis, most carcinomas originate on the anterior third of the vocal cord. The tumor can then extend to the anterior commissure and cross to the contralateral cord. Deep submucosal extension from the cord puts the tumor into the paraglottic fat, with immediate proximity to the thyroid cartilage. Cartilaginous erosion is demonstrated on CT with 1.5

mm contiguous scans, using a special bone algorithm to sharply define the bone. Even in the face of a small soft tissue carcinoma on the cord, the presence of cartilage erosion upgrades the cancer to a T4, rarely cured by radiation alone. These patients usually ultimately require a total laryngectomy. CT is also extremely useful in assessing the neck for lymphadenopathy.

Although other malignancies involve the larynx, they are extremely uncommon, and only two warrant particular mention. Chondrosarcomas[31,33,34] have a virtually pathognomonic appearance on CT. The tumor arises from the posterior cricoid cartilage and presents as an exophytic soft tissue mass extending into the larynx and subglottic region. The most characteristic aspect of this tumor is the extensive bone formation that occurs within it, in association with rather extensive destruction of the underlying posterior cricoid cartilage. On occasion, it can extend through the cartilages and lie within the soft tissues of the neck. The only other lesion having a similar appearance is a chondroma, which can only be differentiated from the sarcomatous variety by biopsy.

Lymphoma[33,35] accounts for 2.8% of all malignancies involving the larynx and is seen as either a primary or secondary tumor. Although not definitively diagnosed radiologically, there are some features that raise a high index of suspicion. The tumor usually is extensive at the time of diagnosis and appears to be homogenously hypodense. It is usually significantly less dense than a squamous cell carcinoma, but definitive diagnosis requires histologic confirmation. Although there may be bilateral lymphadenopathy disproportionate to what one usually sees with squamous cell carcinoma, lymphoma can also occur in the larynx without lymphadenopathy.

2. Inflammatory lesions

Acute inflammatory disease of the laryngotracheobronchial tree secondary to bacterial or viral infections usually produce diffuse nonspecific edematous change.[31,36] Imaging is rarely required to either make the diagnosis or follow the progression of the disease. However, in the instance of nonresponse to antibiotics, imaging is occasionally required to exclude underlying pathology. Secondary infection of a thyroglossal duct cyst, mucous retention cyst, or laryngocele occasionally present as acute inflammatory masses within the larynx.

Thyroglossal duct cysts (Fig. 2-16) arise along the embryologic course of the thyroglossal duct, extending from the foramen cecum at the base of the tongue down to the position of the normal thyroid gland in the neck. Remnants of the cyst may contain secretory epithelium that results in collections of fluid. These may become secondarily infected and present with a soft tissue mass within the supraglottic larynx, producing significant airway obstruction. Fifteen percent of thyroglossal duct cysts occur in or around the hyoid bone, 20% occur in the

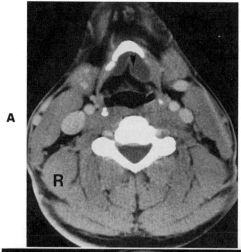

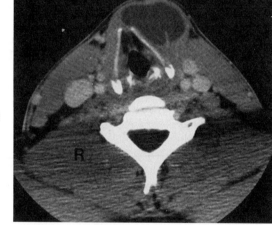

Fig. 2-16. A, *Thyroglossal duct cyst.* Contrast-enhanced axial CT scan reveals cystic mass in the preepiglottic space *(arrow)* with mild airway narrowing. **B,** Location of the inferior aspect of the cyst, now seen extrinsic to thyroid cartilage, is typical of thyroglossal duct cyst.

suprahyoid region up to the base of the tongue, and the remaining 65% occur inferior to the hyoid.[22] In less than 1% of patients, papillary carcinoma of the thyroid may occur within a thyroglossal duct cyst.[2] Either CT or MRI will demonstrate the extent and location of the tract and the intralaryngeal narrowing of the airway.

Mucous secreting glands occur throughout the respiratory epithelium. Occasionally, they may obstruct with the development of mucous retention cysts that may present acutely or with a more indolent history of respiratory symptoms. These cysts, unlike laryngoceles (Fig. 2-17), remain within the larynx and tend to have a thin capsule around a fluid-filled cyst. They can be occasionally confused with an internal laryngocele that is obstructed and filled with fluid. However, a laryngocele can be traced down to the laryngeal ventricle from which it originates, a feature not seen with mucous retention cysts. The common occurrence of a mixed

variety of laryngocele with both external (extending through the thyrohyoid membrane) and internal components is a characteristic feature seen only with laryngoceles.

Chronic inflammatory processes are much less common in the larynx but do on occasion present diagnostic difficulties, since radiologically they cannot be differentiated from malignancies. As the cricoarytenoid and cricothyroid joints are synovial joints, they can be involved with active rheumatoid arthritis and present with relatively large soft tissue masses and cartilage destruction. Although the mucosa overlying the soft tissue mass is intact, the strong suspicion of malignancy is always entertained. Multiple deep biopsies and the appropriate clinical history are essential to make this diagnosis.

Systemic sarcoidosis involves the larynx in 1% to 3% of patients.[36] The involvement, usually of the supraglottic larynx, is nonspecific and requires biopsy for diagnosis. Similarly, chronic granulomatous disease such as Wegener's granulomatosis can produce laryngeal airway narrowing, usually in the subglottic larynx.[36] The imaging characteristics are nonspecific, demonstrating only diffuse soft tissue narrowing the airway. Biopsy of the lesion is required.

I. THE PEDIATRIC TRACHEA

1. Congenital lesions

Tracheal atresia is extremely rare. Patients do not survive to imaging unless esophageal-bronchial fistulae are present. Webs and fibrous strictures may result in fixed focal stenosis of tracheal segments despite lack of adjacent cartilaginous abnormalities. Fixed tracheal stenosis is also seen in association with segmental lack of the membranous portion of the posterior tracheal wall.[37] Diffuse progressive tracheal stenosis has also been described with MPS disorders such as Hurler's and Hunter's syndromes.[18] Evaluation of the entire tracheobronchial tree is necessary in the presence of stenosis, since the surgical prognosis is related to the total extent of tracheal narrowing and whether there is involvement of the mainstem bronchi. Axial CT to measure the diameter and length of the involved segment has replaced bronchography in the evaluation of tracheal narrowing. Tracheal compression and stenosis occurring in association with vascular rings, such as double aortic arch, and pulmonary artery slings are currently best evaluated with MRI.[38]

Tracheomalacia may be focal or diffuse, isolated, or associated with other congenital or acquired cartilaginous disorders. Tracheomalacia has been described following chronic endotracheal intubation and positive pressure ventilation for prematurity and in association with congenital cartilage disorders, such as chondromalacia and Larsen's disease, and in systemic disorders affecting cartilage such as Wegener's granulomatosis or

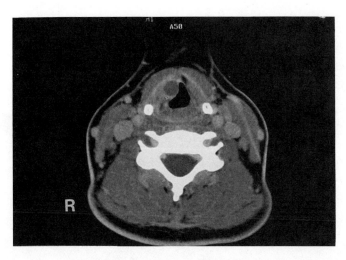

Fig. 2-17. *Internal laryngocele.* Contrast-enhanced axial CT images show cystic mass arising in the laryngeal ventricle. Both the appearance and location are typical for an obstructed internal laryngocele.

polychondritis. Focal tracheomalacia has also been described in 30% of patients with tracheoesophageal fistula and also in association with innominate artery compression.[38]

J. THE ADULT TRACHEA

1. Neoplasms

Benign neoplasms, which comprise less than 10% of tracheal tumors, include papillomas, salivary gland adenomas, and mesenchymal tumors such as hamartomas.[39] These lesions tend to be smooth, round, and well-defined and are generally small, less than 2 cm in diameter. An intratracheal soft tissue mass may be seen on plain film examination, but this will be better demonstrated by CT. The appearance is generally nonspecific, although, if fat is visualized, a hamartoma should be considered.

The commonest primary malignant tumors of the trachea are squamous cell carcinoma and adenoid cystic carcinoma.[40,41] Adenoid cystic carcinoma (Fig. 2-18) usually arises in the trachea or mainstem bronchi, less commonly in the lobar airways, and accounts for approximately 25% of primary malignant tracheal tumors.[42] It occurs most frequently in middle-aged patients, without sex predominance. Since it grows quite slowly, it is often misdiagnosed for years as asthma. The tumor tends to grow in a polypoid fashion into the airway lumen and spreads submucosally, often quite far from the main tumor mass. It may directly metastasize to mediastinal lymph nodes and to more distant sites, including the lungs. Despite metastatic spread, however, patients frequently have a prolonged course. Approximately 75% of patients are disease free 5 years after surgery.

Radiographically, both squamous cell carcinoma (Fig. 2-19) and adenoid cystic carcinoma may appear as intraluminal masses with smooth, irregular, or lobulated margins, causing a variable degree of narrowing of the airway lumen.[43,44] CT demonstrates thickening of the tracheal wall and evidence of extratracheal tumor mass. However, it has been shown that CT underestimates the degree of submucosal extension, with tumor being found in portions of the trachea appearing normal on CT.[43,45]

Mucoepidermoid carcinoma and carcinoid tumors occur infrequently in the trachea, both being more common in the larger airways.[46] Because of the vascular nature of carcinoid tumors, CT may demonstrate marked enhancement following the injection of intravenous contrast material.[47]

Secondary involvement of the trachea by tumor is usually by direct invasion from tumors of the thyroid gland, esophagus, larynx, and lung, or, less commonly, by hematogenous spread of melanoma, colon, breast carcinoma, and tumors of the genitourinary tract. These lesions usually manifest as a focal area of thickening of the tracheal wall. Lymphoma, usually from extracapsular extension from adjacent mediastinal nodes, may cause focal tracheal narrowing. In the absence of direct invasion, respiratory compromise can occur from the mass effect on the trachea.

Bronchogenic carcinoma can directly invade the mediastinum to involve the trachea. This may lead to tracheal displacement or narrowing. If the narrowing is severe, the patient is susceptible to complete collapse of the trachea if given a general anesthetic. This situation, therefore, must always be considered in a patient with a large tumor mass adjacent to the mediastinum in whom mediastinoscopy and/or thoracotomy is about to be

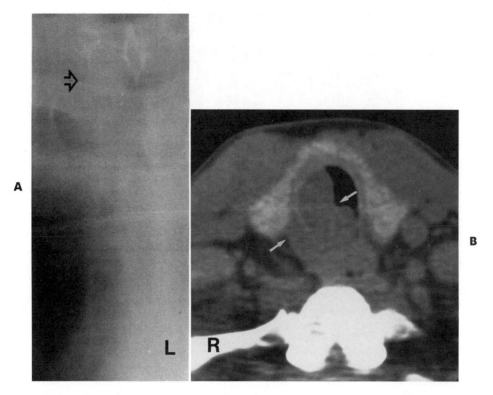

Fig. 2-18. A, *Adenoid cystic carcinoma of the trachea.* This coned radiograph reveals soft tissue mass arising from the right lateral wall of the upper trachea *(arrow)*. **B,** The contrast-enhanced CT image clearly reveals marked thickening of the right lateral and posterior aspects of the wall of the trachea *(arrows)* with narrowing of the lumen.

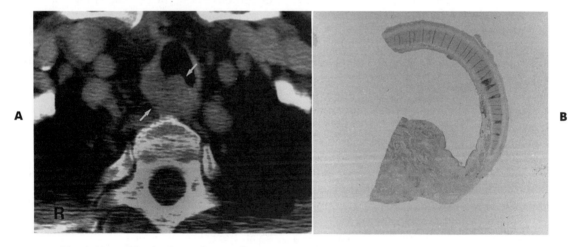

Fig. 2-19. A, *Tracheal squamous cell carcinoma.* Contrast-enhanced axial CT scan reveals significant thickening of right lateral and posterior aspects of the tracheal wall *(arrows)*, with mild narrowing of tracheal lumen. **B,** There is good correlation with the gross pathologic specimen (portion of lateral wall removed for histologic examination).

performed. If such a mass is noted and there is any suspicion of tracheal involvement, CT should be performed for more accurate assessment. If significant narrowing is seen, proper airway support must be established prior to deep anesthesia.

Enlarged mediastinal nodes may be due to a large number of causes. These include neoplastic disease (Hodgkin's and non-Hodgkin's lymphoma, metastases [Fig. 2-20], infection, tuberculosis [TB], fungal disease, chronic bacterial infection as seen in cystic fibrosis),

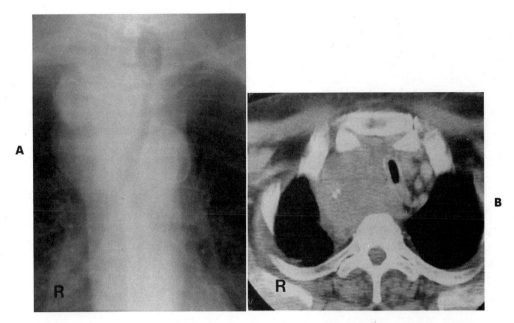

Fig. 2-20. A, *Metastatic lymphadenopathy.* This 67-year-old man presented with superior vena caval syndrome and was found to have metastatic testicular seminoma involving multiple mediastinal nodes. Posteroanterior (PA) chest radiograph reveals marked enlargement of right paratracheal nodes that are causing significant displacement of trachea to the left, with narrowing of the lumen. **B,** Contrast-enhanced axial CT scan reveals marked high right paratracheal lymphadenopathy with significant narrowing of tracheal lumen and displacement to the left. There is loss of fat plane between nodes and tracheal wall.

occupational exposure (silicosis), and chronic inflammatory (fibrosing alveolitis, sarcoidosis) and infiltrative (amyloidosis) diseases. These may cause both tracheal displacement and narrowing, which may require airway support under certain circumstances. A thyroid goiter is also a common cause of tracheal displacement and narrowing (Fig. 2-21).

2. Inflammatory lesions

Patients with active cavitary tuberculosis may develop infection of the trachea itself.[48] It initially causes ulceration of the tracheal mucosa, especially posterolaterally, which may progress to involve deeper layers of the trachea, resulting in a fixed fibrotic stricture (Fig. 2-22). The trachea may also become involved by direct spread from adjacent infected lymph nodes, especially in children. Some fungal diseases, such as histoplasmosis, can cause similar findings.

The trachea is rarely involved in patients with sarcoidosis. When involvement does occur, it generally affects the subglottic region almost always coincident with involvement in other body regions.[49] Involvement may manifest as intrinsic granulomatous lesions in the tracheal wall or compression by adjacent enlarged nodes. CT scanning may reveal thickening of the tracheal wall with primary tracheal disease or luminal narrowing by enlarged nodes.

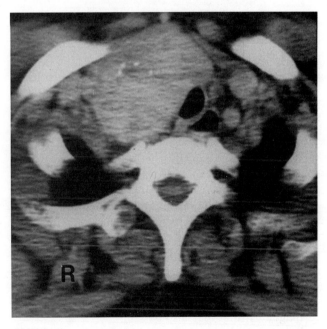

Fig. 2-21. *Goiter.* This 61-year-old woman has pathologically proven nodular hyperplasia of the thyroid. Contrast-enhanced axial CT scan reveals a large goiter that is causing slight narrowing of tracheal lumen and significant displacement to the left.

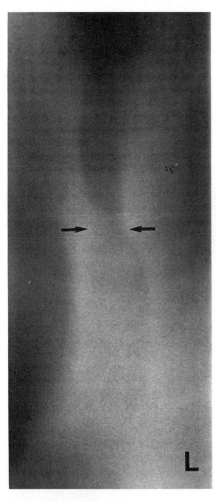

Fig. 2-22. *Tuberculosis.* The patient is a 49-year-old woman with previous history of pulmonary TB. This anteroposterior (AP) tomogram reveals significant narrowing of the mid portion of the trachea *(arrows)* secondary to previous tuberculous involvement of airway wall.

Wegener's granulomatosis is an idiopathic condition characterized by granulomatous inflammation and vasculitis in multiple organ systems, especially the upper and lower respiratory tracts and the kidneys. The entire trachea may be affected, although most commonly the upper trachea is involved.[50] Tracheal involvement is now known to be more common than previously thought and is no longer felt to be a late manifestation of the disease. The trachea may be noted to be narrowed with thickened walls on CT scanning. Abnormal calcification of the cartilaginous rings may also be seen.

Relapsing polychondritis, peaking between 40 and 60 years, is characterized by inflammation and destruction of cartilage in numerous sites, including the earlobes, nose, joints, ribs, larynx, and tracheobronchial tree.[51] The etiology is unknown, although it is generally felt to be an autoimmune disorder. Pathologically, an inflammatory infiltrate causes destruction of cartilage with subsequent fibrosis and stricture, or tracheomalacia. The disorder tends to wax and wane over time. The larynx and trachea are involved in about half of the cases. Tracheobronchial involvement may cause dyspnea, and patients may develop recurrent pneumonias, which constitute the most common cause of death. Radiographically, there may be narrowing of the trachea and large central bronchi. Calcification may be seen in the earlobes. CT may reveal airway deformity and wall thickening.[51]

Some patients with ulcerative colitis may develop tracheobronchitis, which may be associated with fibrosis in the submucosal regions of the trachea, leading to airway narrowing.[52] Both the membranous and cartilaginous portions of the trachea may be involved. The tracheal walls may be noted to be thickened on CT, causing irregular narrowing of the lumen.

3. Trauma

Of particular interest is the group of patients with the postinjured airway.[53] The posterior membranous portion of the trachea may be disrupted by excessive external force that compresses it against the vertebral column. As well, patients may develop a transverse tear of the trachea between cartilaginous rings, most commonly just superior to the carina. These tears may manifest radiographically by the presence of subcutaneous emphysema, pneumothorax, and/or pneumomediastinum.

The injury may be diffuse, as from inhalation of smoke or chemicals, or more focal, often secondary to prolonged endotracheal intubations. The radiologic appearances are virtually identical, differing only in the extent of the pathology, with the postintubation injury usually being more focal. The commonest site of mucosal injury after prolonged endotracheal intubation (greater than 10 days) is the posterior glottis, due to the cricoid ring being the narrowest part of the upper airway.[54] Ulceration of the mucosa rendered ischemic from tube pressure allows secondary bacterial infection with reparative granulation tissue, fibrosis, and, ultimately, scar tissue. Whited[55] reports an incidence of 6% stenosis in the posterior glottis in a prospective study of 200 intubated patients, while other authors report the incidence to be 14%.[56] The true incidence is difficult to ascertain, but postintubation injury definitely results in long-term management problems and significant disability for the patient.

In the postintubation injury, although most of the abnormality is at the glottic and subglottic level, there are diffuse changes in the supraglottic larynx as well. Interestingly, although the imaging appearance is that of diffuse swelling of the epiglottis and aryepiglottic folds

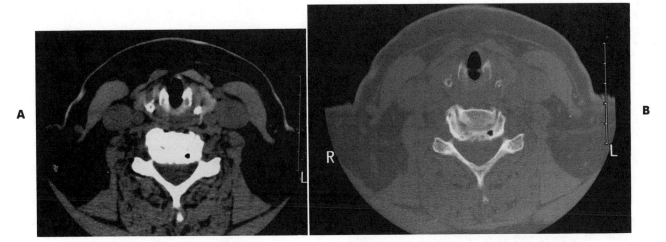

Fig. 2-23. A, *Subglottic soft tissue web.* Soft tissue windows on axial CT scan fail to demonstrate the thin web of soft tissue in the subglottis. **B,** The posterior web is seen only if bone window settings are done.

down to the vocal cords, this can not be appreciated by endoscopy where the mucosa is seen to be intact and the fullness of the aryepiglottic folds is not appreciated. At the level of the vocal cords, several abnormalities can exist, including cricoarytenoid dislocation, vocal cord fixation, extensive posterior soft tissue glottic scar, and simple posterior glottic webs. The injuries tend to be localized to the posterior aspect of the glottis, sparing the anterior commissure. In the subglottic larynx and upper trachea, intraluminal soft tissue extends for a variable length. The soft tissue may be circumferential or more localized but usually is contiguous. The role of imaging is to accurately measure the length of airway involvement. This requires 1.5 mm contiguous axial CT scans so that the segment of pathologic trachea can be determined for the surgeon. By the time imaging is done on these patients, many have had a long course of multiple failed tracheal dilatations.

If surgical resection of the involved segment becomes the treatment of choice, CT imaging is necessary for accurate measurement of the abnormal segment. CT also gives an indication of the possibility of underlying tracheomalacia, since the configuration of the trachea and the contour of the tracheal cartilages can be assessed. Glottic and subglottic webs are more difficult to demonstrate and require 1.5 mm cuts with photography at very high window settings in order to demonstrate the small soft tissue web (Fig. 2-23).

4. Miscellaneous

Although secondary amyloidosis is more common than primary, the latter is more likely to be associated with pulmonary and tracheobronchial involvement. However, local amyloidosis, a third type, is the usual form that affects the trachea. Men are more commonly involved than women, with an average age at diagnosis of 53 years. Sixty-five percent of patients die of their tracheal, bronchial, or pulmonary disease. Usually there is smooth narrowing of the entire trachea, although sometimes the thickening can be nodular (Fig. 2-24). Less commonly there is a single focus of mucosal thickening. Calcification may be seen, especially at CT.

Tracheobronchopathia osteochondroplastica is a rare condition of unknown etiology characterized by the presence of submucosal nodules of cartilage and bone in the trachea and bronchi. The nodules occur in the portions of the airway walls that normally contain cartilage and therefore spare the membranous portion. These nodules cause irregular narrowing of the tracheal lumen from the anterior and lateral walls and may extend into the mainstem bronchi. Most patients are asymptomatic, although some may develop dyspnea, hoarseness, productive cough, or hemoptysis. Tissue obtained at bronchoscopy is generally sufficient for making the diagnosis. Radiographically, the tracheal lumen is irregularly narrowed (Fig. 2-25). On CT, nodular thickening of the tracheal wall with sparing of the membranous portion is evident. Calcification may or may not be present. There may be signs of recurrent bronchial obstruction, including atelectasis and recurrent pneumonia.

Tracheomalacia is due to weakening of the tracheal walls, either due to a congenital deficiency of the cartilage or to acquired causes such as trauma, recurrent infections, intubation, chronic obstructive pulmonary disease, or relapsing polychondritis. Patients are generally elderly and present with dyspnea and wheezing. The diagnosis is made when the tracheal diameter is seen to collapse by more than 50% on CT

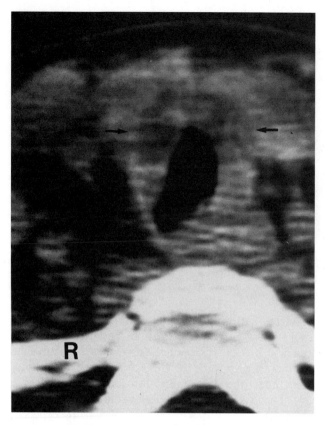

Fig. 2-24. *Amyloidosis.* This 51-year-old female had amyloidosis diagnosed at the time of a partial tracheal resection. Contrast-enhanced axial CT image reveals significant thickening of tracheal wall over most of the circumference *(arrows)*, with distortion of tracheal lumen.

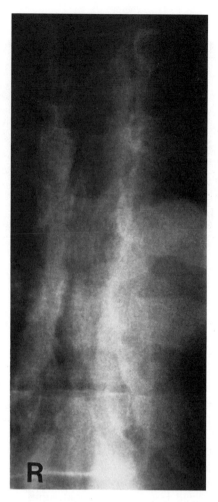

Fig. 2-25. *Tracheobronchopathia osteochondroplastica.* The coned radiograph of the trachea reveals irregular thickening of tracheal wall, with distortion of the lumen and extension of the process into the proximal mainstem bronchi.

scanning. Ultrafast and cine, CT may detect the disorder in some patients in whom the trachea appears normal on standard CT.

Saber sheath trachea is characterized by narrowing of the tracheal diameter in the coronal plane and widening in the sagittal plane, so the coronal diameter becomes less than half that of the sagittal (Fig. 2-26). The narrowing frequently extends over the entire length of the intrathoracic trachea, from the carina up to the thoracic inlet, where there is an abrupt change in the airway caliber back to normal. This abnormality tends to occur in elderly patients, usually men, with chronic obstructive pulmonary disease.

Fibrosing mediastinitis, whether due to histoplasmosis or idiopathic, may cause significant narrowing of the trachea. Radiographically, the tracheal narrowing may be easily visualized on plain films. CT scanning may reveal the adjacent mediastinal calcified fibrous plaques that are characteristic of this disease.

As can be seen from the above discussion, most tracheal diseases have a nonspecific radiographic appearance. The value of imaging, therefore, is in determining the severity and extent of the tracheal narrowing, rather than establishing a specific cause of the abnormality.

It is well known that tracheal lesions can be easily missed by chest radiography and are much more readily seen at CT. In one study, the sensitivity for detection of lesions of the trachea and main bronchi was 66% for chest radiography but 91% to 97% for CT.[57] Most of the lesions missed by radiography were less than 1 cm in diameter; CT missed abnormalities in the main bronchi only, so that its sensitivity for the trachea was actually 100%. They were both quite accurate at determining if the disease was focal or diffuse—correct by chest radiography in 91% of cases and by CT in 97%. However, they were only fair at determining if visible abnormalities represented benign or malignant disease, both having an accuracy of about 80%. As well, they were quite poor at determining the etiology of the lesion, the correct

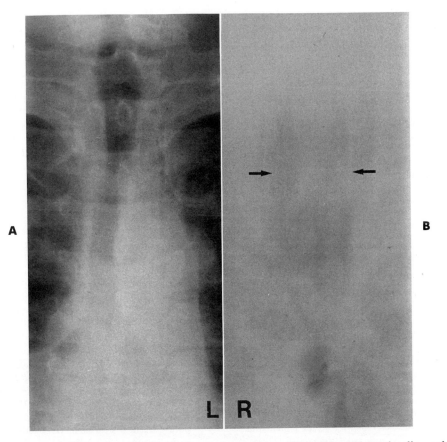

Fig. 2-26. A, *Saber-sheath trachea.* PA view. **B,** Lateral view. These PA and lateral radiographs of the trachea reveal significant narrowing of trachea on PA view with widening of the lumen on lateral view *(arrows).* Narrowing extends over the entire length of intrathoracic trachea with a return to normal caliber at the level of thoracic inlet.

diagnosis being included in the top three differential diagnoses being considered in about 60% of cases for both radiography and CT.

REFERENCES

1. Bannister CM, Kashab M, Dagestani H et al: Nasal endotracheal intubation in a premature infant with a nasal encephalocele, *Arch Dis Child* 69:81, 1993.
2. Reede DL, Bergeron RT, Osborn AG: CT of the soft tissues of the neck. In Som PM, Bergeron RT, editors: *Head & Neck Imaging,* ed 2, St Louis, 1991, Mosby-Year Book.
3. Marty-Ane CH, Alauzen M, Alric P et al: Descending necrotizing mediastinitis: advantage of mediastinal drainage with thoracotomy, *J Thorac Cardiovasc Surg* 107:55, 1994.
4. Cole RR, Myer CM, Bratcher GO: Congenital absence of the nose: a case report, *Int J Pediatr Otorhinolaryngol* 17:171, 1989.
5. Hengerer AS, Newburg JA: Congenital malformations of the nose and paranasal sinuses. In Bluestone CD, Stool SE, editors: *Pediatric otolaryngology,* ed 2, Philadelphia, 1990, WB Saunders.
6. Hengerer AS, Strome M: Choanal atresia: a new embryologic theory and its influence on surgical management, *Laryngoscope* 92:913, 1982.
7. Tadmor R, Ravid M, Millet D et al: Computed tomographic demonstration of choanal atresia, *AJNR Am J Neuroradiol* 5:743, 1984.
8. Carpenter LM, Merten DF: Radiographic manifestations of congenital anomalies affecting the airway, *Radiol Clin North Am* 29:219, 1991.
9. Dunham ME, Miller RP: Bilateral choanal atresia associated with malformation of the anterior skull base: embryogenesis and clinical implications, *Ann Otol Rhinol Laryngol* 101:916, 1992.
10. Conigio JU, Manzione JV, Hengerer AS: Anatomic findings and management of choanal atresia and the CHARGE association, *Ann Otol Rhinol Laryngol* 97:448, 1988.
11. Devine P, Bhan I, Feingold M et al: Completely cartilaginous trachea in a child with Crouzon syndrome, *Am J Dis Child* 138:40, 1984.
12. Barkovich AJ, Vandermarck P, Edwards MS et al: Congenital nasal masses: CT and MR imaging in 16 cases, *AJNR Am J Neuroradiol* 12:105, 1991.
13. Stanievich JF, Lore JM: Tumors of the nose, paranasal sinuses, and nasopharynx. In Bluestone CD, Stool SE, editors: *Pediatric otolaryngology,* ed 2, Philadelphia, 1990, WB Saunders.
14. Wiessman JL, Tabor EK, Curtin HD: Sphenochoanal polyps: evaluation with CT and MR imaging, *Radiology* 178:145, 1991.
15. Som PM, Lawson W, Lidov MW: Simulated aggressive skull base erosion in response to benign sinonasal disease, *Radiology* 180:755, 1991.

16. Belenky WM: Nasal obstruction and rhinorrhea. In Bluestone CD, Stool SE, editors: *Pediatric otolaryngology,* ed 2, Philadelphia, 1990, WB Saunders.

17. Stompro BE, Bunkis J: Surgical treatment of nasal obstruction secondary to craniofacial fibrous dysplasia, *Plast Reconstr Surg* 85:107, 1990.

18. Sasaki CT, Ruiz R, Gaito R et al: Hunter's syndrome: a study in airway obstruction, *Laryngoscope* 97:280, 1987.

19. Brodsky L, Koch RJ: Anatomic correlates of normal and diseased adenoids in children, *Laryngoscope* 102:1268, 1992.

20. Dodds B, Maniglia AJ: Peritonsillar and neck abscesses in the pediatric age group, *Laryngoscope* 98:956, 1988.

21. Chen MY, Elster AD: MR imaging of fatal atlantoaxial dislocation caused by retropharyngeal abscess, *AJNR Am J Neuroradiol* 11:992, 1990.

22. Batsakis JG: Tumors of the head and neck. In *Clinical and Pathological Considerations,* ed 2, Baltimore, 1979, Williams & Wilkins.

23. Fritsch DE, Klein DG: Ludwig's angina, *Heart Lung* 21:39, 1992.

24. Civen R, Vaisanen ML, Finegold SM: Peritonsillar abscess, retropharyngeal abscess, mediastinitis, and nonclostridial anaerobic myonecrosis: a case report, *Clin Infect Dis* 1:S299, 1993.

25. Headley DB, Dolan KS: Infratemporal fossa abscess, *Ann Otol Rhinol Laryngol* 100:516, 1991.

26. Patel KS, Ahmad S, O'Leary G et al: The role of computed tomography in the management of peritonsillar abscess, *Otolaryngol Head Neck Surg* 107:727, 1992.

27. Cotton RT, Reilly JS: Congenital malformations of the larynx. In Bluestone CD, Stoel SE, editors: *Pediatric otolaryngology,* ed 2, Philadelphia, 1990, WB Saunders.

28. Morrison JD: Otolaryngological diseases. In Katz J, Steward DJ, editors: *Anesthesia and uncommon pediatric diseases,* Philadelphia, 1987, WB Saunders.

29. Macpherson RI: Radiologic aspects of airway obstruction. In *The pediatric airway,* Philadelphia, 1991, WB Saunders.

30. Zaw-Tun HI: Development of congenital laryngeal atresias and clefts, *Ann Otol Rhinol Laryngol* 97:353, 1988.

31. Rosai J: *Ackerman's Surgical Pathology,* ed 6, Vol. 1, St Louis, 1981, Mosby.

32. Thedinger BA, Cheney ML, Montgomery WW et al: Leiomyosarcoma of the trachea: case report, *Ann Otol Rhinol Laryngol* 100:337, 1991.

33. Felson B: Neoplasms of the trachea and main stem bronchi, *Semin Roentgenol* 18:23, 1983.

34. Nicalai P, Sasaki CT, Ferlito A et al: Laryngeal chondrosarcoma: incidence, pathology, biological behavior, and treatment, *Ann Otol Rhinol Laryngol* 99:515, 1990.

35. Wiggins J, Sheffield E, Green M: Primary B cell malignant lymphoma of the trachea, *Thorax* 43:497, 1988.

36. Choplin RH, Wehunt WD, Theros EG: Diffuse lesions of the trachea, *Semin Roentgenol* 18:38, 1983.

37. Schild JA: Congenital malformations of the trachea and bronchi. In Bluestone CD, Stool SE, editors: *Pediatric otolaryngology,* ed 2, Philadelphia, 1990, WB Saunders.

38. Strife JL: Upper airway and tracheal obstruction in infants and children, *Radiol Clin North Am* 26:309, 1988.

39. Kwong JS, Muller NL, Miller RR: Diseases of the trachea and main-stem bronchi: correlation of CT with pathologic findings, *Radiographics* 12:645, 1992.

40. Gibbons HC: Congenital lesions, neoplasms, and injuries of the trachea. In Sabiston DC Jr, Spencer FC, editors: *Gibbons surgery of the chest,* ed 4, Vol. 1, Philadelphia, 1983, WB Saunders.

41. Houston HE, Payne WS, Harrison EG et al: Primary cancers of the trachea, *Arch Surg* 99:132, 1969.

42. Olmedo G, Rosenberg M, Fonseca R: Primary tumors of the trachea: clinicopathologic features and surgical results, *Chest* 81:701, 1982.

43. Morency G, Chalaoui J, Samson L et al: Malignant neoplasms of the trachea, *J Can Assoc Radiol* 40:198, 1989.

44. Li W, Ellerbroek NA, Libshitz HI: Primary malignant tumors of the trachea. A radiologic and clinical study, *Cancer* 66:894, 1990.

45. Spizarny DL, Shepard JO, McLoud TC et al: CT of adenoid cystic carcinoma of the trachea, *AJR Am J Roentgenol* 146:1129, 1986.

46. Briselli M, Mark GJ, Grillo HC: Tracheal carcinoids, *Cancer* 42:2870, 1978.

47. Aronchick JM, Wexler JA, Christen B et al: Computed tomography of bronchial carcinoid, *J Comput Assist Tomogr* 10:71, 1986.

48. Ip MSM, So SY, Lam WK et al: Endobronchial tuberculosis revisited, *Chest* 89:727, 1986.

49. Dennie CJ, Coblentz CL: The trachea: pathologic conditions and trauma, *J Can Assoc Radiol* 44:157, 1993.

50. Stin MG, Gamsu G, Webb WR et al: Computed tomography of diffuse tracheal stenosis in Wegener's granulomatosis, *J Comput Assist Tomogr* 10:868, 1986.

51. Mendelson DS, Som PM, Crane R et al: Relapsing polychondritis studied by computed tomography, *Radiology* 157:489, 1985.

52. Wilcox P, Miller R, Miller G et al: Airway involvement in ulcerative colitis, *Chest* 92:18, 1987.

53. Wito JG: Tracheobronchial trauma, *Semin Roentgenol* 18:15, 1983.

54. Maddaus MA, Toth JL, Gullane PJ et al: Subglottic tracheal resection and synchronous laryngeal reconstruction, *J Thorac Cardiovasc Surg* 104:1443, 1992.

55. Whited RE: Posterior commissure stenosis post long-term intubation, *Laryngoscope* 93:1314, 1983.

56. Weymuller EA Jr, Bishop MJ, Santos PM: Problems associated with prolonged intubation in the geriatric patient, *Otolaryngol Clin North Am* 23:1057, 1990.

57. Kwong JS, Adler BD, Padley SPG et al: Diagnosis of diseases of the trachea and main bronchi: chest radiography vs CT, *AJR Am J Roentgenol* 161:519, 1993.

Chapter 3

PHYSICS AND MODELING OF THE AIRWAY

D. John Doyle
Kevin O'Grady

I. THE GAS LAWS

A. IDEAL GASES

Understanding the fundamentals of basic fluid mechanics is essential in grasping the concepts of airway flow (air is a fluid). Since air is also a gas, it is important to understand the laws that govern its gaseous behavior. Gases are usually described in terms of pressure, volume, and temperature. Pressure is most often quantified in terms of mm Hg or torr, volume in ml, and temperature in Celsius or Kelvin scale ($273.16 K = 0°C$). Perhaps the most important law of gas flow in airways is the Ideal (or Perfect) Gas Law which can be written as[1]:

$$PV = nRT \qquad (1)$$

where
  P = pressure of gas (Pascals or mm Hg)
  V = volume of gas (m^3 or cm^3 or ml)
  n = number of moles of the gas in volume V
  R = gas constant (8.3143 J g-mol^{-1}K^{-1}, assuming P in Pascals, V in m^3)
  T = absolute temperature (K)
A mole of gas contains 6.023×10^{23} molecules, and this quantity is represented as Avogadro's number. One mole of an ideal gas takes up 22.4138 liters at standard temperature and pressure (STP) (STP–273.16 K at 1 atmosphere [760 mm Hg]).[1] Avogadro also stated that equal volumes of all ideal gases at the same temperature and pressure contain the same number of molecules.

The Ideal Gas Law incorporates the laws of Boyle and Charles.[1] Boyle's law states that, at a constant temperature, the product of pressure and volume is equal to a constant, that is, $P \times V =$ Constant (at constant T). Hence, P is proportional to $1/V$. Gases do not obey Boyle's law at temperatures approaching their point of liquefaction (the state where the gas becomes a liquid). Note that the critical temperature is the temperature above which an increase in pressure cannot yield liquefaction, that is, $N_2O = 36.5°$ C, $CO_2 = 31.1°$ C, $O_2 = -118°$ C[2]. Boyle's law concerns perfect gases and is not obeyed by real gases over a wide range of pressures. However, at infinitely low pressures, all gases obey Boyle's law. Boyle's law does not apply to anesthetic gases and many other gases because of the van der Waals attraction between molecules.

Charles' law states that, at a constant pressure, volume is proportional to temperature, that is, V is proportional to T (at constant P). Gay-Lussac's law states that, at a constant volume, pressure is proportional to temperature, that is, $P \propto T$ (at constant V).[1] Often, Charles' law and Gay-Lussac's law are shortened for convenience to Charles' law. When a gas obeys both Charles' law and Boyle's law, it is said to be an ideal gas and obeys the Ideal Gas Law.

In clinical situations, gases are typically mixtures of several "pure" gases. Quantifiable properties of mixtures may be determined using Dalton's law of partial pressures, which states that the pressure exerted by a mixture of gases is the sum of the individual pressures exerted by each "pure" gas.[1,3] This may be stated mathematically as:

$$P_{total} = P_A + P_B + P_C + \ldots + P_N \qquad (2)$$

where P_A, P_B, and P_C are the partial pressures of "pure" ideal gases.

B. NONIDEAL GASES: THE VAN DER WAALS EFFECT

Ideal gases have no forces of interaction. Real gases, however, have intramolecular attraction, which requires that the pressure-volume gas law be written as[1,3]:

$$\left(P + \frac{a}{V^2}\right) \times (V - b) = nRT \qquad (3)$$

where
  P = pressure of gas (Pascals or mm Hg)
  V = volume of gas (m^3 or cm^3 or ml)
  n = number of moles of the gas in volume V
  R = gas constant (8.3143 J g-mol^{-1}K^{-1} assuming P in Pascals, V in m^3)
  T = absolute temperature (K)
  a,b = physical constants for a given gas
The terms a and b for a given gas may be found in physical chemistry textbooks and other sources.[1,3,4,5] This formulation, provided by van der Waals, accounts for intramolecular forces fairly well.

C. DIFFUSION OF GASES

Graham's law states that the rate of diffusion of gases through certain membranes is inversely proportional to their molecular weight. A more commonly used relation is Fick's first law of diffusion, which states that the rate of diffusion of a gas across a barrier is proportional to the concentration gradient for the gas. Clinically, this law is applicable to gas flows across lung and placental membranes. Fick's law may be expressed mathematically as[6]:

$$Flux = -D\frac{\Delta C}{\Delta X} \qquad (4)$$

where the flux is the number of molecules/cm^2/s crossing the membrane, ΔC is the concentration gradient (molecules/cm^3), ΔX is the diffusion distance (cm), and D is the diffusion coefficient (cm^2/s) whose value is generally inversely proportional to the gas's molecular weight.

Since gases dissolve when they come into contact with liquid, Henry's law becomes important in some instances. It states that the mass of a gas dissolved in a given amount of liquid is proportional to the pressure of

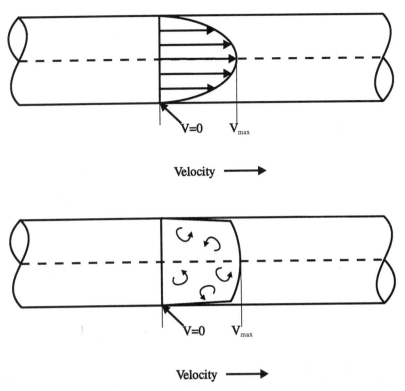

Fig. 3-1. Laminar and turbulent flow. Laminar flow *(top)* in a long smooth pipe is characterized by smooth and steady flow with little or no fluctuations. Flow profile is parabolic in nature, with fluid traveling most quickly at the center of the tube and stationary at the edges. Turbulent flow *(bottom)* is characterized by fluctuating and agitated flow. Its flow profile is essentially flat with all fluid traveling at the same velocity except at tube edges.

the gas at constant temperature, that is, gas concentration (in solvent) = constant × pressure (at constant T).[1]

D. PRESSURE, FLOW, AND RESISTANCE

The laws of fluid mechanics dictate an intricate relationship among pressure, flow, and resistance. Pressure is defined as a force per unit area and, as mentioned previously, is usually measured clinically as mm Hg (torr). However, it is also commonly measured in Pascals (newtons force per square meter). Flow (or the rate of flow) is equal to the change in pressure (pressure drop or pressure difference) divided by the resistance experienced by the fluid. For example, if the flow is 100 ml/s at a pressure difference of 100 mm Hg, the resistance is 100 mm Hg/100 ml/s = 1 mm Hg/ml/s. In *laminar* flow systems only, the resistance is constant, independent of flow.[7,8]

An important relation which quantifies the relationship of pressure, flow, and resistance is given by the Hagen-Poiseuille equation. Poiseuille's law states that the fluid flow rate through a horizontal straight tube of uniform bore is proportional to the pressure gradient and the fourth power of the radius and is related inversely to the viscosity of the gas and the length of the tube. This law, *which is valid for laminar flow only*, may thus be stated as[7,8]:

$$\Delta P = \frac{8\mu L}{\pi r^4} \times \text{Flow} \qquad (5)$$

where μ is the fluid viscosity (poise [g/cm · s]) and L is the length of the tube (cm). See Section II.A for further details.

When the flow rate exceeds a *critical velocity* (the flow velocity below which flow is laminar), the flow loses its laminar parabolic velocity profile, becomes disorderly, and is termed *turbulent* (Fig. 3-1). When turbulent flow exists, the relationship between pressure drop and flow is no longer governed by the Hagen-Poiseuille equation. Instead, the pressure gradient required (or the resistance encountered) during turbulent flow varies as the square of the flow rate. See Section II.B for further details.

Viscosity, μ, characterizes the resistance within a fluid to the flow of one layer of molecules over another (shear characteristics).[7] Blood viscosity is influenced primarily by hematocrit, so that at low hematocrit blood flow is easier. The critical velocity at which turbulent flow begins depends on the ratio of viscosity (μ) to density (ρ), which is defined as the *kinematic viscosity* (ν), that is, $\nu = \mu/\rho$ (Section II.B.1 illustrates this in an example).[7,8,9] The units for viscosity are g/cm · s (poise).

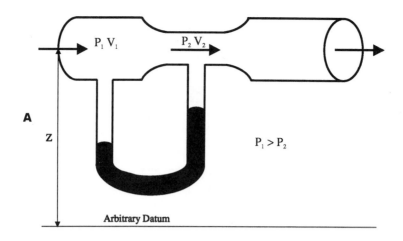

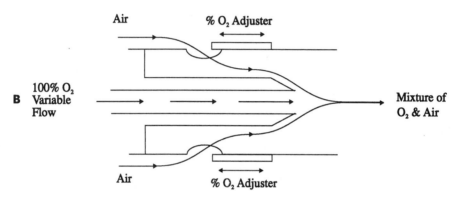

Fig. 3-2. Bernoulli effect. **A,** Diagram shows fluid flow through a tube with varying diameters. At point of flow constriction, fluid pressure is less than at distal end of the tube, as indicated by height of the manometer fluid column. This effect is described by the Bernoulli equation. Note that, in the case of a horizontal pipe, Z_1 and $Z_2 = Z$, where Z_1 and Z_2 are distances between the centerline of the pipe at two different points and an arbitrary datum. **B,** A venturi. The lower pressure caused by the Bernoulli effect entrains air to mix with oxygen.

Typical units for kinematic viscosity are cm^2/s. The viscosity of water is 0.01 poise at 25° C and 0.007 poise at 37° C. The viscosity of air is 183 micropoise at 18° C. Its density (dry) is 1.213 g/L.[4]

Density is defined as mass per unit volume (g/cm^3 or g/ml). The density of water is 1 g/ml. The general relation for the density of a gas is given by:

$$D = D_0 \left(\frac{T_0 P}{T P_0} \right) \qquad (6)$$

where D_0 is a known density of the gas at temperature T_0 and pressure P_0 and D is the density of the gas at temperature T and pressure P. For dry air at 18° C and 760 mm Hg, D = 1.213 g/L.[4]

The fall in pressure at points of flow constriction (where the flow velocity is higher) is known as the Bernoulli effect (Fig. 3-2).[7,8] This phenomenon is used in apparatus employing the Venturi principle, for

example, gas nebulizers, Venturi flowmeters, and some oxygen face masks. The lower pressure due to the Bernoulli effect sucks in (entrains) air to mix with oxygen.

One final consideration that is important in the study of the airway is Laplace's law for a sphere (Fig. 3-3). It states that, for a sphere with one air-liquid interface (e.g., an alveolus), the equation relating the transmural pressure difference, surface tension, and sphere radius is[10]:

$$P = \frac{2T}{R} \qquad (7)$$

where
   P = transmural pressure difference ($dynes/cm^2$)
   T = surface tension (dynes/cm)
   R = sphere radius (cm)
The key point in Laplace's law is that the smaller the sphere radius, the higher the transmural pressure. However, real (in vivo) alveoli do *not* obey Laplace's law

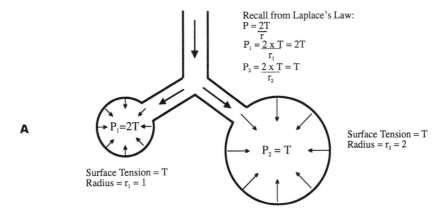

Recall from Laplace's Law:
$$P = \frac{2T}{r}$$
$$P_1 = \frac{2 \times T}{r_1} = 2T$$
$$P_2 = \frac{2 \times T}{r_2} = T$$

Surface Tension = T
Radius = r_2 = 2

$P_1 = 2T$

$P_2 = T$

Surface Tension = T
Radius = r_1 = 1

A

a) Ideal Alveoli: $P_1 > P_2$

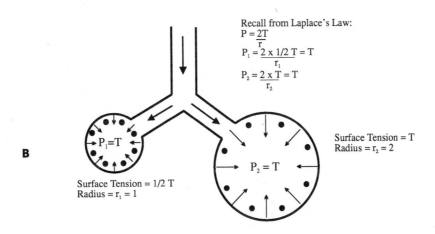

Recall from Laplace's Law:
$$P = \frac{2T}{r}$$
$$P_1 = \frac{2 \times 1/2\, T}{r_1} = T$$
$$P_2 = \frac{2 \times T}{r_2} = T$$

Surface Tension = T
Radius = r_2 = 2

$P_1 = T$

$P_2 = T$

Surface Tension = 1/2 T
Radius = r_1 = 1

B

b) Real Alveoli: $P_1 = P_2$ with pulmonary surfactant

Fig. 3-3. Laplace's law for a sphere. **A,** Laplace's law dictates that for two alveoli of unequal size but of equal surface tension, the smaller alveolus will experience a larger intraalveolar pressure than the larger alveolus. This will cause air to pass into the larger alveolus and cause the smaller alveolus to collapse. **B,** Collapse of smaller alveolus is prevented through action of pulmonary surfactant. Surfactant serves to decrease alveolar surface tension in the smaller alveolus, which results in equal pressures in both alveoli.

because of the action of pulmonary surfactant, which acts to decrease the surface tension disproportionately than what is predicted using physical principles. (Note: 1 dyne/cm^2 = 0.1 Pa = 0.000 751 torr). When pulmonary surfactant is missing from the lungs, the lungs take on the behavior described by Laplace's law.

E. EXAMPLE: APPLICATION OF ENGINEERING ANALYSIS TO TRANSTRACHEAL JET VENTILATION (*THE VALUE OF KNOWING CATHETER RESISTANCE FOR TRANSTRACHEAL JET VENTILATION*)

Transtracheal jet ventilation (TTJV) has been advocated as a means to oxygenate and ventilate patients who would otherwise perish because of a lost airway.[11] A number of systems have been described, usually using equipment commonly available in the operating room, and often using the 50 psi wall oxygen source.[11-14] In this example, we present an approach to the design of TTJV systems that is potentially more rational than the method of simply utilizing commonly available components.

Analysis:

The gas flow through a transtracheal catheter depends on both the resistance of the catheter-connection hose assembly and the driving pressure applied to it. If the resistance of the catheter-connection hose assembly is R, then the flow from the catheter is $F = P_d / R$ where P_d is the pressure difference between the ends of the

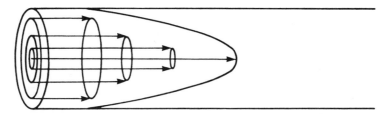

Fig. 3-4. Laminar flow. Laminar gas flow through long straight tube of uniform bore has a velocity profile that is parabolic in shape, with the gas traveling most quickly at center of tube. Conceptually, it is helpful to view laminar gas flow as a series of concentric cylinders of gas, with the central cylinder moving most rapidly. (From Nunn JF: *Nunn's applied respiratory physiology,* ed 4, Stoneham, Mass, 1993, Butterworth-Heinemann.)

catheter-connection assembly. R itself will certainly depend on F when the flow becomes turbulent, but the above relationship still holds. However, P_d is very close to the driving pressure P applied to the ventilation catheter, since the lung offers little relative back pressure. (At back pressures over 100 cm H_2O the lung will likely burst, while P is often chosen to be 50 psi or about 3500 cm H_2O.) Thus the above relationship may be simplified to F = P/R.

Next, suppose that it is desired to deliver through the TTJV catheter a sequence of "jet pulses" each resulting in a given tidal volume (e.g., 500 ml). Then (ignoring entrained air effects) the delivered tidal volume = catheter flow × pulse duration. If we choose a catheter flow of 30 liters/minute, then a jet pulse of 1 second duration will result in a tidal volume of 30 liters/min × 1/60 min = 0.5 liters. Thus, if the desired flow rate of a jet pulse is to be F, and if at this flow the system resistance is R, then the driving pressure needed is P = F × R. If F is chosen, for example, as 30 liters/min, then we need only know R in order to choose P.

In a TTJV setup consisting of a 14-gauge angiocath connected to a regulated oxygen source by a 4.5-foot polyvinyl chloride (PVC) tube of 7/32 inch inside diameter (ID), for oxygen flows between 10 and 60 1/min, the resistance was relatively constant between 0.6 and 0.8 psi/L/min.[15]

Many systems for TTJV choose 50 psi for convenience (50 psi being the oxygen wall outlet pressure), although a regulator could be used to permit lower pressures. However, 50 psi may not be an "optimal" pressure choice for TTJV. Instead, we offer the above approach to selecting the oxygen driving pressure from known catheter-connection hose resistance characteristics and desired jet pulse flow characteristics. Reference to such data will allow driving pressure selection for various TTJV setups and desired jet pulse flows. As an example, if the setup resistance is taken as 0.7 psi/L/min and the desired flow rate is 30 l/min, the driving pressure should be 0.7 × 30 = 21 psi. Similar analyses can be carried out for other arrangements from experiments to obtain resistance data.

II. GAS FLOW

A. LAMINAR FLOW

In laminar flow, fluid particles flow along smooth paths in layers, or laminas, with one layer gliding smoothly over an adjacent layer.[7] Any tendencies toward instability and turbulence are damped out by viscous shear forces that resist the relative motion of adjacent fluid layers. Under laminar flow conditions through a tube, the flow velocity is greatest at the center of the flow and zero at the inner edge of the tube (Figs. 3-1 and 3-4). The flow profile has a parabolic shape. Under these conditions in a horizontal tube, the relation between flow, tube, and gas characteristics is given by the Hagen-Poiseuille equation[7,8,9]:

$$\dot{V} = \frac{\pi \Delta P r^4}{8 \mu L} \qquad (8)$$

where

$\dot{V}$ = flow rate [cm³/s]
$\pi \approx 3.1416$
P = pressure gradient [Pascals]
r = tube radius [cm]
L = tube length [cm]
μ = gas viscosity [g/cm · s]

Typical units are shown in square brackets above. The dot in $\dot{V}$ indicates "rate of change." As V represents volume, $\dot{V}$ represents the *rate of change of volume* or *flow rate.* Another way in which the above concept may be viewed, is that, under conditions of laminar flow through a tube of known radius, the pressure difference across the tube is given by the following proportionality:

$$\Delta Pressure \propto \frac{Flow \times Viscosity \times Length}{Radius^4} \qquad (9)$$

That is, the pressure gradient through the airway increases proportionately with flow, viscosity, and tube length but increases exponentially as the tube radius decreases.

The conditions under which flow through a tube is predominantly laminar can be estimated from *critical*

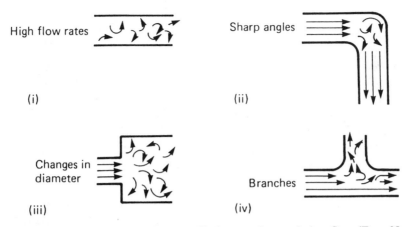

High flow rates

(i)

Sharp angles

(ii)

Changes in diameter

(iii)

Branches

(iv)

Fig. 3-5. Turbulent flow. Four circumstances likely to produce turbulent flow. (From Nunn JF: *Nunn's applied respiratory physiology* ed 4, Stoneham, Mass, 1993, Butterworth-Heinemann.)

flow rates. The critical flow is the flow rate below which flow is predominantly laminar in a given airflow situation (*vide infra*).

1. Laminar flow example

A tube of uniform bore is 1 cm in radius and 100 cm in length. A pressure difference of 10 cm H_2O exists between the ends of the tube, and air is the fluid flowing through the tube. Assuming laminar flow, what flow rate should we expect to get?

Answer:

Using the centimeter-gram-second (CGS) system of units, we have:

$r = 1.0$ cm

$L = 100.0$ cm

$\mu = 183$ micropoise $= 183 \times 10^{-6}$ poise $= 183 \times 10^{-6}$ g/(cm · s)

$\Delta P = 10$ cm $H_2O = 7.35$ mm Hg $= 9800$ dynes/cm^2

Using the Hagen-Poiseuille equation for laminar flow, we determine:

$$\dot{V} = \frac{\pi \times 9800 \times 1^4}{8 \times 183 \times 10^{-6} \times 100} = 210\,298 \text{ cm}^3/\text{s} \approx 21.03 \text{ L/s} \quad (10)$$

B. TURBULENT FLOW

Flow in tubes below the critical flow rate remains mostly laminar. However, at flows above the critical flow rate, the flow becomes increasingly turbulent. Under turbulent flow conditions, the parabolic flow pattern is lost, and the resistance to flow increases with flow itself. Turbulence may also be created when sharp angles, changes in diameter, and branches are encountered (Fig. 3-5). The flow-pressure drop relationship is given approximately by[7,8]:

$$V \propto \sqrt{\Delta P} \quad (11)$$

where

V = mean fluid velocity [cm/s]

P = pressure [Pascals]

1. Reynolds number calculation example

The Reynolds number (Re) represents the ratio of inertial forces to viscous forces.[7,8,9] It is useful because it characterizes the flow through a long, straight tube of uniform bore. It is a dimensionless number having the form of:

$$\text{Re} = \frac{V \times D \times \rho}{\mu} = \frac{V \times D}{v} = \frac{2 \times \dot{V} \times \rho}{\pi \times r \times \mu} \quad (12)$$

where

Re = Reynolds number

$\dot{V}$ = flow rate [ml/s]

ρ = density [g/ml]

μ = viscosity [poise or g/cm · s]

r = radius [cm]

v = kinematic viscosity [cm^2/s] $= \mu/\rho$

D = diameter [cm]

V = mean fluid velocity [cm/s]

Typical units are shown in brackets above. For tubes that are long compared to their diameter (i.e., L/D > $0.06 \times$ Re),[8] the flow is laminar when the Re number is below 2000. Flow will be turbulent at Re numbers as low as 280 for shorter tubes.

When a tube's radius exceeds its length, it is an orifice; flow through an orifice is always turbulent. Under these conditions, the flow is influenced by density rather than the viscosity of the fluid.[2] This is why Heliox (70% He, 30% O_2) flows better in a narrow edematous glottis: helium has a very low density and presents less resistance to flow through an orifice.

How can we predict whether a given gas flow through an endotracheal tube (ET) is laminar or turbulent? One approach is first to identify the physical conditions, for example:

$L = 27$ cm

$r = 0.3$ cm (size 6 mm ET)

flow ($\dot{V}$) = 60 liters/min = 1000 ml/sec

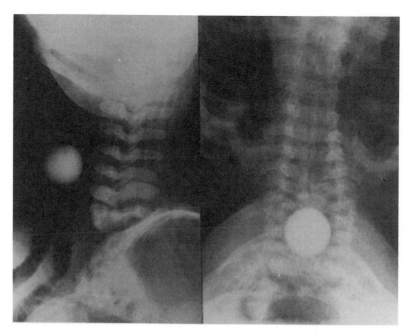

Fig. 3-6. Airway obstruction. Anterior-posterior and lateral radiograph of 18-month-old infant who had swallowed a marble. Presence of this esophageal foreign body caused acute airway obstruction by causing extrinsic compression of the trachea. (From Badgwell JM, McLeod ME, Friedberg J: *Can J Anaesth* 34(1):90, 1987.)

viscosity (μ) = 183 micropoise = 183×10^{-6} g/cm · s (air at 18° C)

density (ρ) = 1.21 g/L = 0.001213 g/ml (dry air at 18° C)

and then calculate the Re number:

$$Re = \frac{2 \times 1000 \times 0.001213}{\pi \times 0.3 \times 183 \times 10^{-6}} = 1.41 \times 10^4 \quad (13)$$

Since this number greatly exceeds 2000, flow is likely quite turbulent.

C. CRITICAL VELOCITY

The critical velocity is the point at which the transition from laminar to turbulent flow begins. The critical velocity is reached when the Re number becomes the critical Re number Re_{crit}. Critical velocity, the flow velocity below which flow is laminar, is given by[8]:

$$V_{crit} = V_c = \frac{Re_{crit} \times Viscosity}{Density \times Diameter} \quad (14)$$

where $Re_{crit} \approx 2000$ for circular tubes. As can be seen, the critical velocity is proportional to the viscosity of the gas and is related inversely to the density of the gas and the tube radius. Viscosity dimensions are force per unit area per second $(N \times s/m^2)$. The critical velocity at which turbulent flow begins depends on the ratio of viscosity to density, that is, μ/ρ. This ratio is known as the *kinematic viscosity, ν,* and has typical units of square centimeters per second (cm^2/s). The actual measure-

ment of viscosity of a fluid is carried out using a viscometer, which consists of two rotary cylinders with the test fluid flowing between.

1. Critical velocity calculation example

Using the same data as the previous Re number calculation, we can calculate the critical velocity at which laminar flow starts to become turbulent:

$$V_c = \frac{(2000) \times (183 \times 10^{-6} \text{ poise})}{(0.001213 \text{ g/cm}^3) \times (2 \times 0.3 \text{ cm})} \quad (15)$$

$$V_c = 502.8 \frac{\text{poise}}{(\text{g/cm}^3) \times \text{cm}} = 502.8 \frac{\text{cm}}{\text{s}}$$

D. FLOW THROUGH AN ORIFICE

Flow through an orifice (defined as involving flow through a tube whose length is smaller than its radius) is always somewhat turbulent.[2] Clinically, airway obstructing conditions such as epiglottis or swallowed obstructions are often best viewed as breathing through an orifice (Fig. 3-6). Under such conditions, the approximate flow across the orifice varies inversely with the square root of the gas density:

$$\dot{V} \propto \frac{1}{\sqrt{\text{Gas Density}}} \quad (16)$$

This is in contrast to laminar flow conditions, where gas flow varies inversely with gas viscosity. The viscosity

Table 3-1. Viscosity and density differences of anesthetic gases[4,5]

	Viscosity @ 300 K	Density @ 20° C
Air	18.6 μPa $\times$ s	1.293 g/L
Nitrogen	17.9 μPa $\times$ s	1.250 g/L
Nitrous oxide	15.0 μPa $\times$ s	1.965 g/L
Helium	20.0 μPa $\times$ s	0.178 g/L
Oxygen	20.8 μPa $\times$ s	1.429 g/L

Table 3-2. Gas flow rates through an orifice

	%	Density (g/L)	Density$^{ims_{1/2}}$ (g/L)$^{ims_{1/2}}$	Relative flow
Air	100	1.293	0.881	1.0
Oxygen	100	1.429	0.846	0.96
Helium (He)	100	0.179	2.364	2.68
He-oxygen	20/80	1.178	0.922	1.048
He-oxygen	60/40	0.678	1.215	1.381
He-oxygen	80/20	0.429	1.527	1.73

From Rudow M, Hill AB, Thompson NW et al: *Can Anaesth Soc J* 33:498, 1986.

values for helium and oxygen are similar, but their densities are very different (Table 3-1). Table 3-2 provides useful data to allow comparison of gas flow rates through an orifice.[16]

1. Helium-oxygen mixtures

The low viscosity of helium allows it to play a significant clinical role in the management of some forms of airway obstruction.[17,18,19,20] For instance, Rudow et al.[16] describe the use of helium-oxygen mixtures on a patient with severe airway obstruction due to a large thyroid mass (see Clinical Vignette below for details).

The usual available mixtures of helium and oxygen are 20% O_2: 80% He and 30% O_2: 70% He and are usually administered by a rebreathing face mask in patients who face an increased work-of-breathing effort because of the presence of airway pathology (e.g., edema) but in whom endotracheal intubation is preferably withheld at this time.

2. Clinical vignette

Rudow et al.[16] provide the following story. A 78-year-old woman with both breast cancer and ophthalmic melanoma developed airway obstruction from a thyroid carcinoma that extended into her mediastinum and compressed her trachea. She had a 2-month history of worsening dyspnea, especially when positioned supine. On examination, inspiratory and expiratory stridor was present. Noted on the chest x-ray were a large superior mediastinal mass and pulmonary metastases. A solid mass was identified on a thyroid ultrasound scan. Computed tomography revealed a large mass at the thoracic inset and extending caudally. Clinically, the patient was exhausted and in respiratory distress.

Almost instant relief was obtained by giving the patient a mixture of 78% He: 22% O_2, with improvements in measured tidal volume and oxygenation. Later, a thyroidectomy was carried out to relieve the obstruction. Here, anesthesia was conducted by applying topical anesthesia to the airway with awake laryngoscopy and intubation performed in the sitting position. Once the airway was secured using an armored tube, the patient was given a general anesthetic with an intravenous induction. Following the surgery, extubation occurred without complication.

E. PRESSURE DIFFERENCES

From the analysis of equations governing laminar flow and turbulent flow, the pressure drop along the noncompliant portion of the airway is given approximately by the Rohrer equation[21]:

$$\Delta P = K_1 \dot{V} + K_2 \dot{V}^2 \qquad (17)$$

where K_1 and K_2 are known as Rohrer constants. Physical interpretation of this equation is as follows: airway pressure is governed by the sum of two terms:

1. effects proportional to gas flow (laminar flow effects)
2. effects proportional to the square of the gas flow (turbulent flow effects)

It can be seen that the lowest pressure loss ΔP across the airway would be expected when $\dot{V}$ is small, that is, predominantly laminar flow. However, it is known that, under conditions of laminar flow, K_1 is largely influenced by viscosity and not density, while K_2 (the turbulent term) is influenced primarily by density and not viscosity.

F. RESISTANCE TO GAS FLOW

When pressure readings are taken at each end of a horizontal tube with a fluid flowing through it, one notices that the pressure measurements at either end are not identical, the pressure at the distal end of the tube being less than the pressure at the proximal end (fluid flowing from the proximal to the distal end). In this case, the pressure loss is attributable to frictional losses incurred by the fluid when in contact with the inside of the tube. This is analogous to heat losses incurred by resistors in an electrical circuit (Fig. 3-7). Frictional losses are irreversible; that is, the energy lost cannot be recovered by the fluid and is mostly lost as heat. Note that, if the tube is not horizontal, pressure differences are also attributable to height differences. The most common relation that describes the flow in a tube is the

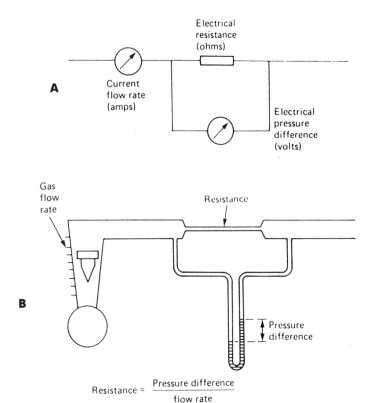

Fig. 3-7. Electrical analogy of gas flow. Analogy between laminar gas flow and flow of electricity through a resistor. **A,** Gas: flow in volume/sec (e.g., ml/s), pressure difference in force/area (e.g., dynes/cm^2), and resistance described by Poiseuille's law. **B,** Electricity: flow in current (amperes), pressure difference in voltage (volts), and resistance described by Ohm's law. Note that for gases, pressure difference = flow rate × resistance, and for electricity, potential difference (voltage) = current × resistance. (From Nunn JF: *Nunn's applied respiratory physiology,* ed 4, Stoneham, Mass, 1993, Butterworth-Heinemann.)

Bernoulli equation, which is valid for both laminar and turbulent flow[8]:

$$\frac{V_1^2}{2g} + \frac{P_1}{\rho g} + Z_1 = \frac{V_2^2}{2g} + \frac{P_2}{\rho g} + Z_2 + h_f \qquad \textbf{(18)}$$

where

V = velocity [m/s]

g = gravitational constant [9.81 m/s^2 or 9.81 N/kg]

P = pressure [Pascals or N/m^2]

ρ = density of fluid [kg/m^3]

Z = height from an arbitrary point (datum) [m]

h_f = frictional losses [m]

Typical units are shown in square brackets above. Note that the above equation is in the units of meters and is termed "meters of head loss." This is typical of fluid mechanics equations. As mentioned previously, the Bernoulli equation is valid for both laminar and turbulent flow.

1. Endotracheal tube resistance

Endotracheal tubes (ETs), like all tubes, offer resistance to fluid flow (Fig. 3-8). However, ETs do not add external resistance to the normal airway, but rather, act as a substitute for the normal resistance of the airway from the mouth to the trachea, which accounts for 30% to 40% of normal airway resistance.[22] This is important because, although mechanical ventilators can overcome impedance to inspiratory flow during extended periods of artificial respiration, they do not augment passive exhalation. Resistance to exhalation through long, small-diameter ET, which is compounded by turbulence, can seriously constrain ventilation rate and tidal volume.[23,24]

The use of the ET influences respiration in a number of ways. First, it decreases effective airway diameter and therefore increases the resistance to breathing. Resistance is further increased by the curved nature of the tube; resistance measurements are typically about 3% higher than if the tubes were straight.[25] Note that the passage from the mouth to the larynx is not a smooth curve and may create additional turbulence.

Second, studies show that intubated patients experience decreased peak flow rates (inspiratory and expiratory), decreased forced vital capacity, and forced expiratory volume in one second (FEV$_1$).[26] However, the tube may paradoxically increase peak flow rates during

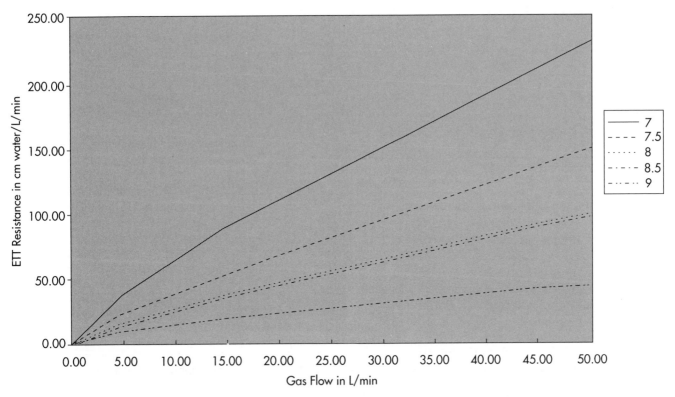

Fig. 3-8. ET resistance dependence on flow. The data provided by Hicks in Table 3-3 can be used to show how endotracheal tube resistance increases nonlinearly with flow (because of turbulence effects). For pure laminar flow, resistance would be constant, regardless of flow.

forced expiration through the prevention of dynamic compression of the trachea.[26] Finally, the tube may cause mechanical irritation of the larynx and trachea that may lead to a reflex constriction of the airway distal to the tube.[27]

The combination of tube and connector may cause higher resistance than the tube alone. Moreover, because of turbulence at component connections, the total resistance of a system is not necessarily the sum of the resistances of its component parts, especially where sharp-angled connectors are used (Fig. 3-5).[28,29] In addition, humidified gases contribute to slightly higher resistances because of the increased density of moist gas.[30] The resistance of single-lumen tubes is generally lower than that of double-lumen tubes.[30]

The resistance associated with ET may be reduced by increasing tube diameter, decreasing tube length or by decreasing the gas density (hence the occasional use of helium-oxygen mixtures). It has been suggested that the presence of the ET may double the work of breathing in chronically intubated adults and lead to respiratory failure in some infants.[25] Therefore, it is important to use as large an ET as is practical in patients who exhibit respiratory dysfunction.

ET resistance can be measured in the laboratory using differential pressure and flow measurement techniques,[31,32] the most common method of which is described by Gaensler et al.[33] Theoretical estimates of resistance under laminar flow conditions can also be obtained using the Poiseuille equation. *In vivo* resistance measurements are generally higher than *in vitro* measurements of ET perhaps because of secretions, head or neck position, tube deformation, or increased turbulence.[34,35]

Airway resistance may be established from first principles using Poiseuille's law when the gas flow is laminar. When gas flow is turbulent, resistance is no longer independent of material properties, and empirical measurements become the only feasible means of characterizing resistance. Intrinsic airway resistance is determined by measuring the transairway pressure, that is, the pressure drop between the airway opening and the alveoli. The following relationship applies[36]:

$$R = \frac{P_{airway} - P_{alveolar}}{\dot{V}} \qquad (19)$$

where

R = airway resistance [cm H_2O/L/sec]

P_{airway} = proximal airway pressure [cm H_2O]

Table 3-3. Coefficients for airway resistance computations

Tube	a	b
7.0	9.78	1.81
7.5	7.73	1.75
8.0	5.90	1.72
8.5	4.61	1.78
9.0	3.90	1.63

From Hicks GH: *Problems in Respiratory Care* 2(2):191, 1989.

$P_{alveolar}$ = alveolar pressure [cm H_2O]
$\dot{V}$ = gas flow rate [L/sec]

Typical units used are shown in brackets above. In clinical practice, airway resistance is easiest to determine using a whole body plethysmograph. Unfortunately, it is an apparatus unsuitable for critically ill patients.

An alternate method of presenting airway resistance is provided by Hicks[36] in which the following equation and constants are used:

$$\Delta P = a\dot{V}^b \qquad (20)$$

where

ΔP = pressure difference [cm H_2O]
$\dot{V}$ = gas flow [L/min]
a,b = empirical constants provided in Table 3-3

Fig. 3-8 depicts the effect of tube diameter and flow rate on ET resistance. Note that resistance is increased as a result of increasing turbulence caused by decreasing ET diameter and increasing flow rate.

III. WORK OF BREATHING

Breathing is comprised of a two-part cycle: inspiration and expiration. During normal breathing, inspiration is an active, energy consuming process, while expiration is ordinarily a passive process in which the diaphragm and intercostal muscles relax (Figs. 3-9 and 3-10). However, expiration becomes an active process during forced expiration, as during exercise or during expiration against a resistance load. Several studies have examined the work of breathing in some clinical settings.[37-42]

Considering only normal breathing, the work of breathing is given by:

Work = Force × Distance
Force = Pressure × Area
Distance = Volume / Area
Work = (Pressure × Area) × (Volume/Area)
    = Pressure × Volume

Since the air pressure in the lung varies with lung volume, and pressure measurements are obtained distal to the end of the ET, work may be expressed as:[43]

$$WORK_{INSPIRATION} = \int_{FRC}^{FRC+TV} P \, dV \qquad (21)$$

where

P = airway pressure [cm H_2O]
dV = (infinitesimal) volume of gas added to the lung [ml]
FRC = functional residual capacity of the lungs [ml]
TV = tidal volume breathed in during respiration [ml]

When the pressure varies as a function of time, the above equation may be integrated in the following manner:

$$LET \ dV = \frac{dV}{dt} \times dt = \dot{V} \, dt \qquad (22)$$

Changing the limits of integration yields:

$$WORK_{INSPIRATION} = \int_{t_1}^{t_2} P(t) \, \dot{V}(t) \, dt \qquad (23)$$

where

t_1 = time at the beginning of inspiration [s]
t_2 = time at the end of inspiration [s]
P = pressure measured at a point of interest in the airway (e.g., at the tip of the ET or at the carina) [cm H_2O]
$\dot{V}$ = flow [ml/s]

The above equation is cumbersome to integrate quickly. However, it is sometimes reasonable to assume that the pressure during inspiration remains fairly constant. Under these circumstances, integration of the original work equation during constant pressure inspiration yields the following approximation:

$$WORK_{INSPIRATION} = P_{AVE} \times TV \qquad (24)$$

where

P_{AVE} = mean airway pressure during inspiration [cm H_2O]
TV = tidal volume of inspiration [ml]

During anesthesia, an ET is often inserted, and additional energy is required to overcome the friction effects of the ET. The added work of breathing presented by an ET is given by:

$$WORK_{ETT} = \int_{FRC}^{FRC+TV} \Delta P \, dV \qquad (25)$$

where ΔP is the pressure drop across the tube. Often, the pressure gradient ΔP is relatively constant during inspiration, and hence:

$$WORK_{ETT} = \Delta P \int_{FRC}^{FRC+TV} dV = \Delta P \times \Delta V \qquad (26)$$

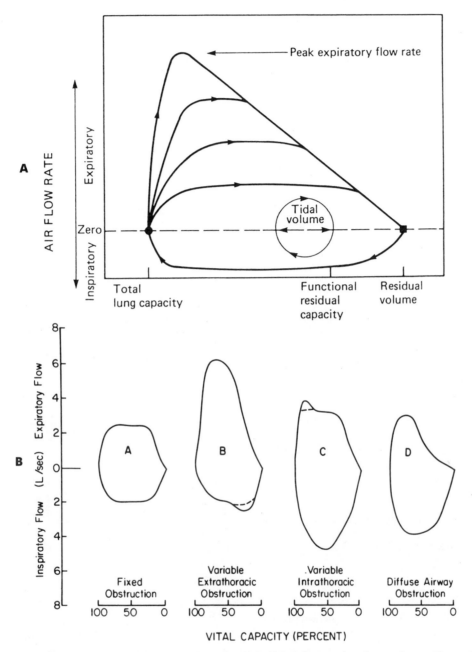

Fig. 3-9. Flow-volume curves. **A,** A flow-volume consists of a plot of gas flow against lung volume. Shown here are four loops corresponding to four different levels of expiratory effort. As can be seen, peak expiratory flow is effort dependent, but towards the end of expiration the curves converge (flow limited by dynamic airway collapse). From a diagnostic viewpoint, the expiratory portion of the loop is of more value than the inspiratory portion. (From Nunn JF: *Nunn's applied respiratory physiology,* ed 4, Stoneham, Mass, 1993, Butterworth-Heinemann. Reproduced with permission.) **B,** Maximum inspiratory and expiratory flow-volume curves (flow-volume loops) in four types of airway obstruction. (From Gal TJ: *Anesthesia,* ed 2, New York, 1986, Churchill Livingstone.)

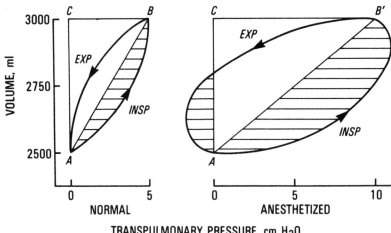

VOLUME, ml

TRANSPULMONARY PRESSURE, cm H₂O

Fig. 3-10. The work of breathing. Lung volume plotted against transpulmonary pressure in a pressure-volume diagram for an awake *(normal)* and anesthetized patient. Total area within the oval and triangles has the dimensions of pressure multiplied by volume and represents the total work of breathing. Hatched area to the right of lines AB and AB′ represents active inspiratory work necessary to overcome resistance to airflow during inspiration *(INSP).* The hatched area to the left of the triangle AB′C represents active expiratory work necessary to overcome resistance to airflow during expiration *(EXP).* Expiration is passive in the normal subject because sufficient potential energy is stored during inspiration to produce expiratory airflow. The fraction of total inspiratory work necessary to overcome elastic resistance is shown by triangles ABC and AB′C. The anesthetized patient has decreased compliance and increased elastic resistance work *(triangle AB′C)* compared with the normal patient's compliance and elastic resistance work *(triangle ABC).* The anesthetized patient shown has increased airway resistance to both inspiratory and expiratory work. (From Benumof JL, *Anesthesia,* ed 2, New York, 1986, Churchill Livingstone.)

where

ΔP = pressure drop across ET during inspiration [mm Hg]

ΔV = volume added to lungs = tidal volume [ml]

Hence, the total work done, measured in joules $(kg \times m^2/s^2)$, is:

$$WORK_{TOTAL} = WORK_{ETT} + WORK_{INSPIRATION} \quad (27)$$

IV. PULMONARY BIOMECHANICS

A. THE RESPIRATORY MECHANICS EQUATION

Approximately 3% of the body's total energy is required to maintain normal respiratory function.[10] Energy is required to overcome three main forces: (1) the elastic resistance of the lungs, which restores the lungs to their original size after inflation, (2) the force required to move the rib cage, diaphragm, and appropriate visceral contents, and (3) the dissipative resistance of the airway and any breathing apparatus.[44] The respiratory system is commonly modeled as the frictional airway R_L that is in series with the lung compliance C_L. Such a model is analogous to a resistor and capacitor in series that form a resistive-capacitive (RC) circuit (Fig. 3-11).

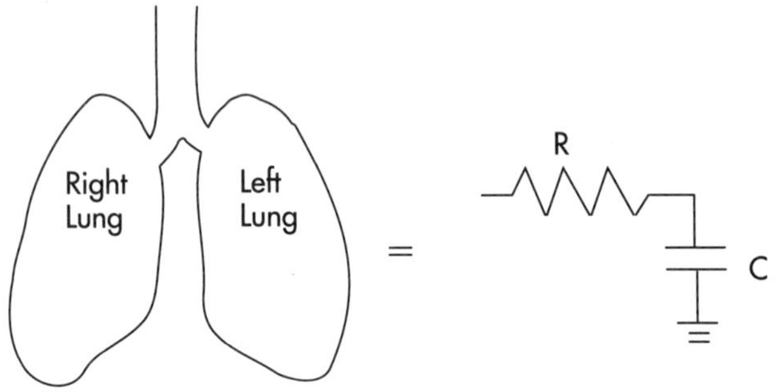

R = Resistance = $\dfrac{\text{Pressure Change}}{\text{Flow Rate}}$

C = Compliance = $\dfrac{\text{Volume Change}}{\text{Pressure Change}}$

Fig. 3-11. Resistance-compliance (RC) model of the lungs. Resistance of lungs to airflow and its natural ability to resist stretch (or compliance) enables lungs to be modeled as an electric circuit. A resistor of resistance, *R*, placed in series with a capacitor of charge, *C*, is a simple and convenient analogy upon which to base pulmonary biomechanics.

A transmural (P_{TM}) pressure gradient exists between the airway at the mouth (at atmospheric pressure) and the pressure inside the pleural cavity. This pressure gradient is responsible for the lungs "hugging" the thoracic cavity as the chest enlarges during inspiration. The presence of an external breathing apparatus causes a further pressure loss (P_{EXT}). Hence, the total pressure drop between the atmosphere and the pleural cavity is given by the respiratory mechanics equation and may be modeled as[44]:

$$P_{TOTAL} = P_{EXT} + P_{TM} = R_{EXT}\,\dot{V} + \frac{V}{C_L} + R_L\,\dot{V} \quad (28)$$

$$P_{EXT} = R_{EXT}\,\dot{V} \quad (29)$$

$$P_{TM} = \frac{V}{C_L} + R_L\,\dot{V} \quad (30)$$

where
  P_{TOTAL} = pressure drop between atmosphere and pleural cavity
  P_{EXT} = pressure drop across external breathing apparatus
  P_{TM} = transmural pressure gradient
  R_{EXT} = external apparatus resistance (e.g., an ET)
  $\dot{V}$ = dV/dt = gas flow rate into the lungs
  C_L = lung compliance
  R_L = airway resistance
  V = volume of gas above the functional residual capacity in the lungs

Thus, the pressure required to inflate the lungs depends both on the lung compliance and gas flow rate. The time required to inflate the lungs is measured in terms of a pulmonary time constant. This time constant (τ) is simply the product $R_L \times C_L$. However, determination of the time constant is not a trivial matter, and attention is now turned to that determination.

1. The pulmonary time constant

Using the previous formula in the case where no external resistance exists, one can show that, during passive expiration, the volume in the lungs in excess of functional residual capacity (FRC) takes on the form[45]:

$$V = V_0 e^{-t/\tau} \quad (31)$$

where V_0 is the volume taken in during inspiration and $\tau = R_L C_L$ is the time constant for the lungs. Flow from the lungs is obtained by differentiating the above equation with respect to time:

$$\dot{V} = \frac{dV}{dt} = V_0 \frac{d(e^{-t/\tau})}{dt} = V_0 e^{-t/\tau}\left(-\frac{1}{\tau}\right) = -\frac{V_0}{\tau} e^{-t/\tau} \quad (32)$$

Tau (τ) may be now estimated by dividing the above equation by the first one:

$$\frac{\dot{V}}{V} = \frac{V_0 e^{-t/\tau}\left(-\frac{1}{\tau}\right)}{V_0 e^{-t/\tau}} = -\frac{1}{\tau} \quad (33)$$

Tau (τ) can be estimated as the negative of the reciprocal of the average slope of the plot of flow ($\dot{V}$) against volume (V) during expiration. Another means of estimating τ is by taking the natural logarithm of the volume equation $V = V_0 e^{-t/\tau}$:

Tau can also be estimated as the negative of reciprocal of the average slope of the natural logarithm of the lung volume plotted against time.

$$\ln V = \ln(V_0) - \frac{t}{\tau} \qquad \frac{d(\ln V)}{dt} = -\frac{1}{\tau} \quad (34)$$

2. Determination of Rohrer's constants

A more complete approach to modeling the pressure-flow relationship of the respiratory system assumes that a single time constant τ may be inadequate to describe pulmonary biomechanics in some situations and goes from the classic form[21]:

$$\frac{V}{\dot{V}} = -\tau = C_L \times R_L \quad (35)$$

to a more elaborate form of:

$$\frac{V}{\dot{V}} = -C_L(K_1 + K_2\dot{V}) \quad (36)$$

where K_1 and K_2 are known as Rohrer's constants and ($K_1 + K_2\dot{V}$) is a form of R_L. In this situation, the resistance of the pulmonary system is not assumed to be constant, but rather, is assumed to be flow dependent:

$$R = K_1 + K_2\dot{V} \quad (37)$$

When this equation is expressed as:

$$\frac{V}{C_L\dot{V}} = -(K_1 + K_2\dot{V}) \quad (38)$$

K_1 and K_2 may be determined as the intercept and slope, respectively, of a plot of $V/C_L\dot{V}$ against $\dot{V}$.

3. Compliance

Pulmonary compliance measurements reflect the elastic properties of the lungs and thorax and are influenced by factors such as degree of muscular tension, degree of interstitial lung water, degree of pulmonary fibrosis, degree of lung inflation, and alveolar surface tension.[46] Total respiratory system compliance is given by[36]:

$$C = \frac{\Delta V}{\Delta P} \quad (39)$$

where

ΔV = change in lung volume

ΔP = change in airway pressure

This total compliance may be related to lung compliance and thoracic (chest wall) compliance by the relation:

$$\frac{1}{C_T} = \frac{1}{C_L} + \frac{1}{C_{Th}} \qquad (40)$$

where

C_T = total compliance (typically 100 ml/cm H_2O)

C_L = lung compliance (typically 200 ml/cm H_2O)

C_{Th} = thoracic compliance (typically 200 ml/cm H_2O)

Values in brackets above are some typical normal adult values that can be used for modeling purposes.[36] Elastance is the reciprocal of compliance and offers notational advantage over compliance in some physiological problems. However, its use has not been popular in clinical practice.

Compliance may be estimated using the pulmonary time constant τ. If a linear resistance of known value ΔR is added to the patient's airway, the time constant will then change, becoming[21]:

$$\tau' = (R_L + \Delta R) \times C_L = \tau + C_L \times \Delta R = \tau + \Delta \tau \qquad (41)$$

Thus, if ΔR is known and τ and τ' are determined experimentally, one can then solve for C_L and then for R_L:

$$C_L = \frac{\tau' - \tau}{\Delta R} = \frac{\Delta \tau}{\Delta R} \qquad R_L = \tau \times \frac{\Delta R}{\Delta \tau} = \frac{\tau \times \Delta R}{\tau' - \tau} \qquad (42)$$

B. AN ADVANCED FORMULATION OF THE RESPIRATORY MECHANICS EQUATION

An alternate equation, the advanced respiratory mechanics (ARM) equation, to the elementary respiratory mechanics equation may be used to describe the physical behavior of the lungs. The original formulation of the equation was carried out by Rohrer during World War I, but the first completely correct formulation is due to Gaensler et al.[33] and is of the form:

$$P = \frac{V}{C} + K_1 \dot{V} + K_2 \dot{V}^2 \qquad (43)$$

where

P = airway pressure

V = lung volume

$\dot{V}$ = gas flow rate into (out of) lung

C = compliance of the pulmonary system

K_1, K_2 = empirical Rohrer's constants

This equation is more advanced than the elementary RM equation, since it is able to account for flow losses attributable to turbulence. Since turbulent flow conditions are most likely to exist during anesthesia, the $\dot{V}^2$ term is very important in accurately quantifying the pressure losses of respiration. In addition, it combines the resistance losses into the constants K_1 and K_2, which requires only empirical determination.

V. ANESTHESIA AT MODERATE ALTITUDE

The parameters that govern the administration of anesthesia are altered slightly when the elevation above sea level is increased. Generally, a change in the atmospheric (or barometric) pressure is responsible for these differences. This section briefly examines the consequences of a moderate change in altitude.

The approximate Alveolar Gas Equation is a useful tool in quantifying the differences that occur at higher elevations[47]:

$$PAo_2 = Pio_2 - \frac{Paco_2}{R} \qquad Pio_2 = (P_B - 47) \times Fio_2 \qquad (44)$$

where

PAo_2 = alveolar oxygen tension

Pio_2 = inspired oxygen tension partial pressure

$Paco_2$ = arterial carbon dioxide tension

R = 0.8 $\Rightarrow$ gas exchange coefficient: CO_2 produced/O_2 consumed

P_B = barometric pressure (760 mm Hg at sea level)

47 = water vapor pressure at 37° C

Fio_2 = fraction of inspired oxygen = 0.21 at all altitudes (room air)

All tensions are in mm Hg (torr).

A. ALTERED PARTIAL PRESSURE OF GASES

The effect of altitude is very apparent on the partial pressure of administered gases. The partial pressure of oxygen is given by $Pio_2 = (P_B - P_{H_2O}) \times 0.21$. At 1524 m (5000 feet) above sea level, Pio_2 is reduced to 128 mm Hg from 158 mm Hg at sea level, so that the maximum PAo_2 is about 83 mm Hg (assuming $Paco_2 = 36$).[48] At 3048 m (10,000 feet), Pio_2 is 111 mm Hg, and the maximum PAo_2 is 65 mm Hg.[48] In order to counteract the effects of the hypoxia, ventilation is increased, so that at 5000 feet $Paco_2 = 36$ mm Hg, and, at 3048 m, $Paco_2 = 34$ mm Hg on average.[48] The effectiveness of N_2O decreases with altitude because of an absolute reduction of its partial pressure (tension).

B. OXYGEN ANALYZERS

There are five main types of oxygen analyzers: paramagnetic, fuel cell, oxygen electrodes, mass spectrometers, and Raman spectrographs. All respond to oxygen partial pressure (not concentration) so that the output changes with barometric pressure. At 1524 m, an analyzer set to measure 21% O_2 at sea level will read 17.4%. If these devices were to calculate the amount of oxygen in terms of partial pressure, the scale readings would reflect the true state of oxygen availability, but clinical practice dictates that a percentage scale be used anyway.

C. CO_2 ANALYZERS AND VAPOR ANALYZERS

Absorption of infrared radiation by gas is the usual analytic method to determine the amount of CO_2 in a gas mixture, although other methods (e.g., Raman spectrographs) work well. This type of method measures partial pressures, not percentages. To operate accurately, these machines must either be calibrated using known CO_2 concentrations at the correct barometric pressure or have the scale converted to read partial pressures.

Similar arguments apply to modern vapor analyzers, all of which respond to partial pressures, not concentrations, despite the fact that the output of these devices, by clinical custom, is usually calculated in percentages.

D. VAPORS AND VAPORIZERS

Practically speaking, the saturated vapor pressure of a volatile agent depends only on its temperature. Thus, at a given temperature, the concentration of a given mass of vapor increases as barometric pressure decreases, but its partial pressure remains unchanged. Similarly, the output of calibrated vaporizers will be altered with changes in barometric pressure. Only the concentration of the vapor will change; the partial pressure will remain the same, as will the patient response at a given setting as compared to sea level. This assumes that the vaporizer characteristics do not change with altered density and viscosity of the carrier gases.

E. FLOWMETERS

Most flowmeters measure the drop in pressure that occurs when a gas passes through a resistance and correlate this pressure drop to flow. The pressure drop is dependent on gas density and viscosity. When the resistance is an orifice, resistance depends primarily on gas density. For laminar flow through a tube, viscosity determines resistance (Hagen-Poiseuille equation). Some flowmeters employ a floating ball or bobbin supported by the stream of gas in a tapered tube. The float is fluted so that it will remain in the center of the flow. At low flow, the device depends primarily on laminar flow, and, as the float moves up the tube, the resistance behaves progressively more like an orifice. The density of a gas changes, of course, with barometric pressure, but the viscosity changes little, being primarily dependent on temperature. Gas flow through an orifice is inversely proportional to the square root of gas density, so that, as the density falls, flow increases (orifice size constant). Thus, at high altitude, the actual flowmeter flow will be greater than that indicated by the float position:

Table 3-4. Gram molecular weights (GMW) for some common and anesthetic gases

Name	Symbol	GMW
Hydrogen	H	1.00797
Helium	He	4.0026
Nitrogen (molecular)	N_2	28.0134
Oxygen (molecular)	O_2	31.9988
Neon	Ne	20.183
Argon	Ar	39.948
Xenon	Xe	131.30
Halothane	$CF_3CClBrH$	197
Isoflurane	CF_2H-O-$CHClCF_3$	184.5
Enflurane	CF_2H-O-CF_2CFHCl	184.5
Nitrous oxide	N_2O	44.013

$$\text{Actual flow} = \text{Nominal flow} \times \sqrt{\frac{760 \text{ mm Hg}}{P_B}} \quad (45)$$

F. FLOWMETER CALIBRATION

The calibration of standard flowmeters, such as the Thorpe tube, depends on gas properties. Usually, a particular flowmeter is calibrated for a particular gas, such as oxygen or air. The factor used to convert nominal flow measurements to actual flow measurements is given by[47]:

$$k = \frac{\sqrt{\text{GMW}_A}}{\sqrt{\text{GMW}_B}} \quad (46)$$

where A is the gas for which the flowmeter is originally designed, B is the gas actually used, and GMW is the gram molecular weight of the gas in question. A list of common anesthetic gases and their respective *GMW*s are presented in Table 3-4.

Example Calculation 1

Determine the actual flow rate of a 70%:30% helium-oxygen mixture if it is passed through an oxygen flowmeter that reads 10 L/min.

Answer:

$$\text{GMW}_{O_2} = 32 \text{ g/gmol} \quad (47)$$

$$\text{GMW}_{Heliox} = 0.3(32) + 0.7(4) = 12.4 \text{ g/gmol} \quad (48)$$

The actual flow rate of Heliox is given by:

$$\text{Actual flow rate} = 10 \times \frac{\sqrt{\text{GMW}_{O_2}}}{\sqrt{\text{GMW}_{Heliox}}} = \quad (49)$$

$$10 \times \frac{\sqrt{32}}{\sqrt{12.4}} = 16.1 \text{ L/min}$$

Example Calculation 2

Determine the appropriate multiplier if oxygen is passed through an airflow meter.

Table 3-5. Variations in MAC that occur at various altitude levels, with the comparative values for MAPP

Agent	MAC (%)			MAPP	
	Sea level	5000 feet	10,000 feet	(kPa)	(mm Hg)
Nitrous oxide	105.0	126.5	152.2	106.1	798.0
Ethyl ether	1.92	2.31	2.78	1.94	14.6
Halothane	0.75	0.90	1.09	0.76	5.7
Enflurane	1.68	2.02	2.43	1.70	12.8
Isoflurane	1.2	1.45	1.73	1.22	9.1

MAPP = MAC × 0.01 × 760 mm Hg
Adapted from James MFM, White JF: *Anesth Analg* 63:1097, 1984.

Answer:

$$\text{Multiplier} = \frac{\sqrt{GMW_{AIR}}}{\sqrt{GMW_{O_2}}} = \frac{\sqrt{0.21\,(32) + 0.79\,(28)}}{\sqrt{32}} = 0.95 \tag{50}$$

G. ANESTHETIC IMPLICATIONS

At 3048 m (10,000 feet), a 30% O_2 mixture has the same partial pressure as a 20% O_2 mixture at sea level.[48] In addition, the reduction in partial pressure of N_2O that occurs seriously impairs the effectiveness of the agent and may be of no benefit to administer. The concept of minimum alveolar concentration (MAC) does not apply at higher altitudes and should be substituted by the concept of minimal alveolar partial pressure (MAPP) (Table 3-5). The use of this concept would eliminate many of the problems identified above.

VI. ESTIMATION OF GAS RATES

A. ESTIMATION OF CARBON DIOXIDE PRODUCTION RATE

The carbon dioxide (CO_2) production rate ($\dot{V}_{CO_2}$) of a patient may be estimated in the following manner. The CO_2 production rate can be described as the product of the amount of CO_2 produced per breath and the number of breaths per minute. The CO_2 production rate hence has typical units of milliliters per minute (ml/min). Hence, $\dot{V}_{CO_2}$ may be expressed as:

$$\dot{V}_{CO_2} = CO_2 \text{ Produced Per Breath} \times \tag{51}$$
$$\text{Number Of Breaths Per Minute}$$

$$\dot{V}_{CO_2} = V_{CO_2} \times BPM \tag{52}$$

The amount of CO_2 produced per breath is calculated as follows:

$$V_{CO_2} = \int_{t=0}^{t=t_{end\,expiration}} C_{CO_2}(t) \times Q(t) \times \gamma \, dt \tag{53}$$

where
$C_{CO_2}(t)$ = capnogram signal [mm Hg]

$Q(t)$ = gas flow rate signal [ml/min]
γ = scaling factor to switch dimensions from mm Hg to concentration % = $\frac{100\%}{760 \text{ mm Hg}}$ = 0.1312

B. ESTIMATION OF OXYGEN CONSUMPTION RATE

The oxygen consumption rate may be estimated in a manner very similar to that of $\dot{V}_{CO_2}$. The oxygen consumption rate can be expressed as the product of oxygen consumed per breath and the number of breaths per minute. Mathematically, this may be written as:

$$\dot{V}_{O_2} = O_2 \text{ Produced Per Breath} \times \tag{54}$$
$$\text{Number Of Breaths Per Minute}$$

$$\dot{V}_{O_2} = V_{O_2} \times BPM \tag{55}$$

The amount of O_2 produced per breath can now be expressed as:

$$V_{O_2} = \int_{t=0}^{t=t_{end\,expiration}} (Pio_2 - Co_2) \times Q(t) \times \gamma \, dt \tag{56}$$

where
Pio_2 = inspiratory oxygen pressure = $(P_B - 47) \times F_1O_2$ [mm Hg]
$C_{O_2}(t)$ = oxygen signal [mm Hg]
Q = gas flow rate signal [ml/min]
γ = scaling factor = 0.1312

C. INTERPRETATION OF CARBON DIOXIDE PRODUCTION AND OXYGEN CONSUMPTION RATES

The rates $\dot{V}_{O_2}$ and $\dot{V}_{CO_2}$ are linked by the respiratory exchange coefficient RQ ($RQ = \dot{V}_{CO_2}/\dot{V}_{O_2}$), which is governed largely by diet, some diets producing less CO_2 than others (RQ smaller). Typically, RQ = 0.8. $\dot{V}_{O_2}$ and $\dot{V}_{CO_2}$ both go up with increases in metabolism, perhaps related to one of several factors (fever, sepsis, light anesthesia, shivering, malignant hyperthermia, thyroid storm, etc.). Decreases in $\dot{V}_{CO_2}$ and $\dot{V}_{O_2}$ may be due to many causes as well (hypothermia, deep anesthesia, hypothyroidism, etc.).

VII. MATHEMATICAL MODELING RELATED TO THE AIRWAY

A. OVERVIEW

In this section, the role of "ready-to-use" numeric analysis software for physiologic model building is discussed, using the respiratory system as a basis for discussion. Using well-established physiologic principles, it can be shown that some "what if" physiologic questions can be answered. These questions could not have been answered in the past because of experimental complexity or because of ethical considerations. Since the model is based upon simple equations accepted by the physiologic community, the obtained results are directly credible, and many of the difficulties of direct experimentation are avoided.

The model concept is explored through a discussion of four oxygen transport problems, some of which are too complex in experimental design for empirical study to be practical. However, considerable insight can be obtained using numerical methods alone.

B. BACKGROUND

Some physiologic systems are especially well suited to physiologic modeling. For example, physiologic modeling of the cardiopulmonary system may be performed to examine issues such as the determinants of pulmonary gas exchange. For instance, both Doyle[49] and Viale et al.[50] have written custom software to explore the determinants of the arterial-alveolar oxygen tension ratio, while Torda[51] has explored the determinants of the alveolar-arterial oxygen tension difference in a similar manner. Prior to the common use of digital computers, graphic techniques were sometimes used for solving respiratory physiologic models, early work by Kelman et al. on the influence of cardiac output on arterial oxygenation being a well-known example.[52] Central to the construction of such a mathematic model is the existence of a number of equations relating physiologic parameters. Examples of physiologic relationships in the respiratory system well-described by equations include (1) the alveolar gas equation,[47,53] (2) the pulmonary shunt equation,[54] (3) the blood oxygen content equation,[54] and (4) various equations describing the oxyhemoglobin dissociation curve.[55-59]

C. PROBLEMS IN MODEL SOLVING

Although many physiologic problems are readily solved by direct analytic methods, frequently their solution is hampered by nonlinearities, self-referencing (circular) equations, or other complexities. (An example of a nonlinearity is the equation $y = x^2$; an example of a self-referencing equation set is the equation pair $y = 1/x$; $x = y + 1$.) Experience has shown that early conventional spreadsheet programs were poorly equipped to solve systems of this kind, since they are not generally designed for iterative equation-solving methods. Newer spreadsheets usually contain an iterative solver of some kind.

Some authors have applied successive approximation methods with custom-written software to solve equation sets of this kind.[49] However, this approach may involve considerable effort, even to experienced computer programmers. Furthermore, many physiologists have limited experience and training in writing computer programs. In the next section we show how equation-solving computer programs can be used to advantage to solve complex physiologic modeling equations. TK SOLVER is the equation-solver package used in most of the examples shown below, but many other packages could also have been used.

D. DESCRIPTION OF TK SOLVER

TK SOLVER (the TK stands for "tool kit") is a software package for equation solving.[60-64] While intended primarily for engineering applications, TK SOLVER functions well in a variety of other application areas. On start-up, TK SOLVER displays two "sheets" or tables out of a total of thirteen (Fig. 3-12). The Variable Sheet is presented on the top "window," while the Rule Sheet goes on the bottom. Equations are then entered in the Rule Sheet using a built-in editor; the variables associated with the equations are then automatically entered in the variable sheet by TK SOLVER. Errors such as unmatched parentheses are automatically detected. (Fig. 3-12 shows sample Rule and Variable Sheets for a pulmonary exchange model.)

Once the equations are entered, TK SOLVER is ready to find solutions. In some cases, the equation set can be solved in "direct-solver" mode, but complex equation sets generally must be solved in "iterative-solver" mode based on initial guesses for all variables. A discussion of the methods used to obtain solutions is presented by Konopasek et al.[63] A book reviewing TK SOLVER from a users' viewpoint is also available.[64]

E. EXAMPLE 1: APPLICATION OF MATHEMATICAL MODELING TO THE STUDY OF GAS EXCHANGE INDICES

Gas exchange indices are commonly used in anesthesia and critical care medicine to assess pulmonary function from an oxygen transport viewpoint. While the determination of pulmonary shunt would be viewed by many as a "gold standard" preferable to any index, measurement of true pulmonary shunt requires pulmonary artery catheterization—a relatively expensive

```
========================= RULE SHEET ===============================
S  Rule
---------
    PaO2=PAO2-(Cav*(Z/(1-Z))-1.34*Hb*(ScO2-SaO2))/0.0031
    SaO2=PaO2^a/(PaO2^a+P50^a)
    ScO2=PAO2^a/(PAO2^a+P50^a)
    Cav=VO2/(10*CO)
    Sav=(Cav-0.0031*(PaO2-PvO2))/(1.34*Hb)
    SvO2=SaO2-Sav
    PvO2=P50*(SvO2/(1-SvO2))^(1/a)
    CaO2=1.34*Hb*SaO2+0.0031*PaO2
    CvO2=CaO2-Cav
    CcO2=1.34*Hb*ScO2+0.0031*PAO2

========================= VARIABLE SHEET ==========================:

St  Input   Name    Output    Unit   Comment
---------   ----    -------   -----  -------
    50      PAO2              mmHg   Alveolar Oxygen Tension
            PaO2    46.602925 mmHg   Arterial Oxygen Tension
            PvO2    29.722228 mmHg   Mixed Venous Oxygen Tension
            SaO2    .80944994 none   Arterial Saturation (%)
            ScO2    .83656560 none   End Pulmonary Capillary Saturation (%)
            SvO2    .56329721 none   Mixed Venous Saturation (%)
            Sav     .24615273 none   Arterio-Venous Saturation Difference
    250     VO2               ml/min Oxygen Consumption
    5       CO                L/min  Cardiac Output
    .1      Z                 none   Pulmonary Shunt Fraction
            Cav     5         vol%   Arterio-venous O2 Content Diff
    15      Hb                g/dl   Hemoglobin Concentration
    2.65    a                 none   Hill's coefficient
    27      P50               mmHg   PO2 for 50% Saturation
            CaO2    16.414413 vol%   Arterial Oxygen Content
            CvO2    11.414413 vol%   Mixed Venous Oxygen Content
            CcO2    16.969968 vol%   End Pulmonary Capillary Oxygen Content
```

Fig. 3-12. TK SOLVER Sheets. *Top,* TK SOLVER Rule Sheet; *bottom,* Sample Variable Sheet. Sample Rule Sheet and Variable Sheet for TK SOLVER. In this case, equations relate factors that determine arterial oxygen tension (PaO$_2$). All variables are defined in comment section of variable sheet. First equation in the Rule Sheet is from Torda and Doyle.[49,51] Second and third equations are Hill equation.

and risky procedure that is not always clinically warranted. Four gas exchange indices which are in common use are:

1. alveolar-arterial oxygen tension difference (P[A-a]O$_2$)[51,64-66]
2. arterial-alveolar oxygen tension ratio (a/A PO$_2$)[49,50,67-69]
3. respiratory index (RI) = P[A-a]O$_2$/PAO$_2$[70,71]
4. PaO$_2$/FiO$_2$ ratio[72]

The importance of these indices and the controversies surrounding their use in clinical practice are reflected in the many publications concerning their use and limitations.[72-76]

1. Analysis

The pulmonary shunt equation is used as a foundation upon which arterial oxygenation and gas exchange indices can be studied. It may be expressed as:

$$\frac{Qs}{Qt} = \frac{Cc'o_2 - Cao_2}{Cc'o_2 - C\overline{v}o_2} \qquad (57)$$

where

$Cc'o_2$ = end-pulmonary capillary oxygen content
Cao_2 = arterial oxygen content
$C\overline{v}o_2$ = mixed venous oxygen content

By algebraic manipulation of the shunt equation, it is possible to relate arterial oxygen tension to its influencing factors[49,51]:

$$Pao_2 = PAo_2 - \qquad (58)$$

$$\frac{Ca-\overline{v}o_2 \times \dfrac{\dfrac{Qs}{Qt}}{1 - \dfrac{Qs}{Qt}} - 1.34 \times (Sc'o_2 - Sao_2) \times Hb}{0.0031}$$

where PAo$_2$ (mm Hg) is the alveolar oxygen tension;

Ca-$\bar{v}o_2$ (vol%) is the arterial-mixed venous oxygen content difference ($= Cao_2 - C\bar{v}o_2$), $Sc'o_2$ is end-pulmonary capillary fractional saturation, Sao_2 is the arterial saturation, and Hb is the blood hemoglobin concentration (g/dL). The full alveolar gas equation is used to determine PAo_2:

$$PAo_2 = (P_B - P_{H_2O}) \times Fio_2 - Paco_2 \times \left(Fio_2 + \frac{1 - Fio_2}{R} \right) \tag{59}$$

where P_B is the barometric pressure (assumed to be 760 mm Hg), P_{H_2O} is the patient's water vapor pressure (assumed to be 47 mm Hg), $Paco_2$ is the arterial CO_2 tension (usually assumed to be 40 mm Hg) and R is the gas exchange ratio (assumed to be 0.8).

Equation (58) does not explicitly show the influence of P_{50} on arterial oxygen tension; such influences are mediated indirectly, principally through the Sao_2 term. To make explicit the influence of Pao_2 and P_{50} on Sao_2, we use the relationship given by Hill[59]:

$$Sao_2 = \frac{Pao_2^n}{Pao_2^n + P_{50}^n} \tag{60}$$

where n is an empirical constant (generally taken as 2.65). A similar expression relates PAo_2, P_{50}, and $Sc'o_2$.

The arterial oxygen tension, the alveolar-arterial oxygen tension difference, and the arterial-alveolar oxygen tension ratio can then be obtained using equations (58), (59), and (60) for specific choices of physiologic variables. Unfortunately, equation (58) is not easily solved because it requires the solution of two simultaneous nonlinear equations (i.e., equations [58] and [60]). In the past, a custom, computer-based successive approximation method was employed to obtain a solution. This amounted to iteratively making successively more accurate estimates of Pao_2 levels that met both equations (58) and (60). In the case of Doyle,[49] equation (58) was solved in this way to an accuracy of 0.1 mm Hg for various values of Hb, Ca-$\bar{v}o_2$, Fio_2, $Paco_2$, and Qs/Qt. The process is considerably simplified when TK SOLVER is used, as can be seen by examining the equation sheets presented in Fig. 3-12.

F. EXAMPLE 2: THEORETICAL STUDY OF HEMOGLOBIN CONCENTRATION EFFECTS ON GAS EXCHANGE INDICES

It is both of theoretic and clinical interest to know what changes in gas exchange indices might be expected with changes in blood hemoglobin concentration when other physiologic parameters are kept constant. Fig. 3-13 shows the results of varying hemoglobin concentration with the following parameters held constant: alveolar oxygen tension (PAo_2) = 100 mm Hg; cardiac output (CO) = 5 l/min; oxygen consumption ($\dot{V}_{O_2}$) = 250 ml/min; shunt fraction (Qs/Qt) = 0.1; P_{50} (oxygen tension corresponding to 50% hemoglobin saturation) = 27 mm Hg.

As can be seen in Fig. 3-13, increasing blood hemoglobin concentration would be expected to improve arterial oxygen tension and improve the gas exchange indices under study. Such data would be almost impossible to obtain experimentally because of the difficulty of varying blood hemoglobin concentration independent of other physiologic factors such as cardiac output.

G. EXAMPLE 3: MODELING THE OXYGENATION EFFECTS OF P_{50} CHANGES AT ALTITUDE

It is well known that the oxyhemoglobin dissociation curve may shift in response to physiologic changes. For example, acidosis, hypercarbia, increased temperature, and increased levels of 2,3-DPG all shift the curve to the right, reducing hemoglobin affinity for oxygen and thereby facilitating its release into tissues. Also, with chronic anemia, intraerythrocyte 2,3-DPG levels increase, yielding a right-shifted oxyhemoglobin curve.[77] Since such a shift apparently increases oxygen release into tissues, teleologically it would also appear to be an appropriate response to high altitude hypoxemia. In fact, however, the opposite appears to be true. Animals that have successfully adapted to high altitude hypoxemia have left-shifted curves,[78,79] as do Sherpas.[80,81] In this example, we use computer modeling to develop a possible explanation for this finding.

It is proposed here that the reason that a left-shifted curve is beneficial in high-altitude hypoxemia is that it increases arterial oxygen content by virtue of increasing end-pulmonary capillary oxygen content. To demonstrate this, first suppose that a person has a pulmonary shunt fraction Qs/Qt. Then from rearranging the shunt equation above, we can show that:

$$Cao_2 = Cc'o_2 - \frac{\frac{Qs}{Qt}}{1 - \frac{Qs}{Qt}} \times Ca\bar{v}o_2 \tag{61}$$

Thus, at constant pulmonary shunt and arteriovenous oxygen content difference, increases in end-pulmonary capillary oxygen content will increase arterial oxygen content.

Now the end-pulmonary capillary oxygen content, $Cc'o_2$, consists of two terms, the first being the oxygen bound to hemoglobin, and the second being the oxygen dissolved in plasma:

$$Cc'o_2 = 1.34 \, Hb \, Sc'o_2 + 0.0031 \, PAo_2 \tag{62}$$

where

Hb = hemoglobin concentration [g/dL]

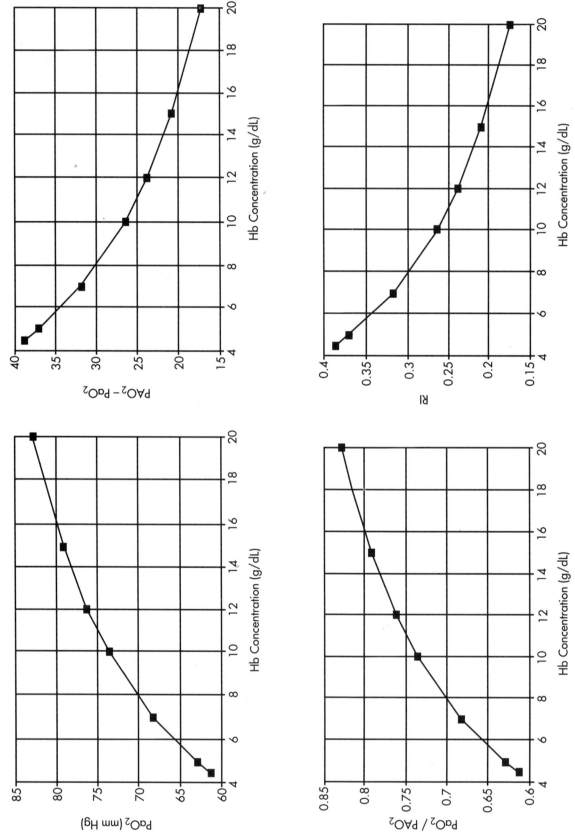

Fig. 3-13. Effect of hemoglobin concentration on various gas exchange indices. Effect of hemoglobin concentration on various gas exchange indices according to TK SOLVER model. *Top left,* effect on arterial oxygen tension (PaO_2); *top right,* effect on alveolar-arterial oxygen tension difference (PAO_2-PaO_2); *bottom left,* effect on arterial-alveolar oxygen tension ratio (PaO_2/PAO_2); *bottom right,* effect on the respiratory index (RI).

Sc'O_2 = end-pulmonary capillary hemoglobin saturation

PAO_2 = alveolar oxygen tension [mm Hg]

PAO_2 is determined only by the alveolar gas equation and is independent of the oxyhemoglobin curve position.[54] Thus, the dissolved oxygen portion of Cc'O_2 is also independent of the curve position. However, the Sc'O_2 term does vary with curve position and increases with a left-shifted curve. Thus, Cc'O_2 also increases with a left

Table 3-6. Oxygenation effects of P_{50} changes at altitude

Oxygen variable	Altitude case*		Shunt case	
	$P_{50} = 27$	$P_{50} = 18$	$P_{50} = 27$	$P_{50} = 18$
PaO_2	46.6	43.3	46.9	33.1
P$\bar{v}O_2$	29.7	23.3	29.8	20.6
SaO_2	0.809	0.911	0.812	0.834
S$\bar{v}O_2$	0.563	0.665	0.566	0.587
ScO_2	0.837	0.937	0.970	0.989
CaO_2	16.41	18.44	16.47	16.87
C$\bar{v}O_2$	11.41	13.44	11.47	11.87
Cc'O_2	16.99	19.00	19.80	20.20

*Detailed figures for altitude case (PAO_2 = 50 mm Hg) and for shunt case (Qs/Qt = 0.4). Other parameters are given in the text. Note that a shift from a P_{50} of 27 to a P_{50} of 18 significantly increases arterial oxygen content (CaO_2) in the altitude case but not in the shunt case.

shift and takes on a maximum value of:

$$[Cc'O_2]_{max} = 1.34 \text{ Hb} + 0.0031 \text{ PA}O_2 \tag{63}$$

This analysis demonstrates that a left-shifted curve increases arterial oxygen content by increasing end-pulmonary capillary oxygen content.

1. Situation A

Consider a patient with high altitude hypoxemia as a result of an alveolar oxygen tension (PAO_2) of 50 mm Hg. With a cardiac output of 5 liters/min, hemoglobin concentration (Hb) of 15 g/dL, oxygen consumption ($\dot{V}O_2$) of 250 ml/min and shunt fraction (Qs/Qt) of 0.1, it can be shown (Table 3-6) that CaO_2 goes from 16.41 vol% with a P_{50} of 27 mm Hg to 18.44 vol% with a P_{50} of 18 mm Hg, a significant increase.

2. Situation B

Consider a patient with a large pulmonary shunt (Qs/Qt = 0.4), a normal alveolar oxygen tension (PAO_2 = 100 mm Hg), and other parameters as in Situation A. Here CaO_2 goes from 16.47 vol% with a P_{50} of 27 mm Hg to 16.87 vol% with a P_{50} of 18 mm Hg, an insignificant change.

Fig. 3-14 illustrates this concept in more detail, where the two examples are studied for P_{50} values from 10 to 50.

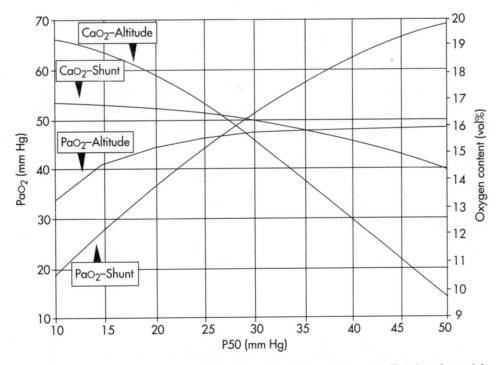

Fig. 3-14. PaO_2 and CaO_2 as a function of P_{50}. Arterial oxygen tension (PaO_2) and arterial oxygen content (CaO_2) as a function of P_{50} for situations depicted in Situations A and B. Notice that in altitude hypoxemia case a decrease in P_{50} (left-shifted curve) significantly increases oxygen content, but not in the shunt hypoxemia case. (From Doyle DJ: *Can J Anaesth* 39 (5II):A89, 1992.)

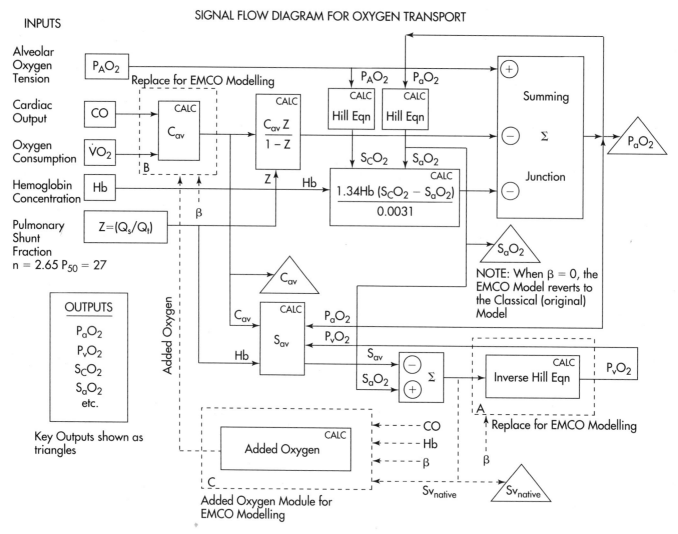

Fig. 3-15. Schematic diagram for venovenous ECMO model. Schematic conceptual diagram for venovenous ECMO. Nomenclature: Svo_2, mixed oxygen saturation; Sao_2, arterial oxygen saturation; ScO_2, end pulmonary capillary oxygen saturation; Qs/Qt (Z), pulmonary shunt fraction; CO, cardiac output; $\dot{V}O_2$, oxygen consumption; PAo_2, alveolar oxygen tension (mm Hg); Pao_2, arterial oxygen tension (mm Hg); Hb, hemoglobin concentration (g/dL).

The numbers provided in Situations A and B and in Fig. 3-14 were obtained using the above mathematical computer model of the oxyhemoglobin dissociation curve. Hill's equation relating saturation, tension, and P_{50}[59] was used in conjunction with Doyle's equation for arterial oxygen tension[49] and solved using TK SOLVER.

These two example situations demonstrate that a left-shift to the oxyhemoglobin dissociation curve significantly improves arterial oxygen content in the case of high-altitude hypoxemia but not in the case of large shunts. This observation is consistent with the fact that, with right-to-left shunts, such as those in cyanotic heart disease, a right-shifted curve is the general finding.[55] The reason that in this latter case a left-shifted curve is not

beneficial is that only a trivial improvement in end-pulmonary capillary oxygen content (and thus arterial oxygen content) is obtained. Teleologically, it may be argued that, in the presence of hypoxemia, at approximately equal arterial contents, the body prefers higher oxygen tensions (right-shift preferred), but, if arterial oxygen content can be significantly improved, despite a decrease in oxygen tension, a left-shift is preferred.

H. EXAMPLE 4: MATHEMATICAL/COMPUTER MODEL FOR EXTRACORPOREAL MEMBRANE OXYGENATION

Extracorporeal membrane oxygen (ECMO) is sometimes used to treat respiratory failure refractory to more

```
alpha=2.65      ; Hill's constant
beta= 0.75        ; beta is the ratio of ECMO flow to cardiac output
CO=5             ; cardiac output
Hb=15             ; hemoglobin concentration
VO2=250         ; oxygen consumption
PAO2=200      ; alveolar oxygen tension
Z=0.6             ; pulmonary shunt
; P50=27          ; a resonable value for P50
; consider oxygen added to body by ECMO machine
; added02 = beta*CO*10*(1.34*Hb*(1-Sv02native))
Cav=(VO2 - (beta*CO*13.4*Hb*(1-Sv02native)))/(10*CO)
Sv02=Sa02 - (Cav - 0.0031*(Pa02-Pv02))/(1.34*Hb)
Pa02=PA02 - (Cav*(Z/(1-Z)) - 1.34*Hb*(SA02-Sa02))/0.0031
Pa02:=85
Sv02native:=0.7
Cav:=0.8
SA02=PA02^alpha / (PA02^alpha + 27^alpha)  ; Hill's equation
Sa02=Pa02^alpha / (Pa02^alpha + 27^alpha)  ; Hill's equation
Pv02=27*(Sv02 /(1-Sv02))^(1/alpha)   ; augmented mixed-venous P02
Pv02native=27*(Sv02native/(1-Sv02native))^(1/alpha)
Sv02native=(Sv02-beta)/(1-beta)    ; Sv02 entering ECMO
Pv02>=Pv02native
PA02>Pa02 >0
Sv02>=Sv02native>0
Sv02native<1
```

Fig. 3-16. Equations for venovenous ECMO model. Equations for venoveno ECMO problem, this time using EUREKA, an equation solver similar to TK SOLVER, but somewhat easier to learn. First seven lines indicate the values of physiological parameters that are held constant. Next three lines are comments to user and are not used by EUREKA. Lines 11-13 and 17-21 list basic equations to be solved. Lines 22-25 give some physiologic constraints that cannot be violated (e.g., arterial oxygen tension must be less than alveolar oxygen tension). Lines 14-16 provide initial estimates for EUREKA's iterative solver. (EUREKA is also available in a "shareware" version known as Mercury, which runs under MS-DOS.) (Adapted from Doyle DJ: *Can J Anaesth* 39 (5II):A34, 1992.)

conservative measures.[82] Unfortunately, clinical experience with ECMO is limited, so that even clinicians familiar with ECMO may disagree about its potential benefits in a particular clinical setting. This is especially true when the patient has a high cardiac output (e.g., 20 liters/min) while the ECMO pump is limited to much smaller flows (e.g., 5 liters/min). In this example, we describe how a computer model may be designed to facilitate management decisions for patients being considered for venovenous ECMO.

A mathematic model of the venovenous ECMO situation may be developed based on the shunt equation,[50] the Hill model for the oxyhemoglobin dissociation curve,[51] Doyle's equation for arterial oxygen tension as a function of cardiorespiratory parameters,[52] and the schematic diagram for venovenous ECMO shown in Fig. 3-15. The relevant equations are given in Fig. 3-16. The model may be solved for various hypothetical clinical circumstances using an equation solver package. In this instance, we used EUREKA, a DOS-based commercial computer software package for solving systems of equations.

Some sample results are shown in Fig. 3-17. Here, the patient parameters are CO = 5 liters/min; $\dot{V}o_2$ = 250 ml/min; Hb = 15 g/dL; Qs/Qt = 0.5; PAo_2 = 200 mm Hg; and an oxygenator oxygen tension output that results in complete hemoglobin saturation.

I. DISCUSSION

There are many questions in physiology that are not easily answered by direct experimentation, either because it is impractical, or impossible, to control all the pertinent variables or because of ethical considerations. In the case of studying the influence of blood hemoglobin concentration on pulmonary gas exchange indices, it would be difficult to rigorously control cardiac output, total body oxygen consumption, and other variables to experimentally study the issue. The approach presented here offers several advantages.

1. It relies on well-established physiologic relationships (e.g., alveolar gas equation, pulmonary shunt equation).
2. It permits insight into physiologic issues not generally attainable in other ways.
3. It is inexpensive.
4. It potentially reduces the need to carry out animal experimentation.

Three drawbacks to the method exist:

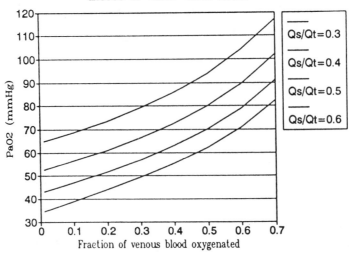

Arterial Oxygenation
Effect of veno–veno ECMO

Fig. 3-17. Sample results for venovenous ECMO model. Sample results from venovenous ECMO model for various levels of relative flow through ECMO oxygenator. Plot of arterial oxygen tension (Pao₂) as function of fraction of venous blood that passes through ECMO oxygenator for various values of pulmonary shunt fraction (Qs/Qt [Z]). (Adapted from Doyle DJ: *Can J Anaesth* 39 (5II):A34, 1992.)

1. The method is no better than the equations upon which it is based.
2. The method may not be convincing to some physiologists who may only be satisfied by confirmatory experimental results.
3. Errors can occur in model building.

One potential difficulty with such modeling methods is that the obtained results depend critically on the equations used. In cases where the equations are known from first principles (e.g., alveolar gas equation, pulmonary shunt equation), this is not an issue, but, where an equation is empirical, alternative equations may possibly produce differing results. An example here is the equation for the oxyhemoglobin dissociation curve, which has many competing formulations.[55-59] In this example we used the formulation given by Hill.[59]

J. UTILITY

Where can such a model be useful? In a particular patient with severe adult respiratory distress syndrome (ARDS) and resulting severe hypoxemia, clinicians might be interested in knowing, for instance, how ECMO would be expected to improve oxygenation. From pulmonary artery catheterization and arterial blood samples one can obtain the following and other data relevant to carrying out oxygen transport modeling:

1. Hemoglobin concentration
2. Cardiac output
3. P_{50} on dissociation curve
4. Arterial and mixed venous (arterial blood gas, ABG) data

Based on a model constructed for that time point, one could explore, for example, the effect of augmenting cardiac output and mixed venous oxygen tension in the ECMO situation. Without a model to describe this problem, the best we can do is fit empirical curves to experimental data. However, with a model, one can easily ask "what if" questions: for example, what happens when the ratio of pump oxygenator flow to cardiac output is set at a particular value.[77]

A good example is one question in respiratory physiology: How does a patient's alveolar-arterial oxygen tension difference change with reduced inspired oxygen tension? The first attempt at this question used pulse oximetry to infer arterial oxygen tension in volunteers subjected to controlled hypoxia by rebreathing.[78] A subsequent study took a more direct approach by cannulating the radial artery of elderly respiratory patient volunteers and drawing off serial arterial blood samples as the patients were subjected to hypoxemia in a hypobaric chamber.[79] This latter study is sufficiently invasive (and even, perhaps, sufficiently risky) that many hospital ethics committees would not approve it under existing guidelines.

Where more than one set of equations exists to describe a physiologic relationship, one can explore the effect of equation choice. One would expect, however, that, if several equations existed that all did a good job of representing the underlying data, equation choice would not have a great influence on obtained results. In the case of a few days (or even a few hours), one can obtain meaningful information about the interaction of several physiologic variables, provided that the relationships describing the variables are available in equation form. By contrast, actual experimentation takes time, funds, and effort that may not always be available. In fields such as oxygen transport, many relevant equations are simple well-known physiologic principles written in equation form, such as those listed below:

1. Alveolar gas equation
2. Pulmonary shunt equation
3. Oxyhemoglobin dissociation curve
4. Oxygen transport parameter definitions

To the extent that one accepts these physiologic principles, the results obtained should also be credible (provided that model design and implementation have been done correctly). In this respect, three issues exist:

1. How meaningful are the equations used? Are they a mathematical form of a well-known physiologic principle?
2. How accurate are the equations in describing the data they are based on?
3. Has the model been appropriately designed and implemented?

K. SOFTWARE

Several platforms exist to do such computations in the IBM-PC environment. TK SOLVER is still available (in a "Plus" form) from software distributors but has nowhere near the market share of MATHCAD, a widely available, popular mathematic modeling package with strong graphical features. MATHCAD has equation solving features similar to TK SOLVER that would make it appropriate for mathematic model building. Another suitable package would be Mercury, a shareware equation solver derived from EUREKA (Borland). All these packages take some effort to master. In particular, the manner in which each package handles convergence to solution will greatly affect ease-of-use and reliability. In general, the three packages mentioned (TK SOLVER, MATHCAD, and Mercury) work reasonably well with some effort. However, it is more difficult to do this modeling using ordinary computer spreadsheets (e.g., early releases of Lotus 1-2-3): first, because it is somewhat awkward for working with equations; and, second, because most spreadsheets are not set up to handle complicated iterative equation solving.

Source: TK SOLVER is available from Universal Technical Systems, Inc., 1220 Rock Street, Rockford, Illinois USA Tel: (815) 963-2220 Fax: (815) 963-8884.

L. COMPUTATIONAL FLOW DIAGRAMS

The representation of mathematic models for complex physiologic systems can sometimes be facilitated by representing the relevant equations using a Computational Flow Diagram. The concept is most easily understood by reviewing the examples mentioned previously.

EXAMPLE 1. Computation of the alveolar-arterial oxygen tension gradient

EXAMPLE 2. Computation of alveolar oxygen tension

EXAMPLE 3. Computation of arterial oxygen tension

EXAMPLE 4. Modeling the effects of veno veno ECMO

Note that where the examples involve feedback (examples 3 and 4), special iterative methods are necessary to obtain a solution. Not all spreadsheets are able to do this.

VIII. SELECTED DIMENSIONAL EQUIVALENTS

Discussions regarding physics in anesthesia may be confusing because of a variety of units used in clinical literature. The following list is a compilation of the units and their equivalents that one is likely to encounter.

Length

$1 \text{ m} = 3.2808 \text{ foot} = 39.37 \text{ in}$

$1 \text{ foot} = 0.3048 \text{ m}$

$1 \text{ m} = 100 \text{ cm} = 1000 \text{ mm} = 1\,000\,000 \text{ } \mu\text{m} = 10,000\,000 \text{ Å} = 10^{-3} \text{ km}$

$1 \text{ km} = 0.621 \text{ mi}$

$1 \text{ in} = 2.54 \text{ cm} = 0.254 \text{ m}$

Volume

$1 \text{ US gal} = 0.133\,68 \text{ foot}^3 = 3.785\,541 \text{ liters}$

$1 \text{ Imp gal} = 4.546\,092 \text{ liters}$

$1 \text{ m}^3 = 1000 \text{ liters}$

$1 \text{ ml} = 1 \text{ cm}^3$

Mass

$1 \text{ kg} = 1000 \text{ g} = 2.2046 \text{ lbm} = 0.068\,521 \text{ slugs}$

$1 \text{ lbm} = 0.453\,592 \text{ kg}$

$1 \text{ slug} = 1 \text{ lbf} \times \text{s}^2/\text{foot} = 32.174 \text{ lbm}$

Force

$1 \text{ lbf} = 4.448\,222 \text{ N} = 4.448 \times 10^5 \text{ dynes}$

$1 \text{ N} = 1 \text{ kg} \times \text{m/s}^2 = 10,000 \text{ dynes} = 10\,000 \text{ g} \times \text{cm/s}^2$

Pressure

$1 \text{ N/m}^2 = 10 \text{ dynes/cm}^2 = 1 \text{ Pa} = 0.007\,501 \text{ mm Hg}$

$1 \text{ atmosphere} = 1013.25 \text{ millibars} = 760 \text{ mm Hg} = 101\,325 \text{ Pa} = 14.696 \text{ lbf/in}^2$

$1 \text{ cm H}_2\text{O} = 0.735 \text{ mm Hg}$

$1 \text{ lbf/in}^2 = 51.71 \text{ mm Hg}$

$1 \text{ dyne/cm}^2 = 0.1 \text{ Pa} = 145.04 \times 10^{-7} \text{ lbf/in}^2$

$1 \text{ bar} = 10^5 \text{ N/m}^2 = 14.504 \text{ lbf/in}^2 = 10^6 \text{ dynes/cm}^2$

Viscosity

$1 \ kg/(m \times s) = 1 \ N \times s/m^2 = 0.6729 \ lbm/(foot \times s) = 10 \ poise$

Energy

$1 \ joule \ (J) = 1 \ kg \times m^2/s^2$

$1 \ Btu = 778.16 \ foot \times lbf = 1055.056 \ J = 252 \ cal = 1.055 \times 10^{10} \ ergs$

$1 \ cal = 4.1868 \ J$

Power

$1 \ watt \ (W) = 1 \ kg \times m^2/s^3 = 1 \ J/s$

$1 \ hp = 550 \ foot \times lbf/s = 745.699 \ W$

REFERENCES

1. Mahan BM, Myers RJ: *University chemistry,* ed 4, Don Mills, Ontario, 1987, Benjamin/Cummings.
2. Hill DW: Physics applied to anaesthesia. VI. gases and vapours, *Brit J Anaesth* 38(2):753, 1966.
3. Reynolds WC, Perkins HC: *Engineering thermodynamics,* ed 2, New York, 1977, McGraw-Hill.
4. Weast RC, editor: *CRC handbook of chemistry and physics: student edition,* Boca Raton, Fla, 1988, CRC Press.
5. Boltz RE, Tuve GL, editors: *CRC handbook of tables for applied engineering science: second edition,* Cleveland, Ohio, 1973, CRC Press.
6. Askeland DR: *The science and engineering of materials,* ed 2, Boston, Mass, 1989, PWS-Kent.
7. Streeter VL, Wylie EB: *Fluid mechanics,* ed 8, New York, 1985, McGraw-Hill.
8. White FM: *Fluid mechanics,* ed 2, New York, 1986, McGraw Hill.
9. Zuck D: Osborne Reynolds, 1842-1912, and the flow of fluids through tubes, *Brit J Anaesth* 43:1175, 1971.
10. Sherwood L: *Human physiology: from cells to systems,* ed 2, St Paul, Minn, 1993, West Publishing.
11. Benumof JL, Scheller MS: The importance of transtracheal jet ventilation in the management of the difficult airway, *Anesthesiology* 71:769, 1989.
12. Meyer PD: Emergency transtracheal jet ventilation, *Anesthesiology* 73:787, 1990.
13. Sprague DH: Transtracheal jet oxygenator from capnographic monitoring components, *Anesthesiology* 73:788, 1990.
14. Delaney WA, Kaiser RE: Percutaneous transtracheal jet ventilation made easy, *Anesthesiology* 74:952, 1991.
15. Doyle DJ, Zawacki J: Importance of catheter resistance in transtracheal jet ventilation, *Can J Anaesth* 40(5II):A37, 1993.
16. Rudow M, Hill AB, Thompson NW et al: Helium-oxygen mixtures in airway obstruction due to thyroid carcinoma, *Canadian Anaesthesia Society Journal* 33:498, 1986.
17. Lu TS, Ohmura A, Wong KC et al: Helium-oxygen in treatment of upper airway obstruction, *Anesthesiology* 45:678, 1976.
18. Duncan PG: Efficacy of helium-oxygen mixtures in the management of severe viral and postintubation croup, *Canadian Anaesthesia Society Journal* 26:206, 1979.
19. Skyrinskas GJ, Hyland RH, Hutcheon MA: Using helium-oxygen mixtures in the management of acute upper airway obstruction, *Can Med Assoc J* 128:555, 1983.
20. Kemper KJ, Ritz RH et al: Helium-oxygen mixture in the treatment of postextubation stridor in pediatric trauma patients, *Crit Care Med* 19(3):356, 1991.
21. Gottfried SP, Emili JM: Noninvasive monitoring of respiratory mechanics. In Nochomovitz ML, Cherniac NS, editors: *Noninvasive respiratory monitoring,* New York, 1986, Churchill Livingstone.
22. Ferris BG, Mead J, Opie LH: Partitioning of respiratory flow resistance in man, *J Appl Physiol* 19:653, 1964.
23. Boretos JW, Battig CG, Goodman L: Decreased resistance to breathing through a polyurethane pediatric endotracheal tube, *Anesthesia and Analgesia* 51(2):292, 1972.
24. Weissman C, Askanazi J, Rosenbaum SH et al: Response to tubular airway resistance in normal subjects and postoperative patients, *Anesthesiology* 64:353, 1986.
25. Wall MA: Infant endotracheal tube resistance: effects of changing length, diameter, and gas density, *Crit Care Med* 8(1):38, 1980.
26. Gal TJ: Pulmonary mechanics in normal subjects following endotracheal intubation, *Anesthesiology* 52:27, 1980.
27. Nadel JA: Mechanisms controlling airway size, *Arch Environ Health* 7:179, 1963.
28. Hingorani BK: The resistance to airflow of tracheostomy tubes, connections and heat and moisture exchangers, *Brit J Anaesth* 37:454, 1965.
29. Heinonen J, Poppius H: The resistance to airflow caused by heat and moisture exchanger and by artificial airways, *Annales Chirurgiae et Gynaecologiae Fenniae* 58:32, 1969.
30. Aalto-Setala M, Heinonen J: Resistance to gas-flow of endobronchial tubes, *Annales Chirurgiae et Gynaecologiae Fenniae* 62:271, 1973.
31. Holst M, Striem J, Hedenstierna G: Errors in tracheal pressure recording in patients with a tracheostomy tube: a model study, *Intensive Care Med* 16:384, 1990.
32. Michels A, Landser FJ, Cauberghs M et al: Measurement of total respiratory impedence via the endotracheal tube: a model study, *Bull Eur Physiopathol Respir* 22:615, 1986.
33. Gaensler EA, Maloney JV, Bjork VO: Bronchospirometry. II. Experimental observations and theoretical considerations of resistance breathing, *J Lab Clin Med* 39:935, 1952.
34. Wright PE, Marini JJ, Bernard GR: In vitro versus in vivo comparison of endotracheal tube airflow resistance, *Am Rev Respir Dis* 140:10, 1989.
35. Gal TJ, Suratt PM: Resistance to breathing in healthy subjects following endotracheal intubation under topical anesthesia, *Anesth Analg* 59:270, 1980.
36. Hicks GH: Monitoring respiratory mechanics, *Problems in Respiratory Care* 2(2):191, 1989.
37. Petros AJ, Lamond CT, Bennett D: The Bicore pulmonary monitor: a device to assess the work of breathing while weaning from mechanical ventilation, *Anaesthesia* 48(11):985, 1993.
38. Mullins JB, Templer JW, Kong J et al: Airway resistance and work of breathing in tracheostomy tubes, *Laryngoscope* 103(12):1367, 1993.
39. Ooi R, Fawcett WJ, Soni N et al: Extra inspiratory work of breathing imposed by cricothyrotomy devices, *Br J Anaesth* 70(1):17, 1993; 70(4):494, 1993 (errata).
40. Fawcett WJ, Ooi R, Riley B: The work of breathing through large-bore intravascular catheters, *Anesthesiology* 76(2):323, 1992.
41. Beatty PC, Healy TE: The additional work of breathing through Portex Polar Blue-Line preformed paediatric tracheal tubes, *Eur J Anaesthesiol* 9(1):77, 1992.
42. Shikora SA, Bistrian BR, Borlase BC et al: Work of breathing: reliable predictor of weaning and extubation, *Crit Care Med* 18(2):157, 1990.
43. Bolder PM, Healy TEJ et al: The extra work of breathing through adult endotracheal tubes, *Anesth Analg* 65:853, 1986.
44. Hill DW: *Physics applied to anaesthesia,* ed 3, London, England, 1976, Butterworths.
45. Zin WA, Pengelly LD, Millic-Emili J: Single breath method for measurement of respiratory mechanics in anaesthetized animals, *J Appl Physiol* 52:1266, 1982.

46. Murray JF: *The normal lung: the basis for diagnosis and treatment of pulmonary disease,* ed 2, Philadelphia, 1986, WB Saunders.

47. Lough MD, Chathurn R, Schrock WA: In Medical Publishers: *Handbook of respiratory care,* Chicago, 1983, Year Book.

48. James MFM, White JF: Anesthetic considerations at moderate altitude, *Anesth Analg* 63:1097, 1984.

49. Doyle DJ: Arterial/alveolar oxygen tension ratio: a critical appraisal, *Can Anaesth Soc J* 33:471, 1986.

50. Viale JP, Carlisle CJ, Annat G et al: Arterial-alveolar oxygen partial pressure ratio: a theoretical reappraisal, *Crit Care Med* 14:153, 1986.

51. Torda TA: Alveolar-arterial oxygen tension difference: a critical look, *Anaesth Intensive Care* 9:326, 1981.

52. Kelman GR, Nunn JF, Prys-Roberts C: The influence of cardiac output on arterial oxygenation: a theoretical study, *Br J Anesth* 39:450, 1967.

53. Pappenheimer JR, Comroe JH, Cournand A et al: Standardization of definitions and symbols in respiratory physiology, *Fed Proc* 34:315, 1950.

54. Jones N: *Blood gases and acid-base physiology,* New York, 1980, Thieme-Stratton.

55. Kelman RG: Digital computer subroutine for the conversion of oxygen tension into saturation, *J Appl Physiol* 21:1375, 1966.

56. Lobdell DD: An invertible simple equation for computation of blood O_2 dissociation relations, *J Appl Physiol: Respirat Environ Exercise Physiol* 50:971-973, 1981.

57. Severinghaus JW: Simple accurate equation for human blood O_2 dissociation computations, *J Appl Physiol: Respirat Environ Exercise Physiol* 46:599, 1979.

58. Aberman A, Cavanilles JM, Trotter J et al: An equation for the oxygen-hemoglobin dissociation curve, *J Appl Physiol* 35:750, 1973.

59. Schnider AJ, Stockman JA, Oski FA: Transfusion nomogram: an application of physiology to clinical decisions regarding the use of blood, *Crit Care Med* 9:469, 1981.

60. Miller AR: TK solver, *Byte,* 9:263, Dec 1984.

61. Rodgers E: TK Solver: a new concept in problem solving software, *PC World* 1(4):93, 1983.

62. Zachmann M: The versatile variables of TK Solver, *PC Magazine* 2(4):489, Sept, 1983.

63. Konopasek M, Jayaraman S: Constant and declarative languages for engineering applications: the TK Solver contribution, *Proceedings of the IEEE* 73:1791, 1985.

64. Konopasek M, Jayaraman S: *The TK Solver book: a guide to problem-solving in science, engineering, business and education,* Berkeley, Calif, 1984, Osborne/McGraw-Hill.

65. Farhi LE, Rahn HA: A theoretical analysis of the alveolar-arterial O_2 difference with special reference to the distribution effect, *J Appl Physiol* 7:699, 1955.

66. Kanber GJ, King FW, Eschar YR et al: The alveolar-arterial oxygen gradient in young and elderly men during air and oxygen breathing, *Am Rev Respir Dis* 97:376, 1968.

67. Shapiro AR, Virgilio RW, Peters RM: Interpretation of alveolar-arterial oxygen tension difference, *Surg Gynecol Obstet* 144:547, 1977.

68. Gilbert R, Keighley JF: The arterial/alveolar oxygen tension ratio: an index of gas exchange applicable to varying inspired oxygen concentrations, *Am Rev Respir Dis* 109:142, 1974.

69. Gilbert R, Auchincloss JH, Kuppinger M et al: Stability of the arterial/alveolar oxygen partial pressure ratio: effects of low ventilation/perfusion regions, *Crit Care Med* 7:267, 1979.

70. Perez LV, Boix JH, Salom JV et al: Clinical use of the arterial/alveolar oxygen tension ratio, *Crit Care Med* 11:999, 1983.

71. Goldfarb MA, Ciurej TF, McAslan TC et al: Tracking respiratory therapy in the trauma patient, *Am J Surg* 129:255, 1975.

72. Hegyi T, Hiatt IM: Respiratory index: a simple evaluation of severity of idiopathic respiratory distress syndrome, *Crit Care Med* 7:500, 1979.

73. Covell HD, Nessan VJ, Tuttle WK: Oxygen derived variables in acute respiratory failure, *Crit Care Med* 11:646, 1983.

74. Herrick IA, Champion LK, Froese AB: A clinical comparison of indices of pulmonary gas exchange with changes in the inspired oxygen concentration, *Can J Anaesth* 37:69, 1990.

75. Rasanen J, Downs JB, Malec DJ et al: Oxygen tensions and oxyhemoglobin saturations in the assessment of pulmonary gas exchange, *Crit Care Med* 15:1058, 1987.

76. Zetterstrom H: Assessment of the efficiency of pulmonary oxygenation: the choice of oxygenation index, *Acta Anaesthesiol Scand* 32:579, 1988.

77. Torrance J, Jacobs P, Restrepo A et al: Intraerythrocytic adaptation to anemia, *New Engl J Med* 283:165, 1970.

78. Eaton JW, Skelton TD, Berger E: Survival at extreme altitude: protective effect of increased hemoglobin-oxygen affinity, *Science* 183:743, 1974.

79. Monge C, Wittembury J: Increased hemoglobin-oxygen affinity at extremely high altitudes, *Science* 186:843, 1974.

80. Morpurgo G, Arese P, Bosia A et al: Sherpas living permanently at high altitude: a new pattern of adaptation, *Proc Natl Acad Sci U S A* 73:747, 1976.

81. Hebbel RP, Eaton JW, Kronenberg RS et al: Human llamas: adaptation to altitude in subjects with high hemoglobin oxygen affinity, *J Clin Invest* 62:593, 1978.

82. Zapol W, Snider MT, Hill JD et al: Extracorporeal membrane oxygenation in severe acute respiratory failure: a randomized prospective study, *JAMA* 242:2193, 1979.

Chapter 4

AIRWAY PHARMACOLOGY

David O. Warner

I. INTRODUCTION

Many drugs can affect airway function. Agents such as bronchodilators may be administered specifically to produce therapeutic effects on the airways. Other drugs, primarily targeted to other organ systems, may also affect the airways. For example, many general anesthetic agents profoundly depress the function of the striated muscles of the upper airway, requiring that much of modern anesthetic practice be directed toward maintaining airway patency. Numerous drugs used in anesthetic practice may also affect the smooth muscle of the lower airway. Thus, an understanding of the pharmacology of drugs with effects on the airways is critical to optimal airway management and the safe conduct of anesthesia.

This chapter will review the pharmacology of drugs commonly administered in the perioperative period that may affect the airways. Both the upper airway (from nares to glottis) and the lower airway (from glottis to terminal bronchiole) will be considered.

II. UPPER AIRWAY
A. CLINICAL CONCERNS

Two aspects of upper airway function are of primary clinical concern. First, the coordinated activity of the striated muscles of the upper airway is critical to maintaining airway patency. Sedation and anesthesia interfere with this activity to an extent that may compromise the integrity of the upper airway. Second, artificial support of the upper airway, such as that provided by an endotracheal tube, is often required to manage this problem. It is often necessary to provide topical anesthesia of the upper airway to permit such instrumentation.

B. PHARMACOLOGIC EFFECTS ON THE FUNCTION OF UPPER AIRWAY MUSCLES

1. Physiology of the upper airway

The patency of the upper airway is controlled by a complex arrangement of muscles.[1,2] Gas enters and exits the airways either via the mouth or the nose, as controlled by the muscles of the soft palate. An intricate system of pharyngeal constrictors and muscles that insert on the tongue and hyoid bone regulate pharyngeal caliber, allowing the pharynx to serve multiple functions, including the conduct of respiratory gases, deglutition, and speech. The position and caliber of the larynx is controlled by muscles both intrinsic and extrinsic to the laryngeal cartilages.

During breathing, activity in several upper airway muscles is crucial to maintain upper airway patency. Many upper airway muscles that surround the pharynx demonstrate phasic activity during inspiration. These muscles include the genioglossus, stylopharyngeus, and styloglossus muscles.[3] All of them help maintain pharyngeal patency during the negative upper airway pressures generated by inspiratory flow. In the absence of their activity, even modest negative upper airway pressures can markedly narrow the upper airway of normal subjects (Fig. 4-1).[4]

Laryngeal muscles are also important in the maintenance of airway patency during breathing. The glottis widens during inspiration and narrows during expiration in human subjects, primarily due to phasic activation of the posterior cricoarytenoid muscle, a vocal cord

abductor.[5-8] This activity decreases during expiration; the resulting glottic narrowing may serve to retard and control expiratory flow.[6,9] Phasic expiratory activity in vocal cord adductors such as the thyroarytenoids also controls expiratory flow.[10] Other laryngeal muscles, such as the cricothyroid muscle, may also demonstrate respiratory activity.[11] Although the interaction among these muscles is not fully understood, it is likely that the coordinated activity of all these muscles is necessary to maintain normal upper airway caliber.

There are two characteristics that distinguish the control of upper airway muscles (Fig. 4-2). First, afferent information plays an important role in the control of these muscles. Receptors in both the lung and the walls of the upper airway provide the bulk of this sensory information. These receptors, which respond to changes in airway pressure and a variety of mechanical and chemical stimuli (including volatile anesthetics),[12] play an important role in modulating the activities of upper airway muscles. They mediate reflex closure of the glottis, involving contraction of multiple upper airway muscles, which serves an important protective function to prevent aspiration of material into the lungs.[13,14] Second, the activity of upper airway muscles is very dependent on the state of arousal.[15] The most familiar example of this dependence is the increase in upper airway resistance that accompanies natural sleep,

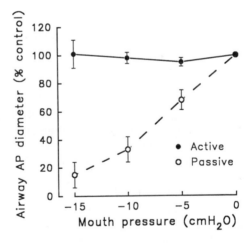

Fig. 4-1. Anterior-posterior *(AP)* diameter of upper airway of six human subjects during negative mouth pressure generated by inspiring against an externally occluded airway ("active" upper airway muscles) or external suction at the mouth during voluntary glottic closure with no inspiratory effort ("passive" upper airway muscles). Note that active muscles are required to prevent airway narrowing during negative mouth pressures, such as those generated by inspiratory effort. This data demonstrates that upper airway muscle activity is crucial to maintenance of upper airway patency. Values are mean ± SE. (Modified from Wheatley JR, et al: *J Appl Physiol* 70:2242, 1991.)

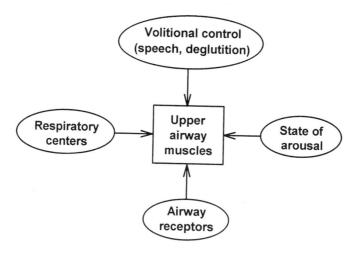

Fig. 4-2. Influences modulating activity of upper airway muscles.

which often produces an audible manifestation (snoring).[16]

2. Effects of anesthesia and sedation

In most experimental animal preparations, anesthesia and sedation depress the activity of upper airway muscles.[12,17-20] Several reports have documented that the sensitivity of upper airway muscles to anesthetic-induced depression differs from that of other respiratory muscles, such as the diaphragm.[12,18-20] Halothane, enflurane, diazepam, and thiopental all produce a greater depression of hypoglossal nerve activity compared with phrenic nerve activity in paralyzed, ventilated, vagotomized cats.[12,19] Measurements of respiratory muscle activity in intact anesthetized cats breathing spontaneously show similar results; electromyogram activity in the diaphragm is more resistant to depression by halothane compared with the genioglossus muscle (Fig. 4-3).[20] This differential suppression may be less pronounced after ketamine administration,[18,19,21] suggesting that it is not a property common to all general anesthetics. Other reports also have noted an apparent preservation of upper airway motoneuron activities in animals anesthetized with ketamine.[17,21] This observation is consistent with the clinical impression that upper airway patency is better preserved with ketamine anesthesia, although firm experimental evidence to support this assertion is lacking.

Because the activity of upper airway motoneurons is highly dependent on inputs from the reticular activating system (Fig. 4-2), it is possible that the sensitivity of this activity to anesthetics is related to anesthetic-induced depression of the reticular activating system. In other words, anesthetic effects may be mediated, not only by a direct effect on motoneurons, but indirectly via changes in the state of arousal. Consistent with this idea, some of the changes in upper airway activity caused by anesthesia mimic those seen during some stages of natural sleep, although there are also important differences that depend on sleep state.[16]

Alterations in airway reflexes that normally protect the laryngeal inlet may also affect perioperative upper airway function. These reflexes are impaired by many anesthetic drugs,[22,23] including the benzodiazapines.[22,24] The mechanism of this depression is unknown. Paradoxically, reflex irritability apparently is increased during some stages of anesthesia and may produce laryngospasm; this phenomenon, though clinically significant, is poorly understood.[13,14] This reflex irritability requires that great care be exercised to minimize airway stimulation during the induction and emergence of anesthesia. Of interest, the inhalation of volatile anesthetics, especially the ethers, may initially stimulate airway receptors, leading to coughing, alterations in respiratory pattern, and cardiovascular stimulation.[12,25,26] This reflex irritability significantly limits the use of agents such as desflurane and isoflurane as inhalation induction agents.[27] Another ether, sevoflurane, is apparently less irritating and is more suitable for this purpose.[26,28]

How changes in the activity of upper airway muscles produced by anesthesia and sedation may influence upper airway caliber is uncertain. Based on early studies in human subjects, it is often assumed that anesthesia and sedation cause a posterior displacement of the tongue that produces airway obstruction at an oropharyngeal level.[29,30] However, a more recent study using ultrasonography could not confirm this finding.[31] In the absence of airflow, the most consistent site of obstruction is at the nasopharyngeal level, where the soft palate

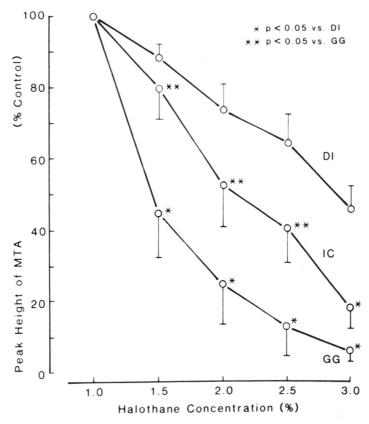

Fig. 4-3. Phasic inspiratory muscle activity, expressed as peak height of a moving time average *(MTA)* value of the electromyogram, during halothane anesthesia in cats. Note that the genioglossus *(GG)*, an upper airway muscle, is most sensitive to anesthetic-induced depression, followed by the internal intercostal muscle *(IC,* a muscle of the rib cage), and the diaphragm *(DI)*. Values are mean ± SEM. (From Ochiai R, Guthrie RD, Motoyama EK: *Anesthesiology* 70:812, 1989.)

becomes approximated to the posterior pharynx (Fig. 4-4).[32] This site is also prone to obstruction in patients with obstructive sleep apnea.[33,34] The epiglottis and supralaryngeal tissues may also participate in upper airway narrowing.[35] Under these conditions, efforts by the diaphragm and other respiratory muscles of the chest wall actually encourage upper airway collapse. These inspiratory efforts decrease airway pressures and produce narrowing at multiple levels, including the base of the tongue.[32]

There is not a consistent relationship between phasic electromyogram activity of upper airway muscles and upper airway resistance. Drummond found that thiopental produced alterations in the amount and pattern of activity in neck and tongue muscles measured with surface electrodes in human subjects.[36] However, reductions in activity could not be related directly to the onset of airway obstruction; rather, activity was often increased, presumably in an attempt to overcome partial obstruction. Also, although benzodiazepines appear to increase upper airway resistance in human subjects,[37]

they decrease genioglossus activity only in older,[38] not in younger, subjects. Thus airway obstruction may not be caused by a simple diminution of activity but by disruption of the normal coordination of activity of muscles controlling different segments of the airways.[39]

It is possible that anesthetics could produce tonic activity in upper airway constrictors, which would explain the clinical observation that pharmacologic paralysis frequently decreases upper airway resistance following induction of anesthesia with thiopental. Factors not directly involving the upper airway muscles may also affect upper airway resistance during anesthesia. For example, the position of the head and neck may change as normal postural muscle tone decreases with the onset of anesthesia. Decreases in the functional residual capacity (FRC) produced by anesthesia may also increase upper airway resistance.[40]

3. Effects of neuromuscular blockade

Drugs that block the neuromuscular junction are frequently used in clinical practice to inhibit respiratory

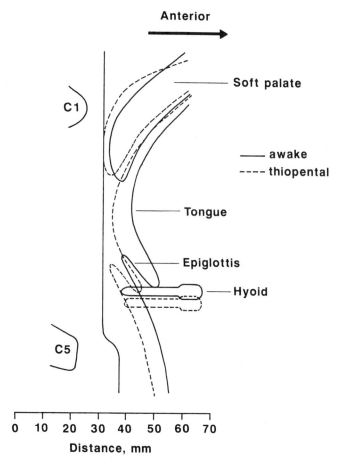

Anterior

C1

Soft palate

— awake
--- thiopental

Tongue

Epiglottis

Hyoid

C5

0 10 20 30 40 50 60 70

Distance, mm

Fig. 4-4. Effect of thiopental anesthesia on airway dimensions. Note that primary site of obstruction is at level of soft palate. (Modified from Nandi PR, et al: *Br J Anaesth* 66:157, 1991.)

muscle function, both to facilitate endotracheal intubation and to eliminate respiratory efforts during mechanical ventilation. These drugs may affect the respiratory muscles differently than other skeletal muscles. This observation becomes clinically relevant during partial neuromuscular blockade with nondepolarizing agents, a situation frequently encountered in the postanesthesia recovery area.

Greater doses of vecuronium,[41-43] atracurium,[41] and pancuronium[44] are required to achieve a given degree of neuromuscular block in the diaphragm compared to the adductor pollicis, although the onset of block is more rapid in the diaphragm. This relative sparing of the diaphragm permits the maintenance of respiratory effort even during complete paralysis of peripheral muscles (Fig. 4-5).[45,46] The adductor muscles of the larynx may be even more resistant to the effects of nondepolarizing drugs than the diaphragm.[47] However, other upper airway muscles may not behave similarly. The susceptibility of the masseter to block appears to be equal to or greater than that of the adductor pollicis. The mechanisms responsible for this differential sensitivity are unknown. Nevertheless, it is apparent that upper airway

patency may be compromised at levels of paralysis that otherwise permit maintenance of normal ventilation (Fig. 4-5).[48]

This differential sensitivity may assume great clinical importance in the postoperative period. If residual neuromuscular blockade is present, the patient with an endotracheal tube or other airway support in place may be able to maintain adequate ventilation. However, once the endotracheal tube is removed, upper airway obstruction may develop. For this reason, adequacy of the reversal of neuromuscular blockade must always be assured before removal of artificial airway support.

4. Effects of hypoxia and hypercarbia

Like the diaphragm and other chest wall muscles, the upper airway muscles also respond to the stresses of hypoxia and hypercarbia.[49] In humans, the inspiratory activity of the upper airway muscles initially increases with both hypoxia and hypercarbia, presumably to maintain airway patency during concurrent increases in minute ventilation.[50] However, these increases cannot be sustained during prolonged hypoxia,[51,52] and airway patency may be compromised.

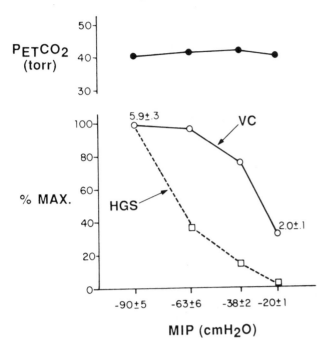

Fig. 4-5. Hand grip strength *(HGS)*, vital capacity *(VC,* with absolute values noted at extremes of measurement), and end-tidal carbon dioxide *($P_{ET}CO_2$)* as a function of maximum inspiratory pressure *(MIP)* developed at the mouth during maximum inspiration against an occluded airway at rest and during increasing degrees of paralysis with d-tubocurare in human subjects. Mandibular elevation was necessary at MIP $\geq -39 \pm 5$ cmH$_2$O to prevent upper airway obstruction. This study demonstrates that ventilation can be maintained by the diaphragm at levels of neuromuscular blockade that cause upper airway collapse. (From Pavlin EG, Holle RH, Schoene RB: *Anesthesiology* 70:381, 1989.)

C. PHARMACOLOGIC EFFECTS OF LOCAL ANESTHETICS ON SENSORY FUNCTION

The upper airway is richly endowed with sensory nerves that normally serve as the afferent limbs of powerful reflexes that protect the airways from the aspiration of foreign material. To instrument the upper airway, this sensory function must be attenuated. This topic is also covered in Chapter 9; here we briefly review the pharmacology of local anesthetics commonly used to provide topical airway anesthesia.

1. Agents

Local anesthetics reversibly block nerve conduction, disrupting the propagation of action potentials by binding to sodium channels and interfering with their function.[53] Chemically, local anesthetics usually consist of a lipophilic group connected to an ionizable group (usually a tertiary amine) by either an ester or amide link (Fig. 4-6).[54]

They are weak bases and are usually formulated as salts. Local anesthetics are metabolized in the liver (amides) or plasma (esters) to water-soluble metabolites

and excreted in the urine. Adequate drug diffusion through mucous membranes to the sensory nerves is necessary for topical efficacy. Almost every local anesthetic agent has some effects when applied to the mucous membranes of the upper airways, although some are too irritating or toxic for this use.

Lidocaine remains the prototypic agent for topical use. Available formulations for upper airway use include a 2% viscous gel and solutions ranging in concentration from 2% to 10%. There are few data concerning any dose-response relationship for intensity or duration of anesthesia within this range of concentration. The duration of action is quite variable, ranging from approximately 10 to 30 minutes.

Benzocaine is poorly soluble in water and thus is poorly absorbed into the systemic circulation. It is available in 20% solution for topical use. Chemically, it differs from most other local anesthetics in that it is an ester of paraaminobenzoic acid that lacks a terminal amino group (Fig. 4-6). The duration of action is from approximately 10 to 30 minutes.

Bupivicaine has been used for topical airway anesthesia in concentrations ranging from 1% to 4%. In animal models, these concentrations provide durations of anesthesia that exceed that provided by lidocaine (up to 75 min).[55] However, the potential for toxicity from systemic absorption engenders limited enthusiasm for this application.

Sodium benzonatate is a nonopioid antitussive that is a long-chain polyglycol derivative of procaine. When applied orally, it provides rapid topical anesthesia suitable for awake oral intubation.[56]

Cocaine, in solutions from 1% to 10%, provides excellent topical anesthesia. It has the advantage of providing vasoconstriction due to its sympathomimetic actions, which may be useful in preventing epistaxis during nasotracheal intubation. However, its potential to be abused limits its clinical use.

2. Systemic absorption and toxicity

Varying amounts of local anesthetic are absorbed into the systemic circulation when topically applied. Most reports show that systemic absorption of topically applied lidocaine is limited. Chinn et al.[57] found plasma lidocaine levels of 0.44 µg/ml after inhalation of 400 mg of nebulized lidocaine. Similarly, Baughman et al.[58] found that patients breathing 4 mg/kg of aerosolized lidocaine developed plasma levels of less than 0.5 µg/ml. Oral lidocaine produces even lower plasma levels,[59] probably because much of the dose is swallowed and subjected to first-pass metabolism by the liver. Lidocaine applied directly to the trachea and bronchi results in higher plasma levels. Viegus and Stoelting[60] found plasma levels of 1.7 µg/ml 9 minutes following tracheal installation of 2 mg/kg lidocaine; similar results have

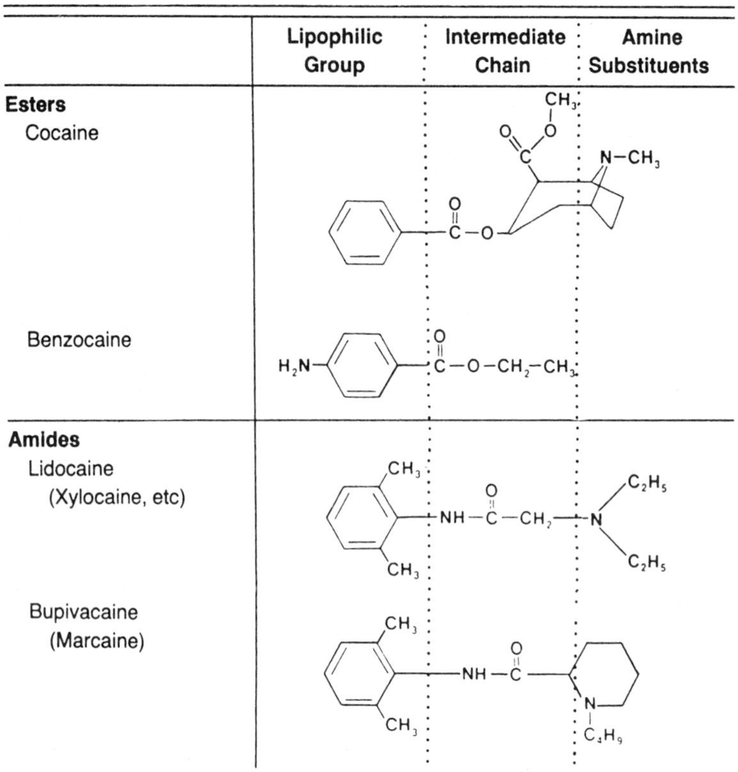

	Lipophilic Group	Intermediate Chain	Amine Substituents
Esters			
Cocaine			
Benzocaine			
Amides			
Lidocaine (Xylocaine, etc)			
Bupivacaine (Marcaine)			

Fig. 4-6. Structure of local anesthetics used for topical airway anesthesia.

been reported by others.[61,62] Sutherland and Williams[63] used a standardized topical anesthesia protocol for awake fiberoptic intubation, combining 4% lidocaine aerosol, topical 2% viscous lidocaine gel, and direct installation of lidocaine via the bronchoscope. Despite a large total dose of lidocaine (5.3 ± 2.1 mg/kg), the mean peak arterial plasma lidocaine concentration was low (0.6 ± 2.1 µg/ml). All of these levels are well below the reported toxic range for lidocaine (> 5 to 6 µg/ml), so that the administration of doses less than the commonly cited limit for parenteral administration of lidocaine (4 mg/ml) should be associated with minimal risk of toxicity.

Prominent toxic reactions related to systemic absorption involve the central nervous system, ranging from irritability to convulsions, and the cardiovascular system, leading in the extreme to cardiovascular collapse. Allergic reactions to amide local anesthetics are extremely rare. Ester agents are metabolized to ρ-aminobenzoic acid derivatives, which may produce hypersensitivity reactions in some patients. Absorbed benzocaine may produce methemoglobinemia[64,65]; because absorption is variable, the threshold dose needed to produce this complication is unclear. Methemoglobinemia is detectable by pulse oximetry, although its magnitude may be underestimated.[66,67] Treatment includes supplemental oxygen and intravenous methylene

blue. Benzocaine should probably be avoided in infants and in patients with anemia or other disorders in which oxygen transport may be impaired.[68]

3. Effects of topical anesthesia on upper airway patency

Topical anesthesia may also affect upper airway patency because upper airway reflex mechanisms play an important role in its maintenance. Topical anesthesia of the upper airway can produce airway obstruction in both normal subjects[69] and subjects with obstructive sleep apnea.[70] Furthermore, instrumentation of the upper airway is often facilitated by the use of sedatives, such as benzodiazepines, which themselves may depress upper airway muscle function. Thus, airway patency must be carefully monitored until an artificial airway is secured or until the effects of local anesthesia and sedation have dissipated.

III. LOWER AIRWAYS
A. CLINICAL CONCERNS

Although the physiologic function of airway smooth muscle remains obscure, there is no doubt that its constriction can produce serious morbidity in the perioperative period. Airway instrumentation during perioperative airway management is a potent stimulus for reflex bronchoconstriction. Other interventions, such as the administration of drugs that may release histamine or other inflammatory mediators, may also trigger bronchospasm. Patients with diseases characterized by heightened airway reactivity, such as asthma and some forms of chronic obstructive pulmonary disease, are thought to be at particular risk to develop perioperative bronchoconstriction.[71] Asthma is one of the most common chronic diseases, affecting over 10 million Americans, and its incidence continues to increase.[72] Thus, proper management of drugs affecting lower airway function will continue to be an important factor in perioperative airway management. It is also important to realize that many instances of perioperative bronchospasm occur in patients without any history of heightened airway reactivity.[73-75] Principal concerns include optimization of preoperative therapy for patients with hyperreactive airways and the prevention and treatment of intraoperative and postoperative bronchospasm. Achievement of these goals requires a thorough understanding of the pharmacology of drugs with primary actions on the lower airways. This section will review the clinical pharmacology of each class of agents, then discuss their rational use in perioperative airway management.

B. DRUGS THAT ATTENUATE THE INFLAMMATORY RESPONSE

Until recently, asthma and other diseases characterized by heightened airway reactivity were regarded as manifestations of abnormalities of airway smooth muscle. However, current understanding regards asthma as a chronic inflammatory disease of the airways.[76,77] This inflammation causes symptoms of reversible airway obstruction, as inflammatory mediators constrict airway smooth muscle (Fig. 4-7). Furthermore, chronic inflammation thickens the airway wall, narrowing the airway and amplifying the effects of smooth muscle shortening. The appreciation of the importance of inflammation to the pathogenesis of asthma has shifted the emphasis of therapeutic strategies from bronchodilators per se, which act directly to relax smooth muscle, to drugs that ameliorate the inflammatory response.

1. Cromolyn sodium and nedocromil

a. MECHANISM OF ACTION

Cromolyn sodium (disodium cromoglycate) and nedocromil prevent the release of inflammatory mediators from various cell types associated with asthma.[78-80] One effect of potential benefit is thought to be suppression of IgE-provoked mediator release from lung mast cells. These drugs may also have multiple other antiinflammatory actions, such as inhibition of the release of other mediators from several other types of inflammatory cells. Pretreatment with these agents inhibits

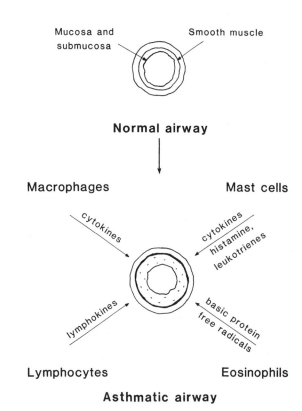

Fig. 4-7. Changes in cross-sectional anatomy of normal and asthmatic airways, with some of the inflammatory cell types and mediators that may be responsible for these changes. Note thickening of smooth muscle and submucosa, associated with infiltration of inflammatory cells.

bronchospasm produced by antigen and by exercise, concurrently attenuating the production of chemotactic factors associated with mast cell activation.

b. PHARMACOKINETICS AND TOXICITY

These drugs are poorly absorbed and are administered by inhalation of powdered drug via a metered-dose inhaler. Absorbed drug is not significantly metabolized and is excreted in urine and bile. Significant side effects or toxicity is rare and include oropharyngeal irritation or symptoms such as cough, caused by the direct irritant effect of the powder. Anaphylaxis is rare but has been reported.

c. CLINICAL USE

Because of their mechanism of action, these drugs are useful only in the prevention of bronchospasm, not in the treatment of established bronchospasm. They may be useful both as a single preventative treatment before exercise or exposure to antigens and as chronic therapy. Efficacy in individual patients varies widely, and, at present, a therapeutic trial is the only way of determining which patients will benefit. Although nedocromil is more potent in preventing some forms of acute bronchoconstriction in some studies, its efficacy in clinical use does not appear to differ sig-

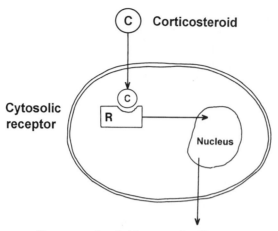

Fig. 4-8. Possible mechanisms of action of corticosteroids in asthma. Corticosteroids bind to cytosolic receptors, which are translated into the nucleus where they control gene expression and regulate activity of many cell types.

nificantly from that of cromolyn sodium.[80] Neither agent has been studied as an adjunct to airway management in the perioperative period.

2. Corticosteroids

a. MECHANISM OF ACTION

These drugs are the most effective antiinflammatory agents for the treatment of asthma.[77,81,82] The multiple possible sites of action in interrupting inflammation probably accounts for their usefulness in all forms of asthma. After binding to receptors within the cytoplasm, corticosteroids are translocated to the nucleus where they regulate the function of steroid-responsive genes (Fig. 4-8). This regulation may increase or decrease the formation of specific proteins.[83] In particular, corticosteroids may inhibit the formation of several cytokines that are important mediators of the inflammatory response; this effect may be most important on T lymphocytes.[84] This inhibition may lead to reductions in the numbers of mast cells[85] and decreases in neutrophil survival.[86] Corticosteroids may also reduce plasma exudation from pulmonary vessels[87] and inhibit the secretion of mucous glycoprotein.[88] As a result of these actions, corticosteroids reduce the immediate and late phase responses to allergens[89] and also reduce nonspecific airway reactivity when administered chronically.[77] Chronic administration improves airway wall inflammation assessed by bronchial biopsy.[90] Corticosteroids may also have actions in addition to direct effects on inflammation. For example, they increase the number of

Table 4-1. Aerosol corticosteroids

Generic	Brands	Dose per puff
Beclomethasone	Beclovent, Vanceril	42μg
Triamcinolone acetonide	Azmacort	100μg
Dexamethasone	Decadron Respihaler	84μg
Flunisolide	Aerobid	250μg

β-receptors and so may increase sensitivity to β_2-receptor agonists.[91]

b. PHARMACOKINETICS

Corticosteroids may be administered by oral, parenteral, or inhaled routes.[92] Oral absorption is rapid and complete. Parenteral administration may be necessary to administer high doses or if the patient cannot take oral medications. The use of inhaled corticosteroids represents a significant advance in asthma therapy, since high, local concentrations of steroids can be achieved in the airway while minimizing the side effects associated with systemic administration. These topical steroids have enhanced topical antiinflammatory potency (due to high affinity for glucocorticoid receptors), with low systemic potency (reflecting their rapid biotransformation in the liver into inactive metabolites).[93] Examples of these compounds include *beclomethasone dipropionate, triamcinolone acetonide, dexamethasone,* and *flunisolide* (Table 4-1). There is little evidence for clinically significant

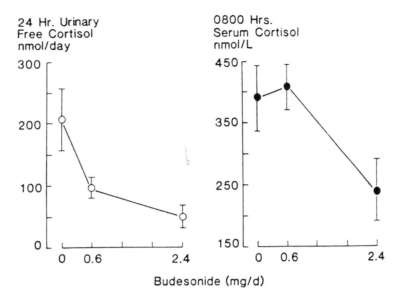

Fig. 4-9. Effect of budesonide, an inhaled corticosteroid, on cortisol production in 10 subjects. Evidence of adrenal suppression from systemic absorption of budesonide is seen in the most sensitive index of cortisol production (24-hour urinary free cortisol) even at relatively low doses of inhaled corticosteroid. (Adapted from Toogood JH, et al: *Am Rev Respir Dis* 138:57, 1988.)

differences in efficacy among the currently available agents. These agents are rapidly and extensively absorbed from the lung and the gut.[93] Drug absorbed from the gut is subject to first-pass hepatic metabolism and is largely inactivated.[94] However, that absorbed from the lung is active systemically.

Like endogenous cortisol, these compounds are significantly protein bound. They are removed from the circulation by the liver, where they are reduced and conjugated to form water-soluble compounds that are excreted into the urine.

c. ADVERSE EFFECTS

Prolonged use of systemic corticosteroids can produce weight gain, muscle wasting, growth retardation, cataracts, diabetes, osteoporosis, avascular necrosis of the hip, and other well-known side effects. In low doses, inhaled corticosteroids are usually free of such clinical effects. However, even low doses may cause detectable abnormalities in sensitive assays of hypothalamic-pituitary-adrenal axis function, such as 24-hour free urinary cortisol output (Fig. 4-9).[95] The clinical significance of these adrenal changes is uncertain. High-dose therapy produces more profound suppression of adrenal activity, with decreases in morning serum cortisol and peripheral eosinophil count.[95] The definition of "low" and "high" doses varies among agents. For most formulations, total daily doses less than 16 to 20 "puffs" of a metered-dose inhaler constitutes a low dose (e.g., approximately 600 to 800 μg/daily of beclomethasone). There is little evidence to support the need for preoperative systemic corticosteroid supplementation in the patient receiving low-dose inhaled corticosteroids.[96] Local effects of inhaled corticosteroids include oropharyngeal candidiasis and dysphonia.[97]

d. CLINICAL USE

Inhaled corticosteroids are often considered as first-line therapy for the chronic management of newly diagnosed asthma.[76,77] More severe asthma may require the chronic use of systemic corticosteroids. Oral doses equivalent to 60 mg of prednisone daily may be required, with dose decreased gradually as tolerated. High-dose inhaled corticosteroids (doses greater than the equivalent of 1 mg daily of beclomethasone) may also be effective in more severe asthma, with fewer systemic side effects. Systemic therapy is effective in the treatment of acute exacerbations of asthma, with parenteral administration sometimes required. No good dose-response data for the use of steroids in asthma exacerbations or status asthmaticus exists, but there is little evidence that doses greater than the equivalent of 60 mg prednisone every 6 hours confers additional benefit.[82] Several hours may be necessary for clinical benefit to occur after administration. If patients are switched from parenteral to inhaled corticosteroids, this transition must be made gradually to prevent symptoms of steroid withdrawal and severe asthma relapse.[93]

3. Methylxanthines

a. CHEMISTRY AND MECHANISM OF ACTION

Caffeine, theophylline, and *theobromine* are methylated xanthines and are found naturally. Their solubility is low and is enhanced by the formation of complexes with

> **BOX 4-1**   **Possible mechanisms of action of methylxanthines in cardiorespiratory disease**
>
> - Inhibition of phosphodiesterase
> - Antagonism of adenosine
> - Stimulation of endogenous catecholamine release
> - Antiinflammatory actions
> - Improved mucociliary clearance
> - Stimulation of ventilatory drive
> - Increased diaphragm contractility
> - Diuresis
> - Positive inotropy
> - Reductions in preload and afterload

other compounds. *Aminophylline* is a complex of theophylline and ethylenediamine. Other preparations, such as salts of theophylline (e.g., *oxytriphylline*) or covalently modified derivatives (e.g., *dyphylline*), also find clinical use.

Theophylline and other methylxanthines have multiple mechanisms of action, and the effect of primary importance remains controversial (Box 4-1).[98] Traditionally, theophylline was thought to work primarily by inhibiting phosphodiesterases that metabolize cyclic adenosine monophosphate (cAMP). This inhibition would increase intracellular cAMP, causing bronchodilation. However, the drug concentrations needed to demonstrate this effect in vitro exceed those present at therapeutic levels in vivo,[99] other phosphodiesterase inhibitors are not efficacious in asthma,[100] and theophylline-induced relaxation of airway smooth muscle in vitro occurs without changes in intracellular cAMP levels.[101] Inhibition of cyclic guanine monophosphate (cGMP) phosphodiesterase by theophylline, demonstrable in vitro,[102] also does not appear to contribute to clinical effects. Other mechanisms demonstrable in laboratory preparations, including antagonism of adenosine and stimulation of endogenous catecholamine release, also do not appear significant to the clinical action of theophylline.[103,104] Recent evidence supports an antiinflammatory role for theophylline in asthma.[98] Xanthines reduce the activity of many of the inflammatory cells implicated in the pathogenesis of asthma.[105] Theophylline increases the activity and numbers of suppressor T cells, which may play an important role in airway inflammation.[106] This indirect evidence awaits confirmation.

Some of the therapeutic actions of methylxanthines may be due to actions other than the relaxation of smooth muscle. These drugs may improve mucociliary clearance, stimulate ventilatory drive,[107] and increase diaphragm contractility,[108,109] actions that all may be beneficial in the patient with reactive airways disease. They also have significant cardiovascular effects, including direct positive chronotropic and inotropic effects on the heart, reductions in pre- and after-load, and diuresis,[110] which may be beneficial in patients with cardiovascular disease.

b. PHARMACOKINETICS

The methylxanthines are readily absorbed after oral administration. Aminophylline, containing 85% anhydrous theophylline by weight, is used for intravenous administration because of greater aqueous solubility.[111] Methylxanthines are eliminated primarily by hepatic metabolism.[112] The plasma clearance varies widely even among healthy subjects; the half-life ranges from approximately 3 hours in children to 8 hours in adults. The half-life may be prolonged in patients with hepatic disease or low cardiac output and may be reduced in smokers.

c. TOXICITY

Areas of primary concern include the central nervous system (CNS) and cardiovascular system. CNS effects include stimulation, insomnia, and tremor, leading to convulsions at toxic plasma levels (considered to be > 20 μg/ml). In the cardiovascular system, toxic levels may produce ventricular and atrial dysrhythmias. Methylxanthines may also produce gastrointestinal disturbances ranging from epigastric discomfort to nausea and vomiting.

d. CLINICAL USE

Given recent therapeutic advances in other drugs used in asthma, some have questioned the continued role of methylxanthines in the management of patients with reactive airways.[113] However, when properly used, these drugs remain safe and efficacious for the chronic management of asthma and some patients with chronic obstructive pulmonary disease.[114]

There is a multitude of methylxanthine preparations available for clinical use. Most vary the physical preparation of theophylline rather than chemically modify it. Several forms of anhydrous theophylline are available in microcrystalline form to enhance rapid and reliable absorption. Sustained release forms are also currently popular, providing dosing convenience and (perhaps) less fluctuation in blood levels. Regardless of the preparation chosen, plasma concentrations of theophylline should be monitored to ensure that levels are in the therapeutic range (approximately 5 to 20 μg/ml).

Aminophylline is usually given to patients requiring parenteral administration of methylxanthines. The initial loading dose is approximately 5 mg/kg, administered over 30 minutes to minimize toxicity. After this loading dose, an infusion of 0.7 mg/kg/hr provides therapeutic levels in most patients. This loading dose and rate may need to be increased in smokers and decreased in patients with liver disease or congestive heart failure. All dose recommendations are guidelines, and patients must be monitored with plasma theophylline concentrations.

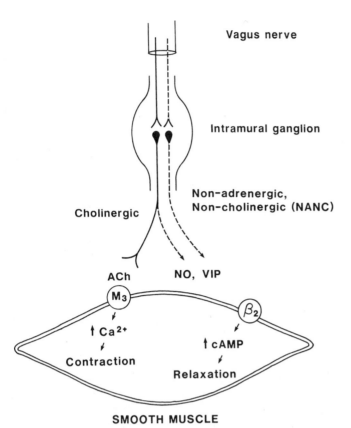

Fig. 4-10. Systems controlling airway smooth muscle activity in humans. Note that β_2-adrenergic receptors on airway smooth muscle are not innervated. It is not known if the nonadrenergic, noncholinergic system utilizes distinct neural pathways (depicted by dashed lines) or whether its putative mediators nitric oxide *(NO)* or vasoactive intestinal peptide *(VIP)* are cotransmitters released with acetylcholine *(ACh)* from postganglionic nerves.

C. DRUGS THAT AFFECT THE AUTONOMIC NERVOUS SYSTEM

1. Neural control of airway smooth muscle

Autonomic nerves control not only airway smooth muscle tone but may also influence vascular blood flow and permeability in the airways, secretion from glands in the airway wall, and the function of inflammatory cells.[115] Human airways are predominantly controlled by cholinergic fibers traveling in the vagus nerve (Fig. 4-10). Stimulation of these parasympathetic pathways causes bronchoconstriction, mucus secretion, and bronchial vasodilatation. Although an abundant supply of adrenoreceptors (β_2 subtype) is found in human airway smooth muscle, there is little, if any, innervation of these receptors by sympathetic nerves.[116] Rather, the activity of these receptors is regulated by circulating epinephrine. Sympathetic nerves innervate bronchial vessels and submucosal glands and cause increased blood flow and mucus secretion.

Other systems less well defined may also affect airway function. In human airways, a neurally mediated bronchodilator pathway is antagonized by neither atropine nor propranolol and has been referred to as the nonadrenergic, noncholinergic (NANC) system.[117] Candidates for neurotransmitters include vasoactive intestinal peptide and nitric oxide (NO).[118,119] NANC effects may be caused by the release of these substances as cotransmitters from cholinergic nerves, rather than as a distinct neural pathway.[120] Neuropeptides from sensory nerves also may be released by stimulation of afferent receptors.[121]

Neurotransmission in nerves innervating the airways may be modulated at multiple sites. For example, β-adrenoreceptor agonists (referred to hereafter as β-agonists) may cause bronchodilation in part by inhibiting acetylcholine release from cholinergic nerves.[122] The physiologic significance of most of these interactions remains poorly understood.[115] However, it is clear that the complexity of the system may make it difficult to predict the effect of any single drug that affects autonomic function.

2. Sympathomimetic agents

a. MECHANISM OF ACTION

The classic mechanism of action of sympathomimetic drugs involves their binding to an adrenoreceptor on the smooth muscle cell (β_2 subtype), which stimulates adenyl cyclase and increases the intracellular concentration of cAMP (Fig. 4-10).[123] The exact mechanism of action of cAMP is unclear, but it probably decreases intracellular calcium concentration[124] and directly affects systems regulating the cellular contractile apparatus[125]; both effects produce bronchodilation. In addition to these "classic" mechanisms, sympathomimetic drugs may also provide beneficial effects by modulating neurotransmission in the cholinergic and perhaps other neural systems,

Table 4-2. Aerosol β_2-agonists

Generic	Brands	Dose per puff
Albuterol	Proventil, Ventolin	90 μg
Bitolterol	Tornalate	370 μg
Isoetharine	Bronkometer	340 μg
Metaproterenol	Alupent, Metaprel	650 μg
Pirbuterol	Maxair	200 μg
Terbutaline	Brethine	200 μg

affecting the function of inflammatory cells, modulating bronchial blood flow, stimulating mucociliary transport, and influencing the composition of mucous secretions.[126]

b. MIXED AGONISTS

These agents have effects on both β_1 and β_2 subtype adrenergic receptors.

Epinephrine can be given subcutaneously, intravenously, or via a metered-dose inhaler or nebulizer. The onset of action is rapid, making it often the first drug administered in an ambulatory emergency setting, providing acute therapy until long-term measures can be instituted. The usual dose is 0.4 ml of a 1:1000 solution in adults (0.005 ml/kg in pediatric patients), which may be repeated at 15 minute intervals. Cardiovascular side effects produced by stimulation of β_1 subtype receptors, such as hypertension, tachycardia, and dysrhythmias, may complicate therapy.

Isoproterenol can be inhaled as a nebulized solution or given via metered-dose inhaler, or administered intravenously. When nebulized, the adult dose is 0.5 ml of a 0.5% solution diluted in 2.5 ml of water. Cardiovascular side effects may also occur.

c. SELECTIVE AGONISTS

These agents have varying degrees of selectivity for the β_2 subtype adrenoreceptors, increasing specificity for the lung and presumably decreasing undesired side effects, especially in the cardiovascular system. However, like most other "selective" receptor agonists, these agents are *relatively* selective, with specificity decreasing as dose increases.

There is a bewildering array of clinical formulations available for use. There are few consistent clinical differences in efficacy among these agents, although the responses of individual patients may vary.[126,127] New, inhaled β_2 agonists with a longer duration of action are in common use elsewhere, but not yet widely used in the United States.[128] Available formulations include metered-dose inhalers, solutions for nebulization with water or saline, parenteral solutions for subcutaneous injection, tablets for oral use, and suspensions or syrups for pediatric use. The following list of selective agonists is representative, not exhaustive (Table 4-2).

Albuterol (also known as salbutamol) is currently a popular agent most often administered as a metered-

dose inhaler in outpatients, with one puff delivering 90 μg of drug. The usual dose in ambulatory patients is 2 puffs 4 times daily or immediately before exposure to exercise or other known stimuli. It is also available as a solution for nebulization, in tablet form (including a sustained-release preparation), and as a syrup for pediatric use.

Metaproterenol, another popular agent, is also available as a metered-dose inhaler, a solution for nebulization, tablets, or syrup.

Terbutaline is available as an aerosol inhaler or tablets. It is the only selective β_2 agonist that is available in a formulation for parenteral use, with the usual dose similar to that of epinephrine (0.25 to 0.5 mg subcutaneously). When used in this fashion, its duration of action exceeds that of epinephrine, and it may have cumulative effects on repeated administration.

Isoetharine and *pirbuterol* are available as aerosol inhalers and solutions for nebulization.

Bitolterol may have a longer duration of action than other available agents (6 to 8 hours versus 4 to 6 hours), although the duration of response in individual patients varies considerably. It is available as an aerosol inhaler (0.37 μg/ml) and as a solution for nebulization.

d. ADVERSE EFFECTS AND CLINICAL USE

Side effects related to stimulation of adrenergic receptors in the cardiovascular system are more prominent with mixed agonists, although they may also occur with selective β_2 agonists, especially at higher doses. Possible manifestations include hypertension, tachycardia, and dysrhythmias. Other side effects encountered in the outpatient setting include tremor, nervousness, and nausea. Significant hypokalemia is rare, especially with inhaled agents.

Recently, concern has been expressed regarding the safety of these agents in the chronic treatment of bronchospasm.[129] Despite increased use of antiasthma medications in recent years, the morbidity and mortality associated with asthma continues to rise, a condition referred to as the "asthma paradox."[130] The increased use of sympathomimetic agents has been implicated as one of the factors responsible for this paradox.

Several studies have shown that sole therapy with β_2-agonists over treatment times ranging from 15 days to 1 year may actually enhance airway reactivity.[131-133] Others have found that the regular use of inhaled β_2-agonist bronchodilators is associated with an increased risk of death or near death in asthmatics.[129,134] Whether β_2-agonists are responsible for this increased risk, or whether their use is simply a marker for severe asthma, remains to be determined. It has been suggested that the chronic use of β_2-agonists may relieve symptoms without treating the underlying chronic inflammatory process that is apparently responsible for asthma.[130] This process can lead to irreversible thickening of the

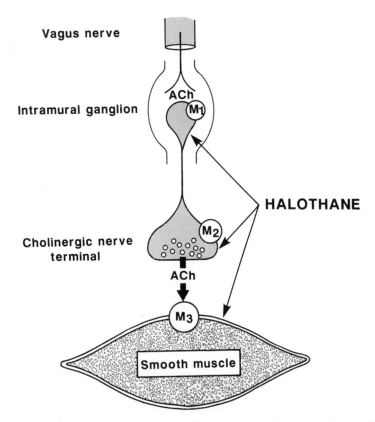

Fig. 4-11. Demonstrated sites of action of halothane on vagal motor pathway. Halothane depresses ganglionic transmission, acetylcholine *(ACh)* release from cholinergic nerve terminals, and directly depresses smooth muscle cell contractility. Also shown are locations of muscarinic (M) receptor subtypes in the vagal motor pathway. M_1 receptors facilitate ganglionic transmission, M_2 receptors inhibit release of ACh, and M_3 receptors mediate smooth muscle contraction.

airway wall, which ultimately worsens hyperreactivity. Although this hypothesis is speculative, and a cause and effect relationship between the use of β_2-agonists and worsening of asthma has not been established, heavy use of these agents should alert the clinician to the possibility of an increased incidence of severe perioperative bronchospasm. Also, it may suggest that drugs that inhibit the inflammatory response, such as inhaled corticosteroids, may be preferable for chronic use.[76]

3. Muscarinic antagonists
a. MECHANISM OF ACTION
These drugs compete with acetylcholine for binding at the muscarinic receptor. At least three subtypes of muscarinic receptors are present in human airways (see Fig. 4-11).[115] Muscarinic receptors of the M_3 subtype produce contraction of airway smooth muscle, vasodilation, and mucous secretion; antagonism of these effects may be beneficial. M_1 subtype muscarinic receptors facilitate ganglionic transmission in parasympathetic pathways innervating airway smooth muscle, and antagonism of this effect should also be beneficial. M_2 subtype muscarinic receptors inhibit the release of acetylcholine

from postganglionic nerves; antagonism of this effect may increase acetylcholine release and thus actually increase airway responsiveness. The net effect of muscarinic antagonists depends on the balance of these physiologic effects and, importantly, on the mechanisms causing bronchoconstriction. For example, these agents should improve or prevent reflex bronchospasm mediated by parasympathetic activation. Conversely, they may have little effect in bronchospasm produced by release of inflammatory mediators (i.e., anaphylactoid or anaphylactic responses to drugs). Because mechanisms producing bronchospasm may vary widely among patients, so also does the efficacy of these agents.

b. SPECIFIC AGENTS
Atropine, the prototypic muscarinic antagonist, may decrease airway resistance and attenuate airway reactivity when given parenterally or when inhaled. Systemic side effects have limited its use specifically as a bronchodilator.

Ipratropium bromide is a quaternary ammonium derivative of atropine. Because it is poorly absorbed and does not readily cross the blood-brain barrier, it can be administered at higher dose and with few systemic side

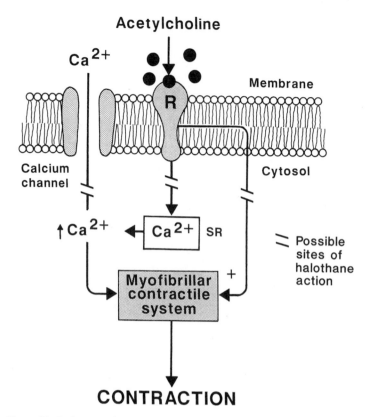

Fig. 4-12. Sites of halothane action in depressing smoothmuscle contractility. Halothane may block calcium influx, impair intracellular calcium release from the sarcoplasmic reticulum *(SR)*, or disrupt mechanisms that sensitize the myofibrillar contractile system to calcium.

effects compared with atropine. It does not appear to be as efficacious as β_2-agonists in asthmatics. However, in patients with chronic obstructive pulmonary disease that includes a reversible component of bronchospasm, ipratropium may have benefits over β_2-agonists, including a longer duration of action and efficacy in some patients in whom β_2-agonists have little effect.[135] It is available as a metered-dose inhaler (18 μg/puff). The usual dose is 2 puffs 4 times daily.

D. ANESTHETICS AND ANESTHETIC ADJUVANTS

Many other drugs administered during the perioperative period may affect the function of the lower airways. Some effects may be beneficial, others deleterious.

1. General anesthetics

Just as most anesthetic agents depress the activity of the striated muscles of the upper airways, most also depress contractility of the smooth muscle of the lower airways. This side effect can prove useful in the perioperative management of patients with reactive airways. On the other hand, to the extent that normal tone in airway smooth muscle helps regulate the matching of ventilation to perfusion, this suppression of normal airway smooth muscle tone may contribute to impaired gas exchange in the perioperative period.

a. VOLATILE ANESTHETICS

Volatile anesthetics are potent bronchodilators. They reduce responses to bronchoconstricting stimuli in both humans and animals.[136-140] They also reduce baseline airway resistances in animals.[141,142] Effects on baseline airway resistances in human subjects are more difficult to interpret due to confounding influences, such as endotracheal intubation and decreases in lung volume associated with general anesthesia, but it appears that these agents may also reduce resting airway smooth muscle tone in humans.[143,144] Because of these bronchodilating effects, volatile anesthetics have been used to treat status asthmaticus, although their efficacy in this condition is not firmly established.[145,146]

Multiple mechanisms contribute to the relaxation of airway smooth muscle produced by volatile anesthetics. These agents attenuate reflex bronchoconstriction in part by depressing neural pathways that mediate these reflexes.[136,147-149] This action has been localized in the vagal motor pathway to a depression of parasympathetic ganglionic transmission and, at higher concentrations of volatile anesthetic, attenuation of acetylcholine release from postganglionic nerves (Fig. 4-11).[147] These agents

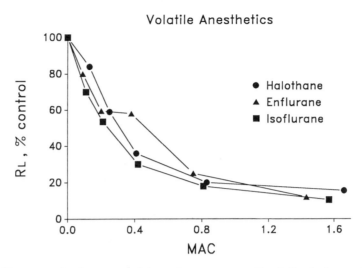

Fig. 4-13. Response of pulmonary resistance to vagus nerve stimulation in dogs as function of expired anesthetic concentration expressed in MAC. All volatile agents studied profoundly depress this response.

may also depress afferent and central integrative portions of airway reflex pathways.

Volatile anesthetics also produce dose-dependent bronchodilation by directly relaxing airway smooth muscle.[136,150] Several mechanisms contribute to this direct relaxation (Fig. 4-12). Halothane attenuates increases in intracellular calcium concentration during the initiation of airway smooth muscle contraction[151] and decreases intracellular calcium concentration during the maintenance of airway smooth muscle contraction.[152,153] Effects during force initiation imply a depression of pathways that mobilize calcium from intracellular stores, whereas effects during force maintenance imply a depression of extracellular calcium influx via calcium channels. Evidence for both of these mechanisms exists in vascular smooth muscle,[154,155] but they have not yet been directly confirmed in the airways. In addition to these effects on intracellular calcium, halothane may also decrease the amount of force developed by the smooth muscle for a given level of intracellular calcium (i.e., halothane depresses the "calcium sensitivity" of the airway smooth muscle).[156] This finding implies that halothane interferes with regulatory pathways that control calcium sensitivity, pathways that can be of crucial importance in the regulation of smooth muscle contraction. The effect of halothane on airway smooth muscle is not mediated by airway epithelium,[157] β-adrenergic effects,[136] or pertussis-sensitive G proteins.[158]

The relative importance of neurally mediated and direct effects of volatile anesthetics to their bronchodilating actions should depend on the mechanism producing bronchoconstriction.[136] During reflex bronchoconstriction, such as that produced in response to airway instrumentation, depression of neural pathways would probably be most significant. During bronchoconstriction produced by the release of mediators from inflammatory cells, such as during anaphylactic or anaphylactoid reactions, direct effects would assume greater importance.

Although ether, halothane, enflurane, and isoflurane all can produce bronchodilation, some differences among agents have been identified. The ability of halothane, enflurane, and isoflurane to attenuate neurally mediated increases in pulmonary resistance produced by electrical stimulation of the vagus nerve does not differ in animals at any concentrations of volatile anesthetic (Fig. 4-13).[138] However, halothane has been shown to be more effective than isoflurane in dilating histamine-constricted airways at concentrations less than 1.2 minimum alveolar concentration (MAC).[159] Above this concentration, effects were similar. This result is consistent with another study finding that the halothane causes greater relaxation of isolated airway smooth muscle compared with isoflurane at similar MAC.[150] In clinical practice, the ethers isoflurane and desflurane are more irritating than the hydrocarbon halothane.[27] This stimulation of airway receptors may produce coughing, breath holding, and laryngospasm, limiting the usefulness of these agents for the induction of anesthesia by inhalation. For desflurane, stimulation of airway receptors may also be responsible for the hypertension and tachycardia observed after its acute administration.[160] Of interest is that irritation by sevoflurane appears to be minimal, making it a more suitable agent for inhalation induction.[28]

In addition to these effects on airway smooth muscle, the volatile anesthetics may also depress mucociliary

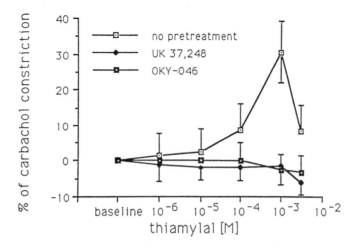

Fig. 4-14. Contraction of segment of guinea pig trachea, expressed as percentage of maximal contraction to carbachol, produced by thiamylal in absence or presence of two thromboxane synthase inhibitors. These results suggest that thiobarbiturates can produce airway constriction mediated by the production of thromboxane. (From Curry C, et al: *Anesthesiology* 75:679, 1991.)

function. Although some of this effect may be attributed to the inhalation of dry gases,[161] halothane and other anesthetics may interfere with ion transport in airway epithelial cells and directly depress ciliary function.[162-165] Both effects may impair the ability of the airways to clear secretions and contribute to postoperative respiratory complications.

b. INTRAVENOUS ANESTHETICS

The intravenous anesthetics also may affect airway reactivity. The barbiturates depress neural portions of the airway reflex pathway in animals, including centers in the CNS and parasympathetic ganglia in the vagal motor pathway.[166-168] Reported effects of barbiturates directly on the smooth muscle have varied, ranging from relaxation to no effect to constriction.[169-171] In a recent study, Lenox et al.[172] found that thiopental produced a dose-dependent constriction of guinea pig trachea. This constriction was not observed with oxybarbiturates, such as methohexital,[173] and was shown to be caused by thromboxane A_2 (Fig. 4-14). Thiopental has also been reported to cause bronchospasm by releasing histamine[174]; other studies have not demonstrated an association between bronchospasm and barbiturate administration.[71,74] Although thiopental releases histamine from skin mast cells, this effect has not been experimentally demonstrated in the lung.[172]

Ketamine also depresses neural airway reflex pathways and directly relaxes airway smooth muscle by mechanisms that are unknown.[175,176] Ketamine-induced release of endogenous catecholamines may also contribute to its bronchodilating effects.[177] Ketamine has been used successfully to treat status asthmaticus,[178-180] although, like volatile anesthetics, its efficacy for this indication is not fully established.

Propofol also apparently blunts airway reflexes, since propofol induction of anesthesia permits insertion of the laryngeal mask airway without apparent reflex responses.[181] One report suggests that, like ketamine, it may directly relax airway smooth muscle,[176] although another study could find little evidence for effects on peripheral airway reactivity.[182]

2. Neuromuscular blocking drugs

There are at least three properties of neuromuscular blocking drugs that could affect airway function.

Some agents, including tubocurarine, atracurium, and mivacurium, can produce a dose-dependent release of histamine that could constrict airway smooth muscle. Atracurium enhances increases in pulmonary resistance caused by vagus nerve stimulation in the dog,[138] although it is not known if histamine release is responsible for this effect. There are case reports of bronchospasm following atracurium administration,[183] and one study found a mild transient decrease in specific airway conductance (the reciprocal of airway resistance) after atracurium (but not tubocurarine).[184] Other studies have also found no effect of tubocurarine on airway tone.[185,186]

Some neuromuscular blocking drugs act as competitive antagonists at muscarinic receptors and so can affect airway reactivity. Pancuronium, but not vecuronium, at lower doses (less than 0.14 mg/kg) also enhances increases in pulmonary resistance caused by vagus nerve stimulation in the dog,[138] probably by blocking prejunctional M_2 subtype muscarinic receptors that normally inhibit acetylcholine release from postganglion parasympathetic nerves. It is not known if this action is clinically significant.

Finally, because succinylcholine is closely related to acetylcholine, it potentially can occupy muscarinic receptors and interact with cholinesterases and so affect airway reactivity. Succinylcholine increases smooth muscle tone in the trachea of dogs.[187] The increase in tracheal tone appears to be mediated by parasympathetic stimulation, since it is abolished by vagotomy and is not present in studies of excised airway smooth muscle. Succinylcholine increases peripheral airway reactivity to acetylcholine,[188] perhaps by competing for plasma cholinesterase. Although case reports have attributed bronchospasm to succinylcholine,[189-191] the widespread clinical use of succinylcholine in asthmatic patients makes the clinical significance of these observations uncertain.

Reversal of neuromuscular blockade by neostigmine and other cholinesterase inhibitors could theoretically cause bronchospasm. However, when coadministered with the anticholinergic drugs atropine or glycopyrrolate, neostigmine does not significantly change specific airway conductance.[192]

3. Narcotics

Opioids may have several effects on airway function. Opioid administration may release histamine, which could potentially produce bronchoconstriction. However, this effect has not been demonstrated. There is evidence in animals that opioid receptors may inhibit cholinergic neurotransmission in the airways of some species.[193] Opioids may also inhibit tachykinin release from sensory nerves and may inhibit other aspects of sensory nerve function.[115] These actions would suggest that opioids should reduce airway reactivity, and evidence exists that morphine can attenuate vagally mediated bronchoconstriction in asthmatics.[194] However, fentanyl and morphine have been found to increase baseline tracheal smooth muscle tone as measured by tracheal cuff pressures in humans anesthetized with thiopental and nitrous oxide.[195] This increase could be abolished by atropine, suggesting an increase in vagal nerve activity. Two other studies have also documented apparent increases in airway resistance caused by fentanyl during barbiturate (but not propofol) anesthesia in humans[196,197] that could be partially blocked by atropine. The clinical significance of these findings is uncertain. Thus, there is currently little evidence to suggest that the use of these agents should be restricted in patients with reactive airways.

4. Benzodiazepines

Receptors for the neurotransmitter γ-aminobuteric acid (GABA) are present in airway nerves and may modulate neurotransmission.[198] Thus, benzodiazepines, which modulate neurotransmission mediated by GABA, have the potential to attenuate reflex bronchoconstriction. In addition, benzodiazepines may relax

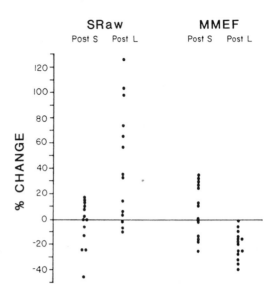

Fig. 4-15. Changes in specific airway resistance *(SRaw)* and maximal midexpiratory flows *(MMEF)* after inhalation of nebulized saline *(S)* or 1% lidocaine *(L)*. Note that lidocaine tended to increase SR and decrease MMEF, suggestive of bronchoconstriction. (From Miller WC, Awe R: *Am Rev Respir Dis* 111:739, 1975.)

airway smooth muscle by a direct effect.[199] Finally, the benzodiazepines produce bronchodilation in dogs by actions on centers in the CNS that control airway smooth muscle tone.[200] As with the narcotics, the clinical significance of these effects are unknown but suggest, at least, that these agents should not contribute to increases in airway smooth muscle tone and may be beneficial.

5. Lidocaine

Given intravenously, lidocaine will antagonize both irritant (reflex) and, to a lesser extent, antigen-induced bronchospasm in dogs with hyperreactive airways.[201,202] Lidocaine also directly relaxes airway smooth muscle in high concentrations,[203,204] although it is not clear that this effect occurs at concentrations of lidocaine achieved in vivo. Intravenous lidocaine has been employed, apparently successfully, to treat intraoperative bronchospasm.[205] Inhaled lidocaine attenuates reflex-induced bronchoconstriction, presumably by interrupting reflex afferents.[206] However, Downes and Hirshman[206] found that nebulized lidocaine was ineffective in antagonizing antigen-induced bronchoconstriction in dogs. Also, several reports have documented significant bronchoconstriction in asthmatics following nebulized lidocaine (Fig. 4-15).[207-210] These effects are not present in normal subjects. Bronchoconstriction can be reversed with aerosolized atropine or isoproterenol,[208] which suggests that it probably represents a reflex bronchoconstriction produced by the locally irritating effects of aerosol administered to the airways.

These bronchoconstrictor effects raise concerns regarding the use of topical lidocaine to permit airway manipulation in awake patients with heightened airway reactivity. However, it is likely that the stimulus for reflex bronchospasm produced by manipulation of an unanesthetized airway would far exceed any bronchoconstricting effects of the lidocaine aerosol itself. Thus, the use of topical lidocaine can be employed in these patients when necessary, with the recognition that lidocaine aerosol may initially cause some degree of bronchoconstriction.[209,210] These reports also call into question the practice of utilizing intratracheal lidocaine as an adjunct to endotracheal intubation in asthmatics following the induction of general anesthesia.

6. Antihistamines

Many atopic patients utilize antihistamines. These drugs are also used in the perioperative period to reduce the volume and acidity of gastric secretions by actions on the H_2 subtype histamine receptor. At least three subtypes of histamine receptors are present in the lung.[211] Specific antagonists of H_1 subtype receptors, which mediate bronchoconstriction, can reduce airway reactivity in some asthmatic subjects.[212] Some studies have found that antagonists of the H_2 subtype receptor, such as cimetidine and ranitodine, can increase airway reactivity.[213,214] Other studies have not been able to confirm this finding.[215,216] This increase in reactivity was originally thought to result from block of receptors that inhibited airway neural transmission. However, it is now clear that neural transmission is modulated by H_3 subtype receptors,[211] so that the mechanisms by which cimetidine and other H_2 agonists might increase airway reactivity are unclear. Clinically, bronchospasm has not been attributed to the use of these agents in the perioperative period, so that they may be utilized in asthmatic patients when appropriate.

E. RESPIRATORY GASES

Several respiratory gases may have important effects on lower airway function.

1. Carbon dioxide

In general, both hypocapnia and hypercapnia cause bronchoconstriction in the lung. Hypocapnic bronchoconstriction probably is caused at least in part by a direct effect smooth muscle, since it is present after vagotomy or atropine under most conditions.[217,218] The mechanism for this direct effect is not known but may involve changes in intracellular pH.[219] This response may assist in the matching of ventilation to perfusion, diverting gas flow away from overventilated regions of the lung.[220] Of interest is that halothane attenuates hypocapnic bronchoconstriction by directly affecting smooth muscle.[221,222] The attenuation of this normal homeostatic mechanism may contribute to ventilation-perfusion mismatch observed during halothane anesthesia.

Hypercapnia produces airway constriction in intact animals by reflex mechanisms, because this bronchoconstriction can be eliminated by vagotomy.[223] In denervated airway smooth muscle, hypercapnia directly relaxes airway smooth muscle.[221,224,225]

2. Oxygen

The effect of hypoxia on the lower airways is controversial. Most studies in humans show that hypoxia does not affect pulmonary resistance, although concurrent changes in lung volume may make these results difficult to interpret. Hypoxia has been reported to increase pulmonary resistance in dogs. A recent study suggests that hypoxia in fact produces bronchodilation,[226] a finding consistent with in vitro studies showing a direct relaxing effect of hypoxia in isolated tissues mediated by opening of potassium channels.[227] Hypoxia may also enhance airway reactivity without changing baseline lung resistance, perhaps by increasing the synthesis of leukotrienes.[228]

3. Nitrogen oxides

Nitrogen oxides (NO_x) are ubiquitous endogenous compounds with important physiologic roles in virtually every vertebrate organ system. Since the proposal that endothelium-derived relaxing factor, a crucial mediator of vascular tone, was the nitric oxide free radical, interest in these compounds has increased exponentially. These compounds may play an important role in the pathogenesis of many diseases affecting the lungs, including asthma, the adult respiratory distress syndrome, and pulmonary hypertension.[229] The family of NO_x contains elemental nitrogen in one of five oxidation states and includes nitroxyl anion (NO^-), the nitric oxide free radical ($NO\cdot$), nitrite (NO_2^-), nitrogen dioxide (NO_2; cd), and nitrate (NO_3^-).

The metabolic machinery needed to synthesize NO_x, based on the enzyme nitric oxide synthase (NOS), is present in the lung. NO_x can be classified as respiratory gases, since they are present in the expired gas of normal subjects.[230] NOS has been found in alveolar macrophages.[231] Other possible sources in the lung include mast cells, neurons, airway epithelium, vascular endothelium, or airway smooth muscle.[229]

Nitroso compounds such as nitroglycerin, which act as nitric oxide donors, have been studied for many years as therapy for bronchospasm with varying results.[232] In isolated preparations, a variety of these compounds directly relax airway smooth muscle.[233] The mechanism of action appears to be primarily via activation of guanylyl cyclase, which increases cGMP concentrations and relaxes the muscle.[234] However, other mechanisms

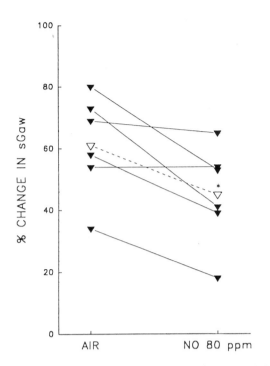

Fig. 4-16. Change in specific airway conductance *(sGaw)* produced by methacholine challenge in asthmatic subjects breathing air or nitric oxide *(NO)* 80 parts per million *(ppm)*. Individual data is shown with closed symbols; open symbols represent mean values. NO produced small but significant decrease in response to methacholine. (From Högman M, et al: *Am Rev Respir Dis* 148:1474, 1993.)

may also operate. NO· may also play a role in the nonadrenergic, noncholinergic system innervating airway smooth muscle.[235,236] Studies of intact animals and humans have shown that inhaled NO· can produce bronchodilation,[237,238] although the effect in humans is modest (Fig. 4-16). Also, inhibition of endogenous NOS enhances airway reactivity,[239] suggesting its role in modifying baseline airway tone.

As in other vascular beds, where it serves as an endothelium-derived relaxing factor, NO· may play an important role in the regulation of pulmonary vascular tone.[240] For example, it has been proposed as mediator of the regional matching of ventilation and perfusion. Disruption of its function may contribute to hypoxemia observed in a variety of pulmonary diseases. Inhalation of exogenous NO· can improve oxygenation in diseases such as adult respiratory distress syndrome (ARDS).[241] This therapy can also act as a selective pulmonary vasodilator because rapid scavenging by hemoglobin prevents any absorbed NO· from reaching the systemic circulation.[240,242]

Although the therapeutic effects of these compounds are promising, any potentially beneficial effects must be balanced against the potential for these highly reactive compounds to stimulate airway inflammation and edema.[243] Indeed, these compounds may be important mediators of lung inflammation and are found in increased concentration in the expired gas of asthmatics.[244] Future therapeutic use of these compounds will be guided by an increased understanding of their biochemical mechanisms of action in the airways, their potential toxicity, and controlled trials demonstrating improvements in clinical outcomes.

IV. APPROACH TO THE PERIOPERATIVE AIRWAY MANAGEMENT OF THE PATIENT WITH INCREASED AIRWAY REACTIVITY

A detailed discussion of all aspects of perioperative management of patients with reactive airway diseases such as asthma and some forms of chronic obstructive pulmonary disease (COPD) is beyond the scope of this chapter and is the subject of recent reviews.[245,246] This section instead will be limited to an extension of previously discussed pharmacologic principles to the airway management of these patients. Primary areas of concern include prophylaxis to prevent bronchospasm and pharmacologic therapy of established bronchospasm. Of course, these principles also apply to patients without a history of increased airway reactivity, who may also develop perioperative bronchospasm.[73-75]

A. INHALATION THERAPY

Inhaled therapy of antiinflammatory agents and bronchodilators has the advantage of producing the greatest local effect on airway smooth muscle with lesser potential for systemic toxicity. In other words, the ratio between therapeutic effect and side effects such as cardiovascular or CNS stimulation may be lower for oral and parenteral formulations as compared to the inhaled methods of administration. Delivery of drug to the airway mucosa by inhaled therapy depends on many factors, including the pattern of breathing, the geometry of lungs and airways (often altered in patients with lung disease), and the size of the aerosol particles. Particles below approximately 1 μm in size generally do not impact on the mucosa and are exhaled, whereas the inertia of particles greater than approximately 5 μm causes them to be deposited in the delivery devices and the upper airway (Fig. 4-17).[247] Because much of the delivered dose may be contained in these larger particles, only approximately 10% to 20% of the delivered dose actually reaches the lung under optimal conditions in patients whose tracheas are not intubated.[248,249] The deposition of particles in the lung can be enhanced by breath holding in inspiration following drug inhalation.[250] The deposition of larger particles in the oropharynx, which are systemically absorbed and may cause side effects, can be reduced by the use of "spacer" devices between the mouth and the drug delivery systems.[249] These devices slow aerosol flow and encourage impac-

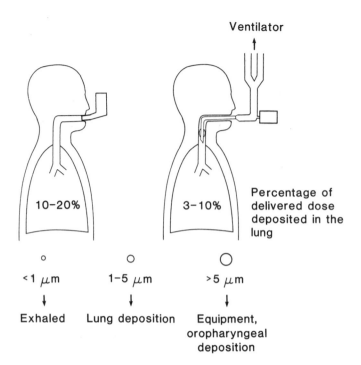

Fig. 4-17. Factors controlling deposition of inhaled aerosol particles, including route of administration (spontaneous inhalation vs. delivery via positive pressure through endotracheal tube) and particle size.

BOX 4-2   Prophylaxis of perioperative bronchospasm

- Ensure optimal preoperative pharmacotherapy, continued up to the morning of surgery
- Adequate corticosteroid preparation
- Adequate preoperative anxiolysis
- Inhaled β₂-agonists immediately before induction
- Regional anesthesia if feasible
- General anesthetic techniques based on the volatile anesthetics
- Adequate anesthesia of the airway before instrumentation
- Intravenous lidocaine, narcotics, and ketamine as adjuncts

---

tion of these large particles in the spacer, rather than in the mouth.

In the perioperative period, it may be necessary to deliver aerosols via an endotracheal tube. Delivery devices can include jet nebulizers, more sophisticated ultrasonic nebulizers, and metered-dose inhalers using fluorocarbon propellants, which are connected to the endotracheal tube via a variety of adapters.[251-255] Several studies have shown that the efficiency of drug delivery is less than that achieved in nonintubated patients, with most of the delivered dose being deposited in the breathing circuit and endotracheal tube. As little as 1% to 2% of the delivered dose actually reaches the lungs

with some systems, with most averaging between 3% and 10% delivery.[251-255] Delivery to the lungs can be enhanced by actuating metered-dose inhalers during inspiratory flow,[255] by increasing tidal volume and prolonging inspiration, and by using larger diameter endotracheal tubes.[253,254] Ultrasonic nebulizers may promote more efficient delivery by providing a more consistent and appropriate particle size.[253] However, it is still necessary to increase the delivered dose (e.g., by giving more puffs of metered dose inhalers) to provide an equivalent dose of drug to the lung during mechanical ventilation, compared with inhalation during spontaneous breathing.

B. PROPHYLAXIS OF BRONCHOSPASM (BOX 4-2)

Based on the understanding of asthma as a chronic inflammatory disease, preoperative pharmacotherapy should strive to minimize airway inflammation. A stepwise approach based on the adequacy of control as assessed by symptoms and spirometric values such as peak expiratory flow is currently recommended (Table 4-3). For mild, intermittent asthma, short-acting β₂-agonists as necessary often suffice. With moderate symptoms, chronic therapy with inhaled antiinflammatory agents such as corticosteroids or cromolyn is instituted. As a next step, the dose of inhaled corticosteroids can be increased and a long-acting bronchodilator such as theophylline added. For severe asthma, defined in part as a limitation of activities with severe

Table 4-3. Asthma therapy

Mild	Moderate		Severe
Step 1	**Step 2**	**Step 3**	**Step 4**
$\beta_2$agonist prn,* or cromolyn prn	inhaled corticosteroids or cromolyn, necrodomil β_2-agonist prn	inhaled corticosteroids long-acting bronchodilator (β_2-agonists anticholinergic, theophylline) β_2-agonist prn	inhaled corticosteroids (high dose) long-acting bronchodilators oral corticosteroids β_2-agonist prn

*Prn, Pro re nata (as circumstances may require).

exacerbations despite medication, systemic corticosteroids may be necessary. With each step, inhaled β_2-agonists can be used as necessary but should not be taken more than 3 or 4 times daily. It would seem prudent to postpone elective surgery until optimal control is achieved, although objective data supporting this approach is lacking.

Patients receiving chronic inhaled or systemic corticosteroids should receive these drugs until immediately before surgery. Those patients taking systemic corticosteroids should receive an increased dose preoperatively, both to ensure adequate protection against adrenocortical suppression and to ensure that airway inflammation is minimized. Because asthma may be exacerbated by emotional distress, adequate preoperative anxiolysis should be provided. The administration of an inhaled β_2-agonist immediately before anesthetic induction may be helpful. The use of intravenous or inhaled muscarinic antagonists should theoretically be useful in ameliorating reflex bronchospasm, but their use in the perioperative period has not been investigated.

Tradition favors the use of regional anesthetic techniques in these patients when feasible, to avoid the upper airway instrumentation often required during general anesthesia. However, firm evidence demonstrating improved perioperative outcomes is lacking. If awake airway manipulation is necessary, every effort must be made to ensure adequate topical airway anesthesia, with the recognition that this topical anesthesia may tend to increase airway resistances in these patients. Avoidance of endotracheal intubation is preferable.

Because of their excellent bronchodilating properties, volatile anesthetics are the foundation of general anesthetic techniques. As previously discussed, halothane, enflurane, and isoflurane are equally efficacious in attenuating neurally mediated bronchoconstriction in animals; data are not yet available for desflurane and sevoflurane. Although halothane may be a more potent bronchodilator under some experimental conditions and has the advantage of being less pungent, Forrest et al.[256] found no difference in the incidence of bronchospasm among patients anesthetized with halothane, enflurane, or isoflurane in a large multicenter study. However, the

incidence of bronchospasm was increased in patients anesthetized with fentanyl-N_2O, confirming the usefulness of volatile anesthetics. For the intravenous induction of anesthesia, thiopental has been implicated in causing bronchospasm; ketamine, and perhaps propofol, may be useful alternatives.

Regardless of the technique employed, the most important principle to prevent bronchospasm is to provide adequate anesthesia of the airway before instrumentation. One useful technique is to induce anesthesia with an intravenous agent, then ventilate the lungs with a volatile anesthetic over a period of time to allow for significant uptake (at least 10 min). Other adjuncts, such as intravenous lidocaine and narcotics, may be useful in attenuating airway reflexes, although their clinical efficacy for this purpose is not established. Intratracheal lidocaine should be avoided, since any aerosol instilled into the trachea may itself cause bronchospasm. Extubation of the trachea during deep levels of anesthesia may be desirable, although this approach should be avoided if there are any doubts as to the ability to maintain airway patency. Again, adjuncts such as intravenous lidocaine and narcotics may be useful in blunting airway reflexes during emergence.

C. TREATMENT OF BRONCHOSPASM (BOX 4-3)

The proper diagnosis of bronchospasm is paramount. Although usually not difficult in the awake patient, many other conditions may mimic bronchospasm in the anesthetized patient. Signs include wheezing, diminished breath sounds, prolonged expiration, and increased airway pressures during positive-pressure ventilation. Common conditions that must be excluded include mechanical airway obstruction at any site, tension pneumothorax, aspiration, and pulmonary edema.

Once the diagnosis is firmly established, the first consideration is to increase anesthetic depth by increasing the inspired concentration of volatile anesthetic. Intravenous adjuncts such as ketamine, propofol, and lidocaine may also be useful. The role of intravenous aminophylline in treating intraoperative bronchospasm is limited. In an animal model of asthma,

---

BOX 4-3   Treatment of perioperative bronchospasm

- Confirm diagnosis
- Deepen anesthesia with a volatile agent
- Consider ketamine, intravenous lidocaine, propofol to further deepen anesthesia
- Inhaled β_2-agonists
- Avoid aminophylline
- Parenteral corticosteroids
- Adjust ventilatory parameters to avoid gas trapping and barotrauma

---

aminophylline provides no additional protection against airway constriction beyond that provided by halothane.[257] Further, aminophylline may produce dysrhythmias, especially when combined with volatile anesthetics (especially halothane) and the hypercarbia that may accompany bronchospasm. Unlike aminophylline, β_2-agonists do provide benefit beyond that afforded by the volatile anesthetics in an animal model of asthma.[258] Inhaled β_2-agonists may be nebulized into the endotracheal tube, recognizing that doses well above those required in ambulatory patients may be needed to compensate for a decreased efficiency of drug delivery to the lung. Intravenous adrenergic agonists such as epinephrine may be necessary, particularly as inadequate tidal volumes may preclude significant delivery of inhaled drugs to the lung. Parenteral corticosteroids may be administered, but a period of several hours is required for significant benefit. Parameters of mechanical ventilation may need to be altered to minimize airway pressures and prolong expiration to minimize gas trapping. (See Box 4-3 and Chapter 5.)

REFERENCES

1. Van Lunteren E, Strohl KP: Striated respiratory muscles of the upper airways, *Lung Biol* 35:87, 1988.
2. Warner DO: Respiratory muscle function. In Biebuyck JF, Lynch C III, Maze M et al., editors: *Anesthesia: biologic foundations,* vol II, part 3, *Respiratory System,* New York, in press, Raven Press.
3. Sauerland EK, Harper RM: The human tongue during sleep: electromyographic activity of the genioglossus muscle, *Exp Neurol* 51:160, 1976.
4. Wheatley JR et al: Pressure-diameter relationships of the upper airway in awake supine subjects, *J Appl Physiol* 70:2242, 1991.
5. Brancatisano T, Collett PW, Engel LA: Respiratory movements of the vocal cords, *J Appl Physiol* 54:1269, 1983.
6. Brancatisano TP, Dodd DS, Engel LA: Respiratory activity of posterior cricoarytenoid muscle and vocal cords in humans, *J Appl Physiol* 57:1143, 1984.
7. Kuna ST, Smickley JS, Insalaco G: Posterior cricoarytenoid muscle activity during wakefulness and sleep in normal adults, *J Appl Physiol* 68:1746, 1990.
8. Brancatisano A, Dodd DS, Engel LA: Posterior cricoarytenoid activity and glottic size during hyperpnea in humans, *J Appl Physiol* 71:977, 1991.
9. England SJ, Bartlett D Jr: Changes in respiratory movements of the human vocal cords during hyperpnea, *J Appl Physiol* 52:780, 1982.
10. Insalaco G, Kuna ST, Cibella F et al: Thyroarytenoid muscle activity during hypoxia, hypercapnia, and voluntary hyperventilation in humans, *J Appl Physiol* 69:268, 1990.
11. Wheatley JR, Brancatisano A, Engel LA: Respiratory-related activity of cricothyroid muscle in awake normal humans, *J Appl Physiol* 70:2226, 1991.
12. Nishino T et al: Responses of recurrent laryngeal, hypoglossal, and phrenic nerves to increasing depths of anesthesia with halothane or enflurane in vagotomized cats, *Anesthesiology* 63:404, 1985.
13. Rex MAE: A review of the structural and functional basis of laryngospasm and a discussion of the nerve pathways involved in the reflex and its clinical significance in man and animals, *Br J Anaesth* 42:891, 1970.
14. Sasaki CT, Buckwalter J: Laryngeal function, *Am J Otolaryngol* 5:281, 1984.
15. Orem J, Lydic R, Norris P: Experimental control of the diaphragm and laryngeal abductor muscles by brain stem arousal systems, *Respir Physiol* 38:203, 1977.
16. Iscoe SD: Central control of the upper airway. In Mathew OP, Sant'Ambrogio G, editors: *Respiratory function of the upper airway,* New York, 1988, Marcel Dekker.
17. Hershenson M et al: The effect of chloral hydrate on genioglossus and diaphragmatic activity, *Pediatr Res* 18:516, 1984.
18. Hwang J-C, St. John WM, Bartlett D Jr: Respiratory-related hypoglossal nerve activity: influence of anesthetics, *J Appl Physiol* 55:785, 1983.
19. Nishino T et al: Comparison of changes in the hypoglossal and the phrenic nerve activity in response to increasing depth of anesthesia in cats, *Anesthesiology* 60:19, 1984.
20. Ochiai R, Guthrie RD, Motoyama EK: Effects of varying concentrations of halothane on the activity of the genioglossus, intercostals, and diaphragm in cats: an electromyographic study, *Anesthesiology* 70:812, 1989.
21. Rothstein RJ et al: Respiratory-related activity of upper airway muscles in anesthetized rabbit, *J Appl Physiol* 55:1830, 1983.
22. Murphy PJ et al: Effect of oral diazepam on the sensitivity of upper airway reflexes, *Br J Anaesth* 70:131, 1993.
23. Nishino T, Hiraga K, Yokokawa N: Laryngeal and respiratory responses to tracheal irritation at different depths of enflurane anesthesia in humans, *Anesthesiology* 73:46, 1990.
24. Drummond GB: Upper airway reflexes, *Br J Anaesth* 70:121, 1993.
25. Sant'Ambrogio FB et al: Effects of halothane and isoflurane in the upper airway of dogs during development, *Respir Physiol* 91:237, 1992.
26. Doi M, Ikeda K: Airway irritation produced by volatile anaesthetics during brief inhalation: comparison of halothane, enflurane, isoflurane and sevoflurane, *Can J Anaesth* 40:122, 1993.
27. Taylor RH, Lerman J: Induction, maintenance and recovery characteristics of desflurane in infants and children, *Can J Anaesth* 39:6, 1992.
28. Naito Y et al: Comparison between sevoflurane and halothane for paediatric ambulatory anaesthesia, *Br J Anaesth* 67:387, 1991.
29. Morikawa S, Safar P, DeCarlo J: Influence of the head-jaw position upon upper airway patency, *Anesthesiology* 22:265, 1961.
30. Safar P, Escarraga LA, Chang F: Upper airway obstruction in the unconscious patient, *J Appl Physiol* 14:760, 1959.
31. Abernethy LJ, Allan PL, Drummond GB: Ultrasound assessment of the position of the tongue during induction of anaesthesia, *Br J Anaesth* 65:744, 1990.
32. Nandi PR et al: Effect of general anaesthesia on the pharynx, *Br J Anaesth* 66:157, 1991.

33. Hudgel DW, Hendricks C: Palate and hypopharynx—sites of inspiratory narrowing of the upper airway during sleep, *Am Rev Respir Dis* 138:1542, 1988.

34. Shepard JW Jr, Thawley SE: Localization of upper airway collapse during sleep in patients with obstructive sleep apnea, *Am Rev Respir Dis* 141:1350, 1990.

35. Boidin MP: Airway patency in the unconscious patient, *Br J Anaesth* 57:306, 1985.

36. Drummond GB: Influence of thiopentone on upper airway muscles, *Br J Anaesth* 63:12, 1989.

37. Montravers P, Dureuil B, Desmonts JM: Effects of i.v. midazolam on upper airway resistance, *Br J Anaesth* 68:27, 1992.

38. Leiter JC et al: The effect of diazepam on genioglossal muscle activity in normal human subjects, *Am Rev Respir Dis* 132:216, 1985.

39. Bartlett D Jr, Leiter JC, Knuth SL: Control and actions of the genioglossus muscle. In Issa FG, Suratt PM, Remmers JE, editors: *Sleep and Respiration,* New York, 1990, Wiley-Liss.

40. Begle RL et al: Effect of lung inflation on pulmonary resistance during NREM sleep, *Am Rev Respir Dis* 141:854, 1990.

41. Laycock JRD et al: Potency of atracurium and vecuronium at the diaphragm and the adductor pollicis muscle, *Br J Anaesth* 61:286, 1988.

42. Lebrault C et al: Relative potency of vecuronium on the diaphragm and the adductor pollicis, *Br J Anaesth* 63:389, 1989.

43. Donati F, Meistelman C, Plaud B: Vecuronium neuromuscular blockade at the diaphragm, the orbicularis oculi, and adductor pollicis muscles, *Anesthesiology* 73:870, 1990.

44. Donati F, Antzaka C, Bevan DR: Potency of pancuronium at the diaphragm and the adductor pollicis muscle in humans, *Anesthesiology* 65:1, 1986.

45. Gal TJ, Goldberg SK: Diaphragmatic function in healthy subjects during partial curarization, *J Appl Physiol* 48:921, 1980.

46. Gal TJ, Goldberg SK: Relationship between respiratory muscle strength and vital capacity during partial curarization in awake subjects, *Anesthesiology* 54:141, 1981.

47. Donati F, Meistelman C, Plaud B: Vecuronium neuromuscular blockade at the adductor muscles of the larynx and adductor pollicis, *Anesthesiology* 74:833, 1991.

48. Pavlin EG, Holle RH, Schoene RB: Recovery of airway protection compared with ventilation in humans after paralysis with curare, *Anesthesiology* 70:381, 1989.

49. Önal E, Lopata M, O'Connor TD: Diaphragmatic and genioglossal electromyogram responses to CO_2 rebreathing in humans, *J Appl Physiol* 50:1052, 1981.

50. Oliven A, Odeh M, Gavriely N: Effect of hypercapnia on upper airway resistance and collapsibility in anesthetized dogs, *Respir Physiol* 75:29, 1989.

51. Salomone RJ, Van Lunteren E: Effects of hypoxia and hypercapnia on geniohyoid contractility and endurance, *J Appl Physiol* 71:709, 1991.

52. Okabe S et al: Upper airway muscle activity during sustained hypoxia in awake humans, *J Appl Physiol* 75:1552, 1993.

53. Courtney KR: Mechanism of frequency-dependent inhibition of sodium currents in frog myelinated nerve by the lidocaine derivative GEA 968, *J Pharmacol Exp Ther* 195:225, 1975.

54. Covino BG: Pharmacology of local anaesthetic agents, *Br J Anaesth* 58:701, 1986.

55. Ford DJ et al: Duration and toxicity of bupivacaine for topical anesthesia of the airway in the cat, *Anesth Analg* 63:1001, 1984.

56. Mongan PD, Culling RD: Rapid oral anesthesia for awake intubation, *J Clin Anesth* 4:101, 1992.

57. Chinn WM, Zavala DC, Ambre J: Plasma levels of lidocaine following nebulized aerosol administration, *Chest* 71:346, 1977.

58. Baughman VL et al: Lidocaine blood levels following aerosolization and intravenous administration, *J Clin Anesth* 4:325, 1992.

59. Greenblatt DJ et al: Lidocaine plasma concentrations following administration of intraoral lidocaine solution, *Arch Otolaryngol* 111:298, 1985.

60. Viegas O, Stoelting RK: Lidocaine in arterial blood after laryngotracheal administration, *Anesthesiology* 43:491, 1975.

61. Pelton DA et al: Plasma lidocaine concentrations following topical aerosol application to the trachea and bronchi, *Can Anaesth Soc J* 17:250, 1970.

62. Curran J, Hamilton C, Taylor T: Topical analgesia before tracheal intubation, *Anaesthesia* 30:765, 1975.

63. Sutherland AD, Williams RT: Cardiovascular responses and lidocaine absorption in fiberoptic-assisted awake intubation, *Anesth Analg* 65:389, 1986.

64. Potter JL, Hillman JV: Benzocaine-induced methemoglobinemia, *JACEP* 8:26, 1979.

65. Townes PL, Geertsma MA, White MR: Benzocaine-induced methemoglobinemia, *Am J Dis Child* 131:697, 1977.

66. Anderson ST, Hajduczek J, Barker SJ: Benzocaine-induced methemoglobinemia in an adult: accuracy of pulse oximetry with methemoglobinemia, *Anesth Analg* 67:1099, 1988.

67. Barker SJ, Tremper KK, Hyatt J: Effects of methemoglobinemia on pulse oximetry and mixed venous oximetry, *Anesthesiology* 70:112, 1989.

68. Severinghaus JW, Xu F-D, Spellman MJ Jr: Benzocaine and methemoglobin: recommended actions, *Anesthesiology* 74:385, 1991.

69. McNicholas WT et al: Upper airway obstruction during sleep in normal subjects after selective topical oropharyngeal anesthesia, *Am Rev Respir Dis* 135:1316, 1987.

70. Chadwick GA et al: Obstructive sleep apnea following topical oropharyngeal anesthesia in loud snorers, *Am Rev Respir Dis* 143:810, 1991.

71. Shnider SM, Papper EM: Anesthesia for the asthmatic patient, *Anesthesiology* 22:886, 1961.

72. Yunginger JW et al: A community-based study of the epidemiology of asthma, *Am Rev Respir Dis* 146:888, 1992.

73. Forrest JB et al: Multicenter study of general anesthesia. III. Predictors of severe perioperative adverse outcomes, *Anesthesiology* 76:3, 1992.

74. Olsson GL: Bronchospasm during anaesthesia: a computer-aided incidence study of 136,929 patients, *Acta Anaesthesiol Scand* 31:244, 1987.

75. Cheney FW, Posner KL, Caplan RA: Adverse respiratory events infrequently leading to malpractice suits, *Anesthesiology* 75:932, 1991.

76. International Consensus Report on Diagnosis and Treatment of Asthma, *Eur Respir J* 5:601, 1992.

77. Barnes PJ: Effect of corticosteroids on airway hyperresponsiveness, *Am Rev Respir Dis* 141:S70, 1990.

78. Hoag JE, McFadden ER Jr: Long-term effect of cromolyn sodium on nonspecific bronchial hyperresponsiveness: a review, *Ann Allergy* 66:53, 1991.

79. Thomson NC: Nedocromil sodium: an overview, *Respir Med* 83:269, 1989.

80. Parish RC, Miller LJ: Nedocromil sodium, *Ann Pharmacother* 27:599, 1993.

81. Barnes PJ: A new approach to the treatment of asthma, *N Engl J Med* 321:1517, 1989.

82. Rowe BH, Keller JL, Oxman AD: Effectiveness of steroid therapy in acute exacerbations of asthma: a meta-analysis, *Am J Emerg Med* 10:301, 1992.

83. Miesfeld RL: Molecular genetics of corticosteroid action, *Am Rev Respir Dis* 141:S11, 1990.

84. Guyre PM et al: Glucocorticoid effects on the production and actions of immune cytokines, *J Steroid Biochem* 30:89, 1988.

85. Laitinen LA, Laitinen A, Haahtela T: A comparative study of the effects of an inhaled corticosteroid, budesonide, and a β$_2$-agonist, terbutaline, on airway inflammation in newly diagnosed asthma: a randomized, double-blind, parallel-group controlled trial, *J Allergy Clin Immunol* 90:32, 1992.

86. Her E et al: Eosinophil hematopoietins antagonize the programmed cell death of eosinophils: cytokine and glucocorticoid effects on eosinophils maintained by endothelial cell-conditioned medium, *J Clin Invest* 88:1982, 1991.

87. Boschetto P et al: Corticosteroid inhibition of airway microvascular leakage, *Am Rev Respir Dis* 143:605, 1991.

88. Shimura S et al: Direct inhibitory action of glucocorticoid on glycoconjugate secretion from airway submucosal glands, *Am Rev Respir Dis* 141:1044, 1990.

89. Cockcroft DW, Murdock KY: Comparative effects of inhaled salbutamol, sodium cromoglycate and beclomethasone diproprionate on allergen-induced early asthmatic responses, late asthmatic responses, and increased bronchial responsiveness to histamine, *J Allergy Clin Immunol* 79:734, 1987.

90. Lundgren R et al: Morphological studies of bronchial mucosal biopsies from asthmatics before and after ten years treatment with inhaled steroids, *Eur Respir J* 1:883, 1988.

91. Fraser CM, Venter JC: Beta-adrenergic receptors: relationship of primary structure, receptor function, and regulation, *Am Rev Respir Dis* 141:S22, 1990.

92. Greenberger PA: Corticosteroids in asthma: rationale, use, and problems, *Chest* 101:418S, 1992.

93. Toogood JH: Complications of topical steroid therapy for asthma, *Am Rev Respir Dis* 141:S89, 1990.

94. Ryrfeldt A et al: Pharmacokinetics and metabolism of budesonide, a selective glucocorticoid, *Eur J Respir Dis* 63 (suppl 122): 86, 1982.

95. Toogood JH et al: Effect of high-dose inhaled budesonide on calcium and phosphate metabolism and the risk of osteoporosis, *Am Rev Respir Dis* 138:57, 1988.

96. Kehlet H, Binder C: Adrenocortical function and clinical course during and after surgery in unsupplemented glucocorticoid-treated patients, *Br J Anaesth* 45:1043, 1973.

97. Toogood JH et al: Candidiasis and dysphonia complicating beclomethasone treatment of asthma, *J Allergy Clin Immunol* 65:145, 1980.

98. Milgrom H, Bender B: Current issues in the use of theophylline, *Am Rev Respir Dis* 147:S33, 1993.

99. Polson JB et al: Analysis of the relationship between pharmacological inhibition of cyclic nucleotide phosphodiesterase and relaxation of canine tracheal smooth muscle, *Biochem Pharmacol* 28:1391-1395, 1979.

100. Persson CGA: The profile of action of enprofylline, or why adenosine antagonism seems less desirable with xanthine antiasthmatic. In Morley J, Rainsford KD, editors: *Pharmacology of asthma,* Basel, Switzerland, 1983, Birkhäuser Verlag.

101. Kolbeck RC et al: Apparent irrelevance of cyclic nucleotides to the relaxation of tracheal smooth muscle induced by theophylline, *Lung* 156:173, 1979.

102. Murad F: Effects of phosphodiesterase inhibitors and the role of cyclic nucleotides in smooth-muscle relaxation. In Andersson KE, Persson CGA, editors: *Anti-asthma xanthines and adenosine,* Amsterdam, 1985, Excerpta Medica.

103. Londos C, Wolff J: Two distinct adenosine-sensitive sites on adenylate cyclase, *Proc Natl Acad Sci U S A* 74:5482, 1977.

104. Lunell E et al: A novel bronchodilator xanthine apparently without adenosine receptor antagonism and tremorogenic effect, *Eur J Respir Dis* 64:333, 1983.

105. Pauwels R, Persson CGA: Xanthines, *Lung Biology in Health and Disease* 49:503, 1991.

106. Shohat B, Volovitz B, Varsano I: Induction of suppressor T cells in asthmatic children by theophylline treatment, *Clin Allergy* 13:487, 1983.

107. Stroud MW et al: The effects of aminophylline and meperidine alone and in combination on the respiratory response to carbon dioxide inhalation, *J Pharmacol Exp Ther* 114:461, 1955.

108. Aubier M et al: Aminophylline improves diaphragmatic contractility, *N Engl J Med* 305:249, 1981.

109. Dureuil B et al: Effects of aminophylline on diaphragmatic dysfunction after upper abdominal surgery, *Anesthesiology* 62: 242, 1985.

110. Cohn JN, Franciosa JA: Vasodilator therapy of cardiac failure (second of two parts), *N Engl J Med* 297:254, 1977.

111. Rall TW: Central nervous system stimulants. In Gilman AG, Goodman LS, Gilman A, editors: *The pharmacological basis of therapeutics,* ed 6, New York, 1980, Macmillan.

112. Hendeles L, Weinberger M, Bighley L: Disposition of theophylline after a single intravenous infusion of aminophylline, *Am Rev Respir Dis* 118:97, 1978.

113. Newhouse MT: Is theophylline obsolete? *Chest* 98:1, 1990.

114. Fragoso CA, Miller MA: Review of the clinical efficacy of theophylline in the treatment of chronic obstructive pulmonary disease, *Am Rev Respir Dis* 147:S40, 1993.

115. Barnes PJ: Modulation of neurotransmission in airways, *Physiol Rev* 72:699, 1992.

116. Richardson J, Béland J: Nonadrenergic inhibitory nervous system in human airways, *J Appl Physiol* 41:764, 1976.

117. Barnes PJ: The third nervous system in the lung: physiology and clinical perspectives, *Thorax* 39:561, 1984.

118. Gao Y, Vanhoutte PM: Attenuation of contractions to acetylcholine in canine bronchi by an endogenous nitric oxide-like substance, *Br J Pharmacol* 109:887, 1993.

119. Ward JK et al: Modulation of cholinergic neural bronchoconstriction by endogenous nitric oxide and vasoactive intestinal peptide in human airways in vitro, *J Clin Invest* 92:736, 1993.

120. Palmer JBD, Cuss FMC, Barnes PJ: VIP and PHM and their role in nonadrenergic inhibitory responses in isolated human airways, *J Appl Physiol* 61:1322, 1986.

121. Uddman R, Sundler F: Neuropeptides in the airways: a review, *Am Rev Respir Dis* 136:S3, 1987.

122. Ito Y, Tajima K: Dual effects of catecholamines on pre- and post-junctional membranes in the dog trachea, *Br J Pharmacol* 75:433, 1982.

123. Torphy TJ, Hay DWP: Biochemical regulation of airway smooth-muscle tone: an overview. In Agrawal DK, Townley RG, editors: *Airway smooth muscle: modulation of receptors and response,* Boca Raton, Fla, 1990, CRC Press.

124. Felbel J et al: Regulation of cytosolic calcium by cAMP and cGMP in freshly isolated smooth muscle cells from bovine trachea, *J Biol Chem* 263:16764, 1988.

125. de Lanerolle P et al: Increased phosphorylation of myosin light chain kinase after an increase in cyclic AMP in intact smooth muscle, *Science* 223:1415, 1984.

126. Nelson HS: Adrenergic therapy of bronchial asthma, *J Allergy Clin Immunol* 77:771, 1986.

127. Habib MP et al: A comparison of albuterol and metaproterenol nebulizer solutions, *Ann Allergy* 58:421, 1987.

128. Tattersfield AE: Clinical pharmacology of long-acting β-receptor agonists, *Life Sci* 52:2161, 1993.

129. Spitzer WO et al: The use of β-agonists and the risk of death and near death from asthma, *N Engl J Med* 326:501, 1992.

130. Page CP: Beta agonists and the asthma paradox, *J Asthma* 30:155, 1993.

131. Vathenen AS et al: Rebound increase in bronchial responsiveness after treatment with inhaled terbutaline, *Lancet* 1:554, 1988.

132. Van Schayck CP et al: Increased bronchial hyperresponsiveness after inhaling salbutamol during one year is not caused by subsensitation to salbutamol, *J Allergy Clin Immunol* 86:793, 1990.

133. Kraan J et al: Changes in bronchial hyperreactivity induced by four weeks of treatment with anti-asthmatic drugs in patients with allergic asthma: a comparison between budesonide and terbutaline, *J Allergy Clin Immunol* 76:628, 1985.

134. Beasley R et al: Asthma mortality and inhaled beta agonist therapy, *Aust N Z J Med* 21:753, 1991.

135. Braun SR, Levy SF: Comparison of ipratropium bromide and albuterol in chronic obstructive pulmonary disease: a three-center study, *Am J Med* 91(suppl 4A):28S, 1991.

136. Warner DO et al: Direct and neurally mediated effects of halothane on pulmonary resistance in vivo, *Anesthesiology* 72:1057, 1990.

137. Hirshman CA, Bergman NA: Halothane and enflurane protect against bronchospasm in an asthma dog model, *Anesth Analg* 57:629, 1978.

138. Vettermann J et al: Actions of enflurane, isoflurane, vecuronium, atracurium, and pancuronium on pulmonary resistance in dogs, *Anesthesiology* 69:688, 1988.

139. Hirshman CA et al: Mechanism of action of inhalational anesthesia on airways, *Anesthesiology* 56:107, 1982.

140. Waltemath CL, Bergman NA: Effects of ketamine and halothane on increased respiratory resistance provoked by ultrasonic aerosols, *Anesthesiology* 41:473, 1974.

141. Watney GCG, Jordan C, Hall LW: Effect of halothane, enflurane and isoflurane on bronchomotor tone in anaesthetized ponies, *Br J Anaesth* 59:1022, 1987.

142. Brown RH et al: Direct in vivo visualization of bronchodilation induced by inhalational anesthesia using high-resolution computed tomography, *Anesthesiology* 78:295, 1993.

143. Heneghan CPH et al: Effect of isoflurane on bronchomotor tone in man, *Br J Anaesth* 58:24, 1986.

144. Lehane JR, Jordan C, Jones JG: Influence of halothane and enflurane on respiratory airflow resistance and specific conductance in anaesthetized man, *Br J Anaesth* 52:773, 1980.

145. Johnston RG et al: Isoflurane therapy for status asthmaticus in children and adults, *Chest* 97:698, 1990.

146. O'Rourke PP, Crone RK: Halothane in status asthmaticus, *Crit Care Med* 10:341, 1982.

147. Brichant J-F et al: Halothane, enflurane, and isoflurane depress the peripheral vagal motor pathway in isolated canine tracheal smooth muscle, *Anesthesiology* 74:325, 1991.

148. Korenaga S, Takeda K, Ito Y: Differential effects of halothane on airway nerves and muscle, *Anesthesiology* 60:309, 1984.

149. Shah MV, Hirshman CA: Mode of action of halothane on histamine-induced airway constriction in dogs with reactive airways, *Anesthesiology* 65:170, 1986.

150. Yamamoto K et al: Factors influencing the direct actions of volatile anesthetics on airway smooth muscle, *Anesthesiology* 78:1102, 1993.

151. Jones KA et al: Halothane alters cytosolic calcium transient in tracheal smooth muscle, *Am J Physiol* 265:L80, 1993.

152. Yamakage M et al: Inhibitory effects of four inhaled anesthetics on canine tracheal smooth muscle contraction and intracellular Ca^{2+} concentration, *Anesth Analg* 77:67, 1993.

153. Yamakage M: Direct inhibitory mechanisms of halothane on canine tracheal smooth muscle contraction, *Anesthesiology* 77:546, 1992.

154. Sill JC et al: Halothane inhibits agonist-induced inositol phosphate and Ca^{2+} signaling in A7r5 cultured vascular smooth muscle cells, *Mol Pharmacol* 40:1006, 1991.

155. Buljubasic N et al: Effects of halothane and isoflurane on calcium and potassium channel currents in canine coronary arterial cells, *Anesthesiology* 76:990, 1992.

156. Jones KA et al: Effects of halothane on the relationship between cytosolic calcium and force in airway smooth muscle, *Am J Physiol* 266:L199, 1994.

157. Sayiner A et al: Bronchodilation by halothane is not modulated by airway epithelium, *Anesthesiology* 75:75, 1991.

158. Morimoto N et al: Halothane and pertussis toxin-sensitive G proteins in airway smooth muscle, *Anesth Analg* 78:328, 1994.

159. Brown RH, Zerhouni EA, Hirshman CA: Comparison of low concentrations of halothane and isoflurane as bronchodilators, *Anesthesiology* 78:1097, 1993.

160. Ebert TJ, Muzi M: Sympathetic hyperactivity during desflurane anesthesia in healthy volunteers: a comparison with isoflurane, *Anesthesiology* 79:444, 1993.

161. Hirsch JA et al: Effects of dry air and subsequent humidification on tracheal mucous velocity in dogs, *J Appl Physiol* 39:242, 1975.

162. Forbes AR, Gamsu G: Depression of lung mucociliary clearance by thiopental and halothane, *Anesth Analg* 58:387, 1979.

163. Forbes AR: Halothane depresses mucociliary flow in the trachea, *Anesthesiology* 45:59, 1976.

164. Manawadu BR, Mostow SR, LaForce FM: Impairment of tracheal ring ciliary activity by halothane, *Anesth Analg* 58:500, 1979.

165. Pizov R et al: Halothane inhibition of ion transport of the tracheal epithelium, *Anesthesiology* 76:985, 1992.

166. Jackson DM, Richards IM: The effects of pentobarbitone and chloralose anaesthesia on the vagal component of bronchoconstriction produced by histamine aerosol in the anaesthetized dog, *Br J Pharmacol* 61:251, 1977.

167. Skoogh B-E et al: Barbiturates depress vagal motor pathway to ferret trachea at ganglia, *J Appl Physiol* 53:253, 1982.

168. Holtzman MJ et al: Selective effect of general anesthetics on reflex bronchoconstrictor responses in dogs, *J Appl Physiol* 53:126, 1982.

169. Fletcher SW, Flacke W, Alper MH: The actions of general anesthetic agents on tracheal smooth muscle, *Anesthesiology* 29:517, 1968.

170. Edney SM, Downes H: Contractor effect of barbiturates on smooth muscle, *Arch Int Pharmacodyn Ther* 217:180, 1975.

171. Okumura F, Denborough MA: Effects of anaesthetics on guinea pig tracheal smooth muscle, *Br J Anaesth* 52:199, 1980.

172. Lenox WC, Mitzner W, Hirshman CA: Mechanism of thiopental-induced constriction of guinea pig trachea, *Anesthesiology* 72:921, 1990.

173. Curry C et al: Contractile responses of guinea pig trachea to oxybarbiturates and thiobarbiturates, *Anesthesiology* 75:679, 1991.

174. Clarke RSJ et al: Adverse reactions to intravenous anaesthetics, *Br J Anaesth* 47:575, 1975.

175. Wilson LE, Hatch DJ, Rehder K: Mechanisms of the relaxant action of ketamine on isolated porcine trachealis muscle, *Br J Anaesth* 71:544, 1993.

176. Pedersen CM, Thirstrup S, Nielsen-Kudsk JE: Smooth muscle relaxant effects of propofol and ketamine in isolated guinea-pig trachea, *Eur J Pharmacol* 238:75, 1993.

177. Hirshman CA et al: Ketamine block of bronchospasm in experimental canine asthma, *Br J Anaesth* 51:713, 1979.

178. Rock MJ et al: Use of ketamine in asthmatic children to treat respiratory failure refractory to conventional therapy, *Crit Care Med* 14:514, 1986.

179. Fisher MM: Ketamine hydrochloride in severe bronchospasm, *Anaesthesia* 32:771, 1977.

180. Jahangir SM, Islam F, Aziz L: Ketamine infusion for postoperative analgesia in asthmatics: a comparison with intermittent meperidine, *Anesth Analg* 76:45, 1993.

181. Wilkins CJ et al: Comparison of the anesthetic requirement for tolerance of laryngeal mask airway and endotracheal tube, *Anesth Analg* 75:794, 1992.

182. Mehr EH, Lindeman KS: Effects of halothane, propofol, and thiopental on peripheral airway reactivity, *Anesthesiology* 79:290, 1993.

183. Siler JN, Mager JG Jr, Wyche MQ Jr: Atracurium: hypotension, tachycardia and bronchospasm, *Anesthesiology* 62:645, 1985.

184. Simpson DA, Wright DJ, Hammond JE: Influence of tubocurarine, pancuronium and atracurium on bronchomotor tone, *Br J Anaesth* 57:753, 1985.

185. Crago RR et al: Respiratory flow resistance after curare and pancuronium measured by forced oscillations, *Can Anaesth Soc J* 19:607, 1972.

186. Gerbershagan HU, Bergman NA: The effect of d-tubocurarine on respiratory resistance in anesthetized man, *Anesthesiology* 28:981, 1967.

187. Koga Y et al: Mechanism of tracheal constriction by succinylcholine, *Anesthesiology* 55:138, 1981.

188. Kaise A et al: Succinylcholine potentiates responses to intravenous acetylcholine in the canine lung periphery, *J Appl Physiol* 69:1137, 1990.

189. Matthews MD, Ceglarski JZ, Pabari M: Anaphylaxis to suxamethonium—a case report, *Anaesth Intensive Care* 5:235, 1977.

190. Katz AM, Mulligan PG: Bronchospasm induced by suxamethonium: a case report, *Br J Anaesth* 44:1097, 1972.

191. Bele-Binda N, Valeri F: A case of bronchospasm induced by succinylcholine, *Can Anaesth Soc J* 18:116, 1971.

192. Hammond J, Wright D, Sale J: Pattern of change of bronchomotor tone following reversal of neuromuscular blockade: comparison between atropine and glycopyrrolate, *Br J Anaesth* 55:955, 1983.

193. Toda N, Hatano Y: Contractile responses of canine tracheal muscle during exposure to fentanyl and morphine, *Anesthesiology* 53:93, 1980.

194. Eschenbacher WL et al: Morphine sulfate inhibits bronchoconstriction in subjects with mild asthma whose responses are inhibited by atropine, *Am Rev Respir Dis* 130:363, 1984.

195. Yasuda I et al: Tracheal constriction by morphine and by fentanyl in man, *Anesthesiology* 49:117, 1978.

196. Cigarini I et al: Comparison of the effects of fentanyl on respiratory mechanics under propofol or thiopental anaesthesia, *Acta Anaesthesiol Scand* 34:253, 1990.

197. Cohendy R et al: Effect of fentanyl on ventilatory resistances during barbiturate general anaesthesia, *Br J Anaesth* 69:595, 1992.

198. Tamaoki J, Graf PD, Nadel JA: Effect of gamma-aminobutyric acid on neurally mediated contraction of guinea-pig trachealis smooth muscle, *J Pharmacol Exp Ther* 243:86, 1987.

199. Koga Y et al: Comparison of the relaxant effects of diazepam, flunitrazepam and midazolam on airway smooth muscle, *Br J Anaesth* 69:65, 1992.

200. Haxhiu MA et al: Benzodiazepines acting on ventral surface of medulla cause airway dilation, *Am J Physiol* 257:R810, 1989.

201. Downes H, Gerber N, Hirshman CA: I.V. lignocaine in reflex and allergic bronchoconstriction, *Br J Anaesth* 52:873, 1980.

202. Downes H, Hirshman CA, Leon DA: Comparison of local anesthetics as bronchodilator aerosols, *Anesthesiology* 58:216, 1983.

203. Downes H, Loehning RW: Local anesthetic contracture and relaxation of airway smooth muscle, *Anesthesiology* 47:430, 1977.

204. Kai T et al: Effects of lidocaine on intracellular Ca^{2+} and tension in airway smooth muscle, *Anesthesiology* 78:954, 1993.

205. Brandus V et al: Bronchial spasm during general anaesthesia, *Can Anaesth Soc J* 17:269, 1970.

206. Downes H, Hirshman CA: Lidocaine aerosols do not prevent allergic bronchoconstriction, *Anesth Analg* 60:28, 1981.

207. Miller WC, Awe R: Effect of nebulized lidocaine on reactive airways, *Am Rev Respir Dis* 111:739, 1975.

208. Fish JE, Peterman VI: Effects of inhaled lidocaine on airway function in asthmatic subjects, *Respiration* 37:201, 1979.

209. McAlpine LG, Thomson NC: Lidocaine-induced bronchoconstriction in asthmatic patients: relation to histamine airway responsiveness and effect of preservative, *Chest* 96:1012, 1989.

210. Prakash GS, Sharm SK, Pande JN: Effect of 4% lidocaine inhalation in bronchial asthma, *J Asthma* 27:81, 1990.

211. Barnes PJ: Histamine receptors in the lung, *Agents Actions* 33:103, 1991.

212. Cookson WOCM: Bronchodilator action of the anti-histaminic terfenadine, *Br J Clin Pharmacol* 24:120, 1987.

213. Tashkin DP et al: Effect of orally administered cimetidine on histamine- and antigen-induced bronchospasm in subjects with asthma, *Am Rev Respir Dis* 125:691, 1982.

214. Nathan RA et al: The effects of H_1 and H_2 antihistamines on histamine inhalation challenges in asthmatic patients, *Am Rev Respir Dis* 120:1251, 1979.

215. Eiser NM et al: The role of histamine receptors in asthma, *Clin Sci* 60:363, 1981.

216. Nogrady SG, Bevan C: H2 receptor blockade and bronchial hyperreactivity to histamine in asthma, *Thorax* 36:268, 1981.

217. O'Cain CF et al: Pattern and mechanism of airway response to hypocapnia in normal subjects, *J Appl Physiol* 47:8, 1979.

218. Severinghaus JW et al: Unilateral hypoventilation produced in dogs by occluding one pulmonary artery, *J Appl Physiol* 16:53, 1961.

219. Wray S: Smooth muscle intracellular pH: measurement, regulation and function, *Am J Physiol* 254:C213, 1988.

220. Domino KB et al: Effect of inspired CO_2 on ventilation and perfusion heterogeneity in hyperventilated dogs, *J Appl Physiol* 75:1306, 1993.

221. Lau H-P et al: Halothane alters the response of isolated airway smooth muscle to carbon dioxide, *Respir Physiol* 87:255, 1992.

222. Coon RL, Kampine JP: Hypocapnic bronchoconstriction and inhalation anesthetics, *Anesthesiology* 43:635, 1975.

223. Nadel JA, Widdicombe JG: Effect of changes in blood gas tensions and carotid sinus pressure on tracheal volume and total lung resistance to airflow, *J Physiol* 163:13, 1962.

224. Twort CHC, Cameron IR: Effects of P_{CO_2}, pH and extracellular calcium on contraction of airway smooth muscle from rats, *Respir Physiol* 66:259, 1986.

225. Sterling GM, Holst PE, Nadel JA: Effect of CO_2 and pH on bronchoconstriction caused by serotonin vs acetylcholine, *J Appl Physiol* 32:39, 1972.

226. Wetzel RC et al: Hypoxic bronchodilation, *J Appl Physiol* 73:1202, 1992.

227. Lindeman KS et al: Role of potassium channels in hypoxic relaxation of porcine bronchi in vitro, *Am J Physiol* 266:L232, 1994.

228. D'Brot J, Ahmed T: Hypoxia-induced enhancement of nonspecific bronchial reactivity: role of leukotrienes, *J Appl Physiol* 65:194, 1988.

229. Gaston B et al: The biology of nitrogen oxides in the airways, *Am J Respir Crit Care Med* 149:538, 1994.

230. Gustafsson LE et al: Endogenous nitric oxide is present in the exhaled air of rabbits, guinea pigs and humans, *Biochem Biophys Res Commun* 181:852, 1991.

231. Jorens PG et al: L-arginine-dependent production of nitrogen oxides by rat pulmonary macrophages, *Eur J Pharmacol* 200:205, 1991.

232. Goldstein JA: Nitroglycerin therapy of asthma, *Chest* 85:449, 1984.

233. Gruetter CA et al: Comparison of relaxation induced by glyceryl trinitrate, isosorbide dinitrate, and sodium nitroprusside in bovine airways, *Am Rev Respir Dis* 139:1192, 1989.

234. Jansen A et al: The relaxant properties in guinea pig airways of S-nitrosothiols, *J Pharmacol Exp Ther* 261:154, 1992.

235. Belvisi MG, Stretton D, Barnes PJ: Nitric oxide as an endogenous modulator of cholinergic neurotransmission in guinea-pig airways, *Eur J Pharmacol* 198:219, 1991.

236. Belvisi MG et al: Nitric oxide is the endogenous neurotransmitter of bronchodilator nerves in humans, *Eur J Pharmacol* 210:221, 1992.

237. Dupuy PM et al: Bronchodilator action of inhaled nitric oxide in guinea pigs, *J Clin Invest* 90:421, 1992.

238. Högman M et al: Inhalation of nitric oxide modulates adult human bronchial tone, *Am Rev Respir Dis* 148:1474, 1993.

239. Shore SA, Romero L: Effect of a nitric oxide synthase inhibitor on bronchoconstriction induced by intravenous histamine, *Am Rev Respir Dis* 147:A445, 1993.

240. Frostell C et al: Inhaled nitric oxide: a selective pulmonary vasodilator reversing hypoxic pulmonary vasoconstriction, *Circulation* 83:2038, 1991.

241. Rossaint R et al: Inhaled nitric oxide for the adult respiratory distress syndrome, *N Engl J Med* 328:399, 1993.

242. Pepke-Zaba J et al: Inhaled nitric oxide as a cause of selective pulmonary vasodilatation in pulmonary hypertension, *Lancet* 338:1173, 1991.

243. Morrow PE: Toxicological data on NO_x: an overview, *J Toxicol Environ Health* 13:205, 1984.

244. Gaston B et al: Expired nitric oxide (NO) concentrations are elevated in patients with reactive airways disease, *Endothelium* 1:87, 1993.

245. Hirshman CA, Bergman NA: Factors influencing intrapulmonary airway calibre during anaesthesia, *Br J Anaesth* 65:30, 1990.

246. Gal TJ: Bronchial hyperresponsiveness and anesthesia: physiologic and therapeutic perspectives, *Anesth Analg* 78:559, 1994.

247. Brain JD, Valberg PA: Deposition of aerosol in the respiratory tract, *Am Rev Respir Dis* 120:1325, 1979.

248. Dolovich M et al: Clinical evaluation of simple demand inhalation MDI aerosol delivery device, *Chest* 84:36, 1983.

249. Kim CS, Eldridge MA, Sackner MA: Oropharyngeal deposition and delivery aspects of metered-dose inhaler aerosols, *Am Rev Respir Dis* 135:157, 1987.

250. Newman SP et al: Deposition of pressurised aerosols in the human respiratory tract, *Thorax* 36:52, 1981.

251. Bishop MJ, Larson RP, Buschman DL: Metered dose inhaler aerosol characteristics are affected by the endotracheal tube actuator/adapter used, *Anesthesiology* 73:1263, 1990.

252. Fuller HD et al: Pressurized aerosol versus jet aerosol delivery to mechanically ventilated patients, *Am Rev Respir Dis* 141:440, 1990.

253. Thomas SHL et al: Delivery of ultrasonic nebulized aerosols to a lung model during mechanical ventilation, *Am Rev Respir Dis* 148:872, 1993.

254. O'Doherty MJ et al: Delivery of a nebulized aerosol to a lung model during mechanical ventilation, *Am Rev Respir Dis* 146:383, 1992.

255. Crogan SJ, Bishop MJ: Delivery efficiency of metered dose aerosols given via endotracheal tubes, *Anesthesiology* 70:1008, 1989.

256. Forrest JB, Rehder K, Cahalan MK et al: Multicenter study of general anesthesia. III. Predictors of severe perioperative adverse outcomes, *Anesthesiology* 76:3, 1992.

257. Cheek DBC et al: Aminophylline does not inhibit bronchoconstriction during halothane anesthesia, *Anesthesiology* 65:A270, 1986.

258. Tobias JD, Hirshman CA: Attenuation of histamine-induced airway constriction by albuterol during halothane anesthesia, *Anesthesiology* 72:105, 1990.

Chapter 5

PHYSIOLOGIC AND PATHOPHYSIOLOGIC RESPONSES TO INTUBATION

Michael J. Bishop
Robert F. Bedford
Hae K. Kil

I. INTRODUCTION

Manipulation of the airway, particularly laryngoscopy and endotracheal intubation, alters cardiovascular and respiratory physiology both via reflex responses and by the physical presence of an endotracheal tube (ET). While the reflex responses may be of short duration and of little consequence in the majority of patients, they may produce serious complications in patients with underlying abnormalities, such as coronary artery disease,[1,2] reactive airways,[3,4] or intracranial neuropathology.[5,6]

II. CARDIOVASCULAR RESPONSES DURING AIRWAY MANIPULATION

A. THE CARDIOVASCULAR REFLEXES

Both the sympathetic and parasympathetic nervous systems mediate cardiovascular responses to endotracheal intubation. Bradycardia, often elicited in infants and small children during laryngoscopy or intubation, is the autonomic equivalent of the laryngospasm response. While only rarely seen in adults, this reflex results from an increase in vagal tone at the sinoatrial node and is virtually a monosynaptic response to a noxious stimulus in the airway.

In adults and adolescents, the more common responses to endotracheal intubation are hypertension and tachycardia, mediated by sympathetic efferents via the cardioaccelerator nerves and sympathetic chain ganglia. The polysynaptic nature of the pathways from the vagal and glossopharyngeal afferents to the sympathetic nervous system via the brain stem and spinal cord results in a diffuse autonomic response that includes widespread release of norepinephrine from adrenergic nerve terminals and secretion of epinephrine from the adrenal medulla. Some of the hypertensive response to endotracheal intubation also results from activation of the renin-angiotensin system, with release of renin from the renal juxtaglomerular apparatus, an end-organ innervated by β-adrenergic nerve terminals.

In addition to activation of the autonomic nervous system, endotracheal intubation stimulates central nervous system activity, as evidenced by increases in electroencephalographic activity, cerebral metabolic rate, and cerebral blood flow (CBF). In patients with compromised intracranial compliance, the increase in CBF may result in elevated intracranial pressure (ICP), which, in turn, may result in herniation of brain contents and severe neurologic compromise.

The effects of endotracheal intubation on the pulmonary vasculature are probably less well understood than the responses elicited in the systemic circulation. They are often coupled with changes in airway reactivity associated with intubation. Thus, acute bronchospasm or a mainstem bronchial intubation will result in a marked maldistribution of perfusion to poorly ventilated lung units (in these situations hyper-expanded lungs have higher pulmonary vascular resistance than poorly ventilated lungs), causing desaturation of pulmonary venous blood and subsequent reduction in systemic arterial oxygen tension. In addition, institution of positive end-expiratory pressure following endotracheal intubation causes a reduction in cardiac output due to impaired venous return to the left heart from the pulmonary circulation. The impact of these changes can be profound in patients with severely compromised myocardial function or intravascular volume depletion.

B. INTUBATION IN THE PRESENCE OF CARDIOVASCULAR DISEASE

The neuroendocrine responses to endotracheal intubation that lead to hypertension and tachycardia can cause a variety of complications in patients with cardiac disease. Probably the most common adverse cardiovas-

cular problem related to intubation is myocardial ischemia in patients with coronary artery insufficiency. Since two of the major determinants of myocardial oxygen demand are heart rate and blood pressure,[2] the increase in myocardial oxygen demand created by the hypertensive-tachycardic response to endotracheal intubation must be met by an increase in the flow of oxygenated blood through the coronary circulation. However, when one or more occlusive coronary lesions result in relatively fixed coronary blood flow, the ability to increase myocardial blood flow during periods of increased demand is minimal, and an abrupt increase in myocardial oxygen demand can result in tissue ischemia that may lead either to myocardial dysfunction or to overt tissue infarction. Furthermore, ischemia induced by arterial hypertension may be compounded by an increase in left ventricular end-diastolic pressure, resulting in further compromise of perfusion to subendocardial tissues. This set of circumstances is responsible for episodes of electrocardiogram (ECG) ST segment depression and increased pulmonary artery diastolic pressure that may be seen when endotracheal intubation is performed in patients with arteriosclerosis; occasionally, these episodes presage the occurrence of a perioperative myocardial infarction.[2]

Patients with vascular anomalies that cause weakening of the lining of major arteries are also at risk during endotracheal intubation. In particular, the integrity of cerebral and aortic aneurysms is largely a function of transmural pressure. A sudden increase in blood pressure can lead to rupture of the affected vessel and abrupt deterioration in the patient's status. Leaking aortic aneurysms are partially tamponaded by intraabdominal pressure but can suddenly expand into the retroperitoneal space during arterial hypertension. This results both in significant blood loss for the anesthesiologist to replace and additional technical problems for the surgeon trying to resect the lesion and insert a vascular prosthesis.

C. IMPLICATIONS FOR PATIENTS WITH NEUROVASCULAR DISEASE

Intracranial aneurysms often present with a small "sentinel hemorrhage" that serves as a warning of worse things to come. These lesions are prone to rebleed, particularly in the face of elevated arterial pressure, resulting in sudden and permanent neurologic injury. Many neurosurgeons operate on these lesions early after hospitalization, specifically in an effort to minimize the risks of rebleeding. The risk of this approach, however, is that the patient comes to the operating room at a time when the clot tamponading the aneurysmal rupture is particularly delicate. Thus, even a small increase in arterial transmural pressure may result in a devastating rebleed. During the course of neurosurgical anesthesia, this is most likely to occur when arterial pressure and pulse rate increase in response to endotracheal intubation.[4]

D. INTUBATION IN NEUROPATHOLOGIC DISORDERS

Reflex responses to endotracheal intubation are also a potential hazard to patients with compromised intracranial compliance resulting from neuropathologic processes. Uncontrolled coughing can result in a marked increase in intrathoracic and intraabdominal pressure that may result in a transient increase in cerebrospinal fluid (CSF) pressure and impairment of cerebral perfusion (CPP). In patients with impaired cerebral autoregulation (brain trauma, cerebrovascular accidents, neoplasms) the normal tendency for cerebral blood flow (CBF) to remain constant over the mean blood pressure from 50 to 150 mm Hg is lost. When endotracheal intubation causes an increase in arterial pressure, there is a marked increase in CBF and cerebral blood volume, which, in turn, can cause dangerous increases in ICP.[5] This effect is magnified by the fact that noxious stimuli such as airway manipulation result in increased CBF, which summates with the hypertensive blood pressure response to cause occasional profound increases in ICP (Fig. 5-1).

E. NEUROMUSCULAR BLOCKING DRUGS AND CARDIOVASCULAR RESPONSES

Endotracheal intubation is infrequently performed in the absence of neuromuscular blockade. Accordingly, it is appropriate to consider the cardiovascular and cerebrovascular responses to the administration of the neuromuscular blocking agents that are given to facilitate the process. Indeed, the hypertensive-tachycardic response to endotracheal intubation was not identified[7] until neuromuscular blocking agents were introduced into clinical practice because, before this time, intubation was only performed under such deep levels of anesthesia that there was relatively little cardiovascular response generated.

The depressor effects of d-tubocurarine and, to a lesser extent, metocurine, atracurium, and mivacurium, are known to be mediated by histamine release. On one hand, this effect could be looked upon as a potential antagonist to the pressor response to endotracheal intubation. In the case of patients at risk for intracranial hypertension, however, histamine-induced cerebral vasodilation may produce increases in ICP even as the blood pressure falls.[8] Pancuronium, on the other hand, is capable of initiating a hyperdynamic cardiovascular state that may potentiate the usual cardiovascular responses seen following endotracheal intubation in lightly anesthetized patients.

At the present time, succinylcholine is the muscle relaxant used most commonly to facilitate endotracheal intubation. Although occasionally associated with bradycardia in children, it is a cardiovascular stimulant in adults. This phenomenon is often associated with activation of the electroencephalogram (EEG)[9] and patients with brain tumors may sustain marked increases in ICP following succinylcholine,[10] particularly when intracranial compliance is compromised and cerebrovascular autoregulation is impaired. Studies in dogs suggest that succinylcholine increases afferent central nervous system (CNS) input as a result of activation of muscle spindles at the time of muscle fasciculations.[11] These studies suggest that, unless defasciculating doses of nondepolarizing agents are used to counteract the effects of succinylcholine, there is likely to be augmentation of the adverse cardiovascular and cerebrovascular effects of endotracheal intubation whenever succinylcholine is used to facilitate airway manipulation.

F. CARDIOPULMONARY CONSEQUENCES OF POSITIVE PRESSURE VENTILATION

Immediately following endotracheal intubation under general anesthesia, positive pressure ventilation is instituted, usually because complete neuromuscular blockade has been previously induced. Positive pressure ventilation results in an increase in mean intrathoracic pressure, which, in turn, impairs cardiac filling and results in a decrease in cardiac output and arterial pressure. Patients with decreased intravascular volume or impaired myocardial contractility are particularly sensitive to this phenomenon, and it is not at all uncommon for a patient to become acutely hypotensive shortly after endotracheal intubation and institution of

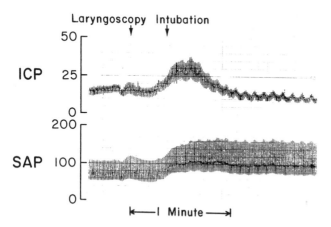

Fig. 5-1. Increases in systemic arterial pressure *(SAP)* and intracranial pressure *(ICP)* in response to endotracheal intubation in patient with a small brain tumor. Note minimal response to rigid laryngoscopy. With intubation there is sustained increase in SAP but only transient increase in ICP, which returns to normal as cerebrovascular autoregulation becomes operative. (From Bedford RF: Circulatory responses to tracheal intubation, *Problems in Anesthesia* 2:201, 1988.

positive pressure ventilation. In some instances, the hypotension is aggravated by intravascular volume depletion secondary to surgical bowel preparation or vigorous diuretic therapy. In other cases, the hypovolemia may be part of the disease process that has brought the patient to the operating room, that is, active bleeding or extravascular fluid accumulation in the peritoneal cavity. Thus, one common clinical scenario is a patient who may respond to endotracheal intubation with a brisk increase in blood pressure and who then suddenly develops acute hypotension as positive pressure ventilation is instituted. In such a case, rapid use of the head-down position to augment venous return, discontinuation of potent anesthetic agent, and prompt instillation of appropriate vascular volume expanders usually suffices to correct the situation. Patients with suspected coronary artery disease may respond more favorably to judicious administration of an α-adrenergic agent, such as phenylephrine, which may increase diastolic pressure and maintain coronary filling pressures. Usually, the adrenergic stimulus of the surgical incision will then suffice to maintain arterial pressure for the duration of the operation.

III. PREVENTION OF CARDIOVASCULAR RESPONSES

A. DEPTH OF ANESTHESIA

In the era prior to the introduction of neuromuscular blocking agents, the hypertensive-tachycardic response to endotracheal intubation was unknown, probably because patients were only intubated under deep cyclopropane or diethyl ether anesthesia and their cardiovascular responses were obtunded. Shortly after the introduction of d-tubocurarine, however, it was recognized that simply increasing anesthetic depth afforded considerable protection from these responses.[8]

The anesthetic dose that blocks the hemodynamic and ICP responses to endotracheal stimulation has remained elusive. In the case of etomidate, it appears to be a dose that results in cerebral metabolic depression as indicated by a burst-suppression pattern on the EEG.[12] Since etomidate supports blood pressure at such deep levels of anesthesia, it is probably the only contemporary agent that, by itself, can achieve suppression of cardiovascular responses to intubation without first producing undue arterial hypotension and compromise of coronary and cerebral perfusion. By contrast, barbiturates, propofol, and benzodiazepines all have been shown to cause profound hypotension at doses that suppress the hemodynamic and ICP responses to intubation.[13,14,15]

With regard to inhalational anesthetics, endotracheal intubation in the minimum alveolar concentration (1-MAC) dose range results in marked cardiovascular stimulation during halothane-nitrous oxide (N_2O) and N_2O-morphine anesthetic techniques.[16] In contrast, N_2O-enflurane and N_2O-fentanyl-droperidol techniques prevented increases above awake control values, although increases in blood pressure occurred above the values determined just before intubation. It should not be surprising that 1-MAC is insufficient, since it is known that approximately 1.5 to 1.6 MAC is needed to block the adrenergic and cardiovascular responses to a simple surgical incision.[17] However, the dose of anesthetic required to prevent coughing during endotracheal intubation, "MAC-ei," is approximately 30% greater than the traditional value of MAC for halothane and enflurane.[18,19] In the case of sevoflurane, however, MAC-ei may exceed MAC by a factor of 2.86.[20] By extrapolation, then, if "MAC-bar-ei" were 50% greater than MAC-ei, the dose of volatile anesthetic required to block the cardiovascular response to endotracheal intubation would be an inordinately deep level of inhalational anesthetic that results in profound cardiovascular depression prior to endotracheal intubation.[21]

From a cerebrovascular point of view, this approach is totally impractical, since high doses of volatile anesthetics cause cerebral vasodilation and marked increases in intracranial pressure in patients with compromised intracranial compliance. Furthermore, from a cardiovascular point of view, the arterial hypotension induced before intubation would be entirely unacceptable for all but the most fit patients.

Since it is impractical to achieve a sufficient depth of inhalational anesthetic for preventing a hyperdynamic response to intubation, a variety of adjuvants have been utilized to potentiate the light anesthetic techniques currently in vogue. Fentanyl appears to give a graded response to blunting hemodynamic responses: 2 μg/kg intravenous (IV) only partially prevents hypertension and tachycardia during a rapid-sequence intubation after thiopental and succinylcholine; 6 μg/kg is considerably more effective in this situation.[22] Chen et al.[23] noted almost complete suppression of hemodynamic response to intubation at both 11 and 15 μg/kg of IV fentanyl, whereas higher doses (30 to 75 μg/kg IV) allowed only a very occasional response to intubation. In doses that prevent hemodynamic response to intubation, however, fentanyl is not a short-acting agent, and the risk of prolonged postoperative respiratory depression must be weighed against the advantages of perioperative cardiovascular stability. Alfentanil has a smaller steady-state distribution volume and a resultant shorter terminal elimination half-life than fentanyl.[24] Ausems et al.[25] demonstrated that an alfentanil plasma concentration of 600 ng/ml effectively prevented hemodynamic responses to intubation during induction of nitrous oxide anesthesia. This was achieved by a 30-second infusion of alfentanil, 150 μg/kg, followed by a 1.5 to 2.5 min infusion at 50 μg/kg/hr. During this induction period, nitrous oxide and succinylcholine were also adminis-

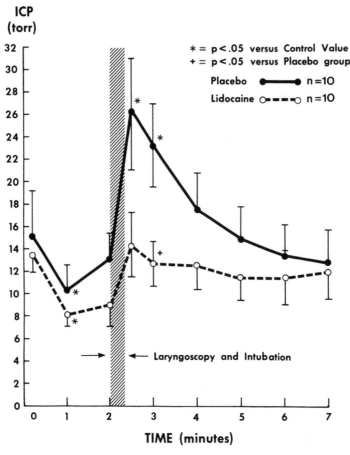

Fig. 5-2. Impact of IV lidocaine 1.5 mg/kg on ICP response to tracheal intubation in brain tumor patients after a rapid-sequence intubation with thiopental 3 mg/kg IV, and succinylcholine 1.5 mg/kg IV. (From Bedford RF et al: Lidocaine prevents increased ICP after endotracheal intubation. In Shulman K, Marmarou A, Miller JD, et al, editors: *Intracranial Pressure IV,* 1980, Berlin, Springer-Verlag.)

tered. Only 5 of the 35 patients sustained an increase in heart rate or blood pressure greater than 15% above preinduction values.

B. INTRAVENOUS LIDOCAINE

Intravenously administered lidocaine is another drug that has long been known to be an effective suppressant of the cough reflex.[26,27] When given in a bolus of 1.5 mg/kg, it adds approximately 0.3 MAC of anesthetic potency.[28] Significant reductions in hemodynamic response to endotracheal intubation have been noted when lidocaine (3 mg/kg) was used as an adjunct to morphine[29] or fentanyl[30] anesthesia and during other light anesthetic techniques such as thiopental nitrous oxide-oxygen-(N_2O-O_2).[31]

The general anesthetic properties of lidocaine tend to reduce cerebral metabolic rate for oxygen and CBF, thus lowering intracranial pressure in patients with compromised intracranial compliance.[32] Furthermore, lidocaine effectively prevents increases in intracranial pressure when used as an adjunct prior to endotracheal intuba-

tion in patients prone to intracranial hypertension[33] (Fig. 5-2).

C. TOPICAL AND NERVE BLOCK ANESTHESIA

Topical anesthesia to the upper airway is also effective in blunting hemodynamic responses to endotracheal intubation[34,35] but, almost invariably, topical anesthesia of the airway has proven to be less effective than systemic administration of lidocaine. During general anesthesia, rigid laryngoscopy and instillation of lidocaine solution initiates the same adverse reflexes caused by placement of an ET[36] (Figs. 5-3 and 5-4). Furthermore, laryngotracheal spray of lidocaine solution may, in itself, produce profound cardiovascular stimulation in adults,[37] or, in children, it may produce the same sort of bradycardic response associated with endotracheal intubation.[38]

While topical anesthesia of the airway appears to be of little benefit, regional nerve blocks involving the sensory pathways from the airway are capable of preventing hemodynamic responses to intubation.

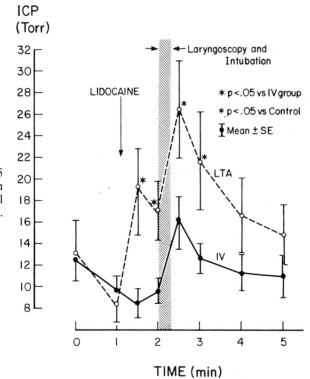

Fig. 5-3. Comparison of effects of IV and intratracheal lidocaine 1.5 mg/kg on ICP response to laryngoscopy and endotracheal intubation in 22 brain tumor patients. Note early elevation of ICP from intratracheal lidocaine instillation followed by augmented response from intubation. (From Hamill JF et al: *Anesthesiology* 55:578, 1981.)

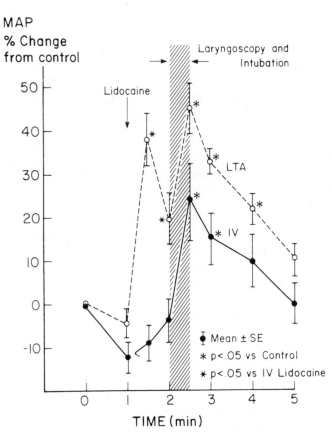

Fig. 5-4. Mean arterial pressure *(MAP)* response to endotracheal intubation after either IV or intratracheal lidocaine instillation, as in Fig. 5-3. (From Hamill JF et al: *Anesthesiology* 55:578, 1981.)

Blockade of the superior laryngeal nerve is the most common method of blunting hemodynamic responses to endotracheal intubation using regional anesthesia. With a deposit of local anesthetic on each cornu of the hyoid bone, awake patients will not only tolerate an ET well, but they will exhibit little response as the ET is inserted. Blockade of the glossopharyngeal nerve (sensory distribution above the level of the epiglottis) potentiates this effect by decreasing the stimulus of laryngoscopy.[39]

Excellent topical anesthesia of the airway performed before awake flexible fiberoptic endotracheal intubation was responsible for reports suggesting that there was less cardiovascular stimulation after this procedure than after intubation with a rigid laryngoscope.[40] Subsequent studies performed under general anesthesia, however, have demonstrated that there is no difference between the two modes of intubation with regard to hemodynamic impact.[41,42,43,44]

D. INTRAVENOUS VASOACTIVE DRUGS

A final means for modifying the cardiovascular responses to endotracheal intubation is to administer vasoactive substances that impact directly on the cardiovascular system. This approach was introduced by DeVault et al.[45] who found that pretreatment with phentolamine, 5 mg IV, prevented the hypertensive and tachycardic response to endotracheal intubation during light barbiturate-succinylcholine anesthetic technique. Subsequently, a large number of articles have appeared advocating the use of both vasodilators and adrenergic blocking agents as pretreatment before endotracheal intubation. Among those described are hydralazine,[46] nitroprusside,[47] nitroglycerin,[48] labetalol,[49] esmolol,[50] and clonidine.[51] Virtually all of these agents appear to be effective when compared to placebo. However, no meaningful studies have been done to date comparing the efficacy of these vasoactive agents against each other; thus, an optimal agent cannot be recommended at this time.

With regard to the patient at risk for intracranial hypertension, it is important that agents used to control cardiovascular responses to intubation also have minimal adverse impact on ICP. During anesthetic induction, therefore, most neuroanesthetists use an IV sleep dose of barbiturate, propofol or etomidate, followed by small doses of opioid (fentanyl 1 to 2 μg/kg IV), IV lidocaine (1.5 mg/kg), and hyperventilation to a $PaCO_2$ of approximately 30 mm Hg while a paralyzing dose of nondepolarizing muscle relaxant takes effect. Often an adrenergic blocking agent such as labetalol (5 to 10 mg IV) is also given prior to endotracheal intubation. Agents that act as cerebral vasodilators, such as volatile anesthetics, nitroglycerin, nitroprusside, or hydralazine, are generally avoided if there is a serious risk of intracranial hypertension.

It should be emphasized that the hypertensive, tachycardic response to endotracheal intubation is a manifestation of light general anesthesia. The first line of prevention should be induction of a sufficient depth of anesthesia before endotracheal intubation is performed. Patients with ischemic coronary artery disease, arterial vascular anomalies, and compromised intracranial compliance require special management and meticulous hemodynamic monitoring in order to optimize their care during this most stressful of anesthetic procedures. (See also Chapter 4.)

IV. AIRWAY EFFECTS OF ENDOTRACHEAL INTUBATION

A. UPPER AIRWAY REFLEXES

Since the upper airway protects the respiratory gas exchange surface from noxious substances, it is appropriate that the nose, mouth, pharynx, larynx, trachea, and carina have an abundance of sensory nerve endings and brisk motor responses. Anesthesiologists are especially familiar with the glottic closure reflex (laryngospasm), which is invariably encountered early in their training. The sneeze, cough, and swallow reflexes are equally important upper airway reflexes.

Afferent pathways for laryngospasm and the cardiovascular responses to endotracheal intubation are initiated by the glossopharyngeal nerve when stimuli occur superior to the anterior surface of the epiglottis and by the vagus nerve when stimuli occur from the level of the posterior epiglottis down into the lower airway. Since the laryngeal closure reflex is mediated by vagal efferents to the glottis, it is virtually a monosynaptic response, occurring primarily when a patient is lightly anesthetized as vagally innervated sensory endings in the upper airway are stimulated and conscious respiratory efforts cannot override the reflex.

B. DEAD SPACE

Patients with severe chronic lung disease often find it easier to breathe following intubation or a tracheostomy. The improvement is most likely due to reduced dead space. The normal extrathoracic anatomic dead space, based on cadaver measurements, is approximately 70 to 75 ml.[52] The exact volume of the ET is easily calculated as the volume (V) of a cylinder using the formula $V = r^2 l$ where r is the radius of the tube and l is the length. Thus, an 8 mm inner diameter ET that is 25 cm in length will have a volume of 12.6 ml. Intubation would therefore result in a reduction in dead space of approximately 60 ml.

Tracheostomy tubes are shorter than oral ETs and have an even smaller dead space. In normal individuals, such a reduction in dead space is negligible compared to the normal tidal volume, thus offering little benefit. In a patient with severe restrictive lung disease, such as in end-stage kyphoscoliosis, tidal volume may be as low as 100 ml. Thus, intubation can confer a major benefit. Similarly, patients with emphysema changed from mouth breathing to tracheostomy demonstrate a reduction in minute volume required and a decrease in total body oxygen consumption, presumably due to a decreased work of breathing.[53] The decreased volume required likely more than compensates for the slight increase in resistance (see following).

The decreases in dead space described above refer only to the volume of the tracheal tube alone and would be applicable only during breathing when there is no additional apparatus dead space. Any extensions added to the breathing circuit and attached to the ET must also be added to the total.

C. UPPER AIRWAY RESISTANCE

Anesthesiologists are well aware that, in most anesthetized patients, adequate ventilation can be maintained with an ET as small as 6 mm inside diameter (ID) in place. Intensivists caring for a patient with respiratory failure, however, often insist that a minimum ET ID be 8 mm. It should be recognized that the above tube sizes are each appropriate for the clinical situations described. The high resistance of the 6 mm ET is inconsequential for the low minute ventilation (usually with positive pressure ventilation) required under general anesthesia. By contrast, the high flow rates required for patients with respiratory failure (who often have some spontaneous ventilation) may render the resistance of a small ET prohibitive.

The ET creates a mechanical burden for a spontaneously breathing patient in the form of a fixed upper airway resistance, since it decreases airway caliber and increases resistance to breathing. Gas flow across an ET is determined by the pressure difference across the tube and the resistance of the ET. Gas flows whenever there is a pressure difference across the ET, whether caused by subatmospheric pressure generated during spontaneous breathing or by positive pressure generated from a mechanical ventilator.

The apparent resistance of an ET is influenced both by the shape of the tube and by two types of friction: the friction among the gas molecules, and the friction between the tube wall and the gas molecules.[54,55] Irregular surfaces created by secretions or by ridges from wire reinforcement may create greater friction and greater resistance.[56] Tracheal tubes or tracheostomies have a higher resistance than the normal upper respiratory tract.[57,58] The relationship between pressure difference and flow rate depends on the nature of the flow: laminar, turbulent, or a mixture of the two. In an ET, turbulent flow predominates. During turbulent flow, the measured resistance is not a constant but will vary with flow rate, becoming markedly higher at high flow

rates. Instead of the laminar flow relationship of pressure being directly proportional to flow, the pressure required to move the gas through an ET with turbulent flow is proportional to the square of the flow. The relationship is thus described by a parabolic curve as in Fig. 5-5. The apparent resistance of a tube is proportional to the fourth power of the radius during laminar flow (Poiseuille's law), but the fifth power during turbulent flow. Assuming turbulent flow, the relative resistance of a 6 mm ET versus an 8 mm ET would be $(4^5/3^5)$, or 4.2 times as great. However, as flow patterns are not entirely predictable, exact respiratory pressure-flow relationships may not be predictable without empiric determination. Such determinations are depicted in Fig. 5-5. The slope of the pressure-flow graph is the apparent resistance. The parabolic shape of the graphs demonstrates the primarily turbulent nature of the flow through an ET. Although the resistance of the ET may be several times greater than the resistance of the normal human upper airway, this is of relatively little consequence at low minute ventilation.[59] With a typical peak inspiratory flow of 25 to 30 L/min, approximately 0.5 cm H_2O pressure must be generated to overcome the resistance of the upper respiratory tract. This represents approximately 10% of the total work of breathing. Even a doubling or tripling of that resistance by placement of an ET does not result in a clinically worrisome increase in the total work of breathing.[60,61]

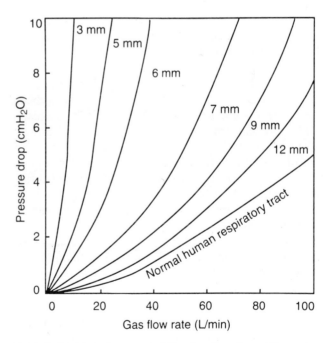

Fig. 5-5. Pressure drop across ETs of various sizes at flow rates from 0 to 100 L per minute. Note wide disparity between 6 mm and 7 mm tubes as flow rate increases to the range typically seen in respiratory failure patients. (From Nunn JF: *Applied respiratory physiology,* ed 3, Boston, 1987, Butterworths.)

As flow rates increase, however, flow becomes more turbulent, and then tube resistance may become a problem. For flow rates above 15 L/min, flow through any tube less than 10 mm diameter becomes turbulent.[62] At the high flows required by patients in respiratory failure, however, the resistance of smaller tubes becomes prohibitive.[63] At the time of weaning patients with respiratory failure from mechanical ventilation, the importance of tube size often becomes a critical factor, with a common question being whether to change from a 7 mm ET to an 8 mm ET. As Fig. 5-5 demonstrates, the difference between the two is negligible at flows below 40 L/min. At a flow of 60 L/min, however, the difference of 3 cm H_2O pressure becomes consequential. Furthermore, one should consider how much less is the resistance of the patient's own airway. Thus, if the patient is close to successful weaning, a more reasonable approach may be to attempt extubation rather than to change ETs. If not, pressure support ventilation might be used to compensate for the added work of breathing through the smaller tube until extubation is warranted.

Tracheostomy tubes have lower resistance than endotracheal tubes of comparable diameters because they are shorter. This difference is generally not of much consequence but may explain the anecdotal observation that patients being weaned from mechanical ventilation are sometimes more rapidly weaned after a tracheostomy is performed.

D. LOWER AIRWAY RESISTANCE

Bronchospasm following induction of anesthesia is a relatively uncommon but well-recognized event, often thought to be related to a reflex response to tracheal intubation. Several studies provide some evidence regarding the frequency of bronchospasm. The American Society of Anesthesiologists closed claims study has been reviewing malpractice claims since 1985. Adverse respiratory events were involved in 762 of 2046 claims, of which bronchospasm accounted for 2% of the cases.[64,65] Only half of the patients had a prior history of asthma or obstructive lung disease. Bronchospasm occurred during induction in 70% of the cases, further supporting the possibility that intubation is a trigger. Tiret et al. studied complications at the time of induction and noted that bronchospasm accounted for 5.3% of fatal or near fatal periinduction complications.[66] The study with the largest denominator was reported by Olsson[67] who noted 246 cases of bronchospasm out of a total of 136,929 for an incidence of 1.7/1000 anesthetics. However, the exact number undoubtedly depends substantially on the patient population.

While the incidence of overt clinical bronchospasm is low, a reflex increase in airway resistance may occur much more often. Receptors in the larynx and upper

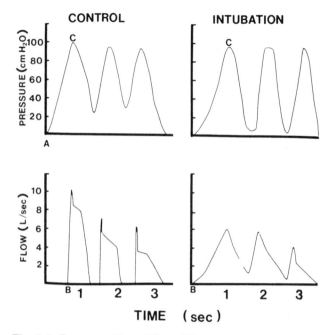

Fig. 5-6. Pressure *(A)* and flow *(B)* curves generated during burst of three successive coughs *(C)* by a volunteer prior to and following tracheal intubation. Note that flow and pressures generated are only modestly diminished following intubation. (From Gal TJ: *Problems in Anesthesia:* 2:191, 1988.)

trachea may cause large airway constriction distal to the tube, which, in turn, may extend to the smaller peripheral airways.[68] Support for this hypothesis comes from the work of Gal, who found an increase in lower airway resistance in a series of volunteers whose tracheas were intubated following topical anesthesia (Fig. 5-6).[69]

Bronchoconstriction also occurs following tracheal intubation of normal subjects who have received thiopental-narcotic anesthesia.[70] In a series of patients pretreated prior to anesthesia with either a β-adrenergic agonist (albuterol) or an inhaled anticholinergic agent (ipratropium bromide), measured airway resistance following intubation is markedly lower as compared to placebo treated patients (Fig. 5-7).

Increases in airway resistance may result from changes in intrinsic smooth muscle tone, airway edema, or intraluminal secretions. These factors are, in turn, controlled by a series of intracellular and extracellular events, including neural and hormonal factors. Rapid changes in airway caliber following airway instrumentation are thought to result largely from parasympathetic nervous system activation of airway smooth muscle.[71,72] Cholinergic innervation predominates in the larger central airways, with efferent nerves arising in the vagal nuclei of the brain stem and synapsing with ganglia in the airway walls. Postganglionic parasympathetic nerves release acetylcholine, activating muscarinic receptors on airway smooth muscle that lead to smooth muscle

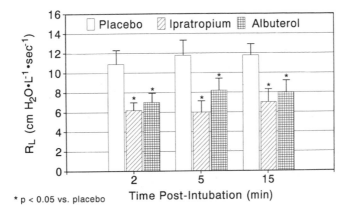

Fig. 5-7. Lung resistance at 2, 5, and 15 minutes following intubation in patients pretreated with either placebo, β-adrenergic agonist albuterol, or anticholinergic drug ipratropium bromide. Either drug markedly diminished lung resistance for at least 15 minutes following tracheal intubation under thiopental-narcotic anesthesia. (From Kil HK et al: *Anesthesiology* 81:43, 1994.)

constriction. Such responses can be blocked via muscarinic blockade, using either systemic or inhaled anticholinergic agents.

Tracheal intubation also may induce bronchospasm by causing coughing. A cough will reduce lung volume, which, in turn, markedly increases bronchoconstriction in response to a stimulus.[73] In the patient with known reactive airways, preventing coughing at the time of tracheal intubation by using either a deep level of anesthetic or a muscle relaxant may help to minimize the likelihood of bronchospasm.

E. THE ET RESISTANCE AND EXHALATION

In normal patients breathing at a moderately elevated minute ventilation, exhalation is usually completed well before the next inhalation begins. By contrast, patients with obstructive airways disease may not complete full exhalation prior to the start of the next inhalation. In this situation, inhalation begins before exhalation to functional residual capacity (FRC), resulting in persistent positive pressure in the alveoli. This phenomenon has been called auto positive end-expiratory pressure (auto-PEEP), or dynamic hyperinflation, and results in air trapping, elevated intrathoracic pressure, and hemodynamic compromise.[74]

Auto-PEEP most commonly occurs in patients with obstructive lung disease and high minute ventilation, but it may also rarely occur in patients with relatively normal airways who are ventilated at very high minute ventilation. This has been observed in patients with burns or sepsis who may require as much as 30 to 40 liters of minute ventilation. Under these circumstances, the resistance of the ET may limit expiratory flow so that full exhalation does not occur. This has been demonstrated experimentally, with the magnitude of the auto-PEEP

correlating directly with the resistance of the ET.[75] Under anesthesia, major resistance to exhalation by the ET is of no consequence in routine cases and is only rarely seen in critically ill patients. However, low levels of auto-PEEP due to tube resistance probably occur frequently in patients with high minute ventilation.[76]

F. FUNCTIONAL RESIDUAL CAPACITY

The effect of endotracheal intubation on FRC has been a subject of considerable controversy in recent years. Intensivists are well aware of patients recovering from respiratory failure in whom oxygenation has improved following extubation. The improvement has been attributed to "physiologic PEEP"—the presumption that there is normally a small positive pressure created by the glottis, which, in turn, leads to breathing at a higher lung volume. The assumption is that an ET removes the glottic barrier and may, therefore, lower lung volume. The existence of positive intratracheal pressure, however, has never been documented, and, in a study of volunteers who underwent awake intubation, no consistent change in FRC could be measured.[77,78,79]

By contrast, a different conclusion was reached in a series of patients just before and after extubation following recovery from respiratory failure. In this situation, both FRC and PaO$_2$ were found to increase following extubation, supporting the concept that the presence of an ET tends to decrease FRC.[80] Resolution of these disparate results is suggested by a rabbit study, where normal rabbits did not demonstrate a difference in oxygenation or tracheal pressure following intubation, but, after respiratory failure was induced, tracheal intubation worsened oxygenation.[81] These results suggest that the rabbits compensated for respiratory failure by using glottic closure to maintain a positive intratracheal pressure and that the effect of an ET on FRC depends on that underlying respiratory state. Based on this work, we suggest that routine addition of PEEP to increase FRC following intubation probably makes sense only when patients are suspected of breathing at a low lung volume prior to intubation.

G. COUGH

While it is widely recognized that cough efficiency is reduced whenever an ET is in place, it is a common observation that a disconnected ET is likely to produce a plug of sputum whenever the patient is stimulated to cough. In awake intubated volunteers, peak airway flow was reduced but still adequate to enable secretion clearance (Fig. 5-6).[82] The ET, however, prevented collapse of the trachea by acting as a stent. Thus, while secretions could be moved to the central airways, the ET prevented maximum efficiency of expectoration. Large airway collapse is important for producing maximum force against secretions, and this explains why moving secretions from the trachea out through the ET often requires assistance with a suction catheter.

H. HUMIDIFICATION OF GASES

Under normal circumstances, the upper airway warms, humidifies, and filters between 7000 and 10,000 L of inspired air daily, adding up to 1 L of moisture to the gases. When the upper airway is bypassed following intubation, the gas must be warmed and humidified in the trachea if it is not adequately humidified prior to inhalation. In an anesthetized patient breathing dry gases, up to 10% of the average metabolic rate may be required to perform these tasks.[83] Delivery of cool, dry gases may also have a significant effect on mucociliary transport, a critical defense mechanism of the respiratory tract. Inhalation of unconditioned gas rapidly leads to abnormal mucosal ciliary motion, with subsequent encrustation and inspissation of tracheal secretions.[84,85] These changes occur as early as 30 minutes following intubation and, theoretically, may lead to an increase in postoperative complications in patients with limited chest excursion. Accordingly, assurance of adequate gas conditioning should be standard in all but very brief tracheal intubations.

V. CONTROL AND TREATMENT OF THE RESPIRATORY RESPONSES TO INTUBATION
A. UPPER AIRWAY RESPONSES

Cough and laryngospasm in response to intubation appear to be sound protective reflexes by the body. Under most circumstances, the body needs to prevent further intrusion by a foreign body and to expel it from the airway. These responses can be troublesome, however, during induction of anesthesia or at the time of extubation. Cough can lead to bronchospasm as lung volume is reduced and can also result in desaturation as the lung volume drops to residual volume. Laryngospasm may result in life-threatening abnormalities of blood gases. Consequently, the anesthesiologist routinely will try to prevent these responses using medications delivered either topically, via inhalation, or intravenously.

1. Preventing upper airway reflexes

When intubation of the trachea takes place under deep anesthesia with muscle relaxants, no further obtundation of reflexes is usually needed. However, when circumstances prevent this, the clinician must give consideration to how best to prevent discomfort, gagging, coughing, and laryngospasm.

2. Regional and topical anesthesia

The surfaces of the mouth and/or nose are easily anesthetized with topical anesthetic sprays or gels. Lidocaine is equally effective as cocaine, is less toxic, and can be combined with a vasoconstrictor to give equivalent intubating conditions.[86,87,88] Administration of an antisialagogue 30 to 60 minutes prior to application of the topical anesthetic results in better anesthesia and better intubating conditions. The lack of secretions probably minimizes dilution of the applied anesthetic and also results in better intubating conditions.

The mouth and pharynx derive their sensory innervation from the trigeminal and glossopharyngeal nerves. Although nerve blocks can be used, they are not easy to perform and are far less comfortable for the patient than application of topical anesthesia.

The supraglottic larynx derives its sensory innervation from the superior laryngeal nerve (SLN), a branch of the vagus, and intubation can be facilitated by blocking it bilaterally.[89] The nerve block relies on the consistent relationship of the SLN to the lateral horns of the hyoid bone. When combined with topical anesthesia of the nose or mouth and adequate anesthesia of the infraglottic larynx, the nerve block provides excellent intubating conditions, and most patients will accept a tube without cough, gag, or laryngospasm. Despite the success of this block, the authors have largely abandoned its use because of equal success with careful spraying of the larynx with topical anesthesia. A nasal trumpet helps ensure that solution reaches the larynx. Topical anesthesia spares the patient two injections.

The infraglottic larynx derives sensory innervation from the recurrent laryngeal nerves that run along the posterolateral surfaces of the trachea. Again, topical anesthesia rather than nerve block is the method of choice for obtunding reflexes. Several ml of 4% lidocaine injected via the cricothyroid membrane routinely results in excellent blockade of sensation.

The efficacy of topical and nerve block anesthesia at suppressing airway reflexes during intubation is evident.

Several recent studies document that topical anesthesia applied preoperatively (for brief cases) or intraoperatively can suppress cough and laryngospasm at the time of extubation.[90] A randomized study of patients undergoing tonsillectomy found that the incidence of stridor or laryngospasm at the time of extubation could be reduced from 12% to 3% by application of topical lidocaine at the time of intubation.[91] A recently marketed ET named LITA (Laryngotracheal Instillation of Topical Anesthetic, Sheridan Corp., Argyle, NY) contains a small channel that can be used to spray the upper airway while an ET is in place. Using this method to spray the ET prior to extubation, coughs were reduced by more than 60%, and the severity of the coughing decreased.[92]

3. Intravenous agents

Given a high enough dose, virtually all agents used as IV anesthetics will suppress the cough response to intubation. However, different agents appear to vary in their ability to inhibit upper airway reflexes when judged on the basis of equal potency in depressing consciousness and in depressing the cardiovascular system. Propofol-narcotic anesthesia may be adequate for intubating the trachea in some patients[93] even without the use of muscle relaxants. On the other hand, ketamine clinically appears to enhance laryngeal reflexes at doses that provide adequate anesthesia for surgery.

IV lidocaine is frequently used to prevent cough and/or laryngospasm at the time of intubation or extubation. Although the studies are not uniform in documenting efficacy, the preponderance of evidence supports the use of lidocaine.[94,95] Studies that did not document efficacy are sometimes flawed by the lack of documentation that adequate serum levels were reached. The maximal efficacy of IV lidocaine occurs 1 to 3 minutes after injection and requires a dose of 1.5 mg/kg or greater. This corresponded to a plasma level in excess of 4 μg/ml.

The ability of IV lidocaine to suppress cough appears to be due to factors beyond induction of general anesthesia, since cough suppression occurs at levels routinely seen in awake patients being treated with the drug. A comparison of the antitussive effects of lidocaine compared with meperidine and thiopental demonstrated that severe respiratory depression occurs with the latter drugs to achieve the same antitussive efficacy that can be achieved with lidocaine with virtually no respiratory depression.[96]

Whether IV lidocaine suppresses laryngospasm remains controversial. A study in which tonsillectomy patients were given 2 mg/kg of IV lidocaine and then extubated 1 minute later found suppression of laryngospasm.[97] Another study of tonsillectomy patients given 1.5 mg/kg found no clear effect.[98] A major difference in the latter was the authors' design of not extubating the

patient until swallowing had begun. Thus, there may have been a significant difference in the anesthetic depth at which the children were extubated.

B. PREVENTING BRONCHOCONSTRICTION

Following tracheal intubation, bronchoconstriction appears to result routinely. As noted earlier, in normal subjects this appears to be of moderate degree. However, the exaggerated response seen in patients with hyperactive airways may be life threatening. Prevention or treatment of this response can be performed using topical or IV agents. Inhaled anesthetic agents also inhibit the response, whether because of direct absorption by smooth muscle or via absorption in inhibition of reflexes.

1. Topical anesthesia

The studies of Gal and Surratt[77] demonstrated a doubling of lower airway resistance following tracheal intubation of awake volunteers under topical anesthesia. The bronchoconstrictive response must, indeed, be a powerful one if local anesthesia sufficient to permit volunteers to be intubated was not sufficient to prevent the reflex bronchoconstriction. There are no other human studies of topical anesthesia. However, a lidocaine aerosol given to dogs prior to a challenge with inhaled citric acid did attenuate the response to this irritant.[99] The efficacy of the inhaled aerosol lidocaine may, in part, be due to IV absorption of the drug. In addition, the aerosol itself produces a slight increase in lung resistance. Given the time required to administer the aerosol and the efficacy of IV drugs or other inhaled drugs, topical administration may not be the ideal route to use.

2. Intravenous drugs

A variety of drugs has been studied for bronchodilating properties. While IV β-agonists clearly produce bronchodilation, there is no benefit to parenteral administration of these drugs rather than inhalational administration. Among the drugs used for induction of anesthesia, ketamine and propofol appear to have significant inhibitory effect on the bronchoconstrictive response to tracheal intubation.[100,101] The thiobarbiturates do not appear to be significantly effective in preventing this response. In a study of asthmatics induced with either thiopental, methohexital, or propofol at equipotent doses, none of the asthmatic patients wheezed following tracheal intubation when propofol was used, whereas both of the barbiturates resulted in significant incidences of wheezing (Fig. 5-8).

IV lidocaine as a preventive measure for bronchoconstriction has not been studied in humans. However, in dogs, IV lidocaine at blood levels of 1.5 to 2.5 μg/ml substantially inhibited the response to an irritative citric

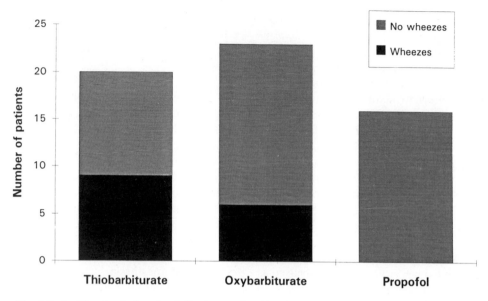

Fig. 5-8. Incidence of wheezing following tracheal intubation in asthmatics when induction is performed with either an oxybarbiturate, a thiobarbiturate, or propofol. (p < 0.05 for either thiobarbiturate or oxybarbiturate versus propofol). (Data from Pizov et al: *Anesthesiology* 82:1111, 1995.)

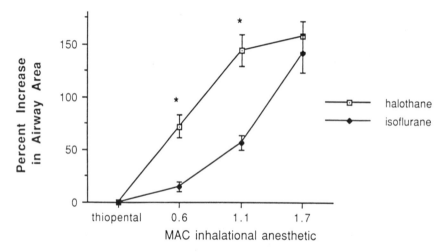

Fig. 5-9. Relative bronchodilating efficacy of halothane and isoflurane following histamine-induced bronchoconstriction in dogs. Notice that, at low concentrations, halothane appears to be more effective in increasing airway cross-sectional area, but the two are equally effective at higher concentration. (*p < 0.001 for halothane versus isoflurane.) (From Brown RH et al: *Anesthesiology* 78:1097, 1993.)

acid aerosol.[102] These data strongly suggest a role in the prevention of the response to the irritation from the tracheal tube.

The role of theophylline in preventing the broncho-constrictive response to tracheal intubation has not been studied. However, in most studies of the treatment of patients with bronchospasm, theophylline appears to add little to inhaled β-agonists nor does it supplement the bronchodilating effects of inhaled halothane.[103]

3. Inhaled agents

The classic dictum for anesthesiologists treating patients with hyperactive airways is to intubate the trachea only after achieving deep inhalation anesthesia. Halothane, isoflurane, and enflurane all have significant bronchodilating properties,[104,105] but recent studies suggest that, under some circumstances, the bronchodilation afforded by halothane may exceed that provided by isoflurane[106] (Fig. 5-9).

Pretreatment of patients with either inhaled β_2-adrenergic agonists or an inhaled anticholinergic markedly reduced lung resistance following tracheal intubation[70] and should be used routinely in patients known to have reactive airways. (See also Chapter 4.)

REFERENCES

1. Loeb HS et al: Effects of pharmacologically induced hypertension on myocardial ischemia and coronary hemodynamics in patients with fixed coronary obstruction, *Circulation* 57:41, 1978.
2. Slogoff S, Keats A: Does perioperative myocardial ischemia lead to postoperative myocardial infarction? *Anesthesiology* 55:212, 1981.
3. Nadel JA, Widdicombe JG: Reflex effects of upper airway irritation on total lung resistance and blood pressure, *J Appl Physiol* 17:861, 1962.
4. Dohi S, Gold MI: Pulmonary mechanics during general anesthesia, *Br J Anaesth* 51:205, 1979.
5. Fox EJ et al: Complications related to the pressor response to endotracheal intubation, *Anesthesiology* 47:524, 1977.
6. Shapiro HM et al: Acute intraoperative intracranial hypertension in neurosurgical patients: mechanical and pharmacological factors, *Anesthesiology* 37:399, 1972.
7. King BD et al: Reflex circulatory responses to direct laryngoscopy and tracheal intubation performed during general anesthesia, *Anesthesiology* 12:556, 1951.
8. Tarkkanen L, Laitinen L, Johansson G: Effects of d-Tubocurarine on intracranial pressure and thalamic electrical impedance, *Anesthesiology* 40:247, 1974.
9. Mori K, Iwabuchi K, Fujita M: The effects of depolarizing muscle relaxants on the electroencephalogram and the circulation during halothane anesthesia in man, *Br J Anaesth* 45:605, 1973.
10. Minton MD et al: Increases in intracranial pressure from succinylcholine: prevention by prior nondepolarizing blockade, *Anesthesiology* 65:165, 1986.
11. Lanier WL, Milde JH, Michenfelder JD: Cerebral stimulation following succinylcholine in dogs, *Anesthesiology* 64:551, 1986.
12. Modica PA, Tempelhoff R: Intracranial pressure during induction of anaesthesia and tracheal intubation with etomidate-induced EEG burst suppression, *Can J Anaesth* 39:236, 1992.
13. Moss E et al: Effects of tracheal intubation on intracranial pressure following induction of anaesthesia with thiopentone or althesin in patients undergoing neurosurgery, *Br J Anaesth* 50:353, 1978.
14. Ravussin P et al: Effect of propofol on cerebrospinal fluid pressure and cerebral perfusion pressure in patients undergoing craniotomy, *Anaesthesia Supplement* 43:37, 1988.
15. Giffin JP et al: Intracranial pressure, mean arterial pressure and heart rate following midazolam or thiopental in humans with brain tumors, *Anesthesiology* 60:491, 1984.
16. Bedford RF, Marshall WK: Cardiovascular response to endotracheal intubation during four anesthetic techniques, *Acta Anaesthesiol Scand* 28:563, 1984.
17. Roizen MF, Horrigan RW, Frazer BM: Anesthetic doses that block adrenergic (stress) and cardiovascular responses to incision—MAC-BAR, *Anesthesiology* 54:390, 1981.
18. Yakaitis RW, Blitt CD, Angiulo JP: End-tidal enflurane concentration for endotracheal intubation, *Anesthesiology* 50:59, 1979.
19. Yakaitis RW, Blitt CD, Angiulo JP: End-tidal halothane concentration for endotracheal intubation, *Anesthesiology* 47:386, 1977.
20. Kimura T et al: Determination of end-tidal sevoflurane concentration for tracheal intubation and minimum alveolar anesthetic concentration in adults, *Anesth Analg* 79:378, 1994.
21. Zbinden AM, Petersen-Felix S, Thomson DA: Anesthetic depth defined using multiple noxious stimuli during isoflurane/oxygen anesthesia, *Anesthesiology* 80:261, 1994.
22. Kautto HM: Attenuation of the circulatory response to laryngoscopy and intubation by fentanyl, *Acta Anaesth Scand* 26:217, 1982.
23. Chen CT et al: Fentanyl dosage for suppression of circulatory response to laryngoscopy and endotracheal intubation, *Anesthesiology Review* 13:37, 1986.
24. Scott JC, Ponganis KV, Stanski DR: EEG quantitation of narcotic effect: the comparative pharmacodynamics of fentanyl and alfentanil, *Anesthesiology* 62:234, 1985.
25. Ausems ME et al: Plasma concentrations of alfentanil required to supplement nitrous oxide anesthesia for general surgery, *Anesthesiology* 65:362, 1986.
26. Steinhaus JE, Howland DE: Intravenously administered lidocaine as a supplement to nitrous oxide thiobarbiturate anesthesia, *Anesth Analg* 37:40, 1958.
27. Yukioka H et al: Intravenous lidocaine as a suppressant of coughing during tracheal intubation in elderly patients, *Anesth Analg* 77:309, 1993.
28. Himes RS Jr, DiFazio CA, Burney RG: Effects of lidocaine on the anesthetic requirements for nitrous oxide and halothane, *Anesthesiology* 47:437, 1977.
29. Denlinger JK et al: *Effect of intravenous lidocaine on the circulatory response to tracheal intubation.* Abstracts of Scientific Papers, Annual Meeting of the American Society of Anesthesiologists, Chicago p. 43, 1975.
30. Dasten GW, Owens E: Evaluation of lidocaine as an adjunct to fentanyl anesthesia for coronary artery bypass graft surgery, *Anesth Analg* 65:511, 1986.
31. Abou-Madi MN, Keszler H, Yacoub JM: Cardiovascular reactions to laryngoscopy and tracheal intubation following small and large intravenous doses of lidocaine, *Can Anaesth Soc J* 24:12, 1977.
32. Bedford RF et al: Lidocaine or thiopental for rapid control of intracranial hypertension? *Anesth Analg* 58:435, 1980.
33. Bedford RF et al: Intracranial pressure response to endotracheal intubation: efficacy of intravenous lidocaine pretreatment for patients with brain tumors. In Shulman, Marmarou, Miller et al., editors: *Intracranial pressure IV,* New York, 1980, Springer-Verlag.
34. Stoelting RK: Circulatory response to laryngoscopy and tracheal intubation with or without prior oropharyngeal viscous lidocaine, *Anesth Analg* 56:618, 1977.
35. Stoelting RK: Circulatory changes during direct laryngoscopy and tracheal intubation: influence of duration of laryngoscopy with or without prior lidocaine, *Anesthesiology* 47:381, 1977.
36. Youngberg JA, Graybar G, Hutchings D: Comparison of intravenous and topical lidocaine in attenuating the cardiovascular responses to endotracheal intubation, *South Med J* 76:1122, 1983.
37. Hamill JF et al: Lidocaine before endotracheal intubation: intravenous or laryngotracheal? *Anesthesiology* 55:578, 1981.
38. Mirakhur RK: Bradycardia with laryngeal spraying in children, *Acta Anaesth Scand* 26:130, 1982.
39. Rovenstine EA, Papper EM: Glossopharyngeal nerve block, *Am J Surg* 75:713, 1948.
40. Hawkyard SJ et al: Attenuating the hypertensive response to laryngoscopy and endotracheal intubation using awake fiberoptic intubation, *Acta Anaesthesiol Scand* 36:1, 1992.
41. Smith JE: Heart rate and arterial pressure changes during fiberoptic tracheal intubation under general anesthesia, *Anaesthesia* 43:629, 1988.
42. Finfer SR et al: Cardiovascular responses to tracheal intubation:

a comparison of direct laryngoscopy and fiberoptic intubation, *Anaesth Intensive Care* 17:44, 1989.

43. Schaefer HG, Marsch SC: Comparison of orthodox with fiberoptic orotracheal intubation under total IV anaesthesia, *Br J Anaesth* 66:608, 1991.

44. Smith JE, Mackenzie AA, Scott-Knight VC: Comparison of two methods of fiberscope-guided tracheal intubation, *Br J Anaesth* 66:546, 1991.

45. De Vault M, Greifenstein FE, Harris LC Jr: Circulatory responses to endotracheal intubation in light general anesthesia: the effect of atropine and phentolamine, *Anesthesiology* 21:360, 1960.

46. Davies MJ, Cronin KD, Cowie RW: The prevention of hypertension at intubation: a controlled study of intravenous hydralazine on patients undergoing intracranial surgery, *Anaesthesia* 36:147, 1981.

47. Stoelting RK: Attenuation of blood pressure response to laryngoscopy and tracheal intubation with sodium nitroprusside, *Anesth Analg* 58:116, 1979.

48. Gallagher JD et al: Prophylactic nitroglycerin infusions during coronary artery bypass surgery, *Anesthesiology* 64:785, 1986.

49. Van Aken H, Puchstein C, Hidding J: The prevention of hypertension at intubation, *Anaesthesia* 37:82, 1982.

50. Gold MI et al: Heart rate and blood pressure effects of esmolol after ketamine induction and intubation, *Anesthesiology* 64:718, 1986.

51. Ghignone M et al: Effects of clonidine on narcotic requirements and hemodynamic response during induction of fentanyl anesthesia and endotracheal intubation, *Anesthesiology* 64:36, 1986.

52. Nunn JF, Campbell EJM, Peckett BW: Anatomical subdivisions of the volume of respiratory dead space and effect of position of the jaw, *J Appl Physiol* 14:174, 1959.

53. Cullen JH: An evaluation of tracheostomy in pulmonary emphysema, *Ann Intern Med* 58:953, 1963.

54. Habib MP: Physiologic implications of artificial airways. *Chest* 96:180, 1989.

55. Hirshman CA, Bergman MJ: Factors influencing intrapulmonary airway calibre during anaesthesia, *Br J Anaesth* 65:30, 1990.

56. Kil HK, Bishop MJ: Head position and oral vs nasal route as factors determining endotracheal tube resistance, *Chest* 105:1794, 1994.

57. Cavo J et al: Flow resistance in tracheostomy tubes, *Ann Otol Rhinol Laryngol* 82:827, 1973.

58. Yung MW, Snowdon SL: Respiratory resistance of tracheostomy tubes, *Arch Otolaryngol* 110:591, 1984.

59. Colgan FS, Lian JQ, Borrow RE: Non-invasive assessment by capacitance respirometry of respiration before and after extubation, *Anesth Analg* 54:807, 1975.

60. Nunn JF: *Applied respiratory physiology,* ed 3, Boston, 1987, Butterworths.

61. Bolder PM et al: The extra work of breathing through adult endotracheal tubes, *Anesth Analg* 65:853, 1986.

62. Hill DW: Properties of liquids, gases and vapours. In: *Physics applied to anaesthesia,* ed 4, London, 1980, Butterworths & Co.

63. Shapiro M et al: Work of breathing through different sized endotracheal tubes, *Crit Care Med* 14:1028, 1986.

64. Caplan RA et al: Adverse respiratory events in anesthesia: a closed claims analysis, *Anesthesiology* 72:828, 1990.

65. Cheney FW, Posner KL, Caplan RA: Adverse respiratory events infrequently leading to malpractice suits, *Anesthesiology* 75:932, 1991.

66. Tiret L et al: Complications associated with anaesthesia: a prospective survey in France, *Can Anaesth Soc J* 33:336, 1986.

67. Olsson GL: Bronchospasm during anaesthesia: a computer-aided incidence study of 136,929 patients, *Acta Anaesthesiol Scand* 31:244, 1987.

68. Nadel JA: Mechanisms controlling airway size, *Arch Environ Health* 7:179, 1963.

69. Gal TJ: Pulmonary mechanics in normal subjects following endotracheal intubation, *Anesthesiology* 52:27, 1980.

70. Kil HK et al: Effect of prophylactic bronchodilator treatment on lung resistance after tracheal intubation, *Anesthesiology* 81:43, 1994.

71. Hirshman CA: Airway reactivity in humans, *Anesthesiology* 58:170, 1983.

72. Boushey HA et al: Bronchial hyperreactivity, *Am Rev Respir Dis* 121:389, 1980.

73. Ding DJ, Martin JG, Macklem PT: Effects of lung volume on maximal methacholine-induced bronchoconstrictions in normal humans, *J Appl Physiol* 62:1324, 1987.

74. Marini JJ, Pepe PE: Occult positive end-expiratory pressure in mechanically ventilated patients with airflow obstruction, *Am Rev Respir Dis* 126:166, 1982.

75. Scott LR, Benson MS, Bishop MJ: Relationship of endotracheal tube size to auto-PEEP at high minute ventilation, *Respir Care* 31:1080, 1986.

76. Davis K et al: Changes in respiratory mechanics following tracheostomy, *Crit Care Med* 21:S211, 1993 (abstract).

77. Gal TJ, Surratt PM: Resistance to breathing in healthy subjects after endotracheal intubation under topical anesthesia, *Anesthesiology* 59:270, 1980.

78. Rodenstein DO, Stanescue DC, Francis C: Demonstration of failure of body plethysmography in airway obstruction, *J Appl Physiol* 52:949, 1982.

79. Gal TJ, Arora NS: Respiratory mechanics in supine subjects during progressive partial curarization, *J Appl Physiol* 52:57, 1982.

80. Quan SF, Falltrick RT, Schlobohm RM: Extubation from ambient or expiratory positive airway pressure in adults, *Anesthesiology* 55:53, 1984.

81. Smith RA et al: Laboratory and animal investigations: influence of glottic mechanism on pulmonary function after acute lung injury, *Chest* 98:206, 1990.

82. Gal TJ: Effects of endotracheal intubation on normal cough performance, *Anesthesiology* 52:324, 1980.

83. Bickler PE, Sessler DI: Efficiency of airway heat and moisture exchangers in anesthetized humans, *Anesth Analg* 71:415, 1990.

84. Casthely P, Chalon J: Tracheobronchial cytologic changes during prolonged cannulation, *Anesth Analg* 59:759, 1980.

85. Klainer AS, Turndorf H: Surface alterations due to endotracheal intubation, *Am J Med* 58:674, 1975.

86. Goodell JA, Gilroy G, Huntress JD: Reducing cocaine solution use by promoting the use of a lidocaine-phenylephrine solution, *Am J Hosp Pharm* 45:2510, 1988.

87. Sessler CN et al: Comparison of 4% lidocaine/0.5% phenylephrine with 5% cocaine: which dilates the nasal passage better? *Anesthesiology* 64:274, 1986.

88. Gross JB, Hartigan ML, Schaffer DW: A suitable substitute for 4% cocaine before blind nasotracheal intubation: 3% lidocaine–0.25% phenylephrine nasal spray, *Anesth Analg* 63:915, 1984.

89. Gotta AW, Sullivan CA: Anaesthesia of the upper airway using topical anaesthetic and superior laryngeal nerve block, *Br J Anaesth* 53:1055, 1981.

90. Viguera M et al: Efficacy of topical administration of lidocaine through a Malinckrodt Hi-Lo Jet tube in lessening cough during recovery from general anesthesia, *Rev Esp Anestesiol Reanim* 39:316, 1992.

91. Staffel JG et al: The prevention of postoperative stridor and laryngospasm with topical lidocaine, *Arch Otolaryngol Head Neck Surg* 117:1123, 1991.

92. Gonzalez R et al: Prevention of coughing during emergence from general anesthesia: comparison of intravenous versus topical

lidocaine delivered via a new type of endotracheal tube, *Anesthesiology* 79:A553, 1993 (abstract).

93. Scheller MS, Zornow MH, Saidman LJ: Tracheal intubation without use of muscle relaxants: a technique using propofol and varying doses of alfentanil, *Anesth Analg* 75:788, 1992.

94. Yukioka H et al: Intravenous lidocaine as a suppressant of coughing during tracheal intubation in elderly patients, *Anesth Analg* 77:309, 1993.

95. Mulholland D, Carlisle RJ: Intubation with propofol augmented with intravenous lignocaine, *Anaesthesia* 46:312, 1991.

96. Steinhaus JE, Gaskin L: A study of intravenous lidocaine as a suppressant of cough reflex, *Anes* 24:285, 1963.

97. Baraka A: Intravenous lidocaine controls extubation laryngospasm in children, *Anesth Analg* 57:506, 1978.

98. Leicht P, Wisborg T, Chraemmer-Jorgensen B: Does intravenous lidocaine prevent laryngospasm after extubation in children? *Anesth Analg* 64:1193, 1985.

99. Downes H, Hirshman CA: Lidocaine aerosols do not prevent allergic bronchoconstriction, *Anesth Analg* 60:28, 1981.

100. Pizov R et al: Wheezing during induction of general anesthesia in patients with and without asthma: a randomized, blind trial, *Anesthesiology* 82:1111, 1995.

101. Hirshman CA et al: Ketamine block of bronchospasm in experimental canine asthma, *Br J Anaesth* 51:713, 1979.

102. Downes H, Gerber N, Hirshman CA: I.V. lignocaine in reflex and allergic bronchoconstriction, *Br J Anaesth* 52:873, 1980.

103. Tobias JD, Lubos KL, Hirshman CA: Aminophylline does not attenuate histamine-induced airway constriction during halothane anesthesia, *Anesthesiology* 71:723, 1989.

104. Hirshman CA, Bergman NA: Factors influencing intrapulmonary airway calibre during anesthesia, *Br J Anaesth* 65:30, 1990.

105. Brichant JF et al: Halothane, enflurane and isoflurane depress the peripheral vagal motor pathway in isolated canine tracheal smooth muscle, *Anesthesiology* 74:325, 1991.

106. Brown RH, Zerhouni EA, Hirshman CA: Comparison of low concentrations of halothane and isoflurane as bronchodilators, *Anesthesiology* 78:1097, 1993.

Part II

THE DIFFICULT AIRWAY: DEFINITION, RECOGNITION, AND THE ASA ALGORITHM

Chapter 6

DEFINITION AND INCIDENCE OF THE DIFFICULT AIRWAY

Jonathan L. Benumof

I. INTRODUCTION
II. DEFINITION AND CLASSIFICATION OF AIRWAY
   DIFFICULTY
III. INCIDENCE OF EACH DEGREE OF AIRWAY
   DIFFICULTY
IV. INCIDENCE OF COMPLICATIONS WITH EACH
   DEGREE OF AIRWAY DIFFICULTY

I. INTRODUCTION

The fundamental responsibility of an anesthesiologist is to maintain adequate gas exchange. In order to do this, the airway must be managed in such a way that it is almost continuously patent. Failure to maintain a patent airway for more than a few minutes results in brain damage or death. Thus, it is not surprising that more than 85% of all respiratory-related closed malpractice claims involve a brain-damaged or dead patient,[1] and it has been estimated that inability to successfully manage very difficult airways has been responsible for as many as 30% of deaths totally attributable to anesthesia.[2,3]

In any patient, the greater the degree of difficulty in maintaining airway patency, the greater the risk of brain damage or death. Before discussing the specific management of a difficult airway (Chapters 11 to 35), we must (1) define what is meant by a "difficult airway", (2) classify the degrees of difficulty experienced in maintaining a patent airway, (3) determine the incidence of each degree of airway difficulty, and (4) determine the

incidence of major and minor complications as a function of the degree of airway difficulty. In this discussion, it is always assumed that a reasonably well-trained anesthesiologist is attempting to maintain airway patency.

II. DEFINITION AND CLASSIFICATION OF AIRWAY DIFFICULTY

There are three common ways of maintaining airway patency and gas exchange. First, inspired gas is delivered to the face via a mask that is sealed to the patient's face, while the natural airway from the face to the vocal cords is kept patent with or without external jaw thrust maneuvers or internal upper airway devices (mask ventilation) (Chapter 12). Second, the inspired gas is delivered to a mask that covers the larynx; this mask is known as the laryngeal mask airway. Since the laryngeal mask airway is extensively described in Chapter 19, it will not be specifically considered in this chapter, and, for the purpose of this discussion, the laryngeal mask airway may be considered a face mask applied to the larynx, which may have varying degrees of goodness of fit (see Chapter 19). Third, the airway is kept open to the inspired gas by some sort of tube passed from the environment to some point below the vocal cords (endotracheal intubation).

In terms of degree of difficulty, mask ventilation can range from zero to infinite (Fig. 6-1, *top*). Zero degree of mask ventilation difficulty means that no external effort and/or internal upper airway device is required to maintain airway patency; that is, mask ventilation is

DEFINITION OF DIFFERENT DEGREES OF A DIFFICULT AIRWAY

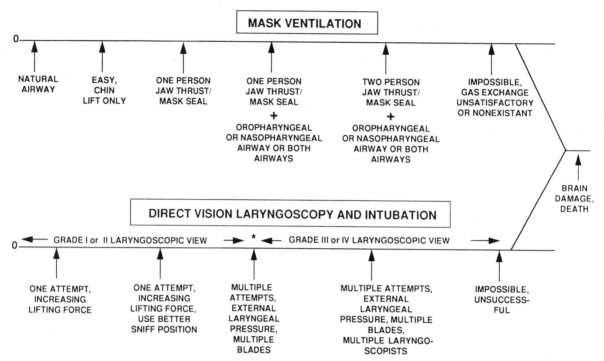

Fig. 6-1. Definition of difficult airway. Airway refers to either mask ventilation or endotracheal tube (ET) intubation by direct vision laryngoscope. The degree of difficulty can range from zero, which is extremely easy, to infinity, which is impossible. When both mask ventilation and direct vision laryngoscopy are impossible, and no other maneuver is successful, brain damage and/or death will ensue. Between these extremes, there are several well-defined, commonly encountered degrees of difficulty. Grade of laryngoscopic view is represented as an approximate continuum above the discrete progressive indicies of laryngoscopic difficulty. (From Benumof JL: *Anesthesiology* 75:1087, 1991.)

extremely easy and occurs *via* the natural airway. Next, there are several specific, reproducible, and progressive degrees of mask ventilation difficulty: these consist of one-person jaw thrust-mask seal, insertion of an oropharyngeal or nasopharyngeal airway, one-person jaw thrust and insertion of one or both airway(s), and two-person jaw thrust–mask seal (see next paragraph) and both airways. Whenever an airway is used, it is likely that jaw thrust will also be used, and, therefore, these indices of difficulty are shown in Fig. 6-1 as occurring together. Infinite degree of mask ventilation difficulty means that, despite maximal two-person external effort (see next paragraph) and full use of oropharyngeal and nasopharyngeal airways, adequate airway patency cannot be maintained; that is, mask ventilation is impossible. Of course, in any given patient the degree of difficulty with mask ventilation may change with time.

When two persons combine to effect jaw thrust and mask seal, they must interact in an additive-synergistic way. Ideally, the primary anesthetist stands at the head of the patient and the left hand effects jaw thrust at the angle of the left mandible and left-sided mask seal, while the right hand compresses the reservoir bag; this is the standard position for the primary anesthetist (Fig. 6-2). The secondary (helping) person should stand at the patient's side, at the level of the patient's shoulder, facing the primary anesthetist. The right hand of the secondary anesthetist should cover the left hand of the primary anesthetist and contribute to left-sided jaw thrust and mask seal, and the left hand of the secondary person should achieve right-sided jaw thrust and mask seal. In this way, all four hands are doing something important and do not interfere with one another, and there is almost no redundant effort. With this positioning, the secondary person can additionally continuously watch the monitors and provide external laryngeal manipulation to the patient and hand equipment to the primary anesthetist.

The difficulty of intubation under direct vision can also range from zero to infinity (Fig. 6-1, *bottom panel*). Zero degree of difficulty with intubation means that an endotracheal tube (ET) can be inserted into a fully

TWO-PERSON MAXIMUM MASK VENTILATION EFFORT

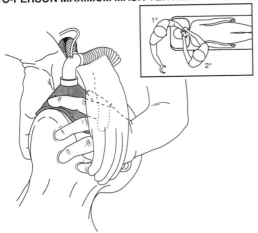

Fig. 6-2. Optimal two-person mask ventilation effort. Primary anesthetist stands at head of patient and uses left and right hands in standard-classical fashion. Secondary (helping) person stands facing the primary anesthetist at level of patient's shoulder and uses right hand to help achieve left-sided jaw thrust and mask seal, while left hand achieves right-sided jaw thrust and mask seal.

visualized laryngeal aperture (Fig. 6-3, *grade I laryngoscopic view*[4,5]) with little effort. Next, there are several specific, reproducible, and progressive degrees of intubation difficulty; these consist of visualization of progressively less of the laryngeal aperture (Figs. 6-1 and 6-3, *grades II and III laryngoscopic views*[4,5]). As the view worsens, increasing anterior lifting force with the laryngoscope blade, optimal sniff position, multiple attempts, external laryngeal manipulation (see Chapter 14 and Fig. 14-8), multiple blades, and laryngoscopists may be required to achieve intubation. External laryngeal manipulation (see Chapter 14 and Fig. 14-8) may be required to push the larynx more posteriorly and cephalad into better view (thereby decreasing the laryngoscopic view from a higher to a lower grade) (see following). Similarly, it should be recognized that anatomy that results in a high-grade laryngoscopic view for an inexperienced individual with a given laryngoscopic blade may result in a lower laryngoscopic grade for a more experienced or skillful individual with perhaps a different blade. Whenever multiple attempts are required, it is likely that external laryngeal manipulation will also be applied; therefore, these indices of difficulty are shown occurring together. Although a severe grade III (tip epiglottis) and a grade IV (Figs. 6-1 and 6-3, just soft palate) laryngoscopic view[4,5] may result in a successful "blind" intubation, these views will often result in an impossible intubation. An infinitely difficult intubation means that the trachea cannot be intubated under direct vision, despite full paralysis and optimal head and neck positioning, very forceful anterior elevation of the laryngoscope blade, use of multiple attempts,

Laryngoscopic View Grading System

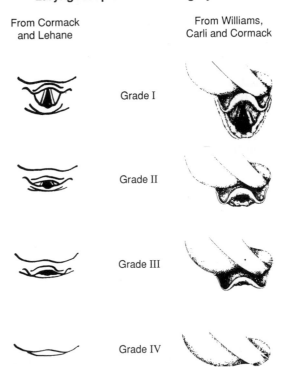

Fig. 6-3. Four grades of laryngoscopic view. Grade I is visualization of entire laryngeal aperture; grade II is visualization of just the posterior portion of laryngeal aperture; grade III is visualization of only the epiglottis; and grade IV is visualization of just the soft palate. It is assumed that care has been taken to get the best possible view of the vocal cords (see text). (Adapted from Cormack RS, Lehane J: *Anaesthesia* 39:1105, 1984, [*left column*] and Williams KN, Carli F, Cormack RS: *Br J Anaesth* 66:38, 1991, [*right column*]).

laryngoscope blades, and laryngoscopists, and external posterior and cephalad displacement of the larynx; that is, tracheal intubation through a nonvisualized larynx is impossible. Of course, in any given patient, the degree of tracheal intubation difficulty can be independent of the degree of mask ventilation difficulty and can progressively increase and approach the impossible extreme.

In order for studies on difficult laryngoscopy to be reliable and the above laryngoscopic grading system to be helpful, it is necessary that the reported grades are the best view that was obtainable, which, in turn, depends on the best possible performance of laryngoscopy. The components of best performance of laryngoscopy consist of the optimal sniff position, good complete muscle relaxation, firm forward traction on the laryngoscope, and, if necessary, firm external laryngeal manipulation. For example, the application of external laryngeal pressure may reduce the incidence of grade III view from 9% to 5.4 − 1.3%.[6] In doubtful cases the anesthetist, while performing the laryngoscopy with his left hand,

Table 6-1. Incidence of difficult intubation according to degree of difficulty

Degree of difficulty with intubation (Fig. 6-1)	Range of incidence		Reference
	Per 10,000	%	
ET intubation successful but multiple attempts and/or blades may be required; probable grade II or III	100-1800	1-18	5, 9-13
ET intubation successful but multiple attempts and/or blades and/or laryngoscopists required; grade III	100-400	1-4	4, 6, 7, 14, 15, 16
ET intubation not successful; grade III or IV	5-35	0.05-0.35	4, 5, 7, 14, 17-19
Cannot ventilate by mask plus cannot intubate; transtracheal jet ventilation, tracheostomy, brain damage, or death	0.01-2.0	0.0001-0.02	2, 3, 20-22

should quickly apply external pressure over the hyoid-thyroid-cricoid cartilages with his right hand. The location of external laryngeal pressure that affords the best laryngeal view can be determined in just several seconds. Having found the position that gives the best view, the assistant should be asked to carefully press on exactly the same spot. Reproducing the identical external laryngeal pressure by the assistant must be under the complete direction of the laryngoscopist, and this recommendation is advisable even if the assistant is fully trained. The best performance of laryngoscopy avoids awkward high-arm postures, positioning the laryngoscope blade over part of the tongue, gripping the laryngoscope at the junction of the handle and blade with rotation about a horizontal axis, choice of wrong blade size, and wrong blade placement. Theoretically, if the above components of best performance of laryngoscopy are used and the pitfalls avoided, all laryngoscopists (novice and expert) should have close to the same laryngoscopy view.

Difficult laryngoscopy (as defined by a grade III or IV view)[4,5] is synonymous with difficult intubation in the vast majority of patients. However, there are four relatively uncommon exceptions to this contention. First, some grade II patients have a trachea that may be intubated at the first or second attempt, if the distal end of the ET is appropriately curved by a malleable stylet (hockey stick shape) or a small curved introducer is used (e.g., a gum elastic bougie). Therefore, tracheal intubation depends a little bit more on the skill of the individual than does laryngoscopy, and therefore a degree of inconsistency may arise between the difficulty of laryngoscopy and tracheal intubation. Consequently, studies of incidence of difficulty of tracheal intubation will depend on the dexterity of the intubationists involved and some variability in results are inevitable. Second, grade III laryngoscopic view has been variously described as seeing only the palate and all of the epiglottis[5,6,8] and as seeing only the palate and just the tip of the epiglottis.[4,8] These different definitions of

grade III may respond differently to adjustments, such as optimal external laryngeal pressure, and therefore may differ initially and subsequently with respect to difficulty of tracheal intubation. Third, a grade III view with a curved blade placed in the vallecula (due to a long floppy epiglottis) may be a lower grade (I or II) if either a curved or straight blade is placed posterior to the epiglottis and lifted anteriorly. Fourth, pathologic conditions, such as laryngeal web, laryngeal tumors, tracheal stenosis, etc., may disassociate ease of laryngoscopy from difficulty of tracheal intubation.

III. INCIDENCE OF EACH DEGREE OF AIRWAY DIFFICULTY

The incidence of airway difficulty in the general surgical population varies greatly depending on its degree (Table 6-1). A grade II or III laryngoscopic view requiring multiple attempts and/or blades (and presumably external laryngeal pressure) is relatively common and occurs in 100 to 1800 of 10,000 patients, or 1% to 18%.[5,9-13] As the degree of difficulty increases to a definite grade III laryngoscopic view, then the incidence is generally slightly less and ranges from 100 to 400 of 10,000 patients, or 1% to 4%.* The incidence of failed endotracheal intubation (presumably a severe grade III or grade IV view) is still less and ranges from 5 to 35 of 10,000 patients, or 0.05% to 0.35%†; the high and low ends of this range are associated with obstetric and other surgical patients, respectively. There are no data available regarding the incidence of difficulty with mask ventilation alone. However, the incidence of completely failed mask ventilation *and* ET intubation can be estimated because such an airway failure combination heretofore frequently resulted in brain damage or death and has ranged from 0.01 to 2.0 of 10,000 patients.[2,3,20-22] The incidence of brain damage, cardiac arrest, and death appears to be decreasing.[21,22]

*References 4, 6, 7, 14, 15, 16.
†References 4, 5, 7, 14, 17-19.

IV. INCIDENCE OF COMPLICATIONS WITH EACH DEGREE OF AIRWAY DIFFICULTY

Anesthesia in a patient with a difficult airway can lead both to direct airway trauma and morbidity from hypoxia and hypercarbia. Direct airway trauma occurs because the management of the difficult airway often involves the application of more physical force to the patient's airway than is normally used (but not necessarily). The most common consequence is probably a chipped or broken tooth. Direct trauma may involve any part of the face, teeth, and upper airway, resulting in hemorrhage, lacerations, and subsequent tissue emphysema and infection, fracture-subluxation of the cervical spine, and trauma to the eye. Much of the morbidity specifically attributable to managing a difficult airway comes from an interruption of gas exchange (hypoxia and hypercapnia), which may then cause brain damage and cardiovascular activation or depression. Directly mediated reflexes (laryngovagal [airway spasm, apnea, bradycardia, arrhythmia, or hypotension], and laryngospinal [coughing, vomiting, or bucking]) provide the final source for morbidity. Both direct trauma and morbidity from airway obstruction can range from minor (trivial or nuisance value) to major (life-threatening or death).

It is reasonable to postulate that the more difficult the airway is to manage, the greater will be the use of physical force, the number of attempts to establish the airway, and the incidence of complications. Only one study[16] has directly addressed this question, and its data strongly support this contention. In this study, the incidence of relatively minor upper airway complications (posterior pharyngeal and lip lacerations and bruises) with laryngoscopy and intubation under direct vision in patients with normal airways was 5%.[16] In patients in whom tracheal intubation was anticipated to be difficult, the incidence of minor trauma to the upper airway increased to 17%.[16] In patients in whom tracheal intubation was actually found to be difficult (multiple attempts at laryngoscopy but ultimately successful), the incidence of upper airway complications was 63%. Of course, when it has been impossible to manage the airway, the incidence of complications may further increase because of the inclusion of some cases of brain damage or death.[20]

REFERENCES

1. Caplan RA, Posner KL, Ward RJ et al: Adverse respiratory events in anesthesia: a closed claims analysis, *Anesthesiology* 72:828, 1990.
2. Benumof JL, Scheller MS: The importance of transtracheal jet ventilation in the management of the difficult airway, *Anesthesiology* 71:769, 1989.
3. Bellhouse CP, Doré C: Criteria for estimating likelihood of difficulty of endotracheal intubation with Macintosh Laryngoscope, *Anaesth Intensive Care* 16:329, 1988.
4. Samsoon GLT, Young JRB: Difficult tracheal intubation: a retrospective study, *Anaesthesia* 42:487, 1987.
5. Cormack RS, Lehane J: Difficult tracheal intubation in obstetrics, *Anaesthesia* 39:1105, 1984.
6. Wilson ME, Spiegelhalter D, Robertson JA et al: Predicting difficult intubation, *Br J Anaesth* 61:211, 1988.
7. Williams KN, Carli F, Cormack RS: Unexpected, difficult laryngoscopy: a prospective survey in routine general surgery, *Br J Anaesth* 66:38, 1991.
8. Williamson R: Grade III laryngoscopy—which is it? *Anaesthesia* 43:424, 1988.
9. Aro L, Takki S, Aromaa U: Technique for difficult intubation, *Br J Anaesth* 43:1081, 1971.
10. Mallampati SR, Gatt SP, Gugino LD et al: A clinical sign to predict difficult tracheal intubation: a prospective study, *Can J Anaesth* 32:429, 1985.
11. Phillips OC, Duerksen RL: Endotracheal intubation: a new blade for direct laryngoscopy, *Anesth Analg* 52:691, 1973.
12. Finucane BT, Santora AH: Difficult intubation, *Principles of airway management*, Philadelphia, 1988, Davis Co.
13. Deller A, Schreiber MN, Gramer J et al: Difficult intubation: incidence and predictability: a prospective study of 8,284 adult patients, *Anesthesiology* 73:A1054, 1990 (abstract).
14. Glassenburg R, Vaisrub N, Albright G: The incidence of failed intubation in obstetrics: is there an irreducible minimum? *Anesthesiology* 73:A1061, 1990 (abstract).
15. Cohen SM, Laurito CE, Segil LJ: Oral exam to predict difficult intubations: a large prospective study, *Anesthesiology* 71:A937, 1989.
16. Hirsch IA, Reagan JO, Sullivan N: Complications of direct laryngoscopy: a prospective analysis, *Anesthesiology Review* 17:34, 1990.
17. Bellhouse CP: An angulated laryngoscope for routine and difficult tracheal intubation, *Anesthesiology* 69:126, 1988.
18. Lyons G: Failed intubation, *Anaesthesia* 40:759, 1985.
19. Lyons G, MacDonald R: Difficult intubation in obstetrics, *Anaesthesia* 40:1016, 1985 (letter).
20. Tunstall ME: Failed intubation in the parturient, *Can J Anaesth* 36:611, 1989 (editorial).
21. Keenan RL, Boyan CP: Decreasing frequency of anesthetic cardiac arrests, *J Clin Anesth* 3:354, 1991.
22. Eichhorn JH: Documenting improved anesthesia outcome, *J Clin Anesth* 3:351, 1991.

Chapter 7

RECOGNITION OF THE DIFFICULT AIRWAY

The physician must be able to tell the antecedents, know the present and foretell the future—must mediate these things, and have two special objects in view with regard to diseases, namely, to do good or to do no harm.

HIPPOCRATES

S. Rao Mallampati

I. INTRODUCTION

Although medicine has changed immeasurably in scope and in practice since the times of Hippocrates, the goals remain the same, namely, to do no harm and to do good to the disabled and ill. To achieve these goals, health care providers, including anesthesiologists, should preserve and protect the individual's usual state of health and strive to apply state-of-the-art remedies, surgical or otherwise, to alleviate the infirmity or cure the illness. Less-than-satisfactory results in most instances may be traced to an array of factors; in clinical anesthesiology these may include, among others, inad-

equate level of assessment of systems, failure to anticipate or recognize the problem, inadequate vigilance, insufficient preparedness to address the adverse situations encountered, and suboptimal skill, particularly under stressful conditions. These are likely to result in iatrogenic injury, reversible or irreversible, to the patient, which may constitute a significant proportion of the overall morbidity and mortality in clinical practice.

Adverse anesthetic outcomes in a number of instances have been traced partly or totally to airway difficulties or mismanagement. Keenan and Boyan[1] reported that failure to provide adequate ventilation was responsible for 12 of 27 cardiac arrests during the operative period. Caplan et al.[2] reported that 34% of 1541 liability claims were for adverse respiratory events, which constituted the single largest source of adverse outcome in the American Society of Anesthesiologists closed claims study. Appropriately, 75% of these undesirable events were attributed to three mechanisms of injury: inadequate ventilation (38%), esophageal intubation (18%), and difficult tracheal intubation (17%). Cheney et al.[3] in their analysis of 300 liability claims for less common but important categories of ventilation-related adverse outcomes identified recurrent themes of management error or patterns of injury: airway trauma, pneumothorax, airway obstruction, aspiration, and bronchospasm. These and other similar retrospective analyses serve well to reflect on the magnitude of the problem, though not the precise mechanism of causation or solution.

It is plausible that the causation is multifactorial, but the ultimate contributor to airway-related morbidity and mortality is inadequate effective ventilation in the vast majority of circumstances. Unanticipated airway difficulty could have been a compromising factor in a large percentage of these morbid events. An anesthesiologist subjected to sudden and unexpected stress as a consequence of a totally unforeseen airway difficulty could find himself or herself in a taxing situation: he or she may be unprepared to face the crisis; all the resources may not be handy; a state of apprehension may cloud his or her mind and impair his or her decision-making power. Gripped by worry and fear over the endangered life of the patient, the anesthesiologist may not be able to alert or direct his or her surgical colleagues until very late into the crisis about the need for the surgical airway. Often stimulation of the airway from repeated unsuccessful attempts at laryngoscopy and intubation, in light of compromised or inadequate ventilation by bag-mask leading to hypoxemia, hypercarbia, respiratory acidosis, and endogenous release of catecholamines, may precipitate cardiac dysrhythmias. Heightened awareness of potential for risk based upon a thorough and objective assessment should help to prevent such airway-related morbidity and mortality in clinical practice. Guidelines for appropriate management strategies and their clinical execution have been addressed in recent publications.[4] The paramount step fundamental to the safe conduct of airway management is airway evaluation and recognition of potential for difficulty; the objective is to move the patient from the risky path to the safe path.

Unarguably the single most important function of a clinical anesthesiologist is to establish and maintain a patent airway in the anesthetized state and in any circumstance that predisposes the individual to an unprotected or compromised airway. The unique role played by the clinical anesthesiologist in rendering patients unconscious and free from pain, either in the form of regional anesthesia or general anesthesia to facilitate surgical procedures, has an inherent element of risk. As a result of rapid-acting, almost instantaneously effective neurodepressants and muscle relaxants used in contemporary clinical practice and the attendant physiologic changes and protective reflexes, respiratory function, hemodynamics, and acid-base status are subdued or interfered with. These functions are bound to suffer further if oxygenation should be compromised during induction or maintenance of the anesthetized state. Accordingly, the foremost responsibility of the anesthesiologist is to safeguard the patency of the airway, that is, to preserve and protect it during induction, mainte-

nance, and recovery from the state of anesthesia. In the event of patency deterioration or loss, it should be promptly reestablished by instrumentation or surgery before the subject suffers irreversible injury from respiratory compromise. The technologic innovations—pulse oximetry, capnography, carbon dioxide detectors—are undoubtedly useful as monitors to indicate the state of well-being of the patient and alert the clinician when the well-being is unsound or threatened. But they are not a substitute for comprehensive clinical evaluation and anticipation of any problem such as a potentially difficult airway.

In daily clinical usage, the term *airway* refers to the upper airway, which may be defined as the extrapulmonary air passage, consisting of the nasal and oral cavities, pharynx, larynx, trachea, and principal bronchi. In health, the airway performs a variety of functions, the principal one being conduction of air to and from the lungs for gaseous exchange between pulmonary alveoli and capillaries; airway patency is ensured by bones, cartilages, ligaments, and tone of the surrounding muscles. The nose, mouth, larynx, and trachea, equipped with rigid and semirigid bones and cartilages, are naturally patent. But the oropharynx, in contrast, due to the absence of such rigid elements in its wall, is dependent on the tone of the surrounding muscles, particularly genioglossus and mylohyoid, and ligaments for its patency. These muscles do so by mooring the tongue, directly or indirectly, to the mandible and hyoid bone through their reflexly maintained tone. Since the ultimate regulator of this tone adjustment, the central nervous system, is depressed during induction and maintenance of the anesthetized state, the tongue passively gravitates down into the hypopharynx, particularly in the supine position, occluding the pharynx and causing supraglottic obstruction. The greater the proximity of the glottic inlet to the base of tongue, particularly when the latter is disproportionately big, the greater the likelihood of severe or unrelievable obstruction. It is under these circumstances that maneuverability of the airway is crucial. However, in spite of appropriate maneuvers (sniff position, jaw thrust, etc.) and upper airway devices (oropharyngeal and nasopharyngeal airways), one may find it difficult to relieve this obstruction quickly and effectively in a small minority of patients; that is, the maneuverability of the upper airway is curtailed or poor, and consequently the obstruction is not easily relievable. Under such circumstances it is essential to secure a patent airway by translaryngeal placement of an orotracheal tube. In a small group of patients, exposure of the laryngeal inlet by direct laryngoscopy is nearly impossible, either because it is significantly masked by a disproportionately large base of tongue or because of associated pathologic conditions. These two concepts—maneuverability of airway and accessibility of laryngeal inlet—are crucial to our understanding of sleep disorders, such as sleep apnea, and a majority of difficulties experienced during the perioperative period. In fact, it is possible to explain the difficulty in a vast majority of circumstances, albeit not pinpointing the exact degree of difficulty, on the basis of "decreased maneuverability of airway" or "decreased accessibility of laryngeal inlet" or both. This chapter explores the anatomic variations, morphologic characteristics, and pathologic conditions that variously influence these two aspects of airway difficulties to help the clinician recognize the potential difficulty. Management options and strategies are discussed elsewhere in this book.

II. GLOBAL OBSERVATION

Although the primary focus of airway evaluation ought to be on the topography of the airway, an anatomically complex arena, a general inspection of the body habitus and the head and neck yields valuable information to the practitioner. A glance from a trained eye, more often than not, would spot many reliable clues as to potential airway difficulty. Trainees should be encouraged to view the head and neck frontally and in profile and take into consideration the body build as well. The short, muscular, and thick neck that is very often associated with difficult laryngoscopy and poor visualization of the laryngeal inlet is well known. Airway difficulties tend to be more common among short and stumpy individuals than among tall and lean individuals; this is particularly true with gravid women, perhaps also as a result of fluid retention during pregnancy. Obesity, particularly the so-called morbid obesity, could compromise the airway by means of excessive redundant tissue in the paratonsillar and paraglottic areas; this could mask the visibility and the accessibility of the glottis during laryngoscopy in the awake and in the anesthetized state. Many anatomic parameters can be screened as the patient walks into the office or during a conversational encounter—mobility of the mandible at temporomandibular joints, mobility of the head at atlanto-occipital joint, length, size, and muscularity of neck, size and configuration of palate, size of mandible in relation to face, and prominence or overbite of maxillary teeth in relation to mandibular teeth. It is also important to focus attention on the most prominent point of the thyroid cartilage, the Adam's apple, and visually gauge its approximate proximity to the mentum and the angle of the mandible. The vocal cords are located at the level of the midpoint of the anterior margin of the thyroid cartilage. By visually locating the position of Adam's apple with head maximally extended at the atlanto-occipital joint or in the sniff position, one can gauge roughly the anatomic closeness of glottis to the mandible and the base of tongue.

III. DENTITION

In individuals with difficult airways, dental injury as a consequence of difficult or excessive manipulations during laryngoscopy is a common cause of professional liability to the clinician; oftentimes this is also a cause of dissatisfaction to the patient. A few timely observations and precautions would serve to prevent potentially serious trauma and complications, including dislodgment of teeth to become foreign bodies in airway and subsequent aspiration. Aside from the general condition and strength, teeth should be examined with focus on their potential, not only for possible damage and dislodgment during airway management, but, more importantly, for possible impedance of axis alignment. If teeth are found to be shaky and too precarious, they should be extracted preoperatively for safety.

Prominent upper incisors or canines, with or without overbite (maxillary incisors are anterior to mandibular incisors), can impose a variable degree of limitation on alignment of oral, pharyngeal, and laryngeal axes during laryngoscopy and intubation; this is because the oral axis can be tilted upward only up to the tip of maxillary teeth, while the laryngoscopist or intubator standing behind the patient focuses his vision into the oropharnx. Unless the extensibility of head at atlanto-occipital joint is extremely favorable to compensate for this limitation, axis alignment is bound to be restricted, particularly when the airway is anything but class I (see following). When the thyromental distance is unsatisfactory (< 6 cm) and the airway is class II or III, the degree of laryngoscopic difficulty imposed by the relatively larger base of tongue is greatly compounded by the overbite. It is in these potentially difficult airways that the overbite is likely to be a significant limiting factor during laryngoscopy. In addition, overbite represents a disproportionate growth on the maxillary teeth relative to the mandibular teeth, but overbite may also be associated with micrognathia. In contrast, the edentulous state obviously offers less hindrance to axis alignment.

IV. COMPROMISED AIRWAY

The concept of evaluation is an integral element in the art of medical practice. Evaluation of cardiovascular and other parameters in the form of monitoring is a constant process during the intraoperative period to modulate the risks and therapeutic benefits. By applying this concept prior to subjecting the individual to elective (and as much as feasible in emergency) surgery and anesthesia, we hope to foresee the potential risks and life-threatening complications during the perioperative period. American Society of Anesthesiologists (ASA) physical status classification and New York Heart Association Cardiovascular status classification are often used as evaluation methods. However, there has been very little emphasis on the all-important airway

Table 7-1. Airway compromising conditions

Group	Pathologic condition	Principal pathologic/clinical features
I. Congenital:	A. *Supralaryngeal*	
	1. Pierre Robin syndrome	Micrognathia, macroglossia, cleft soft palate
	2. Treacher Collins syndrome	Auricular and ocular defects; malar and mandibular hypoplasia
	3. Goldenhar's syndrome	Auricular and ocular defects; malar and mandibular hypoplasia; occipitalization of atlas
	4. Down syndrome	Poorly developed or absent bridge of the nose; macroglossia
	5. Klippel-Feil syndrome	Congenital fusion of a variable number of cervical vertebrae; restriction of neck movement
	B. *Sublaryngeal*	
	1. Goiter	Compression of trachea, deviation of larynx-trachea
II. Acquired:	A. *Infections*	
	1. Supraglottitis	Laryngeal edema
	2. Croup	Laryngeal edema
	3. Abscess (intraoral, retropharyngeal)	Distortion of the airway and trismus
	4. Ludwig's angina	Distortion of the airway and trismus
	B. *Arthritis*	
	1. Rheumatoid arthritis	Temporomandibular joint ankylosis, cricoarytenoid arthritis, deviation of larynx, restricted mobility of cervical spine
	2. Ankylosing spondylitis	Ankylosis of cervical spine; less commonly, ankylosis of temporomandibular joints; lack of mobility of cervical spine
	C. *Benign tumors*	Stenosis or distortion of the airway
	1. Ex: cystic hygroma, lipoma, adenoma, goiter	
	D. *Malignant tumors*	Stenosis or distortion of the airway; fixation of larynx or adjacent tissues secondary to infiltration or fibrosis from irradiation
	1. Ex: Carcinoma of tongue, carcinoma of larynx, carcinoma of thyroid	
	E. *Trauma*	Edema of the airway, hematoma, unstable fracture(s) of the maxillae, mandible, and cervical vertebrae
	1. Ex: Facial injury, cervical spine injury, laryngeal-tracheal trauma	
	F. *Obesity*	Short, thick neck; redundant tissue in the oropharynx; sleep apnea
	G. *Acromegaly*	Macroglossia; prognathism
	H. *Acute burns*	Edema of airway

status, notwithstanding the fact that the morbidity and mortality from airway-related problems have been unacceptably high as shown in ASA closed claims analyses.

This chapter attempts to shed light on the anatomically compromised airway, with the hope that a good conceptual framework will lead to easier recognition and management of potentially difficult airways. Although it is difficult to give a succinct definition for a compromised airway, particularly in the absence of any visible adverse functional impact, for practical purposes it may be defined as one which has impaired structural integrity; i.e., an airway that is less than ideal in size, shape, proportionality of tissues, and mobility, regardless of whether the functional status is adversely affected or not. Structural integrity of the airway may be affected by a broad spectrum of conditions leading to changes in size, shape, proportionality, and mobility; when the airway is significantly compromised in any of these aspects, the result is likely to be an inadequate airway leading to impairment in its dynamics, particularly under stressful circumstances. The airway may be anatomically compromised by any of a broad array of factors at any phase of life, including the prenatal period; these may be best classified on the basis of etiology. Table 7-1 illustrates the conditions commonly encountered in clinical practice. The degree of anatomic compromise, regardless of its mechanism, may or may not be of functional significance in the awake state in a healthy individual, owing to protection from unhindered neurogenic and reflex-mediated compensatory mechanisms. For example, a patient with Ludwig's angina, by adopting the most favorable posture, may be able to maintain a patent airway to a sufficient degree without any visible evidence of respiratory distress; however, an unrelievable airway obstruction might result following conventional induction of anesthesia, since the compensatory mechanisms are subdued or abolished by the induction process.

In clinical situations wherein spontaneous or controlled ventilation by bag-mask is found to be difficult or impossible, ventilation by way of an endotracheal tube is the most practical means available, notwithstanding the

Table 7-2. Anatomic causes and mechanisms of difficult laryngoscopy

Cause	Example(s)	Primary mechanism
1. Disproportion	Mallampati class III airway Pierre robin syndrome Down Syndrome	Disproportionately increased size of the base of tongue
	Receding chin Very short thyromental distance Very short hyomental distance	Larynx relatively anterior to the rest of the upper airway structures

2. Distortion
    from intrinsic factors
 	
    from extrinsic factors
	Carcinoma of larynx
	Laryngeal edema
	Goiter
	Carcinoma of the base of tongue
	Postoperative hematoma in the neck
		Stenosis and deviation from intrinsic or extrinsic factors or both

3. Decreased mobility of joints	Klippel-Feil syndrome Ankylosing spondylitis Rheumatoid arthritis	Impedance of axis alignment
4. Dentition overbite	Likely to be a significant factor particularly in association with Mallampati class II and class III airway	Impedance of axis alignment

fact that surgical airway (cricothyrotomy or tracheostomy) may be more appropriate and safer in a small subgroup of patients with extremely compromised airways. Since orotracheal intubation entails visualization of laryngeal inlet during direct laryngoscopy by adequate displacement of the base of tongue and proper alignment of oral, pharyngeal, and laryngeal axes, the central focus of airway evaluation should be on recognition of anatomic conditions that are prone to render glottic visualization difficult or impossible. The amount of laryngoscopic difficulty, subjectively experienced or objectively anticipated, varies in accordance with the extent of anatomic compromise as a result of anatomic variations or pathologic conditions. The following are the primary causes of difficulty; these may act singly or in combination:

1. Disproportion, particularly between the base of tongue and oropharyngeal space
2. Distortion, anywhere in the airway
3. Decreased mobility of any or all joints (atlanto-occipital, cervical, and temporomandibular joints)
4. Dental overbite

Table 7-2 illustrates these causes and their mechanisms of difficult direct laryngoscopy.

In clinical terms, the degree of adverse effect any of these causes may have on the airway may be obvious and easily recognizable or very subtle and not easily discernible. Nevertheless, a seemingly negligible impact in the awake state might result in a profoundly difficult airway in the anesthetized state owing to loss of tone of the supporting muscles and ensuing passiveness. It is particularly under these circumstances that, not only greater skill is called for on the part of the caregiver, but also greater preparedness to function under stressful circumstances, including the ability to enlist all the available resources and adopt effective alternative methods.

Many authors have identified anatomic characteristics in difficult intubations as having an influence on the mechanics of direct laryngoscopy. The basis of difficulty is explainable by one or more of the aforementioned four primary causes of difficulty, namely, disproportion, distortion, decreased mobility of joints, and dental overbite. Cass, James, and Lines[5] directed attention to the short, muscular neck with a full set of teeth; a receding mandible with obtuse mandibular angles; protruding maxillary incisor teeth because of relative overgrowth of premaxilla; poor mobility of temporomandibular joint; a long, high-arched palate; and increased alveolar-mental distance. White and Kander[6] discovered, by radiographic studies, that the posterior depth of mandible (distance between the alveolus immediately behind third molar tooth and the lower border of mandible) was a significant factor in determining the ease or difficulty of direct laryngoscopy. Nichol and Zuck[7] placed emphasis on the atlanto-occipital distance as the major factor that determines the range of motion at the atlanto-occipital joint and ease of exposure of larynx. Bannister and MacBeth[8] stressed the significance of optimal position for alignment of axes of mouth, pharynx, and larynx. The most optimal position can be accomplished by flexion of the neck and extension of the head at the atlanto-occipital joint, so-called sniff position.[9] A faulty technique on the part of the intubator or failure to bring about optimal axis alignment is a common cause of failure in direct laryngoscopy.[10]

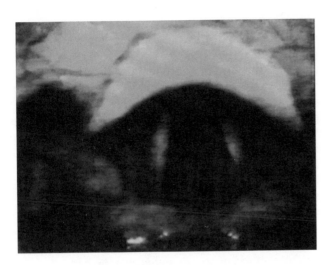

Fig. 7-1. Grade I view of larynx.

V. OBJECTIVE EVALUATION

Experienced clinicians apply a variety of criteria based upon previous personal experiences with varying degrees of success and reliability in identifying potentially difficult airways in surgical patients. However, conceptually sound and objectively defined clinical methods and criteria are far more desirable for descriptive and practical purposes; they also serve as better communication yardsticks among members of the professional community. As these method(s) are needed and applied to evaluate the airway with regard to potential for difficult orotracheal intubation and/or mask ventilation, any objectively designed clinical method is bound to have some limitations and generate bias among clinicians on account of the fact that almost all parts of the airway are mobile, the notable exception being the hard palate. It is inevitable that there will be some interobserver variability; oftentimes, it can be significant because parts of the airway are apt to vary significantly in size and, to some extent, in shape. They also are under central neurogenic and voluntary control of the patient who can arch the tongue or elevate the soft palate, for example, at will. The patient also may not appreciate the full significance of the test and so fail to cooperate well. Notwithstanding these drawbacks, the underlying conceptual basis is expected to prevail and contribute immensely to patient safety. Clinical methods also are simple and free of cost in comparison to radiologic methods and magnetic resonance imaging scans, which are costly, time consuming, and cannot be routinely employed. Their use, however, may be warranted sporadically to evaluate pathologic conditions of the airway.

Maintenance of the airway in the patent state at all times, for the purpose of uncompromised oxygenation, is the most vital part of the anesthesiologists' role. There are two methods of maintaining airway patency, namely, mask ventilation and tracheal intubation. With both methods, the degree of difficulty can range from none to an infinite degree.

Exposure of laryngeal inlet by direct laryngoscopy entails displacement of the base of tongue and alignment of oral, pharyngeal, and laryngeal axes to bring the laryngeal aperture into the path of vision as the laryngoscopist performs standing behind the head of the patient; optimal alignment is achieved by placing the head in the sniff position (flexion of neck and extension of head at the atlanto-occipital joint). If the tongue size is normal relative to the capacity of the oropharynx, it would be easily maneuverable during laryngoscopy. Axis alignment would be unimpeded if the mobility of joints of cervical spine, particularly the extensibility at the atlanto-occipital joint, is normal. Under these favorable circumstances, the laryngeal inlet would be fully visualized (grade I laryngoscopic view), facilitating easy insertion of endotracheal tube (ET). Fig. 7-1 illustrates laryngoscopic view in grade I. As the tongue size gets progressively bigger relative to oropharynx, with or without a restriction in the mobility of cervical spine and temporomandibular joints, the laryngoscopic view correspondingly diminishes, leading to grade II (visualization of just the posterior portion of laryngeal inlet), grade III (visualization of just the corniculate cartilages or epiglottis), and grade IV (visualization of just the hypopharynx and soft palate).[11]

Since the base (posterior part) of the tongue is in close proximity to the laryngeal inlet and optimal degree of axis alignment is necessary for unimpeded direct laryngoscopy, design of evaluation methods ought to focus primarily on these two elements. The basic question these methods should address is: Are these two favorable or unfavorable for mask ventilation and endotracheal intubation? To date there is no single method available that is capable of evaluating both aspects. Most airway-related catastrophes have occurred when difficulty was unanticipated.[12,13,14] These are preventable by predicting the potential for difficulty.

VI. EVALUATION OF TONGUE SIZE RELATIVE TO PHARYNX SIZE

The tongue is the largest occupant of the cavity of oropharynx; its base (posterior part) is in close proximity to the laryngeal inlet. Its anatomic relation to larynx in terms of closeness and relative size is of practical significance to laryngoscopists and intubators and, when assessed objectively, yields valuable information. This author previously propounded a hypothesis[15] that, when the base of the tongue is disproportionately large relative to the capacity of the oropharyngeal cavity, it would render laryngoscopy and intubation difficult. Conceptually, the difficulty results perhaps because the angle between the base of the tongue and the larynx is more acute and not conducive for easy exposure of laryngeal inlet, or because the larynx is overshadowed by the larger tongue, or both. Anatomically, a large base of the tongue would not only overshadow the larynx but also mask the visibility of the posterior part of soft palate where the uvula is an easily identifiable landmark. Because it is not possible to measure the volume or determine the size of the base of the tongue, relative to the capacity of the oropharyngeal cavity, it is quite logical to infer that the base of the tongue is disproportionately large when it is able to mask the visibility of the faucial pillars and uvula. Elicitation of this sign is easy; the patient remains seated with head in the neutral position and is asked to open the mouth as widely as possible and to protrude the tongue as far out as possible. Although some degree of phonation (saying "ah") is inevitable at times, the patient should not be encouraged to actively phonate to avoid a spuriously positive picture of the pharynx. This can be largely prevented by encouraging the patient to stretch the masseter muscles as maximally as possible and simultaneously protrude the tongue forcefully. In order to avoid a false-positive or false-negative picture, it is desirable that this be repeated at least twice. The observer then relates the size of the base of the tongue to the pharyngeal structures, namely, the uvula, faucial pillars, and soft palate. If the tongue base is proportional in size relative to oropharynx, it can be reasoned that exposure of laryngeal inlet would not be difficult, provided there are no other factors—anatomic or pathologic—at play, such as ankylosing spondylitis; this is because the tongue could be easily maneuvered inside a roomy pharynx and the fact that the base of the tongue is not bulky enough to overshadow the larynx. In contrast, a disproportionately large base of the tongue overshadows the larynx and possibly renders the angle between the two more acute; this anatomic relation is not conducive for easy exposure of the larynx.

This method of assessment is also the basis of airway classification into three classes, according to the extent that the base of the tongue is able to mask the visibility of pharyngeal structures[16]:

Class I: uvula, faucial pillars, soft palate visible
Class II: faucial pillars, soft palate visible
Class III: only soft palate visible

Figs. 7-2 and 7-3 illustrate the conceptual basis of the hypothesis and the classification, respectively. In Sam-

Conceptual Basis of Mallampati Airway Classification

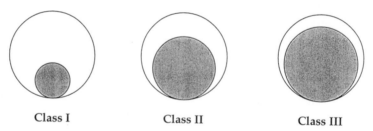

Class I   Class II   Class III

Fig. 7-2. Conceptual basis of the Mallampati Airway Classification is determining size of the tongue *(shaded area)* relative to size of the pharyngeal cavity *(open circle).*

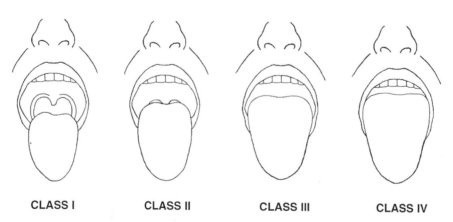

CLASS I   CLASS II   CLASS III   CLASS IV

Fig. 7-3. Samsoon and Young[12] modification of the Mallampati Airway Classification. See text for precise definition of classes.

soon and Young's modification[12] of the Mallampati classification, the size of the tongue relative to the pharynx is divided into four classes, the fourth class (class IV) reflecting an extreme form of Mallampati class III in which the soft palate is completely masked by the tongue; only the hard palate is visible. Fig. 7-4 illustrates a schematic representation of the classification that shows that the uvula is at the posterior level, and the soft palate at the anterior level. As the tongue size progressively increases, it occupies more and more room inside the oropharyngeal cavity—a concept that is the hallmark of the classification. A study by this author[16] (Table 7-3) demonstrated significant correlation between airway class and degree of ease of exposure of laryngeal inlet by direct laryngoscopy; in class I ease of exposure is the rule, whereas in class III it is significantly difficult. Similar findings were demonstrated by Samsoon and

Young.[12] The practical significance of this method stems from the fact that it would alert the clinician to potential airway difficulty, almost inevitable in class III airway, and likely in class II, particularly in association with other unfavorable factors, including short thick neck, receding jaw, decreased mobility of cervical and atlanto-occipital joints, and thyromental distance of less than 6 cm. Since this method is based on assessment of mobile parts of the airway, some amount of interobserver variability[17] is bound to creep into the classification—a limitation that can be eliminated as one's experience grows. It can also be rendered negligible by eliciting the sign in the seated position, with head not flexed toward chest but in the neutral position, not encouraging the patient to phonate (to say "ah"), which spuriously improves the view, and avoiding the arching of the tongue that obscures the uvula. However, in incapacitated patients, supine position during elicitation of the sign is unlikely to make much difference if phonation is avoided.[18]

VII. EVALUATION OF THE MANDIBULAR SPACE

The mandible provides the skeleton for the floor of the mouth and a housing compartment for the tongue and larynx; the greater the space in this compartment, the less compact the structures will be. Apart from the overall size and shape, the two most important dimensions that determine the capacity of this compartment are the horizontal length and width of the mandible.

The concept of mandibular space helps to explain a number of difficulties encountered in difficult laryngoscopy and intubation. When the space is relatively small, the tongue mass and larynx have to be compressed together to fit into this small compartment; these are likely to be much more compact if the tongue is not proportionately smaller. In other words if the tongue

Schematic representation of Mallampati Airway Classification

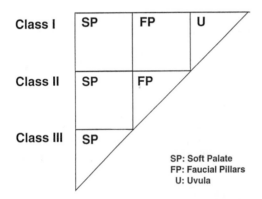

Fig. 7-4. Schematic representation of the Mallampati Airway Classification according to structures visualized. Right-hand side of schematic corresponds to posterior part of pharynx, and left-hand side of the schematic to anterior part of pharynx.

Table 7-3. Correlation between visibility of faucial pillars, soft palate, and uvula and exposure of glottis by direct laryngoscopy

Visibility of structures* No. of pts. (%)	Laryngoscopy grade			
	Grade 1 No. of pts. (%)	Grade 2 No. of pts. (%)	Grade 3 No. of pts. (%)	Grade 4 No. of pts. (%)
Class 1 155 (73.8%)	125 (59.5%)	30 (14.3%)	—	—
Class 2 40 (19%)	12 (5.7%)	14 (6.7%)	10 (4.7%)	4 (1.9%)
Class 3 15 (7.14%)	—	1 (0.5%)	9 (4.3%)	5 (2.4%)

*Class 1, Faucial pillars, soft palate, and uvula could be visualized. Class 2, Faucial pillars and soft palate could be visualized, but uvula was masked by the base of the tongue. Class 3, Only soft palate could be visualized. Grade 1, Glottis (including anterior and posterior commissures) could be fully exposed. Grade 2, Glottis could be partly exposed (anterior commissure not visualized). Grade 3, Glottis could not be exposed (corniculate cartilages only could be visualized). Grade 4, Glottis including corniculate cartilages could not be exposed. No. of pts., Number of patients.

base is relatively larger, they are so compact that the larynx is relatively anterior to the base of tongue. Also during development, the tongue base is likely to overshadow and envelope the larynx from above and behind. Pierre Robin syndrome, characterized by both micrognathia and macroglossia, exemplifies this anatomic topography. The concept of mandibular space also serves to explain the ease of axis alignment. At laryngoscopy, it is the area bounded by the plane of the line of vision and the mandibular arch in front.[19] In the case of smaller mandibular space, the laryngeal axis will make a more acute angle with the pharyngeal axis, necessitating greater extensibility at the atlanto-occipital joint to bring about alignment between these two axes.

It is clinically easy to measure the space anterior to the larynx with the head in the maximally extended position at the atlanto-occipital joint by means of a ruler or in terms of finger breadths and to express the length as the thyromental or hyomental distance and/or the horizontal length of the mandible. This author prefers thyromental distance because the Adam's apple (the thyroid cartilage) is an easily recognizable and palpable landmark in the neck and the vocal cords are slightly below the level of the middle of the anterior margin of thyroid cartilage. The thyromental distance and horizontal length of the mandible have been found to inversely correlate well with the class of airway described above.[20,21] The correlation with airway classification is so strong that a thyromental distance greater than 6 cm and a horizontal length of the mandible greater than 9 cm are strongly suggestive of relatively easy direct laryngoscopy.[14,20,21] The most significant obstacle in the path of vision (between the laryngoscopist's eye and the target, namely, the laryngeal inlet) is the posterior part of the tongue: the larger the tongue the greater the obstacle. This would be augmented by prominent maxillary teeth or overbite and anterior displacement of larynx when the neck is in extension rather than flexion.[11]

VIII. EVALUATION OF THE EXTENT OF MOBILITY OF THE JOINTS

The skeleton of the thorax provides a hermetically sealed cavity that encloses and protects the lungs, while the skeleton of the head and neck provides a framework that provides stability and flexibility to the upper airway in its passage towards the lungs. Apart from the mobility of the mandible at the temporomandibular joints, the dimensions of the upper airway are governed by excursions of the head and neck, largely at the atlanto-occipital joint. The atlas facilitates flexion and extension of the head by virtue of the absence of its spinous process, which is rudimentary in humans; the diminutive size of the spinous process obviates interference with the movements between the atlas and the skull.

It is common knowledge that joggers prefer to keep the head in the neutral or slightly extended position at the atlanto-occipital joint while jogging; this is because the airway is more patent in this position than when the head is flexed toward chest. This principle is crucial in understanding the mechanics of the airway and its management in clinical anesthesiology. Extension of the head at the atlanto-occipital joint while the neck is moderately flexed (25 to 35 degrees) brings the oral, pharyngeal, and laryngeal axes into almost a straight line (sniff, or Magill position). Nichol and Zuck[7] directed attention to the atlanto-occipital distance (distance between the occiput and the rudimentary spinous process of the cervical vertebra C1) as the major factor that determines the range of motion at the atlanto-occipital joint. The C1-C2 interspinous gap is also a governing albeit less significant, factor in this respect. Naturally, when these two gaps are less than normal or when the C1 spinous process is more prominent, the degree of extension of head at the atlanto-occipital joint, which is naturally 35 degrees, would be curtailed. This range of motion can be restricted in short, thick necks and in individuals with congenital prominence of C1 spinous process or reduced atlanto-occipital gap. In the face of such restriction, vigorous attempts to extend the head at the atlanto-occipital joint will make laryngoscopic visualization of glottis difficult by rendering the cervical spine more convex anteriorly, which will push the larynx forwards.

Evaluation of atlanto-occipital extension can be carried out visually at bedside, expressing any reduction in extension as a fraction of normal and grading it accordingly as described by Bellhouse and Dore.[19] When the airway class is unfavorable, as in class III, a normal range of motion at the atlanto-occipital joint would help to lessen the difficulty at laryngoscopy through greater axis alignment. Ironically, more often than not, reduction in extensibility at the atlanto-occipital joint tends to coexist with difficulty posed by airway class, compounding the problem. A two-variable analysis of intubation difficulty proposed by Bellhouse and Dore indicates the two factors tend to additively interact.[19] By assessing the relative tongue-pharyngeal size (airway class), neck mobility, and mandibular space, one can anticipate the difficult intubation in nearly all instances.[19,21,22,23]

IX. RECOGNITION OF POTENTIAL AIRWAY DIFFICULTY

Ability to provide effective pulmonary ventilation either by bag-mask or through an endotracheal tube is a vital clinical task performed by anesthesiologists in medical practice; this is also crucial for other physicians such as otolaryngologists and emergency room physicians who are often involved in managing the human airway in emergency situations.

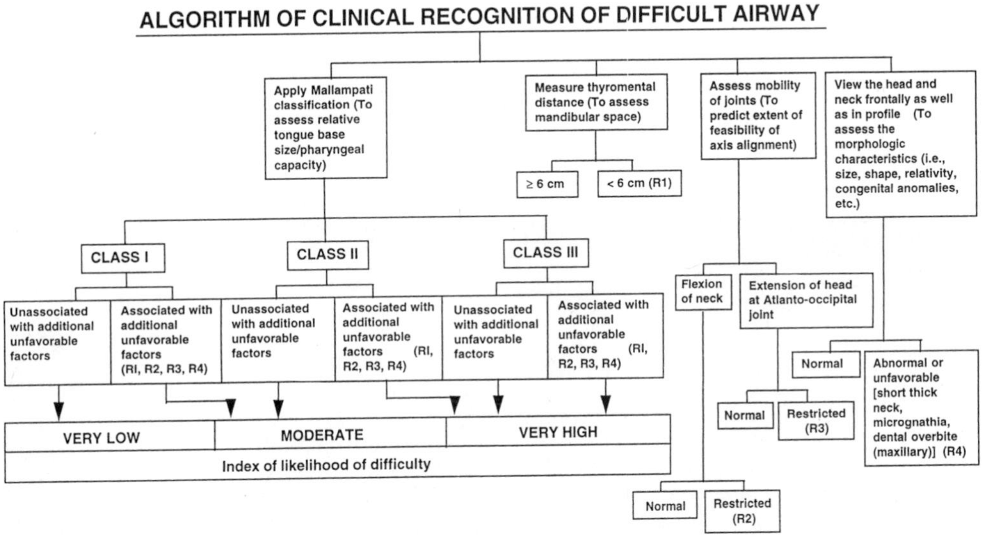

ALGORITHM OF CLINICAL RECOGNITION OF DIFFICULT AIRWAY

Fig. 7-5. Algorithm for recognition of the difficult airway emphasizes the primary use of oropharyngeal classification, measurement of thyromental distance, range of motion of head and neck, and neck morphology. *R1,* Thyromental distance < 6 cm; *R2,* restricted neck flexion; *R3,* restricted extension of the head; *R4,* short, thick neck.

In order to ensure unhindered and effective ventilation by bag-mask, the laryngeal inlet ought to be freely accessible to the airflow generated during the ventilation process. In the absence of traumatic and pathologic conditions, the ease or difficulty of airflow in the supralaryngeal part of the airway is a function of the size of the conduit and compliance of the tissues: the greater the size of the conduit and compliance, the lower the resistance to airflow and easier the ventilation by bag-mask. Theoretically, any condition that renders the passageway narrower and decreases the compliance of tissues would increase difficulty with ventilation by bag-mask. The nasal part of the airway is not of serious concern in this respect because it is naturally supported by rigid elements in its walls and is noncollapsible, as is the case with the oral part that is bounded superiorly by the hard palate. The pharyngeal part of the airway, on the other hand is predisposed to collapse and obstruction by the tongue during sleep and in the anesthetized state, since it lacks skeletal framework in its walls. However, it is usually manageable by means of appropriate position and upper airway support devices: oropharyngeal and nasopharyngeal airways. In contrast, resistance to ventilation in the immediate vicinity of laryngeal inlet is more ominous; in the absence of an obstructive lesion such as a pedunculated polyp in the glottis, it is a direct result of obstruction of laryngeal inlet by the posterior part of the tongue and perhaps also by the epiglottis. Naturally the size of these structures relative to oropharynx is crucial: the more disproportionately larger they are relative to oropharnx, the greater the likelihood of laryngeal obstruction. Notable contributing factors include significant reduction in the tone of supporting muscles during induction, lack of tissue compliance, and existence of redundant fatty tissue in the perilaryngeal areas. Tissue compliance might be inherently poor or rendered unfavorable by pathologic factors such as edema, prior radiation, or tumor invasion. Resistance to ventilation in these adverse circumstances can be mild or moderate and relievable or severe and unrelievable; if the latter situation is followed by extremely difficult or impossible exposure of glottis and failed intubation, it would be tantamount to the so-called cannot-ventilate-and-cannot-intubate situation, which may prove lethal to the subject unless it is immediately followed by surgical airway or other modality of ventilation, such as transtracheal jet ventilation. Although it is fortunately uncommon, the cannot-ventilate-and-cannot-intubate scenario is extremely dangerous and may carry high morbidity and mortality even in skilled hands, despite appropriate position, physical maneuvers, and therapeutic interventions. It is always better to err on the side of defensiveness and safety rather than on the side of danger.

As the airway dynamics are altered during induction and converted into a passive state, one should be able to maneuver the airway into the most favorable position that would augment not only the patency of the conduit but also the accessibility of larynx for emergency intubation; any position or technique that is not conducive for patency and accessibility of larynx ought to be immediately recognized and replaced by a more fruitful method. Maneuverability of the airway—ease of movements of the airway joints, including the atlanto-occipital joint, the joints of the cervical spine, and the temporo-

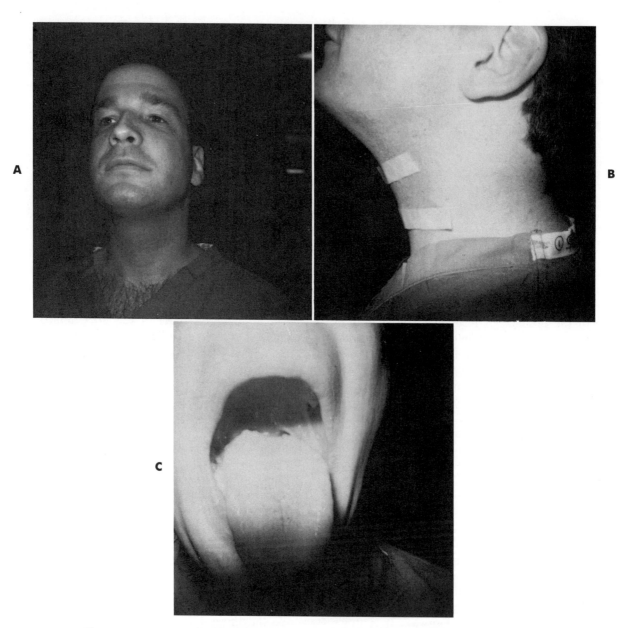

Fig. 7-6. A, C, A 25-year-old male with normal anatomic features, class I airway, thyromental distance of 10 cm, unrestricted mobility of head and neck, and full normal dentition. **B,** Tapes on neck indicate location of hyoid bone and thyroid cartilage, respectively. Since vocal cords lie at level of middle of anterior margin of thyroid cartilage, the thyromental distance correlates well with airway class. No difficulty is anticipated.

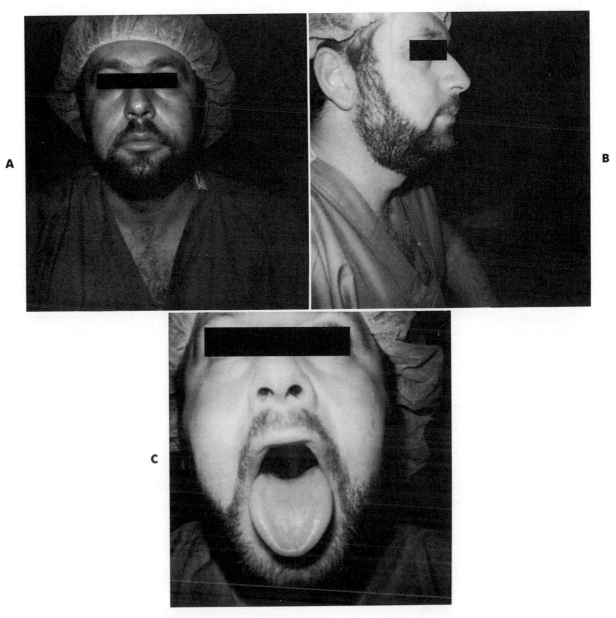

Fig. 7-7. A, B, A 35-year-old male with unremarkable orofacial features, class I airway, thyromental distance of 8 cm, unrestricted mobility of head and neck, and full dentition without overbite. **C,** At maximal protrusion of tongue, pharyngeal structures (soft palate, faucial pillars, and uvula) are fully visible. Only noteworthy feature is appearance of double chin and muscular neck. Since this is a class I airway, no difficulty is anticipated.

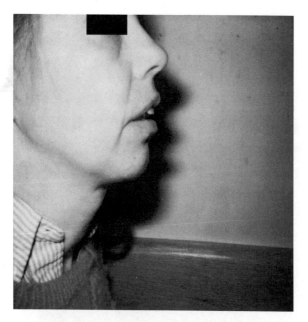

Fig. 7-8. A 35-year-old woman has normal orofacial features but has maxillary overbite that is quite significant when viewed in profile. She was found to have a class I airway, a thyromental distance of 8 cm, and unrestricted mobility of head and neck. At laryngoscopy and intubation following induction with thiopental and succinylcholine, grade II laryngoscopic view was observed and orotracheal intubation was accomplished with ease. Since this was a class I airway, the limitation in axis alignment posed by dental overbite was not significant. If she possessed a class II airway, intubation would have been at least moderately difficult.

mandibular joints—is essential to facilitating the manipulations during ventilation and laryngoscopy. Particularly important is extensibility of head at the atlanto-occipital joint to facilitate axis alignment. Mobility of joints may be inherently restricted or adversely affected by congenital or acquired factors such as congenital fusion of cervical vertebrae, inflammation of joints, or scarification of tissues.

For practical purposes, a difficult airway may be succinctly defined as one that, by virtue of disproportionate anatomy, or preexisting pathology, is likely to offer a moderately severe or very severe degree of difficulty to bag-mask ventilation (that is, to experience significant upper airway resistance to ventilation) or to direct laryngoscopy (that is, to experience significant difficulty in visualizing the laryngeal inlet) for the purpose of orotracheal intubation or both. Mask ventilation also might be rendered difficult by easily recognizable factors that include a thick beard, massive jaw, lack of teeth (edentulous state), extreme sensitivity of skin to motion or friction (burns, skin grafts, or epidermolysis bullosa), and the presence of massive facial dressings. Since these conditions are easily recognized before anesthetic induction, they have not been

responsible for many anesthesia-related catastrophes (brain damage or death).[12,13] Nevertheless, they may contribute significantly to morbidity and mortality by compounding the difficulty when they coexist with subtle conditions that were unanticipated and also increase the difficulty with the airway.

The above concepts form the ladder for a routine evaluation of a patient's airway, assuming that the patient has no pathologic airway problem; the primary purpose is to guide the evaluator in identifying the ease of accessibility of laryngeal inlet and the degree of maneuverability of head and neck. The ultimate objective is to recognize the potential for difficult airway as a result of curtailed accessibility of laryngeal inlet and limited maneuverability of head and neck secondary to restricted mobility of joints and perhaps also due to a thick, muscular neck. The algorithm of clinical recognition of difficult airway (Fig. 7-5) is designed to facilitate this evaluation process; it is simple in structure, easy to memorize and apply, and free of cost. Its clinical application calls for four steps:

1. Application of Mallampati classification
2. Measurement of thyromental distance digitally or by means of a ruler
3. Assessment of mobility of joints
4. Viewing the head and neck frontally and in profile

The following eight case examples illustrate the use of the algorithm in Fig. 7-5 on p. 135 and the principles associated in this chapter (Figs. 7-6 to 7-13, pp. 136 to 141).

It is also advised that other sources of information be judged critically. In the case of a previous airway difficulty, it is desirable to examine the medical record for the nature and intensity of the problem and, if possible, get firsthand information from the anesthesia provider. Attention to body habitus (build) is to be part and parcel of the total evaluation picture; it is often neglected, particularly by our trainees. This author prefers to look at the feasibility of sniff position while the patient is in supine position prior to anesthetic induction, particularly in short, stumpy, and obese individuals. In morbidly obese individuals, supine posture is likely to diminish compliance of airway tissues and augment airway obstruction.

As our ultimate goal is to have a live patient at the end of every surgical procedure, it is of paramount importance to evaluate in detail systemic diseases, clinically evident or otherwise, such as coronary artery disease, congestive heart failure, respiratory failure, and bleeding diathesis that might impose limitations on, or require special precautions during, induction or intubation, such as increased fraction of inspired oxygen (FiO_2) and prevention of sympathetic nervous system stimulation leading to tachycardia and hypertension. In some uncertain situations, it may be necessary, fol-

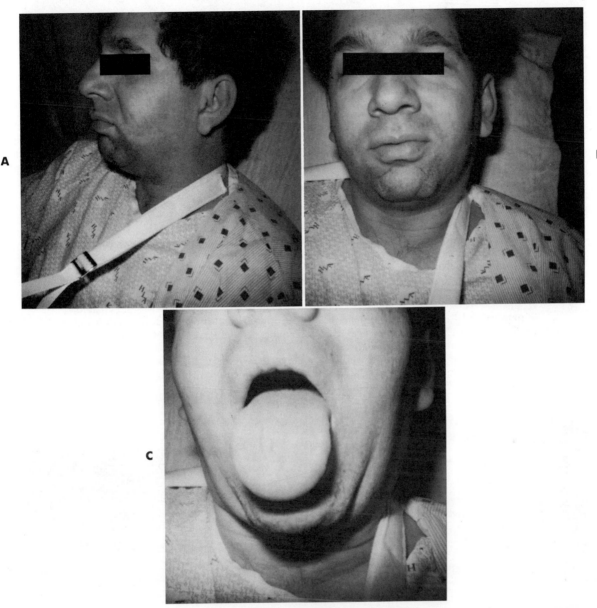

Fig. 7-9. A, B, A 36-year-old male required multiple attempts at laryngoscopy and intubation. He was informed by his anesthesiologist and surgeon that they could accomplish intubation only with utmost difficulty; it is not known whether they could visualize any part of glottis at all. **C,** On examination, he was found to have a class II airway (uvula completely masked by base of tongue), thyromental distance of 5.5 cm, normal mobility of head and neck, and full dentition. In light of known intubation difficulty, he opted to have regional anesthesia for a surgical procedure on the hand. Physically, he is a well-built individual with a muscular neck.

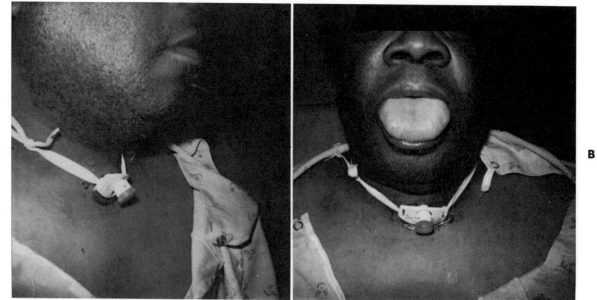

Fig. 7-10. A, A 40-year-old male with history of sleep apnea was advised to undergo uvulopalatoplasty (UPP). An experienced anesthesiologist recognized potential for airway difficulty by classifying the airway, measuring the thyromental distance, assessing the mobility of head and neck, and noting his body build. **B,** Only anterior part of soft palate was barely visible on maximal protrusion of tongue with mouth widely open in the seated position (class III airway). Thyromental distance was 5 cm. Very high degree of difficulty was anticipated. Patient was advised of the need for awake tracheal intubation; orotracheal intubation was carried out uneventfully under topical anesthesia and sedation. Patient was tracheostomized prior to UPP. Three days postoperatively, he developed hemorrhage in the vicinity of tracheal stoma. Following successful orotracheal intubation under topical anesthesia and sedation, tracheostomy tube was removed and bleeding point identified and ligated. By direct laryngoscopy, laryngeal inlet could not be visualized.

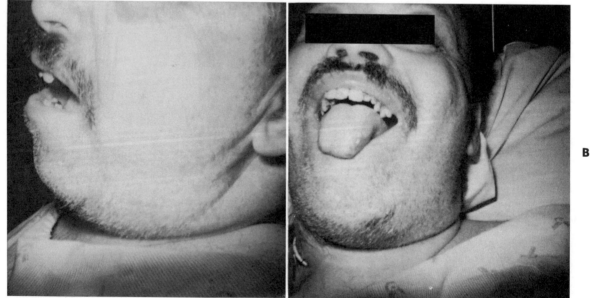

Fig. 7-11. A, B, A 45-year-old man with very short neck, class III airway (only soft palate was visible on maximal protrusion of tongue), thyromental distance of about 6 cm, and somewhat reduced (probably by one-third) extensibility of head at atlanto-occipital joint, with full dentition. At laryngoscopy laryngeal inlet could not be visualized; however, he could be ventilated following thiopental and succinylcholine and intubated after multiple attempts with multiple blades and maximal laryngeal pressure.

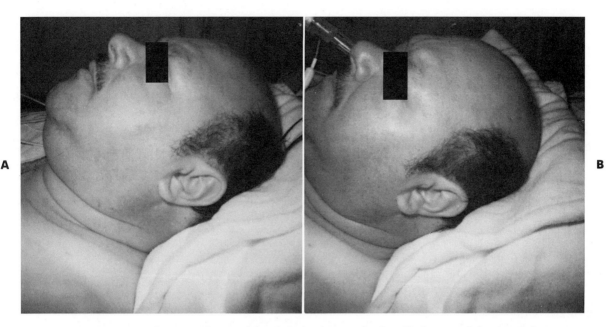

Fig. 7-12. A, A 50-year-old man with relatively short neck, class II airway and thyromental distance of 5.8 cm, and full normal dentition. The remarkable feature in this case is that the occiput was almost in line with the posterior surface of neck; extensibility of head at the atlanto-occipital joint was almost negligible. This made laryngoscopy following adequate muscle relaxation impossible, but not ventilation. **B,** Awake nasotracheal intubation subsequently was carried out uneventfully.

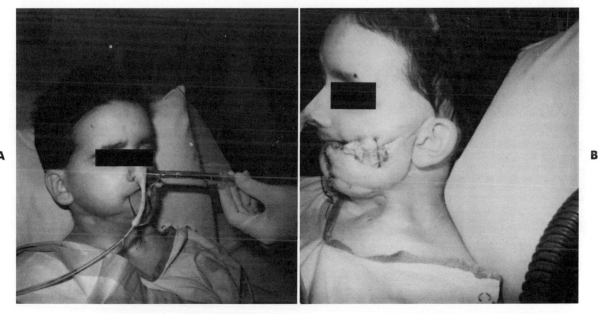

Fig. 7-13. A, B, A teenage boy has undergone surgery for malignant lesion in the submandibular region. This postsurgical state has produced so much distortion and restricted mobility that the inter-incisor interval was hardly 2 cm. When he required cosmetic surgery, he was intubated nasally, fiberoptically, under topical anesthesia without complications.

lowing appropriate preparation, to carry out awake direct laryngoscopy to help ascertain intubation difficulty. If the epiglottis and vocal cords can be visualized, it is very likely, but not certain, that direct laryngoscopy will permit uneventful intubation during induction and paralysis.

The upper airway is an anatomically complex structure and has many variables. As a result of this simple, yet comprehensive, evaluation methodology, a clinician can uncover the hidden potential for difficulty and place the patient on the path of safety. Occurrence of difficulty for mask ventilation or intubation or both is a result of either anatomic factors or pathologic conditions or a combination thereof. If a very high degree of airway difficulty is recognized, then airway patency should be secured (usually by intubation and occasionally by surgical airway) before subjecting the patient to anesthesia and paralysis.

REFERENCES

1. Keenan RL, Boyan CP: Cardiac arrest due to anesthesia, *JAMA* 252(16):2373, 1985.
2. Caplan RA, Posner KL, Ward RJ et al: Adverse respiratory events in anesthesia: a closed claims analysis, *Anesthesiology* 72:828, 1990.
3. Cheney FW, Posner KL, Caplan RA: Adverse respiratory events infrequently leading to malpractice suits: a closed claims analysis, *Anesthesiology* 75:932, 1991.
4. Benumof JL: Management of the difficult adult airway, *Anesthesiology* 75:1087, 1991.
5. Cass NM, James NR, Lines V: Difficult direct laryngoscopy complicating intubation for anesthesia, *BMJ* 1:488, 1956.
6. White A, Kander PL: Anatomical factors in difficult direct laryngoscopy, *Br J Anaesth* 47:74, 1975.
7. Nichol HC, Zuck D: Difficult laryngoscopy—the "anterior" larynx and the atlanto-occipital gap, *Br J Anaesth* 55:141, 1983.
8. Bannister FB, MacBeth RG: Direct laryngoscopy and intubation, *Lancet* 2:651, 1944.
9. Gillespie NA: Endotracheal anesthesia, ed 2, Madison, 1950, University of Wisconsin Press.
10. Salem MR, Mathrubhutham M, Bennett EJ: Difficult intubation, *N Engl J Med* 295:879, 1976.
11. Cormack RS, Lehane J: Difficult tracheal intubation in obstetrics, *Anaesthesia* 39:1105, 1984.
12. Samsoon GLT, Young JRB: Difficult tracheal intubation: a retrospective study, *Anaesthesia* 42:487, 1987.
13. King TA, Adams AP: Failed tracheal intubation, *Br J Anaesth* 65:400, 1990.
14. Finucane BT, Santora AH: Evaluation of the airway prior to intubation. In *Principles of airway management,* Philadelphia, 1988, FA Davis.
15. Mallampati SR: Clinical sign to predict difficult tracheal intubation (hypothesis), *Can J Anaesth* 30:316, 1983.
16. Mallampati SR, Gatt SP, Gugino LD et al: A clinical sign to predict difficult tracheal intubation: a prospective study, *Can J Anaesth* 32:429, 1985.
17. Wilson ME, John R: Problems with the Mallampati sign, *Anaesthesia* 45:486, 1990.
18. Tham EJ, Gilldersleve CD, Sanders LD et al: Effects of posture, phonation, and observer on Mallampati classification, *Br J Anaesth* 68:32, 1992.
19. Bellhouse CP, Dore C: Criteria for estimating likelihood of difficulty of endotracheal intubation with Macintosh laryngoscope, *Anaesth Intensive Care* 16:329, 1988.
20. Mathew M, Hanna LS, Aldretre JA: Preoperative indices to anticipate a difficult tracheal intubation, *Anesth Analg* 68:S187, 1989.
21. Patil VU, Stehling LC, Zaunder HL: *Fiberoptic endoscopy in anaesthesia,* Chicago, 1983, Year Book Medical.
22. Wilson ME, Spiegelhalter D, Robertson JA et al: Predicting difficult intubation. *Br J Anaesth* 61:211, 1988.
23. Frerk CM: Predicting difficult intubation, *Anaesthesia* 46:1005, 1991.

Chapter 8

THE AMERICAN SOCIETY OF ANESTHESIOLOGISTS' MANAGEMENT OF THE DIFFICULT AIRWAY ALGORITHM AND EXPLANATION-ANALYSIS OF THE ALGORITHM

Jonathan L. Benumof

I. INTRODUCTION

The literature provides strong evidence that specific strategies facilitate the management of the difficult airway. Specific strategies can be linked together to form more comprehensive treatment plans or algorithms. The purpose of the American Society of Anesthesiologists' (ASA) Algorithm on the Management of the Difficult Airway is to facilitate the management of the difficult airway and to reduce the likelihood of adverse outcomes. The principal adverse outcomes associated with the difficult airway include (but are not limited to): death, brain injury, myocardial injury, and airway trauma.

The ASA Algorithm on the Management of the Difficult Airway was developed over a 2-year period by the ASA Task Force on Guidelines for Management of the Difficult Airway. The task force consisted of Robert A. Caplan, M.D. (chairman); Jonathan L. Benumof, M.D.; Frederic A. Berry, M.D.; Casey D. Blitt, M.D.; Robert H. Bode, M.D.; Frederick W. Cheney, M.D.; Richard T. Connis, Ph.D. (health services research methodologist); Orin F. Guidry, M.D.; and Andranik Ovassapian, M.D., and therein included academicians, private practitioners, airway experts, adult and pediatric anesthesia generalists, and a statistical methodologist. The algorithm was approved by the ASA House of Delegates, October 21, 1992, and became effective July 1, 1993.

The Task Force developed the algorithm principally by conducting an extensive, structured literature search and a meta-analysis of this literature. Agreement between the Task Force members and the methodologist with respect to the literature was established by inter-rater reliability testing. The findings of the literature analysis were supplemented by opinion from Task Force members and 50 consultant anesthesiologists with recognized interest in airway management and guidelines. Finally, the algorithm was presented and discussed at an open forum with the anesthesia community at a large anesthesia meeting; anesthesiologists from academia, private practice, and industry were invited and were well represented at the open forum.

This chapter presents and explains the ASA Algorithm on the Management of the Difficult Airway. The algorithm is concerned with the maintenance of airway patency at all times. Special emphasis is placed on an operating room setting (although the algorithm can be extrapolated to the intensive care unit and the ward). The algorithm assumes that a fully trained anesthesiologist is attempting to maintain airway patency. Adherence to the principles of the difficult airway management algorithm and the widespread adoption of a precise plan for management of airway difficulties should result in reduction of respiratory catastrophes and a decrease in anesthesia morbidity and mortality.

II. THE ASA ALGORITHM ON THE MANAGEMENT OF THE DIFFICULT AIRWAY

The management of the difficult airway will follow the algorithm shown in Figs. 8-1[1] and 8-2.[2] Fig. 8-2, which was published as a medical intelligence article on the algorithm,[2] is arranged in a manner that best shows the total algorithm and the flow of the algorithm. Fig. 8-1, which is contained within the official ASA guideline statement,[1] is arranged slightly differently (but has the same intellectual content). Fig. 8-2 contains some specifics that are not included in Fig. 8-1, and vice versa.

The algorithm begins with the most basic question of whether or not the presence of a difficult airway is recognized (see Chapter 7). Obviously, if the potential for difficulty is recognized, then one can make proper mental and physical preparation, and the chance of a successful-good outcome is increased, whereas failure to recognize the potential for difficulty means, by definition, that the actual difficulty will be unexpected, proper mental and physical preparation will be minimized, and a chance of a successful-good outcome decreased.

The following plan for routine evaluation of a patient's airway, assuming that the patient has no obvious pathologic airway problem, is a reasonable one (see Chapter 7 for a complete discussion of preoperative evaluation). (1) The medical record should be examined for a history of previous difficulty with managing the patient's airway. (2) Patients should be asked to open their mouths as widely as possible and extend their tongues. The mandibular opening (measured by ruler, if there is doubt about limitation) and pharyngeal anatomy (uvula, tonsillar pillars, etc.) are observed. (3) The length of the submental space (mandible to hyoid or thyroid cartilage distance) should be noted (measured by ruler, if there is a doubt). (4) Patients should be viewed from the side to see their ability to assume the sniff position (flexion of the neck on chest and extension of the head on the neck). The lateral view should also reveal any degree of maxillary overbite. (5) The patency of the nostrils must be assessed. (6) Systemic diseases, such as respiratory failure and coronary artery disease, that might place limits on or require special attention during awake intubation, such as increased fraction of inspired oxygen (FiO_2) and prevention of sympathetic nervous system stimulation, respectively, should be noted. (7) In a few patients, an awake direct laryngoscopy (after adequate preparation; see following) may be indicated to help determine intubation difficulty. If the epiglottis and vocal cords can be seen, it is likely, but not certain, that direct laryngoscopy will reveal the vocal cords and permit successful intubation during anesthesia and paralysis.

If it is recognized that the intubation or mask ventilation is going to be difficult because of the presence of a pathologic factor(s) or a combination of anatomic factors (large tongue site, small mandibular space, or restricted atlanto-occipital extension), then airway patency should be secured and guaranteed (usually by intubation) while the patient remains awake.

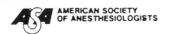

DIFFICULT AIRWAY ALGORITHM

1. Assess the likelihood and clinical impact of basic management problems:

   A. Difficult Intubation

   B. Difficult Ventilation

   C. Difficulty with Patient Cooperation or Consent

2. Consider the relative merits and feasibility of basic management choices:

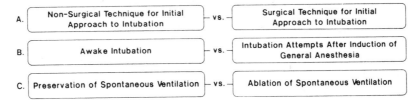

   A. [Non-Surgical Technique for Initial Approach to Intubation] — vs. — [Surgical Technique for Initial Approach to Intubation]

   B. [Awake Intubation] — vs. — [Intubation Attempts After Induction of General Anesthesia]

   C. [Preservation of Spontaneous Ventilation] — vs. — [Ablation of Spontaneous Ventilation]

3. Develop primary and alternative strategies:

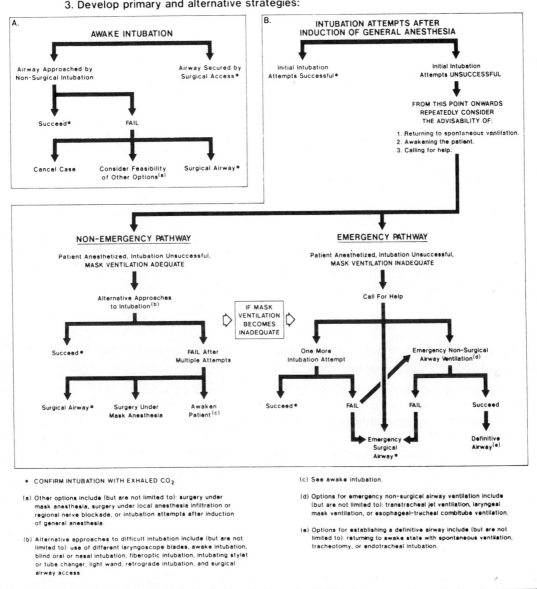

A. AWAKE INTUBATION

Airway Approached by Non-Surgical Intubation — Airway Secured by Surgical Access*

Succeed* — FAIL

Cancel Case — Consider Feasibility of Other Options(a) — Surgical Airway*

B. INTUBATION ATTEMPTS AFTER INDUCTION OF GENERAL ANESTHESIA

Initial Intubation Attempts Successful* — Initial Intubation Attempts UNSUCCESSFUL

FROM THIS POINT ONWARDS REPEATEDLY CONSIDER THE ADVISABILITY OF:
1. Returning to spontaneous ventilation.
2. Awakening the patient.
3. Calling for help.

NON-EMERGENCY PATHWAY

Patient Anesthetized, Intubation Unsuccessful, MASK VENTILATION ADEQUATE

Alternative Approaches to Intubation(b)

IF MASK VENTILATION BECOMES INADEQUATE

Succeed* — FAIL After Multiple Attempts

Surgical Airway* — Surgery Under Mask Anesthesia — Awaken Patient(c)

EMERGENCY PATHWAY

Patient Anesthetized, Intubation Unsuccessful, MASK VENTILATION INADEQUATE

Call For Help

One More Intubation Attempt — Emergency Non-Surgical Airway Ventilation(d)

Succeed* — FAIL — FAIL — Succeed

Emergency Surgical Airway* — Definitive Airway(e)

* CONFIRM INTUBATION WITH EXHALED CO_2

(a) Other options include (but are not limited to): surgery under mask anesthesia, surgery under local anesthesia infiltration or regional nerve blockade, or intubation attempts after induction of general anesthesia.

(b) Alternative approaches to difficult intubation include (but are not limited to): use of different laryngoscope blades, awake intubation, blind oral or nasal intubation, fiberoptic intubation, intubating stylet or tube changer, light wand, retrograde intubation, and surgical airway access.

(c) See awake intubation.

(d) Options for emergency non-surgical airway ventilation include (but are not limited to): transtracheal jet ventilation, laryngeal mask ventilation, or esophageal-tracheal combitube ventilation.

(e) Options for establishing a definitive airway include (but are not limited to): returning to awake state with spontaneous ventilation, tracheotomy, or endotracheal intubation.

Fig. 8-1. The American Society of Anesthesiologists' (ASA) difficult airway algorithm. See text for full explanation. (From a report by ASA Task Force on Management of the Difficult Airway: *Anesthesiology* 78:597, 1993.)

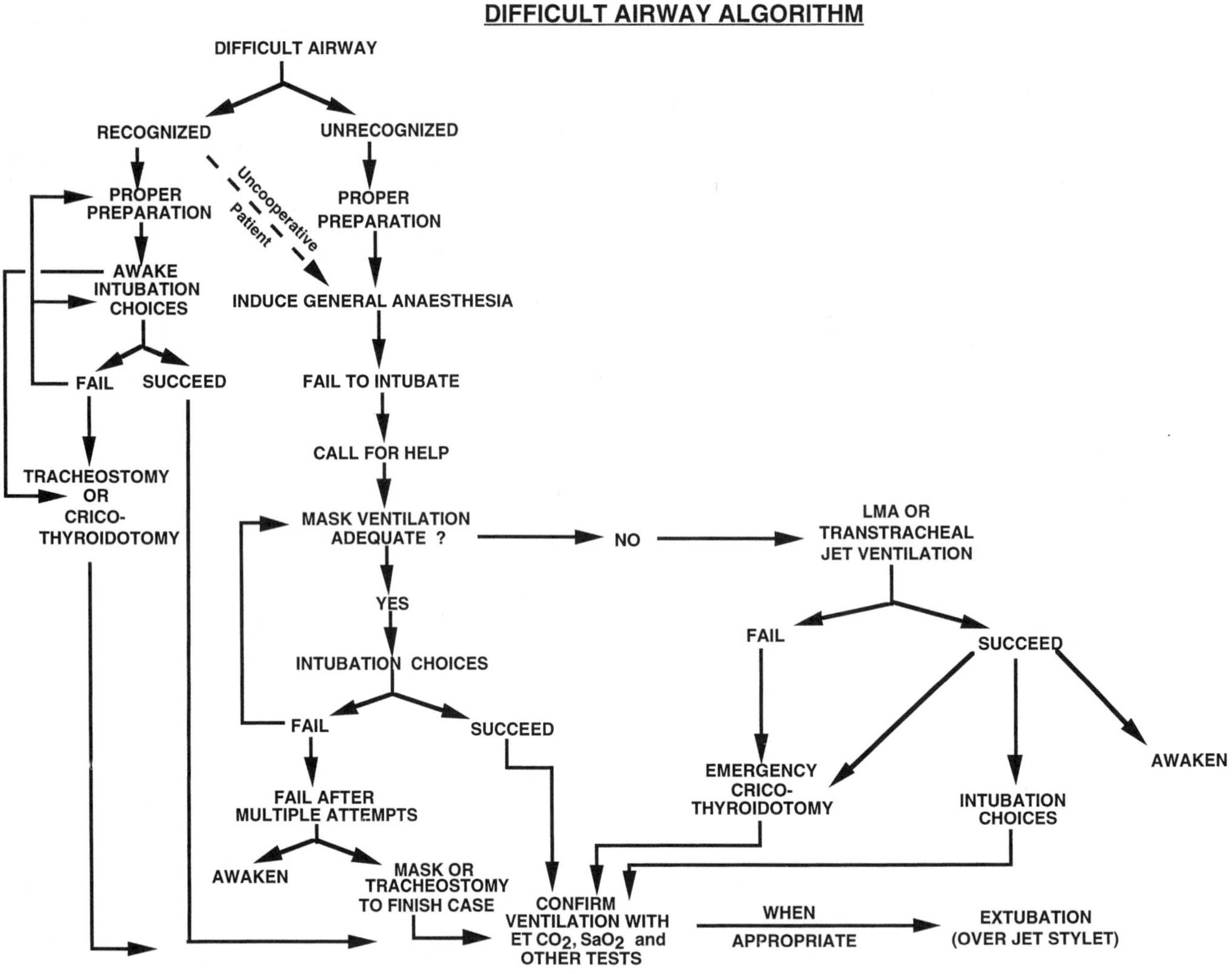

DIFFICULT AIRWAY ALGORITHM

Fig. 8-2. This difficult airway management algorithm is same as in Fig. 8-1. See text for full explanation. (From Benumof JL: *Anesthesiology* 75:1087, 1991, which was a preliminary presentation of the ASA algorithm in the form of a Medical Intelligence Article.)

A. AWAKE TRACHEAL INTUBATION

When management of the airway is expected to be difficult, either because of the presence of a pathologic factor(s) and/or a combination of anatomic factors, an endotracheal airway should be guaranteed while the patient is awake. Although awake intubation is generally much more time consuming for the anesthesiologist and a more unpleasant experience for the patient, there are several compelling reasons why intubation should be done while a patient with a recognized difficult airway is still awake. First, and most important, the natural airway will be better maintained in most patients when they are awake ("no bridges are burned"). Second, in the awake patient enough muscle tone is maintained to keep the relevant upper airway structures (the base of the tongue, vallecula, epiglottis, larynx, esophagus, and posterior pharyngeal wall) separated from one another and much easier to identify. In the anesthetized and paralyzed

patient, loss of muscle tone tends to cause these structures to collapse toward one another (e.g., the tongue moves posteriorly), which distorts the anatomy.[3,4] Third, the larynx moves to a more anterior position with the induction of anesthesia and paralysis, which makes conventional intubation more difficult.[5] Thus, if a difficult intubation is anticipated, awake tracheal intubation is indicated.

Crucial to the success of an awake tracheal intubation is proper preparation of the patient (see Chapter 9); most intubation techniques will work well in most patients when they are quiet and cooperative and have a larynx that is nonreactive to physical stimuli. The components of proper preparation for an awake intubation consist of psychological preparation (awake intubation will proceed more easily in the patient who knows and agrees with what is going to happen); appropriate monitoring (electrocardiogram, noninvasive blood pres-

---

BOX 8-1   Suggested contents of the portable storage unit for difficult airway management

IMPORTANT: The items listed in this box represent suggestions. The contents of the portable storage unit should be customized to meet the specific needs, preferences, and skills of the practitioner and healthcare facility.

1. Rigid laryngoscope blades of alternate design and size from those routinely used.
2. Endotracheal tubes of assorted size.
3. Endotracheal tube guides. Examples include (but are not limited to) semirigid stylets with or without hollow cores for jet ventilation, light wands, and forceps designed to manipulate the distal portion of the endotracheal tube.
4. Fiberoptic intubation equipment.
5. Retrograde intubation equipment.
6. At least one device suitable for emergency nonsurgical airway ventilation. Examples include (but are not limited to) a transtracheal jet ventilator, a hollow jet ventilation stylet, the laryngeal mask, and the esophageal-tracheal Combitube.
7. Equipment suitable for emergency surgical airway access (e.g., cricothyrotomy).
8. An exhaled CO_2 detector.

BOX 8-2   Techniques for difficult airway management

IMPORTANT: This box displays commonly cited techniques. It is not a comprehensive list. The order of presentation is alphabetical and does not imply preference for a given technique or sequence of use. Combinations of techniques may be employed. The techniques chosen by the practitioner in a particular case will depend upon specific needs, preferences, skills, and clinical constraints.

I.   Techniques for difficult intubation

Alternative laryngoscope blades
Awake intubation
Blind intubation (oral or nasal)
Fiberoptic intubation
Intubating stylet-tube changer
Light wand
Retrograde intubation
Surgical airway access

II.   Techniques for difficult ventilation

Esophageal-tracheal combitube
Intratracheal jet stylet
Laryngeal mask
Oral and nasopharyngeal airways
Rigid ventilating bronchoscope
Surgical airway access
Transtracheal jet ventilation
Two-person mask ventilation

---

sure, pulse oximetry, and capnography) and oxygen supplementation (nasal prongs, nasal catheter, insufflate oxygen down the suction channel of a fiberoptic proctoscope, transtracheal needle for transtracheal jet ventilation in rare cases)[6-9]; administration of a drying agent, topical anesthesia, and judicious sedation; performance of nerve blocks (e.g., block of the lingual branch of the glossopharyngeal nerve [IX] and superior laryngeal nerve); aspiration prevention-prophylaxis (see Chapter 10); and having the appropriate airway equipment available. Box 8-1 lists the suggested (ASA guidelines) contents of a portable airway management cart.

There are numerous ways to intubate the trachea and/or ventilate the patient (see Chapters 11-28). Box 8-2 shows a list of the techniques contained within the ASA guidelines. The techniques chosen will depend, in part, upon the anticipated surgery, the condition of the patient, and the skills and preferences of the anesthesiologist.

Occasionally, all attempts at intubation fail. Prior to abandoning the awake intubation procedure, canceling surgery, or performing an elective tracheostomy, three responses seem reasonable in most patients. First, the patient may need to be better prepared for an awake intubation. This may mean repeating topical local anesthesia, local nerve block, or intravenous sedation-analgesia. Second, it may be prudent to change the intubation technique. For example, if any one of the several techniques listed in Box 8-2 has not been successful, any one of the remaining techniques may be successful. Third, combining several intubation techniques (e.g., use laryngoscope blade with fiberoptic instrument or passing a retrograde wire up the suction port of a fiberoptic bronchoscope) may increase the success rate. However, when all of the above fail and cancellation of surgery is not appropriate, a surgical airway (see Chapter 26) is indicated.

Elective tracheostomy is often the best first intubation choice in conditions such as (1) laryngeal fracture or disruption, (2) upper airway abscesses located along, and distorting, the route of intubation, and (3) basilar skull fractures with cerebrospinal fluid leak and/or nasal fractures or deformity that contraindicate a nasotracheal tube and a requirement for arch bars and jaw wiring that contraindicate an orotracheal tube.

B. THE ANESTHETIZED PATIENT WHOSE TRACHEA IS DIFFICULT TO INTUBATE

There are three general situations in which an anesthesiologist will be required to intubate the trachea of an unconscious or anesthetized patient whose airway is difficult to manage. First, the patient may already be unconscious (e.g., posttrauma) or anesthetized (e.g., drug overdose). Second, the patient may absolutely refuse or not tolerate awake intubation (e.g., a child, a mentally retarded patient, or an intoxicated combative patient [see dashed line, Fig. 8-2]). Third, and perhaps most commonly, the anesthesiologist may fail to recognize intubation difficulty on the preoperative evaluation. Of course, even in the first and second situations above, the preoperative airway evaluation is very important because the findings may dictate the choice of intubation technique. In all three of the situations above, the patient may, in addition, have a full stomach.

All of the intubation techniques that are described for the awake patient[1,2] can be used in the unconscious or anesthetized patient without modification. However, direct and fiberoptic laryngoscopy may be slightly more difficult in the paralyzed, anesthetized patient compared to the awake patient because the larynx may become more anterior relative to other structures due to relaxation of oral and pharyngeal muscles.[5] In addition, and more importantly, the upper airway structures may coalesce into a horizontal plane instead of separating out in a vertical plane.[3,4]

In the anesthetized patient whose trachea has proven to be difficult to intubate, it is necessary to try to maintain gas exchange between intubation attempts by mask ventilation and also during intubation attempts whenever possible. Positive pressure ventilation may be continuously maintained during fiberoptic endoscopy-aided orotracheal intubation by using an anesthesia mask that has a special fiberoptic instrument port that is covered by a self-sealing diaphragm (instead of standard mask) along with an airway intubator (instead of the standard oropharyngeal airway) (see Chapter 16)[4,10] or by using a laryngeal mask airway as the conduit for the fiberscope (see Chapter 19).[11]

It is extremely important to realize that the amount of laryngeal edema and bleeding will very likely increase after every forceful intubation attempt. Although laryngeal edema and bleeding can occur with any intubation method, it is most common after use of a laryngoscope or retraction blade. Consequently, if there does not appear to be anything really new or different that can be atraumatically and quickly tried (better sniff position, external laryngeal manipulation, new blade, new technique, much more experienced laryngoscopist, etc.) after a few failed intubation attempts, and ventilation by mask can still be maintained, it is prudent to cease attempting to intubate the trachea and to awaken the patient, continue anesthesia via mask ventilation, or perform a tracheostomy or cricothyrotomy before the ability to ventilate the lungs via mask is lost (Figs. 8-1 and 8-2). In fact, the most common scenario in the respiratory catastrophes in the ASA closed-claims study was the development of progressive difficulty in ventilating via mask between persistent and prolonged failed intubation attempts; the final result was inability to ventilate via mask and provide gas exchange (see Chapter 46).[12] If the surgical procedure is not urgent, awakening the patient and doing the procedure another day will allow for better planning. Still, many other cases may be done (and may have to be done) via mask ventilation (e.g., cesarean section) if it is reasonably easy. Finally, in some cases, the trachea will have to be intubated by tracheostomy or cricothyrotomy (e.g., thoracotomy, intracranial-head-neck cases, and cases in the prone position).

If regurgitation or vomiting occurs at any time during attempts at endotracheal intubation in an anesthetized patient, then there are a number of therapeutic steps that must be taken. First, the patient must be put in the Trendelenburg position, and the head, and perhaps the body, turned to the left. Second, the mouth and pharynx should be suctioned with a large bore catheter. Tracheal intubation may then be tried with the patient on his or her left side; the advantage of this maneuver is that the tongue may be more out of the way, but the disadvantage is that this intubation position may be unfamiliar to most anesthesiologists. If the endotracheal tube (ET) has been passed into the esophagus, it may be left there; the advantage is that the endotracheal tube may decompress the stomach and perhaps guide (by negative example) future intubation attempts. However, the disadvantage is that it may be harder to obtain a satisfactory mask seal between intubation attempts, even if the esophageal endotracheal tube is sharply bent off to the side by the rim of the mask. Once the airway is secured and aspiration of gastric contents is believed to have occurred, standard treatment consists of suctioning, mechanical ventilation, positive end-expiratory pressure, fiberoptically guided saline lavage, and suction and perhaps steroids and appropriate antibiotics after specific cultures and sensitivities are available (see Chapter 10).

C. THE PATIENT WHOSE LUNGS CANNOT BE VENTILATED BY MASK AND WHOSE TRACHEA CANNOT BE INTUBATED

In rare cases, it is impossible either to ventilate the lungs of a patient via mask or to intubate the trachea. Under these circumstances, unless there is an alternative ventilation method immediately available, death will rapidly ensue. In the past few years, three alternative ventilation methods have been described that can be instituted blindly and quickly and that appear to have a low risk/benefit ratio. These are the esophageal tracheal Combitube (ETC) (see Chapter 22), laryngeal mask airway (LMA) (see Chapter 19), and transtracheal jet ventilation (TTJV) (see Chapter 23). It should be realized that both the ETC and LMA are supraglottic ventilatory devices.

D. TRACHEAL EXTUBATION OF A PATIENT WITH A DIFFICULT AIRWAY

The anesthesiologist should have a preformulated strategy for extubation of the difficult airway. This strategy will depend upon the surgery, the condition of the patient, and the skills and preferences of the anesthesiologist. The preformulated extubation strategy should include a consideration of the relative merits of awake extubation versus extubation before the return of consciousness; an evaluation for general clinical factors that may produce an adverse impact on ventilation after the patient has been extubated; and the formulation of an airway management plan that can be implemented if the patient is not able to maintain adequate ventilation after extubation.

If tracheal extubation of a patient with a known difficult airway is followed by respiratory distress, then reintubation and ventilation may be difficult or impossible. Thus, the ideal method of extubation is one that permits a withdrawal from the airway that is controlled, gradual, step-by-step, and reversible at any time. Extubation over a jet stylet closely approximates this ideal (see Chapter 40).

A jet stylet is a small inside diameter (ID), hollow, semirigid catheter that is inserted into an in situ ET prior to extubation. After the ET is withdrawn over the jet stylet, the small-ID hollow catheter may then be used as a means of ventilation (i.e., the jet function) and/or as an intratracheal guide for reintubation (i.e., the stylet function). The jet function may safely allow additional time to assess the need for the reintubation stylet function (see Chapter 40).

E. FOLLOW-UP CARE

The anesthesiologist should document the presence and nature of the airway difficulty in the medical record. The intent of this documentation is to guide and facilitate the delivery of future care. Aspects of documentation that may prove helpful include (but are not limited to): (1) a description of the airway difficulties that were encountered. If possible, the description should distinguish between difficulties encountered in mask ventilation and difficulties encountered in tracheal intubation; and (2) a description of the various airway management techniques that were employed. The description should indicate the extent to which each of the techniques played a beneficial or detrimental role in management of the difficult airway.

The anesthesiologist should inform the patient (or responsible person) of the airway difficulty that was encountered. The intent of this communication is to provide the patient (or responsible person) with information in guiding and facilitating the delivery of future care. The information conveyed may include (but is not limited to): the presence of a difficult airway, the apparent reasons for difficulty, and the implications for future care. Finally, the anesthesiologist should strongly consider dispensing-advising a Medic-Alert Bracelet for the patient (see Chapter 44).

The anesthesiologist should evaluate and follow the patient for potential complications of difficult airway management. These complications include (but are not limited to): airway edema, bleeding, tracheal and esophageal perforation, pneumothorax, and aspiration.

III. SUMMARY OF THE ASA ALGORITHM

Difficulty in managing the airway is the single most important cause of major anesthesia-related morbidity and mortality. Successful management of a difficult airway begins with recognizing the potential problem. All patients should be examined for their ability to open their mouth widely and for the structures visible upon mouth opening, the size of the mandibular space, and ability to assume the sniff position. If there is a good possibility that intubation and/or ventilation by mask will be difficult, then the airway should be secured while the patient is still awake. In order for an awake intubation to be successful, it is absolutely essential that the patient be properly prepared; otherwise, the anesthesiologist will simply fulfill a self-defeating prophecy. Once the patient is properly prepared, it is likely that any one of a number of intubation techniques will be successful. If the patient is already anesthetized and/or paralyzed and intubation is found to be difficult, many repeated forceful attempts at intubation should be avoided because progressive development of laryngeal edema and hemorrhage will develop and the ability to ventilate the lungs via mask consequently may be lost. After several attempts at intubation, it may be best to awaken the patient, do a semielective tracheostomy, or proceed with the case using mask ventilation. In the event that the ability to ventilate via mask is lost and the patient's lungs still cannot be ventilated, either the LMA or TTJV should be instituted immediately. If the LMA does not provide adequate gas exchange, either TTJV or a surgical airway should be instituted immediately. Tracheal extubation of a patient with a difficult airway over a jet stylet permits a controlled, gradual, and reversible (in that ventilation and reintubation is possible at any time) withdrawal from the airway.

BOX 8-3   ASA difficult airway algorithm take home messages

1. If suspicious of trouble → Secure the airway awake
2. If you get into trouble → Awaken the patient
3. Have a plan B, C, immediately available/in place = think ahead
4. Intubation choices → Do what you do best

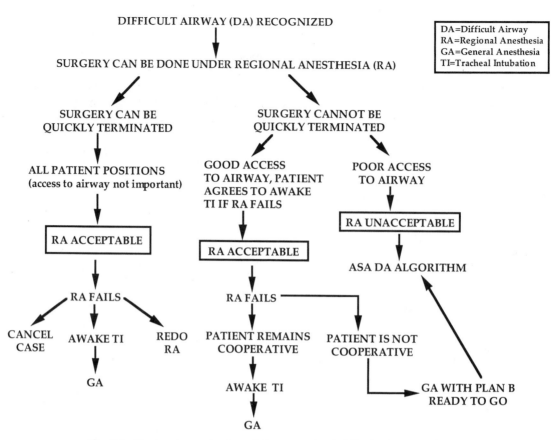

Fig. 8-3. Regional anesthesia and the recognized difficult airway algorithm.

Four concepts emerge from the preceding discussion, four very important, take-home messages on the ASA difficult airway algorithm as presented in Box 8-3.

IV. PROBLEMS WITH THE ASA ALGORITHM AND LIKELY FUTURE DIRECTIONS

The ASA difficult airway algorithm has been before the anesthesia community, in one form or another, since 1991. Within the 5 years to date, a number of new issues have emerged that will certainly require either modification of, inclusion in, or exclusion from the ASA difficult airway algorithm. These issues, discussed in following sections, include: (A) Use of regional anesthesia and the difficult airway; (B) Choice of duration of action of muscle relaxant; (C) Definition of optimal-best attempt at conventional laryngoscopy; (D) More realistic definition of difficult endotracheal intubation; (E) Definition of optimal-best attempt at conventional mask ventilation; (F) Confirmation of endotracheal intubation during cardiac arrest; (G) Appropriate options for the cannot-ventilate-cannot-intubate situation; and (H) Communication of a difficult airway experience to future caretakers.

A. USE OF REGIONAL ANESTHESIA AND THE DIFFICULT AIRWAY

Use of regional anesthesia in the patient with a recognized difficult airway does not solve the problem of the difficult airway; it is still there. Obviously, if regional anesthesia fails in a patient with a known difficult airway and general anesthesia is induced, the risk of losing the airway and harming the patient is directly proportional to the degree of perceived difficulty. If surgery can be quickly terminated and if regional anesthesia fails (irrespective of patient position), the case can be canceled, the patient intubated awake (if cooperative and after proper preparation) and then general anesthesia induced, or the regional anesthesia redone (left panel-column of Fig. 8-3). No respiratory bridges are burned with this approach.

When surgery cannot be quickly terminated, it is acceptable to do regional anesthesia in a patient with a known difficult airway if a preoperative contract (firm agreement) has been made with the patient that an awake endotracheal intubation will be done if regional anesthesia fails (middle panel-column of Fig. 8-3). Obviously, in order for this plan to work, there must be good access to the patient's airway. In order for awake

Table 8-1. Advantages and disadvantages of muscle relaxants with different duration of action

Muscle Relaxant	Advantages	Disadvantages
Succinyldicholine	1. Permits the awaken option at the earliest time possible	1. A period of poor ventilation (either spontaneous or with positive pressure) may occur as the drug wears off 2. Does not permit a smooth transition to Plan B (such as use of a fiberoptic bronchoscope[4]), etc.
Nondepolarizing	1. Permits a smooth transition to Plan B, etc., provided mask ventilation is adequate	1. Does not allow awake option at an early time

endotracheal intubation to succeed under such conditions, it is essential that the patient is kept in meaningful contact with the anesthesiologist (i.e., rational, oriented, and responsive to commands), fully cooperative and not oversedated or disinhibited. Finally, if general anesthesia has to be induced in a patient with a known difficult airway and a failed regional anesthetic and there is good access to the patient's airway, an alternate plan (Plan B) should be immediately available and ready to go (e.g., the elective preinduction placement of the suitable TTJV catheter, or an appropriately gloved surgeon with scalpel in hand and neck prepared). It is unacceptable to do regional anesthesia with a known difficult airway when surgery cannot be terminated rapidly and there is poor access to the patient's head (right panel-column of Fig. 8-3).

B. CHOICE OF DURATION OF ACTION OF MUSCLE RELAXANT

In patients presenting for elective surgery who end up in a cannot-ventilate-cannot-intubate situation, the following is a common story. Preoperatively, the anesthesiologist does not recognize a difficult airway or feels the difficult airway is questionable and induces general anesthesia with an intravenous drug and paralyzes the patient with succinyldicholine. Mask ventilation is initiated without difficulty, but endotracheal intubation with conventional laryngoscopy fails (Figs. 8-1 and 8-2). Appropriately, gas exchange is controlled by mask ventilation for a second time, and then, after some adjustment, endotracheal intubation with conventional larngoscopy is attempted and fails for a second time. Mask ventilation controls gas exchange for a third time but is now perceptibly more difficult than before. After some adjustment (see Section C following), endotracheal intubation with conventional laryngoscopy is attempted for the third time and fails. At this point, approximately 5 to 8 minutes have passed since the administration of succinyldicholine. Although the anesthesiologist may want to exercise the awake option, the patient is not breathing spontaneously; mask ventilation is now attempted for a fourth time but is extremely

difficult and may be impossible because the chest wall is rigid due to the patient sustaining a forceful exhalation mode and the presence of laryngospasm and edema due to the prior three laryngoscopies and perhaps endotracheal intubation attempts. Now a race begins: will the patient resume adequate spontaneous ventilation (awaken) before he/she experiences severe hypoxemia causing organ damage? The answer is not certain and depends on many pharmacologic and physiologic variables.

From this common story in patients who have ended up in a cannot-ventilate-cannot-intubate situation, the advantages and disadvantages of muscle relaxants with different duration of action become obvious (Table 8-1).

Thus, use of succinyldicholine in a patient either with a recognized or questionable difficult airway may not be the best choice, particularly if it is thought that mask ventilation will be possible and it will be desirable to have a smooth transition to Plan B (e.g., fiberoptic bronchoscopy[4]), C, D, etc. The key elements in the choice of a nondepolarizing muscle relaxant is the decision that mask ventilation will be adequate (i.e., two-person, good mask seal, jaw thrust [see Section E following], and patient anatomy and a ready Plan B).

C. DEFINITION OF OPTIMAL-BEST ATTEMPT AT CONVENTIONAL LARYNGOSCOPY

The problem with multiple repeated attempts at conventional laryngoscopy is the creation of laryngeal edema and bleeding, which will impair mask ventilation and subsequent endotracheal intubation attempts, thereby creating a cannot-ventilate-cannot-intubate situation. Thus, it is imperative that the anesthesiologist makes his/her optimal-best attempt at laryngoscopy as early as possible, and, if that fails, Plan B should be activated so that no further risk, without likely benefit, will be incurred.

What is an optimal-best attempt at conventional laryngoscopy?[13] First, a reasonably experienced person should perform the laryngoscopy. In my experience, the learning curve for laryngoscopy for most anesthesiologists becomes flat after 3 full years of experience;

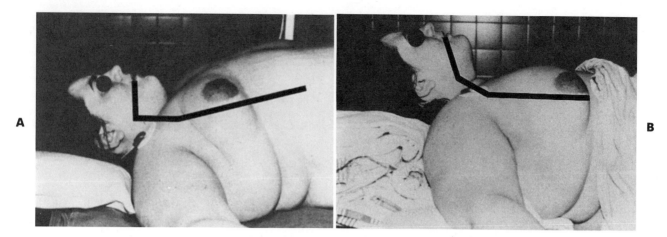

Fig. 8-4. Getting the patient in an optimal sniff position prior to the induction of general anesthesia will occasionally (e.g., with very obese patients) take a great deal of work. **A,** Just head on pillow. **B,** Scapula, shoulder, nape of neck, and head support results in the sniff position. (Modified from Davis JM, Weeks S, Crone LA: *Can J Anaesth* 36:668, 1989.)

thereafter I consider anesthesiologists to be reasonably experienced.

Second, the patient should always be in an optimal sniff position (slight flexion of the neck on the head and severe extension of the head on the neck),[13] which aligns the oral, pharyngeal, and laryngeal axis into more of a straight line. In some patients (such as the obese) obtaining an optimal sniff position takes a great deal of work (Fig. 8-4), such as placing pillows and blankets under the scapula, shoulders, nape of the neck, and head, and this kind of positioning is extremely hard to do when anesthesia and paralysis have made the patient a massive (dead) weight. Thus an endotracheal intubation attempt should not be wasted because of failure to have the patient in an optimal sniff position prior to the induction of general anesthesia.

Third, if the laryngoscopic grade is either II (just arytenoids), III (just epiglottis), or IV (just soft palate), then optimal external laryngeal manipulation (OELM) should be used (Fig. 8-5).[13,15] OELM is *not* cricoid pressure (Fig. 8-5) and can be achieved in 5 to 10 seconds.[15] OELM very frequently can improve the laryngoscopic view by at least one whole grade and should be an inherent part of laryngoscopy and an instinctive and reflex response to a poor laryngoscopic view.[15] Thus, an endotracheal intubation attempt should not be wasted because of failure to use OELM.

Fourth, the proper function of both a Macintosh and Miller blade is dependent on using an appropriate length of blade. In order to lift the epiglottis out of the line of sight, the Macintosh blade must be long enough to put tension on the glossoepiglottic ligament, and the Miller blade must be long enough to trap the epiglottis against the tongue. Thus, in some patients it may be appropriate

DETERMINING OPTIMAL EXTERNAL LARYNGEAL MANIPULATION WITH FREE (right) HAND

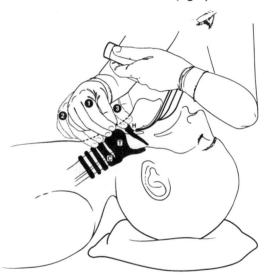

Fig. 8-5. Optimal external laryngeal manipulation (OELM) should be an inherent part of laryngoscopy and an instinctive and reflex response to a poor laryngoscopic view.[15] OELM consists of quickly pressing posteriorly and cephalad over the thyroid, hyoid, and cricoid cartilages. Ninety percent of the time, the best view will be obtained by pressing over the thyroid cartilage.[15]

to change the length of the blade one time in order to obtain proper blade function.

Fifth, in some patients a Macintosh blade may provide a superior view or intubating conditions than a Miller blade, and vice versa. A Macintosh blade is generally regarded as a better blade whenever there is little upper airway room to pass the endotracheal tube (e.g., small narrow mouth, palate, oropharynx),

TWO-PERSON MASK VENTILATION

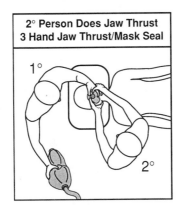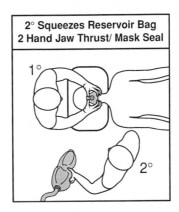

Fig. 8-6. Optimal mask ventilation. *Left panel,* two-person effort when second person knows how to perform jaw thrust; *right panel,* two-person effort when second person can only squeeze the reservoir bag.

and a Miller blade is generally regarded as a better blade in patients who have a small mandibular space (anterior larynx), large incisors, or a long, floppy epiglottis.

In summary, an optimal-best attempt at laryngoscopy can be defined as: (1) laryngoscopist is reasonably experienced (at least 3 full recent years); (2) use of optimal sniff position; (3) use of optimal external laryngeal manipulation; (4) change of length of blade one time; and (5) change of type of blade one time. With this definition, and with no other confounding considerations, optimal-best attempt at laryngoscopy may be achieved on the first attempt and should not take more than a maximum of four attempts.

D. MORE REALISTIC DEFINITION OF DIFFICULT TRACHEAL INTUBATION

At present, the ASA difficult airway algorithm defines difficult endotracheal intubation as "(1) proper insertion of the endotracheal tube with conventional laryngoscopy requires *more than three attempts* and/or (2) proper insertion of the endotracheal tube with conventional laryngoscopy requires *more than ten minutes.*"[1] (It should be noted that difficult laryngoscopy is appropriately defined according to laryngoscopic view.) This definition of difficult endotracheal intubation is illogical because an optimal-best attempt at laryngoscopy may be achieved on the first attempt (see Section C preceding), and within 30 seconds, and reveals a grade IV view (whether due to inherent anatomy and/or massive pathology) that results in an esophageal intubation. Thus, difficult endotracheal intubation may be readily apparent to a reasonably experienced intubationist on the very first attempt and therefore be both number of attempts and time independent. A more logical definition would be based on optimal-best attempt

laryngoscopic view and periglottic and subglottic pathology and retain number of attempts and time of attempt as maximal boundary airway conditions.

E. DEFINITION OF OPTIMAL-BEST ATTEMPT AT CONVENTIONAL MASK VENTILATION

If the patient cannot be intubated, then gas exchange is dependent on mask ventilation. If the patient cannot be ventilated by mask, then a cannot-ventilate-cannot-intubate situation exists, and immediate organ-lifesaving maneuvers must be instituted (see Section G following). Since each of the acceptable responses to a cannot-ventilate-cannot-intubate situation has its own risks, the decision to abandon mask ventilation should be made after the anesthesiologist has made an optimal-best attempt at mask ventilation.

The first component of optimal-best attempt at conventional mask ventilation is that it should be a two-person effort (Fig. 8-6) because far better mask seal, jaw thrust, and therefore tidal volume can be achieved with two persons versus one person. The left-hand panel of Fig. 8-6 shows a proper two-person mask ventilation effort when the second person knows how to perform jaw thrust, and the right-hand panel of Fig. 8-6 shows a proper two-person mask ventilation effort when the second person is only capable of squeezing the reservoir bag.

The second component of optimal-best attempt at conventional mask ventilation is to use large oropharyngeal and/or nasopharyngeal airways. If mask ventilation is very poor or nonexistent with a vigorous two-person effort in the presence of large artificial airways, then it is time to move on to a potentially organ-lifesaving Plan B (see Figs. 8-1 and 8-2 and Section G following).

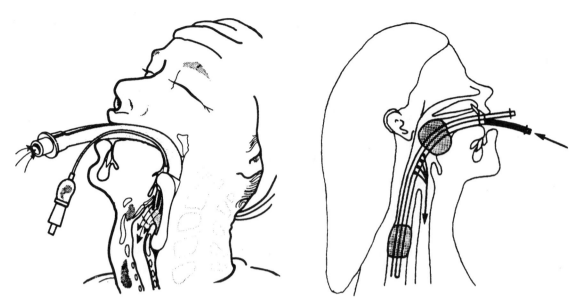

Fig. 8-7. Both the laryngeal mask airway *(left panel)* and Combitube *(right panel)* are supraglottic ventilatory devices.

F. CONFIRMATION OF TRACHEAL INTUBATION DURING CARDIAC ARREST

Cardiac arrest may occur in a cannot-ventilate-cannot-intubate situation, and with cardiac arrest (i.e., no pulmonary blood flow) $P_{ET}CO_2$ decreases to zero. Thus, capnography cannot be used to confirm subsequent endotracheal intubation during cardiac arrest. If the endotracheal tube cannot be visualized passing through the vocal cords (even with depressing the pharyngeal part of the endotracheal tube posteriorly, which, in turn, pulls the larynx posteriorly) and a fiberscope cannot quickly reveal endotracheal intubation, then no fail-safe method of confirming endotracheal intubation is available (all other methods are subject to considerable error). However, the esophageal detector device has been recently and convincingly introduced as very nearly a fail-safe device for detecting esophageal and endotracheal intubation.[16] If the endotracheal tube is in the esophagus, the previously collapsed bulb of the esophageal detector device fails to immediately expand, and, if the endotracheal tube is in the trachea, the previously collapsed bulb of the esophageal detector device immediately expands. The only false-negative endotracheal intubation conditions are with a collapsible trachea, obstructing tracheal masses-fluids, obstructed endotracheal tube, severe bronchospasm, and very low lung volume states; the only (theoretical) false-positive tracheal intubation condition (endotracheal tube in the esophagus) is with a gas-filled esophagus.[16]

G. APPROPRIATE OPTIONS FOR THE CANNOT-VENTILATE-CANNOT-INTUBATE SITUATION

In the past 5 years, anesthesiologists in the United States have become familiar with the laryngeal mask airway[17] and the Combitube[18] and have found that the laryngeal mask airway works well in elective situations and both the laryngeal mask airway and combitube have worked very well as ventilatory devices in the cannot-ventilate-cannot-intubate situation.[11,17,18] The laryngeal mask airway, in addition, has proven also to be an excellent conduit to the larynx for a fiberscope.[11,17] Although the ASA difficult airway algorithm presently lists these two devices, along with TTJV, as appropriate nonsurgical solutions for the cannot-ventilate-cannot-intubate situation (see Figs. 8-1 and 8-2), they both deserve higher prominence and ranking in the minds of many anesthesiologists for the following four reasons. First, they will likely work as ventilatory mechanisms. Second, they both can be inserted blindly, quickly, and with a relatively low level of skill. Third, so far they have been associated with few complications. Fourth, although TTJV is also rapidly instituted with a low level of skill and will very likely work well if the practitioner has prepared in advance, there is still a significant risk of barotrauma (too large tidal volume, too short exhalation, letting go of the catheter with subsequent dislodgment). However, it must be remembered and clearly understood that both the laryngeal mask airway and Combitube are supraglottic ventilatory mechanisms (Fig. 8-7) (the

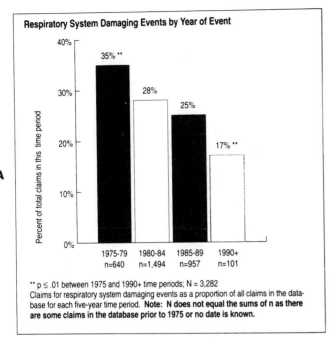

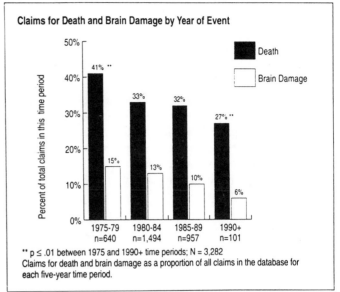

Fig. 8-8. The incidence of respiratory system damaging events *(panel A)* and brain death and death *(panel B)* has significantly decreased in the last 4 years. (From Cheney FW: *American Society of Anesthesiologists' News Letter,* June 1994.)

Combitube enters the esophagus 99% of the time), and that is the inherent weakness of these devices: that is, they cannot solve a truly glottic (e.g., spasm, massive edema, tumor, abscess etc.) or subglottic problem.[11] With a truly glottic or subglottic problem, the solution will be to get the ventilatory mechanism below (distal to) the lesion (e.g., TTJV, endotracheal tube, surgical airway).

H. COMMUNICATION OF A DIFFICULT AIRWAY EXPERIENCE TO FUTURE CARETAKERS

There are several ways to communicate a near organ-life-taking difficult airway experience to future caretakers. First, a detailed note in the chart can be written. However, the old chart may not be available years later, in a different hospital, or in an emergency, and it may not be asked for if the patient does not have a clear understanding of his/her problem (probably the majority of patients). Second, a detailed note can be given to the patient, but the note may likely be stuck in a drawer and forgotten about and certainly will not be available in an emergency. Third, close relatives may be informed of the problem, but this method of communication suffers from all the limitations inherent in the first two methods. Fourth, and far best of all in terms of being fail safe, is to dispense to the patient a Medic-Alert Bracelet.[19] Although this may seem overdone to some, a moment's reflection upon the consequence of failing to

communicate a near organ-life-taking difficult airway experience, just as with malignant hyperthermia, should convince one that this is an appropriate action to take. The telephone number to call to enter the patient in the Medic-Alert system is 1-(800)-344-3226.

In summary, the ASA difficult airway algorithm has worked well over the past 5 years. In fact, there has been a very dramatic decrease (30% to 40%) in the number of respiratory-related malpractice law suits, brain damage, and death attributable to anesthesia in just the last 4 years (Fig. 8-8).[20] However, a number of issues have emerged that indicate that the ASA difficult airway algorithm can be improved. First, the algorithm mentions regional anesthesia but does not define when its use is prudent or imprudent, and this discussion makes a strong suggestion in that regard. Second, the algorithm mentions ablation of spontaneous ventilation with muscle relaxants but does not discuss the great clinical management implications of muscle relaxants that have different durations of action. Third, fourth, and fifth, definition of optimal-best attempts at conventional laryngoscopy, mask ventilation, and difficult endotracheal intubation is important because it provides an end point at which clinicians may quit this approach (limit risk) and move on to something that has a better chance of working (gain benefit). Sixth, although the algorithm advises confirmation of endotracheal intubation, the usefulness of capnography for this purpose is limited during cardiac arrest (which is not an uncommon consequence of a cannot-ventilate-cannot-intubate situation), whereas the esophageal detector device is not. Seventh, although the algorithm mentions the laryngeal mask airway and Combitube in connection with the cannot-ventilate-cannot-intubate situation, perhaps they should be mentioned with more prominence (i.e., promoted) because of their good track record of the last 5 years. Finally, the algorithm should consider communicating a near organ-life-taking difficult airway experience by dispensing a Medic-Alert Bracelet to the patient so that future caretakers will not unwittingly reproduce the same experience and risk. Consideration of these issues should make the ASA difficult airway algorithm still more clinically specific and functional.

REFERENCES

1. American Society of Anesthesiologists Task Force on Management of The Difficult Airway: Practice guidelines for management of the difficult airway: a report, *Anesthesiology* 78:597, 1993.
2. Benumof JL: Management of the difficult airway: with special emphasis on awake tracheal intubation, *Anesthesiology* 75:1087, 1991.
3. Fink RB: *Respiration, the human larynx: a functional study,* New York, 1975, Raven Press.
4. Rogers S, Benumof JL: New and easy fiberoptic endoscopy aided tracheal intubation, *Anesthesiology* 59:569, 1983.
5. Sivarajan M, Fink RB: The position and the state of the larynx during general anesthesia and muscle paralysis, *Anesthesiology* 72:439, 1990.
6. Benumof JL, Scheller MS: The importance of transtracheal jet ventilation in the management of the difficult airway, *Anesthesiology* 71:769, 1989.
7. McLellan J, Gordon P, Khawaja S et al: Percutaneous transtracheal high frequency jet ventilation as an aid to difficult intubation, *Can J Anaesth* 35:404, 1988.
8. Baraka A: Transtracheal jet ventilation during fiberoptic intubation under general anesthesia, *Anesth Analg* 65:1091, 1986.
9. Dallen L, Wine R, Benumof JL: Spontaneous ventilation via transtracheal large bore intravenous catheter is possible, *Anesthesiology* 75:531, 1991.
10. Patil V, Stehling LC, Zauder HL et al: Mechanical aids for a fiberoptic endoscopy, *Anesthesiology* 57:69, 1982.
11. Benumof JL: Laryngeal mask airway: indications and contraindications, *Anesthesiology* 77:843-846, 1992 (editorial).
12. Caplan RA, Posner KL, Ward RJ et al: Adverse respiratory events in anesthesia: a closed claims analysis, *Anesthesiology* 72:828, 1990.
13. Benumof JL: Difficult laryngoscopy: obtaining the best view, *Can J Anaesth* 41:361, 1994 (editorial).
14. Davis JM, Weeks S, Crone LA: Difficult intubation in the parturient, *Can J Anaesth* 36:668, 1989.
15. Benumof JL, Cooper SD: Quantitative improvement in laryngoscopic view by optimal external laryngeal manipulation, *J Clin Anesth* (in press).
16. Salem R, Baraka A: Confirmation of tracheal intubation. In Benumof JL, editor: *Airway management: principles and practice,* chap. 27, St Louis, 1995, Mosby.
17. Joshi GP, Smith I, White PF: Laryngeal mask airway. In Benumof JL, editor: *Airway management: principles and practice,* chap. 19, St Louis, 1995, Mosby.
18. Frass M: The combitube. In Benumof JL, editor: *Airway management: principles and practice,* chap. 22, St Louis, 1995, Mosby.
19. Mark L, Schauble J, Gordon G et al: Effective dissemination of critical airway information: the Medical Alert National Difficult Airway/Intubation Registry. In Benumof JL, editor: *Airway management: principles and practice,* chap. 44, St Louis, 1995, Mosby.
20. Cheney FW: ASA Newsletter, June 1994, 58(6):7-10, Committee on Professional Liability-Overview, *American Society of Anesthesiologists News Letter,* June 1994.

Part III

PREINTUBATION-
VENTILATION
PROCEDURES

Chapter 9

PREPARATION OF THE PATIENT FOR AWAKE INTUBATION

Antonio Sanchez
Narendra S. Trivedi
Debra E. Morrison

4. **Translaryngeal (transtracheal) anesthesia:**
   cautions, complications, contraindications
5. **Spray as you go**
6. **Labat technique**

I. BACKGROUND

A. HISTORY

"He sat in bed supporting himself with stiffened arms; his head was thrown forward, and he had the distressed anxiety so characteristic of impending suffocation depicted on his countenance. His inspirations were crowing and laboured. . . . He complained of intense pain . . . and begged that something should be done for his relief."

The preceding is from Dr. Macewend's 1880 account in the *British Medical Journal* of the first awake endotracheal intubation and describes a patient suffering from glottic edema. This patient underwent an *awake manual* endotracheal intubation using a *metallic* endotracheal tube (ET). This technique was performed without benefit of anesthesia and *without topical or regional blocks, sedatives or analgesics*. The ET was kept in place with the patient in an awake state for 35 hours.[1] Although we may perceive this as brutal, Dr. Macewend was aware over 100 years ago that in spite of the patient's discomfort, the safest method for securing the airway was to perform an awake intubation rather than to provide comfort at the risk of compromising the airway totally.

There have been myriad subsequent reports of awake intubation (AI) with favorable results,[2-10] yet many of us still hesitate to perform AI. It does appear that AI has been more readily accepted in the United States than in the European community.[11] In one large series from a single institution in the United States, 35% of all patients intubated and 21% of all patients anesthetized were intubated while awake.[10] The latter cannot, of course, be construed as indicative of the frequency of AI in the United States; this is unknown. Awake intubations in Europe are performed only in specialized centers.

B. THE ASA ALGORITHM: A MILESTONE, "AWAKE INTUBATION"

In 1992, the American Society of Anesthesiologists (ASA) formed the Difficult Airway Task Force (DATF), which looked at closed-claims malpractice suits and found that "inability to successfully manage very difficult airways has been responsible for as many as 30% of deaths totally attributable to anesthesia."[12] In the majority of these cases, patients did not display gross signs of airway difficulty, such as large tumors deviating the trachea of a patient in extremis, but had unrecognized difficult airways.[13] This implies that we are in need

of more accurate predictors[14,15] of airway difficulty (fewer false positives and fewer false negatives within the predicted parameters) and that we must become better detectives. The DATF constructed an algorithm (see Chapter 8), which used as its cornerstone AI as the most prudent choice when an anesthesiologist is faced with a difficult airway. The difficult airway (DA) is defined as "the clinical situation in which a conventionally trained anesthesiologist experiences difficulty with mask ventilation, difficulty with tracheal intubation, or both."[16]

C. PHYSICIAN RELUCTANCE TO PERFORM AWAKE INTUBATION

There seems to be an overall general hesitancy within the anesthesia community to perform AI.[11] At the present time there are no surveys to verify this statement,[17] but some of the reasons why there may be physician reluctance to perform awake intubation include lack of a personal association with an airway disaster; AI is too stressful emotionally and physically for the patient; the physician may lack training; and fear of litigation or that the patient will refuse the procedure.

Although the majority of the reservations represented by these statements are addressed in other chapters of this textbook, we will discuss patient refusal in the section on the preoperative visit.

D. INDICATIONS AND CONTRAINDICATIONS FOR AWAKE INTUBATION

The ASA algorithm stresses the concept that formulation of a strategy for intubation should include the feasibility of three basic options: surgical versus nonsurgical techniques, preservation versus ablation of spontaneous ventilation, and AI versus intubation after induction of general anesthesia.[16] It is the opinion of most of the consultants of the DATF and expressed in the literature[5,7-10,12,16,18-24] that the safest method for a patient who requires endotracheal intubation and has a DA is for that individual to undergo AI for the following reasons:

1. The natural airway is preserved. (Patency of the airway is maintained via upper pharyngeal muscle tone.)
2. Spontaneous breathing is maintained (maintaining oxygenation and ventilation).
3. A patient who is awake and well topicalized is easier to intubate. (The larynx after induction of anesthesia moves to a more anterior position when compared with the larynx in the awake patient.)
4. The patient can still protect his/her airway from aspiration.
5. Patients are able to monitor their own neurologic symptoms (for example, the patient with potential cervical pathology).[2,10,12]

BOX 9-1   Indications for awake intubation[2,10,22,24,25]

1. Previous history of difficult intubation
2. Anticipated DA (assessment on physical examination) as follows:
    Prominent protruding teeth
    Small mouth opening (scleroderma, temporomandibular joint pathology, anatomic variant)
    Narrow mandible
    Micrognathia
    Macroglossia
    Short muscular neck
    Very long neck
    Limited range of motion of the neck
    Congenital airway anomalies
    Obesity
    Pathology involving the airway (tracheomalacia)
    Malignancy involving the airway
    Upper airway obstruction
3. Trauma to the following:
    Face
    Upper airway
    Cervical spine
4. Anticipated difficult mask ventilation
5. Severe risk of aspiration
6. Respiratory failure
7. Severe hemodynamic instability

General indications for AI are compiled in Box 9-1.[2,10,22,24,25] There are no absolute contraindications to AI other than patient refusal, a patient who is unable to cooperate (such as a child, a mentally retarded patient, or an intoxicated, combative patient), or a patient with documented true allergy to all local anesthetics.[12]

II. THE PREOPERATIVE VISIT

Since in the majority of the cases in the closed-claims malpractice study the DA was unanticipated, we will focus on elective patients, where there is time to evaluate the airway and communicate with the patient. In the setting of an emergency, which in itself should increase the probability of airway difficulty, especially with a patient in extremis,[26] the physician may not have time nor can he/she be expected to be able to perform the detailed investigation of the airway to be described in this chapter.

A. THE DETECTIVE IN ALL OF US: REVIEWING OLD CHARTS

Whenever possible, previous anesthetic records (records, not just a record!) should be examined, since they may provide useful information.[16,27] Obviously the most important are those records involving intubation, especially the most recent. Other records documenting

ease of mask ventilation and tolerance of drugs are also valuable. One should be alert for evidence of reactions to local anesthetics and of apnea with minimal doses of narcotics. Another reason for checking as many operating room (OR) records as possible, including noting the surgical procedure involved, is that the last intubation may have been routine but the three previous ones may have been difficult, or the last intubation may have been routine but the operation then performed may have rendered the airway difficult.

When reading through a chart, one should focus on four important features.

1. Degree of difficulty of the endotracheal intubation (the difficulty encountered and the method used)
2. The positioning of the patient during laryngoscopy (sniffing position, other position)
3. The equipment used (Even if the intubation was performed routinely in one attempt, a Bullard blade or a fiberoptic bronchoscope, neither of which requires the alignment of the three axes, may have been used.)
4. Whether the technique that was used is previously familiar to you (One should not attempt to learn a new technique on a DA.)

Once the medical records have been reviewed, the preoperative interview should address the possibility of events having occurred since the last anesthetic (such as weight gain in the obese patient, laryngeal stenosis from previous airway intervention, suicide attempt with lye ingestion, motor vehicle accident, outpatient plastic surgery procedure such as chin implants, or worsening rheumatoid arthritis).

B. INTERVIEWING SKILLS

Dorland's Medical Dictionary defines empathy as the *intellectual* and *emotional* awareness and understanding of another person's thoughts, feelings, and behavior, even those that are distressing and disturbing. Although the anesthesiologist may participate in 1000 operations a year, few patients undergo more than five in a lifetime.[25] The patient's perception of empathy from the physician is the cornerstone of the patient's acceptance of an AI. Empathy helps the interviewer establish effective communication, which is important for accurate diagnosis and patient management.[28] Two facets of medical education limit the clinician's development of empathy: the traditional format of interviewing training and the social ethos of medical training and medical practice, which stresses clinical detachment.[28,29] With empathy and the ability to communicate it, the physician can perform the interview in a more patient-oriented rather than disease-oriented fashion, resulting in better data gathering and patient *compliance*.[30]

Plato recognized that "a life unexamined is not worth living." We as physicians must examine ourselves for

Table 9-1. Incidence of recall in patients undergoing awake intubation

Reference	No. of AIs	Complete amnesia	Partial recall	Unpleasant memories
Thomas[2]	25	6	14	5
Kopman et al.[10]	249	213	19	17
Mongan and Culling[6]	40	35	5	0
Ovassapian et al.[3]	129	89	37	3
Total	443	343 (77%)	75 (17%)	25 (6%)

biases[31] and unrecognized negative feelings towards an individual patient (such as the patient with morbid obesity, drug addiction, or simply the need to remain in control), which could be detrimental to effective communication and ultimately patient compliance.[31,32]

Once we have determined that AI is in order, we should in a careful, unhurried manner describe to the patient the conventional intubation contrasted with AI. Focusing on the fact that the former is easier and less time-consuming, but that the latter is safer in light of the patient's own anatomy and/or condition, we must communicate to the patient that the knowledgeable, caring physician is willing to take extra measures to ensure patient safety. Recommendations should be presented to the patient with conviction, but at the same time allowing the patient the option of the conventional method of intubation as a *last resort.*[22]

Complications of AI should be presented, including local anesthetic toxicity, specific complications of technique planned, discomfort, and recall. We should strive to develop sufficient skill in the techniques of AI in order to honestly communicate to the patient that he/she will experience a minimum of discomfort and unpleasantness, although he/she may or may not recall the intubation. Patient recall after AI using different methods of sedation, analgesia, or local anesthetics has not been studied in a controlled fashion. While episodes of explicit awareness during general anesthesia are rare (incidence is 0.2% to 3% and depends on both the depth of anesthesia and specific agents administered), it is anticipated that incidence of recall of AI using minimal levels of sedation would be higher.[25] In reviewing 443 cases of AI (Table 9-1) where various combinations of sedation and analgesia were utilized (11 patients had no sedation), 17% (mean of four studies) of the patients had partial recall and 6% (mean of four studies) had recall with unpleasant memories.[2,3,6,10]

If the patient refuses AI, the anesthesiologist still has the option to discuss the case with the primary care physician and/or the surgeon in order to recruit them in helping to convince the patient. If this, as well as

subsequent discussion with the patient, is unsuccessful, the anesthesiologist should then document these data in the chart.

III. PREMEDICATION

A small percentage of patients requiring awake intubation need pharmacologic support to relieve anxiety and fear even after an effective preoperative visit. The primary goals for use of premedications are to relieve anxiety, to provide a clear and dry airway, to protect against aspiration and to provide adequate topicalization of the airway. The commonly used medications in the preoperative period include sedatives, aspiration prophylaxis agents, antisialogogues, and mucosal vasoconstrictors.

A. SEDATIVES

Since patient cooperation is of utmost importance, sedation should be titrated to the minimum amount needed to provide adequate relief from anxiety. Sedatives should be used only when a patient is closely monitored by the anesthesiologist. The heavily sedated patient may not be able to protect his/her airway or to maintain adequate oxygenation and respiration.

The benzodiazepines (diazepam, midazolam, and lorazepam) are the drugs most commonly used to relieve anxiety and provide adequate amnesia. Oral diazepam (0.1 to 0.2 mg/kg) is rapidly absorbed with peak effect in 55 minutes and elimination half-life of 21 to 37 hours.[33] Parenteral midazolam (0.1 mg/kg IM, 1 to 2.5 mg IV) has a rapid onset of action with elimination of half life of 1 to 4 hours. Midazolam provides greater amnesia and less postoperative sedation as compared with diazepam. Oral lorazepam is slowly absorbed from the gastrointestinal (GI) tract with peak effects in 2 to 4 hours.[34] All three agents provide adequate sedation and relief of anxiety for awake intubation, but midazolam is preferred because of its rapid onset and short duration.

If a patient becomes heavily sedated, flumazenil, a specific and exclusive benzodiazepine antagonist, can reverse the effects of benzodiazepines in doses of 8 to 15 μg/kg without major side effects.[35]

Other medications less commonly used for sedation are narcotics, ketamine, and droperidol. Fentanyl citrate and alfentanil are excellent narcotic agents that can provide mild sedation and analgesia even in low doses but can be associated with respiratory depression and chest wall rigidity. Respiratory depression can easily be reversed with an opioid-specific antagonist (naloxone 1 to 5 μg/kg). Chest wall rigidity can be relieved by a small dose of short-acting muscle relaxant (succinylcholine 0.2 to 0.3 mg/kg), but the respiration may need to be supported and awareness of paralysis must be treated.[36] The newer opioid agent, remifentanil, has rapid onset of action and an elimination half-life of 3 to 5 minutes. It provides sedation with excellent analgesia. This drug has not been studied extensively, but it appears that it may be an excellent drug for shorter procedures.[37] Ketamine in low doses (0.2 to 0.5 mg/kg) can be used for sedation but can produce excessive secretions; hallucinations, and mild respiratory depression.[38] Droperidol (50 to 70 µg/kg), a butyrophenone derivative with longer duration of action, used alone or with fentanyl, can provide sedation but causes respiratory depression, extrapyramidal symptoms, and confusion.[39]

B. ASPIRATION PROPHYLAXIS

A small percentage of patients requiring awake intubation may require prophylaxis against aspiration as they may have a full stomach (e.g., trauma victims) and/or be obese with difficult airway. Preoperative administration of nonparticulate antacids like bicitra (sodium citrate and citric acid) provides effective buffering of gastric acid pH.[40] Polycitra (sodium citrate, potassium citrate, and citric acid) is also a nonparticulate antacid with better buffering capacity than bicitra.[41] A single dose of antacid increases gastric volume. This effect is offset by an increase in the pH of gastric fluid, such that if aspiration occurs, morbidity and mortality are significantly lower.[42]

H_2-receptor antagonists (cimetidine and ranitidine) are selective and competitive antagonists that block secretion of Hydrogen ion (H^+) by gastric parietal cells and also decrease the secretion of gastric fluid. With IV administration of cimetidine (100 mg) or ranitidine (50 mg), peak effects are achieved within 30 to 60 minutes, which increase gastric pH and decrease gastric volume.[43]

Metoclopramide is a dopamine antagonist that stimulates motility of the upper GI tract and increases lower esophageal sphincter tone. The net effect is accelerated gastric clearance of liquids and solids in the patent GI tract.[44]

For complete aspiration prophylaxis, a combination of nonparticulate antacid, H_2-receptor blocking agent, and metoclopramide may be used.

C. ANTISIALOGOGUES

Anticholinergic drugs (atropine, scopolamine hydrobromide, and glycopyrrolate) are excellent agents for drying the secretions in the airway to facilitate awake intubation. Scopolamine produces excellent antisialogogue effects with good sedation. Glycopyrrolate, which does not cross the normal blood-brain barrier, provides a moderate antisialogogue effect with no sedation. Atropine provides a mild antisialogogue effect with mild sedation but is the most likely to cause tachycardia.[45] The anticholinergics can cause delirium, restlessness, confusion, tachycardia, relaxation of lower esophageal sphincter tone, mydriasis, and cycloplegia.[46]

Each of the three agents provides satisfactory drying of the airway.

D. NASAL MUCOSAL VASOCONSTRICTORS

The nasal mucosa and nasopharynx are highly vascular. When a patient requires awake nasal intubation, adequate anesthesia of this area, along with vasoconstriction, is essential. Agents commonly used are 4% cocaine and 2% lidocaine with 1% phenylephrine.[47] Once these agents are applied appropriately to the nasal area, adequate anesthesia and vasoconstriction can be achieved in 10 to 15 minutes, which will facilitate awake nasal intubation (see Nerve Blocks).

It is helpful to begin the process of vasoconstriction preoperatively by using nasal decongestants. When the patient is called to the OR, the floor nurse can be asked to apply 0.025% to 0.05% oxymetazoline hydrochloride nasal solution (Afrin spray), sprayed twice in each nostril, which vasoconstricts the anterior half of the nasal cavity. When the patient arrives in the holding area, the anesthesiologist repeats the process, allowing the solution to reach the posterior half of the nasal cavity.

IV. PREOPERATIVE PREPARATIONS
A. GENERAL PREOPERATIVE PREPARATIONS

The preparation of the patient for an AI begins, as discussed, with verbal communication to allay fear and appropriate premedication. The preparation for AI includes assembling necessary equipment, as discussed later, and arranging *in advance* for needed assistance. Patient acuity must be considered when arranging transport to OR.

The decision must be made (1) to secure the airway at once (the patient in extremis who warrants a bedside emergency airway procedure), (2) to transport the patient to the OR with appropriate monitors (electrocardiogram [ECG] pulse oximeter, and automated blood pressure cuff) and supplemental oxygen, accompanied by anesthesiologist and/or surgeon, or (3) to call for routine transport to the OR. In the elective scenario, supplemental oxygen should be provided if appropriate (high-dose oxygen may be detrimental in some patients, such as those who rely on hypoxic respiratory drive),[25] and position should be considered. (e.g., The morbidly obese patient may experience dramatic physiologic changes when supine and should be transported in a wheelchair or on a gurney in a semirecumbant position.)[48,49,50]

B. OPERATING ROOM PREPARATIONS
1. Staff

There should be "at least one additional individual who is immediately available to serve as an assistant in difficult airway management."[16] Preferred whenever possible is a secondary anesthesiologist who can assist in monitoring and ventilation of the patient (two-person ventilation and assistance in mask ventilation while the primary anesthesiologist performs fiberoptic intubation). In cases of the patient in extremis or a patient who refuses AI, a surgeon trained in performing a surgical airway should be at hand with a tracheostomy-cricothyrotomy tray, ready to perform an emergency surgical airway.

2. Monitors

During awake intubation the routine use of ECG, noninvasive blood pressure monitor, pulse oximetry, capnography, and a precordial stethoscope is required as part of standard basic intraoperative monitoring. Depending on the complexity of the surgery and the patient's condition, monitoring may include more sophisticated and often invasive monitors.

ECG is a continuous display of the patient's cardiac activity during the intraoperative period and helps in diagnosis and necessary treatment of changes seen in heart rate and rhythm, as well as heart blocks and ischemia. An audible indicator for each QRS complex allows the anesthesiologist to carry on with tasks in the operating room while listening to cardiac rate and rhythm changes. ECG is usually monitored in lead II and lead V_5 for detection of myocardial ischemia and dysrhythmia.[51,52] Electrolyte changes, particularly those of potassium and calcium, can frequently be diagnosed with ECG.

Blood pressure is usually measured noninvasively by oscillometric method during awake intubation. Devices automatically measure blood pressure at intervals of 1, 2.5, or 5 minutes and give accurate measurement of mean arterial pressure even in hypotensive conditions.[53] The blood pressure cuff width should be about 40% of the circumference of the arm. If the patient's general condition or the complexity of the operation demands, arterial blood pressure may be recorded continuously by the "invasive" method by placement of an arterial catheter in the radial artery.

The precordial stethoscope is commonly placed on the suprasternal notch or over the left side of the chest under the clavicle area to monitor heart sounds and breath sounds continuously during the awake intubation procedure. This device can help in detection of bronchospasm or obstructed airway.

Pulse oximetry is essential for detection of arterial oxygen saturation changes during awake intubation, allowing early detection of hypoxemia so that the patient can be ventilated with 100% oxygen. Oxygen saturation values obtained by the pulse oximeter reading may not be accurate in the presence of hypotension, hypothermia, motion, OR lights, electrocautery interference, or peripheral vasoconstriction.[54]

Capnography measures carbon dioxide (CO_2) levels

BOX 9-2   Suggested contents of the portable unit for difficult airway management

1. Rigid laryngoscope blades of alternate designs and sizes from those routinely used.
2. Endotracheal tubes of assorted sizes.
3. Endotracheal tube guides. Examples include (but are not limited to) semirigid stylets with or without hollow core for jet ventilation, light wands, and forceps designed to manipulate the distal portion of the endotracheal tube.
4. Fiberoptic intubation equipment.
5. Retrograde intubation equipment.
6. At least one device for emergency nonsurgical airway ventilation. Examples include (but are not limited to) a transtracheal jet ventilation stylet, the laryngeal mask, and the esophageal-tracheal Combitube.
7. Equipment suitable for emergency surgical airway access (cricothyrotomy).
8. An exhaled CO_2 detector.
9. Pulse oximetry unit.
10. Portable O_2 tank.

Important: The items listed in this table represent suggestions. The contents of the portable storage unit should be customized to meet the specific needs, preferences, and skills of the practitioner and health-care facility.

Modified from Practice guidelines for management of the difficult airway, *Anesthesiology* 78:597, 1993.

---

in inhaled and exhaled gases of the patient. Upon achievement of awake intubation the presence of three consecutive wave forms of end-tidal CO_2 confirms tracheal intubation. The absence of end-tidal CO_2 wave form on the monitoring device detects esophageal intubation and alerts the anesthesiologist. Capnography also helps to diagnose other problems such as disconnection of anesthesia delivery system, obstruction in the airway, exhausted carbon dioxide absorber, and malfunctioning inspiratory or expiratory valve.[55]

3. Supplemental oxygen

Administration of supplemental oxygen (O_2) should be considered during the entire process of DA management, which includes topicalization, intubation, and extubation.[16] Arterial hypoxemia has been well documented during bronchoscopy (an average decrease in Pao_2 of 20 to 30 mm Hg in patients breathing room air) and has been associated with cardiac dysrhythmias.[56] Daos et al.[57] have shown that the use of supplemental oxygen delayed circulatory arrest resulting from local anesthetic toxic effects in animals but did not show statistically significant improvement in the incidence of respiratory arrest.[57] Considering the advantage of improving patient safety, the use of supplemental oxygen

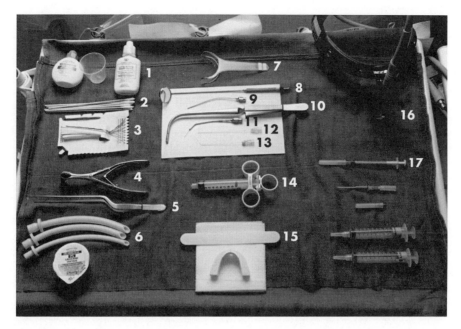

Fig. 9-1. The top surface of our airway cart is used as a workstation for topicalization and nerve blocks. *1,* Nasal vasoconstrictors and container for local anesthetics. *2,* Long cotton-tipped applicators. *3,* Neuropledgets. *4,* Nasal speculum. *5,* Bayonet forceps. *6,* Nasal trumpets in various sizes with viscous lidocaine. *7,* Cheek retractor. *8,* Indirect mirror. *9,* Modified Labat needle. *10,* Krause's forceps. *11,* Tonsillar needle. *12,* Straight 25-gauge spinal needle for glossopharyngeal nerve block. *13,* Angled 25-gauge spinal needle for sphenopalatine nerve block. *14,* Three-ring syringe. *15,* Tongue blade and mouth guard for glossopharyngeal nerve block. *16,* Light source. *17,* 25-gauge needle for superior laryngeal nerve block, 20-gauge angiocatheter for translaryngeal block, and syringes for local anesthetic.

must be encouraged in all patients undergoing awake intubation.

In addition to the standard methods of supplementing oxygen (nasal prongs, face mask, and binasal airways), there are nonconventional methods for increasing the fractional concentration of oxygen in inspired gas (FiO_2): delivering O_2 through the suction port of the fiberoptic bronchoscope,[12] delivering O_2 through the atomizer during topicalization,[60] or elective transtracheal jet ventilation (TTJV) in the patient in extremis.[12,48,58-60]

4. Airway equipment

Consultants of the DATF agreed strongly that "preparatory efforts enhance success and minimize risk to the patient" (fewer adverse outcomes).[16] The concept of preassembled carts for emergency situations is not new ("crash carts" for cardiac arrest on every floor and malignant hyperthermia carts in every OR area). DATF recommendations are that *every anesthetizing location* should be equipped with a DA cart. (If the main operating room is in a different location from the outpatient surgical center, two carts are necessary.) The DA cart should be a portable storage unit that contains specialized equipment for managing the DA. This cart should be customized to the individual *group* of anesthesiologists who will be using it (Box 9-2). For example,

only *one* physician in the group may be familiar with a specific cricotome for establishing a surgical airway. The options are to either train the rest of the staff in the mechanics of that particular instrument or supply the cart with various equipments sufficient to satisfy *all* staff preferences and expertise. At our institution we have chosen the latter approach.

On top of our cart we have dedicated capnograph and pulse oximeter, since we are frequently asked to manage difficult airways outside of the OR setting in locations such as the burn unit of the Surgical Intensive Care Unit (SICU). The top surface of the cart is used as a workstation for preparation of fiberoptic equipment and laying out equipment for topicalizing the airway and for nerve blocks (Fig. 9-1). The first drawer is for drugs (including flumazenil and naloxone) and ancillary fiberoptic equipment (Fig. 9-2). The fiberoptic bronchoscopes themselves are suspended on the outside of the cart (Fig. 9-3), with tubes designated for clean or used bronchoscopes. The second drawer is for specialized blades, lighted stylets, and laryngeal mask airways (Fig. 9-4). Below the drawers, space is available for the fiberoptic light source, different sizes of endotracheal tubes, and other ancillary equipment. On the *outer wall* of the airway cart we hang, on clips, emergency airway equipment such as cricotomes, retrograde kits, jet stylets,

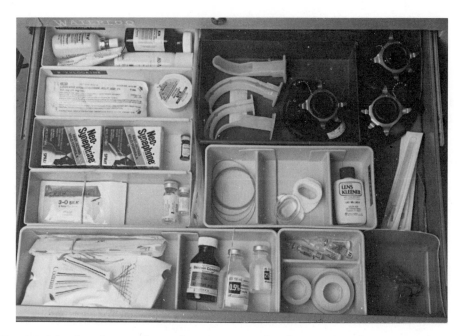

Fig. 9-2. The first drawer of our airway cart contains drugs and ancillary equipment for fiberoptic bronchoscope (fiberoptic masks and oral airways).

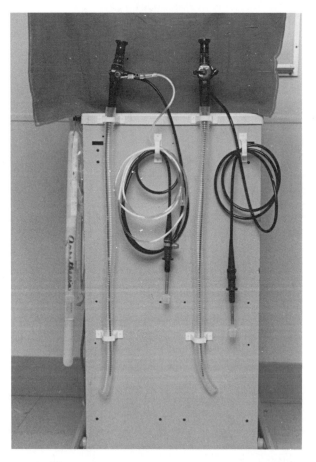

Fig. 9-3. Fiberoptic bronchoscope suspended on the outside of the cart for easy access. Scope on the left has a triple stopcock and air hose to deliver oxygen as well as to administer local anesthetic through the suction port of the scope.

Combitubes and portable jet ventilator equipment (Fig. 9-5). Critical airway equipment can easily be obtained in a "pop-off" manner with one hand.

In addition to the equipment on the cart, on every OR anesthetic machine we have a designated Combitube, gum elastic bougie, and jet ventilator with preassembled transtracheal kit. There are multiple acceptable TTJV systems available (see Chapter 23). We are currently using an injector (blowgun) powered by a regulated central wall oxygen pressure unit with a universal adapter to the oxygen wall outlet.[58] Taped to the jet ventilator is a kit containing a 14-gauge angiocatheter (for adult patients), an 18-gauge angiocatheter (for pediatric patients), and a 20-ml syringe. As part of our machine check the jet ventilator is set at 40 to 50 psi[12,58,61] for adults and 5 psi[35] for pediatric patients as starting pressures, to minimize the incidence of barotrauma.[12,13,28,63]

V. TOPICALIZATION

Awake intubation with airway instrumentation causes discomfort unless adequate topical anesthesia of the respiratory tract is performed, rendering the process painless. It is important to know the onset of action and mechanism of action, optimal concentration, and maximum amount of a drug that can be used safely.[62] The rate and amount of topical drug absorption usually varies depending on the site of application, the amount of the drug applied locally, hemodynamic status of the patient, and patient individual variation.[63] The rate at which the drug is absorbed from the respiratory tract is more rapid from the alveoli than from the tracheobronchial tree,

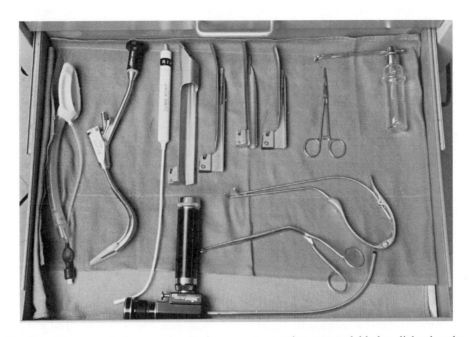

Fig. 9-4. The second drawer of our airway cart contains assorted blades, lighted stylet, instruments to bend or manipulate endotracheal tubes, and laryngeal mask airways.

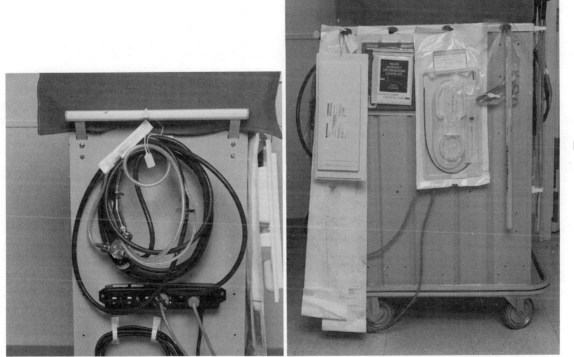

Fig. 9-5. A and **B,** Suspended on outside of cart for easy access is emergency equipment (Combitube, jet stylet, cricotome, retrograde kit, and jet ventilator).

which is more rapid than from the pharynx. It is still controversial whether the addition of vasoconstrictor to these drugs really prolongs the duration of action or slows the rate of absorption.[62]

The most commonly used drugs for topical anesthesia are cocaine, benzocaine, lidocaine, and tetracaine.

A. COCAINE

Cocaine is a natural alkaloid that causes local anesthesia and vasoconstriction when applied topically; thus cocaine is widely used in otolaryngologic surgical procedures.[64] The vasoconstrictive properties of cocaine result from interference with the reuptake of circulating catecholamine by the adrenergic nerve endings.[65] Cocaine should be used with caution in patients with known hypersensitivity, coronary artery disease, hypertension, pseudocholinesterase deficiency, pregnancy with hypertension (preeclampsia), hyperthyroidism, as well as with children, elderly patients, and patients receiving monoamine oxidase (MAO) inhibitors. Following topical application of cocaine to the nasal mucosa, peak plasma level is achieved within an hour and the drug persists in plasma for 5 to 6 hours.[66] The metabolism of cocaine is mainly by plasma cholinesterase, with hepatic and renal excretion. The signs and symptoms of cocaine overdose include tachycardia, cardiac dysrhythmia, hypertension, and fever. It is important to remember that cocaine does have addictive properties because of cortical stimulation resulting in euphoria, excitement, feeling "high," and increased muscle activity. Severe complications include convulsions, respiratory failure, coronary spasm, stroke, and death.

Cocaine is available in two preparations, 4% and 10% solutions, for topical application. The 10% solution is not used because of a very high incidence of toxic effects. The dosage varies and depends on the area to be anesthetized, vascularity of the tissue, individual tolerance, and the technique of anesthesia. The dosage should be reduced in children and in elderly and debilitated patients. The maximum dose should not exceed 200 mg.

B. BENZOCAINE

Benzocaine (ethyl aminobenzoate) is a water-insoluble ester-type local anesthetic agent that is mainly useful for topical application. The onset of action is rapid (less than 1 minute) with effective duration of about 10 minutes. Benzocaine is available for use as 10%, 15%, and 20% solutions. To prolong duration of action, it is usually mixed with 2% tetracaine. Topical application is usually nontoxic, although methemoglobinemia has been reported in adult patients taking sulfonamides and in pediatric patients.[67]

Benzocaine 20% spray (Hurricaine, Beutlich Pharmaceuticals, Waukegan, IL) contains 200 mg/ml; thus 0.5 ml is equal to the toxic dose, which is 100 mg. A half-second spray delivers approximately 0.15 ml, or 30 mg.

Cetacaine is a topical application spray containing benzocaine 14%, tetracaine 2%, butyl aminobenzoate 2%, benzalkonium chloride, and cetyldimethyl ethyl ammonium bromide, which has been shown to be effective for topicalizing the airway. Combining these agents hastens onset of action and prolongs duration of action. Interestingly, there are case reports of methemoglobinemia occurring immediately following application of this spray. Of the preceding compounds, only benzocaine has been implicated. In the patient who develops this complication, cyanosis appears first (at a methemoglobin level of as low as 2.5%), and clinical symptoms (fatigue, weakness, headache, dizziness, and tachycardia) appear later (at methemoglobin levels of 20% to 50%). Treatment is with intravenous methylene blue (1mg/kg body weight).[68-70]

C. LIDOCAINE

Lidocaine is an amide local anesthetic agent that is widely used. It is available in various preparations including aqueous (1%, 2%, and 4%) and viscous (1%) solutions, ointment (1%), and aerosol preparation. Xylocaine 10% metered-dose oral spray (Astra) delivers 10 mg per spray and rapidly anesthetizes the upper airway.

Once in the plasma, lidocaine is metabolized mainly by the hepatic microsomal system. In awake patients the toxic plasma level of lidocaine is 5 µg/ml.[55] In most of the clinical situations where lidocaine is used as a local anesthesic agent for topicalization, the peak plasma level measured has been far below the 5 or 6 µg/ml level;[70,71] thus severe toxic reactions secondary to lidocaine are uncommon in the context of airway management. Symptoms of severe lidocaine toxicity include convulsions, respiratory failure, and circulatory collapse.

D. TETRACAINE

Tetracaine is an amide local anesthetic agent with a longer duration of action than lidocaine and cocaine. It is available as 0.5%, 1%, and 2% solutions for local use. It is metabolized via hydrolysis by plasma cholinesterase. Tetracaine has been shown to have higher toxic effects when used as an aerosol with doses as small as 40 mg because absorption of the drug from the respiratory tract and GI tract is fast.[72] Severe toxic reactions following tetracaine overdose include convulsions, respiratory arrest, and circulatory collapse.[76] Fatalities have been reported with topical application of tetracaine 100 mg used to anesthetize mucous membrane.[73]

E. APPLICATION TECHNIQUES

1. Atomizers

Sprays and atomizers with long delivery systems are available to deliver local anesthesia to the larynx and

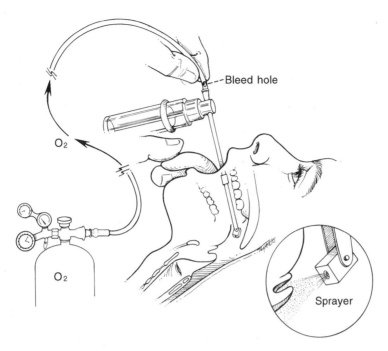

Fig. 9-6. Atomizer hooked up to an oxygen (O₂) tank. A bleed hole is made close to the operator's hand, allowing for intermittent spraying. Inset shows the tip of atomizer as it is angulated to spray toward the glottic opening. (From UCI Department of Anesthesia: *D.A. Teaching Aids.*)

trachea. Tetracaine (0.3% to 0.5% with epinephrine 1:200,000), maximum 20 ml, or lidocaine (4%), maximum 10 ml, is placed in an atomizer (Fig. 9-6), connected to the oxygen tank (flow, 8 to 10 L/min), and sprayed in the oropharynx for 10-second periods with 20-second rest intervals for about 20 minutes. Any residual agents from the oropharynx must be suctioned out to reduce absorption from the GI tract. This is, relatively, a safe and simple method to provide adequate anesthesia of the airway.

2. Nebulizers

The ultrasonic nebulizer utilizes 5 ml of 4% lidocaine to be nebulized with oxygen (6 to 8 L/min). The size of the droplet depends on the flow of oxygen and the type of nebulizer. With oxygen flow of less than 6 L per minute, droplet size of 30 to 60 μ can be achieved, which coats the mucosa up to the trachea. The advantages of this technique include ease of application and safety. This is a difficult technique to use in small children and uncooperative patients. This approach is especially advantageous in patients with increased intracranial pressure (ICP), open eye injury and severe coronary artery disease.[74]

Other less commonly used techniques for topical anesthesia include use of lozenges (amethocaine lozenges 60 mg) and gargle with 4% lidocaine gel,[79] neither of which are routinely used since they provide limited anesthesia.

VI. NERVE BLOCKS

Because of the multitude of nerves innervating the airway (see Chapter 1), there is no single anatomic site where a physician can perform a nerve block and anesthetize the entire airway. Even though topicalization of the mucosa serves, in the majority of patients, to adequately anesthetize the entire airway, some patients require supplementation to ablate sensation in those nerve endings running deep to the mucosal surface such as the periosteal nerve endings of the nasal turbinates and the stretch receptors at the base of the tongue, which are involved in gagging. The following nerve blocks are remarkable for their ease of performance, their minimal risk to the patient, the density of the block (complete ablation of sensory fibers), and speed of onset.

A. NASAL CAVITY AND NASOPHARYNX[22-24,27,75-82]

1. Anatomy

The nasal cavity is innervated by a plethora of sensory fibers with multiple origins. The majority of the innervation is derived from two sources: the sphenopalatine ganglion and the anterior ethmoidal nerve.

The sphenopalatine ganglion (pterygopalatine, nasal, or Meckel's ganglion) is located in the pterygopalatine fossa (Fig. 9-7, *A* and *B*) posterior to the middle turbinate. It is covered by a 1- to 5-mm layer of connective tissue and mucous membrane. The ganglion is a 5-mm triangular or heart-shaped structure compris-

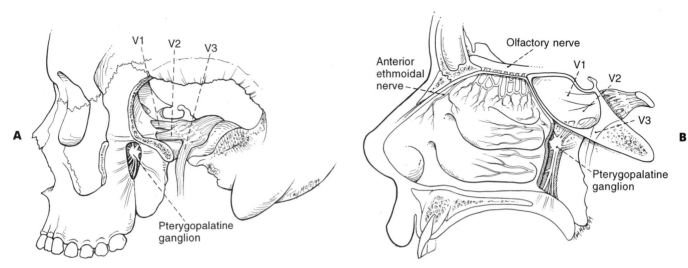

Fig. 9-7. A, Left lateral view of the skull with temporal bone removed depicting the gasserian ganglion with the three branches (V1 to V3) of the trigeminal nerve. V2 is the major contributor to the pterygopalatine ganglion (shown as it sits in the pterygopalatine fossa). **B,** Left lateral view of the right nasal cavity depicting the anterior ethmoidal nerve, olfactory nerve, gasserian ganglion, and the trigeminal nerve (V1 to V3). The pterygopalatine ganglion lies just beneath the mucosal surface on the caudad surface of the sphenoid sinus (and forms the roof of the pterygopalatine fossa). (From UCI Department of Anesthesia, *D.A. Teaching Aids.*)

ing branches primarily from the gasserian ganglion via the trigeminal nerve (V2). Although it sends out multiple branches, two nerves in particular, the greater and lesser palatine nerves, provide sensory innervation to the nasal turbinates and to two thirds of the posterior nasal septum (including the periosteum).

The anterior ethmoidal nerve is one of the branches of the ciliary ganglion, which is located within the orbital cavity and inaccessible to nerve blocks. The anterior ethmoidal nerve (Fig. 9-7, *B*) gives sensory innervation to one third of the anterior portion of the nares.

2. Sphenopalatine nerve block:
  oral approach[24,27,75-78,82]

With the patient in the supine position, the physician stands facing the patient on the contralateral side of the nerve to be blocked. Using the left index finger, the greater palatine foramen (GPF) is identified. The GPF (Fig. 9-8, *A* and *B*) is located between the second and third maxillary molars approximately 1 cm medial to the palatogingival margin and usually can be palpated as a small depression near the posterior edge of the hard palate. In approximately 15% of the population the foramen is closed and inaccessible. A 25-gauge spinal needle, bent 2 to 3 cm proximal to the tip to an angle of 120 degrees, is used. Pain on insertion of the needle can be avoided by application of 2% viscous lidocaine with a cotton-tipped applicator for 1 to 2 minutes or digital pressure over the foramen. The 25-gauge spinal needle is then inserted into the greater palatine foramen in a superior and slightly posterior direction (to a depth of 2 to 3 cm). An aspiration test is performed to ascertain that the sphenopalatine artery has not been cannulated, and 1 to 2 ml of 2% lidocaine with epinephrine 1:100,000 is injected. The epinephrine is used as a vasoconstrictor for the sphenopalatine artery, which runs parallel to the nerves, and further decreases the incidence of epistaxis. The injection of the local anesthetic should be performed in a slow continuous fashion (preventing acute increases in pressure within the fossa) in order to decrease sympathetic stimulation. This injection anesthetizes the anterior, middle, and posterior palatine nerves, as well as the nasociliary and nasopalatine nerves. Complications are bleeding, infection, nerve trauma, intravascular injection of local anesthetics, and hypertension.

3. Sphenopalatine nerve block:
  nasal approach[24,80-84,87]

Two noninvasive nasal approaches to the sphenopalatine ganglion have been described, both of which take advantage of the ganglion's shallow position beneath the nasal mucosa. The *first* involves the application of long cotton-tipped applicators (one may also use neuropledgets using bayonet forceps) soaked in either 4% cocaine or 4% lidocaine with epinephrine 1:200,000 over the mucosal surface overlying the ganglion (Fig. 9-9). The applicator is passed along the upper border of the middle turbinate (at an approximately 45 degree angle to the hard palate) and directed back and down

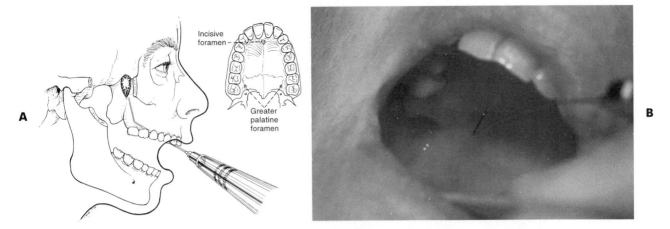

Fig. 9-8. A, Inferior view of the hard palate showing location of the greater palatine foramen. Right lateral view of the head with zygomatic arch and coronoid process of the mandible removed exposing the pterygopalatine fossa (containing the pterygopalatine ganglion) with angulated spinal needle in place. **B,** Right sphenopalatine nerve block. (From UCI Department of Anesthesia, *D.A. Teaching Aids.*)

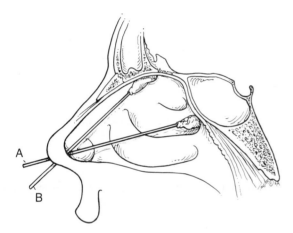

Fig. 9-9. Left lateral view of the right nasal cavity, showing long cotton-tipped applicators soaked in local anesthetic with vasoconstrictors. *A,* Applicator angled at 45 degrees to the hard palate with cotton swab over mucosal surface overlying the sphenopalatine ganglion. *B,* Applicator placed parallel to the dorsal surface of the nose, blocking anterior ethmoidal nerve. (From UCI Department of Anesthesia, *D.A. Teaching Aids.*)

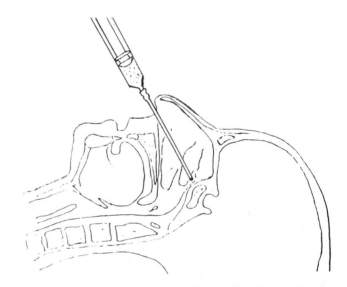

Fig. 9-10. Left lateral view of the right nasal cavity. Angiocatheter with syringe angled at 45 degrees to the hard palate aiming for the sphenopalatine ganglion. (Modified from Boudreaux AM: *Am Soc Crit Care Anesthesiologists* 6(3):8, 1994.)

until the upper posterior wall of the nasopharynx (sphenoid bone) is reached. The applicators are then left in place for approximately 5 to 10 minutes. The *second* method involves using the plastic sheath of a 20-gauge angiocatheter placed along the same path as described previously (Fig. 9-10). The anesthetic solution (4 ml of 4% lidocaine containing 3 mg of phenylephrine) is then rapidly injected. Allow about 2 minutes for the anesthetic to take effect.

4. Nasal pledgets and trumpets[22-24,80-82]

Regardless of which technique is used to anesthetize the nasal cavity, the nares should first be inspected for a

deviated septum using a nasal speculum and the patient asked to breathe deeply through each individual nare (occluding the opposite nare). Patency can also be determined by passing multiple long, cotton-tipped applicators soaked in either 4% cocaine or 4% lidocaine with epinephrine 1:200,000 along the floor of the nasal cavity. The applicators are applied deep, to the level of the posterior nasal pharyngeal wall. The added benefits of this technique are that additional topicalization is applied to the airway, the angle of ET insertion can be predicted, and dilation of the nasal cavity is initiated. The applicators are then followed by nasal trumpets (in

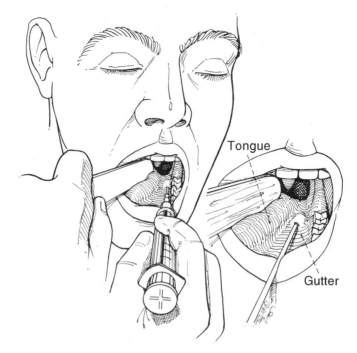

Fig. 9-11. Anterior approach, left-sided glossopharyngeal nerve block. Tongue displaced medially forming a gutter (glossogingival groove), which ends distally in a cul-de-sac. 25-gauge spinal needle placed at the base of the palatoglossal fold. (From UCI Department of Anesthesia, *D.A. Teaching Aids.*)

increasing diameters) soaked in 2% viscous lidocaine, which further dilate the nasal cavity and allow approximation of ET size (nasal trumpet French (F) size 36F predicts easy passage of 7.0 I.D. [inner diameter] ET).

5. Anterior ethmoidal nerve block[22,78,80,82]

The anterior ethmoidal nerve is blocked by the insertion of a long cotton-tipped applicator, soaked in either 4% cocaine or 4% lidocaine with epinephrine 1:200,000, that is placed parallel to the dorsal surface of the nose until it meets the anterior surface of the cribriform plate (Fig. 9-9). The applicator is held in position for 5 to 10 minutes.

B. OROPHARYNX*

1. Anatomy

The somatic and visceral afferent fibers of the oropharynx are supplied by a plexus derived from the vagus, facial, and glossopharyngeal nerves. The glossopharyngeal nerve (GPN) emerges from the skull through the jugular foramen and passes forward between the internal jugular and carotid vessels, traveling anteriorly along the lateral wall of the pharynx. It supplies sensory innervation to the posterior third of the tongue (lingual branch), vallecula, anterior surface of the epiglottis, posterior and lateral walls of the pharynx,

*References 12, 24, 25, 56, 75, 76, 78, 82-94.

and the tonsillar pillars. Its only motor innervation in the pharynx is to the stylopharyngeus muscle (one of the muscles of deglutition).

In the majority of patients, topicalization of the mucosa of the oropharynx is sufficient to allow instrumentation of the airway, such as placement of a fiberoptic oral airway. In some patients the gag reflex is so pronounced that no amount of topicalization allows for a stationary, quiet field for intubation. The gag arises from stimulation of deep pressure receptors, found in the posterior third of the tongue, which cannot be reached by the diffusion of local anesthetics through the mucosa. There are various measures for minimizing this problem: instructing the patient to breathe in a nonstop panting fashion, avoiding pressure on the tongue (nasal intubation), administration of narcotics, and glossopharyngeal nerve block.[24,92] The GPN block is easy to perform and highly effective in abolishing the gag reflex and decreasing the hemodynamic response to laryngoscopy, including awake laryngoscopy. The anterior and posterior approaches are described.

2. Glossopharyngeal nerve block: anterior approach (palatoglossal fold)

The oropharynx is topicalized as previously described. The patient is placed in the sitting position with the physician facing the patient on the *contralateral* side of the nerve to be blocked. The patient is asked (Figs. 9-11

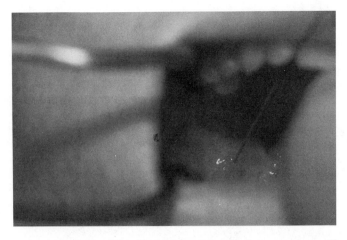

Fig. 9-12. Anterior approach, right-sided glossopharyngeal nerve block. Cheek retractor displacing cheek laterally for better view, tongue displaced medially. Spinal needle in place, 1.5 ml of local injected: Translucency of the mucosa is formed by the local anesthetic. (From UCI Department of Anesthesia, *D.A. Teaching Aids.*)

and 9-12) to open his/her mouth wide and to protrude the tongue anteriorly. A right-hand dominant physician holding a tongue blade with the left hand displaces the tongue medially, forming a gutter or trough along the floor of the mouth between the tongue and the teeth. The gutter ends in a cul-de-sac formed by the base of the palatoglossal arch. (In its tented state it resembles a hammock or U-shaped structure.) A 25-gauge spinal needle is inserted at the base of the cul-de-sac (where the gutter meets the base of the palatoglossal arch) and advanced 0.25 to 0.5 cm. An aspiration test is performed: if air is aspirated, the needle has been advanced too deep (the tip has gone all the way through the thin membrane) and should be withdrawn until no air can be aspirated. If blood is aspirated, the needle should be redirected more medially. Two ml of 1% to 2% lidocaine is injected, and the procedure is repeated on the other side. The spinal needle allows for an unobstructed view of the very narrow field of view in the oral cavity, which would be obstructed by the syringe were a shorter needle to be used.

The block is intended to isolate the lingual branch of the GPN, although in one study using methylene blue it was shown that in some cases retrograde submucosal tracking occurs, blocking the primary trunk of the nerve (pharyngeal and tonsillar branches).[12]

3. Glossopharyngeal nerve block: posterior approach (palatopharyngeal fold)

The posterior approach is a technique that is used frequently by the otolaryngologist for tonsillectomies; it blocks the nerve more proximally, closer to its origin than the anterior approach. It blocks both the sensory fibers (pharyngeal, lingual, and tonsillar branches) and the motor branch innervating the stylopharyngeus muscle.

The patient is placed in the sitting position with the physician facing the patient on the *ipsilateral* side of the nerve to be blocked. The patient is asked to open his/her mouth wide (Figs. 9-13 and 9-14). Using a tongue depressor held in the non-dominant hand, the tongue is displaced caudad and medially exposing the soft palate, uvula, palatoglossal arch, tonsillar bed, and palatopharyngeal arch. This maneuver stretches both the palatoglossal arch and the palatopharyngeal arch, making them more accessible. The dominant hand then holds a 23-gauge tonsillar needle attached to a three-ring syringe containing 3 ml of 2% lidocaine with epinephrine 1:200,000. The tonsillar needle is placed behind the palatopharyngeal arch at its midpoint and inserted into the lateral wall of the oropharynx to the maximum depth allowed by the 1-cm needle shaft. An aspiration test is performed to prevent intravascular injection. A test dose of 0.25 to 0.5 ml is performed while looking for hemodynamic changes and local anesthetic toxic effects. If blood is aspirated or the patient complains of headache, the needle should be removed and repositioned. The remainder of the local anesthetic is injected, and the procedure is repeated on the opposite side.

4. Cautions, complications, contraindications

Potential complications have been cited: headache, pharyngeal abscess, paralysis of the pharyngeal muscles with airway obstruction, hematoma, dysrhythmias, seizures, and intraarterial injection. The potential for intraarterial injection is greater for the posterior approach because of proximity of the carotid artery in this region. One study reported 823 patients who had block by the posterior approach, of which two had self-limited hematomas.[83] A second study using the posterior approach reported 0.8% incidence of headache, believed to be due to intravascular injection; 0.4% incidence of seizures; and 1% incidence of dysrhythmias (supraven-

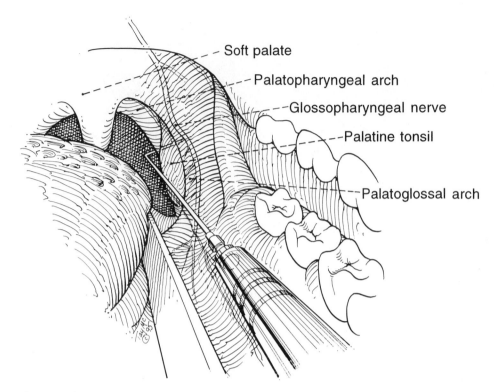

Soft palate

Palatopharyngeal arch

Glossopharyngeal nerve

Palatine tonsil

Palatoglossal arch

Fig. 9-13. Posterior approach, left glossopharyngeal nerve block. Tonsillar needle (or a 25-gauge spinal needle bent at right angle) is placed behind the midportion of the palatoglossal fold, allowing blocking of the nerve at a more proximal position. (From UCI Department of Anesthesia, *D.A. Teaching Aids.*)

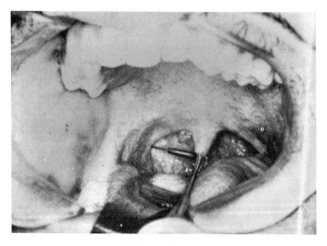

Fig. 9-14. Posterior approach, right glossopharyngeal nerve block. (From UCI Department of Anesthesia, *D.A. Teaching Aids.*)

tricular tachycardia and bigeminy). Of the patients with dysrhythmias, one required treatment with propranolol.[88] Some believe that the tachycardia may result from blocking the afferent nerve fibers of the GPN that arise from the carotid sinus.[84] There have been no reported cases of airway obstruction secondary to laxity of the pharynx resulting from paralysis of the pharyngeal musculature. There have been no reported cases of complications with the anterior approach. One would

expect potential complications to be bleeding, infection, and intravascular injection of local anesthetics.

C. LARYNX*

1. Anatomy

The general nerve supply of the laryngeal inlet is primarily via the superior laryngeal nerve (SLN). The SLN supplies sensory innervation to the base of the tongue, vallecula, epiglottis, aryepiglottic folds, arytenoids, and down to but excluding the vocal cords. The SLN originates as a branch of the vagus nerve, lying deep to the carotid artery. It then travels anteriorly and at the level of the cornu of the hyoid bone branches into the internal branch, which is sensory, and the external branch, which is motor (cricothyroid muscle). The internal branch subsequently pierces the thyrohyoid ligament (membrane) along with the accompanying superior laryngeal artery and vein. The nerve then enters the space just beneath the mucosa covering the pyriform fossa and preepiglottic space (Fig. 9-15).

2. Superior laryngeal nerve block: position and landmarks

The patient is placed in the supine position, head slightly extended, with the physician standing on the *ipsilateral* side of the neck. The two main anatomic

*References 2, 6, 12, 21-27, 56, 76, 77, 82, 83, 88, 91-99.

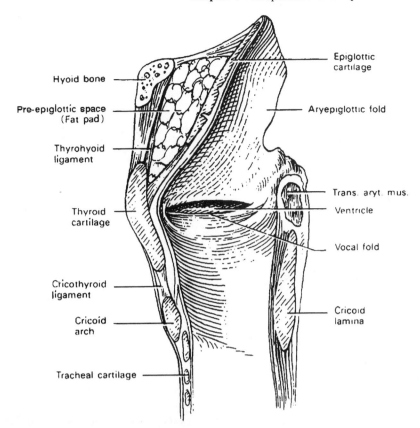

Fig. 9-15. Mid-sagittal view of the larynx showing the preepiglottic space containing adipose tissue or fat pad (see **C** in Fig. 9-16).

structures that should be identified are the cornu of the hyoid bone and the superior cornu of the thyroid cartilage. *The cornu of the hyoid bone* lies beneath the angle of the mandible and anterior to the carotid artery. It can be palpated transversely with the thumb and index finger on the sides of the neck as a bilateral, rounded structure. One side can be made more prominent by displacing the contralateral side toward the side being blocked. The *superior cornu of the thyroid cartilage* can be recognized by palpating the thyroid notch (Adam's apple) and tracing the upper edge of the thyroid cartilage posteriorly, and can be palpated as a smaller bilateral, rounded structure lying just underneath the superior cornu of the hyoid bone.

Four approaches to the block have been described: three external approaches and one internal approach.

After administration of the local anesthetic from the external approaches, SNL block is achieved in approximately 1 minute. The internal approach takes longer. The success rate of the SLN blocks has been reported to be as high as 92%.[97]

3. Superior laryngeal nerve block: techniques

a. EXTERNAL APPROACH: CORNU OF THE HYOID

Aseptic technique should be used in the external approach. In a right-hand dominant physician the left index finger is used to depress the carotid artery laterally and posteriorly. With the right hand, a 2.5-cm, 25-gauge needle and syringe combination is walked off the cornu of the hyoid bone (Fig. 9-16) in an anterior-caudad direction aiming toward the middle of the thyrohyoid ligament. A slight resistance will be felt as the needle is advanced through the ligament usually at a depth of 1 to 2 cm (2 to 3 mm deep to the hyoid bone). The needle at this point has entered a closed space between the thyrohyoid membrane laterally and the laryngeal mucosa medially. Aspiration through the needle should be attempted. If air is aspirated, the needle has gone too deep and may have entered the pharynx, and should be withdrawn until no air can be aspirated. If blood is aspirated, the needle has cannulated either the superior laryngeal artery or vein or has cannulated the carotid artery; the needle should be directed more anteriorly. The space, when found, is injected with 1.5 to 2.0 ml of 2% lidocaine with epinephrine 1:200,000, as the needle is withdrawn. The block is repeated on the opposite side.

b. EXTERNAL APPROACH: CORNU OF THE THYROID

This is the same technique as stated previously but uses the cornu of the thyroid as the landmark. The benefit of this technique is that in many patients these structures are easier to palpate, and palpating them is less painful to the patient. A 4-cm, 25-gauge needle is

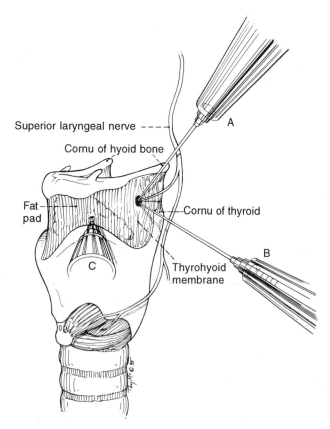

Fig. 9-16. Superior laryngeal nerve block. External approach, *A*, using the cornu of the hyoid bone as landmark; *B*, using the cornu of the thyroid cartilage as landmark; and *C*, using the thyroid notch as landmark. (Fat pad is found in the preepiglottic space.) (From UCI Department of Anesthesia, *D.A. Teaching Aids.*)

walked off the cornu of the thyroid cartilage (Fig. 9-16) in a superior-anterior direction aiming toward the lower third of the thyroid ligament; the same precautions as before are taken. The block is repeated on the opposite side.

c. EXTERNAL APPROACH: THYROID NOTCH

The easiest landmark to identify in many of the patients, especially males, is the thyroid notch (Adam's apple). The thyroid notch is palpated, and the upper border of the thyroid cartilage is traced posteriorly for approximately 2 cm (Fig. 9-16). Using a 2.5-cm, 25-gauge needle, the thyrohyoid ligament is directed posterior and cephalad and entered to a depth of 1.0 to 1.5 cm. This corresponds to the preepiglottic space, which normally contains the terminal branches of the SLN imbedded in a fat pad. The area is injected with the same solution, using precautions as previously described, but the entire volume is injected into the preepiglottic space before the needle is withdrawn. The block is repeated on the opposite side. An added benefit of this approach is the decreased likelihood of blocking the motor branch of the SLN.

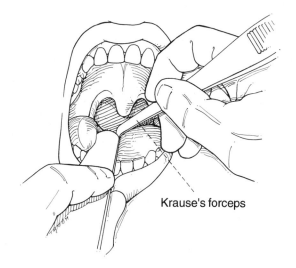

Fig. 9-17. Superior laryngeal nerve block. External approach. Krause's forceps advanced over tongue toward pyriform sinus. (From UCI Department of Anesthesia, *D.A. Teaching Aids.*)

d. INTERNAL APPROACH: PYRIFORM FOSSA

A noninvasive SLN block can be performed by applying local anesthetic to the pyriform fossa. (The internal branch of the SLN lies just superficial to the mucosa.) After local anesthetic is applied topically to the tongue and pharynx, the patient is placed in the *sitting* position with the physician standing on the *contralateral* side of the nerve to be blocked. The patient is asked to open his/her mouth wide with tongue protruded. The tongue is grasped with the left hand using a gauze pad (or depressed with a tongue blade) and gently pulled anteriorly. With the right hand a Jackson (Krause) forceps armed with cottonoids soaked in 4% cocaine is advanced (Fig. 9-17) over the lateral posterior curvature of the tongue (along the downward continuation of the tonsillar fossa). The tip of the forceps is advanced until it meets resistance (Fig. 9-18) and cannot be advanced any further: at this point, the handle of the forceps should be in a horizontal position. The position of the tip of the forceps may be checked by palpating the neck lateral to the posterior-superior aspect of the thyroid cartilage. The forceps are kept in this position for at *least* 5 minutes, and the process is repeated on the opposite side.

4. Cautions, complications, contraindications

When performing the block from the external approaches, caution should be exercised in order not to insert the needle into the thyroid cartilage, since there is a possibility of injecting the solution at the level of the vocal cords, causing edema and airway obstruction. The carotid artery should be identified and displaced posteriorly to minimize the risk of intravascular injection: even small amounts of local anesthetics (0.25 to 0.5 ml) can induce seizures. On rare occasions (reported inci-

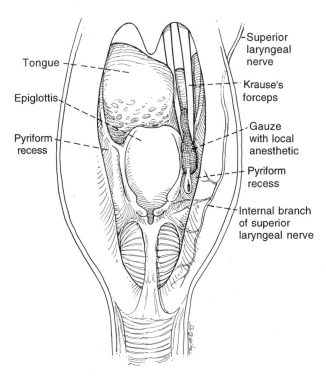

Tongue

Epiglottis

Pyriform
recess

Superior
laryngeal
nerve

Krause's
forceps

Gauze
with local
anesthetic

Pyriform
recess

Internal branch
of superior
laryngeal nerve

Fig. 9-18. Superior laryngeal nerve block. External approach. Posterior view of the larynx showing tip of Krause's forceps at the level of the pyriform sinus. (From UCI Department of Anesthesia, *D.A. Teaching Aids.*)

dence of 2.7%), hypotension and bradycardia have been associated with SLN blocks. A number of possible causes of this reaction have been postulated: (1) apprehension and subsequent vasovagal reaction due to painful stimulation, (2) digital pressure on the sensitive carotid sinus, (3) excessive manipulation of the larynx causing vasovagal reaction, (4) large doses of or accidental intravascular administration of local anesthetic drugs, and (5) direct neural stimulation of the branch of the vagus nerve by the needle. Therefore it is recommended that anticholinergics be administered before the block is performed. The drying agent given before initiation of AI should suffice. Complications of the external approach also include hematoma (reported incidence of 1.4%), pharyngeal puncture, and rupture of the ET cuff in patients already intubated. Contraindications to the external approach are poor anatomic landmarks, local infections, local tumor growth, coagulopathy, and patients at risk for aspiration of gastric contents due to a depressed sensorium. The last is also a contraindication to the internal approach.

D. TRACHEA AND VOCAL CORDS*

1. Anatomy

The sensory innervation of the trachea and vocal cords is supplied by the vagus nerve via the recurrent

*References 2, 3, 6, 12, 22, 23, 25-27, 56, 77, 82, 89-94, 98, 100-102.

laryngeal nerves (RLN). The right RLN originates at the level of the right subclavian artery; the left originates at the level of the aortic arch (distal to the ligamentum arteriosum). Both ascend along the tracheoesophageal groove to supply sensory innervation to the tracheobronchial tree (up to and including the vocal cords), as well as supplying motor nerve fibers to the intrinsic muscles of the larynx (except the cricothyroid muscle). Because both the sensory and motor fibers run together, nerve blocks cannot be performed since this would result in bilateral vocal cord paralysis and complete airway obstruction. The only alternative is topicalization of the mucosa. In addition to the use of nebulizers and atomizers to topicalize the trachea, there are three other techniques: translaryngeal anesthesia (transtracheal), "spray as you go" technique via the fiberoptic bronchoscope, and the Labat technique.

2. Translaryngeal (transtracheal) anesthesia: positioning and landmarks

The ideal position for translaryngeal anesthesia is in the supine position with the neck hyperextended. In this position the cervical vertebrae push the trachea and cricoid cartilage anteriorly and displace the strap muscles of the neck laterally. As a result the cricoid cartilage and the structures above and below it are easier to palpate.

3. Translaryngeal (transtracheal) anesthesia: technique

Using aseptic technique, a right-hand dominant person should stand on the left side of a supine patient. The patient is asked not to talk, swallow, or cough until instructed. Using a tuberculin syringe, a small skin wheal is raised over the intended puncture site but not through the cricothyroid membrane (CTM). The left hand then is used to stabilize the trachea by placing the thumb and third digit on either side of the thyroid cartilage. The index finger of the left hand is used to identify the midline of the CTM and the upper border of the cricoid cartilage. The right hand then grasps the 20-gauge angiocatheter[27] and 10-ml syringe containing 4 to 5 ml local anesthetic like a pencil; the fifth digit is used to brace the right hand on the patient's lower neck. The needle is aimed at a 45-degree angle (Fig. 9-19, *A* to *D*) in a caudad direction. As the needle passes through the CTM, resistance will be felt, and at that point aspiration for air should be attempted to verify placement in the lumen of the airway. (The needle should not be advanced any further.) The sheath of the angiocatheter is advanced, the needle is removed and syringe carefully reattached, and the aspiration test is again performed. The patient is asked to take a vital capacity breath, and at end of inspiration, 4 ml of either 2% or 4% lidocaine is injected. We leave the sheath of the angiocatheter in

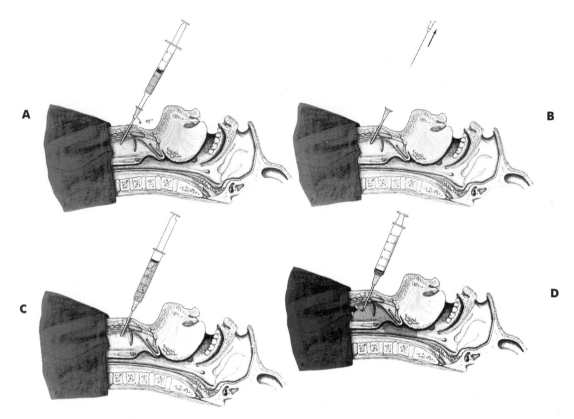

Fig. 9-19. A, Midsagittal view of the head and neck (translaryngeal anesthesia). Angiocatheter aimed at 45 degrees to the cricothyroid membrane. Aspiration test performed to verify position of tip of needle in tracheal lumen. **B,** Midsagittal view of the head and neck (translaryngeal anesthesia). Needle is removed from angiocatheter. **C,** Midsagittal view of the head and neck (translaryngeal anesthesia). Aspiration test repeated. **D,** Midsagittal view of the head and neck (translaryngeal anesthesia). Patient is asked to take a vital capacity breath and asked to cough. At end inspiration the local anesthetic is injected, resulting in coughing and nebulization of the local anesthetic (stippled area). (From UCI Department of Anesthesia, *The Retrograde Cookbook.*)

place until the intubation is completed in case more local anesthetic is needed, and to decrease the likelihood of subcutaneous emphysema (see Chapter 17). The coughing helps to nebulize the local anesthetic so that the inferior and superior surfaces of the vocal cords can be anesthetized.[92,94]

Whether the entry site is above or below the cricoid cartilage, a significant amount of local anesthetic bathes the tracheobronchial tree, false cords, true cords, epiglottis, vallecula, tongue, and posterior pharyngeal wall.[106] The success of translaryngeal anesthesia has been found to be as high as 95% and is attributed to both topicalization of the airway and systemic absorption.[22,103-106] After translaryngeal anesthesia using 5 mg/kg of a 10% lidocaine solution, therapeutic serum levels of lidocaine (greater than 1.4 μg/ml) were reached in a mean time of 5.1 minutes (±3.2 minutes).[103]

4. Translaryngeal (transtracheal) anesthesia: cautions, complications, contraindications

The technique has been described using a 25-gauge needle, but we discourage this because of the possibility of breaking the needle as a result of the cricoid cartilage moving cephalad when the patient is coughing.[102] The tip of the needle should *not* be aimed in a cephalad direction, since the tip of the angiocatheter sheath would then be advanced above the level of the vocal cords, resulting in local anesthetic above but not below the vocal cords. Coughing is a known factor in elevation of mean arterial pressure (MAP), heart rate, intracranial pressure (ICP), and intraocular pressure (IOP). In a series of 186 AI patients using translaryngeal anesthesia, 34.8% coughed slightly, 47.5% coughed moderately severely, and 16.7% coughed severely (only two patients did not cough). The MAP and heart rate rose minimally during translaryngeal anesthesia: maximum increase in MAP (average 10 mm Hg above baseline) occurred during placement of the ET through the nares, and peak heart rate occurred as the ET entered the trachea.[3] In a study of 22 patients with brain tumors randomized to either intravenous lidocaine or laryngotracheal lidocaine anesthesia, the laryngotracheal group showed higher ICP ("in excess of 40 torr") after laryngoscopy. Patients receiving laryngotracheal anesthesia, however, received

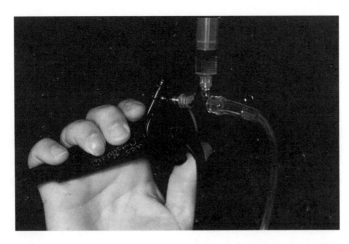

Fig. 9-20. "Spray-as-you-go" technique. Oxygen hose and triple stopcock attached to the suction port of a fiberoptic bronchoscope with syringe attached containing local anesthetic; injected intermittently in aliquots of 0.2 to 1.0 ml. (From UCI Department of Anesthesia, *D.A. Teaching Aids.*)

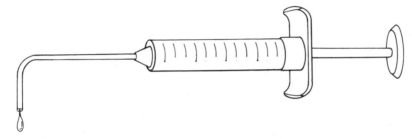

Fig. 9-21. Labat needle for dripping local anesthetic over vocal cords. (From UCI Department of Anesthesia, *D.A. Teaching Aids.*)

the transtracheal lidocaine *after* laryngoscopy, suggesting that the elevation of ICP may have been due to laryngoscopy and not to the transtracheal administration of lidocaine. In another study, 20 patients (11 of whom had either cervical pathology or head and neck malignancy), were given translaryngeal anesthesia without undesirable side effects.[6] Complications and contraindications are similar to those for retrograde intubation (see Chapter 17). Potential complications are bleeding (subcutaneous and intratracheal), infection, subcutaneous emphysema, pneumomediastinum, pneumothorax, vocal cord damage, and esophageal perforation. These complications are rare, as illustrated by Gold and Buechael's study[102] of 17,500 cases of translaryngeal punctures with an incidence of complications of less than 0.01%.[102] Translaryngeal anesthesia is contraindicated in patients at risk for elevated ICP and IOP; in those with severe cardiac disease, chronic cough, or unstable cervical fracture (unless adequate stabilization has been achieved); and in patients at risk for aspiration of gastric contents.

5. Spray as you go[12,22,80,107]

In addition to using a nebulizer or an atomizer to anesthetize the vocal cords and trachea, a technique

called "spray as you go" via the fiberoptic bronchoscope can be performed. The technique is noninvasive and involves injecting local anesthetics through the suction port of the fiberoptic bronchoscope. Two methods have been described. The *first* requires attaching a triple stopcock (Fig. 9-20) to the proximal portion of the suction port in order to connect oxygen tubing from a regulated oxygen tank set to flow at 2 to 4 L/min. Under direct vision through the bronchoscope, targeted areas are sprayed with aliquots of 0.2 to 1.0 ml of 2% to 4% lidocaine. The physician then waits 30 to 60 seconds before advancing to deeper structures and repeating the maneuver. The flow of oxygen allows for higher Fio_2 delivery; keeps the fiberoptic bronchoscope lens clean; disperses mucous secretions away from the lens, allowing a better view; and aids in nebulizing the local anesthetic. The *second* method involves passing a long angiographic or epidural catheter (internal diameter of 0.5 to 1.0 mm) through the suction port of an adult fiberoptic bronchoscope. The catheter is cut short by 5 mm to prevent obstruction of the fiberoptic lens and allow more accurate placement of the local anesthetic (which flows as a stream instead of dribbling on the field). These techniques are especially useful in patients who are at risk for aspirating gastric contents, since the topical anesthetic is applied only seconds before the intubation is accomplished and allows the patient to maintain his/her airway reflexes as long as possible.

6. Labat technique[108-110]

The Labat technique is an antiquated method of anesthetizing the vocal cords and trachea. This technique requires a laryngeal mirror, a head lamp, and a Labat needle (Fig. 9-21). The patient is placed in the sitting position and asked to open his/her mouth wide. The tongue is pulled outward and an assistant is asked to hold the tongue with a gauze pad. In a right-hand dominant physician the left hand holds the laryngeal mirror over the oropharynx in order to identify the vocal cords. The right hand then holds the Labat needle and syringe (Fig. 9-21) and drips local anesthetic (4 ml of 2% lidocaine) over the vocal cords. We use this technique only to illustrate to our residents that ear, nose, and throat surgeons frequently make claim to an easy *direct* laryngoscopy because they were indeed, able to visualize the vocal cords using this same method. This is misleading, since it doesn't take into account the three-axis alignment required for direct laryngoscopy using a standard anesthesia laryngoscope.

ACKNOWLEDGMENTS

I would like to thank Tay McClellan for her medical illustrations and Kim Bass for her administrative support.

REFERENCES

1. Macewend EM: Clinical observations on the introduction of tracheal tubes by the mouth instead of performing tracheostomy or laryngotomy, *Br Med J* July 24, 1880, p. 122.
2. Thomas JL: Awake intubation: indications, techniques and a review of 25 patients, *Anaesthesia* 24:28, 1969.
3. Ovassapian A, Yelich SJ, Dykes MH et al: Blood pressure and heart rate changes during awake fiberoptic nasotracheal intubation, *Anesth Analg* 62:951, 1983.
4. Dundee JW, Haslett WHK: The benzodiazepines: a review of their actions and uses relative to anesthetic practice, *Br J Anaesth* 42:217, 1970.
5. Sidhu VS, Whitehead EM, Ainsworth QP et al: A technique of awake fibreoptic intubation: experience in patients with cervical spine disease, *Anaesthesia* 48(10):910, 1993.
6. Mongan PD, Culling RD: Rapid oral anesthesia for awake intubation, *J Clin Anesth* 4(2):101, 1992.
7. Meschino A, Devitt JH, Koch P et al: The safety of awake tracheal intubation in cervical spine injury, *Can J Anaesth* 39(2):114, 1992.
8. Ovassapian A, Krejcie TC, Yelich SJ et al: Awake fibreoptic intubation in the patient at high risk of aspiration, *Br J Anaesth* 62(1):13, 1989.
9. Sinclair JR, Mason RA: Ankylosing spondylitis: the case for awake intubation, *Anaesthesia* 39(1):3, 1984.
10. Kopman AF, Wollman SB, Ross K et al: Awake endotracheal intubation: a review of 267 cases, *Anesth Analg* 54(3):323, 1975.
11. Latto IP: *Awake intubation.* First International Symposium on the Difficult Airway, Newport Beach, Calif, Sept 16, 1993.
12. Benumof JL: Management of the difficult airway, *Anesthesiology* 75:1087, 1991.
13. Benumof JL: First International Symposium on the Difficult Airway, Newport Beach, Calif, Sept 16, 1993.
14. Mallampati SR, Gatt SP, Gugino LD et al: A clinical sign to predict difficult tracheal intubation: a prospective study, *Can J Anaesth* 32:429, 1985.
15. Frerk CM: Predicting difficult intubation, *Anaesthesia* 56:1005, 1991.
16. American Society of Anesthesiologists Task Force: Practice guidelines for management of the difficult airway, *Anesthesiology* 78(3):597, 1993.
17. Le P, Ovassapian A, Benumof JL: Survey of university training programs: residency training in Airway Management (unpublished data).
18. Shibutani T, Hirota Y, Niwa H et al: Cerebral arterial blood flow velocity during induction of general anesthesia: rapid intravenous induction versus awake intubation, *Anesth Prog* 40(4):122, 1993.
19. Hawkyard SJ, Morrison A, Doyle LA et al: Attenuating the hypertensive response to laryngoscopy and endotracheal intubation using awake fibreoptic intubation, *Acta Anaesthesiol Scand* 36(1):1, 1992.
20. Sutherland AD, Williams RT: Cardiovascular responses and lidocaine absorption in fiberoptic-assisted awake intubation, *Anesth Analg* 65(4):389, 1986.
21. Gotta AW, Sullivan CA: Superior laryngeal nerve block: an aid to intubating the patient with fractured mandible, *J Trauma* 24(1):83, 1984.
22. Reed AF, Han DG: Preparation of the patient for awake intubation: *Anesthesiol Clin North Am* 9(1):69, 1991.
23. Reed AF: Preparation for awake fiberoptic intubation. *ASA refresher course: workshop on the management of the difficult airway,* Orlando, Fla, Nov 5, 1994.
24. Difficulties in tracheal intubation. In Latto IP, Rosen M, editors: Latto IP: *Management of difficult intubation,* Balliere Tindall, 1984.
25. Miller DM: *Anesthesia,* ed 3, New York, Churchill Livingstone, 1990.
26. Norton ML, Brown ACD: *Atlas of the difficult airway,* St. Louis, 1991, Mosby.
27. Barash PG, Cullen BF, Stoelting RK: *Clinical Anesthesia,* Philadelphia, 1989, Lippincott.
28. Evans BJ, Stanley RO, Burrows GD: Measuring medical students' empathy skills, *Br J Med Psychol* 66:121, 1993.
29. Block MR, Coulehan JL: Teaching the difficult interview in a required course on medical interviewing, *Education* 62(1):35, 1987.
30. Farsad P, Galliguez P, Chamberlin R et al: Teaching interviewing skills to pediatric house officers, *Pediatrics* 61(3):384, 1978.
31. Breytspraak LM, McGee J, Conger JC et al: Sensitizing medical students to impression formation processes in the patient interview, *J Med Educ* 52(1):47, 1977.
32. Smith RC: Teaching interviewing skills to medical students: the issue of "countertransference," *J Med Educ* 59(7):582, 1984.
33. Frumin MJ, Herekar VR, Jarvik ME: Amnestic actions of diazepam and scopolamine in man, *Anesthesiology,* 45:406, 1976.
34. Fragan RJ, Caldwell N: Lorazepam premedication: lack of recall and relief of anxiety, *Anesth Analg* 55:792, 1976.
35. White PF, Shafer A, Boyle WA et al: Benzodiazepine antagonism does not provoke a stress response, *Anesthesiology* 70:636, 1989.
36. Shafer SL, Varvel JR: Pharmacokinetics, pharmacodynamics, and rational opioid selection, *Anesthesiology* 74:53, 1991.
37. Egan TD, Lemmens HJM, Fiset P et al: The pharmacokinetics of the new short-acting opioid Remifentanil in healthy adult male volunteers, *Anesthesiology* 79:881, 1993.
38. White PF, Way WL, Trevor AJ: Ketamine: its pharmacology and therapeutic uses, *Anesthesiology* 56:119, 1982.
39. Tornetta FJ: A comparison of droperidol, diazepam and hydroxyzine hydrochloride as premedication, *Anesth Analg* 56:496, 1977.
40. Eyler SW, Cullen BF, Murphy ME et al: Antacid aspiration in

rabbits: a comparison of mylanta and bicitra, *Anesth Analg* 61:288, 1982.

41. Conklin KA, Ziadlou-Rad F: Buffering capacity of citrate antacids, *Anesthesiology* 58:391, 1983.

42. James CF, Modell JH, Gibbs CP et al: Pulmonary aspiration effects of volume and pH in the rats, *Anesth Analg* 63:665, 1984.

43. Feldman M, Burton ME: Histamine receptor antagonists, *N Engl J Med* 323:1672, 1990.

44. Schulze-Delrieuer RT: Drug therapy: metoclopramide, *N Engl J Med* 305:28, 1981.

45. Mirakhur RK: Anticholinergic drugs and anesthesia, *Can J Anaesth* 35:443, 1988.

46. Mirakhur RA, Clarke RSJ, Dundee JW et al: Anticholinergic drugs in anesthesia: a survey of their present position, *Anesthesia* 33:133, 1978.

47. Gross JB, Hartigan ML, Schaffer DW: A suitable substitute for 4% cocaine before blind nasotracheal intubation: 3% lidocaine–0.25% phenylephrine nasal spray, *Anesth Analg* 63:915, 1984.

48. Tsueda K, Debrand M, Zeok SS et al: Obesity supine death syndrome: reports of two morbidly obese patients, *Anesth Analg* 58:4, 1979.

49. Paul DR, Hoyt JL, Boutros AR: Cardiovascular and respiratory changes in response to change of posture in the very obese, *Anesthesiology* 45:73, 1976.

50. Vaughan RW: *Obesity: implications in anesthetic management and toxicity. ASA Refresher Course in Anesthesiology,* vol 9, Philadelphia, 1981, Lippincott.

51. Slogoff S, Keats AS, David Y et al: Incidence of perioperative myocardial ischemia detected by different electrocardiographic systems, *Anesthesiology* 73:1074, 1990.

52. Bertrand CA, Steiner NV, Jameson AG et al: Disturbances of cardiac rhythm during anesthesia and surgery, *JAMA* 216:1615, 1971.

53. Ramsey M: Blood pressure monitoring: automated oscillometric devices, *J Clin Monit* 7:56, 1991.

54. Barker SJ, Tremper KK: Pulse oximetry: applications and limitations, *Int Anesthesiol Clin* 25:155, 1987.

55. Bhavani-Shanker K, Mosely H, Kumar AY et al: Capnometry and anesthesia, *Can J Anesth* 39:617, 1992.

56. Zupan J: Fiberoptic bronchoscopy in anesthesia and critical care. In Benumof JL, editor: *Clinical procedures in anesthesia,* Philadelphia, 1992, Lippincott.

57. Daos FG, Lopez L et al: Local anesthetic toxicity modified by oxygen and by combination of the agents, *Anesthesiology* 23:755, 1962.

58. Benumof JL, Scheller MS: The importance of transtracheal jet ventilation in the management of the difficult airway, *Anesthesiology* 71:769, 1989.

59. Ravussin P, Bayer-Berger M, Monnier P et al: Percutaneous transtracheal ventilation for laser endoscopic procedures in infants and small children with laryngeal obstruction, *Can J Anaesth* 34(1):83, 1987.

60. Boucek CD, Gunnerson HB, Tullock WC: Percutaneous transtracheal high-frequency jet ventilation as an aid to fiberoptic intubation, *Anesthesiology* 67:247, 1987.

61. Yealy DM, Stewart RD, Kaplan RM: Myths and pitfalls in emergency translaryngeal ventilation: correcting misimpressions, *Ann Emerg Med* 17(7):690, 1984.

62. Adriani J, Zepernick R, Arens J et al: The comparative potency and effectiveness of topical anesthetics in man, *Clin Pharmacol Ther* 5:49, 1964.

63. Perry LB: Topical anesthesia for bronchoscopy, *Chest* 73:691, 1978.

64. Schenck NL: Local anesthesia in otolaryngology, *Ann Otol Rhinol Laryngol* 84:65, 1975.

65. Anderton JM, Nassar WY: Topical cocaine and general anes-thesia: an investigation of the efficacy and side effects of cocaine on the nasal mucosa, *Anaesthesia* 30:809, 1975.

66. Van Dyke C, Barash PG, Jatlow P et al: Cocaine: plasma concentrations after intranasal application in man, *Science* 191:859, 1976.

67. Murphy TM: Somatic blockade of head and neck. In Cousins MJ, Bridenbaugh PO, editors: *Neural blockade in clinical anaesthesia and management of pain,* ed 2, Philadelphia, 1988, Lippincott.

68. Sandza JG, Roberts RW et al: Symptomatic methemoglobinemia with a commonly used topical anesthetic, Cetacaine, *Ann Thorac Surg* 30:187, 1980.

69. Douglas WW, Fairbanks VF: Methemoglobinemia induced by a topical anesthetic spray (Cetacaine), *Chest* 71:587, 1977.

70. Kotler RL, Hansen-Flaschen J et al: Severe methemoglobinemia after flexible fibre optic broncoscopy, *Thorax* 44:234, 1989.

71. Rosenberg PH, Heinonen J et al: Lidocaine concentration in blood after topical anesthesia of the upper respiratory tract, *Acta Anesthesiol Scand* 24:125, 1980.

72. Weisel W, Anthony Tella R: Reaction to tetracaine used as topical anesthetic in broncoscopy, *JAMA* 147:218, 1951.

73. Adriani J, Campbell D: Fatalities following topical application of local anesthetic to the mucous membrane, *JAMA* 162:1527, 1956.

74. Bourke DL, Katz J, Tonneson A: Nebulized anesthesia for awake endotracheal intubation, *Anesthesiology* 63:690, 1985.

75. Raj PP: *Handbook of regional anesthesia,* New York, 1985, Churchill Livingstone.

76. Roberts JT: Anatomy and patient positioning for fiberoptic laryngoscopy, *Anesthesiol Clin North Am* 9(1):53, 1991.

77. Katz J: *Atlas of regional anesthesia,* ed 2, New York, 1994, Appleton & Lange.

78. Adriani J: *Nerve blocks: a manual of regional anesthesia for practioners of medicine,* Springfield, Ill, 1954, Charles C Thomas.

79. Boudreaux AM: Simple technique for fiberoptic bronchoscopy, *Am Soc Crit Care Anesthesiologist* 6(3):8, 1994.

80. Ovassapian A: *Fiberoptic airway endoscopy in anesthesia and critical care,* New York, 1990, Raven.

81. Reed AP: Preparation of the patient for awake flexible fiberoptic bronchoscopy, *Chest* 101:244, 1992.

82. Clemente CD: *Gray's Anatomy,* ed 13, Philadelphia, 1985, Lea & Febiger.

83. Cooper M, Watson RL: An improved regional anesthetic technique for peroral endoscopy, *Anesthesiology* 43:372, 1975.

84. Kazuhisa K, Norimasa S, Takanori M et al: Glossopharyngeal nerve block for carotid sinus syndrome, *Anesth Analg* 75:1036, 1992.

85. Platzer W: *Atlas of topographical anatomy,* Stuttgart, 1985, George Thieme Verlas.

86. Bedder MD, Lindsay D: Glossopharyngeal nerve block using ultrasound guidance: a case report of a new technique, *Reg Anesth* 14(6):304, 1989.

87. Rovenstein EA, Papper EM: Glossopharyngeal nerve block, *Am J Surg* 75:713, 1948.

88. Demeester TR, Skinner DB et al: Local nerve block anesthesia for peroral endoscopy, *Ann Thorac Surg* 24:278, 1977.

89. Snell RS, Katz J: *Clinical anatomy for anesthesiologists,* New York, 1989, Appleton & Lange.

90. Wildsmith JAW, Armitage EN: *Principles and practices of regional anaesthesia,* New York, 1987, Churchill Livingstone.

91. Byron J, Bailey J: Head and neck surgery–otolaryngology: Philadelphia, 1993, Lippincott.

92. Prakash UB: *Bronchoscopy: A text atlas,* New York, 1994, Raven.

93. Finucane TF, Santora HS: *Principles of airway management,* Philadelphia, 1988, Davis.

94. Paparella MM, Shumrick DA, Gluckman JL, editors: *Otolaryngology,* Philadelphia, 1991, WB Saunders.

95. Hunt LA, Boyd GL: Superior laryngeal nerve block as a

supplement to total intravenous anesthesia for rigid laser bronchoscopy in a patient with myasthenic syndrome, *Anesth Analg* 75(3):458, 1992.

96. Wiles JR, Kelly J, Mostafa SM: Hypotension and bradycardia following superior laryngeal nerveblock, *Br J Anaesth* 63(1):125, 1989.

97. Gotta AW, Sullivan CA: Anaesthesia of the upper airway using topical anaesthetic and superior laryngeal nerve block, *Br J Anaesth* 53(10):1055, 1981.

98. Gotta AW, Sullivan CA: Anaesthesia of the upper airway using topical anaesthetic and superior laryngeal nerve block, *Br J Anaesth* 53:1055, 1981.

99. Hast Malcolm: Otolaryngology. In English GM, editor: *Anatomy of the larynx,* vol 3(14), Philadelphia, 1987, Harper & Row.

100. Bonica JJ: Transtracheal anesthesia for endotracheal intubation, *Anesthesiology* 10:736, 1949.

101. Walts LF, Kassity KJ: Spread of local anesthesia after upper airway block, *Arch Otolaryngol* 81:77, 1965.

102. Gold MI, Buechael DR: Translaryngeal anesthesia: a review, *Anesthesiology* 20:181, 1959.

103. Boster SR, Danzl DF, Madden RJ et al: Translaryngeal absorption of lidocaine, *Ann Emerg Med* 11(9):461, 1982.

104. Viegas O, Stoelting RK: Lidocaine in arterial blood after laryngotracheal administration, *Anesthesiology* 43:491, 1975.

105. Chu SS, Rah KH, Brannan MD et al: Plasma concentration of lidocaine after endotracheal spray, *Anesth Analg* 54:438, 1975.

106. Hamill JF, Bedford RF et al: Lidocaine before endotracheal intubation: intravenous or laryngotracheal? *Anesthesiology* 5:578, 1981.

107. Hill AJ, Feneck RO et al: The hemodynamic effects of bronchoscopy: Comparison of propofol and thiopentone with and without alfentanil pretreatment, *Anaesthesia* 46:266, 1991.

108. Weisel W, Tella RA: Reaction to tetracaine used as topical anesthetic in bronchoscopy a study of 1000 cases, *JAMA* 147:218, 1951.

109. Snow JC: *Anesthesia in otolaryngology and opthalmology,* London, 1982, Prentice-Hall International.

110. Eriksson E: *Illustrated handbook in local anaesthesia,* London, 1979, Lloyd Luke.

SUGGESTED READINGS

Adriani J: *Labat's regional anesthesia,* ed 4, St Louis, 1985, Warren HJ Green.

Benumof JL: Clinical considerations IV: airway management. *Annual anesthesiology refresher course (UCSD),* San Diego, Calif, May 19, 1989.

Efthimiou J, Higenbottam T et al: Plasma concentration of lignocaine during fibre optic broncoscopy, *Thorax* 37:68, 1982.

McClure JM, Brown DT, Wildsmith JAW: Comparison of IV administration of midazolam and diazepam as sedation during spinal anesthesia, *Br J Anaesth* 55:1089, 1983.

Sanchez AS: *The retrograde cookbook: First International Symposium on the Difficult Airway,* Newport Beach, Calif, Sept 17, 1993.

Stoelting RK: Circulatory response to laryngoscopy and tracheal intubation with or without prior oropharyngeal viscous lidocaine, *Anesth Analg* 56:618, 1977.

Chapter 10

ASPIRATION PREVENTION, PROPHYLAXIS, AND TREATMENT

Mark D. Tasch
Robert K. Stoelting

The pulmonary aspiration of gastric contents, while fortunately an uncommon event, has inspired a great deal of research and recrimination in the anesthesia literature. Aspiration pneumonitis is an anesthetic complication whose consequences can be formidable, whose treatment is essentially nonspecific and supportive, and whose prevention seems, at least from outside the operating room, to be so imminently attainable. Our preoccupation with minimizing gastric contents before anesthetic induction has led to rituals of *nil per os* (NPO), which have recently been challenged with respect to fluids. [1] On the other hand, to observe or to read a description of even one case of aspiration and its dire sequelae may inspire enthusiastic and rigid adherence to conservative NPO standards.

I. PERIOPERATIVE ASPIRATION

A. INCIDENCE

The statistical risk of suffering a perioperative aspiration has been examined in long-term prospective and retrospective case reviews. Others have attempted to determine the incidence of silent aspiration, with or without clinical consequences. LoCicero[2] wrote that "between 16 and 27 percent of all anesthetized patients will have silent aspiration to some extent," often the result of either gastric inflation during ventilation by mask before tracheal intubation or manipulation of the intestines during abdominal surgery. On the other hand, Hardy et al.[3] looked for gastroesophageal reflux (GER) by means of visual inspection of the pharynx and continuous measurement of upper esophageal pH, and found no cases of GER during anesthetic induction in 100 patients.

A multicenter, prospective study of nearly 200,000 operations in France from 1978 to 1982 found the overall incidence of clinically apparent aspiration to be 1.4 per 10,000 anesthetics. In this report, 14 of the 27 aspirations occurred postoperatively.[4] Leigh and Tytler's five-year survey of nearly 110,000 anesthetics found six cases of aspiration requiring unplanned critical care, three of which occurred postoperatively.[45] Warner et al.,[6] retrospectively reviewing over 215,000 general anesthetics from 1985 to 1991, found an incidence of aspiration of 3.1 per 10,000 cases. Olsson et al.,[7] examined the computer-based records of the nearly 177,000 anesthetics administered at the Karolinska Hospital over 13 years and noted an incidence of aspiration of 4.7 per 10,000. Kallar and Everett's multicenter survey[4] of more than 500,000 outpatient anesthetics during 1985 found the incidence of aspiration to be 1.7 per 10,000.

B. RISK FACTORS

These large-scale surveys of anesthetics have found some patient characteristics to cluster around cases of aspiration. Warner et al.[6] noted that the relative risk of aspiration was more than four times as high for emergency as for elective surgery. Higher American Society of Anesthesiologists (ASA) physical status classification was also associated with a higher risk of aspiration. The incidence of aspiration ranged from 1.1 per 10,000 elective anesthetics in ASA group I patients to 29.2 per 10,000 emergency anesthetics in ASA groups IV and V patients. Contrary to conventional wisdom, "[a]ge, gender, pregnancy, . . . concurrent administration of opioids, obesity, . . . experience . . . of anesthesia provider, and types of surgical procedure were not independent risk factors for pulmonary aspiration. . . . The most common predisposing condition in all patients was gastrointestinal obstruction." One third of aspirations occurred during laryngoscopy, but 36% arose at extubation.[6]

Olsson et al.,[7] found that children and the elderly were more likely than others to aspirate perioperatively. Statistically, the risk of aspiration was more than three times as high in emergency surgery as it was in elective operations. The incidence of aspiration was increased more than sixfold when surgery was performed at night rather than during daylight hours. About one half of these aspirations occurred during induction of anesthesia, one eighth intraoperatively, and one fifth during emergence from anesthesia. In accordance with clinical intuition, the authors concluded that "[e]mergency cases

---

BOX 10-1   Risk factors for aspiration of gastric contents

Regurgitation or vomiting
   Hypotension in awake patient
   Opioids in awake patient
   Increased intragastric volume & pressure
   Decreased lower esophageal barrier pressure
Incompetent laryngeal protective reflexes
   Neurologic disease
   Neuromuscular disease
   Central nervous system depressants
   Advanced age or debility

---

anaesthetised in the middle of the night by an inexperienced anaesthetist constitute a high risk group for aspiration."[7]

In Kallar and Everett's outpatient survey,[4] aspiration occurred most frequently in patients less than 10 years of age. "In patients with no other identifiable risk factors, 67% of aspirations occurred after difficulties in airway management or intubation."[4] In the study of Olsson et al.,[7] 15 of 83 aspirations were suffered by patients with no known risk factors. In 10 (67%) of these 15 cases, aspiration accompanied airway problems. No patient aspirated while intubated.[7] Although regional techniques are often favored for the patient at increased risk of aspiration, elderly patients, in particular, have been reported to vomit and aspirate with serious consequences during subarachnoid anesthesia. Hypotension resulting from neuraxial sympathectomy can induce nausea and vomiting, while supplemental analgesics and sedatives given during lengthy operations can seriously obtund protective airway reflexes.[2,7,8]

Patients likely to have gastric contents of increased volume or acidity, elevated intragastric pressure, or decreased tone of the lower esophageal sphincter (LES) are traditionally considered to be at increased risk of perioperative pulmonary aspiration[1,3] (Boxes 10-1 and 10-2). As will be discussed later, pregnancy combines several of these likely risk factors. Although a lengthy NPO period before elective surgery is intended to minimize the volume of gastric contents, up to 90% of fasted patients will have a gastric fluid pH of less than 2.5.[9] Recent ethanol ingestion or hypoglycemic episodes stimulate gastric acid secretion, while tobacco inhalation temporarily lowers LES tone. None of these effects are chronic.[3,9] LES tone has also been found to be reduced by gastric fluid acidity, caffeine, chocolate, and fatty foods.[9,11]

The obese patient is considered at relatively high risk for aspiration due to increases in gastric fluid volume and acidity, intragastric pressure, and the incidence of GER.[12] Patients with connective tissue, neurologic, or

---

BOX 10-2   Factors that increase intragastric volume and pressure

Increased gastric filling
   Air inflation during mask ventilation
   Increased gastric acid production
      Gastrin
      Histamine-$_2$ receptor stimulation
      Recent ethanol ingestion
      Recent hypoglycemic episode
Decreased gastric emptying
   Intestinal obstruction
   Diabetic gastroparesis
   Opioids
   Anticholinergics
   Sympathetic stimulation (pain and anxiety)

BOX 10-3   Pathophysiology of aspiration

Particulate aspiration
   Airway obstruction
   Granulomatous inflammation
Acid aspiration
   Neutrophilic inflammation
   Hemorrhagic pulmonary edema
   Destruction of airway epithelium
   Loss of type I alveolar cells
      Loss of surfactant
         Alveolar instability and collapse
   Disruption of alveolar-capillary membrane
      Plasma leakage from pulmonary capillaries
         Noncardiogenic pulmonary edema
         Hypovolemia

---

neuromuscular diseases may be imperiled by esophageal dysfunction or laryngeal incompetence. Scleroderma and myotonia dystrophica have been specifically mentioned in case reports.[13,15] Diabetic gastroparesis impairs gastric emptying and may also compromise LES function.[10] Advanced age may be associated with attenuated cough or gag reflexes. The presence of a nasogastric tube, while allowing gastric decompression, may also hold open the LES.[9,14] Outpatients have traditionally been thought to present for surgery with gastric contents of expanded volume and reduced pH, possibly due to preoperative anxiety in the absence of premedication. However, clinical studies have failed to consistently confirm this expectation.[4] Furthermore, Hardy et al.[3] contradicted several conventional notions by finding that gastric content volume or pH did not correlate with preoperative anxiety, body mass index, ethanol or tobacco intake, or reflux history.

When aspiration does occur, the subsequent clinical course can range from the benign to the fatal. In the report of Olsson et al.,[7] 18% of patients who aspirated perioperatively required mechanical ventilatory support and 5% died. All those who died of aspiration were noted to have a poor preoperative physical status. Warner et al.[6] reported that 64% of patients did not manifest coughing, wheezing, radiographic abnormalities, or a 10% decrease in arterial oxygen saturation from preoperative room air values during the first two hours after aspiration. These patients who remained asymptomatic for two hours did not develop any respiratory sequelae. Of those patients who did manifest signs or symptoms of pulmonary aspiration within two hours of the event, 54% required mechanical ventilatory support for at least six hours and 25% were ventilated for at least 24 hours. Half of those ventilated for at least 24 hours died, an overall mortality rate of under 5% of all aspirations.

Mortality rates resulting from perioperative pulmonary aspiration have ranged from less than 5% to greater than 80% in different reports. In the studies of Warner et al.[6] and Olsson et al.[6] there were no deaths in healthy patients undergoing elective surgery.[1,9,16] Hickling and Howard[16] retrospectively studied patients in New Zealand from 1982 to 1986 who required mechanical ventilation for aspiration pneumonitis. Of 38 such patients, three (8%) died of ventilatory failure or myocardial infarction.[16] Even in Mendelson's seminal report[17] of peripartum aspiration in 1946, all patients who were not promptly asphyxiated by solid material survived, and "recovery was usually complete with an afebrile and uncomplicated course." In general, most healthy patients who aspirate only gastric fluid can expect to survive without residual respiratory impairment, although sometimes after a stormy postoperative course. On the other hand, as Gardner[18] wrote in 1958, "[a]spiration of vomit is . . . often . . . the *coup de grace* in an ill patient who might otherwise have a chance of survival."

C. PATHOPHYSIOLOGY

When gastric contents enter the lungs, the resultant pulmonary pathology depends on the nature of the material aspirated (Box 10-3). Food particles small enough to enter the distal airways induce a foreign body reaction characterized by peribronchial mononuclear cell inflammation and eventual granuloma formation. The aspiration of particulate antacids produces the same response.[19,21] Acid aspiration induces a neutrophilic inflammatory response that begins within minutes and progressively develops over 24 to 36 hours.[19,22] In 1940, Irons and Apfelbach[23] wrote that the "characteristic microscopic changes are intense engorgement of the alveolar capillaries with erythrocytes, edema and hemorrhage into the alveolar spaces. . . . Another outstanding characteristic is the extensive desquamation of the lining of the bronchial tree with aspiration of the desquamated cells into the alveolar spaces." Subsequent authors have described similar findings, noting hemorrhagic pulmonary edema, intense inflammation, and derangement of the pulmonary epithelium.[11,22,24] The membranous (type I) epithelial cells that produce surfactant are damaged or destroyed by the acid, to be replaced by granular (type II) epithelial cells.[2] As surfactant production fails, lung units progressively collapse. Fibrin and plasma leak from the capillaries into the pulmonary interstitium and alveoli, producing the noncardiogenic pulmonary edema often referred to as the *adult respiratory distress syndrome* (ARDS).[2,12,22,25,26] Although most researchers have found that localized acid exposure leads to localized pathology, one animal study demonstrated that localized aspiration produced generalized pulmonary inflammation, presumably due to "inflammatory mediators" acting at sites distant from the original insult.[16] With effective supportive care, the acute inflammation can diminish, and epithelial regeneration begin, within 72 hours.[11]

The clinical features of aspiration pneumonitis have been well described for a half-century. Even before then, in 1887, Becker referred to bronchopneumonia as a postoperative complication due to the inhalation of gastric contents.[23] Hall, in 1940, published the first description of gastric fluid inhalation in obstetric patients. He distinguished between the aspiration of solid material, which could quickly produce death by suffocation, and the aspiration syndrome produced by gastric fluid, for which he coined the term "chemical pneumonitis."[27] Mendelson,[17] in 1946, described the clinical features of 66 cases of peripartum aspiration observed from 1932 to 1945. Solid food produced airway obstruction, which was quickly fatal in two instances. Otherwise, wheezing, rales, rhonchi, tachypnea, and tachycardia were prominent. Subsequent reports have not found wheezing to be so universal a manifestation, occurring in about one third of aspirations. When present, wheezing is thought to result from bronchial mucosal edema and from a reflex response to acidic airway irritation.[9,22,28]

Refractory hypoxemia can occur almost immediately after pulmonary aspiration of gastric contents as bronchospasm, airway edema, or obstruction, and alveolar collapse or flooding increase the effective intrapulmonary shunt fraction (Box 10-4). The awake patient may experience intense dyspnea and cough up the pink, frothy sputum characteristic of pulmonary edema.[9,21,22] On the other hand, more modest aspirations may not become clinically evident until several hours after the episode.[11,20,21,29]

Hemodynamic derangements can also demand therapeutic attention. As the alveolar-capillary membrane loses its integrity, plasma leaks out of the pulmonary

---

BOX 10-4 Aspiration and hypoxemia

Upper airway obstruction
Increased lower airway resistance
  Obstruction by airway debris
  Airway edema
  Reflex bronchospasm
Alveolar collapse and flooding

---

vasculature. If the leak becomes a flood, the loss of circulating fluid volume can produce hemoconcentration, hypotension, tachycardia, and even shock.[9,11,21] Pulmonary vasospasm may also contribute to right ventricular dysfunction.[9]

The radiographic evidence of pulmonary aspiration may become evident promptly, if aspiration is massive, or only after a delay of several hours. There is no pattern on the chest roentgenogram that is specific for aspiration. The distribution of infiltrates depends on the volume of material inhaled and on the patient's position at the time of the event. Due to bronchial anatomy, aspiration occurring in the supine patient affects the right lower lobe most commonly, the left upper lobe least often.[9,21] If pulmonary aspiration is not complicated by secondary events, improvement in symptomatology can be anticipated within 24 hours, but the radiographic picture may continue to worsen for another day.[11,21]

D. DETERMINANTS OF MORBIDITY

1. pH and volume of aspirated fluid

In his 1946 report of peripartum aspiration pneumonitis, Mendelson[17] also undertook to determine the relationship between gastric fluid acidity and pulmonary morbidity. When Mendelson instilled liquid containing hydrochloric acid (HCl) into the tracheae of rabbits, the animals were seen to develop a syndrome "similar in many respects to that observed in the human following liquid aspiration," with cyanosis, dyspnea, and pink frothy sputum. On the other hand, when neutral liquid was instilled into their tracheas, the rabbits endured a brief symptomatic period, "but within a few hours they [were] apparently back to normal, able to carry on rabbit activities uninhibited."[17] (Mendelson maintained a discreet silence as to the nature of these uninhibited rabbit activities.)

Since Mendelson's report, numerous attempts (and assumptions) have been made to define a "critical" volume and pH of gastric contents necessary to inflict significant damage on the lungs. Such neatly defined threshold values may be illusory objects of desire, rather than features of clinical reality. Nonetheless, almost all researchers in the field of aspiration pneumonitis have made some use of such "critical values" to define the success or failure of drug therapies in the modification of gastric contents.

Teabeaut[30] injected HCI solutions of different volumes and acidities into rabbits' tracheae. He found that solutions with a pH greater than 2.4 caused a relatively benign tissue response similar to that induced by the intratracheal injection of water. As the pH of the injectate was reduced from 2.4 to 1.5, a progressively more severe tissue reaction was elicited. At pH 1.5, the damage was maximal and was thus not more intense at lower pH values. From this 1952 study stemmed the popular concept of pH less than or equal to 2.5 as a threshold for chemical pneumonitis. Other authors have advocated a higher standard, a pH of 3.5, for defining hazardous gastric content acidity. However, arguments for a "critical pH" value higher than 2.5 are generally based on case reports of severe pneumonitis caused by the aspiration of *particulate* gastric contents at higher pH values.[31]

The determination of a "critical volume" of gastric contents required to produce severe aspiration pneumonitis has been even more contentious than that of a "critical pH." Two teams of investigators each found that, in dogs, pulmonary injury became independent of pH as the volume of aspirate was increased from 0.5 to 4.0 ml/kg.[9] A preliminary experiment by Roberts and Shirley, involving gastric fluid instillation into the right mainstem bronchus of a single monkey, led to the acceptance, in some quarters, of 0.4 ml/kg as the volume of gastric fluid which placed the subject "at risk" of developing aspiration pneumonitis.[32,33,34] Subsequent researchers have challenged this number. James et al.[35] demonstrated that aspirate volumes as low as 0.2 ml/kg could induce pulmonary injury if the aspirate pH was reduced to 1.0.[9] On the other hand, Raidoo et al.,[32] studying monkeys, found that the aspiration of 0.4 or 0.6 ml/kg of fluid with a pH of 1.0 produced mild or moderate pulmonary injury, while 0.8 or 1.0 ml/kg at pH 1.0 produced severe pneumonitis, with a 50% mortality rate (3 of 6) at 1.0 ml/kg. Clearly, the volume of aspirate that is considered hazardous depends on how much morbidity or pathology must be produced to be considered significant. Arguments have also been made concerning the experimental instillation of gastric fluid into one lung versus both lungs, as well as the reliability of gastric fluid volume measurements. In addition, even if a "critical volume" for aspiration pneumonitis could be reliably determined, it cannot be known how much fluid must be present in the stomach in order to deposit this "critical volume" into the lung(s).[32,36] However, studies of therapeutic interventions require criteria for success or failure, so threshold values for gastric fluid volume and pH will doubtless continue to be used, regardless of their validity.

2. Particulate matter

Volume and acidity are not, of course, the only determinants of morbidity or mortality when gastric contents enter the lungs. Since the report of Bond et al.[37] in 1979, it has been appreciated that gastric fluid containing particulate antacids can produce severe aspiration pneumonitis, even at near-neutral pH, with wheezing, pulmonary edema, and hypoxemia requiring mechanical ventilatory support. Canine studies have confirmed that acidic gastric contents and particulate antacid solutions carry an equivalent potential for morbidity if aspirated.[20] While blood and digestive enzymes do not appear to induce chemical pneumonitis, feculent gastric contents with a high bacterial density readily produce pneumonitis and death in animals regardless of pH. (Acidic gastric contents are normally sterile.) Another study demonstrated that the mucus present in the gastric fluid of dogs with intestinal obstruction produced diffuse small airway obstruction and pulmonary injury when aspirated.[9]

The clinical challenges of perioperative pulmonary aspiration are prevention, prophylaxis, and treatment. Ideally, gastric contents can be physically prevented from entering the lungs in the first place. Should prevention fail, pharmacologic prophylaxis may modify the volume and character of gastric contents so that they inflict minimal damage on the lungs. Least desirably, aspiration pneumonitis can require intensive medical treatment and ventilatory support.

II. PREVENTION OF ASPIRATION

The nonpharmacologic means of keeping gastric contents out of the lungs are preoperative fasting, gastric decompression, and optimal airway management.

A. PREOPERATIVE FASTING

The commonest first step in keeping gastric contents out of the lungs is to minimize the volume of such contents by means of preoperative fasting. In recent years both the utility and the necessity of adhering to conventional NPO regimens for clear liquids have been challenged. The issue has been studied in both pediatric and adult surgical patients and has become particularly contentious and emotional regarding obstetric anesthesia.

Conventional preoperative fasting can impose notable physical and emotional discomfort on children and their parents and may be difficult to reliably enforce in outpatients. Dehydration in infants and hypoglycemia in neonates may also result from prolonged NPO times.[1,4] The normal stomach, unimpeded by medication or pathology, can empty 80% of a clear liquid load within an hour of ingestion. While the stomach continues to secrete and reabsorb fluid throughout NPO time, ingested clear liquids are completely passed into the duodenum within 2.25 hours.[38] Several researchers have therefore sought to demonstrate that children may safely be allowed to drink clear liquids until just 2 to 3 hours before elective surgery.

Van der Walt et al. and other groups determined that healthy infants could drink limited volumes of clear liquids 3 to 4 hours before surgery without increasing their gastric content volume.[39] Splinter et al.[40] found that healthy infants could drink clear liquids *ad libitem* until 2 hours before anesthetic induction without altering gastric fluid volume or pH. (Gastric fluid pH was quite variable, and mean pH was less than 2.5 in all patient groups studied, regardless of NPO time.) On the other hand, milk or formula intake on the morning of surgery (4 to 6 hours preinduction) was associated with the presence of curds in many of the gastric aspirates. This was considered to represent an unacceptable risk of particulate aspiration. The authors thus concurred with previous recommendations that infants not be allowed milk or formula the morning of surgery.[40]

Schreiner et al.[41] compared the gastric contents of children subjected to conventional preoperative fasting (mean NPO time, 13.5 hours) with those permitted clear liquids until 2 hours before anesthetic induction (mean NPO time, 2.6 hours). Gastric fluid volumes actually tended to be somewhat smaller in the children allowed to drink clear liquids up to 2 hours preoperatively, and almost all children in both groups had gastric content pH values less than or equal to 2.5. The authors concluded that allowing children clear fluids until 2 hours before surgery did not increase the risk of gastric acid aspiration.[41]

Sandhar et al.,[38] studying children 1 to 14 years of age, also found that clear liquid ingestion 2 to 3 hours preoperatively did not significantly increase the mean volume of gastric contents and did not increase the number of patients with gastric contents greater than 0.4 ml/kg. In adolescents, it was also shown that unlimited fluid ingestion until 3 hours before surgery decreased thirst and did not affect gastric contents.[42] Clear liquids, alone, thus appear to pose no demonstrable hazard if taken at least 2 hours before anesthesia by children without gastrointestinal pathology. However, solid or semisolid foods are not cleared from the stomach as rapidly as are clear liquids. Meakin et al.[43] found that a light breakfast of biscuits or orange juice with pulp, taken 2 to 4 hours before induction, did increase the volume of gastric aspirate in healthy children, compared with those who had fasted for at least 4 hours. In all fasted children, and in almost all of those fed, the gastric content pH was less than or equal to 2.5.[43] Hyperosmolar glucose solutions are also associated with delayed gastric emptying.[38]

NPO times are not a reliable indicator of gastric emptying in children who have been injured. Significant trauma is generally considered to effectively terminate gastric emptying; thus the time from last food intake to injury probably represents the actual time during which gastric contents pass into the duodenum. Bricker et al.,[44] studying 110 children (ages 1 to 14 years) undergoing surgery for trauma, found that the volume of gastric aspirate was greater in those in whom the injury occurred within 2 hours of eating than in those whose NPO time before injury was greater than 2 hours. Gastric pH did not differ significantly between these two groups. Gastric content volumes were also higher in children suffering moderate or severe injury than in those with minor injuries. Contrary to other findings in adults, there was no association in this study between opioid administration and the volume of gastric contents. Of note regarding the times at which aspiration may occur, 23 of the children vomited on emergence from anesthesia, none during induction.[44]

In adult surgical patients, too, considerable evidence is accumulating that clear liquid intake within 2 to 3 hours of anesthetic induction does not increase the risk of gastric acid aspiration. It is important to note that these studies typically involve healthy, nonpregnant, nonobese patients, free of known gastrointestinal pathology, not receiving opioids or other medications known to interfere with gastric emptying, undergoing elective surgery. The results of such studies cannot, therefore, be reliably applied to any patient groups thus excluded.[42,45,46]

With adults, as with children, the basic arguments favoring relaxed NPO regimens for clear liquids involve their rapid gastric clearance in the normal state. Over 90% of a 750-ml bolus of isotonic saline has been found to pass from the normal stomach within 30 minutes.[47] After 2 hours of fasting, the fluid in the stomach primarily represents the acid secreted by the stomach, itself. Exogenous clear liquids thus tend to dilute endogenous gastric acid and may even accelerate gastric emptying.[36,41,42] Solids, lipids, and hyperosmotic liquids are thought to delay gastric emptying, and their intake would thus be considered ill-advised on the day of surgery.[36]

Several researchers have sought to determine whether these theoretic considerations translate into clinical reality. Lewis et al.[48] divided healthy adult inpatients scheduled for elective surgery into three groups: those allowed clear liquids less than 5 hours before surgery, those allowed clear liquids until 5 to 8 hours before surgery, and those made NPO after the previous midnight. (Clear liquids included jello and coffee or tea with or without cream or sugar.) Neither gastric pH nor gastric volume differed significantly among these groups, but both values varied widely within each group.[48] Read and Vaughan[49] similarly found that permitting patients to drink water *ad libitem* until 2 hours before surgery had no impact on gastric volume or pH but did decrease preanesthetic anxiety. Many patients had gastric pH values less than or equal to 2.5, regardless of the time elapsed since fluid intake.[49] Phillips et al.[42] also determined that patients allowed to drink clear liquids until 2 hours preoperatively had gastric volume and pH values similar to those fasted for 6 hours.

Maltby et al.[47] studied outpatients who were either kept NPO from the previous midnight or given 150 ml of water 2.5 hours before anesthetic induction. While the mean gastric pH did not differ significantly between the two groups, the mean gastric volume was significantly *less* in the patients who drank than in those who fasted.[47] Other studies have also confirmed that the ingestion of 150 ml of orange juice, coffee, tea, or apple juice 2 to 3 hours before surgery has no detrimental effect on gastric pH or volume in surgical outpatients.[42]

The safety of clear liquid ingestion before surgery does not, of course, imply that solid food may also be taken with impunity. Miller et al.[46] compared 22 adults kept NPO overnight before surgery with 23 adults permitted a "light breakfast" (one slice of buttered toast and tea or coffee with milk) the morning of surgery (mean NPO time, 3.8 hours). The two groups were found not to differ significantly in the mean volume or median pH of their gastric contents, or in the percentage of patients with a gastric pH of less than 3.0. Interestingly, though, in those patients who were not given an opioid premedication, 7 of 8 "fed" patients had a gastric pH of less than 3.0 (median pH, 1.9), while only 2 of 5 fasted patients had a gastric pH of less than 3.0 (median pH, 6.3). In addition, the authors remarked that "[i]t is likely that any large pieces of toast in the stomach would not be aspirated by the tube we used. Thus, the results of the study apply only to liquid in the stomach."[46]

In the past few years, strenuous debate has arisen over the necessity of adhering to conventional NPO regimens for patients in labor. Obstetricians, nurse-midwifes, and psychologists have joined the fray. On the one hand, anesthesiologists have long recognized that advanced gestation increases the risk of gastric content aspiration. The enlarging uterus increases intragastric pressure by compressing the stomach, physically delays gastric emptying by pushing the pylorus cephalad and posteriorly, and promotes GER by altering the angle of the gastroesophageal junction. Progesterone decreases the tone of the LES, while excess gastrin, produced by the placenta, promotes gastric acid secretion.[10,12,21] The alterations in physique typical of late pregnancy can interfere with laryngoscopy and tracheal intubation. Laryngeal and upper airway edema are also common in the parturient, and can be exaggerated by preeclampsia.[50] On the other hand, arguments in favor of liberalizing oral intake for parturients include the infrequency of aspiration pneumonitis in modern prac-

tice, the futility of fasting in ensuring an empty stomach, and detrimental effects of fasting on maternal and fetal well-being. The fashionable pennant of "patient autonomy" has also been raised over this battlefield.

Elkington[51] cited a Washington state survey (1977-1981) in which none of 36 maternal deaths resulted from anesthetic complications and a North Carolina survey (1981-1985) in which only 1 of 40 maternal deaths resulted from aspiration. He did not advocate uninhibited feeding of patients in labor, however, but recommended that "[f]or otherwise uncomplicated parturients, a nonparticulate diet should be allowed as desired," and that "for patients who are not candidates for regional anesthesia . . . intake should be limited to that required for oral comfort, with intravenous fluids after labor is established."[46] This distinction fails, of course, to take into account the patient who may well be a candidate for regional anesthesia, but who nonetheless comes to require a general anesthetic for an emergency cesarean section.

Ludka and Roberts[52] referred to a Michigan survey (1972 to 1984), showing that only 1 of 15 maternal deaths (0.82 per 100,000 live births) resulted from the aspiration of gastric contents, that no deaths were related to regional anesthesia, and that "failure to secure a patent airway was the primary cause of anesthesia-related maternal deaths." They cited other studies indicating that women who ate during labor were less ketotic, required less analgesic medication and oxytocin, and had more active fetuses and neonates with higher Apgar scores than did women who fasted during labor. They also "found that laboring women self-regulated intake. Once active labor began, women usually preferred liquids."[52]

Regarding the inevitability of a full stomach in the parturient, Kallar and Everett[4] referred to an ultrasound study in which nearly two thirds of patients in labor had solid food in the stomach, regardless of how long they had fasted. Elkington[51] cited a report that about one fourth of parturients were "at risk" of aspiration pneumonitis, regardless of the duration of fasting, and that prolonged fasting was actually associated with increased gastric fluid volume at a lower pH. Broach and Newton[53] contended that "[a]dministration of narcotics, not labor itself, appears to be the major factor in delaying stomach emptying."

McKay and Mahan[54] wrote that "[c]oncern about the incidence of maternal aspiration and its effect upon maternal morbidity and mortality has resulted in restricting oral intake of laboring women, although data show maternal death to be rare. Among many factors that can be linked to the occurrence of aspiration, the most important appears to be faulty administration of obstetric anesthesia." The authors further questioned "whether parturients should be kept from eating and drinking or on restricted liquid intake to protect them from what appears to be the basic problem: inadequate anesthesia practices."[54] The apparent implication is that the parturient should eat, drink, and be merry, for if she aspirates, only poor anesthetic care is to blame.

On the other hand, Chestnut and Cohen[55] cited the *Report on Confidential Enquiries into Maternal Deaths in England and Wales* (1982 to 1984), which found that 7 of 19 anesthesia-associated maternal deaths resulted from the aspiration of gastric contents into the lungs, and an ASA review of closed malpractice claims in which "maternal aspiration was the primary reason for 8% of all claims against anesthesiologists for obstetric cases." The authors argued that "[t]hese data hardly suggest that the risk of maternal aspiration is remote" and noted that "[u]nfortunately, there are few data regarding maternal *morbidity* from aspiration."[55]

In his reply to McKay and Mahan, Crawford[56] noted that "[m]ost of the deaths from aspiration prior to the mid-1950s . . . were due to asphyxia, caused by respiratory obstruction with solid or semisolid material—since that time, with introduction of a firm dietary regimen for labor, only 2 of the 146 deaths noted have been in that category." Furthermore, he contended, "There is inevitably an incidence of cesarean section and of general anesthesia in every obstetric population. . . . In an obstetric population the incidence of failed or difficult intubation is roughly one in 300."[56]

Obviously, the pregnant patient with a difficult airway cannot always be avoided, nor can general anesthesia for cesarean section, no matter how aggressively regional analgesia is promoted. Regardless of gastric fluid volume or acidity, the presence of solid food imparts the immediate hazard of asphyxiation. Mendelson,[17] himself, warned that "[m]isinformed friends and relatives often urge the patient to ingest a heavy meal early in labor before going to the hospital" and encouraged "competent administration of general anesthesia with full appreciation of the dangers of aspiration during induction and recovery." Crawford[56] concluded that "[g]rafting good anesthetic technique upon poor preparation of a patient for anesthesia is unjustifiable—there is an essential symbiosis between the two if safety is to be ensured."

B. PREINDUCTION SUCTION OF GASTRIC CONTENTS (OROGASTRIC OR NASOGASTRIC TUBE)

When a patient at increased risk of aspirating gastric contents presents for surgery, the stomach may be emptied, at least in part, by means of suction through an orogastric or a nasogastric tube. Many patients, of course, will have had such a tube already placed for gastric decompression, particularly if intestinal obstruction has been diagnosed. In such cases, the anesthesi-

ologist must decide whether to remove the gastric tube prior to induction. On the other hand, if gastric decompression has not been attempted, the anesthesiologist may wish to insert a gastric tube while the patient's protective airway reflexes remain intact.

It has been argued that the presence of a gastric tube interferes with the sphincter function of the gastroesophageal junction and promotes GER by acting as a "wick."[57] The presence of a foreign body in the pharynx could also interfere with laryngoscopy. These considerations would favor removal of the gastric tube before induction.

However, in a prospective, randomized study by Satiani et al.[58] the incidence of "silent" GER was found to be 12% in anesthetized patients without a nasogastric (NG) tube versus 6% in patients with an NG tube in place (a difference that did not achieve statistical significance). Hardy[59] wrote that "[a] nasogastric tube need not be withdrawn before induction of anesthesia. The tube can act as an overflow valve" and provide "a venting mechanism whereby pressure cannot build up in the stomach."

Dotson et al.[60] prospectively studied the effect of nasogastric tube size on GER in normal subjects. Attempts were made to provoke GER with an "abdominal pressure device" that elevated abdominal pressure stepwise up to 100 mm Hg. In this report, GER "was not detected at any level of abdominal pressure regardless of the presence or size of a nasogastric tube."[60] As will be discussed later, gastric contents entering the lower esophagus can be stopped at the upper esophagus by means of cricoid pressure. Salem et al.[61] demonstrated that "cricoid pressure is effective in sealing the esophagus around an esophageal tube against an intraesophageal pressure up to 100 cm H_2O." The authors also advocated the utility of an NG tube as a "blow-off valve" for increased intragastric pressure during induction.[61]

The studies previously cited would seem to indicate that an NG tube, already inserted, can be safely left in place during induction and may even carry a protective benefit. Gastric decompression during surgery could also reduce the risk of regurgitation and aspiration in the postanesthetic period.[59] The necessity and utility of NG tube insertion just prior to induction are not so well defined. The benefits of awake gastric decompression depend, in part, on how completely the stomach can thereby be emptied. The primary drawback is patient discomfort during NG tube insertion.

Several authors have studied the thoroughness of gastric emptying attainable by gastric tube suctioning, usually in the context of comparing different methods for estimating gastric residual volume. Ong et al.[62] reported that the volume of fluid obtained by orogastric suctioning correlated poorly with the gastric residual volume calculated by a dilution method, "the volume aspirated being frequently much less than the volume calculated." The authors concluded that "[a]spiration through a gastric tube will not empty the stomach completely." Mechanical decompression of the stomach before induction might therefore be of limited reliability and thus provide a false sense of security.[62]

Taylor et al.[63] studied 10 obese patients in whom gastric contents were first aspirated through a 16F multiorificed Salem Sump tube, then "completely" removed via a gastroscope. "The blind aspirated volume underestimated true total gastric volume by an average of 14.7 ml, [which] was statistically significant.... The residual content volume left in the stomach after blind aspiration varied from 4 ml to 23 ml," a maximal discrepancy far less than that found by Ong et al.[62] in 42 patients.

Hardy et al.[64] measured the volume of gastric fluid aspirated through an 18F Salem Sump tube in 24 patients, then directly inspected the stomach and measured the volume of fluid remaining. The residual volume that eluded orogastric suctioning ranged only from 0 to 13 ml. The authors thus concluded "that the volume of aspirated gastric fluid ... is a very good estimate of the volume present in the stomach at the time of induction," and that gastric tube suctioning "could also be suitable to empty the stomach of its liquid contents prior to anaesthesia."[64]

Alessi and Berci[65] reported the results of a cinelaryngoscopic study of postoperative patients with NG tubes. They contended that the "[r]outine use of nasogastric tubes in major surgery is associated with unwarranted risks of aspiration through at least three mechanisms: hypersalivation—allowing pooling of secretions in the hypopharynx, a depressed cough reflex, ... and various laryngeal and pharyngeal abnormalities ... leading to an inability to handle secretions and protect the airway."[65] This study, however, involved patients subjected to prolonged nasogastric intubation after surgery and does not clearly pertain to the immediate preoperative period.

It can be argued that any reduction in intragastric volume and pressure prior to anesthetic induction is desirable and should therefore be attempted. On the other hand, as Satiani et al.[58] conceded, "particulate matter ... [is] impossible to evacuate through the lumen of an ordinary nasogastric tube." Salem et al.[61] concluded that "placement of a nasogastric tube before anesthetic induction seems to be indicated only in patients with overdistention of the stomach." While obvious enteric obstruction will conventionally be treated with gastric decompression prior to anesthetic induction, not every emergency or "at-risk" patient will be subjected to NG tube insertion while awake. There is currently no consensus to dictate preinduction placement of a gastric tube in any set of patients without

intestinal obstruction. In any case, gastric decompression in no way substitutes for proper perioperative management of the airway.

C. CRICOID PRESSURE

For the patient whose stomach is assumed to be full, the anesthesiologist must first, of course, decide whether to secure the airway before or after induction of anesthesia. If anesthetic induction is to precede tracheal intubation, the standard protective maneuver is *effective* cricoid pressure. As described by Sellick[66] in 1961, "[t]he manoeuvre consists in temporary occlusion of the upper end of the oesophagus by backward pressure of the cricoid cartilage against the bodies of the cervical vertebrae.... Extension of the neck and application of pressure on the cricoid cartilage obliterates the oesophageal lumen at the level of the body of the fifth cervical vertebra.... Pressure is maintained until intubation and inflation of the cuff of the endotracheal tube is completed." In his original report[66] of 26 "high-risk" cases, 23 patients neither vomited nor regurgitated at any time near induction, while in the other 3 "release of cricoid pressure after intubation was followed immediately by reflux into the pharynx of gastric or oesophageal contents, suggesting that in these three cases cricoid pressure had been effective."

Sellick,[66] himself, warned against applying cricoid pressure to the patient actively vomiting, lest the resulting increased pressure injure the esophagus. The maneuver, itself, can induce gagging and even vomiting in the awake patient. However, the commonest problem with Sellick's maneuver is the failure to perform it correctly. As Stept and Safar[67] wrote in 1970, "[t]he attempt to close the esophagus by pressing the cricoid cartilage against the cervical vertebrae is rarely applied with proper timing, namely, starting with the onset of unconsciousness and continuing until the tracheal cuff is inflated." Obviously, the safe administration of general anesthesia to the patient at risk of gastric content aspiration mandates the presence of an assistant who understands the importance and the technique of correctly providing cricoid pressure. Properly applied cricoid pressure can prevent passive regurgitation into the pharynx even in the presence of a nasogastric tube.[68]

Although the lower esophageal sphincter (as will be discussed later) has received considerable attention with regard to the pharmacology and pathophysiology of gastroesophageal reflux, there is also effective sphincter tone at the upper end of the esophagus. As described by Vanner et al.,[69] "[t]he upper oesophageal sphincter is formed mainly by the cricopharyngeus, a striated muscle situated behind the cricoid cartilage. The muscle tone of the cricopharyngeus creates a sphincter pressure which prevents regurgitation in the awake state." These authors found that general anesthesia with neuromus-

---

BOX 10-5   Factors that decrease lower esophageal barrier pressure

Gastric fluid components
    Increased acidity
    Lipids
    Hyperosmolar fluid
Progesterone
Pharmacologic agents
    Dopaminergic agonists
    β-adrenergic agonists
    Theophylline and caffeine
    Anticholinergics
    Opioids

BOX 10-6   Factors that increase lower esophageal barrier pressure

Dopaminergic antagonists
    Metoclopramide
    Domperidone
β-adrenergic antagonists
Gastrointestinal cholinergic agonists
    Cisapride
    Metoclopramide

---

cular blockade reduced the upper esophageal sphincter pressure from 38 mm Hg (while awake) to 6 mm Hg, a pressure that would typically permit passive regurgitation. They further found that Sellick's maneuver could exceed the normal awake level of upper esophageal sphincter pressure but was often not applied firmly enough to do so.[69]

III. MEDICAL PROPHYLAXIS OF ASPIRATION
A. LOWER ESOPHAGEAL SPHINCTER TONE AND GASTROESOPHAGEAL MOTILITY

Although patient preparation (rationale NPO strategy and perhaps gastric suctioning) and airway management (rapid sequence induction with cricoid pressure) are the twin pillars of aspiration prevention, pharmacologic prophylaxis has been promoted as adjunctive to patient safety. Since gastric contents must first pass through the esophagus before entering the pharynx and trachea, the lower esophageal sphincter has become a locus of attention. As described by Ciresi,[70] the LES "consists of functionally but not anatomically specialized smooth muscle, about 2 to 4 cm in length, just proximal to the stomach. The sphincteric muscle maintains closure of the distal esophagus through a mechanism of tonic contraction. . . . The state of closure is accompanied by a zone of intraluminal high pressure."[70] Normally, a cholinergic reflex loop acts to increase LES pressure when intragastric or intraabdominal pressure rises.[7,11] The pressure gradient between the LES and the stomach is referred to as the barrier pressure and is responsible for preventing GER[8,71,72] (Boxes 10-5 and 10-6).

LES function is modulated by neurohumoral influences. Dopaminergic and adrenergic stimulation decrease LES tone, while cholinergic stimulation increases LES contractility.[8,15,71] β-adrenergic agents and theophylline have been demonstrated to reduce LES pressure and promote GER, often with symptomatic heartburn in awake patients. LES relaxation due to theophylline can persist for several hours. β-adrenergic blockade has been shown to increase LES pressure.[73] Anticholinergics have often been demonstrated to attenuate LES tone and to counteract the effects of medications given to increase LES barrier pressure.[4,10,20,74,75] Although prochlorperazine raises LES pressure (presumably via an antidopaminergic effect), promethazine lowers LES pressure because of its anticholinergic properties.[8] Among the wide variety of other drugs that may also reduce LES tone are benzodiazepines, opioids, barbiturates, dopamine, tricyclic antidepressants, calcium channel blockers, nitroglycerin, and nitroprusside.[4,10] Although succinylcholine-induced fasciculations can elevate intraabdominal pressure, LES tone also rises, so the barrier pressure is maintained or increased.[4,8] Apart from pharmacologic influences, Rabey et al.[72] demonstrated that "barrier pressure may be reduced after insertion of a laryngeal mask airway during anesthesia with spontaneous ventilation."

In many cases, agents that increase LES contractility also promote forward passage of gastric contents into the duodenum, while those factors that attenuate LES tone also retard gastric emptying. This correlation compounds our pharmacologic opportunities for either protection or mischief. In both children and adults, opioids and anticholinergics have often been shown to inhibit gastrointestinal motility, increasing the volume of gastric contents available for vomiting or regurgitation.[11,75,76] Although pain and anxiety delay gastric emptying via sympathetic stimulation, the administration of an opioid for analgesia causes an even more profound inhibition of gastric content propulsion into the small intestine.[10,71]

1. Metoclopramide
Gastroprokinetic drugs are now available to promote gastric, pyloric, and duodenal activity while simultaneously enhancing LES barrier pressure. Metoclopramide is the prototypical agent in this category. The mechanisms of action proposed for metoclopramide include central antidopaminergic activity and prolactin stimulation, as well as peripheral blockade of dopamine

and facilitation of cholinergic stimulation in the upper gastrointestinal tract. While metoclopramide retains its gastrokinetic effects in the vagotomized subject, atropine has been shown to interfere with these actions.[70,77] The antiemetic property of metoclopramide is said to result, at least in part, from direct inhibition of the chemoreceptor trigger zone.[7] Metoclopramide both raises LES contractility and barrier pressure and accelerates gastric emptying. The latter effect is achieved by increasing the frequency and intensity of gastric longitudinal muscle contraction while relaxing the gastroduodenal sphincter and increasing the coordination of gastrointestinal peristalsis. Metoclopramide has no effect on gastric acid secretion.[20,70]

Metoclopramide has been extensively investigated as a chemoprophylactic agent for aspiration pneumonitis in children and in adults. Several studies of patients given metoclopramide, in a dose of 10 or 20 mg, either orally or intravenously, (with or without a coadministered H_2-receptor blocking agent) have demonstrated the drug's utility in reducing gastric residual volume.[20,78,79] Gonzalez and Kallar[20] wrote that "metoclopramide 10 mg p.o. or i.v., in combination with Bicitra or an H_2-receptor antagonist, provides the most effective control of gastric volume and pH." Given orally, metoclopramide's onset of action reportedly varies from 30 to 60 minutes, with a duration of action of 2 to 3 hours.[20] Ciresi[70] wrote that "[m]etoclopramide administered in a 10 to 20 mg intravenous dose can effectively empty the stomach within a 10 to 20 minute period."

Other researchers, though, have not found metoclopramide to be consistently effective in reducing gastric volume content, especially in the context of opioid coadministration or the recent ingestion of a solid meal.[74] Christensen et al.[80] demonstrated no influence of metoclopramide 0.1 mg/kg on the gastric pH or volume of healthy pediatric patients. As a perioperative antiemetic, metoclopramide is inconsistently useful.[74] Side effects attributed to metoclopramide have included somnolence, dizziness, and faintness. These problems may surface more frequently in elderly or severely ill patients.[20,70] Extrapyramidal reactions pose the most serious problem but reportedly occur in only 1% of subjects.[70]

Metoclopramide has also been investigated in obstetric anesthesia. The drug has been shown to increase LES tone in pregnant women and may thus be a useful prophylactic agent before cesarean section.[74,77] Studies of gastric emptying in the parturient have provided less consistent results. Metoclopramide has been shown to accelerate the gastric emptying of a test meal or of recently ingested food in patients undergoing elective or urgent cesarean section.[77,78] On the other hand, Cohen et al.[77] examined 58 healthy parturients undergoing elective cesarean section after an overnight fast and found that metoclopramide, 10 mg IV, had no significant effect on mean gastric volume or pH or on the proportion of patients with a gastric content volume exceeding 25 ml. The authors suggested that the drug might be more useful in the emergency setting characterized by active labor, recent food intake, pain, and anxiety.[77] Maternal metoclopramide administration does produce detectable and variable neonatal blood levels of the drug, but without reported effects on Apgar scores or neurobehavioral test results.[77,81]

Other gastroprokinetic agents may become available for clinical use in the United States. Domperidone specifically antagonizes the inhibitory actions of dopamine on the upper gastrointestinal tract and may thus be less likely than metoclopramide to induce extrapyramidal side effects. Cisapride reportedly enhances gastrointestinal cholinergic activity, increasing antegrade peristalsis without significant central side effects. None of these agents is recommended for use in the patient with intestinal obstruction.[4,8]

B. REDUCTION OF GASTRIC ACID CONTENT

Chemoprophylaxis of aspiration pneumonitis can also include the inhibition of gastric acid secretion or the neutralization of HCl already in the stomach. The former should increase the pH and reduce the volume of gastric contents but will have no effect on acidic fluid already in the stomach. The latter should elevate gastric fluid pH but may also increase gastric fluid volume. The aspiration of particulate antacids can, as previously described, pose hazards equivalent to those of gastric acid inhalation. Therefore, current oral antacid prophylaxis should include only soluble, nonparticulate agents.

1. Citrates

The clear antacid solutions most commonly studied are sodium citrate, 0.3 molar solution, and Bicitra, a commercial preparation containing sodium citrate and citric acid. The pH of sodium citrate solutions typically exceeds 7.0, whereas that of Bicitra is 4.3.[79] Manchikanti et al.[79] compared surgical outpatients given Bicitra 15 ml or 30 ml orally (PO) with a similar control group. All patients studied were nonobese and NPO for at least 8 hours. Of control patients, 88% had gastric content pH of less than or equal to 2.5, in contrast to 32% of those given Bicitra 15 ml and 16% of those given Bicitra 30 ml. Among the Bicitra-treated patients, low pH values were typically found in those with gastric fluid volumes less than 25 ml, confirming previous findings that the antacid effect was attenuated in patients with more rapid gastric emptying.[79]

Sodium citrate has been evaluated as a sole prophylactic agent in a variety of surgical settings, with inconsistent results. Kuster et al.[82] found that sodium citrate 30 ml, taken shortly before elective surgery, resulted in gastric fluid pH values less than 3.5 in 95% of patients. Colman et al.[83] administered 15 or 30 ml sodium citrate to 30 laboring parturients prior to emergency cesarean section. All 15 patients given 30 ml sodium citrate, and 14 of 15 given 15 ml, had gastric pH values less than or equal to 2.5. In other reports, however, sodium citrate has failed to alter gastric fluid pH in surgical patients. Of a 0.3 molar solution, 30 ml may be more consistently effective than 15 ml but may not have prolonged effects in patients with rapid gastric emptying.[8,84,85] Antacid prophylaxis may thus be adequate at the induction of anesthesia but inadequate at the time of awakening. Failure to neutralize gastric contents at the time of anesthetic induction may represent inadequate mixing of the sodium citrate with gastric fluid. Adequate mixing may require either adequate time for mixing or adequate movement of the patient.[9,82] Larger volumes of sodium citrate can induce nausea, vomiting, or diarrhea.[79]

2. H₂-receptor blockade

Gastric acid production by the parietal cell is strongly influenced by the action of H_2 receptors. H_2-receptor blockade inhibits basal acid secretion, as well as that stimulated by the presence of gastrin or food.[7] Both H_2-antagonists and anticholinergic agents block the neural stimulation of gastric acid secretion.[11,70] However, this beneficial effect of anticholinergic medications is overridden by the inhibition of gastrointestinal motility, so gastric volume is not reduced and gastric pH is elevated only inconsistently.[20] Various H_2-antagonists, most notably cimetidine and ranitidine, have therefore been evaluated in both surgical and obstetric settings, in different doses and routes of administration, with and without other prophylactic medications, to produce an expansive volume of findings.

a. CIMETIDINE

Given prior to elective surgery, a variety of cimetidine regimens can ensure that *most* patients will have gastric fluid volume and/or pH values in the "safe" range, as defined by their investigators. These usually effective regimens include cimetidine 300 mg PO at bedtime followed by 300 mg PO or intramuscularly (IM) the morning of surgery, cimetidine 300 to 600 mg PO 1.5 to 2 hours preoperatively, or cimetidine 200 mg intravenously (IV) 1 hour before surgery. In one study cimetidine most reliably produced gastric content "safety" when combined with preoperative metoclopramide.[4] The reliability of oral cimetidine is generally improved if the drug is administered both the night before and the morning of anesthesia.[9]

Gastric fluid pH of 2.5 or less has been found in around 5% to 35% of patients treated with single 300-mg doses of cimetidine given PO, IM, or IV, in different studies. Significant elevation of gastric pH requires 30 to 60 minutes to become evident following the intravenous administration of cimetidine and 60 to 90 minutes following intramuscular or oral dosing. Effective inhibition of gastric acid secretion persists for 4 to 6 hours.[20,74] Papadimitriou et al.[86] administered cimetidine 400 mg IV to 20 patients facing emergency surgery. Compared with 10 such patients given placebo treatment, those receiving cimetidine demonstrated a reduction of gastric fluid volume that did not achieve statistical significance. Mean gastric acidity was significantly reduced by cimetidine, although the range of pH values was 1.6 to 7.2.[86]

Cimetidine chemoprophylaxis has also been evaluated in obstetric anesthesia. In a study of women scheduled for elective cesarean section, the administration of cimetidine 400 mg PO the night before surgery, followed by 200 mg IM 90 minutes before induction, resulted in a mean gastric fluid pH of 6.2. However, 3 of the 16 patients studied had gastric fluid pH values of less than 2.5.[83] In a study of 100 patients undergoing emergency cesarean section, cimetidine 200 mg IM was administered when surgical delivery was decided upon, followed by oral intake of a 0.3 molar solution of sodium citrate 30 ml just prior to induction. None of these patients had a gastric fluid pH of less than 2.7, and only 1 of 100 had a gastric fluid pH of less than 3.0.[54] Cimetidine administered in this fashion would most likely reduce gastric acidity by the time of extubation. Whereas sodium citrate would be required to neutralize the acid already secreted by the gastric parietal cells.

To achieve both prompt neutralization of gastric HCl and subsequent inhibition of parietal cell activity, cimetidine (800 mg) and sodium citrate (1.8 g) have been combined in tablet form. (Alkalinization of gastric fluid has also been suggested to accelerate the systemic uptake of orally administered cimetidine.[85,87]) This formulation, known as effervescent cimetidine, is not currently available in the United States. In healthy elective surgical patients, a single tablet of effervescent cimetidine has been shown to provide both significant elevation of gastric content pH and significant reduction of gastric content volume when given 2 hours prior to induction, with no patient considered "at risk" of acid aspiration.[88] When given 10 to 50 minutes prior to elective or emergency cesarean section, one-half tablet of effervescent cimetidine achieved gastric pH values greater than 2.5 in 98% to 100% of patients at the times of both induction and extubation.[85,87]

Although cimetidine has a well-established record of safety when administered in the short term, as for perioperative aspiration prophylaxis, there are potential and observed side effects. The rapid intravenous infusion of large doses (e.g., 400 to 600 mg) has reportedly induced both hypotension and dangerous ventricular dysrhythmias.[71,74] Smith et al.[89] found that cimetidine 200 mg, given intravenously over 2 minutes to 20 critically ill patients, resulted in temporary and variable decreases in mean arterial pressure and systemic vascular resistance, not requiring treatment. Heart rate, cardiac output, and cardiac filling pressures were not altered. The authors advised that intravenous cimetidine be infused over at least a 10-minute period.[89] Other side effects sporadically associated with cimetidine include confusion, dizziness, headaches, and diarrhea, although these have not been reported to occur with single-dose preoperative administration. In addition, since H_2-mediated bronchodilation may serve to counterbalance H_1-mediated bronchoconstriction, there has been a speculative concern that H_2-blockade could conceivably exacerbate respiratory dysfunction in the asthmatic patient.[70,71,74]

Cimetidine, with an imidazole ring structure, competitively inhibits the hepatic mixed-function oxidase system (cytochrome P450 enzyme), and also reduces hepatic perfusion.[71,73,74] As a result, cimetidine may elevate the blood concentrations of other drugs that are cleared by the liver, including warfarin, propranolol, diazepam, theophylline, phenytoin, meperidine, bupivacaine, and lidocaine. Clinically, this seems to be a greater concern with long-term than with one-or two-dose administration.[70,74,83]

b. RANITIDINE

After cimetidine, ranitidine emerged as the next option for H_2 blockade. Ranitidine is purported to be nearly devoid of undesirable side effects. Ranitidine also has a longer duration of action (6 to 8 hours) than cimetidine, and its efficacy is greater than or equal to that of the older H_2 blocker. Onset times for the two drugs to exert their effects appear to be similar.[4,20,74,90] The structure of ranitidine is based upon a furan, rather than an imidazole ring. This structural difference is said to account for ranitidine's lesser or minimal inhibition of the hepatic cytochrome P450 enzyme system.[83] Smith et al.[89] reported that ranitidine 50 mg, given intravenously over 2 minutes to 20 critically ill patients, led to variable, transient reductions in mean arterial pressure and systemic vascular resistance. These hemodynamic effects occurred less frequently, and were of lesser degree and duration, than those resulting from cimetidine 200 mg, similarly administered. Previous sporadic case reports associated significant bradycardia with the intravenous administration of either cimetidine or ranitidine.[89]

In a study of adult surgical outpatients by Maltby et al.[47] ranitidine 150 mg PO, given 2.5 hours prior to anesthetic induction, significantly decreased gastric residual volume and significantly increased gastric fluid pH compared to placebo treatment. In no patient was the "at risk" combination of gastric pH less than 2.5 and gastric volume greater than 25 ml found. Kuster et al.[82] administered ranitidine 300 mg PO the night before and 150 mg PO the morning of elective surgery. Gastric fluid pH was greater than 4.0 in all cases on both induction and extubation, "even after delayed or prolonged operations." McAllister et al.[91] treated adult patients with a single oral dose of ranitidine 300 mg 2 hours before surgery and found both a significant increase in mean gastric fluid pH and a significant decrease in mean gastric fluid volume, compared with placebo treatment. Some patients did have gastric fluid pH values less than 2.5, despite this ranitidine regimen, but the incidence of such low pH values was also significantly lower than with placebo. The authors cautioned that "it is unsafe to assume that H_2 antagonists will *always* eliminate the risk of acid aspiration pneumonitis."

In other studies a single oral dose of ranitidine 150 mg, given 2 to 3 hours before anesthetic induction, has been found to produce gastric fluid pH values greater than 2.5 in *most* adult surgical patients. Another report indicated that ranitidine 150 mg PO given both the night before and the morning of surgery, produced gastric fluid pH values greater than 2.5 in all such patients studied. Single-dose intravenous administration of ranitidine, 40 to 100 mg, has also been found to reliably generate gastric fluid pH values greater than 2.5 in adults, manifesting a greater efficacy than that of cimetidine 300 mg IV.[4]

Sandhar et al.[92] evaluated the efficacy of a single oral dose of ranitidine, 2 mg/kg, given 2 to 3 hours before surgery to patients aged 1 to 14 years. While ranitidine significantly reduced both the volume and the acidity of gastric contents, when compared with placebo, 6 of 44 children receiving ranitidine did have gastric fluid pH values less than or equal to 2.5. These findings confirmed those of a similar study by Goudsouzian et al.,[93] although other authors have not demonstrated a consistent reduction in gastric fluid volume.[4,47]

Papadimitriou et al.[86] compared ranitidine 150 mg IV with cimetidine 400 mg IV and with placebo, given 1 hour before anesthetic induction to emergency surgical patients. Ranitidine and cimetidine caused similar reductions in gastric volume and acidity; only the reductions in acidity were statistically significant. Although the mean pH values in the cimetidine and ranitidine groups were similar, only ranitidine consistently produced "safe" gastric pH values (all of which were ≥ 5.0).[86] Vila et al.,[94] evaluating H_2 antagonists in morbidly obese surgical patients, concluded that ranitidine was superior to cimetidine in elevating gastric fluid pH. When such patients were given ranitidine 150 mg PO the night before surgery and again 2 hours prior to induction, all pH values obtained were greater than 2.5.[94] A literature review cited by Gonzalez and Kallar[20] also found that ranitidine more reliably ensures that gastric fluid pH will exceed 2.5 than does cimetidine. Although neither agent consistently reduces gastric fluid volume into the range considered "safe" by given authors, ranitidine also appears to be more reliable than cimetidine in this regard.[20]

The effect of oral ranitidine (150 mg 2 to 3 hours before the scheduled time of surgery) with or without oral metoclopramide (10 mg 1 hour before surgery) and/or sodium citrate (30 ml on call to the operating room) on gastric fluid volume and pH was measured in 196 elective surgical inpatients.[95] Although no combination guaranteed a low gastric fluid volume and increased gastric fluid pH, a single oral dose of ranitidine was as effective as triple prophylaxis.

Ranitidine has also been evaluated for prophylactic use in obstetric anesthesia. Ewart et al.[96] administered ranitidine 150 PO the night before and the morning of elective cesarean section. At both induction and extubation, all gastric aspirate volumes were less than 25 ml. Of patients, 19% had gastric fluid pH values less than 3.5, and 6% had gastric fluid pH values less than 2.5, either at induction or at extubation, or both.[96] Colman et al.[83] administered ranitidine 150 mg PO 8 to 14 hours prior to elective cesarean section, then 50 mg IM 90 minutes before induction. All 20 patients in this study had gastric fluid volumes less than 25 ml and pH values greater than 2.5. A previous study by McAuley et al. demonstrated that 79 of 80 parturients had gastric fluid pH values greater than 2.5 when given ranitidine 150 mg PO 2 to 6 hours prior to elective cesarean section.[83,97]

Colman et al.[83] also studied 60 laboring parturients subjected to emergency cesarean section. All such patients had received ranitidine 50 mg IM every 6 hours during labor. Of 30 such patients who received no further antacid therapy, 5 had gastric fluid pH values less than 2.5 at the time of anesthetic induction, of whom 4 had gastric fluid volumes greater than 25 ml. Of 30 such patients who also received 0.3 molar sodium citrate, 15 or 30 ml, before induction, all had gastric pH values greater than 2.5. The authors concluded that, although ranitidine 50 mg IM every 6 hours significantly reduced gastric fluid volume and acidity, it "cannot be relied on as sole prophylaxis against aspiration pneumonitis."[83] Yau et al.[98] similarly administered ranitidine 150 mg PO every 6 hours to women in labor, followed by sodium citrate just prior to emergency cesarean section. Of their patients, 2% had gastric fluid volumes greater than 25 ml along with pH values less than 2.5. No pH values less than 2.5 were found, however, when at least 2 hours had elapsed since ranitidine administration.[98]

Rout et al.[90] evaluated the efficacy of ranitidine 50 mg IV given to laboring patients when cesarean section was decided upon. A control group received no H_2-antagonist therapy, but all patients were given 0.3 molar sodium citrate, 30 ml, shortly before induction. At the time of induction, 4% of those given only sodium citrate had a gastric fluid volume greater than 25 ml along with a pH less than 3.5, compared with 2.3% of those given both citrate and ranitidine (P = .05). At the time of extubation, 5.6% of those given only sodium citrate were considered "at risk" by the preceding criteria, compared with 0.3% of those given both citrate and ranitidine (P < .05). There was no significant difference between the mean pH values of those parturients given citrate, alone, and those given ranitidine less than 30 minutes before surgery. On the other hand, all gastric fluid pH values exceeded 3.5 in patients who received ranitidine more than 30 minutes prior to induction.[90]

An extensive body of evidence thus voluminously documents the safety and efficacy of short-term cimetidine and ranitidine therapy in reducing the acidity and volume of gastric contents. Newer agents, such as famotidine, have also been evaluated, with generally favorable results.[94] However, the routine preoperative use of H_2 antagonists is not generally considered either essential or cost-effective. As stated by Kallar and Everett,[4] "[I]t has yet to be proven that prophylaxis against acid aspiration changes morbidity or mortality in healthy patients having elective surgery."

Based on the presumably high ratio of benefit to risk, H_2-blocking agents are commonly recommended for surgical patients with an increased likelihood of inhaling gastric contents.[4,36] Because of the relative infrequency of perioperative aspiration pneumonitis, documentation of the actual clinical benefit of such practice has yet to be provided. In the review of Warner et al.[6] of over 215,000 general anesthetics in adults, 35 patients with generally acknowledged risk factors did aspirate perioperatively. Of these 35, 17 had been given prophylactic medication. In this small sample, aspiration prophylaxis produced no discernible difference in the incidence of pulmonary complications.[6]

c. OMEPRAZOLE

Beyond the H_2 antagonists, omeprazole is the newest agent introduced for the suppression of gastric acid production. Acetylcholine, histamine, and gastrin all stimulate HCl secretion by the gastric parietal cell. While these agonists stimulate different populations of receptors, their mechanisms of action all eventually result in the formation of cyclic adenosine monophosphate (cAMP). This cAMP activates the proton pump, H^+-K^+-ATPase, which exchanges intraluminal potassium ion for intracellular hydrogen ions. Hydrogen ions are thereby secreted from the parietal cell into gastric fluids.[91,92] Omeprazole, a benzimidazole derivative, is actually a prodrug, which is absorbed in the small intestine from an enteric-coated granule, and can only be transformed into its active form, sulphenamide, in the highly acidic milieu of the gastric parietal cell. Activated omeprazole then remains in the parietal cell for up to 48 hours, inhibiting the proton pump in a noncompetitive, long-acting manner. Omeprazole thus selectively suppresses the final step of gastric acid secretion.[81,88,96,99] Omeprazole has often been shown capable of prolonged, nearly complete inhibition of gastric acid secretion, with no discernible side effects. A single dose of omeprazole, 20 to 40 mg, reduces gastric acidity for up to 48 hours. Omeprazole 40 mg has been found to reduce gastrin-stimulated acid secretion by 65%, while 90% inhibition is accomplished with an 80-mg dose.[88,100]

Although the use of omeprazole is currently attaining popularity only in the management of acute flareups of peptic ulcer disease, it has also been evaluated as a preoperative agent for the chemoprophylaxis of aspiration pneumonitis. Bouly et al.[88] gave omeprazole 40 mg PO to healthy patients either the evening before or 2 hours prior to elective surgery. Although mean gastric fluid pH was significantly higher with omeprazole treatment than with placebo, gastric acidity was significantly greater with omeprazole than with effervescent cimetidine. Of 30 patients receiving omeprazole, 6 had gastric fluid pH values less than 2.5 at the time of induction. Omeprazole significantly reduced gastric fluid volume when compared with placebo.[88] Wingtin et al.[100] administered either placebo or omeprazole 40 mg PO to healthy, nonobese adults the night before elective surgery. Patients receiving omeprazole had a significantly higher mean gastric fluid pH than did those receiving placebo. The lowest gastric fluid pH observed with omeprazole was 2.4, in contrast to a minimal pH of 1.1 with placebo. Only 4.5% of omeprazole-treated patients had gastric fluid pH values less than 3.5, compared with 50% of those given a placebo.[100]

Omeprazole has also been evaluated in obstetric anesthesia. Yau et al.[98] administered omeprazole 40 mg PO every 12 hours to parturients in labor, then gave sodium citrate to half of those who underwent emergency cesarean section. Seventeen percent of those given omeprazole, alone, and 6% of those given omeprazole and sodium citrate manifested the "at risk" combination of gastric fluid volume greater than 25 ml with gastric fluid pH less than 2.5. In their multifaceted study, the authors also found that two doses of omeprazole 40 mg were superior to two doses of ranitidine 150 mg in producing gastric fluid pH values greater than 3.5 in nonlaboring patients undergoing elective cesarean section. On the other hand, ranitidine was superior to omeprazole in reducing gastric acidity during labor.[98] Orr et al.,[81] administered omeprazole 40 mg PO the night before and the morning of elective cesarean section. Only 1 of 30 such patients had a gastric fluid pH less than 2.5 on induction, and all gastric fluid pH values exceeded 2.5 at the time of extubation. In no case did gastric fluid volume exceed 25 ml with a pH less than 2.5. Of 15 patients who also received metoclopramide 20 mg IM at least 20 minutes before elective cesarean section, all had gastric fluid pH values greater than 2.5, both on induction and at extubation. When omeprazole 80 mg PO was given on the morning of elective cesarean section, 2 of 33 patients had a gastric fluid pH less than 2.5 at induction, 1 of whom also had a gastric fluid volume greater than 40 ml. All gastric fluid pH values were greater than 2.5 at extubation. Of 16 patients who also received metoclopramide 20 mg IM at least 20 minutes before elective cesarean section, 2 had gastric fluid pH values less than 2.5 (with gastric fluid volumes less than 25 ml) on induction, while all gastric fluid pH values exceeded 2.5 at extubation.[81]

Ewart et al.[96] administered omeprazole 40 mg PO the night before and the morning of elective cesarean section. In this report, all gastric fluid pH values were greater than or equal to 3.5, both on induction and at extubation, while all gastric fluid volumes were less than 25 ml. Moore et al.[99] administered omeprazole 80 mg PO the evening before elective cesarean section, with no subsequent morning dose, and noted somewhat less consistent antacid prophylaxis. In their series, 17 of 20 gastric fluid pH values were greater than 2.5 on induction, as well as at the end of surgery. Sixteen of 20 gastric fluid volumes were less than 25 ml on induction, and 19 of 20 were less than 25 ml at the time of extubation. Of 20 gastric fluid samples taken on induction, 1 met the authors' criteria for placing the patient "at risk" of aspiration pneumonitis. They concluded that this single-dose omeprazole regimen was not adequate to guarantee "acceptable gastric pH and volume 12 to 16 hours after administration."[99]

IV. TREATMENT OF ASPIRATION PNEUMONITIS
A. CLEARANCE OF THE AIRWAY

When ill fortune prevails and gastric contents are inhaled, the clinician's efforts must turn from prevention to treatment. Patency of the upper airway must immediately be ensured by clearing the mouth and pharynx of solid and liquid material and, as a rule, promptly intubating the trachea. (In many cases, difficulties in airway management have already been encountered before regurgitation and aspiration occur.) After asphyxiation has been averted, bronchoscopy may then be indicated in order to clear obstructing materials from the lower airways.[9,11] After gastric contents have entered the lungs, any attempts to remove or neutralize the acid are altogether futile. As described by Kirsch and Sanders,[19] "instillation of acidic gastric juice, tagged with methylene blue, into the airways of excised canine lungs shows the appearance of blue dye on the lung surface within 12 to 18 seconds." Other researchers have shown that HCl instilled into the trachea appears in the systemic circulation nearly as rapidly as if it were injected intravenously, with peak plasma concentrations attained within 2 to 3 minutes.[22,25] As Kirsch and Sanders concluded, "the extreme rapidity of acid-induced airway and parenchymal lung damage precludes effective therapy by attempts at neutralization of acid with intratracheal alkaline solutions."[19] As soon as the acid reaches the lung, the primary injury can no longer be prevented. Alkaline or dilutional lavage may only exacerbate the pulmonary insult.[9,11,100]

B. MECHANICAL VENTILATION AND POSITIVE END-EXPIRATORY PRESSURE

The next challenge, one not always easily met, is the maintenance of adequate arterial oxygenation. Mechanical ventilation is often required to overcome the obstacles of bronchospasm, pulmonary edema, and ventilation-perfusion mismatching. Prophylactic application of positive pressure ventilation before respiratory insufficiency occurs may or may not be of value. A study of massive acid aspiration in dogs demonstrated that survival of all subjects could be achieved by immediately instituting mechanical ventilation. Clinical researchers, as well, have advocated "early ventilation" as a cornerstone of management. Other studies, however, including a prospective clinical trial, did not confirm that the outcome was improved when positive pressure ventilation with positive end-expiratory pressure (PEEP) was begun prophylactically.[9,16,22,25] Severe bronchospasm may call for an aminophylline infusion or the inhalation of a β-adrenergic bronchodilator.[101]

Patients who require mechanical ventilation for aspiration pneumonitis may also require substantial levels of PEEP, in order to achieve acceptable arterial oxygenation with a "nontoxic" inspired oxygen fraction (FiO_2). Some researchers have also advocated prophylactic application of PEEP as a means of preserving the compliance and aeration of noninjured lung units.[25] On the other hand, when lung units are overdistended by excessive inflating pressures, damage to the alveolar-capillary membrane may be exacerbated.[22]

Zucker et al.[102] proposed that acute lung injury initiates a pernicious cycle in which pulmonary edema and the loss of surfactant reinforce each other. When pulmonary capillaries leak fluid into the lungs, surfactant is diluted or washed out, and alveolar surface tension rises. This increased surface tension tends to draw still more fluid from the capillaries into the alveoli, washing out still more surfactant. In a canine study of HCl aspiration, the authors demonstrated that the therapeutic inhalation of exogenous surfactant reduced pulmonary edema and pulmonary venous admixture only in those animals in which PEEP (8 cm H_2O) was also applied. The authors concluded that the "addition of PEEP to the ventilator circuit initially recruited alveoli, reduced [venous admixture], and protected against deterioration after surfactant administration."[102]

Sohma et al.[26] evaluated the effects of PEEP, either 10 cm H_2O or 3 cm H_2O, following intratracheal instillation of HCl in rabbits. Although the higher level of PEEP was associated with greater arterial oxygenation and pulmonary compliance than was the lower level, "there were no significant differences between the groups in terms of survival and histological findings."[26] It may be noted that the levels of PEEP evaluated in this study did not differ greatly in magnitude.

Veddeng et al.[24] evaluated the application of PEEP to either one lung or both lungs following unilateral aspiration of HCl. They proposed that, with conventional ventilation or bilateral PEEP, the "more compliant healthy lung receives a larger proportion of the tidal volume leading to alveolar hyperinflation and increased airway pressure, which is transmitted to the tissue around the alveolar capillaries." As a result, pulmonary perfusion is diverted to the more poorly aerated lung, impairing arterial oxygenation. In their study, PEEP applied selectively to the injured lung resulted in a lesser degree of hemodynamic impairment than did PEEP applied to both lungs or to the uninjured lung, alone.[24] From a clinical standpoint, the prolonged maintenance of a double-lumen endotracheal tube in the proper position to permit one-lung PEEP is a considerable challenge to critical care personnel.

C. CORTICOSTEROIDS?

Corticosteroids were once hailed as a promising adjunct in the treatment of aspiration pneumonitis. Proposed beneficial actions included the stabilization of cellular and lysosomal membranes, the maintenance of pulmonary microvascular integrity, the suppression of alveolar and airway inflammation, the preservation of distal airway architecture, and a reduction in pulmonary edema formation.[103,104] In various studies that demonstrated a protective effect of corticosteroids, the medication was administered almost immediately following acid aspiration. Generally, clinical and laboratory reports from 1964 onward have demonstrated no favorable effect of corticosteroids upon the outcome of aspiration pneumonitis. In fact, corticosteroids in some studies have been found to impair the subjects' immunocompetence, increasing the risk of bacterial pneumonia or sepsis.[16,25,104] The current consensus appears to be that, at present, corticosteroids have no role in the treatment of aspiration pneumonitis.[9,16]

D. ANTIBIOTICS?

The antimicrobial treatment of secondary bacterial pneumonia is beyond the scope of this chapter. However, the current consensus is that antibiotics should not be administered prophylactically following aspiration of gastric contents. Routine antibiotic administration is not thought to offer any useful protection against the subsequent development of bacterial pneumonitis, but instead promotes secondary infection with resistant organisms. The possible exception to this standard would be the pulmonary aspiration of grossly infected or feculent material.*

Although bacterial pneumonia is not generally an immediate concern following an episode of aspiration, the injured lung has a diminished resistance to subsequent infection. Bacterial superinfection may develop in up to 40% of such patients.[9] When bacterial infection does complicate aspiration pneumonitis, the predominant organisms are typically oropharyngeal anaerobes if the patient has not been hospitalized for long beforehand. With prolonged antecedent hospitalization or illness, oropharyngeal flora are more likely to include gram-negative bacilli, *Staphylococcus aureus, Pseudomonas organisms,* and *Serratia organisms.*[9,14,21] Acidic gastric contents are normally sterile, but chronic suppression of gastric acid secretion can permit bacterial overgrowth in the stomach.[2]

E. CIRCULATORY SUPPORT

As previously mentioned, the outpouring of fluid from the damaged pulmonary capillary bed can lead to hypovolemic circulatory insufficiency. Large amounts of fluid may need to be infused. The therapeutically prolonged retention of colloid solutions within the intravascular space, as compared with crystalloids, would not be expected to pertain when capillary integrity is disrupted. In the absence of any evidence of a therapeutic advantage to colloid solutions, crystalloid fluids are most often chosen for intravascular volume repletion in this setting.[14]

V. CONCLUSION

Just as the lung reacts to a variety of insults with a limited repertoire of responses, our established methods of treating aspiration pneumonitis are limited to the basic practices of intensive respiratory care and circulatory support. An impressive array of pharmacologic agents can now be employed to promote antegrade gastric emptying, inhibit gastroesophageal reflux, and reduce the acid content of gastric fluids. These drugs have been utilized with an established record of safety and offer us the reasonable expectation of rendering gastric fluid contents less threatening to the lungs. However, due to the relative infrequency of significant perioperative aspiration, it may not be possible to demonstrate statistically that the use of these agents actually improves patient outcome.

It is obviously best to prevent gastric contents from entering the airway in the first place. While this ideal may not always be attainable, even by the most skillful of clinicians, its likelihood would appear to be favored by optimal patient preparation and a carefully executed

*References 9, 14, 15, 22, 25, 101.

well-designed plan for anesthetic induction and airway management. All other techniques and therapies are of secondary importance in ensuring ultimate patient well-being.

REFERENCES

1. Cote CJ: NPO after midnight for children: a reappraisal, *Anesthesiology* 72:589, 1990.
2. LoCicero J: Bronchopulmonary aspiration, *Surg Clin N Am* 69:71, 1989.
3. Hardy J-F, Lepage Y, Bonneville-Chouinard N: Occurrence of gastroesophageal reflux on induction of anaesthesia does not correlate with the volume of gastric contents, *Can J Anaesth* 37:502, 1990.
4. Kallar SK, Everett LL: Potential risks and preventive measures for pulmonary aspiration: new concepts in preoperative fasting guidelines, *Anesth Analg* 77:171, 1993.
5. Leigh JM, Tytler JA: Admissions to the intensive care unit after complications of anaesthetic techniques over 10 years, *Anaesthesia* 45:814, 1990.
6. Warner MA, Warner ME, Weber JG: Clinical significance of pulmonary aspiration during the perioperative period, *Anesthesiology* 78:56, 1993.
7. Olsson GL, Hallen B, Hambraeus-Jonzon K: Aspiration during anaesthesia: a computer-aided study of 185,358 anaesthetics, *Acta Anaesthesiol Scand* 30:84, 1986.
8. Aitkenhead AR: Anaesthesia and the gastro-intestinal system, *Eur J Anaesthesiol* 5:73, 1988.
9. DePaso WJ: Aspiration pneumonia, *Clin Chest Med* 12:269, 1991.
10. Ruffalo RL: Aspiration pneumonitis: risk factors and management of the critically ill patient, *DICP* 24:S12, 1990.
11. Kinni ME, Stout MM: Aspiration pneumonitis: predisposing conditions and prevention, *J Oral Maxillofac Surg* 44:378, 1986.
12. Saleh KL: Practical points in understanding aspiration, *J Post Anesthesia Nursing* 6:347, 1991.
13. Hannon VM, Cunningham AJ, Hutchinson M et al: Aspiration pneumonia and coma: an unusual presentation of dystrophica myotonia, *Can Anaesth Soc J* 33:803, 1986.
14. Khawaja IT, Buffa SD, Brandstetter RD: Aspiration pneumonia, *Postgrad Med* 92:165, 1992.
15. Russin SJ, Adler AG: Pulmonary aspiration, *Postgrad Med* 85:155, 1989.
16. Hickling KG, Howard R: A retrospective survey of treatment and mortality in aspiration pneumonia, *Intensive Care Med* 14:617, 1988.
17. Mendelson CL: The aspiration of stomach contents into the lungs during obstetric anesthesia, *Am J Obstet Gynecol* 52:191, 1946.
18. Gardner AMN: Aspiration of food and vomit, *Q J Med* 27:227, 1958.
19. Kirsch CM, Sanders A: Aspiration pneumonia: medical management, *Otolaryngol Clin N Am* 21:677, 1988.
20. Gonzalez ER, Kallar SK: Reducing the risk of aspiration pneumonitis, *DICP* 23:203, 1989.
21. Hollingsworth HM, Irwin RS: Acute respiratory failure in pregnancy, 13:723, 1992.
22. Dal Santo G: Acid aspiration: pathophysiological aspects, prevention, and therapy, *Int Anesthesiol Clin* 24:31, 1986.
23. Irons EE, Apfelbach CW: Aspiration bronchopneumonia, *JAMA* 115:584, 1940.
24. Veddeng OJ, Myhre ESP, Risoe C et al: Haemodynamic effects of selective positive end-expiratory pressure after unilateral pulmonary hydrochloric acid-aspiration in dogs, *Intensive Care Med* 18:356, 1992.

25. Pennza PT: Aspiration pneumonia, necrotizing pneumonia, and lung abscess, *Emerg Med Clin N Am* 7:279, 1989.

26. Sohma A, Brampton WJ, Dunnill MS et al: Effect of ventilation with positive end-expiratory pressure on the development of lung damage in experimental acid aspiration pneumonia in the rabbit, *Intensive Care Med* 18:112, 1992.

27. Hall CC: Aspiration pneumonitis, *JAMA* 114:728, 1940.

28. Hollingsworth HM: Wheezing and stridor, *Clin Chest Med* 8:231, 1987.

29. Smith BE: Anesthetic emergencies, *Clin Obstet Gynecol* 28:391, 1985.

30. Teabeaut JR: Aspiration of gastric contents, *Am J Pathol* 28:51, 1952.

31. Rocke DA, Brock-Utne JG, Rout CC: At risk for aspiration: new critical values of volume and pH? *Anesth Analg* 76:666, 1993 (letter).

32. Raidoo DM, Rocke DA, Brock-Utne JG et al: Critical volume for pulmonary acid aspiration: reappraisal in a primate model, *Br J Anaesth* 65:248, 1990.

33. Roberts RB, Shirley MA: Reducing the risk of acid aspiration during cesarean section, *Anesth Analg* 53:859, 1974.

34. Roberts RB, Shirley MA: Antacid therapy in obstetrics, *Anesthesiology* 53:83, 1980.

35. James CF, Modell JH, Gibbs CP et al: Pulmonary aspiration— effects of volume and pH in the rat, *Anesth Analg* 63:665, 1984.

36. Goresky GV, Maltby JR: Fasting guidelines for elective surgical patients, *Can J Anaesth* 37:493, 1990.

37. Bond VK, Stoelting RK, Gupta CD: Pulmonary aspiration syndrome after inhalation of gastric fluid containing antacids, *Anesthesiology* 51:452, 1979.

38. Sandhar BK, Goresky GV, Maltby JR et al: Effect of oral liquids and ranitidine on gastric fluid volume and pH in children undergoing outpatient surgery, *Anesthesiology* 71:327, 1989.

39. van der Walt JH, Carter JA: The effect of different pre-operative feeding regimens on plasma glucose and gastric volume and pH in infancy, *Anaesth Intens Care* 14:352, 1986.

40. Splinter WM, Schaefer JD, Bonn GE: Unlimited clear fluid ingestion by infants up to 2 hours before surgery is safe, *Can J Anaesth* 37(4, Pt 2):S95, 1990.

41. Schreiner MS, Triebwasser A, Keon TP: Ingestion of liquids compared with preoperative fasting in pediatric outpatients, *Anesthesiology* 72:593, 1990.

42. Phillips S, Hutchinson S, Davidson T: Preoperative drinking does not affect gastric contents, *Br J Anaesth* 70:6, 1993.

43. Meakin G, Dingwall AE, Addison GM: Effects of fasting and oral premedication on the pH and volume of gastric aspirate in children, *Br J Anaesth* 59:678, 1987.

44. Bricker SRW, McLuckie A, Nightingale DA: Gastric aspirates after trauma in children, *Anaesthesia* 44:721, 1989.

45. Strunin L: How long should patients fast before surgery? Time for new guidelines, *Br J Anaesth* 70:1, 1993.

46. Miller M, Wishart HY, Nimmo WS: Gastric contents at induction of anaesthesia: is a 4-hour fast necessary? *Br J Anaesth* 55:1185, 1983.

47. Maltby JR, Sutherland AD, Sale JP et al: Preoperative oral fluids: is a five-hour fast justified prior to elective surgery? *Anesth Analg* 65:112, 1986.

48. Lewis P, Maltby JR, Sutherland LR: Unrestricted oral fluid until three hours preoperatively: effect on gastric fluid volume and pH, *Can J Anaesth* 37(4, Pt 2):S132, 1990.

49. Read MS, Vaughan RS: Allowing pre-operative patients to drink: effects on patients' safety and comfort of unlimited oral water until 2 hours before anesthesia, *Acta Anaesthesiol Scand* 35:591, 1991.

50. Morgan M: Anaesthetic contribution to maternal mortality, *Br J Anaesth* 59:842, 1987.

51. Elkington KW: At the water's edge: where obstetrics and anesthesia meet, *Obstet Gynecol* 77:304, 1991.

52. Ludka LM, Roberts CC: Eating and drinking in labor, *J Nurse Midwifery* 38:199, 1993.

53. Broach J, Newton N: Food and beverages in labor. II. The effects of cessation of oral intake during labor, *Birth* 15:88, 1988.

54. McKay S, Mahan C: How can aspiration of vomitus in obstetrics best be prevented? *Birth* 15:222, 1988.

55. Chestnut DH, Cohen SE: At the water's edge: where obstetrics and anesthesia meet, *Obstet Gynecol* 77:965, 1991 (letter).

56. Crawford JS: Commentary: setting the record straight, *Birth* 15:230, 1988.

57. Stone SB: *J Trauma* 21:996, 1981 (letter).

58. Satiani B, Bonner JT, Stone HH: Factors influencing intraoperative gastric regurgitation, *Arch Surg* 113:721, 1978.

59. Hardy J-F: Large volume gastroesophageal reflux: a rationale for risk reduction in the perioperative period, *Can J Anaesth* 35:162, 1988.

60. Dotson RG, Robinson RG, Pingleton SK: Gastroesophageal reflux with nasogastric tubes: effect of nasogastric tube size, *Am J Respir Crit Care Med* 149:1659, 1994.

61. Salem MR, Joseph NJ, Heyman HJ et al: Cricoid compression is effective in obliterating the esophageal lumen in the presence of a nasogastric tube, *Anesthesiology* 63:443, 1985.

62. Ong BY, Palahniuk RJ, Cumming M: Gastric volume and pH in out-patients, *Can Anaesth Soc J* 25:36, 1978.

63. Taylor WJ, Champion MC, Barry AW et al: Measuring gastric contents during general anaesthesia: evaluation of blind gastric aspiration, *Can J Anaesth* 36:51, 1989.

64. Hardy J-F, Plourde G, Lebrun M et al: Determining gastric contents during general anaesthesia: evaluation of two methods, *Can J Anaesth* 34:474, 1987.

65. Alessi DM, Berci G: Aspiration and nasogastric intubation, *Otolaryngology* 94:486, 1986.

66. Sellick BA: Cricoid pressure to control regurgitation of stomach contents during induction of anaesthesia, *Lancet* 2:404, 1961.

67. Stept WJ, Safar P: Rapid induction/intubation for prevention of gastric-content aspiration, *Anesth Analg* 49:633, 1970.

68. Marco AP, Furman WR: Anesthetic problems: venous air embolism, airway difficulties, and massive transfusion, *Surg Clin N Am* 73:213, 1993.

69. Vanner RG, O'Dwyer JP, Pryle BJ et al: Upper oesophageal sphincter pressure and the effect of cricoid pressure, *Anaesthesia* 47:95, 1992.

70. Ciresi SA: Gastrointestinal pharmacology review and anesthetic application to the combat casualty, *Military Med* 154:555, 1989.

71. Nimmo WS: Aspiration of gastric contents, *Br J Hosp Med* 34:176, 1985.

72. Rabey PG, Murphy PJ, Langton JA et al: Effect of the laryngeal mask airway on the lower oesophageal sphincter during anaesthesia, *Br J Anaesth* 68:404P, 1992.

73. Barish CF, Wu WC, Castell DO: Respiratory complications of gastroesophageal reflux, *Arch Intern Med* 145:1882, 1985.

74. McCammon RL: Prophylaxis for aspiration pneumonitis, *Can Anaesth Soc S* 33:S47, 1986.

75. Randell T, Saarvinaara L, Oikkonen M et al: Oral atropine enhances the risk for acid aspiration in children, *Acta Anaesthesiol Scand* 35:651, 1991.

76. Todd JG, Nimmo WS: Effect of premedication on drug absorption and gastric emptying, *Br J Anaesth* 55:1189, 1983.

77. Cohen SE, Jasson J, Talafre M-L et al: Does metoclopramide decrease the volume of gastric contents in patients undergoing cesarean section? *Anesthesiology* 61:604, 1984.

78. Shaughnessy AF: Potential uses for metoclopramide, Drug Intell Clin Pharm 19:723, 1985.

79. Manchikanti L, Grow JB, Colliver JA et al: Bicitra (sodium

citrate) and metoclopramide in outpatient anesthesia for prophylaxis against aspiration pneumonitis, *Anesthesiology* 63:378, 1985.

80. Christensen S, Farrow-Gillespie A, Lerman J: Effects of ranitidine and metoclopramide on gastric fluid pH and volume in children, *Br J Anaesth* 65:456, 1990.

81. Orr DA, Bill KM, Gillon KRW et al: Effects of omeprazole, with and without metoclopramide, in elective obstetric anaesthesia, *Anaesthesia* 48:114, 1993.

82. Kuster M, Naji P, Gabi K et al: Die intraoperative, direkte und kontinuierliche pH-messung im magen nach vorbehandlung mit ranitidin oder natriumcitrat, *Anaesthesist* 38:59, 1989.

83. Colman RD, Frank M, Loughnan BA et al: Use of i.m. ranitidine for the prophylaxis of aspiration pneumonitis in obstetrics, *Br J Anaesth* 61:720, 1988.

84. Joyce TH: Prophylaxis for pulmonary acid aspiration, *Am J Med* 83(Suppl 6A):46, 1987.

85. Ormezzano X, Francois TP, Viaud J-Y et al: Aspiration pneumonitis prophylaxis in obstetric anaesthesia: comparison of effervescent cimetidine-sodium citrate mixture and sodium citrate, *Br J Anaesth* 64:503, 1990.

86. Papadimitriou L, Kandiloros A, Lakiotis K et al: Protecting against the acid aspiration syndrome in adult patients undergoing emergency surgery, *Hepato gastroenterol* 39:560, 1992.

87. Ganansia MF, Bouyer L, Guillet JC et al: Aspiration pneumonia prophylaxis: use of oral effervescent cimetidine in obstetric anesthesia, *Anesth Analg* 67:S69, 1988.

88. Bouly A, Nathan N, Feiss P: Comparison of omeprazole with cimetidine for prophylaxis of acid aspiration in elective surgery, *Eur J Anaesth* 10:209, 1993.

89. Smith CL, Bardgett DM, Hunter JM: Haemodynamic effects of the i.v. administration or ranitidine in the critically ill patient, *Br J Anaesth* 59:1397, 1987.

90. Rout CC, Rocke DA, Gouws E: Intravenous ranitidine reduces the risk of acid aspiration of gastric contents at emergency cesarean section, *Anesth Analg* 76:156, 1993.

91. McAllister JD, Moote CA, Sharpe MD et al: Random double-blind comparison of nizatidine, famotidine, ranitidine, and placebo, *Can J Anaesth* 37(4, Pt 2):S22, 1990.

92. Sandhar BK, Goresky GV, Maltby JR et al: Effect of oral liquids and ranitidine on gastric fluid volume and pH in children undergoing outpatient surgery, *Anesthesiology* 71:327, 1989.

93. Goudsouzian NG, Young ET: The efficacy of ranitidine in children, *Acta Anaesthesiol Scand* 31:387, 1987.

94. Vila P, Valles J, Canet J et al: Acid aspiration prophylaxis in morbidly obese patients: famotidine vs. ranitidine, *Anaesthesia* 46:967, 1991.

95. Maltby JR, Elliott RH, Warnell I et al: Gastric fluid volume and pH in elective surgical patients: triple prophylaxis is not superior to ranitidine alone, *Can J Anaesth* 37:650, 1990.

96. Ewart MC, Yau G, Gin T et al: A comparison of the effects of omeprazole and ranitidine on gastric secretion in women undergoing elective caesarean section, *Anaesthesia* 45:527, 1990.

97. McAuley DM, Moore J, McCaughey W et al: Ranitidine as an antacid before elective Caesarean section, *Anaesthesia* 38:108, 1983.

98. Yau G, Kan AF, Gin T et al: A comparison of omeprazole and ranitidine for prophylaxis against aspiration pneumonitis in emergency caesarean section, *Anaesthesia* 47:101, 1992.

99. Moore J, Flynn RJ, Sampaio M et al: Effect of single-dose omeprazole on intragastric acidity and volume during obstetric anaesthesia, *Anaesthesia* 44:559, 1989.

100. Wingtin LN, Glomaud D, Hardy F et al: Omeprazole for prophylaxis of acid aspiration in elective surgery, *Anaesthesia* 45:436, 1990.

101. Ellmauer S: Prophylaxe und therapie des saure-aspirations-syndroms, *Anaesthesist* 36:599, 1987.

102. Zucker AR, Holm BA, Crawford GP et al: PEEP is necessary for exogenous surfactant to reduce pulmonary edema in canine aspiration pneumonitis, *J Appl Physiol* 73:679, 1992.

103. Nagase T, Fukuchi Y, Teramoto S et al: Intravenous bolus of prednisolone decreases 15-hydroxyeicosatetraenoic acid formation in the rat model of acid aspiration, *Crit Care Med* 19:950, 1991.

104. Robertson C: A review of the use of corticosteroids in the management of pulmonary injuries and insults, *Arch Emerg Med* 2:59, 1985.

Part IV

THE AIRWAY
TECHNIQUES

Chapter 11

OXYGEN DELIVERY SYSTEMS, INHALATION THERAPY, AND RESPIRATORY THERAPY

Jeffrey S. Vender
Mary V. Clemency

I. INTRODUCTION

Many patients suffer from acute and chronic dysfunction of the cardiopulmonary system. Appropriate management of the surgical and critical care patient necessitates an understanding of both prophylactic and therapeutic techniques to support gas exchange and pulmonary function. Oxygen therapy is one of the most commonly employed medical interventions. An understanding of the oxygen delivery systems and devices is essential for optimal care. Bronchial hygiene is now a cornerstone in prophylactic care of the perioperative surgical patient. The bronchial hygiene techniques employed are supportive of the natural cough mechanism. Finally, any medications that are specifically intended to treat pulmonary pathophysiology can be delivered by inhalation therapy with both greater efficiency and less toxicity than oral or parenteral methods. This chapter is an overview of the various procedures and techniques employed in the respiratory care of our patients.

II. OXYGEN THERAPY
A. INDICATIONS

Oxygen (O_2) is one of the most common therapeutic substances used in the practice of critical care medicine. This section reviews some of the indications, goals, and modes of O_2 therapy in the adult patient.

Treatment or prevention of hypoxemia is the most common indication for O_2 therapy, and the final goal of effective treatment is the avoidance or resolution of tissue hypoxia. Tissue hypoxia exists when delivery of O_2 is inadequate to meet the metabolic demands of the tissues. O_2 content (Box 11-1) depends on the arterial partial pressure of O_2 (Pao_2), the hemoglobin concentration of arterial blood, and the saturation of hemoglobin with O_2. O_2 delivery (Do_2) is calculated by multiplying cardiac output (L per minute) by the arterial O_2 content. Do_2 is measured in mL O_2 per minute and, for a 70-kg healthy patient, is approximately 1000 (Box 11-2).

Hypoxia may result from a decrement of any of the determinants of Do_2, including anemia, low cardiac output, hypoxemia, or abnormal hemoglobin affinity (e.g., carbon monoxide toxicity). Hypoxia also may arise from a failure of O_2 utilization at the tissue level (e.g., the microvascular perfusion defect of shock) or even at the cell itself (e.g., cyanide poisoning).

Aerobic metabolism requires a balance between Do_2 and O_2 consumption. Breathing-enriched inspired concentrations of O_2 may increase the Pao_2, the percentage of saturation of hemoglobin, and O_2 content, thereby augmenting Do_2 until the underlying cause of the hypoxia can be corrected (e.g., transfusing the anemic patient). The clinical situation in which O_2 therapy is most effective, however, is in the treatment of hypoxemia.

Hypoxemia may be defined as a relative deficiency of O_2 tension in the arterial blood. The most common causes of hypoxemia include true shunt, ventilation-perfusion inequalities, and decreased mixed venous O_2 content Cvo_2).

True intrapulmonary shunting is defined as the condition in which deoxygenated blood from the right heart enters the left heart without the benefit of alveolar gas exchange. True intrapulmonary shunts cause hypoxemia that is poorly responsive to O_2 therapy. The greater the percentage of the cardiac output shunted, the less

---

BOX 11-1   Calculation of arterial oxygen content (Cao_2)

$$Cao_2 = Sao_2 \times Hg \times 1.34 + Pao2 \times 0.0031$$

Cao_2	=	Arterial oxygen content (vol%)
Hg	=	Hemoglobin (g%)
1.34	=	Oxygen-carrying capacity of hemoglobin
Pao_2	=	Arterial partial pressure of oxygen (torr)
0.0031	=	Solubility coefficient of oxygen in plasma

BOX 11-2   Calculation of oxygen delivery (Do_2)

$$Do_2 = Cao_2 \times CO \times 10$$

Cao_2	=	Arterial oxygen content in cc per 100 cc blood (vol%). This value is approximately 20 in the normal adult with a hemoglobin of 15 g%.
CO	=	Cardiac output in l per minute. This value is approxiamtely 5 in the normal 70-kg adult.
Do_2	=	Oxygen delivery in cc per minute. This value is approximately 1000 in the normal 70-kg adult.

---

responsive to O_2 the hypoxemia will be. Therapy for this "oxygen refractory" hypoxemia is aimed at reducing the shunt. Respiratory therapy such as tracheobronchial toilet to remove mucous plugging of a lobar bronchus or adjusting an endotracheal tube that has advanced into a mainstem bronchus may be effective. Positive airway pressure therapy can reduce intrapulmonary shunting in certain disease states associated with a diffuse reduction in functional residual capacity.

Mismatch of ventilation and perfusion (V/Q; shunt effect) causes hypoxemia when mixed venous blood flowing past the alveolar capillary membrane (ACM) takes away O_2 molecules faster than ventilation to that alveolus can replace them. This alveolus receives perfusion in excess of ventilation and is considered an area of "low V/Q." The resultant partial pressure of O_2 in the alveolus (PAo_2) is too low to fully oxygenate the blood flowing past it. When a significant number of the lungs' gas-exchanging units are affected, hypoxemia results.

The easiest way to understand the hypoxemic effect of low PAo_2 is to consider the effect of breathing gas with a subnormal O_2 tension (eg, 100% nitrous oxide). In time, there would be a washout of the O_2 in the alveoli. The PAo_2 would drop and hypoxemia would ensue. Although the critical care clinician is unlikely to encounter this situation, a similar drop in PAo_2 is seen in many other circumstances.

Hypoventilation causes hypoxemia when an increase in alveolar carbon dioxide (CO_2) "crowds out" the oxygen molecules and decreases PAO_2. Clinical entities associated with low PAO_2 include chronic obstructive pulmonary disease (COPD), asthma, retained secretions, sedative or narcotic administration, acute lung injury syndrome, and early or mild pulmonary edema. Breathing enriched inspired concentrations of O_2 under these circumstances increases PAO_2, which increases the O_2 gradient across the alveolar-capillary membrane (ACM), resulting in faster equilibration of mixed venous blood exposed to the ACM and a higher pulmonary venous, left atrial, left ventricular, and arterial PO_2.

Even small increases in inspired O_2 tension can correct hypoxemia when low PAO_2 is the cause. Indeed, drug-induced alveolar hypoventilation resulting in hypoxemia on room air is exquisitely sensitive to increases in inspired O_2 concentration. Appropriate initial management of patients with alteration in mental status includes the use of O_2 therapy, so long as ventilatory needs also are monitored.

Cases of hypoxemia caused by either true shunt of V/Q mismatch share a common phenomenon. Both pathophysiologic mechanisms are enhanced by a decreased mixed venous hemoglobin saturation (low SvO_2). Decreased SvO_2 results in a decreased O_2 content of the mixed venous blood. Low CvO_2 causes hypoxemia by worsening the hypoxemic effect of any existing shunt or areas of low V/Q by presenting more desaturated blood to the left atrium and lowering PaO_2 by binding dissolved O_2 to the desaturated hemoglobin. Decreased CvO_2 arises from low O_2 delivery (e.g., low cardiac output, anemia, or hypoxemia) or increased O_2 consumption (e.g., high fever or increased minute ventilation and work of breathing).

The consequences of untreated hypoxemia include tachycardia and increased myocardial O_2 demand, as well as increased minute volume and work of breathing. By treating hypoxemia, supplemental O_2 restores homeostasis and greatly decreases the stress response and its attendant cardiopulmonary sequelae.

B. OXYGEN DELIVERY SYSTEMS

With the exception of anesthetic breathing circuits, virtually all O_2 delivery systems are nonrebreathing. In nonrebreathing circuits, the inspiratory gas is not made up in any part by the exhaled tidal volume, and the only CO_2 inhaled is that which exists in any entrained room air (RA). In order to avoid rebreathing, exhaled gases must be sequestered by one-way valves and inspired gases must be presented in sufficient volume and flow to allow for the high peak flow rates and minute ventilation demonstrated in critically ill patients. Inspiratory entrainment of RA or the use of inspiratory reservoirs (including the anatomic dead space of the nasopharynx, oropharynx, and non-gas-exchanging portion of the

bronchial tree) and one-way valves typifies nonrebreathing systems and defines them into two groups.[1-3] Low-flow systems depend on inspiration of RA to meet inspiratory flow and volume demands. High-flow systems provide the entire inspiratory atmosphere. High-flow systems use reservoirs or very high flow rates to meet both the large peak inspiratory flow demands and the exaggerated minute volumes found in many critically ill patients.

1. Low-flow oxygen systems

A low-flow–variable-performance system depends on room air (RA) entrainment to meet the patient's peak inspiratory and minute ventilatory demands that are not met by the inspiratory gas flow or oxygen reservoir alone. Low-flow devices include nasal cannulas, simple face masks, partial rebreathing masks, nonrebreathing masks, and tracheostomy collars. Low-flow systems are characterized by the ability to deliver high and low FiO_2. The fraction of inspired oxygen (FiO_2) becomes unpredictable and inconsistent when these devices are used for patients with abnormal or changing ventilatory patterns. Low-flow systems produce FiO_2 values ranging from 21% to 80%. The FiO_2 may vary with the size of the oxygen reservoir, oxygen flow, and the patient's ventilatory pattern (e.g., tidal volume, peak inspiratory flow, respiratory rate, and minute ventilation). With a normal ventilation pattern, these devices can deliver a relatively predictable and consistent FiO_2.

It is imperative to understand and appreciate the fact that low-flow systems do not mean low FiO_2 values. As stated, with changes in tidal volume, respiratory rate, oxygen reservoir size, and so on, the FiO_2 can vary dramatically at comparable oxygen flow rates. The following two examples are theoretical mathematical estimates of an FiO_2 produced by a low-flow system (e.g., nasal cannula) in two different clinical conditions.

The following example for estimation of FiO_2 from a low-flow system is based on the textbook "normal" patient and ventilatory pattern. The following assumptions are used for the FiO_2 calculation: the anatomic reservoir for a nasal cannula consists of nose, nasopharynx, and oropharynx and is approximately one third of the entire normal anatomic dead space (includes trachea)—for example, $1/3 \times 150 \times ml = 50$ ml; a nasal cannula oxygen flow rate of 6 L/min (100 ml/sec); a tidal volume (VT) of 500 ml; a respiratory rate of 20 breaths per minute; inspiratory time (I) of 1 second; and expiratory time (E) of 2 seconds. If the terminal 0.5 seconds of the 2-second expiratory time has negligible gas flow, the anatomic reservoir (50 ml) will completely fill with 100% oxygen, assuming an oxygen flow rate of 100 ml/sec. Using the preceding "normal" variables, the FiO_2 is calculated for a patient with a 500-ml and 250-ml tidal volume.

Example 1

Cannula	6 L/min	V_T, 500 ml
Mechanical reservoir	None	I/E ratio, 1:2
Anatomic reservoir	50 ml	Rate, 20 breaths per min
100% O_2 provided per second	100 ml	Inspiratory time, 1 second
Volume inspired O_2		
Anatomic reservoir	50 ml	
Flow/s	100 ml	
Inspired room air	70 ml	
(0.20 × 350 cc)		
O_2 inspired	220 ml	

$$Fio_2 = \frac{220 \text{ ml } O_2}{500 \text{ ml } V_T} = 0.44$$

Example 2

If V_T is decreased to 250 ml:		
Volume inspired O_2		
Anatomic reservoir	50 ml	
Flow/s	100 ml	
Inspired room air	20 ml	
(0.20 × 100 cc)		
O_2 inspired	170 ml	

$$Fio_2 = \frac{170 \text{ ml } O_2}{250 \text{ ml } V_T} = 0.68$$

The preceding 50% variability in Fio_2 at 6 L/min of oxygen flow clearly demonstrates the effects of a variable ventilatory pattern. In general, the larger the V_T or faster the respiratory rate, the lower the Fio_2. The smaller the V_T or lower the respiratory rate, the higher the Fio_2.

Low-flow oxygen devices are the most commonly employed oxygen delivery systems because of simplicity, ease of use, familiarity, economics, availability, and patient acceptance. In most clinical situations (see High-Flow Oxygen Systems and High-Flow Devices) these systems should be initially employed.

2. High-flow oxygen systems

High-flow–fixed-performance systems are nonrebreathing systems that provide the entire inspiratory atmosphere needed to meet the peak inspiratory flow and minute ventilatory demands of the patient. To meet the patient's peak inspiratory flow, the flow rate and reservoir are very important. Flows in excess of 30 to 40 L/min (or four times the measured minute volume) are often necessary. High-flow devices include aerosol masks and T pieces that are powered by air-entrainment nebulizers or air-oxygen blenders and Venturi masks (see Oxygen Delivery Devices). The advantage of high-flow systems is the ability to deliver predictable, consistent, and measurable high and low Fio_2s, despite the patient's ventilatory pattern, and to control the humidity and temperature of the delivered gases. The primary limitations of these systems are cost, bulkiness, and patient tolerance.

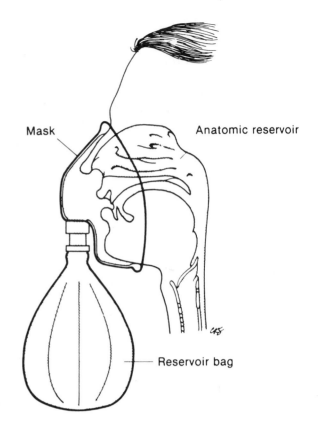

Fig. 11-1. The three reservoirs of low-flow oxygen therapy. (From Vender JS, Clemency MV: Oxygen delivery systems, inhalation therapy, respiratory care. In Benumof JL, editor: *Clinical procedures in anesthesia and intensive care,* Philadelphia, 1992, JB Lippincott.)

There are two primary indications for high-flow oxygen devices:

1. Patients who require a consistent, predictable, minimal Fio_2 to reverse hypoxemia yet prevent hypoventilation because of a dependence on hypoxic ventilatory drive benefit from high-flow oxygen devices.
2. The patient with increased minute ventilation and abnormal respiratory pattern who needs a predictably and consistently high Fio_2 benefits from high-flow oxygen devices.

C. OXYGEN DELIVERY DEVICES

1. Low-flow devices

a. NASAL CANNULAS

Because of their simplicity and the ease with which patients tolerate them, nasal cannulas are the most frequently used oxygen delivery devices. The nasal cannula consists of two prongs, one inserted into each naris, which deliver 100% oxygen. To be effective, the nasal passages must be patent, but the patient need not breathe through the nose. The flow rate settings range from 0.25 to 6 L/min. The nasopharynx serves as the oxygen reservoir (Fig. 11-1). Gases should be humidified

Table 11-1. Approximate F_{IO_2} delivered by nasal cannula*

Flow rate (L/min)	Approximate F_{IO_2}
1	0.24
2	0.28
3	0.32
4	0.36
5	0.40
6	0.44

*Based on normal ventilatory patterns.
F_{IO_2}, Fraction of inspired oxygen.

Table 11-2. Approximate F_{IO_2} delivered by simple face mask*

Flow rate (L/min)	F_{IO_2}
5–6	0.4
6–7	0.5
7–8	0.6

*Based on normal ventilatory patterns.
F_{IO_2}, Fraction of inspired oxygen.

to prevent mucosal drying if the oxygen flow exceeds 4 L/min. For each 1-L/min increase in flow, the F_{IO_2} is assumed to increase 4% (Table 11-1).

Thus, an F_{IO_2} of 0.24 to 0.44 can be delivered predictably if the patient breathes at a normal minute ventilation rate with a normal respiratory pattern. Increasing flows to greater than 6 L/min does not significantly increase the F_{IO_2} above 0.44 and is often poorly tolerated by the patient.

The components needed for nasal cannula assembly include nasal cannula prongs, delivery tubing, adjustable restraining headband, and oxygen flowmeter to provide a controlled gas delivery from a wall outlet; a humidification system increases patient comfort at higher flows (4 L/min or more).

Procedurally, the initiation of any oxygen therapy should be preceded by a review of the chart and documentation of the oxygen concentration and device ordered. If a humidifier is used, it should be filled to the appropriate level with sterile water and connected to the flowmeter.

The nasal prong should be secured in the patient's naris, and the cannula secured around the patient's head by a restraining strap.

Avoidance of undue cutaneous pressure is essential. Gauze may be needed to pad pressure points around the cheeks and ears during prolonged use. The flowmeter should be adjusted to the prescribed liter flow to attain the desired F_{IO_2} (see Table 11-1).

Although nasal cannulas are simple and safe, several potential hazards and complications do exist. Oxygen supports combustion, and any type of oxygen therapy is a fire hazard. Nasal trauma from prolonged use of or pressure from the nasal prongs can cause tissue damage. With poorly humidified, high gas flows, dehydration of the airway mucosal surface can occur. This mucosal dehydration can result in mucosal irritation, nosebleeds, laryngitis, earache, substernal chest pain, and bronchospasm.[1,2,4] Finally, because this is a low-flow system, it is imperative to remember the F_{IO_2} can be inaccurate and inconsistent, leading to the potential for underoxygen-

ation and overoxygenation. This problem is of special concern with overoxygenation in COPD patients with increased hypoxic drive to breathe. Underoxygenation potentiates any problems associated with hypoxemia.

b. SIMPLE FACE MASK

To provide a higher F_{IO_2} than that provided by nasal cannula with low-flow systems, the size of the oxygen reservoir must increase (Fig. 11-1). A simple face mask consists of a mask with two side ports. The mask serves as an additional 100 to 200 ml oxygen reservoir. The sideports allow RA entrainment and exit for exhaled gases. The mask has no valves. An F_{IO_2} of 0.40 to 0.60 can be achieved predictably when patients exhibit normal respiratory patterns. Gas flows greater than 8 L/min do not significantly increase the F_{IO_2} above 0.60 because the oxygen reservoir is filled. A minimum flow of 5 L/min is necessary to prevent CO_2 accumulation and rebreathing. The actual delivered oxygen is dependent on the ventilatory pattern of the patient, similar to the situation with nasal cannulas.

The equipment needed is identical to that used for nasal cannula oxygen administration. The only difference is the use of a face mask. The predicted F_{IO_2} can be estimated from the oxygen flow rate (Table 11-2). Appropriate mask application is needed with all masks to maximize the F_{IO_2} and patient comfort. The mask should be positioned over the nasal bridge and on the forehead, restricting oxygen escape into the patient's eye, which can cause ocular drying and irritation. The use of face masks has the added risk of aspiration because of concealed vomitus. If F_{IO_2} values above 0.60 are required, a partial rebreathing mask, nonrebreathing mask, or high-flow system should be employed. All oxygen devices that deliver higher F_{IO_2} increase the potential of oxygen toxicity (see Complications).

c. PARTIAL REBREATHING MASK

To deliver an F_{IO_2} above 60% with a low-flow system, the oxygen reservoir system must be increased (Fig. 11-1).[1] A partial rebreathing mask adds a reservoir bag with a 600- to 1000-ml capacity. Side ports allow entrainment of RA and the exit of exhaled gases. The distinctive feature of this mask is that the first 33% of the patient's exhaled volume fills the reservoir bag. This volume is from the anatomic dead space and contains

Table 11-3. Approximate Fio_2 delivered by mask with reservoir bag*

Flow rate (L/min)	Fio_2
6	0.6
7	0.7
8	0.8
9	0.8+
10	0.8+

*Based on normal ventilatory patterns.
Fio_2, Fraction of inspired oxygen.

little carbon dioxide. During inspiration the bag should not completely collapse. A deflated reservoir bag will result in a decreased Fio_2 because of entrained RA. With the next breath, the first exhaled gas (which is in the reservoir bag) plus fresh gas are inhaled—thus the name partial rebreather. Fresh gas flows should equal or exceed 8 L/min, and the reservoir bag must remain inflated during the entire ventilatory cycle to ensure the highest Fio_2 and adequate carbon dioxide evacuation. Fio_2 varies, depending on the flow rate (Table 11-3). An Fio_2 of 0.60 to 0.80+ can be delivered with this device if the mask is applied appropriately and the ventilatory pattern is normal. This mask's rebreathing capacity allows oxygen conservation and thus may be useful during transportation, when oxygen supply may be limited. Complications with partial rebreathing oxygen delivery systems are similar to those with other mask devices with low-flow systems.

d. NONREBREATHING MASK

A nonrebreathing mask (Fig. 11-2) is similar to a partial rebreathing mask but adds three unidirectional valves. One valve is located on each side of the mask to permit the venting of exhaled gases and prevent RA entrainment. The third unidirectional valve is situated between the mask and the reservoir bag and prevents exhaled gases from entering the bag.

The bag must be inflated throughout the ventilatory cycle to ensure the highest Fio_2 and adequate carbon dioxide evacuation. Typically, the Fio_2 is 0.80 to 0.90+. Fresh gas flow is usually 15 L/min (range, 10 to 15 L/min). If room air is not entrained, an Fio_2 approaching 1.0 can be achieved. If fresh gas flows do not meet ventilatory needs, many masks have a spring-loaded tension valve that permits RA entrainment if the reservoir evacuates. This is often needed to meet the increased inspiratory drive of critically ill patients. This spring valve is often called a safety valve. The spring valve tension should be periodically checked. If such a valve is not present, one of the unidirectional valves on the mask should be removed to allow RA entrainment if needed to meet ventilatory demands. If the total ventilatory needs are met without RA entrainment, the rebreathing mask performs like a high-flow system. The operational application of a nonrebreathing mask is similar to that of other mask devices. To optimize the system, the mask should fit snugly (without excessive pressure) to avoid air entrainment around the mask, which would dilute the delivered gas and lower the Fio_2. If the mask fit is appropriate, the reservoir bag will respond to the patient's inspiratory efforts. The high flows often employed increase the potential for several problems. Gastric distention, cutaneous irritation, and distention of the venting valves in the open position allowing RA entrainment can all occur with excessive gas flows.

e. TRACHEOSTOMY COLLARS

Tracheostomy collars are used primarily to deliver humidity to patients with artificial airways. Oxygen may be delivered with these devices, but as with the nasal cannula, the Fio_2 is unpredictable, inconsistent, and dependent on ventilatory pattern.

2. High-flow devices

a. VENTURI MASKS

As discussed earlier, high-flow systems have flow rates and reservoirs large enough to provide the total inspired gases reliably. Most high-flow systems use gas entrainment to provide the flow and Fio_2 needs. Venturi masks entrain air via the Bernoulli principle and constant pressure-jet mixing.[5] This physical phenomenon is based on a rapid velocity of gas (e.g., oxygen) moving through a restricted orifice. This produces viscous shearing forces, which create a decreased pressure gradient (subatmospheric) downstream relative to the surrounding gases. This pressure gradient causes room air to be entrained until the pressures are equalized. Fig. 11-3 illustrates the Venturi principle.

By altering the gas orifice or entrainment port size, the Fio_2 will vary. The oxygen flow rate determines the total volume of gas provided by the device. It provides predictable and reliable Fio_2 values of 0.24 to 0.50 that are independent of the patient's respiratory pattern.

These masks come in the following varieties:

1. A fixed Fio_2 model, which requires specific inspiratory attachments that are color-coded and have labeled jets that produce a known Fio_2 with a given flow.
2. A variable Fio_2 model (Fig. 11-4), which has a graded adjustment of the air entrainment port that can be set to allow variation in delivered Fio_2.

To use any air entrainment device properly to control the Fio_2, the standard air-oxygen entrainment ratios and minimum recommended flows for a given Fio_2 must be used (Table 11-4). The minimum total flow requirement should result from entrained RA added to the fresh oxygen flow and equal three to four times the minute ventilation. This minimal flow is required to meet the

Non-Rebreathing Oxygen Mask

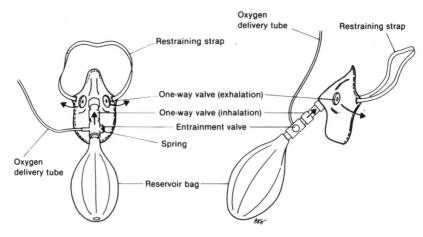

Fig. 11-2. A nonrebreathing oxygen mask. In addition to the exhalation valve, the mask has a one-way inhalation valve. (From Vender JS, Clemency MV: Oxygen delivery systems, inhalation therapy, respiratory care. In Benumof JL, editor: *Clinical procedures in anesthesia and intensive care,* Philadelphia, 1992, JB Lippincott.)

Venturi Principle

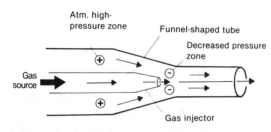

Fig. 11-3. Illustration of the Venturi principle. (From Vender JS, Clemency MV: Oxygen delivery systems, inhalation therapy, respiratory care. In Benumof JL, editor: *Clinical procedures in anesthesia and intensive care,* Philadelphia, 1992, JB Lippincott.)

patient's peak inspiratory flow demands. As the desired FiO_2 increases, the air-oxygen entrainment ratio decreases with a net reduction in total gas flow. Therefore the higher the desired FiO_2, the greater the probability of the patient's needs exceeding the total flow capabilities of the device.

Venturi masks are often useful when treating COPD patients who depend on hypoxic ventilatory drive and accurate FiO_2s.[6] The Venturi mask's ability to deliver a high flow with no particulate H_2O makes it beneficial in treating asthmatics in whom bronchospasm may be precipitated or exacerbated by aerosolized H_2O administration.

Several specific concerns regarding the application of a Venturi mask must be recognized to provide appropriate function. Obstructions distal to the jet orifice can produce back pressure and an effect referred to as "Venturi stall." When this occurs, RA entrainment is compromised, causing a decreased total gas flow and an increased FiO_2. Occlusion or alteration of the exhalation ports could also produce this situation. Aerosol devices should not be used with these devices. Water droplets can occlude the oxygen injector. If humidity is needed, a vapor-type humidity adapter collar should be used.

b. AEROSOL MASKS AND T PIECES WITH NEBULIZERS OR AIR-OXYGEN BLENDERS

FiO_2 greater than 0.40 with a high-flow system are best provided by large-volume nebulizers and wide-bore tubing. Aerosol masks, in conjunction with air entrainment nebulizers or air-oxygen blenders, deliver consistent and predictable FiO_2s, regardless of the patient's ventilatory pattern. A T piece is used in place of an aerosol mask for patients with an artificial airway.

Air entrainment nebulizers can deliver FiO_2s of 0.35 to 1.00 and produce an aerosol. The maximum gas flow through the nebulizer is 14 to 16 L/min. Similar to the Venturi masks, less room air is entrained with higher FiO_2s. As a result, total flow at high FiO_2s is decreased. To meet ventilatory demands, two nebulizers may feed a single mask to increase the total flow, and a short length of corrugated tubing may be added to the aerosol mask side ports to increase the reservoir capacity (Fig. 11-5). If the aerosol mist exiting the mask side ports disappears during inspiration, room air is probably being entrained and flow should be increased.

Circuit resistance can increase from water accumulation or kinking of the aerosol tubing. The increased pressure at the Venturi device decreases RA entrainment, increases FiO_2, and decreases total gas flow. Thus, if a predictable FiO_2 above 0.40 is desired, an air-oxygen blender should be used. Air-oxygen blenders can deliver consistent and accurate FiO_2s from 0.21 to 1.0 and flows

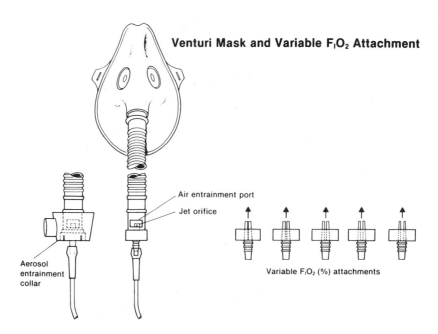

Fig. 11-4. Air entrainment Ventimask. Specific Fio_2 levels are provided by the various jet orifices. (From Vender JS, Clemency MV: Oxygen delivery systems, inhalation therapy, respiratory care. In Benumof JL, editor: *Clinical procedures in anesthesia and intensive care,* Philadelphia, 1992, JB Lippincott.)

Table 11-4. Approximate air entrainment ratio and gas flow (Fio_2)*

Fio_2 (%)	Ratio	Recommended O₂ flow (L/min)	Total gas flow (to port) (L/min)
24	25.3:1	3	79
26	14.8:1	3	47
28	10.3:1	6	68
30	7.8:1	6	53
35	4.6:1	9	50
40	3.2:1	12	50
50	1.7:1	15	41

*Varies with manufacturer.
Fio_2, Fraction of inspired oxygen.

of up to 100 L/min. The higher flows tend to produce excessive noise through the long-bore tubing. They usually are used in conjunction with humidifiers. Air-oxygen blenders are recommended for patients with increased minute ventilation who require a high Fio_2 and for whom bronchospasm may be precipitated or worsened by a nebulized H_2O aerosol.

With artificial airway, a 15- to 20-inch reservoir tube should be added to the Briggs T piece (Hudson, RCI, Temecula, Ca.) to prevent the potential of entraining air into the system.

D. HUMIDIFIERS

Humidity is the water vapor in a gas. When air is 100% saturated at 37° C, it contains 43.8 mg H_2O/L. The amount of water vapor a volume of gas contains depends on the temperature and water availability. The vapor pressure exerted by the water vapor is equal to 47 mm Hg. Alveolar gases are 100% saturated at 37° C. When the inspired atmosphere contains less than 43.8 mg H_2O/L or has a vapor pressure below 47 mm Hg, a gradient exists between the respiratory mucosa and the inhaled gas. This gradient causes water to leave the mucosa and to humidify the inhaled gas.

Room air that has relative humidity of 50% at 21° C has a relative humidity of 21% at 37° C. Under normal conditions the lungs contribute approximately 250 ml/ H_2O per day to saturate inspired air 100%.[1]

The administration of dry oxygen lowers the water content of the inspired air. The upper respiratory tract filters, humidifies, and warms inspired gases. Nasal breathing is more efficient than oral breathing for conditioning inspired gases. The use of an artificial airway bypasses the nasopharynx and oropharynx, where a significant amount of warming and humidification of inspired gases is accomplished. As a result, oxygen administration and the use of artificial airways increase the demand on the lungs to humidify the inspired gases.

This increased demand ultimately leads to mucosal drying, inspissated secretions, and decreased mucociliary clearance. This can eventually result in bacterial infections, atelectasis, and pneumonia. To prevent these complications, a humidifier or nebulizer should be used to increase the water content of the inspired gases.

Indications for humidity therapy include high-flow

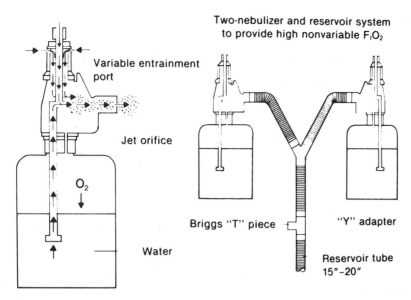

Fig. 11-5. Single-unit and double (tandem)-unit mechanical aerosol systems. (From Vender JS, Clemency MV: In Benumof JL, editor: *Clinical procedures in anesthesia and intensive care,* Philadelphia, 1992, JB Lippincott.)

therapeutic gas delivery to nonintubated patients, delivery of gases via artificial airways, and reduction of airway resistance in asthma. It is generally accepted that low flows (1 to 4 L/min) do not need humidification except in specific individuals and that all O_2 delivered to infants be humidified.

A humidifier increases the water vapor, either heated or unheated, in a gas. This can be accomplished by passing gas over heated water (heated passover humidifier), by fractionating gas into tiny bubbles as gas passes through water (bubble diffusion or jet humidifiers), by allowing gas to pass through a chamber that contains a heated, water-saturated wick (heated wick humidifier), and by vaporizing water and selectively allowing the vapor to mix with the inspired gases (vapor-phase humidifier). Other variations of humidification systems exist but are beyond the scope of this chapter.[7]

Bubble humidifiers can be used with nasal cannulas, simple face masks, partial and nonrebreathing masks, and air-oxygen blenders. They increase the relative humidity of gas from 0% to 70% at 25° C, which is approximately equal to 34% at 37° C.[8,9] Large-volume bubble-through humidifiers are available for use with ventilator circuits or high-gas-flow delivery systems.

A heated humidifier should be used when delivering dry gases to patients with endotracheal tubes, since it allows delivery of gases with an increased water content and relative humidity exceeding 65% at 37° C. When heated humidifiers are used, proximal airway temperature should be monitored to ensure a gas temperature that allows maximum moisture-carrying capacity yet prevents mucosal burns.

Heat and moisture exchangers (HME) are simple, small humidifier systems designed to be attached to an artificial airway. The HMEs are often referred to as an "artificial nose." The efficiency of these devices is quite variable depending on the HME design, tidal volume, and atmospheric conditions. HMEs are typically used for short-term ventilatory support and for humidification during anesthesia. Several noted contraindications include neonatal and small pediatric patients; copious secretions; significant spontaneous breathing, in which the patient's tidal volume exceeds the HME specifications; and large-volume losses through a bronchopleural fistula or leakage around the endotracheal tube.[7]

A nebulizer increases the water content of the inspired gas by generating aerosols (small droplets of particulate water) that become incorporated into the delivered gas stream and then evaporate into the inspired gas as it is warmed in the respiratory tract. There are two basic kinds of nebulizers, pneumatic and electric. Pneumatic nebulizers operate from a pressured gas source and are either jet or hydrodynamic. Electric nebulizers are powered by an electrical source and are referred to as "ultrasonic." There are several varieties of both types of nebulizers, and they depend more on design differences than on the power source. A more in-depth discussion of nebulizers is available elsewhere.[1,4] The resultant humidity ranges from 50% to 100% at 37° C, depending on the device used. If heated, the relative humidity of the gas can exceed 100% at 37° C. Air entrainment nebulizers are used in conjunction with aerosol masks and T pieces.

There are three general purposes for aerosol therapy. First, aerosol therapy increases the particulate and molecular water content of the inspired gases. The aerosol increases the water content of desiccated and retained secretions, enhancing bronchial hygiene. This does not alleviate the need for systemic hydration. Second, delivery of medications is a primary indication for aerosol therapy, for example, β-2-agonists, corticosteroids, anticholinergics, and antiviral-bacterial agents (see Inhalation Therapy). Third, aerosol therapy has also been employed for sputum inductions. The success of aerosol therapy depends on proper technique of administration and an appropriate indication for use.

The aerosol generated by the nebulizer can precipitate bronchospasm of hyperactive airways.[1,2] Prophylactic bronchodilator therapy should be entertained prior to or during the aerosol treatment. Fluid accumulation and overload have been reported. These are more common in pediatrics and with continuous or ultrasonic rather than intermittent or jet therapy. Dry secretions are hydrophilic and can swell because of the absorbed water content. If secretions swell, they can obstruct airways. Mobilization of secretions limits this problem. Aerosol therapy for drug delivery has been reported to precipitate the same side effects as systemic drug delivery. Therapeutic aerosols have been implicated in nosocomial infections.[10] Cross-contamination between patients must be avoided.

E. MANUAL RESUSCITATION BAGS

Manual resuscitation bags are used primarily for resuscitation and manual ventilation of ventilator-dependent patients. These bags can deliver FiO_2 above 0.90 and tidal volumes up to 800 ml when oxygen flows to the bag are 10 to 15 ml/min. Factors that promote the highest FiO_2s include the use of an oxygen reservoir, connection to an oxygen source, and slow rates of ventilation that allow the bag to refill completely. Positive end-expiratory pressure (PEEP) valves should be used for patients who require more than 5 cm H_2O PEEP. Be aware of differing capabilities among various resuscitation bags in delivery of maximum FiO_2.[11-13]

F. COMPLICATIONS

Complications related to oxygen delivery can be divided into two groups: complications related to the oxygen delivery systems (see sections that discuss the specific devices) and pathophysiologic complications related to oxygen therapy.

Pathophysiologic complications related to oxygen therapy can lead to serious consequences. The three major complications encountered in adults are hypoventilation, absorption atelectasis, and oxygen toxicity.

Hypoventilation that is related to oxygen therapy is peculiar to COPD patients who rely on hypoxic ventilatory drive. They typically have a chronically elevated arterial carbon dioxide tension ($PaCO_2$), a normal pH, and a $PaCO_2$ usually below 60 mm Hg. Because the increased $PaCO_2$ is compensated by an increased bicarbonate ion concentration in the arterial blood and the cerebral spinal fluid, the patient may become desensitized to ventilatory stimulation from changes in the $PaCO_2$. Instead, the chemoreceptors in the aortic and carotid bodies control ventilation. They are sensitive to $PaCO_2$ below 60 mm Hg. When worsening hypoxemia is treated with supplemental oxygen, the goal is to raise the $PaCO_2$ just to the patient's chronic level. Thus the minimum FiO_2 needed to accomplish this goal should be delivered. If oxygen administration raises the $PaCO_2$ above this level, the patient's hypoxic drive is blunted and hypoventilation can result. If hypoventilation is not reversed rapidly, respiratory failure necessitating mechanical ventilation ensues.

Absorption atelectasis occurs when high alveolar oxygen concentrations cause alveolar collapse. Nitrogen, already at equilibrium, remains within the alveoli and "splints" alveoli open. When high FiO_2 are administered, nitrogen is washed out of the alveoli, which then are filled primarily with oxygen. In areas of the lung with reduced ventilation-perfusion ratios, oxygen will be absorbed into the blood faster than ventilation can replace it. The affected alveoli become smaller and smaller until surface tension becomes so great as to cause their collapse. Progressively higher fractions of inspired oxygen above 0.50 cause absorption atelectasis in normal individuals. Fractions of inspired oxygen of 0.50 or more may precipitate this phenomenon in patients with decreased ventilation-perfusion ratios.

The third pathophysiologic complication of oxygen therapy, oxygen toxicity, becomes clinically important after 8 to 12 hours of exposure to a high FiO_2. Oxygen toxicity probably results from direct exposure of the alveoli to a high FiO_2. Normal lungs appear to tolerate FiO_2s of less than 0.6. In damaged lungs FiO_2s greater than 0.50 can result in toxic alveolar oxygen concentration. Since most oxygen therapy is delivered at 1 atm barometric pressure, the FiO_2 and the duration of exposure become the determining factors in the development of most clinically significant oxygen toxicity.

The mechanism of oxygen toxicity is related to the significantly higher production of oxygen free radicals including superoxide anions (O_2^-), hydroxyl radicals (OH^-), hydrogen peroxide (H_2O_2), and single oxygen. These radicals affect cell function by inactivating sulfhydryl enzymes, disrupting DNA synthesis, and disrupting cell membranes' integrity. Vitamin E, superoxide dismutase, and sulfhydryl compounds promote normal, protective free-radical scavenging within the lung. During periods of lung tissue hyperoxia, these protective mechanisms are overwhelmed and toxicity results.[14]

The classic clinical manifestations of oxygen toxicity include cough, substernal chest pain, dyspnea, rales, pulmonary edema, progressive arterial hypoxemia, bilateral pulmonary infiltrates, decreasing lung compliance, and atelectasis. These signs and symptoms are nonspecific; thus oxygen toxicity is frequently difficult to distinguish from severe underlying pulmonary disease. Often, only subtle progression of arterial hypoxemia heralds the onset of pulmonary oxygen toxicity.

On pathologic study there are two distinct phases of classic oxygen toxicity. The early, or exudative, phase, observed during the first 24 to 48 hours, is characterized by the destruction of type I pneumocytes and the development of interstitial and intraalveolar hemorrhage and edema. The late or proliferative phase, which begins after 72 hours, is characterized by resorption of early infiltrates, hyperplasia, and proliferation of type II pneumocytes and increased collagen synthesis. Once oxygen toxicity progresses to the proliferative stage, permanent lung damage may result from scarring and fibrosis.

The treatment for oxygen toxicity is prevention. Oxygen therapy should be directed at improving oxygenation with the minimum FiO_2 needed to obtain an SaO_2 of greater than 90%. Inhalation treatments and raised expiratory airway pressure may be useful adjuncts in improving pulmonary toilet, decreasing V/Q mismatch, and improving arterial oxygenation and may be used to maintain adequate oxygenation at an FiO_2 of 0.50 or less.

III. TECHNIQUES OF RESPIRATORY CARE

The provision of adequate pulmonary gas exchange is implicit in our teaching and management of respiratory care. For optimal gas exchange to occur, the airways must be maintained clear of foreign material (secretions). The various therapeutic techniques available are aimed at the mobilization and removal of pulmonary secretions. In addition, various therapies are intended to optimize breathing efficiency.

Critically ill patients have multiple factors contributing to the presence of increased secretion. Alterations in the mucociliary escalator system due to smoking, stress, high FiO_2s, anesthesia, foreign bodies in the trachea (e.g., endotracheal tube), various tracheobronchial diseases, and abnormalities in mucus production are all recognized contributors to retention of airway secretions. To help compensate for these deficiencies, the patient must be able to promote an adequate cough. In the critically ill patient or the individual with an artificial airway, an adequate cough is often absent. If any of these problems is present, there will be an increased tendency to retain secretions.

Retained secretions promote several potential complications. Occlusion of the airway promotes ventilation-perfusion inequalities and eventually absorption atelectasis. This produces a progressively worse hypoxemia that is less responsive to oxygen therapy (see Indications, in Oxygen Delivery Systems). Retained secretions and distal airway occlusion promote an increased incidence of stasis pneumonia. In addition, retained secretions increase the patient's work of breathing because of an increased airway resistance associated with the airway inflammation and partial airway occlusion and result in a reduced pulmonary compliance because of the atelectasis and reduced lung volumes.

Many of the fundamental practices of respiratory care are aimed at the provision of optimal airway care, tracheobronchial toilet, and the prevention and management of retained secretions. Because dehydration is a common cause of retained secretions, adequate hydration and humidification of gas delivery are essential. Humidity and aerosol therapy were discussed in the oxygen (gas) delivery section of this chapter. The remainder of this section addresses other techniques commonly employed in respiratory care. These include airway suctioning, chest physical therapy, and incentive spirometry. Intermittent positive pressure breathing (IPPB) is discussed separately, since it is used for both the promotion of tracheobronchial toilet and the delivery of medication (see Inhalation Therapy).

A. SUCTIONING

Airway suctioning is commonly employed in respiratory care to promote optimal tracheobronchial toilet and airway patency in critically ill patients. Because of the "perceived" simplicity and limited complications, airway suctioning is frequently employed. If proper indications and technique are not appreciated, however, the potential for significant complications does exist!

1. Indications

Suctioning of the airway should not be done without appropriate clinical indications. The audible (auscultatory) or visible presence of airway secretions is the most common indication. Increasing peak inspiratory pressures in mechanically ventilated patients are often indicative of retained secretions. "Routine" prophylactic suctioning is unwarranted except in neonates, in whom the small airway diameters can be acutely obstructed by a small accumulation of secretions.

In addition to removal of secretions, suction catheters are employed as aids in evaluating airway patency. If an artificial airway appears to be occluded, an attempt to pass a lubricated suction catheter can help assess airway patency. Several causes of artificial airway occlusion include mucous plugging, foreign body obstructions, kinking, and cuff herniations. If the suction catheter cannot be passed and ventilation is obstructed, several successive maneuvers are advisable. The cuff should be deflated and the airway repositioned; if improvement is

Side and End Holes of Suction Catheters

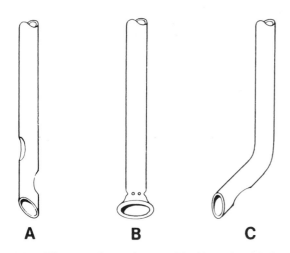

A   B   C

Fig. 11-6. Three suction catheters with side and end holes. **A,** Conventional catheter. **B,** Argyle Aero-Flow catheter (distal orifice and multiple side holes; flared end decreases tissue trauma but increases insertion difficulty). **C,** Coudé angle-tipped catheter (increases cannulation of left mainstem bronchus). (From Vender JS, Clemency MV. In Benumof JL, editor: *Clinical procedures in anesthesia and intensive care,* Philadelphia, 1992, JB Lippincott.)

inadequate, the airway should be provided by air-mask-bag unit (AMBU) and the artificial airway should be replaced.

The actual provision of airway suctioning depends on an appreciation of the available equipment, the appropriate techniques, and the potential complications.

2. Equipment

Numerous commercial suction catheters exist.[1,2,15] The ideal catheter is one that optimizes secretion removal and minimizes tissue trauma. Several specific features of the catheters include the material of construction, frictional resistance, size (length and diameter), shape, and position of the aspirating holes. An opening at the proximal end of the catheter to allow the entrance of room air, neutralizing the vacuum without disconnecting the vacuum apparatus, is ideal. The proximal hole should be larger than the catheter lumen. Tracheal suctioning can occur only with occlusion of this proximal opening.

The conventional suction catheter has both side holes and end holes (Fig. 11-6).

The Argyle Aero-Flo (Sherwood Medical, St. Louis) catheter provides a distal orifice, multiple side holes, and a flared end. Reportedly, this catheter is not as efficacious as the conventional one for removing secretions. The flared tip is to minimize tissue trauma, but it

increases the overall catheter diameter, potentially making insertion more difficult and traumatic. Other catheters are designed with special anatomic or physiologic needs in mind. The Coudé angle-tipped catheter (Bard, Covington, Ga) is shaped to increase the selective cannulation of the left mainstem bronchus. This is facilitated by turning the head to the right during suctioning. Newer systems have been developed to provide a "closed system" for suctioning. These self-contained catheters allow suctioning of the patient without discontinuation of mechanical ventilation. This can limit some of the complications associated with suctioning and ventilatory disconnection.

The length of the typical catheter should pass beyond the distal tip of the artificial airway. The diameter of the suction catheter is very important. The optimal catheter diameter is approximately one-half the internal diameter of the artificial airway. Too large a catheter can produce an excessive vacuum and evacuation of gases distal to the tip of the airway, promoting atelectasis because of inadequate space for entrainment of air around the suction catheter. If too small a catheter is employed, removal of secretions can be compromised.

3. Technique

The technique of suctioning is very important for the optimal removal of secretions and limitation of complications. This is a "sterile" procedure necessitating appropriate care in handling the catheter. Gloves and hand washing are necessary unless a closed system is employed. Other necessary equipment includes a vacuum source, sterile rinsing solution, AMBU-oxygen system, and lavage solution. The optimal vacuum pressure should be adjusted for patient age.

Prior to suctioning, the patient should be preoxygenated by increasing the FiO_2 or by manual resuscitator ventilatory assistance. Preoxygenation minimizes the hypoxemia induced by FiO_2 disconnection and application of the suction vacuum. After preoxygenation, the sterile catheter is advanced past the distal tip of the artificial airway without the vacuum. When the catheter can no longer easily advance, it should be slightly withdrawn and intermittent vacuum pressure applied while the catheter is removed in a rotating fashion. This technique reportedly reduces mucosal trauma and enhances secretion clearance. The vacuum (suction) time should be limited to 10 to 15 seconds, and discontinuation of ventilation and oxygenation should not exceed 20 seconds. After removal of the catheter, reoxygenation and ventilation are essential. Throughout the procedure, patient stability and tolerance should be monitored. If signs of patient distress or dysrhythmia develops, immediately discontinue the procedure and reestablish oxygenation and ventilation. Suctioning is repeated until secretions have been adequately removed. After airway suctioning, oropharyngeal secretions should be suctioned and the catheter should be disposed.

Optimization of secretion removal necessitates adequate hydration and humidification of delivered gases. Occasionally, secretions can become quite viscous. Instillation of 5 to 10 ml of sterile normal saline can aid removal.

In critically ill patients, using a "closed-system" or swivel adapter to allow simultaneous suctioning and ventilation limits the consequences of airway disconnection and enhances sterility. These disposable systems are usually more costly but are used for 24 hours.

When an artificial airway is absent, nasotracheal suctioning techniques are employed. These techniques are technically less effective and more difficult than oral suctioning without an artificial airway, and have the potential for additional complications. After appropriate lubrication the catheter is inserted into a patient's nasal passage (often through a previously placed nasopharyngeal airway). The catheter is advanced into the larynx. Breath sounds from the proximal end of the catheter are often used as an audible guide. Upon the catheter's entry into the larynx, the patient often coughs. The vacuum is connected, and suctioning of the trachea is accomplished as previously described.

4. Complications

Complications of suctioning can be significant.[1,16] Although the suction vacuum is used to remove secretions, it also removes oxygen-enriched gases from the airway. If inappropriately applied and monitored, suctioning can produce significant hypoxemia. The use of arterial oxygen monitors (e.g., pulse oximetry) can often help detect alterations in arterial oxygenation (SaO_2) and heart rate and the presence of dysrhythmias.

Cardiovascular alterations are common. Dysrhythmias and hypotension are the most frequent cardiac complications. Arterial hypoxemia (and eventually myocardial hypoxia) and vagal stimulation secondary to tracheal suctioning are two recognized precipatory etiologies for cardiovascular complications. In addition, coughing induced by stimulation of the airway can reduce venous return and ventricular preload. Avoidance of hypoxemia, prolonged suctioning (greater than 10 seconds), and appropriate monitoring help reduce the incidence and significance of these complications.

As discussed earlier, inappropriate suction catheter size can produce an excessive evacuation of gas distal to the artificial airway because of inadequate space for proximal air entrainment. This leads to hypoxemia and atelectasis. This is best avoided by reducing the catheter size to one-half the internal diameter of the airway. Presuctioning and postsuctioning auscultation of the lungs helps detect significant atelectasis. After suction-

ing, several hyperinflations of the lungs can help reinflate atelectatic lung segments.

Mucosal irritations and trauma are common with frequent suctioning. The incidence and severity of trauma depend on the frequency of suctioning; technique; catheter design; absence of secretions, allowing more direct mucosal contact; and amount of vacuum pressure applied. Blood in the secretions is usually the first sign of tissue trauma. Meticulous technique is essential to limit this common complication. Airway reflexes can be irritated by direct mechanical stimulation. Wheezing resulting from bronchoconstriction can necessitate bronchodilator therapy. Nasotracheal suctioning can induce several additional complications. Nasal irritation, epistaxis, and laryngospasm are all noted complications. Laryngospasm can be life threatening if it is not recognized and appropriately managed.

B. CHEST PHYSICAL THERAPY

Chest physical therapy (CPT) techniques are an integral part of respiratory care. Chest physical therapy plays an important role in the provision of bronchial hygiene and optimization of ventilation. The mucociliary escalator systems and cough can be aided by adjunctive techniques. This section discusses postural drainage techniques, percussion and vibration therapy, and incentive spirometry. Other breathing exercises and coughing techniques are covered in more extensive reviews of respiratory care.

1. Postural drainage

The fundamental goal of postural drainage is to move loosened secretions toward the proximal airway for eventual removal. Pulmonary drainage takes advantage of the fact that liquids flow in the direction of gravity. Flow of secretions is optimized by liquefaction (see Humidifiers).

The primary indications for pulmonary drainage are malfunctioning of normal bronchial hygiene mechanisms and excessive or retained secretions.[1,4,17,18] In patients with ineffective lung volumes and cough, pulmonary drainage can be used prophylactically to prevent accumulation of secretions. Several clinical conditions typically benefiting from pulmonary drainage are bronchiectasis, cystic fibrosis, COPD, asthma, lung abscess, spinal cord injuries, atelectasis, pneumonia, and healing after thoracic and abdominal surgery.

To administer postural drainage appropriately, the practitioner must be able to visualize the location of the involved lung segments and the proper position to optimize drainage into the proximal airway. The lungs are divided into lobes, segments, and subsegments (Table 11-5).

Precise anatomic descriptions of the various pulmonary subsegments and positions are beyond the

Table 11-5. Lung segments

Right side	Left side
Upper lobe	**Upper lobe**
Apical	Apical-posterior
Posterior	Anterior
Anterior	
Middle lobe	**Lingula**
Lateral	Superior
Medial	Inferior
Lower lobe	**Lower lobe**
Superior	Superior
Medial basal	Anterior basal
Anterior basal	Lateral basal
Lateral basal	Posterior basal
Posterior basal	

Dependent Lung Segments

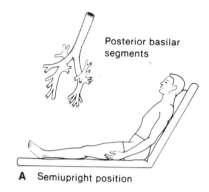

A Semiupright position

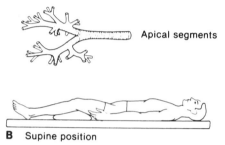

B Supine position

Fig. 11-7. Lung segments typically at risk for retained secretions, atelectasis, and pneumonia that are due to body position during convalescence. **A,** Posterior basilar segment of the lower lobe. **B,** Apical segment of the lower lobe. (From Vender JS, Clemency MV. In Benumof JL, editor: *Clinical procedures in anesthesia and intensive care,* Philadelphia, 1992, JB Lippincott.)

scope of this section. The large posterior and superior basal segments of the lower lobe are commonly involved in hospital patients with atelectasis and pneumonia. In the typical hospital patient these segments are most gravity dependent, causing stasis of secretions. (Fig. 11-7).

Appropriate patient positioning can enhance gravitational flow. This therapy also includes turning or rotating the body around its longitudinal axis. Newer critical care beds have incorporated this feature into their design and function. Commonly employed positions for postural drainage are demonstrated in Fig. 11-8.

Postural drainage should be done several times per day. For optimal results, postural drainage should follow humidity treatments and other bronchial hygiene therapies. Postural drainage should precede meals by 30 to 60 minutes, and the duration of treatment should not exceed 30 minutes.

Postural drainage can produce physiologic and anatomic stresses that are potentially detrimental to specific patients.[19] Alterations in the cardiovascular system from abrupt changes in position are well recognized. Hypotension or congestive heart failure that is due to changes in preload can be induced by positional change. Ventilation-perfusion relationships are altered by changes in position. Ideally, if the diseased pulmonary drainage is in the uppermost position, blood will preferentially flow to the gravity-dependent, non-diseased segments, improving the ventilation-perfusion relationships. The head-down position, which is commonly used, is best avoided in patients with the intracranial disease. The decreased venous return from the head could increase intracranial pressure.

Continual assessment of patient tolerance during the procedure is necessary. Vital signs, oxygenation monitoring, general appearance, level of consciousness, and

subjective comments by the patient are all part of the appraisal process.

2. Percussion and vibration therapy

Percussion and vibration therapy are used in conjunction with postural drainage to loosen and mobilize secretions that are adherent to the bronchial walls.[1,20] Percussion involves a manually produced, rhythmic vibration of varying intensity and frequency. In a "clapping" (cupped hands) motion, a blow is delivered during inspiration and expiration over the affected area while in the appropriate position for postural drainage (Fig. 11-9).

Mechanical energy is produced by compression of the air between the cupped hand and the chest wall. Proper percussion should produce a popping sound (similar to striking the bottom of a ketchup bottle). Proper force and rhythm can be accomplished by placing the hands not further than 5 inches from the chest and then alternating a flexing and extending of the wrists (similar

Postural Drainage: Use of Various Positions to Drain Different Segments

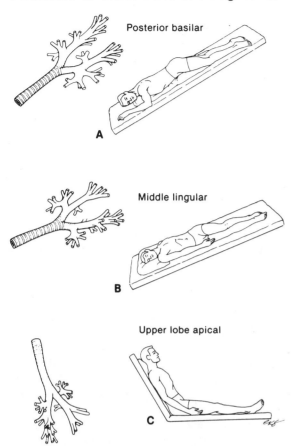

Fig. 11-8. Common position for optimizing postural drainage of, **A,** the posterior basilar, **B,** middle lingular, and, **C,** upper lobe apical segments. (From Vender JS, Clemency MV. In Benumof JL, editor: *Clinical procedures in anesthesia and intensive care,* Philadelphia, 1992, JB Lippincott.)

to a waving motion). The procedure should last 5 to 7 minutes per affected area.

Like all respiratory care, percussion therapy should not be performed without a medical order. Therapy should not be performed over bare skin, surgical incisions, bony prominences, kidneys, and female breasts or with hard objects. If a stinging sensation or reddening of the skin develops, the technique should be reevaluated.

Special care must be given to the "fragile" patient. Fractured ribs, localized pain, coagulation abnormalities, bony metastases, hemoptysis, and empyemas are relative contraindications for percussion therapy.

Vibration therapy is used to promote bronchial hygiene in a fashion similar to chest percussion. Manually or mechanically gentle vibrations are transmitted via the chest wall to the affected area during exhalation. Vibrating frequencies in excess of 200 per minute can be achieved if the procedure is done correctly. In patients

Chest Percussion with Cupped Hand-Clapping Motion

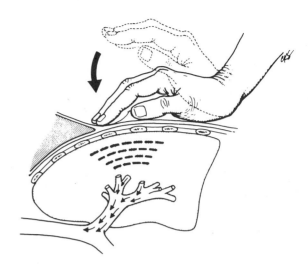

Fig. 11-9. Typical hand position for chest percussion therapy. The hand is cupped and positioned about 5 inches from the chest, and the wrist is flexed. The hand strikes the chest in a waving motion. (From Vender JS, Clemency MV. In Benumof JL, editor: *Clinical procedures in anesthesia and intensive care,* Philadelphia, 1992, JB Lippincott.)

receiving intermittent positive pressure breathing (IPPB), all chest physical therapy procedures should be performed during the IPPB.

3. Incentive spirometry

In the 1970s, alternative methods for prophylactic bronchial hygiene were developed to replace the more costly and controversial use of IPPB. Incentive spirometry (IS) was developed after several techniques utilizing expiratory maneuvers (e.g., blow and glove bottles) and carbon dioxide–induced hyperventilation were found either to be clinically ineffective or to cause other risks.[1,2,4]

Incentive spirometry was developed with an emphasis on sustained maximal inspiration (SMI). Incentive spirometry provides a visual goal or incentive for the patient to achieve SMI. Normal spontaneous breathing patterns have periodic hyperinflations that prevent the alveolar collapse associated with shallow tidal ventilation breathing patterns. Narcotics, sedative drugs, general anesthesia, cerebral trauma, and abdominal or thoracic surgery can all promote shallow tidal ventilation breathing patterns. Complications from this breathing pattern include atelectasis, retained secretions, and pneumonia.

The physiologic principle of SMI is to produce a maximal transpulmonary pressure gradient by generating a more negative intrapleural pressure. This pressure gradient produces alveolar hyperinflation with maximal air flow during the inspiratory phase.[21]

The indications for IS and SMI are primarily related to bronchial hygiene. These techniques should be employed perioperatively in surgical patients at an increased risk of pulmonary complications. Incentive spirometry involves the patient in his/her care and recovery, which can be psychologically beneficial while also being cost-advantageous relative to the equipment and personal costs associated with other forms of respiratory care (e.g., IPPB).

The goals of IS and SMI therapy are to optimize lung inflation to prevent atelectasis, to optimize the cough mechanism by providing larger lung volumes, and to provide a baseline standard to assess the effectiveness of therapy or detect the onset of acute pulmonary disease (as noted by a deteriorating performance). To optimally achieve these goals necessitates patient instruction and supervision. It is now well recognized that preoperative education enhances the effectiveness of postoperative bronchial hygiene therapy (e.g., IS and SMI). The purpose of IS and SMI is not to replace an adequate cough and deep-breathing regimen, but to provide the tool to support the patient who for various reasons is ineffective in spontaneous ability to provide bronchial hygiene. Appropriate instruction for proper breathing techniques can help produce an effective cough mechanism.

Various clinical models of incentive spirometers are available.[4] The devices vary in how they function, guide the therapy, or recognize the achievements. Each manufacturer provides instructions for use that should be followed. The devices are aimed at generating the largest inspiratory volumes during 5 to 15 seconds. The actual device used or rate of flow is not as important as the frequency of use and the attainment of maximal inspiratory volumes and sustained inspiration. Maximal benefit with most devices can be achieved only with user education.

The administration of IS and SMI therapy necessitates a physiologically and emotionally stable patient. Patient cooperation and motivation are very important. To be optimally effective, the patient should be free of acute pulmonary disease and have a forced vital capacity of more than 15 ml/kg and a spontaneous respiratory rate of less than 25 beats per minute. Ideally, the patient should not require a high FiO_2. Therapy should be done hourly while awake. Typically, the patient should do four to five SMIs at a 30- to 60-second interval. The patient should be coached to inspire slowly while attaining maximal inspiratory volumes.

There are no significant complications associated with IS and SMI therapy. The only contraindications are patients who are uncooperative, physically disabled with acute pulmonary disease, or unable to generate minimum volumes for lung inflation (e.g., 12 to 15 ml/kg).

C. INTERMITTENT POSITIVE PRESSURE BREATHING

In the past four decades few respiratory care therapies have been as controversial as intermittent positive pressure breathing (IPPB).[1,2,4,22] Objective data assessing therapeutic benefit relative to cost and alternative therapies have been less than confirmatory.[21,22] Numerous conferences have been sponsored by medical organizations to evaluate literature supporting and opposing IPPB. The inconclusive result of these efforts has significantly reduced (and in some situations, eliminated) the use of IPPB. Alternative techniques (previously discussed) have been substituted. This section is intended to define IPPB, recognize its indications, and describe the technique of administration and potential side effects and complications. An extensive historical and in-depth analysis of IPPB controversies is beyond the scope of this section.

1. Indications

Intermittent positive pressure breathing is the therapeutic application of inspiratory positive pressure to the airway and is distinctly different from intermittent positive pressure ventilation (IPPV) or other means of prolonged, continuous ventilation.

The clinical indications of IPPB are subjective and unproven. It is easier to assess IPPB if the indications are described as clinical goals. The fundamental basis and singular goal of IPPB is to provide larger tidal volume (V_T) than the spontaneously breathing patient in a physiologically tolerable manner. If this goal is achieved, IPPB could be employed (1) to improve and promote the cough mechanism, (2) to improve distribution of ventilation, and (3) to enhance delivery of inhaled medications.

Bronchial hygiene can be compromised in patients with a reduced or inadequate cough mechanism. An adequate vital capacity (15 ml/kg) is necessary to generate the volume and expiratory flow needed to produce an effective cough. Although IPPB can increase V_T significantly, effectiveness still depends on the pressure and flow patterns generated, as well as on an understanding of cough technique. Therefore, if cough is improved, one can indirectly see the benefit of IPPB for removal of secretions and for limiting complications associated with this problem.

The increased V_T produced by IPPB can be used to improve the distribution of ventilation. As in most respiratory care therapies, the efficacy depends on the patient's underlying condition, patient selection, optimal technique, and frequency of application. Continual assessment of the therapy is mandatory. Theoretically, if ventilation increases, atelectasis could be prevented or treated.

In patients who are unable to provide an adequate inspiratory volume, IPPB can enhance drug delivery and distribution. When the patient is capable of an adequate cough and spontaneous deep breath, a hand nebulizer is as efficacious as IPPB. IPPB is rarely used solely for delivery of medication.

2. Administration

The effectiveness of IPPB depends on the individual administering the therapy.[4] It is incumbent for that individual (1) to understand the appropriate operation maintenance and clinical application of the mechanical device employed; (2) to select the appropriate patient; (3) to provide the necessary patient education to optimize the effort; (4) to assess the effectiveness relative to goals and indications; and (5) to identify complications or side effects associated with the therapy.

The generic device uses a gas pressure source, a main control valve, a breathing circuit, and an automatic cycling control. Typically, IPPB is delivered via a pressure-cycled ventilator. Positive pressure (e.g., 30 to 50 cm H_2O) is used to expand the lungs. To be effective, the increase in V_T from the IPPB treatment must exceed the patient's limited spontaneous vital capacity by 100%. A prolonged inspiratory effort to the preset pressure limit should be emphasized. Therapy is typically 6 to 8 breaths per minute, lasting 10 minutes.

Keys to successful therapy include (1) machine sensitivity to the patient's inspiratory effort; (2) a tight seal between the machine and patient, since these are pressure-limited devices; (3) a progressive increase in the inspiratory pressure as tolerated by the patient in an effort to achieve a desired exhaled volume; and (4) a cooperative, relaxed, and well-educated patient.

The physiologic side effects and complications associated with IPPB are well described in the literature.[4] Both hyperventilation and variable oxygenation can result from IPPB therapy. Hypocarbia that is due to an increased V_T and respiratory frequency can produce altered electrolytes (K^+), dizziness, muscle tremors, and tingling and numbness of the extremities. Proper patient instruction and a 5- to 10-minute rest period after therapy can minimize this problem. Hypoxemia and hyperoxia that are due to inaccurate F_{IO_2} values can be a concern in patients who are dependent on "hypoxic respiratory drive" (carbon dioxide retainers).

The use of IPPB can increase mean intrathoracic pressure, resulting in a decreased venous return. Like other forms of positive pressure ventilation, a decreased venous return (preload) can produce a decreased cardiac output and subsequent vital-sign changes (hypotension or tachycardia). In addition to cardiovascular changes, IPPB can impede venous drainage from the head. This is a potential but limited concern in patients with intracranial pressure, if IPPB is appropriately administered in the sitting position.

Barotrauma is a concern with all forms of positive pressure ventilation (PPV). The exact etiologic mechanism of PPV in the development of pneumothorax and ruptured lobes is unclear. Clearly, PPV results in increased intrapulmonary volume and pressure, but these same conditions tend to promote a better cough mechanism that causes sudden marked changes in pressure and lobe rupture. Before proceeding with an IPPB treatment, any chest pain complaints must be evaluated to rule out barotrauma.

Other reported complications include, but are not limited to, gastric insufflation and secondary nausea and vomiting, psychologic dependency, nosocomial infections, altered airway resistance, and adverse reactions to administered medications. The incidence and significance of these adverse effects are often the result of inappropriate administration, patient noncompliance, patient selection, and simple lack of attention to detail. Asthmatics reportedly tolerate IPPB poorly and have an increased airway resistance and a higher incidence of barotrauma.

There are few definite contraindications to IPPB. Relative contraindications of IPPB are focused on its lack of documented efficacy. Untreated pneumothorax is a definite contraindication to IPPB. Good clinical contraindications are lack of a definite indication for IPPB or an available, less expensive alternative therapy.

IV. INHALATION THERAPY

Inhalation therapy is often used synonymously with the term *respiratory care*. In a general context, inhalation therapy can be thought of as the delivery of gases for ventilation and oxygenation, as aerosol therapy, or as a means of delivering therapeutic medications.

Therapeutic aerosols have been employed in the treatment of pulmonary patients with bronchospastic airway disease, chronic obstructive pulmonary disease, and pulmonary infection. The basic goals of aerosol therapy are to improve bronchial hygiene, humidify gases delivered through artificial airways, and to deliver medications. The first two goals were discussed earlier in this chapter.

The advantages of delivering drugs by inhalation are multiple. Easier access, rapid onset of action, reduced extrapulmonary side effects, reduced dosage, coincidental application with aerosol therapy for humidification, and psychologic benefits have all been cited.[1,2,4] In the nonintubated patient, aerosol therapy necessitates patient cooperation and skilled help. The equipment is a potential source of nosocomial infections.[10] Aerosol therapy has many of the same disadvantages noted with humidification. Although drug usage is often reduced, precise titration and dosages are difficult to ascertain because of variable degrees of drug deposition in the airway.

This section provides an overview of inhalation pharmacology. The basic principles, devices for medication delivery, and specific pharmacologic agents that are employed are discussed. For a more comprehensive topic review and specific drug information, one should refer to available reference texts.

A. BASIC PHARMACOLOGIC PRINCIPLES

The basic pharmacology of inhalation therapy necessitates a brief pharmacologic review. A medication is a drug that is given to elicit a physiologic response and is used for therapeutic purposes. Undesired responses (side effects) are also produced. The medication can interact with receptors by direct application (topical effect) or absorption into the bloodstream.

Various routes of pharmacologic administration are used for respiratory care. Subcutaneous, parenteral, gastrointestinal, and inhalation administrations are all commonly employed in the management of pulmonary diseases. Inhalation therapy employs the increased surface area of the lung parenchyma as a route of medication administration. This necessitates the drug reaching the alveolar and tracheobronchial mucosal surfaces for systemic capillary absorption.

Although inhaled medications can have topical effects, the primary reasons for the inhalation of medications are convenience, a safe method for self-administration, and maximal pulmonary benefit with reduced side effects. If the drug depends on systemic absorption, the drug's distribution and blood concentration are important. Blood concentration is altered by several mechanisms, such as dosage, route of administration, absorption, metabolism, and excretion. Alteration in liver and kidney function can produce unexpected drug levels and side effects.

If multiple drugs are employed for respiratory care, various drug interactions can occur. *Potentiation* is the result of one drug with limited activity changing the response of another drug; *synergism* is two drugs with similar action resulting in a greater response than the sum of the individual drugs. If the response of the two drugs is the sum of the individual medications, they are *additive*. *Tolerance* necessitates increasing drug levels to elicit a response, and *tachyphylaxis* results in the inability of larger doses to produce the expected response. Finally, the nomenclature for drug dosages should be understood. Two common methods for expressing drug dosage are *ratio strength* (drug dilutions) and *percentage strength* (percentage solutions). The following facts are necessary to understand this often confusing topic. A *solution* is a homogeneous mixture of two substances. A *solute* is the dissolved drug, and a *solvent* is the fluid in which the drug is dissolved. A gram of water equals 1 ml of water, and 1 g equals 1000 mg. *Ratio strength* is expressed in terms of parts of solute in relation to the total parts of solvent (or grams of solute per grams of solvent). A 1:1000 solution is 1 g of a drug in 1000 g of solvent (or 1000 mg/1000 ml − 1 mg/1 ml). *Percentage strength* is expressed as the number of parts of solute in 100 parts of solvent (or grams of solute per 100 g of solvent). A 1% solution is 1 g of drug in 100 g of solvent.

B. AEROSOLIZED DRUG DELIVERY SYSTEMS

Therapeutic aerosols are commonly employed in respiratory care. As stated earlier, inhalation delivery of drugs can often produce therapeutic drug effects with reduced toxicity. The effectiveness of aerosols is related to the amount of drug delivered to the lungs. Actual pulmonary deposition of aerosolized drugs is a result of drug sedimentation that is due to gravity, inertial impact that is due to airway size, and directional change of air flow and kinetic energy.[1] Aerosol delivery also depends on particle size, pattern of inhalation, and degree of airway obstruction. Particle size should be smaller than 5 μm; otherwise, the upper airway is not penetrated. The preferable route of administration is through the mouth, since the nose acts as a barrier. The ideal pattern of inhalation should be large volume, slow inspiration (5 to 6 seconds), and accentuated by an inspiratory hold (10 seconds). If airway obstruction is significant, adequate deposition of drugs can be limited. If the obstruction is not relieved, larger dosages or increased frequency of administration could be necessary. The most common methods for aerosolized drug delivery are metered-dose inhalers (MDI), small-volume (gas-powered) nebulizers (SVN), dry powder inhalers, and IPPB (discussed earlier).

The MDI is a convenient, self-contained, and commonly employed method of aerosolized drug delivery (Figs. 11-10 and 11-11).[2,4] These prefilled drug canisters are activated by manual compression and deliver a predetermined unit (metered) of medication. Appropriate instruction is necessary for optimal use.[23] With the canister in the upside-down position, the device should be compressed only once per inhalation. A slow maximal inspiration with a breath hold is typically recommended. It is imperative that the tongue not obstruct flow, but it is controversial whether the device should be placed in the mouth or held several centimeters from the lips with the mouth wide open. Concerns for excessive oral deposition of large particles must be offset against consistency of administration when the device is held away from the mouth. Other issues regarding use of MDIs include ideal lung volume for actuation, time of inspiratory hold, and inspiratory flow rate. If multiple doses are prescribed, an interval of several minutes between puffs is advisable.

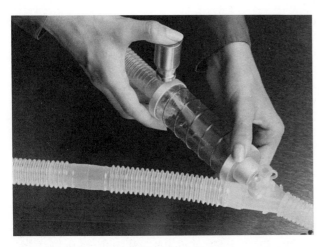

Fig. 11-10. Metered-dose inhaler and circuit inspiratory limb spacer (AeroVent-Monaghan Medical, Plattsburgh, N.Y.).

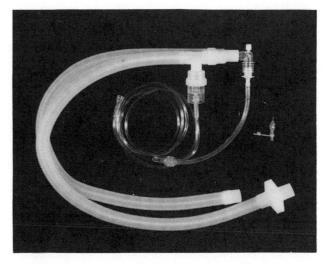

Fig. 11-12. In-line, gas-powered nebulization system.

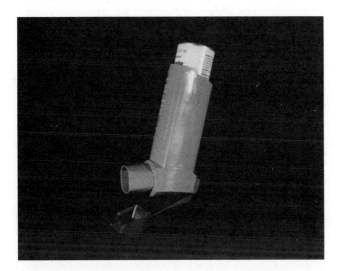

Fig. 11-11. Metered-dose inhaler for handheld use.

Several problems with MDI drug delivery have been previously recognized. Manual coordination is necessary to activate the canister. Arthritis can cause difficulty, as can misaiming the aerosol. Pharyngeal deposition can lead to local abnormalities (e.g., oral candidiasis secondary to aerosolized corticosteroids). Systemic effects that are due to swallowing the drug can be reduced if the pharynx is rinsed after inhalation to reduce pharyngeal deposition.[2] The new MDI devices have been designed to reduce some of these problems. In addition, several spacing devices are available as extensions to MDIs. Spacers are designed to eliminate the need for hand-breath coordination and reduction of large-particle deposition in the upper airway.

The gas-powered nebulizers can be handheld or placed in line with the ventilatory circuit (Fig. 11-12).[2,4] The handheld devices are typically employed on more

acutely ill individuals and as an alternative to an MDI. The full handheld system uses a nebulizer, a pressurized gas source, and a mouthpiece or face mask. The mouthpiece is preferable, since some drugs could be deposited in the lung.

These systems are more expensive, cumbersome, and often less efficient than MDIs. Supervision is usually necessary for appropriate drug preparation and administration. Typically, the drug is diluted in saline. The drug is usually more concentrated, since a majority of the drug is never aerosolized or is lost during exhalation. Only the drug that is inspired could reach the lung.

The total volume to be nebulized is usually 4 to 6 ml (see Pharmacologic Agents) at gas flows of 6 to 8 L/min (device dependent). The treatment time is usually 5 to 10 minutes. During the course of treatment the patient's vital signs and subjective tolerance must be monitored. Aerosolization of medication for drug delivery is different from aerosol therapy for humidification (see Humidifiers).

Both the MDI and the gas-powered nebulizers can be used in line with an artificial airway and/or ventilator circuit (Figs. 11-10 and 11-12). The drug delivery system is positioned in the inspiratory limb, as proximal to the artificial airway as possible. In-line drug delivery is usually less efficient in ventilated patients than in spontaneously breathing, nonintubated patients because of the breathing pattern, drug deposition on the endotracheal tube, and airway disease.

C. PHARMACOLOGIC AGENTS

Numerous drugs are used in the management of pulmonary diseases. Nebulized (aerosolized) drug delivery is commonly employed to improve mucociliary clearance (mucokinetics) and relieve bronchospastic airway disease. The major drugs employed for inhalation therapy can be categorized by their ability to affect these two issues. In addition, certain antiinflammatory, anti-asthmatic, antifungal, antiviral, and antibacterial drugs are given by aerosol. The following reviews some of the commonly employed *aerosolized* drugs and is not meant to be a comprehensive review of respiratory pharmacology. All listed dosages are meant to be representative for adult patients (if needed, specific product literature should be referred to, prior to use).

1. Mucokinetic drugs

Mucokinetic drugs are employed to enhance mucociliary clearance. These agents can be classified according to their mechanism of action. Hypoviscosity agents are the most commonly employed mucokinetic agents. Saline, sodium bicarbonate, and alcohol are the specific agents most commonly used. The mechanism of action for each drug varies but tends to affect mucus viscosity by disrupting the mucopolysaccharide chains that are the primary composition of mucus. The other category of mucokinetic aerosol agents is made up of the mucolytics. The following is a brief synopsis of the various drugs in these two groups.[24]

a. HYPOVISCOSITY AGENTS

Saline is the most commonly employed mucokinetic agent. It can be used as a primary drug or solvent. The mechanism of action is reduced viscosity by dilution of the mucopolysaccharide strands. The indication for use is thick, tenacious mucus secretions. The typical concentration is 0.45% to 0.9% sodium chloride (NaCl). The two major side effects associated with aerosolized saline are overhydration and the promotion of bronchospasm in patients with hyperactive airway disease (especially in newborns).

Alcohol (ethyl alcohol and ethanol) decreases the surface tension of pulmonary fluid. The typical concentration is 30%, and the dosage is 4 to 10 ml. The primary indication is pulmonary edema. This agent should be administered by side-arm nebulization or IPPB but not as a heated aerosol. The contraindication is a hypersensitivity to alcohol or its derivative. Side effects include airway irritation, bronchospasm, and local dehydration.

b. MUCOLYTIC AGENTS

Acetylcysteine 10% (Mucomyst) is an effective mucolytic. The mechanism of action is the lysis of the disulfide bonds in mucopolysaccharide chains reducing the viscosity of the mucus. The indication is the management of viscous, inspissated, mucopurulent secretions. The actual effectiveness in the treatment of mucostasis is inconclusive, and each individual must be monitored to determine the benefit of therapy. The usual dosage is 2 to 5 ml every 6 hours. Hypersensitivity is a contraindication. In general, acetylcysteine is relatively nontoxic. Side effects include unpleasant taste and odor, local irritation, inhibition of ciliary activity, and bronchospasm. For these reasons pretreatment with a bronchodilator is recommended. Other reported side effects include nausea, vomiting, stomatitis, rhinorrhea, and generalized urticaria. Acetylcysteine is incompatible with several antibodies. The drug should be avoided or used with extreme caution in patients with bronchospastic airway disease. Other special concerns are a need for refrigeration, reactivity with rubber, and limited use after opening (96 hours).[25]

2. Bronchodilators and antiasthmatic drugs

Acute and chronic bronchospastic airway diseases afflict many individuals. Many drugs, varying primarily by their mechanism of action and route of delivery, are available to manage this problem. This section deals only with aerosolized drugs that are commonly employed in the therapy of bronchospastic airway disease (Table 11-6).[7,26,27] The drug groups are divided by their mechanism of action: sympathomimetics, anticholinergics, corticosteroids, and cromolyn. A comprehensive review of these drugs, the various mechanisms for bronchodilation, and the management of specific pathophysiologic problems is beyond the scope of this chapter.

a. SYMPATHOMIMETICS

Sympathomimetics include the β-adrenergic agonists and methylxanthines (not available in aerosol). The primary mechanism of action of the β-adrenergic agonists is to stimulate the enzyme adenyl cyclase to increase the conversion of adenosine triphosphate (ATP) to cyclic adenosine monophosphate (cAMP). The cAMP causes bronchial smooth muscle relaxation and inhibits antigen-induced release of medicators that induce some of the pathophysiologic responses seen in allergic asthma. In general, the response of sympathomimetic drugs is classified according to whether the effects are α, β-1, or β-2. β-2 receptors are responsible for bronchial smooth muscle relaxation. The common side effects associated with β-adrenergic agonists are due to their additional β-1 and α effects. β-1 effects cause an increase in heart rate, dysrhythmias, and cardiac contractility; α effects increase vascular tone. Potent β-2 stimulants can produce unwanted symptoms: anxiety, headache, nausea, tremors, and sleeplessness. Prolonged utilization can lead to receptor down-regulation and reduced drug response. Ideally, the more pure the β-2 response, the better the therapeutic benefit relative to side effects. The following sympathomimetics are commonly employed in clinical practice.[1,2,21,25]

Isoetharine hydrochloride 1% (Bronkosol) is available in a 1% solution. Its primary action is β-2 with weak β-1 (therapeutic doses) and not α effects. The nebulized dosage is usually 0.25 to 0.5 ml in 4.0 ml normal saline. The bronchodilatory effects are weaker than isoproter-

Table 11-6. Aerosolized bronchodilators and antiasthmatic drugs

Type of drug	Method	Dosages*	Mechanism
Sympathomimetics (trade)			
Isoetharine hydrochloride 1%	Nebulized	0.25-0.5 ml in 4.0 ml	β-2 agonist increase in cyclic AMP
(Bronkosol)	MDI	2 puffs (340 μg/puff) q.i.d.	
Metaproterenol sulfate 5%	Nebulized	0.3 ml in 2.5 ml	
(Alupent)	MDI	2 puffs (0.65 mg/puff) q.i.d.	
Albuterol	MDI	2 puffs (90 μg/puff) q.i.d.	
(Ventolin, Proventil)	Nebulized	2.5-5.0 mg in 4 ml q.i.d.	
Racemic epinephrine 2.25%	Nebulized	0.5 ml in 3.5 ml	Weak β-2 and mild α mucosal vasoconstrictor
(Vaponepherine)			
Isoproterenol (0.5%)	Nebulized	0.25-0.5 in 3.5 ml	Prototype β-agonist
Isuprel	MDI		Significant β-1 side effects
Anticholinergic			
Ipratropium bromide	MDI	2 puffs (18 μg/puff) q.i.d.	Cholinergic blocker increasing β stimulation
(Atrovent)			
Antiallergy agents			
Cromolyn sodium 1%	Nebulized	20 mg q.i.d. in 2-4 ml	Suppression of mast cell response to Ag-Ab reactions
(Intal)	MDI	2 puffs (800 μg/puff) q.i.d.	Used prophylactically
Beclomethasone acetonide	MDI	2 puffs (42 μg/puff) q.i.d.	Antinflammatory
(Vanceril, Beclovent)			Inhibit leukocyte migration
			Potentiate effects of β-agonists
Dexamethasone sodium phosphate (Decadron)	Nebulized	0.25 ml (1 mg) in 2.5 ml	

*Dosages may vary; references to specific drug inserts are recommended.
MDI, Metered-dose inhaler; *q.i.d.,* four times a day.

enol and last 1 to 3 hours. The drug is available in an MDI. Typical dosage of the MDI is two puffs (340 μg per puff) four times a day.

Metaproterenol sulfate 5% (Alupent) is very similar to isoetharine, but the duration of action is approximately 5 hours. The dosage is 0.3 ml (5%) in 2.5 ml normal saline. Metaproterenol is available in an MDI.

Albuterol (Ventolin, Proventil) is a newer sympathomimetic agent available in an MDI. It has a strong β-2 effect with limited β-1 properties. Its β-2 duration of action is approximately 6 hours.

Racemic epinephrine 2.25% (Vaponephrine) is a mixture of levo and dextro isomers of epinephrine. It is a weak β and mild α drug. The α effects provide mucosal constriction. In the aerosol form, this drug acts as a good mucosal decongestant. The drug does have minimal bronchodilatory action. Cardiovascular side effects are limited. Typical dosage is 0.5 ml (2.25%) in 3.5 ml saline, given as frequently as every hour in adult patients. Racemic epinephrine is commonly mixed with 0.25 ml (1 mg) dexamethasone for the management of postextubation swelling and croup.

Isoproterenol (Isuprel) is the prototype pure β-adrenergic bronchodilator. Bronchodilation depends on adequate blood levels. In addition, isoproterenol is a

pulmonary and mucosal vascular dilator. This causes an increased rate of absorption, higher blood levels, and increased β-1 side effects. These side effects can be quite significant and often reduce the utilization of this agent in patients with cardiac disease; dysrhythmias, myocardial ischemia, and palpitations can all occur. If the pulmonary vasculature vasodilates to areas of low ventilation, the potential to augment ventilation-perfusion mismatch and increase intrapulmonary shunt exists. Typical dosage is 0.25 to 0.5 ml (0.5%) in 3.5 ml saline. The effect lasts 1 to 2 hours. Isoproterenol is also available as an MDI.

b. ANTICHOLINERGIC AGENTS

Anticholinergic drugs play an increasing role in the management of bronchospastic pulmonary disease. These drugs inhibit acetylcholine at the cholinergic receptor site, reducing vagal nerve activity. This produces bronchodilation (preferentially in large airways) and a reduction in mucus secretion. Major side effects include dry mouth, blurred vision, headache, tremor, nervousness, and palpitations.

Ipratropium bromide (Atrovent) is a newer, commercially available anticholinergic. Its effects are primarily β-2. It is available as an MDI. The standard dosage is 36 μg, four times a day (18 μg per puff). Hypersensitivity to the drug is a contraindication. Caution should be exercised in patients with narrow angle glaucoma.

c. ANTIALLERGY AND ASTHMATIC AGENTS

The two main groups of aerosolized agents in this category are cromolyn and corticosteroids. These drugs are often used in concert with other medications.

Cromolyn sodium 1% (Intal) is primarily used prophylactically to prevent bronchospasm in exercise-induced asthma.[2] The drug is not effective in the management of acute bronchospasm. The mechanism of action is suppression of mast cell response to antigen-antibody reactions. Cromolyn sodium is available in a powder (spinhaler), liquid, and MDI for inhalation therapy. The typical dosages are 20 mg four times a day via nebulizer or 2 puffs four times a day (800 μg per puff) with the MDI. The MDI appears to be tolerated best. Hypersensitivity is a contraindication. Side effects include local irritation, allergic symptoms—rash and urticaria—and airway hyperactivity (most common with the powder).

Corticosteroids are commonly used for maintenance therapy in patients with chronic asthma.[28,29] The mechanism of action is attributed to their antiinflammatory properties, reducing leakage of fluids, inhibiting migration of macrophages and leukocytes, and possibly blocking the response to various mediators of inflammation. Recently, corticosteroids have been reported to potentiate the effects of the sympathomimetic drugs.[2]

Dexamethasone sodium phosphate (Decadron) is the prototypic steroid for respiratory care. It is used most often for its antiinflammatory action and for postextubation with racemic epinephrine. The typical dosage is 0.25 ml (1 mg) in 2.5 ml saline. The side effects of corticosteroids are related to their chronicity of use and degree of systemic absorption. Because of its systemic effects, dexamethasone is used on a limited basis as an aerosol.

Beclomethasone dipropionate (Vanceril, Beclovent) is an aerosolized corticosteroid that is highly active topically and that has limited systemic absorption or activity. The typical dosage is 2 puffs (42 μg per puff) three or four times a day. Hoarseness, sore throat, and oral candidiasis are reported side effects. The candidiasis can be managed with topical antifungal drugs. Mild adrenal suppression is reported with high doses, and caution is advised when switching from oral to inhaled corticosteroids.

The preceding pharmacologic agents are representative of those commonly employed by aerosol in respiratory care. Other drugs (e.g., antiviral and antibiotic drugs) are beyond the scope of this chapter. Appropriate pharmacologic management necessitates assessing response to therapy. Objective and subjective relief of symptoms and improvement in pulmonary function while minimizing side effects of these drugs are the end points of good inhalation therapy.

REFERENCES

1. Shapiro BA, Kacmarek RM, Cane RD et al: *Clinical application of respiratory care,* ed 4, St Louis, 1991, Mosby.
2. Kacmarek RM, Stoller JK, editors: *Current respiratory care,* Toronto, 1988, BC Decker.
3. Marini JJ: Postoperative atelectasis: pathophysiology, clinical importance, and principles of management, *Respir Care* 29:516, 1984.
4. Burton GL, Hodgkin JE, editors: *Respiratory care,* ed 2, Philadelphia, 1984, JB Lippincott.
5. Scacci R: Air entrainment masks: jet mixing is how they work; the Bernoulli and Venturi principles are how they don't, *Respir Care* 24:928, 1979.
6. Gibson RL, Comer PB, Beckham RW et al: Actual tracheal oxygen concentrations with commonly used oxygen equipment, *Anesthesiology* 44:71, 1976.
7. Kacmarek RM: Humidity and aerosol therapy. In Pierson DJ, Kacmarek RM, editors: *Foundations of respiratory care,* New York, 1992, Churchill Livingstone.
8. Klein EF, Shah DA, Shah NJ et al: Performance characteristics of conventional and prototype humidifiers and nebulizers, *Chest* 64:690, 1973.
9. Hall TO: Aerosol generators and humidifiers. In Barnes TA, editor: *Respiratory care practice,* Chicago, 1988, Year Book.
10. Craven DE, Goulartet A, Maki BJ: Contaminated condensate in mechanical ventilator circuits: a risk factor for nosocomial pneumonia? *Am Rev Respir Dis* 129:625, 1984.
11. Carden E, Friedman D: Further studies of manually operated self-inflating resuscitation bag, *Anesth Analg* 56:202, 1977.
12. Barnes TA, Watson ME: Oxygen delivery performance of four adult resuscitation bags, *Respir Care* 27:139, 1982.
13. Barnes TA, Watson ME: Oxygen delivery performance of old and new designs of the Laerdal, Vitalograph and AMBU adult manual resuscitators, *Respir Care* 28:1121, 1983.
14. Deneke SM, Fanburg BL: Normobaric oxygen toxicity of the lung, *N Engl J Med* 303:76, 1980.
15. Chapman GA, Kim CS, Frankel J et al: Evaluation of the safety and efficiency of new suction catheter design, *Respir Care* 31:889, 1986.
16. Demers RR: Complications of endotracheal suctioning procedures, *Respir Care* 27:453, 1982.
17. Harris JA, Jerry BA: Indications and procedures for segmental bronchial drainage, *Respir Care* 20:1164, 1975.
18. Zadai CL: Physical therapy for the acutely ill medical patient, *Phys Ther* 61:1746, 1981.
19. Tyler ML: Complications of positioning and chest physiotherapy, *Respir Care* 27:458, 1982.
20. Radford R: Rational basis for percussion: augmented mucociliary clearance, *Respir Care* 27:556, 1982.
21. Ziment I: Why are they saying bad things about IPPB? *Respir Care* 18:677, 1973.
22. Murray JF: Review of the state of the art of intermittent positive pressure breathing therapy, *Am Rev Respir Dis* 110:193, 1974.
23. Self TH, Brooks JB: Necessity of teaching patients correct bronchodilator inhalation technique, *Immunol All Pract* 4:40, 1982.
24. Barton AD: Aerosolized detergents and mucolytic agents in the treatment of stable chronic obstructive pulmonary disease, *Am Rev Respir Dis* 110:104, 1974.
25. Eubanks DH, Bone RC: *Comprehensive respiratory care,* St Louis, 1985, Mosby.

26. Weinberger M, Hendeles L, Ahrens R: Pharmacologic management of reversible obstructive airway disease, *Med Clin North Am* 65:529, 1981.
27. McFadden RR: Aerosolized bronchodilators and steroids in the treatment of airway obstruction in adults, *Am Rev Respir Dis* 122:89, 1980.
28. Morse HG: Mechanisms of action and therapeutic role of corticosteroids and asthma, *J Allergy Clin Immunol* 75:1, 1985.
29. Newhouse MT, Dolovich MB: Control of asthma by aerosols, *N Engl J Med* 315:870, 1986.

SUGGESTED READINGS

American College of Chest Physicians—Heart, Lung and Blood Institute: *National Conference on Oxygen Therapy,* Chest 85:234, 1984.
Fisher AB: Oxygen therapy: side effects and toxicity, *Am Rev Respir Dis* 122:61, 1980.
Martin RJ, Roger RM, Grant BA: The physiologic basis for the use of mechanical aids to lung expansion, *Am Rev Respir Dis* 122:105, 1980.
Vender JS, Clemency MV: Oxygen delivery systems, inhalation therapy, respiratory care. In Benumof JL, editor: *Clinical procedures in anesthesia and intensive care,* Philadelphia, 1992, JB Lippincott.

Chapter 12

NONINTUBATION MANAGEMENT OF THE AIRWAY: MASK VENTILATION

John P. McGee II
Jeffrey S. Vender

I. OVERVIEW

Maintaining a patent airway is the first principle of resuscitation and life support, and airway management is an essential skill for those caring for anesthetised or critically ill patients. Respiratory care, nursing, intensive care, and emergency room physicians should all be competent in the essentials of airway care.

Too frequently, inexperienced personnel believe airway management necessitates intubation of the trachea. The focus of this chapter is twofold: a review of tools and skills of nonintubation airway management and a preliminary discussion of choosing airway management techniques. Other chapters focus on techniques of tracheal intubation and pharyngeal intubation (laryngeal mask airway). Airway management can be divided into the establishment and maintenance of a patent airway and of breathing (respiratory support). Establishing and maintaining a patent airway are achieved by manipulating the head and neck in ways that maximize the anatomic airway or by using artificial airway devices. Respiratory support techniques control the atmosphere the patient breathes and allow for manual ventilatory assistance.

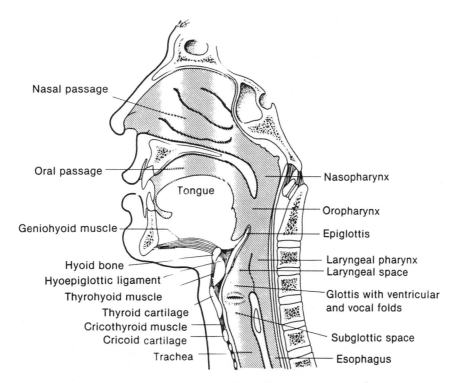

Nasal passage

Oral passage

Tongue

Geniohyoid muscle

Hyoid bone

Hyoepiglottic ligament

Thyrohyoid muscle

Thyroid cartilage

Cricothyroid muscle

Cricoid cartilage

Trachea

Nasopharynx

Oropharynx

Epiglottis

Laryngeal pharynx

Laryngeal space

Glottis with ventricular and vocal folds

Subglottic space

Esophagus

Fig. 12-1. Normal airway anatomy: lateral view of head and neck in neutral position. The various components of the airway and surrounding structures are labeled. Note that (1) the tongue could easily obliterate the airway at the oropharynx by falling backward. The likelihood of the epiglottis sealing against the posterior pharyngeal wall is better seen in the xerograms (Figs. 12-3 and 12-4) and that (2) the muscular line from the mentum to hyoid bone (geniohyoid muscle) to thyroid cartilage (thyrohyoid muscle and membrane) to cricoid (cricothyroid muscle) has a folded and right-angle character *(dotted line)*. This line can be straightened by extending the head and pulling the jaw forward (anteriorly), thus pulling the epiglottis and tongue away from the posterior wall.

A. AIRWAY ANATOMY

The airway is the passageway that air or respiratory gases must track between the outside environment and the alveoli. Nonintubation airway management seeks to produce patency to gas flow through the oropharynx, nasopharynx, and larynx without the use of an artificial airway device that extends into the trachea or laryngopharynx. A thorough understanding of airway anatomy is necessary to appreciate the therapeutic maneuvers and devices employed in airway management (Fig. 12-1). Very detailed reviews of airway anatomy can be found in Chapters 1 and 2 of this book and various atlases and texts.[1-3]

Gas passes to the larynx by two routes. One is through the nares, warmed and humidified by the turbinates, into the nasopharynx via the choanae to the oropharynx, laryngopharynx, and larynx. The nasal passages can be obstructed by choanal atresia, septal deviation, mucosal swelling, or foreign material (e.g., mucus or blood). The entry into the nasopharynx may be blocked by the apposition of the soft palate against the posterior pharyngeal wall. The other route is through the mouth, between the palate and tongue to the oropharynx, laryngopharynx, and larynx. The common pathway, the oropharynx and laryngopharynx, can be occluded by a relaxed tongue or epiglottis protruding posteriorly and caudad against the inferior pharyngeal constrictor and laryngeal introitus. Airway manipulations and devices can treat this cause of obstruction fairly efficaciously in most cases. Laryngeal obstruction that is due to spasm must be treated by positive airway pressure, deeper anesthesia, muscle relaxants, or endotracheal intubation.

Laryngeal closure can occur from intrinsic or extrinsic muscles of the larynx. Tight airway closure (laryngospasm or effort closure) is accomplished by the external laryngeal muscles forcing the mucosal folds of the quadrangular membrane into apposition by contracting the cylindric section of airway from the hyoid bone to the cricoid cartilage (Fig. 12-2). Muscle groups also extend from the thyroid cartilage to the hyoid and cricoid. When they contract, the interior mucosas and soft tissue (ventricular and vocal folds) are forced into the center of the airway and the thyroid shield is

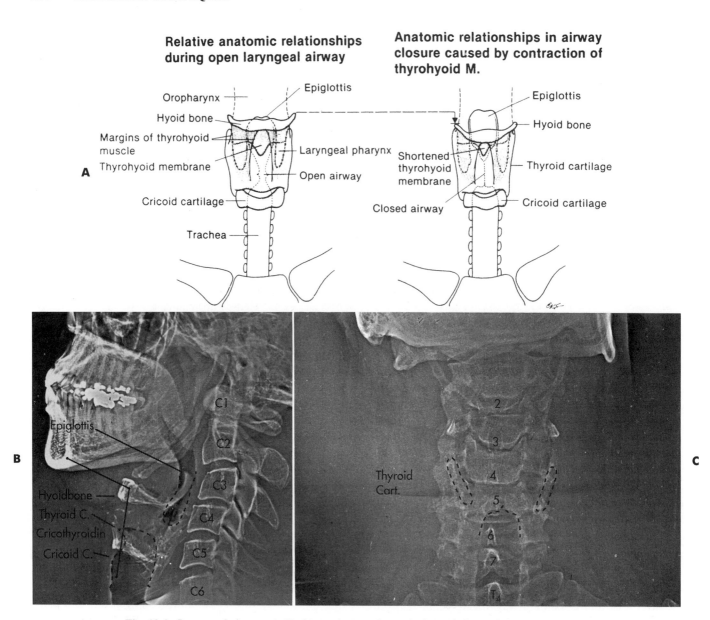

Relative anatomic relationships during open laryngeal airway

Oropharynx
Epiglottis
Hyoid bone
Margins of thyrohyoid muscle
Thyrohyoid membrane
Laryngeal pharynx
Open airway
Cricoid cartilage
Trachea

Anatomic relationships in airway closure caused by contraction of thyrohyoid M.

Epiglottis
Hyoid bone
Shortened thyrohyoid membrane
Thyroid cartilage
Cricoid cartilage
Closed airway

A

B

C

Epiglottis
Hyoidbone
Thyroid C.
Cricothyroidin
Cricoid C.
C1
C2
C3
C4
C5
C6

Thyroid Cart.
2
3
4
5
6
7
T4

Fig. 12-2. Laryngeal closure. **A,** Both panels are schematic frontal views of the airway at the larynx. The left panel shows an open airway with an air column visible centrally and the hyoid bone clearly above the thyroid shield. The right panel shows obliteration of the air column (caused by apposition of the ventricular and vocal folds) and approximation of the hyoid bone to the thyroid cartilage, caused by contraction of the thyrohyoid muscle. **B,** and **C,** Lateral and frontal xerograms during Valsalva-induced laryngeal closure. In the lateral view, note the marked thyrohyoid approximation and in the frontal view, the abrupt airway cutoff and lack of air column within the thyroid shield, which is at the level of C4-5.

deformed (compressed inward), providing a spring to rapidly open the airway once these muscles relax.[1] The larynx closes at the level of the true cords by action of the intrinsic muscles of the larynx (especially interarytenoid and cricothyroid) during phonation, but this closure is not as tight as the laryngeal spasm described earlier.

Opening the larynx is achieved by elongating and unfolding the airway section from the hyoid to the cricoid cartilage.[1,3] Muscles tether the hyoid bone and the tongue to the chin or anterior mandible (geniohyoid, digastric, hyoglossus, and genioglossus). Other muscles tether the cricoid and thyroid cartilages to the sternum and first rib (sternothyroid). The "strap muscles" tether the hyoid bone to the sternum and rib (sternohyoid and omohyoid). When the head is tilted to extend the chin and the mandible is displaced forward on the tempero-mandibular sliding joint (a jaw-thrust maneuver), maximum stretch occurs at the hyoid-thyroid-cricoid area.

The hyoid bone is pulled in an anterior direction along with the epiglottis and root of the tongue, opening up the oropharynx. The ventricular and vocal folds flatten against the sides of the thyroid cartilage, opening the laryngeal airway.[1]

The inferior and middle constrictors close the superior part of the esophagus (cervical sphincter), thus preventing regurgitation. Muscle relaxants open the airway by relaxing the intrinsic and extrinsic laryngeal muscles that close the airway, but they also relax the pharyngeal constrictors, permitting regurgitation (and aspiration) if gas has been forced into the stomach during attempts at ventilation or if the patient has an incompetent lower esophageal sphincter mechanism (hiatus hernia, achalasia, or esophageal dysmotility). These two problems, airway patency versus airway protection, represent the major dilemma of airway management without an endotracheal tube.

B. UPPER AIRWAY OBSTRUCTION

Upper airway obstruction is a common airway emergency necessitating nonintubation airway manipulation and airway devices. Soft tissue obstruction of the pharynx and larynx are the usual causes of upper airway obstruction; lower airway obstruction is not dealt with in this chapter.

The causes of soft tissue upper airway obstruction at the pharynx include hypopharyngeal obstruction that is due to loss of muscle tone from a central nervous system abnormality (anesthesia, trauma, or coma), expanding, space-occupying lesions (tumor, mucosal edema, abscess, and hematoma), and foreign substances (such as teeth, vomitus, or foreign body). Laryngeal obstruction is most often related to increased muscle activity from attempted vocalization or a reaction from foreign substances (secretions, foreign bodies, or tumors). Recognition of upper airway obstruction is essential and is dependent on observation, suspicion, and clinical data.

The presentation of airway obstruction can be partial or complete. *Partial* airway obstruction is recognized by noisy inspiratory sounds. Depending on the magnitude, cause, and location of the obstruction, the tone of the sounds can vary. Snoring is the typical sound of partial airway obstruction in the hypopharynx and generally is most audible during expiration. Stridor or crowing suggests glottic (laryngeal) obstruction or laryngospasm and is heard most often in inspiration. In addition, signs and symptoms of hypoxemia or hypocarbia (or both) should make one suspicious of an airway obstruction.

Complete airway obstruction is a medical emergency. Signs of complete obstruction in the spontaneously breathing individual are inaudible breath sounds or the inability to feel air movement; use of accessory neck muscles; sternal, intercostal, and epigastric retraction

with inspiratory effort and absence of chest expansion on inspiration; and agitation.

Prevention and relief of airway obstruction are the focus of this chapter. Rapid, simple maneuvers should take precedence in the management of this problem.

II. MANAGEMENT OF THE AIRWAY WITHOUT INTUBATION

A. SIMPLE (NONINSTRUMENTAL) AIRWAY MANEUVERS: HEAD TILT, CHIN LIFT, JAW THRUST

The section on airway anatomy and airway obstruction in this chapter, as well as Chapter 1, constitute essential background to the understanding of airway maneuvers. When muscles of the floor of the mouth and tongue relax, the tongue lies close to or on the back wall of the oropharynx, causing soft tissue obstruction.[4,5] It is also possible for the epiglottis to overlie and obstruct the glottic opening or to seal against the posterior pharyngeal wall.[4,6] This is exaggerated by flexing the head and neck and/or opening the mouth (Fig. 12-3). The distance between the mentum (chin) and the thyroid notch is relatively short in the flexed position. Any maneuver that increases the distance will straighten out the mentum-geniohyoid-hyoid-thyroid line, thus elevating the hyoid bone further from the pharynx. The hyoid elevates the epiglottis via the hyoepiglottic ligament. There are two maneuvers to lengthen this anterior neck distance. The first maneuver (head tilt) is to tilt the head back on the atlantooccipital joint while keeping the mouth closed (teeth approximated). This distance may be further augmented by elevating the occiput 1 to 4 inches above the level of the shoulders (sniffing position), so long as the larynx and posterior pharynx stay in their original position.

In some patients the cervical spine is stiff enough that elevating the head also elevates the C4-5 laryngeal area, leaving the airway unchanged. In children under 5 years of age the upper cervical spine is more flexible and can bow upward, forcing the posterior pharyngeal wall upward against the tongue and epiglottis, thereby exacerbating the obstruction. Therefore, a child's airway is usually best maintained by leaving the head in a more neutral position than that described for an adult. The head tilt is the simplest, first airway maneuver in resuscitation (Fig. 12-4). Head tilt may be accomplished by a chin or neck lift. Extreme caution should be exercised in patients with suspected neck injuries or cerebrovascular disease. The head tilt by chin lift is reportedly more effective than the head tilt by neck lift. In the latter, the mouth opens, the geniohyoid is slack, and the hyoid bone (and epiglottis) may remain close to the pharyngeal wall.

The second maneuver (jaw thrust) more directly lifts the hyoid bone and tongue away from the posterior

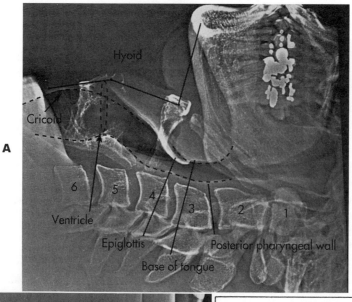

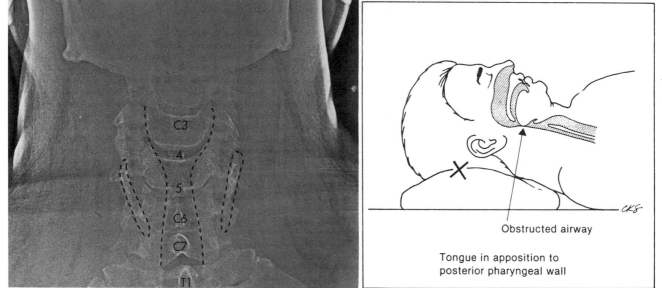

Fig. 12-3. A, Lateral xerogram of the head and neck in neutral position. Patient is awake and supine. Mentum overlies the hyoid bone, the temporomandibular joint is in place, the base of the tongue and the epiglottis are close to the posterior pharyngeal wall, and the thyroid shield and cricoid cartilage are at the level of C5-6. **B,** Frontal view, demonstrating the air column within the thyroid shield with its narrowest site at the level of the vocal cords (C5-6). **C,** Diagram of flexed head with tongue in apposition to posterior pharyngeal wall.

pharyngeal wall by subluxating the mandible forward onto the sliding part of the temporomandibular joint. The occluded teeth prevent the movement of the mandible, so the thumbs depress the mentum while the fingers grip the rami of the mandible and lift it upward to protrude the mandibular teeth in front of the maxillary teeth after the mouth opens slightly. (The insertion of a small airway sometimes makes this procedure easier because it separates the teeth, allowing the teeth to slide.) This is called the jaw thrust maneuver and reliably opens the airway (Fig. 12-5). In most people the mandible is readily drawn back into the joint by elasticity of the joint capsule and masseter muscle; consequently, this position is difficult to maintain with one hand.

Some 20% of patients occlude the nasopharynx with the soft palate during exhalation, when the muscles are relaxed. If the mouth and lips are closed, exhalation is

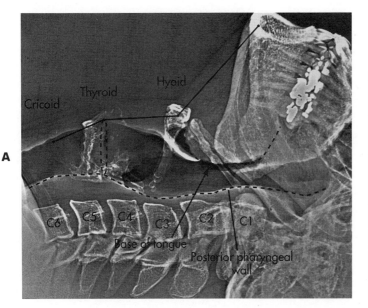

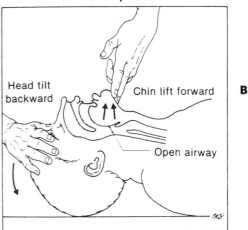

Head tilt and chin lift to obtain extended position

A

B

Fig. 12-4. A, Head and neck in extended position (head tilt). Lateral xerogram with labeling as in Fig. 12-3. Mentum is now superior to the hyoid bone, the temporomandibular joint is still in place (reduced position), the base of the tongue and epiglottis are further off the posterior pharyngeal wall, and the thyroid and cricoid shield are at the level of C4-5. The hyoid bone has been raised and elevated from C3-4 to C2-3. **B,** The drawing shows the head tilted back and the chin lifted forward, both of which contribute to opening the airway.

impeded. In these cases an airway device is required to allow free exhalation. Without an airway device, the mouth must be opened slightly to ensure that the lips are parted. These three maneuvers, done together, are known as the triple airway maneuver (head tilt, jaw thrust, and open mouth) (Fig. 12-5; Box 12-1). The triple airway maneuver is the most reliable manual method to achieve upper airway patency.

B. HEIMLICH MANEUVER

As previously airway maneuvers can help obtain airway patency but do not relieve airway obstruction that is due to foreign material lodged in the upper airway. A foreign body obstruction should be suspected with a witnessed aspiration and when the patient cannot talk, when ventilation is absent, or when positive pressure ventilation meets resistance after routine airway maneuvers have been done. Prior to the insertion of artificial airway devices, a manual effort (finger sweep) should be made to evacuate any foreign material present in the oropharynx. A Heimlich maneuver is indicated when coughing or traditional means are unable to relieve *complete* airway obstruction that is due to foreign material. The intent is to increase intrathoracic pressure sufficiently to stimulate a cough. The Heimlich maneuver (subdiaphragmatic abdominal thrusts) is a recently recommended alternative to back blows (Fig. 12-6; Box 12-2). In emergency situations one technique should not

exclude the other alternatives. The Heimlich maneuver is not advocated by all authorities.[7]

C. ARTIFICIAL AIRWAY DEVICES

When airway maneuvers are inadequate to establish airway patency, it is often necessary to employ artificial airway devices. The following addresses the various available devices and discusses techniques of insertion, maintenance, indications, contraindications, and complications.

1. Oropharyngeal airways

An oral airway can be used as a bite block to prevent occlusion of the teeth, but more often it is used to provide a patent airway. The oral airways range in size from 0 for neonates to 4 for adults. The airways are usually made of either plastic, metal, or rubber. They should be wide enough to contact two or three teeth on the mandible and maxilla and be slightly compressible so that the pressure of a clenched jaw is distributed over all the contacted teeth while the lumen remains patent. The airway is designed with a straight bite section to contact the teeth, a flange at the buccal (proximal) end to prevent swallowing or overinsertion of the airway, and a distal semicircular section to follow the curvature of the mouth, tongue, and posterior pharynx so that the tongue is displaced anteriorly (concave side against the tongue) (Fig. 12-7). In ad-

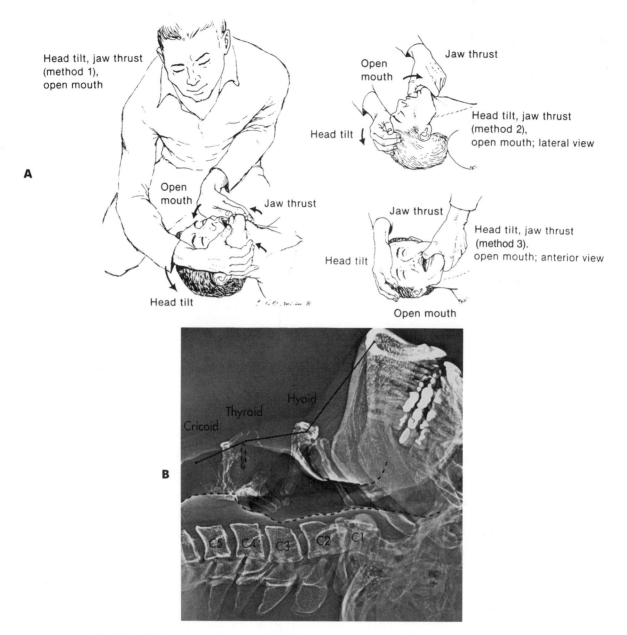

Fig. 12-5. Triple airway maneuver (head tilt, jaw thrust, and open mouth). **A,** Diagram shows, *1,* the head extended on the atlantooccipital joint; *2,* the mouth opened to get the teeth out of occlusion as well as to open the oral fissure; and, *3,* the mandible forced upward, forcing the mandibular condyles to slide anteriorly at the temporomandibular joint. **B,** Lateral xerogram of jaw protrusion (patient awake). In addition to the extended position, the mandibular incisors protrude beyond the maxillary incisors, the teeth are not in occlusion, and the condyles of the mandible are forward, out of the hollow of the temporomandibular joint and onto the sliding portion (subluxated).

dition, an air channel is often provided to facilitate oropharyngeal suctioning.

There are several types of oral airways; all the ones described in the following list have a flange, straight section, and pharyngeal curve (Fig. 12-7).

1. The Guedel airway has a plastic elliptic tube with a central lumen reinforced by a harder inner plastic tube at the level of the teeth and by plastic ridges along the pharyngeal section. Since the airway is completely enclosed, redundant oral and pharyngeal mucosae cannot occlude or narrow the lumen from the side. Because it is oval, the four central incisors usually contact it with great force during masseter spasm.

BOX 12-1   Simple (noninstrumental) airway maneuvers

Head tilt

PROCEDURE
1. With the patient supine and operator at the patient's side, place one hand under the neck and the heel of the other hand on the forehead.
2. Extend the head by displacing the forehead back and lifting the occiput up (neck lift).

INDICATION:	Soft tissue upper airway obstruction
CONTRAINDICATIONS:	Fractured neck
	Basilar artery syndrome
	Infants
COMPLICATIONS:	Sore neck
	Pinched nerve

Chin lift

PROCEDURE:
1. With the patient supine and operator at the head of the patient, place one hand on the forehead, with the first two fingers of the other hand over the underside of the chin.
2. Simultaneously tilt the forehead and exert upward traction on the chin.

INDICATION:	Alternative to neck lift for head tilt
CONTRAINDICATIONS:	Same as head tilt
COMPLICATIONS:	Same as head tilt

Jaw thrust

PROCEDURE:
1. From above the patient's head, place thumbs on the maxilla and fingers behind the angle of the mandible (bilaterally), opening, lifting, and displacing the jaw forward.
2. Retract the lower lip with thumbs.
3. Tilt the head backward (unless contraindicated).

INDICATION:	Head tilt contraindicated (e.g., fractured neck) or ineffective
CONTRAINDICATIONS:	Fractured jaw
	Dislocated jaw
	Awake patient
COMPLICATIONS:	Dislocated jaw
	Damaged teeth

Open mouth

PROCEDURE:
1. Open lips with thumbs after subluxating jaw as part of triple airway maneuver.

INDICATION:	Expiratory obstruction after head tilt
CONTRAINDICATIONS:	Worsening of inspiratory airway
COMPLICATIONS:	None

---

2. The Berman airway consists of two horizontal plates joined by a median ridge. The plates are usually flat and contact more of the teeth than the Guedel airway.
3. The Ovassapian airway has a large anterior flange to control the tongue and a large opening at the level of the teeth, open posteriorly, to allow a fiberscope and endotracheal tube to be passed through it and later disengaged from the airway.
4. The Berman airway has been designed with moveable upper and lower plates and a hinged lower section meant to lift the base of the tongue

(Fig. 12-7). Such airways frequently penetrate deeper into the pharynx, contact the epiglottis, and cause airway reactivity (laryngospasm) in a lightly anesthetized patient (vide infra).

The use of an oral airway seems deceptively simple, but it is essential to do it correctly. The patient should be comatose or adequately anesthetized so that the pharyngeal and laryngeal reflexes are depressed. The mouth is opened and a tongue blade placed at the base of the tongue and drawn upward, lifting the tongue off the posterior pharyngeal wall (Fig. 12-8, *A* on p. 238). The airway is placed so that the oropharyngeal tube is just off

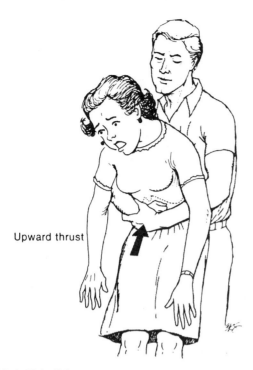

Upward thrust

Fig. 12-6. Heimlich maneuver. Opening an airway obstructed by a laryngeal foreign body by compressing the lungs through external pressure on the abdominal viscera, forcing the diaphragm cephalad. An alternative method to create this "external cough" is by compressing the thorax directly.

BOX 12-2   **The Heimlich maneuver**

PROCEDURE

In the upright patient, wrap both arms around the chest with the right hand in a closed fist in the low sternal-xiphoid area and the left hand on top of the fist. With a rapid forceful thrust, compress upward, increasing subdiaphragmatic pressure and creating an artificial cough.

INDICATION:	Complete upper airway obstruction by a foreign body threatening asphyxia
CONTRAINDICATIONS:	Fractured ribs (relative) Cardiac contusion (relative) Partial airway obstruction
COMPLICATIONS:	Fractured ribs, sternum Liver or spleen trauma

---

the posterior wall of the oropharynx with 1 to 2 cm protruding above the incisors (Fig. 12-8, *B*). (If the flange is at the teeth when the tip is just at the base of the tongue, the airway is too small.) A jaw-thrust maneuver is done with the fingers of both hands to lift the tongue off the pharyngeal wall; the thumbs then tap the airway down the last 2 cm so that the curve of the pharyngeal airway lies behind the base of the tongue (Fig. 12-8, *C* on p. 239). The condyles of the mandible are then allowed to reduce back into the temporomandibular joint. The mouth should be inspected so that neither tongue nor lips are caught between teeth and airway.

An alternative method of insertion is to insert the airway backward (convex side toward the tongue) until the tip is close to the pharyngeal wall of the oropharynx (past the uvula) and then to rotate it 180 degrees (Fig. 12-8, *D*). Rather than pushing the tongue straight downward, the tip rotates and sweeps under from the side. This method is not as reliable as the tongue-blade–assisted method mentioned earlier and has the added risk that the twisting motion can catch gapped teeth and loosen them in patients with poor dentition. If the airway is too short, the tongue may still obstruct the airway at the level of the oropharynx. If it is too long, it may reach to the level of the laryngopharynx, where it contacts the epiglottis. In the lightly anesthetized or awake patient, this stimulation causes coughing or laryngeal spasm. The

best treatment for this problem is to withdraw the airway 1 to 2 cm. A topical anesthetic spray of the pharynx (tetracaine [Cetacaine], 0.5%, lidocaine, 4%) and/or a water-soluble, local anesthetic lubricant on the airway reduces the chance of laryngeal activity but should be used judiciously or avoided in the patient thought to be at risk of aspiration.

Indications for use of an oropharyngeal airway consist of an obstructed upper airway (complete or partial) in the unconscious patient or a need for a bite block in the unconscious patient, and it also may be used as an adjunct for oropharyngeal suctioning. It does not help true laryngospasm or effort closure of the larynx and may worsen it. There are two important caveats in using oral airways. First, awake or lightly anesthetized patients may have reactive airways, and an oral airway may cause retching or vomiting. Second, patients with caps on any of the front four teeth risk fracturing the caps if they bite down hard on the airway. Although the use of the nasopharyngeal airway avoids this risk, it exposes the patient to the risk of epistaxis (discussed later).

There are three major complications with the use of oral airways: trauma, airway hyperactivity, and airway obstruction. Minor trauma, including pinching of the lips and tongue, is common. Potential ulceration and necrosis of oropharyngeal structures from pressure and long-term (days) contact have been reported.[8] These problems necessitate regular intermittent surveillance during use. Dental injury can occur from twisting of the airway, involuntary clenching of the jaw, or direct axial pressure. Dental damage is most common in patients with periodontal disease, dental caries, pronounced degrees of dental proclination, and isolated teeth.[9]

Airway hyperactivity is potentially lethal. Oropharyngeal and laryngeal reflexes can be stimulated by the

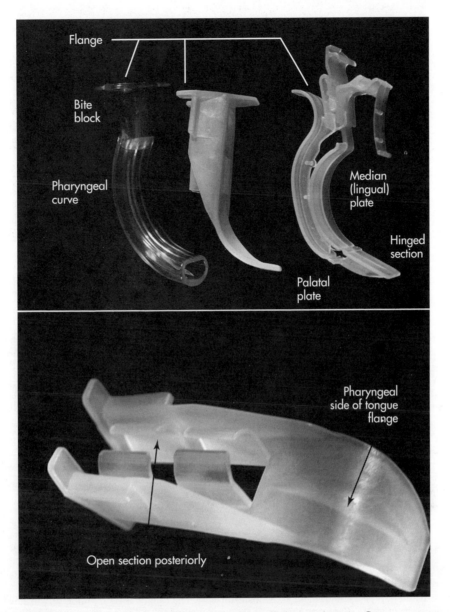

Fig. 12-7. Types of oropharyngeal airways. All oral airways have a flange to prevent overinsertion, a straight bite-block portion, and a pharyngeal curve section. The Guedel airway is a bent cylinder, enclosed at the sides so that soft tissue cannot restrict the central airway. A small suction catheter (less than 14 gauge) can usually be inserted through the Guedel airway into the lower oropharynx, but the oral cavity must still be suctioned around it to remove oral secretions. The Ovassapian airway has a large anterior flange to control the tongue. The airway is open posteriorly so that an endotracheal tube can be inserted through the airway with the fiberoptic technique and the assembly later separated. The absence of a posterior flange allows easier manipulation of the fiberoptic bronchoscope. The Berman airway has anterior and posterior flanges and a central ridge. The open sides of the airway allow secretions to pool toward the center, where a suction catheter inserted down the airway can reach them. The flanges are usually sufficiently close together that soft tissue does not bulge in from the sides. The type shown has a hinged lower plate and a sliding mechanism allowing the lingual flange to slip upward, tilting the lower plate up to elevate the root of the tongue off the pharyngeal wall. Posterior view of Ovassapian airway showing open posterior section.

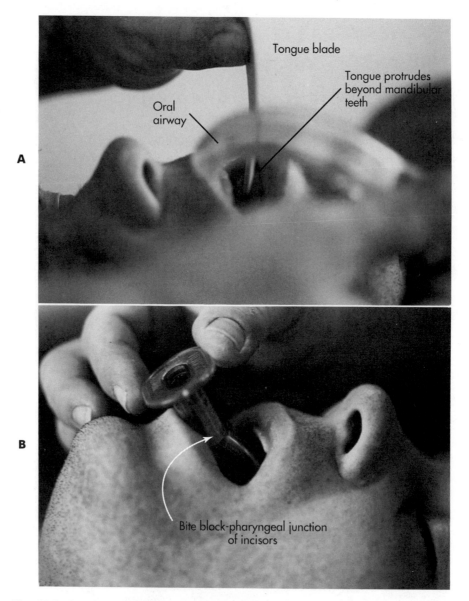

Fig. 12-8. Oropharyngeal airway insertion technique. **A** to **C,** standard technique; **D,** an alternative when no tongue blade is available. **A,** The tongue blade is placed deep into the mouth and depresses the tongue at its posterior half. The tongue is then pulled forward by the tongue blade in an attempt to pull it off the back wall of the pharynx. The airway is inserted with the concave side toward the tongue until the incisors are at the junction of the pharyngeal curve and the bite-block sections. The tongue blade is removed. **B,** The oral airway has been placed by the right hand and the tongue blade removed.   *Continued.*

placement of an artificial airway. Coughing, retching, emesis, laryngospasm, and bronchospasm are common reflex responses. Any oropharyngeal airway (OPA) that contacts the epiglottis or vocal cords can simulate these responses, but the problem is more common with larger oropharyngeal airways. The initial management is to partially withdraw the OPA. If an anesthetic is being administered, deepen the level with an intravenous agent. In cases of laryngospasm it might be necessary to apply mild positive airway pressure and, in trained hands, to cautiously administer small doses of succinylcholine for prompt cessation.

2. Nasopharyngeal airway

The nasopharyngeal airway provides an alternative airway device for treating soft tissue upper airway obstruction. A nasopharyngeal airway (NPA) is less stimulating than an OPA and therefore better tolerated in the awake, semicomatose, or lightly anesthetized patient. In oropharyngeal trauma the nasal airway is often preferable. Nasopharyngeal airways are pliable bent cylinders made of plastic or soft rubber in variable lengths and widths (Fig. 12-9). A flange or moveable disk prevents the outside end from passing beyond the nares and controlling the depth of insertion. The concavity is

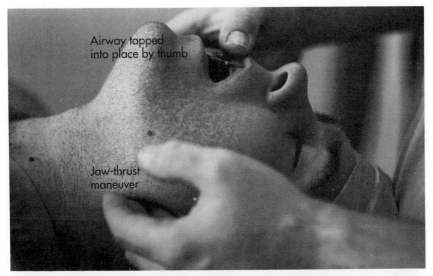

Alternative method of oropharyngeal airway insertion

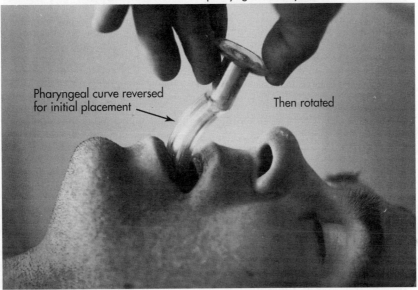

Fig. 12-8. C, A jaw thrust maneuver is done with the fingers at the angle of the jaws (to elevate the posterior tongue) while the thumb taps the airway into place (behind the tongue). When the jaw is allowed to relax, inspect the lips so they are not caught between the teeth and airway. **D,** In an alternate technique the airway is placed in reverse manner (concave toward palate) and then spun into place so that the lower section of the airway rotates between the tongue and posterior pharyngeal wall. The junction of the bite block section and the pharyngeal curve should be near the incisors before the spin move is done.

meant to follow the superior side of the hard palate and posterior wall of the nasooropharynx. The airway is beveled on the left side to aid in following the airway and minimizing mucosal trauma as it advances. A narrow nasopharyngeal tube is often desired to minimize nasal trauma but may be too short to reach behind the tongue. An endotracheal tube of the same diameter may be cut to a longer length and softened in hot water to provide a longer airway. A safety pin or 15-mm adapter should be inserted in the cut endotracheal tube to prevent its migration into the nasopharynx (Fig. 12-9, *A*). A variant of this airway is known as a cuffed nasopharyngeal tube.

It is cut shorter than the endotracheal tube but retains the inflatable cuff. The cuff is blown up in the oropharynx or laryngopharynx and the tube pulled back so that the cuff lies against the soft palate and displaces the base of the tongue forward. This inflatable airway is more stimulating to the patient and the airway than the uncuffed type but is readily managed in an anesthetized patient.[10,11]

The nose should be inspected to determine its size and patency and the presence of nasal polyps or marked septal deviation. Vasoconstriction of the mucous membranes can be accomplished with cocaine or phenyleph-

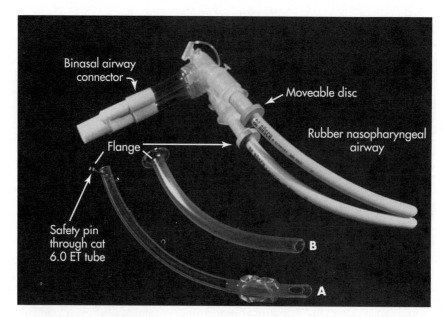

Fig. 12-9. Nasopharyngeal airways. *A,* A size 6.0 endotracheal tube cut at 18 cm with a safety pin through the proximal end to prevent overinsertion. Added length allows tube to go behind the tongue or epiglottis. *B,* Clear nasal airway with flange at proximal end. *C,* Binasal airway. Two standard airways (these have moveable disks to prevent overinsertion) connected to a double-lumen tube adapter.

rine (Neo-Synephrine) drops or spray. Cotton swabs can be saturated in the solution and gently passed parallel to the palate into the nasopharynx. If three cotton swabs can be accommodated in the nasal passage, a size 7.5 airway will usually pass. The airway is generously lubricated with a water-soluble anesthetic ointment. The ointment may also be squirted into the nare. The swabs are removed, and the airway is gently (firmly with gradually increasing force until slow, steady movement is perceived) passed with the concave side against the hard palate (Fig. 12-10) through the nasal passage parallel to the palate, passing under the inferior turbinate, until resistance is felt in the posterior nasopharynx (anterior wall of the retropharyngeal space).

Sometimes it is helpful to rotate the NPA 90 degrees counterclockwise, bringing the open part of the bevel against the posterior nasopharyngeal mucosae, and to resume gentle pressure. As the tube makes the bend (indicated by a relative loss of resistance to passage), it should be rotated back to the original position. If the tube will not pass with moderate pressure, there are three management options: a narrower tube, redilation of the naris, and trying the other naris. If the tube will not pass into the oropharynx, withdraw the tube 2 cm, pass a suction catheter through the nasal airway as a guide, and push the airway forward over the suction tube. If the patient coughs or reacts as the nasal tube is inserted to its full extent, it should be withdrawn 1 to 2 cm. (The tip has probably touched the vocal cords.) If the patient's airway is still obstructed after insertion, the airway

should be checked for obstruction by mucus or kinking by passing a small suction catheter. If the obstruction persists, it is possible that the NPA is too short and the base of the tongue lies at its tip. A longer airway should be tried. A size 6.0 endotracheal tube can be cut at 18 cm to provide this, and a safety pin put through the proximal end as a flange outside the nose if the 14-mm adapter of the endotracheal tube is too bulky to fit under the face mask. If laryngospasm is suspected, withdraw the NPA 1 to 2 cm and manage further as previously described.

The indications for a nasopharyngeal airway consist of upper airway obstruction in awake, semicomatose, or lightly anesthetized patients; in patients who are not adequately treated with oropharyngeal airways; in patients with dental indications or oropharyngeal trauma; and in patients in whom there is a need to facilitate oropharyngeal and laryngopharyngeal suctioning. The contraindications consist of nasal airway occlusion, nasal fractures, marked deviated septum, coagulopathy (risk of epistaxis), prior transphenoidal hypophysectomy or Caldwell-Luc procedures (nose packed), cerebrospinal fluid rhinorrhea, and adenoid hypertrophy (relative, usually in pediatrics).

The complications of nasopharyngeal airways consist of failure of passage of the airway, epistaxis (mucosal tears or avulsion of the turbinate), submucosal tunneling, and pressure sores.[9,12] Epistaxis is usually self-limiting and resolves spontaneously. The problem usually presents itself when the nasal tube is removed, removing the tamponade. Treat anterior plexus bleeding

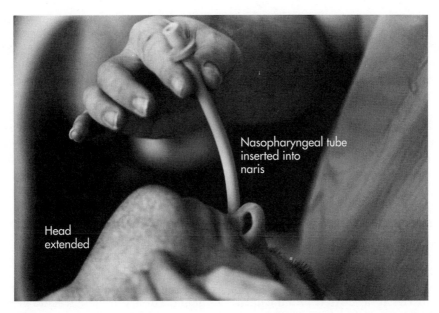

Fig. 12-10. Insertion of nasopharyngeal airway. The airway is oriented concave to the hard palate and inserted straight back. Gripping the airway near the top allows the tube to bend if resistance to passage is extreme. If it is gripped close to the naris, sufficient force can be transmitted to shear off a turbinate.

by applying pressure to the nostrils. If the posterior plexus is bleeding, leave the airway in, suction the pharynx, ventilate the patient, and consider intubating the trachea if the bleeding does not stop rapidly. Position the patient on his or her side to avoid aspiration of blood. A nasal pack or otolaryngology consultation may be necessary. The management of submucosal tunneling in the retropharyngeal space is to withdraw the airway. Once this occurs, it is unlikely that a nasopharyngeal airway can be successfully passed by this route. The other nostril may be tried, or an oropharyngeal airway used. The patient should be periodically observed for pressure sores of the ali nasi or for evidence of sinusitis. Upon extubation some mucosal ulceration may be observed.

3. Binasal airway

The use of two nasopharyngeal airways joined together by an adapter (Fig. 12-9, *C*) has been previously described.[10,13] This technique allows for spontaneous and potentially low positive pressure ventilation if the mouth is occluded. To allow for assisted ventilation, the tubes must be positioned near the larynx and the surrounding soft tissues must help seal the hypopharynx. The use of two tubes provides enough bulk to seal and enough cross-sectional area to minimize airway resistance. (Two 6-mm airways have a cross-sectional area exceeding that of an 8-mm airway.) Although gastric inflation is possible, excessive gas flow can exit the mouth.[13] The laryngeal mask airway (LMA) is likely to be a better management option in any circumstance where this is a potentially useful technique, although a

greater level of anesthesia is probably needed for the LMA insertion (see Chapter 19).

D. NONINTUBATION VENTILATION

Despite a patent airway, ventilation can be inadequate. Ventilatory assistance can be achieved through several alternatives other than intubation. Standard cardiopulmonary resuscitation courses have long taught the effectiveness of mouth-to-mouth and mouth-to-nose ventilation. Mouth-to-artificial-airway ventilation using an S tube (Two Guedel airways with the flanges bonded together) overcomes many of the aesthetic objections to the previous techniques. More sophisticated approaches to ventilatory assistance (as in anesthesia) typically include the use of bag-mask-valve systems. Ventilation of a patient generally requires a sealed interface between the patient and a delivery system that supplies airway gases and can be pressurized. For nonintubation ventilation, this seal is either on the skin of the face (face-mask techniques) or in the hypopharynx (laryngeal mask). A partial seal can be obtained in the hypopharynx or nasopharynx by the binasal airway or the cuffed nasopharyngeal airway so long as the mouth is closed, but the effectiveness of the seal is limited. The most reliable seal, allowing high positive pressures, is at the trachea, but the price is airway and hemodynamic reflex activity.

1. Face masks

Face masks differ in material, shape, type of seal, and transparency. The mask is composed of three parts: the body, seal (or cushion), and connector (or collar). The body is the main structure of the mask. Since the body rises above the face, all face masks increase dead space. A more malleable body allows for a better fit to the face and a reduced dead space. The added dead space is usually not significant when ventilation is spontaneous, and it is never significant if ventilation is controlled. Respiratory gas analysis (capnography) can verify ventilation. The seal is the actual rim of the mask that comes in contact with the face. The two types of seals are a cushion rim that is often inflatable and a rubber or plastic edge that is a noninflatable, flexible extension of the body. The connector is at the top of the body and provides a 22-mm female adapter for a breathing circuit or air-mask-bag unit (AMBU)–bag elbow. A collar with hooks allows for a mask-retaining strap to be attached to help hold the mask to the face. The precise application of the straps (e.g., crossed [ipsilateral strap to contralateral hook] or uncrossed) is a matter of individual preference and is usually the result of a trial-and-error process to find the best seal and airway patency on the individual patient.

The Ohio anatomic face mask has a body contoured to the face, with a sharp notch for the nose, a double curve to fit the malar eminence of the cheek, and a curved chin section (Fig. 12-11). It is made of conductive rubber, is slightly malleable, and has a high-pressure, low-volume cushion. For those whom it fits, it allows the chin to be lifted high into the mask while sealing the sides and maintaining maxillary pressure, providing the best compromise between adequacy of seal and patency of airway. Its disadvantages include poor fit on a face with a broad, flat bridge of the nose and poor malleability to different-sized faces. The correct size is important, and several sizes should be readily available. It is opaque, so vomitus cannot be readily seen, and it requires extensive aeration with the seal cushion collapsed after ethylene oxide sterilization because the ethylene oxide absorbed in the rubber can cause a chemical burn on the skin. Disposable transparent plastic masks have been made with high-volume, low-pressure cushions that seal to the face much more easily. They have little or no chin curve, however, and obtaining a patent airway is slightly more difficult. The base of the body of these transparent masks is flat; the large, flexible cushion fits a wide variety of faces. The cushion may be factory sealed or have a nipple for the injection of air. A progression of this style is the "easy-seal" mask having a reinforced flexible disk for a body and a large, floppy cushion comprising the entire undersurface of the disk except for the 22-mm adapter air passage. This mask is used in arrest situations but has not been commonly used to administer anesthesia.

Properly using a face mask depends on obtaining a good seal between the mask and the patient's face; successfully doing this is fundamental to administering adequate ventilation and inhalation anesthesia. The mask should comfortably fit both the hand of the user and the face of the patient. An anatomic mask (Ohio) is meant to fit at the bridge of the nose, the alveolar ridge of the mandible, and along the malar eminences (the maxillary curve). Although the body of the mask is formed so that a cushion is not essential for a seal much of the time, the cushion should be inflated to equalize pressure all along the contact points of the face. If the mask is too long, the face can be elongated 1 to 2 cm by placing an oral airway. If the mask is too short with the oropharyngeal airway placed, the OPA can be removed and a nasopharyngeal airway placed. The mask can also be moved 1 to 2 cm along the bridge of the nose to make a small mask fit at the chin.

Several methods are described for holding the mask. Regardless of the precise method, multiple trials with close monitoring for leaks are necessary. Our preferred method follows. The left hand grips the mask with the thumb and index finger around the collar (Figs. 12-12 and 12-13). The left side of the mask fits into the palm. The hypothenar eminence of the left hand should extend below the left side of the mask. If it does not, the mask is too big for the user's hand and a smaller mask should be tried. The problem with a large mask is that the left hypothenar eminence cannot pull the patient's cheek against the left side of the mask to maintain a seal if pronation is necessary to seal the right side (vide infra).

The patient may, of course, require a large mask, in which case retaining straps are usually necessary to get a satisfactory seal in all quadrants. The middle finger can be on the mask or chin, depending on the span of the user's hand, the sizes of the mask and face, and the ease of fit. The proximal interphalangeal joints of the fingers and the distal interphalangeal joint of the thumb should be at the midline of the mask, allowing the pads of the fingers to put pressure on the right side of the mask. The mask must be sealed at all four sides. To seal the mask at the bridge of the nose, spread the sides of the mask at its bridge and place it on the bridge of the nose so that the mask does not put pressure on the eyes. The nose will subsequently be sealed by downward pressure of the thumb. Lower the mask onto the face and note where the lower edge of the mask (the chin curve) touches the patient's face. If it touches at the teeth, use a larger mask or slide the current one down the nose 1 to 2 cm. If the chin curve hits the mentum instead of the alveolar ridge, the sides of the mask may not seal to the face (especially with the Ohio anatomic mask). Use an oral airway to "lengthen the face" 1 to 2 cm or use a smaller mask. To seal the chin section, grip the mandible with the fingers and rotate the wrist so as to pull the mandible up into the mask with the fingers while pushing the bridge of the mask down with the thumb. To seal the left side of the mask, gather skin of the cheek against the side of

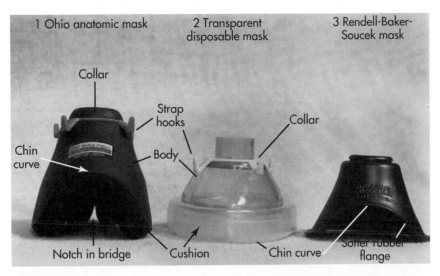

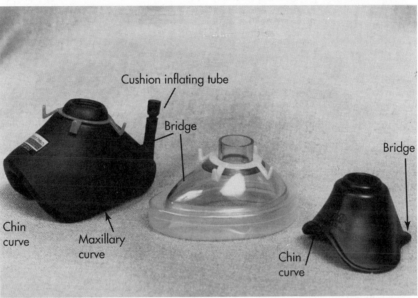

Fig. 12-11. Face masks, front *(top panel)* and side *(bottom panel)* views. *1,* Ohio anatomic mask. *2,* transparent disposable mask. *3,* Rendell-Baker-Soucek mask. The various parts of the masks and different cushions and contours are evident; strap hooks can also be put on the Rendell-Baker-Soucek mask if desired. The use of high-volume, low-pressure cuffs has eliminated the need for an anatomically formed body of the mask to get an adequate seal to the face and has reduced the chances of pressure points over the face. However, this type of mask does little to aid the maintenance of a patent airway, making the use of artificial airways more important.

the mask with the hypothenar eminence. (The user's left elbow must be at his or her side in order to do this.) To seal the right side, pronate the left forearm while pressing the ends of the thumb, index finger, and possibly middle finger onto the right side of the mask.

The sides of the mask are somewhat malleable to adjust to wide or narrow faces. In edentulous patients the cheeks are often too hollow to allow an adequate fit. Edentulous patients also lose a vertical dimension to their face that can be restored by an oral airway. In rare

situations, leave the dentures in place to allow a mask fit, but the dentures could be lost, broken, or dislodged with consequent obstruction. Alternatively, use a large mask so that the chin fits entirely inside the mask with the seal on the caudal surface of the chin, the cheeks fit within the mask, and the sides of the mask seal along the lateral maxilla and mandible. (These maneuvers to make a difficult mask fit possible are often best side-stepped by endotracheal intubation or use of a laryngeal mask airway, but clinical judgment must determine when this

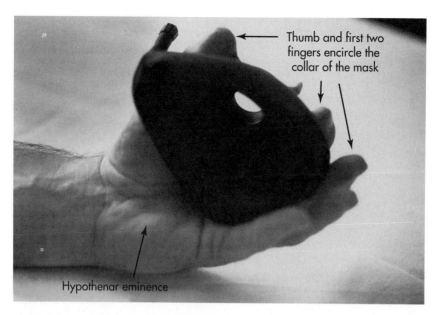

Fig. 12-12. Proper hand grip of face mask. Hypothenar eminence extends down from mask while thumb and two fingers encircle collar.

is the case.) (Box 12-3). Mask-retaining straps can be placed at the occiput and connected to the mask collar to put pressure at various angles to assist the seal. The tension on the straps should be no more than necessary to achieve a seal, and the tension should be released and the mask moved slightly every 15 to 30 minutes to allow perfusion of underlying skin. External gauze sponges may be used to protect the skin from excessive pressure by a strap. When straps or gauze sponges are employed, extreme care must be given to avoid ocular trauma.[5,10] An additional maneuver to compensate for mask leaks is to increase fresh gas flow.

The preceding detailed procedures are important if black Ohio anatomic masks are used. The transparent masks with high-volume, low-pressure cuffs deform to seal more easily and contact a larger surface area of skin, minimizing the chance of pressure ischemia in a case of long duration. The chin and cheek areas seal more easily, but the size of the cushion occasionally results in pressure on the globe of the eye if the mask is high on the bridge of the nose. The thumb can pull the mask caudad to roll the cushion away from the eye. The cushions may be factory sealed or inflatable. The latter should be filled sufficiently so that the edge of the body of the mask does not contact the face. Some masks do not have cushions (Rendell-Baker-Soucek masks), but the rubber or plastic edge is usually tapered and flexible so that it deforms along the face to give a larger area of contact than just the edge.

A face mask is indicated to seal a patient's airway to allow application of a mixture of gases to either ventilate, oxygenate, or anesthetize. These situations include preoxygenation with spontaneous ventilation, ventila-

tion prior to endotracheal intubation (including resuscitation situations), ventilation or oxygenation when placement of an endotracheal tube cannot be achieved (visually or by capnography) and the patient's vital signs deteriorate, and the delivery of anesthetic gases. Mask ventilation is relatively contraindicated in situations requiring general anesthesia but also with a large likelihood of gastric contents soiling the trachea (such as a full stomach, hiatus hernia, esophageal motility disorders, and pharyngeal diverticula (e.g., Zenker's). In addition, whenever there is a likelihood of gas inflating the stomach (such as with a weakened cricopharyngeal sphincter [e.g., with prolonged neuromuscular paralysis or bulbar neurologic disease]), a need for high airway pressures (e.g., decreased compliance of lungs or chest wall, obesity [twice the ideal body weight], marked kyphoscoliosis, or marked bronchospasm), an adverse position (marked headdown or prone) or inability to easily reach the head of the patient (fracture table, lithotripsy, CT scan), use of a mask for positive pressure ventilation must be done cautiously. Mask ventilation is also relatively contraindicated whenever there is a need to avoid the head and neck manipulation (head tilt) that may be necessary to maintain the airway or whenever there is a need to avoid touching the neck (surgery of the head and neck) or an inability to seal the mask (e.g., facial trauma and edentulous mouths with aveolar recession). Lack of integrity of the dermis, resulting in marked bullae from friction (e.g., epidermolysis bullosa) is a contraindication to the use of a face mask. Finally, inability to sustain adequate assisted or spontaneous ventilation is a relative contraindication to further use of a face mask.

Application of mask to face

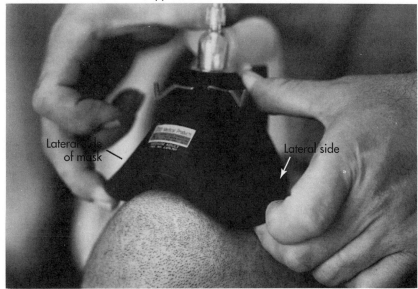

Lateral side of mask

Lateral side

A

Standard one handed grip of mask to face

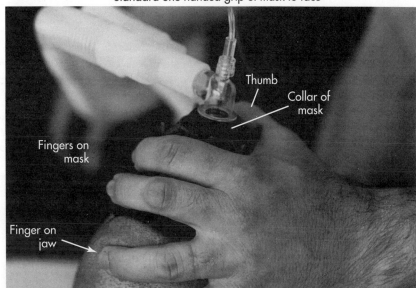

Thumb

Collar of mask

Fingers on mask

Finger on jaw

B

One handed mask grip with jaw-thrust

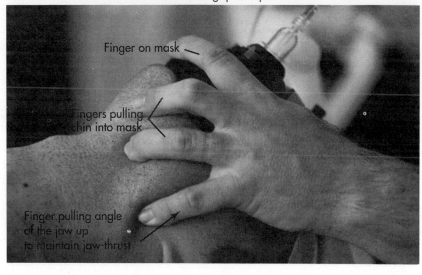

Finger on mask

Fingers pulling chin into mask

Finger pulling angle of the jaw up to maintain jaw-thrust

C

Fig. 12-13. Sealing and holding the mask to the face. **A,** Application of mask to face. Fingers spread the bridge and lateral sides of the mask as it is lowered onto face. **B,** Side view of standard one-handed grip of mask to face. The thumb and first two fingers encircle the collar of the mask while the last two fingers pull mandible up into the mask and extend the head. **C,** One-handed mask grip: maintaining jaw-thrust. Caudad view of handgrip shows little finger at the angle of the jaw maintaining backward and upward pull to maintain jaw thrust. Because of the increased span required of the hand, only the first finger is now on the mask, while the second and third fingers pull the mandible into the face and extend the head. (The exact position of each of the four fingers depends slightly on the size of the left hand.) To prevent teeth from grating on one another, this technique usually requires the prior insertion of an oral airway. The jaw-thrust position is initiated with the usual two-handed maneuver; this one-handed grip can at best only maintain the position. The strong pull on the mandible resulting in friction of the incisors on the bite-block portion of the oral airway does as much to maintain the position as does the little finger at the angle of the jaw.

BOX 12-3 Airway management choices

Mask with oropharyngo-airway

INDICATIONS:	Ventilation preceding tracheal intubation
	Failed tracheal intubation
	Awake patient requires high levels of inspired O_2
ADVANTAGES:	Can be done in awake patient without airway
	Does not require relaxants
	Minimal patient response
DISADVANTAGES:	Requires constant attention (left hand is constantly on patient's face or mask; skill required throughout)
	Gastric inflation and inadequate ventilation if positive pressure consistently over 20 torr
CONTRAINDICATIONS:	Known increased risk of vomiting or regurgitation
	Known significant airway obstruction
COMPLICATIONS:	Lip or dental trauma on airway
	Inadequate airway patency (laryngospasm, pharyngeal obstruction)
	Facial pressure injury (skin, supraorbital, or infraorbital nerves, mental nerves from fingers or mask straps)
	Aspiration risk highest of the three techniques

Laryngeal mask airway

INDICATIONS:	Failed intubation
	Difficult face-mask fit
ADVANTAGES:	Minimal patient response, but does require anesthetic
	Does not require relaxant
	Smooth emergence
	Once placed, hands are free; requires intermediate level of monitoring
	Regurgitation and laryngospasm less likely than with mask
DISADVANTAGES:	Cannot generate airway pressures >20 torr reliably
	Requires anesthetic level; can be misplaced
	Laryngospasm possible
	Regurgitation more likely than with endotracheal tube
CONTRAINDICATIONS:	Known increased risk of vomiting, regurgitation
	High airway pressures required
COMPLICATIONS:	Regurgitation/aspiration
	Inadequate placement and inadequate ventilation
	Hypoglossal nerve palsy
	Pharyngeal trauma

Endotracheal tube airway

INDICATIONS:	Increased risk of vomiting, regurgitation
	High airway pressures anticipated (obese patient)
	Inaccessibility of airway
ADVANTAGES:	Most secure airway, once placed and confirmed
	Skill requirement low after initial placement
	Seals trachea from gastrointestinal tract; high pressure possible
DISADVANTAGES:	Nociceptive response to tracheal foreign body
	Coughing during and after extubation
	Postextubation laryngospasm, noncardiac pulmonary edema
	Usually requires relaxant to place
	Can result in death if esophageal placement unrecognized
CONTRAINDICATIONS:	No capnography available (relative)
	Chance of minor voice changes unacceptable (professional singer-relative)
COMPLICATIONS:	Cough, straining on endotracheal tube or at extubation (suture lines compromised)
	Noncardiac pulmonary edema, croup
	Hypertension, tachycardia
	Bronchospasm in susceptible individual
	Undiscovered esophageal intubation (if no capnograph)
	Hoarseness (usually 24 hours; can be 6 months)

There are several complications from using a face mask. First, a poor mask fit can result in gas leaks that waste gases, prevent the maintenance of positive pressure, collapse the reservoir bag and prevent monitoring of ventilation, and potentially compromise ventilation and oxygenation. Various techniques to manage this problem were described earlier. Second, pressure from a malpositioned mask or too tight a seal, especially with the use of straps, can cause skin, nerve, and ophthalmic injury. Appropriate mask selection, application, and vigilance constitute the best means of avoiding this problem. Gastric distention and aspiration constitute a potentially lethal problem with positive pressure ventilation by mask. Transparent masks allow for earlier recognition of regurgitation. Finally, reactions from the residue of the sterilization process can cause a contact dermatitis. Allergies to the mask material have been reported.

2. Respiratory (resuscitator) bags

The air-mask-bag unit (AMBU) was developed in 1955 by Rubin.[14] The AMBU has provided an alternative means of artificial ventilation to the standard anesthesia bag and circuit. The bag can be used with a mask or endotracheal tube. Its advantage is in being self-inflating, thus avoiding the need for compressed gas. The disadvantages are that the "feel" of the airway (compliance and resistance) is poor and the delivery of high concentrations of oxygen more complex. Various types of hand resuscitator units exist. They use various valve systems to ensure nonrebreathing, and the units vary to a minor or moderate extent in size, weight, percentage of oxygen delivery, volume, reinflation time, cycling rate, and number of parts; this equipment has recently been well reviewed.[15]

Criteria for selection of an AMBU should include easy, fool-proof assembly; a nonsticking valve system to prevent rebreathing while allowing exhalation; a closable pressure pop-off valve with standard 15-22-mm connection; capability to deliver 95% oxygen and 0 to 12 cm H_2O positive end-expiratory pressure (PEEP); airway pressure monitor; capability to be sterilized; and performance under varying common environmental conditions.[15,16] Limited complications have been associated with the use of AMBU equipment. Inaccurate inspired oxygen that is due to inadequate oxygen inflow rate and valve locking that is due to mechanical malfunction or excessive oxygen flow rates are some of the reported problems.

3. Determining the effectiveness of nonintubation ventilation and use of supplemental airway maintenance techniques

The mask seal should be sufficient to permit a 20-cm H_2O positive pressure with a minimal leak. It is important to limit positive airway pressure to 25 cm H_2O to avoid inflating the stomach, which will in turn restrict diaphragmatic movement and increase the chance of regurgitation through the esophageal sphincters.[5,10,16,17] The effectiveness of ventilation should be judged by exhaled tidal volume, movement of the chest, good bilateral breath sounds, vital signs, and available monitors of oxygenation and ventilation. If the patient cannot be ventilated with 25 cm H_2O positive pressure, either the airway is obstructed at the pharynx by the tongue, the airway is obstructed at the larynx by cord spasm, the patient has sufficient muscle tone to prevent chest expansion, or there is a decrease in pulmonary compliance or increased airway resistance. The oral airway corrects the first; a small dose of succinylcholine decreases laryngeal spasm and muscle tone, and definitive treatment of the compliance and resistance issues depends on the etiologic factors. Tracheal tug (caudad movement of the larynx) or paradoxic movement of the chest suggests airway obstruction. A nasopharyngeal or oropharyngeal airway (OPA) may open the pharyngeal airway at the cost of laryngeal spasm, which is again treated with a small dose of succinylcholine. Paralysis should be a temporary expedient in treating laryngeal spasm, with deeper anesthesia being the more definitive treatment. The known presence of anatomic airway obstruction (tumor or polyp) precludes the use of muscle relaxants, since loss of muscle tone may cause nearly untreatable airway obstruction.

Occasionally the airway is sufficiently difficult to require the triple airway maneuver to be maintained during ventilation or anesthesia. Since the jaw tends to slide back into the temporomandibular joint, the force required to maintain the position is large and therefore difficult to maintain constantly, but this must be done. Placement of an OPA as previously described can be helpful in this regard. After the OPA is set in place with the thumbs, the last three fingers of the left hand pull the mandible tightly against the OPA so that the friction of the incisors on the airway is sufficient to prevent the mandible from slipping back into joint. The right hand places the mask at the bridge of the nose while the thumb and first finger of the left hand receive the mask by encircling the collar and adjust the mask to the face. (The other three fingers of the left hand continue to maintain steady pressure on the mandible, holding the teeth firmly against the OPA.) The left hand now squeezes the mandible-OPA-face mask together as a unit. If pressure is relaxed, the jaw can be felt to slide back into joint. (If it does so, the triple airway maneuver is repeated.) The tension on the jaw can be adjusted by grip strength, by backward weight of the anesthetist, or by the left little finger placed below the angle of the jaw to keep the mandible protruded. (This last maneuver usually requires a rather large hand; see Fig. 12-13, C).

This position may not only clear the tongue from the pharynx but also partly treat laryngeal spasm by exerting force on the hyoid bone, elevating the epiglottis and unfolding the vestibular and vocal folds. It is fatiguing to maintain this position, and the pressure required creates a risk of local skin or nerve injury. The cause of the difficulty is partial airway closure caused by a reactive airway; deepening the anesthetic frequently helps the situation. If, however, after 5 to 10 minutes the patient will not maintain the airway without a jaw thrust, the trachea should be intubated (or a laryngeal mask airway used). Positive airway pressure (PEEP or continuous positive airway pressure [CPAP]) can be used throughout the respiratory cycle to lessen soft tissue obstruction. The pop-off valve is closed to maintain about a 15-cm H_2 positive pressure during expiration (no greater than 20 cm). Inspiration can still be assisted at 25 cm H_2O.

The difficulty in maintaining a mask fit and a patent airway with one hand is occasionally so great that the patient's safety is best served if the mask fit and airway are controlled by two hands while a second person ventilates the patient's lungs by squeezing the bag.[16,17] The two-handed airway technique uses the fingers to perform a jaw-thrust maneuver while the thumbs hold the mask in place by pressure on the lateral sides of the mask (Fig. 12-14). This maneuver can be done from the side of the patient, facing the patient's mandible, as well as from behind.

The confirmation of adequate ventilation is of primary importance to patient safety. Vigilant clinical observation is key in the assessment of the airway and ventilation, which can be monitored by several techniques. First, the fingers of the left hand supporting the mandible sense the vibration of air flow in the mouth and pharynx. The distal interphalangeal joint should be at the rim of the mandible so that the pads of the fingers contact the soft tissue at the floor of the mouth. They also sense anesthetic depth (muscle tone and swallowing prior to vomiting). Second, the right hand on the anesthesia reservoir bag senses emptying and filling of the bag during the respiratory cycle. (Assisted ventilation techniques should be used every other breath so that the intervening respiratory cycle can be sensed.) With experience, this technique helps assess airway resistance and compliance. Third, pretracheal (or precordial) stethoscopes are basic monitors that should not be neglected. The stethoscope can be attached to the skin over the sternal notch by double-sided adhesive disks, usually permitting both tracheal sounds and heart tones to be heard. Fourth, a normal capnogram offers positive evidence of ventilation. Occasionally a poor mask fit and a gas leak (with high compensatory flows) prevent a good capnogram, even with adequate ventilation. Placing an aspirating cath-eter into a nasal prong and connecting it to a capnometer can give a trendable index of ventilation, even in a sedated patient. Fifth, the pulse oximeter offers reassurance that the oxygenation is adequate when the pulse oximetry (SpO_2) is above 95%. When below 90%, it indicates that oxygenation is inadequate and inadequate ventilation is probable.

III. SPECIFIC CLINICAL SITUATIONS

Airway maintenance without endotracheal intubation is a necessity of the practice of anesthesia, respiratory care, emergency medicine, and critical care. Occasionally, nonintubation techniques are desirable, since they avoid the foreign body responses to tracheal intubation (tachycardia, hypertension, and coughing). The risks of nonintubation of the airway have been previously discussed. This technique is not well suited to prolonged positive pressure ventilation. Airway maintenance during a prolonged steady state (30 minutes to 3 hours) presents a different set of problems and vigilance requirements from those of airway maintenance in a transitional period between a natural airway and the placement or removal of an endotracheal tube. Three situations requiring airway maintenance without endotracheal intubation that deserve special mention are sedation, transitional periods surrounding endotracheal intubation, and induction and maintenance of a general anesthetic.

A. DURING SEDATION

Sedation is used to allay patient anxiety or minimize discomfort from position or duration of the procedure, when the stimuli of surgery have been largely ablated by a regional anesthetic block or local anesthetic infiltration. Mild sedation during which the patient can converse easily requires no special airway management, although supplemental oxygen per nasal cannulas or clear plastic oxygen insufflation mask should always be used. Sedation to the point of somnolence or stertor requires some intervention to ensure adequacy of ventilation and oxygenation, and moderate patient discomfort often requires sedation to this level. Chin lift or jaw thrust usually results in increased patient awareness and clearing of the stertor, reassuring the anesthetist that the patient is not overly sedated. If stertor returns, turning the head 45 degrees to one side or the other may help. (The epiglottis may be the cause of this stertor,[18] and mild twisting of the neck may open a sufficient airway.) Monitoring with pretracheal stethoscope or pulse oximetry may provide enough reassurance to continue with present conditions. The patient may allow an anesthesia mask (attached to a circle system) to lie over the nose and mouth (secured loosely with a mask-retaining strap). This arrangement permits monitoring of respiration via the reservoir bag, and perhaps

Holding the mask to the face with 2 hands
from above the patient

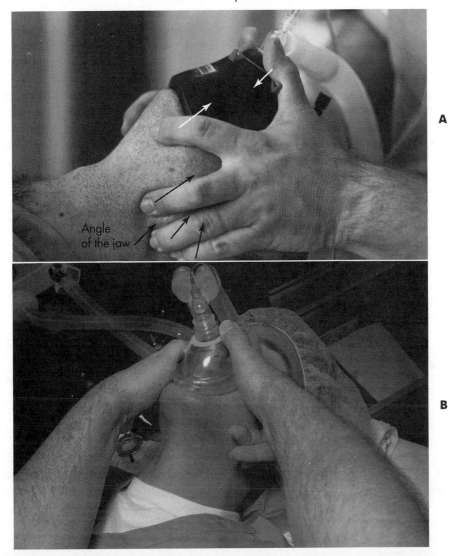

Fig. 12-14. Holding the mask to the face with two hands. **A,** Thumbs are hooked over collar of the mask, with lower fingers maintaining jaw thrust (if needed) and upper fingers pulling mandible into the mask and extending the head. (Arrows indicate direction of force.) A second individual must ventilate the patient. In this figure the airway is maintained from above the head. **B,** The airway and mask fit is maintained from the side of the patient, allowing the person ventilating the patient improved access to the patient. The thumbs maintain downward pressure from the collar of the mask, the thenar eminence maintains lateral pressure on the mask, and the first and second fingers maintain jaw thrust from the angle of the jaw. This position is helpful if the person ventilating the patient is preparing to intubate the patient's trachea under direct vision using a laryngoscope or by fiberoptic bronchoscopy.

capnography, as well as continued sedation with 25% to 50% nitrous oxide. Since a mask or nasal airway used in this way may not have a tight fit to the face, scavenging of nitrous oxide is probably incomplete and controlled ventilation impossible. In patients whom a mask will not fit at all closely (edentulous patients being the most common), sedation can be temporarily deepened, the nares anesthetized, and a small nasopharyngeal airway

inserted, into which a 15-mm adapter (which goes to an oxygen source) has been inserted. A more complete seal and wider airway can be used by using two nasal airways (see Binasal Airway). These techniques have less hemodynamic disturbances than do endotracheal intubation, but they require monitoring and the ability to revise techniques as determined by the level of sedation. Because of field avoidance, mask techniques are usually not feasible during monitored anesthesia care for cataract surgery. An oral airway is usually not successful, since it is more stimulating than the nasal airway and may induce retching with this level of sedation. Complications of mild sedation are usually minimal.

B. TRANSITIONAL AIRWAY TECHNIQUES

Prior to intubation of the trachea, the patient usually has received a neuromuscular blocker or, in the case of cardiopulmonary arrest, has no muscle tone. The larynx is open, and laryngeal spasm is not a consideration. The techniques of airway maintenance (triple airway maneuver, obtainment of mask seal, limitation of ventilatory pressures to 25 cm H_2O, and early use of oropharyngeal airways) are usually sufficient to permit ventilating the patient. Airway maintenance from extubation to smooth, spontaneous ventilation is complicated by the presence of a reactive larynx capable of spasm. Therefore the timing of extubation is an important consideration. Extubation can be either at a deep stage of anesthesia with minimal airway reactivity or during very light anesthesia (nearly or fully awake) so that there is full control of reflex activity (and usually some coughing and straining). The patient extubated during the middle ground of moderate anesthetic depth is at increased risk of laryngospasm. The correct timing is estimated as follows. The patient should be breathing spontaneously and be considered to have an empty stomach. The oropharynx is suctioned (with a flexible suction catheter) to remove pooled secretions. If smooth, spontaneous breathing continues, the tube is moved slightly and the cuff is deflated. If the patient continues to breathe smoothly, the trachea is extubated during inspiration with pressure on the reservoir bag. If, on the other hand, coughing and straining ensue, extubation must be delayed until the patient again breathes smoothly for two or three cycles. In either event, an inspiratory breath is augmented maximally and the endotracheal tube is withdrawn at end-inspiration, allowing rapid expiratory air flow or a cough to clear retained secretions from around the vocal cords. A triple airway maneuver is done immediately (within 5 seconds),[18] spontaneous ventilation is confirmed, and a mask with 100% oxygen is applied to the face. If secretions are copious or intraoral blood is expected, the patient should be put into a position to optimize drainage (head down or lateral).

Laryngeal spasm can be treated with positive pressure if it seems to improve breath by breath.[19,20] A small dose of succinylcholine (10 mg) remedies the situation more completely at the risk of some muscle ache postoperatively. If obstruction continues, laryngoscopy should be performed to investigate the cause, and reintubation should be considered. Special attention must be given to patients with full stomachs, since they are at increased risk of vomiting and aspiration.

During emergence, the patient usually passes through a stage of generalized increased muscle tone, especially masseter spasm. If an oral airway is in place, the force of contraction can put extreme pressure on the central incisors of the mandible and maxilla with damage to caps or teeth with periodontal disease. An airway should never be removed by force, since lateral stresses may dislodge teeth. Either wait for jaw relaxation or open the jaw with firm pressure on the mandibular ramus between the clenched teeth and the buccal mucosae. Two techniques can be used to minimize the the danger to teeth. The first is to have an acrylic tooth guard made by the dental service prior to operation to distribute the forces over more teeth. The other is to place a nasopharyngeal tube prior to extubation of both the oral endotracheal tube and oral airway so that the teeth are in occlusion when the masseter tightening occurs. The disadvantages of this method are the possibility of epistaxis and the risk that the nasopharyngeal airway will be too short to provide an adequate airway.

C. INDUCTION AND MAINTENANCE OF ANESTHESIA WITHOUT MUSCLE RELAXATION

The major difference between airway management during an inhalation anesthetic without muscle relaxation and with muscle relaxation is that the larynx is responsive to irritation and can obstruct by spasm. Spasm can occur in response to irritation of the epiglottis and laryngeal introitus from oropharyngeal or nasopharyngeal airways, pungent anesthetics, secretions, and surgical stimulation if the anesthetic level is inadequate.[20] If the airway must be maintained for more than 30 minutes, anesthesiologist fatigue can be a problem, and vigilance for a sudden change in airway patency is always imperative.

Prophylaxis of aspiration-induced lung injury can be directed toward increasing the pH of gastric contents (0.3 M sodium citrate or H_2-blocking drugs), decreasing secretion volume (ranitidine or cimetidine), or speeding gastric emptying (metoclopramide). These measures are prudent but not required precautions before undertaking an inhalation anesthetic by mask. Control of secretions with an antisialogogue (glycopyrrolate, scopolamine, or atropine) should be done, since secretions can stimulate the larynx to spasm. Mild sedation with a narcotic supresses some cough reflexes, although heavy sedation makes spontaneous ventilation more difficult. Since regurgitation is always a fear with this technique, people with a risk of full stomach or those in whom the esophageal sphincters (cardiac or cricopharyngeal) are weakened (e.g., those with recent food ingestion, hiatus hernia, or pregnancy from 3 months' gestation to 2 weeks postpartum) are not good candidates for mask ventilation. Prolonged muscle paralysis is also a relative contraindication, since the cricopharyngeal sphincter (being striated muscle) is weakened. Patients with an esophageal pouch or Zenker's diverticulum also should not receive an anesthetic by mask, since the contents of the pouch might be regurgitated into the pharynx. Ventilation with more than 20 cm H_2O airway pressure is associated with air passing the cricopharyngeal sphincter and entering the esophagus and stomach.[5] Patients who cannot be ventilated satisfactorily with 20 cm H_2O inspiratory pressures when paralyzed or breathing spontaneously with augmented ventilation (obese, head-down position, bronchospasm, or tense abdominal distention) should have the trachea intubated.

Before beginning, the room and equipment should be arranged to provide all needed material within reaching distance. Because the left hand will be on the patient's face or chin nearly continuously, charting, machine changes, and reaching for drugs will be done with the right hand. The anesthesia machine should be just off the corner of the operating room (OR) table, the anesthetic chart should be taped (or otherwise fixed) to the writing surface, and the anesthetic chart should be immediately behind the anesthetist. All controls and surfaces should be reachable with the right hand while the left hand remains on the headboard of the operating table at the level of the patient's head. Several towels (or a foam head support) should be available to elevate the patient's head, and a head strap (mask-retaining strap) should be on top of the towels.

Equipment for intubation should be checked and ready, as for any anesthetic. A Yankauer or "tonsil" suction should be attached to a suction line for induction and maintenance to allow one-handed manipulation. It may be changed to a soft, 18-gauge flexible suction catheter for emergence, when increasing muscle tone and decreasing levels of anesthesia may preclude the pharyngeal placement of a rigid suction catheter. A selection of masks of at least two sizes and two nasal-bridge configurations should be available. Clear plastic masks are preferable, since the airway can be observed, although the black rubber anatomic models may fit better and be easier to use. Masks must fit both the anesthetist's hand and the patient's face without the use of marked pressure, so having a variety of masks for trial is more important here than when less than 5 minutes of mask ventilation is anticipated prior to endotracheal intubation. An assortment of oral airways (nos. 3, 4, and 5 for most adults) and nasal airways (6.5 to 8.0 mm) should be available. Since commercial nasal airways are occasionally too short, a 6.0- or 6.5-mm endotracheal tube may be cut at 18 cm, a safety pin put through it at the 17-cm mark, and the tube softened in hot irrigating solution prior to use. The balloon may be left deflated and the endotracheal tube used as a long nasopharyngeal airway. The balloon can also be inflated

in the posterior pharynx and the balloon withdrawn back against the soft palate.

All drugs expected to be used should be drawn up in labeled syringes. Those in which repeated small doses may be given throughout the induction period should be fitted with small-gauge needles (22 to 25 gauge) to minimize backup into the syringe if it is left in the intravenous (IV) line. Alternatively, a series of stopcocks can be used to allow several syringes to be connected simultaneously. (Thiopental sodium, propofol, and succinylcholine are the most common drugs used in this way.)

Preoxygenation should be done unless the patient has a strong objection to it. For intravenous induction, thiopental sodium has been the most commonly used drug, although propofol can be used in a similar manner in either of two ways. First, a large-bolus dose (after a 50-mg test dose) of 4 to 5 mg thiopental sodium can be given, an oral airway placed early, and the patient ventilated with increasing concentrations of inhalation anesthetic (up to 2 to 3 minimal anesthetic concentration [MAC] within 2 to 3 minutes delivered in high gas flows to allow rapid changes in inspired concentration). Ventilation is best controlled until incision, when the increased stimulation is usually sufficient to promote spontaneous ventilation. Attempts to achieve spontaneous ventilation before the onset of surgical stimulation usually require such a decrease in anesthesia depth that the level of anesthesia is too low for the patient to lie quietly after the incision. The initial high induction dose of drug allows the oral airway to be placed early without stimulating a laryngeal response.

Second, a small dose of thiopental sodium (2 to 3 mg/kg) or other induction agent can be titrated in 50-mg increments to allow spontaneous or assisted ventilation while the inhalation anesthetic is gradually increased in 0.25- to 0.50-MAC increments until the patient breathes smoothly and the blood pressure has decreased by 20%. This procedure takes time, during which the room should be quiet and the patient should be undisturbed. Hastening the process by rapid escalation of inspired anesthetic concentrations or early instrumentation of the airway usually produces coughing and laryngeal irritation and spasm. Passage through the second stage of anesthesia (delirium or breath-holding) may be hastened by increasing the nitrous oxide concentration to 70% to use the second gas effect, or by using small doses of thiopental sodium. (Equivalent doses of thiopental sodium and propofol are not certain and are subject to experience, but 50 mg of thiopental sodium and 20 mg propofol are reasonable starting points for this purpose.) If mild airway obstruction occurs, head position and neck maneuvers (to test muscle tone) should be tried before inserting artificial airways, as should gentle positive airway pressure (assisted ventilation at no more than 25 cm H_2O and/or constant airway positive pressure of 10 to 15 cm H_2O augmented during inspiration to 20 to 25 cm H_2O). In general, nasal airways are better tolerated than oral, but at the risk of epistaxis. Reactivity to oropharyngeal airways can be lessened by topical anesthesia of the pharynx and epiglottis by preinduction gargling with viscous lidocaine. A post induction spray with 4% lidocaine (200 mg, maximum) or tetracaine (Cetacaine) can be helpful. The mask must not be off the face for more than 20 seconds to avoid rapid decreases in anesthetic level. The fingers of the left hand holding the mandible and mask will perceive muscle tightening as an early sign of lightness or overstimulation, and swallowing as a prelude to vomiting. In general, smaller airways are tried first in nonparalyzed patients to avoid laryngeal irritation. Despite the best plans, laryngeal irritation frequently presents with "crowing," stertor, or obstruction. Crowing can usually be remedied by deepening the anesthetic (thiopental sodium 50 to 100 mg) or increasing the inhalation agent, or both; stertor or obstruction may be from the tongue, necessitating airway maneuvers or devices, but may also be from laryngeal spasm, in which case muscle relaxation (10 to 20 mg succinylcholine) temporarily cures the problem. A succinylcholine infusion can usually be titrated more easily than the bolus injection.

Despite the stated drawbacks, no agent is more effective than succinylcholine in restoring a patent airway if the patient's airway was previously normal. Large airway tumors, especially if pedunculated, can act as a ball-valve with relaxation of the airway musculature; muscle relaxants should not be used in these patients. Occasionally a patient does not breathe smoothly, regardless of depth of anesthesia, or coughs repeatedly unless paralyzed. It is better to intubate the trachea than to continue to administer an anesthetic by mask to a completely paralyzed patient.

An inhalation induction is most commonly performed in children to avoid the discomfort of an awake placement of an IV. In an adult an inhalation induction is occasionally necessary. There are two approaches to this situation. One is to preoxygenate the patient and rapidly turn the vaporizor to 4 to 5 MAC for the minute required to induce anesthesia. This approach is more likely to cause bradycardia and coughing, but frequently works well in children. (The vagal reflex should be blocked with adequate doses of atropine.) The other approach is to preoxygenate the patient and begin a rhythmic monologue while introducing the inhalation agent slowly and in small-concentration increments, encouraging the patient to breathe smoothly and predicting the sensations (dizziness, tingling at the lips, etc.) just as he or she is about to experience them. The anesthetist gradually increases the concentration of the anesthetic from 0.5 MAC to 2 MAC in 10 L/min O_2. As the patient nears the second stage of anesthesia, heralded by uneven respiration and increased muscle tone, the nitrous oxide is rapidly increased to 70% to hasten passage through the second stage. The concentration of volatile inhalation anesthetic is usually raised to 3 to 4 MAC temporarily. As the patient resumes a smooth respiratory pattern, the blood pressure will have decreased by 20% and the fresh gas flows will be reduced to 2 to 4 L/min of N_2O and O_2 with volatile inhalation agent at a concentration of 1 to 2 MAC. After the incision the level is titrated against respiration and blood pressure.

The most important feature of unintubated airway management during the maintenance of anesthesia is monitoring the progress of the operation and the state of the airway. Increasing levels of stimuli must be anticipated and the anesthetic deepened prior to its occurrence, usually by increased concentration of inhaled volatile anesthetic. The use of intravenous narcotics as the major means of deepening anesthetic depth is usually self-defeating, since ventilation decreases and the uptake of inhalation anesthetic decreases. If the increased stimulus is unheeded and laryngeal spasm occurs, succinylcholine is the fastest way to regain control of the airway. Positive pressure on the airway may suffice but often requires high airway pressures leading to gastric inflation (which can in turn cause bradycardia from vagal reflexes, explosive regurgitation from the pent-up pressure, and decreased ventilation because of diaphragmatic pressure from below). The smooth conduct of an inhalation anesthetic by mask requires more vigilance, anticipation, and knowledge of the individual surgeon than does one by endotracheal tube, but the practitioner of the art of anesthesia and the patient can be greatly rewarded.

Fatigue is a common problem if the operation lasts more than 1 hour and the airway is difficult to manage. There are many ways to minimize fatigue. The patient's head should be at a level between the anesthetist's waist and shoulders. The anesthetist should stand or sit on a variable-heighth chair so as to accomplish this. The elbow of the anesthetist's left arm should be kept tucked against his or her left side to minimize shoulder strain, and weight can be substituted for muscle power if the left arm is allowed to extend and the anesthetist leans backward. Resting the elbow on the table next to the patient's head also relaxes the shoulder. The right hand may hold the mask temporarily to give the left hand a rest if the patient is breathing spontaneously. A head strap can assist the anesthetist's forearm muscles. Strapping the mask does not free the left hand for other than the briefest of times (15 to 30 seconds) because the pads of the fingers are irreplaceable monitors. The left hand still provides extension of the head, sometimes required to maintain a patent airway even with artificial airways in place. Vaseline gauze can be placed between the mask and skin to improve the seal or minimize friction on the dermis; this is especially important in cases of epidermolysis bullosa. The length of time for which the inhalation anesthetic can be safely administered depends in great part on the ease of holding the airway.

IV. DECIDING WHICH AIRWAY TECHNIQUE TO USE

Choosing the airway technique is every bit as important a medical decision as choosing the drugs used (see Box 12-3). It is based on a risk-benefit analysis and is individualized for each patient-anesthetist combination. The three airway techniques in common use that allow control of the atmosphere breathed and allow some degree of controlled ventilation are face mask, laryngeal mask, and endotracheal intubation. They vary in the ability to seal the airway, ensure patency, free the hands, evoke patient response, and result in complications.

The airway can be sealed to a delivery system at the face (face mask), in the laryngopharynx (laryngeal mask) or within the trachea (endotracheal tube). The endotracheal tube cuff is capable of the highest pressure seal (albeit at the risk of damage to the tracheal mucosae); the laryngeal mask the least (about 10 to 30 cm of water); and the face mask the most variable level of seal depending on facial anatomy and operator skill. The face mask and LMA are best suited to a spontaneously breathing patient with assisted ventilations. The endotracheal tube is best suited to patients requiring controlled ventilation, especially at high ventilatory pressures. The face mask has the poorest seal between esophagus and trachea, the LMA intermediate, the cuffed endotracheal tube the best.

Patency of the airway is best ensured by an endotracheal tube; the LMA produces intermediate, and the face mask and airway the poorest and most variable airway patency. The LMA in theory can cause laryngeal spasm (although in clinical practice this is rare, since the hyoid-cricoid region is stretched) but bypasses obstruction at the tongue or epiglottis. Freeing the hands and allowing attention to the airway correlates with increasing probability of airway patency. The endotracheal tube is the best, the LMA almost as good, and the face mask the least able to do this by a wide margin. If the patient requires critical care and full attention cannot be given to managing the airway throughout the period, the face mask should be abandoned.

The presence of cardiovascular changes (hypertension or tachycardia) and airway spasm implies patient response to a foreign body. The face mask alone is best tolerated, followed by nasal airway, oral airway, and laryngeal mask airway; the endotracheal tube (by a fairly wide margin) is least tolerated. In most cases the patient "settles" and breathes smoothly when placed on any of these airway arrangements after a period of time to allow extinction of the nociceptive stimulus.

Anticipated complications, especially those that extend beyond the immediate period of airway management, determine the preferred management technique more than any other factor. The catastrophic airway complications involve death and irreversible coma; the next tier, prolonged ventilation and intensive care stay; then unexpected or prolonged hospitalization, followed by prolonged loss of faculties; then emotional or real pain and nuisance discomforts. The mechanisms of such injury related to airway management include the following possibilities.

- For death or irreversible coma: Loss of airway (unrecognized esophageal intubation, laryngeal spasm, ball-valve effect of airway tumor, or soft tissue obstruction of pharynx); inadequate ventilation (soft tissue obstruction, kinked endotracheal tube, poor chest wall/lung compliance as in bronchospasm, or inadequate airway pressures); and regurgitation and aspiration of vomitus (unrecognized hiatus hernia) are possible.
- For prolonged ventilation or intensive care stay: Less severe variants of the preceding; aspiration, bronchospasm, and myocardial infarct related to patient response to nociceptive stimulus such as endotracheal intubation are possibilities.
- Unexpected hospitalization: Any of the preceding in an outpatient; in addition, noncardiac pulmonary edema following extubation and laryngospasm can occur.
- Loss of faculties: Voice hoarseness may be prolonged after vocal cord injury from endotracheal intubation; eye injury can occur if a face mask is strapped on in such a way that the cushion puts pressure on the globe, especially during a case of long duration; dental damage may occur such that a post for a bridge is damaged and a full mouth denture is required.
- Emotional or real pain (but in general a remediable complication): Hoarseness in a singer, dental damage, and corneal abrasion may occur.
- Nuisance problems: Possibilities include sore throat, nausea and vomiting, lip or tongue trauma related to intubation or muscle spasm against an oral airway, and muscle aches if succinylcholine is used to facilitate endotracheal intubation.

The catastrophic complications are rare, the nuisance ones frequent, but the exact frequency of these occurrences are not available even in gross form, much less categorized by airway management technique. Yet the experienced practitioner processes this kind of information from personal and collegial experience to make his or her decisions. It is possible, and in fact probable, that rare complications may differ significantly in different patient populations. A patient known or thought to be at risk of vomiting (in labor or with bowel obstruction) properly has an endotracheal tube placed as the airway management technique used in a general anesthetic. The decision becomes more complex if all of the airway techniques are possible and appropriate for the patient's surgery (herniorrhaphy, knee arthroscopy, cystoscopy, and transurethral resection). For practical purposes, the use of capnography eliminates the unrecognized esophageal intubation. The noncardiac pulmonary edema following endotracheal tube extubation[21] and regurgitation and aspiration under a mask occur at similar frequencies with similar severities in our practice (1 in 5000 to 10,000 cases). It is possible that continuous quality improvement and complex computerized data bases will provide the data needed to make these decisions more rational. For now, the fear of a lost airway or regurgitation and aspiration drives the airway management toward endotracheal intubation for use during a general anesthetic in all but the briefest of general anesthetics for peripheral surgery unless the stimulus of an endotracheal tube will cause unwanted cardiovascular (hypertension or tachycardia) or respiratory (bronchospasm or coughing) response, or if initial attempts at intubation fail and the airway is easily controlled by mask (laryngeal or conventional). It remains to be seen whether the benefits of the laryngeal mask airway will "prove out" in the United States, where paralysis and controlled ventilation are much more common than spontaneous ventilation without relaxants.[22,23] Regardless, transitional airway techniques using the mask and airway will continue to be a necessary prelude and postlude to the more invasive airway management techniques. The patient, the anesthetist's airway skills, and the ability to confirm endotracheal intubation (capnography) interact in any given situation to determine the best approach. Airway skills remain a primary skill of the anesthetist. An understanding of the anatomy, airway maneuvers, and devices and the appropriate use of the bag and mask[24] are essential to the safe administration of anesthesia and care of critically ill patients.

REFERENCES

1. Fink BR, Demerest RJ: *Laryngeal biomechanics,* Cambridge, Mass, 1978, Harvard University.
2. Applebaum EL, Bruce DL: *Tracheal intubation,* Philadelphia, 1976, WB Saunders.
3. Ferner H: *Pernkopf atlas of topographical and applied human anatomy: head and neck,* Philadelphia, 1980, WB Saunders.
4. Standards and guidelines for cardiopulmonary resuscitation and emergency cardiac care, *JAMA* 244:453, 1980.
5. Safar P, Bircher NG: *Cardiopulmonary cerebral resuscitation,* Philadelphia, 1988, WB Saunders.
6. Boidin MP: Airway patency in the unconscious patient, *Br J Anaesth* 57:306, 1985.
7. Redding JS: The choking controversy: critique of evidence on the Heimlich maneuver, *Crit Care Med* 7:745, 1979.
8. Moore W, Rauscher L: A complication of oropharyngeal airway placement, *Anesthesiology* 16:643, 1955.
9. Stauffer JL, Silvestri RL: Complications of endotracheal intubation, tracheostomy, and artificial airways, *Respir Care* 27:417, 1982.
10. Ralston SJ, Charters P: Cuffed nasopharyngeal tube as "dedicated airway" in difficult intubation, *Anaesthesia* 49:133, 1994.
11. Feldman SA, Fauvel NJ, Ooi R: The cuffed pharyngeal airway, *Eur J Anaesthesiol* 8:291, 1991.
12. Zwillich C, Pierson DJ: Nasal necrosis: a complication of nasotracheal intubation, *Chest* 64:376, 1973.
13. Weisman H, Bauer RO, Huddy RA et al: An improved binasopharyngeal airway system for anesthesia, *Anesth Analg* 51:11, 1972.
14. Rubin H: A new non-rebreathing valve, *Anesthesiology* 16:643, 1955.
15. LaBouef LL: Assessment of eight resuscitators, *Respir Care* 80:1136, 1980.
16. Stephenson HE: Cardiopulmonary resuscitation. In Burton GC, Hodgkin JE, editors: *Respiratory care,* Philadelphia, 1984, JB Lippincott.
17. Finucane BT, Santori AH: *Principles of airway management,* Philadelphia, 1988, FA Davis.
18. Hanning CD: Obstructive sleep apnea, *Br J Anaesth* 63:477, 1989.
19. Fink BR: *The human larynx,* New York, 1975, Raven.
20. Fink BR: Etiology and treatment of laryngeal spasm, *Anesthesiology* 17:569, 1956.
21. Hartley M, Vaughan RS: Problems associated with tracheal extubation, *Br J Anaesth* 71:561, 1993.
22. Nagai K, Sakuramoto C, Goto F: Unilateral hypoglossal nerve paralysis following the use of the laryngeal mask airway, *Anaesthesia* 49:603, 1994.
23. Dingley J, Whitehead MJ, Wareham K: A comparative study of the incidence of sore throat with the laryngeal mask airway, *Anaesthesia* 49:251, 1994.
24. McGee JP, Vender JS: Nonintubation management of the airway. In Benumof JL, editor: *Clinical procedures in anesthesia and intensive care,* New York, 1992, JB Lippincott.

SUGGESTED READINGS

Dorsch JA, Dorsch SE: *Understanding anesthesia equipment,* ed 2, Baltimore, 1984, Williams & Wilkins.
Heimlich HJ: A life-saving maneuver to prevent choking, *JAMA* 234:398, 1975.
Morikowa S, Safar P, DeCarlo J: Influence of head position upon upper airway patency, *Anesthesiology* 22:265, 1961.
Pontoppidan J, Gefin B, Lowenstein E: Acute respiratory failure in the adult, *N Engl J Med* 287:690, 1972.
Safar P, Ajuto-Escarraja L, Chang F: A study of upper airway obstruction on the unconscious patient, *J Appl Physiol* 14:760, 1959.

Chapter 13

INDICATIONS FOR
TRACHEAL INTUBATION

Jonathan L. Benumof

I. INTRODUCTION
II. INDICATIONS FOR TRACHEAL INTUBATION OF
   THE AWAKE PATIENT IN RESPIRATORY FAILURE
   A. OBJECTIVE QUANTITATIVE CRITERIA
   B. SUBJECTIVE QUALITATIVE CRITERIA
III. INDICATIONS FOR TRACHEAL INTUBATION OF
   THE GENERALLY ANESTHETIZED PATIENT
   A. PRIMARY NEED FOR A GUARANTEED
      AIRWAY
   B. SECONDARY NEED FOR A GUARANTEED
      AIRWAY
      1. Inadequate mask ventilation
      2. The surgical procedure is changed after the
         induction of anesthesia
      3. A major complication occurs

I. INTRODUCTION

Tracheal intubation achieves four main goals (Box 13-1): it guarantees patency of the upper airway (provided the tracheal tube itself is kept clear of secretions), protects the airway from gastric contents, allows mechanical positive pressure ventilation to be administered, and permits suctioning of the tracheobronchial tree for removal of secretions. Tracheal intubation may be required to achieve one, or any combination, of these four goals.

Two major categories of patients require tracheal intubation; the two categories usually emphasize different tracheal intubation goals. First, awake patients who have impending respiratory failure, or are in respiratory failure, require tracheal intubation (see the next section). In this group of patients the usual purposes of

tracheal intubation, in descending order of importance, are to provide mechanical ventilation, tracheobronchial tree suctioning capability, airway patency, and airway protection. Since the degree of respiratory failure in awake patients is amenable to quantification, the most important indications for tracheal intubation in most of these patients are the objective tests of respiratory function. However, in some patients the gross appearance of the patient alone is sufficient indication (Box 13-2).

Second, generally anesthetized patients who have a primary need for a guaranteed airway (e.g., patients who undergo neurosurgical, cardiothoracic, ear, nose, mouth, and throat procedures and major intraabdominal procedures) or patients who develop a secondary need for a guaranteed airway (e.g., if ventilation via mask is inadequate, the procedure is changed after induction of anesthesia, or a major complication occurs [such as malignant hyperthermia]) require tracheal intubation (see last section in this chapter). In this group of patients the usual purposes of tracheal intubation, in descending order of importance, are to provide airway patency, mechanical ventilation, airway protection, and ability to remove secretions. Airway protection is relatively more important in patients who are thought to have gastric contents (i.e., full stomachs) and in patients undergoing intraabdominal procedures. A severely poisoned patient is equivalent to a generally anesthetized patient with a full stomach and requires tracheal intubation for airway protection, patency, and mechanical ventilation. Since generally anesthetized patients are usually intubated to provide a guaranteed airway, the most important indication for tracheal intubation in these patients is

---

BOX 13-1   Goals of tracheal intubation

Guarantees patency of the upper airway
Protects the airway from gastric contents
Allows mechanical positive pressure ventilation
Permits suctioning of the tracheobronchial tree

BOX 13-2   Signs of respiratory distress and impending fatigue[2-6]

Look of anxiety → Frowning
Signs of sympathetic overactivity → Dilated pupils, forehead sweat
Dyspnea → Decreased talking
Use of accessory muscles → Holds head off pillow
Mouth opens during inspiration → Licking of dry lips
Self PEEP → Pursed lips, expiratory grunting, groaning
Cyanosed lips
Restlessness and fidgeting → Apathy and coma

---

preoperative knowledge of the surgical procedure, and in anesthetized unintubated patients (e.g., patients being ventilated via mask, patients undergoing regional anesthesia, or sedated patients with local anesthesia) intraoperative recognition of the signs of airway obstruction.

II. INDICATIONS FOR TRACHEAL INTUBATION OF THE AWAKE PATIENT IN RESPIRATORY FAILURE

In the absence of frank cardiopulmonary arrest, the diagnosis of impending or actual respiratory failure in awake patients is based on objective quantitative criteria or subjective qualitative criteria, or both. There are many causes of respiratory failure, and detailing them is beyond the scope of this book. For our purposes, it is sufficient to classify the cause of respiratory failure as acute versus chronic lung disease (Fig. 13-1). The treatment of respiratory failure is mechanical ventilation. The following discussion of indications for tracheal intubation of the awake patient in respiratory failure emphasizes this primary goal of tracheal intubation.

A. OBJECTIVE QUANTITATIVE CRITERIA

The three right-hand columns of Table 13-1 describe a deterioration in the results of respiratory function testing from an acceptable range to an unstable, possible intubation status requiring close monitoring and intensive nontracheal intubation support (see Chapters 11 and 12), to probable intubation and mechanical ventilation necessary status.[1] The respiratory function testing is divided into mechanical, oxygenation, and ventilation

categories. In practice, arterial partial pressure of oxygen (Pao_2) and ($Paco_2$) are used most often as indicators of tracheal intubation (see Fig. 13-1), and vital capacity, peak inspiratory force, and respiratory rate are used most often as indicators of tracheal extubation.

The trend of the data in Table 13-1 is as important as the data themselves. For example, progressively increasing $Paco_2$ from a normal $Paco_2$ in a patient without previous lung disease is more important than an already high $Paco_2$ in a patient with emphysema. Thus a Pao_2 of 50 mm Hg and a $Paco_2$ of 65 mm Hg might be normal for a chronic obstructive pulmonary disease (COPD) patient, but these same values would indicate a marked degree of respiratory embarrassment for a previously normal patient. Knowledge of the patient's usual state of health is very helpful in making the decision to intubate the trachea.

B. SUBJECTIVE QUALITATIVE CRITERIA

Fig. 13-1 shows a tracheal intubation logic tree for acute and chronic lung disease. In acute lung disease, hypoxemia is the most important, hypercapnia is the next most important, and the subjective qualitative criteria are the least important indicators for tracheal intubation. Nevertheless, the algorithm shows that each of the three indicators can independently be a primary reason for tracheal intubation. In chronic lung disease, hypercapnia is the most important indicator of tracheal intubation; the other indicators, in order of importance, are hypoxemia and the subjective qualitative criteria. Nevertheless, this algorithm also shows that all three indicators can be independently a primary indication for tracheal intubation. Thus in both of the algorithms presented in Fig. 13-1, tracheal intubation is still indicated in patients with a $Paco_2$ less than 50 to 60 mm Hg and a Pao_2 greater than 45 to 50 mm Hg, provided one of the subjective qualitative criteria is present in sufficient magnitude.

The postoperative patient emerging from anesthesia often has a significant element of several of these objective and subjective indications for continued tracheal intubation and mechanical ventilation. These elements include residual anesthesia and/or paralysis (mental state obtunded, weak breathing muscles, and no swallowing), objective deterioration in lung function, and need for a smooth transition into a postoperative period that will include many other intensive therapies for other major organs.

In Fig. 13-1, medical therapy may include incentive spirometry, coughing routines, frequent tracheal suctioning (even via fiberoptic bronchoscopy), chest physical therapy (chest percussion and vibration in various postures), humidification of the inspired gases, ambulation, increased nutrition, administration of antibiotics, bronchodilators, steroids, diuretics, inotropic drugs, and

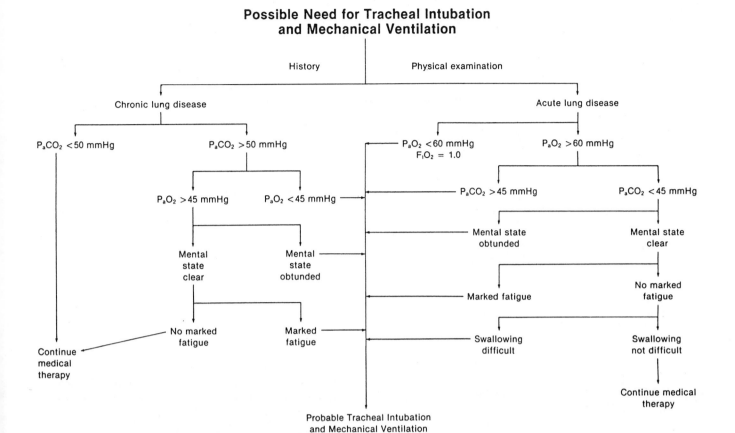

**Possible Need for Tracheal Intubation
and Mechanical Ventilation**

Fig. 13-1. Algorithm for institution of tracheal intubation and mechanical ventilation in patients with acute (right-hand side) and chronic (left-hand side) lung disease. Note that hypoxemia (Pao_2 < 60 mm Hg on Fio_2 of 1.0), hypercapnia ($Paco_2$ > 50 mm Hg), and subjective qualitative signs (obtunded mental state, marked respiratory fatigue, and difficulty in swallowing) can each be independent indications for tracheal intubation and mechanical ventilation. (See text for explanation of medical therapy.) (From Benumof JL, editor: *Clinical procedures in anesthesia and intensive care,* Philadelphia, 1991, JB Lippincott.)

cessation of smoking. These vigorous attempts to improve regional ventilation, together with the controlled administration of oxygen to relieve tissue hypoxia, may be successful in avoiding tracheal intubation in patients who have only marginal indications for tracheal intubation. Indeed, Campbell[7] has reported that only 8 of 70 acutely hospitalized patients with chronic lung disease treated in this manner required tracheal intubation. Similarly, Zwillich et al.[8] have reported that only 26 of 304 patients with chronic airway obstruction and acute respiratory failure treated in this manner required tracheal intubation.

III. INDICATIONS FOR TRACHEAL INTUBATION OF THE GENERALLY ANESTHETIZED PATIENT

A. PRIMARY NEED FOR A GUARANTEED AIRWAY

Many surgical procedures require that the patient be tracheally intubated (Box 13-3). All surgical procedures that are performed with the patient under general anesthesia and that prevent the anesthesiologist from having access to and/or control over the patient's natural airway require tracheal intubation. These procedures consist of all neurosurgical, ear, nose, mouth, and tracheal procedures; all procedures performed with the patient in the prone position; most procedures performed with the patient in the lateral decubitus position; and any procedure that involves turning the patient so that the anesthesiologist is not at the patient's head. Intrathoracic and intraabdominal procedures require tracheal intubation because of both mechanical and physiologic impediments to adequate gas exchange. Surgical procedures of a very long duration usually require tracheal intubation because the ability of one individual to maintain an adequate airway decreases with time. Procedures that require a great deal of the anesthesiologist's attention and time for nonrespiratory matters (e.g., those involving massive blood loss or extensive monitoring) require tracheal intubation so that

Table 13-1. Objective quantitative criteria for tracheal intubation

Respiratory function		Acceptable range	Possible intubation chest PT, oxygen, drugs, close monitoring	Probable intubation and ventilation
Category	Variable			
Mechanics	Vital capacity (ml/kg)	67-75	65-15	<15
	Inspiratory force (ml H_2O)	100-50	50-25	<25
Oxygenation	A-aDO_2 (mm Hg) room air	<38	38-55	>55
	FiO_2 = 1.0	<100	100-450	>450
	PaO_2 (mm Hg) room air	>72	72-55	<55
	FiO_2 = 1.0	>400	400-200	<200
Ventilation	Respiratory rate, (breaths/min)	10-25	25-40 or <8	>40 or <6
	$PaCO_2$ (mm Hg)	35-45	45-60	<60

Adapted from Pontpoppidan H, Geffin B, Lowenstein E: *N Engl J Med* 287:743, 1972.
PT, physical therapy; A-aDO_2, alveolar-arterial partial pressure of oxygen difference; PaO_2 and $PaCO_2$, arterial partial pressure of oxygen and carbon dioxide, respectively; FiO_2, inspired concentration of oxygen.

BOX 13-3 Primary need for a guaranteed airway in the generally anesthetized patient

I. Prevention of loss of control over airway in patients under general anesthesia
   A. Surgical procedures: neurosurgical, ear, nose, mouth, tracheal
   B. Patient position: prone or lateral decubitus position and procedures that require turning the patient so that the anesthesiologist is not at the head of the patient
II. Gas exchange is expected to be impaired
   A. Intrathoracic procedures
   B. Intraabdominal procedures
III. Prolonged general anesthesia
IV. Complicated anesthetics requiring a great deal of nonairway attention

---

the anesthesiologist's hands and attention are not tied to maintaining a nonguaranteed airway. As noted earlier, the patient emerging from anesthesia for a very major surgical procedure often requires continued tracheal intubation and mechanical ventilation for multiple reasons.

B. SECONDARY NEED FOR A GUARANTEED AIRWAY

When a secondary need for a guaranteed airway arises, it is usually unexpected and may not be planned for. For example, ventilation by mask may become inadequate, the surgical procedure may be changed, or

a major surgical or anesthesia complication may occur (Box 13-4). Consequently the difficulty of tracheal intubation under these circumstances may be increased.

1. Inadequate mask ventilation

Airway obstruction is the most common serious cause of inadequate ventilation via a mask, and major airway obstruction unrelieved by such maneuvers as anterior jaw dislocation and insertion of a nasopharyngeal and/or oropharyngeal airway is a strong indication for tracheal intubation; other less certain-to-succeed options include insertion of a laryngeal mask airway (Chapter 19) and a combitube (Chapter 22). The obstruction can be at any level of the airway and may cause preferential ventilation of the esophagus (pathway of least resistance), resulting in distention of the stomach. Stomach distention, in turn, will impair ventilation of the lungs further. Patients under general anesthesia who are breathing via an anesthesia mask make up the largest group with this indication for tracheal intubation. However, respiratory failure patients who are narcotized by carbon dioxide retention, patients who are excessively intravenously sedated or narcotized while under regional anesthesia, patients who are poisoned or have taken or been given (iatrogenically) a drug overdose, and head-injured patients are also in this category.

Total airway obstruction is characterized by lack of breath sounds, which may be coupled with continuing, sometimes strenuous but ineffectual efforts at breathing. Excessive diaphragmatic activity causes abdominal movements and chest retraction, but they do not represent movement of air. The diagnosis is made by absence of breath sounds, failure to observe movement

---

BOX 13-4   Secondary need for a guaranteed airway

1. Mask ventilation is inadequate.
2. Surgical procedure is changed after anesthesia is induced.
3. A major anesthetic or surgical complication occurs.

---

of the breathing bag or failure to feel the movement and warmth of air at the airway outlet, and absence of a carbon dioxide excretion waveform (if an end-tidal CO_2 monitor is being used).

Partial upper airway obstruction is characterized by restriction of air movement with inspiration that prolongs the inspiratory phase; diminished tidal exchange and breath sounds; excessive diaphragmatic activity; retraction of the upper chest; discrepancy between the movements of the breathing bag and the chest wall; and various characteristic sounds. Partial obstruction caused by the tongue causes a rough, irregular, stuttery noise frequently associated with "stertorous" respiration. Preoperatively, one's index of suspicion for partial obstruction of the upper airway by a large tongue falling against the pharynx can be increased by a history of heavy snoring and sleep apnea, and the relative size of the tongue to the oropharynx can be determined by having the patient open his or her mouth widely and say "ah." If the uvula and tonsillar pillars are obscured by the tongue, the tongue is very large in relation to the oropharynx.[9,10] Partial laryngospasm usually causes a high-pitched whistle or squeak. Partial obstruction by the lips is most noticeable during expiration and is accompanied by a low-pitched, rough, fluttery sound. Pharyngeal secretions cause a gurgling, bubbling noise. Partial obstruction at the trachea due to foreign materials and secretions produces a rattly or sloshy noise.

Lower airway obstruction is characterized by diminished tidal exchange, excessive intercostal and diaphragmatic activity, active inspiration and expiration during spontaneous respiration, and most important, adventitious breath sounds consisting of rales, rhonchi, or wheezing. Bronchiolar secretions cause rhonchi, and bronchiolar constriction causes wheezing. Alveolar obstruction may be associated with all types of adventitious sounds, but rales are most common. With lower airway obstruction the breathing bag classically empties and refills slowly, and moderate changes in compliance can be felt by squeezing the reservoir bag.

Very obese patients may be predictably difficult to ventilate by mask because of the difficulty in raising the heavy chest wall and displacing the massive abdominal wall. Dentureless patients may be difficult to ventilate by mask because of large air leaks between the sunken cheeks and the mask. Although such maneuvers as changing the size of the mask, pressing the mask closer to the face, and changing the contour of the patient's face (e.g., placing saline-soaked gauze rolls in the buccal pouches to round out the cheeks) may sometimes diminish or eliminate the air leak, tracheal intubation is often necessary.

2. The surgical procedure is changed after the induction of anesthesia

Change in the planned surgical procedure most frequently follows diagnostic procedures such as conversion of a breast biopsy into a mastectomy, conversion of a dilation and curettage of the uterus to a hysterectomy, and conversion of a bronchoscopy or mediastinoscopy to a lung resection.

3. A major complication occurs

The occurrence of a major anesthetic or surgical complication—such as a high or total spinal anesthetic, massive blood loss, malignant hyperthermia, or wearing off of a regional anesthetic (patient experiences undue pain)—often requires tracheal intubation (along with other important treatments).

In summary, both awake and anesthetized patients may require tracheal intubation. In awake patients, this decision will be based on objective quantitative and subjective qualitative criteria and trends in all of these data. In anesthetized patients the need for tracheal intubation is usually identified preoperatively but may occasionally arise unexpectedly after the induction of anesthesia. Thus tracheal intubation may be either an expected, elective, planned procedure or an unexpected, nonelective, emergency procedure. The exact set of circumstances under which the need for tracheal intubation arises often determines the technique by which tracheal intubation is accomplished. Orotracheal intubation is especially indicated when speed of intubation is the primary consideration. Nasotracheal intubation is especially indicated for many surgical procedures involving the face and mouth; it may also be indicated to increase the comfort of intubations of very long duration (days). Decision-making logic algorithms have been developed to determine the best method of tracheal intubation under all circumstances,[11] especially regarding whether a difficult tracheal intubation is suspected or unsuspected.[11] Chapters 13 to 28 describe all the techniques one may use to accomplish the tracheal intubation.

REFERENCES

1. Pontpoppidan H, Geffin B, Lowenstein E: Acute respiratory failure in the adult (second of three parts), *N Engl J Med* 287:743, 1972.
2. Campbell EJM, Agostini E, Davis EN: *The respiratory muscles: mechanics and neural control*, ed 2, London, 1970, Lloyd Luke.

3. Knelson JH, Howatt WF, Demuth GR: The physiologic significance of grunting respiration, *Pediatrics* 44:393, 1969.

4. Cohen BM: The interrelationship of the respiratory functions of the nasal and lower airways, *Bull Physiopathol Respir* 7:895, 1971.

5. Mueller RE, Petty TL, Filley GF: Ventilation and arterial blood-gas changes induced by pursed-lips breathing, *J Appl Physiol* 28:784, 1970.

6. Schmidt RW, Wasserman K, Lillington GA: The effect of air flow and oral pressure on the mechanics of breathing in patients with asthma and emphysema, *Am Rev Respir Dis* 90:564, 1964.

7. Campbell EJM: The J. Burns Amberson Lecture: the management of acute respiratory failure in chronic bronchitis and emphysema, *Am Rev Respir Dis* 96:626, 1967.

8. Zwillich CW, Pierson DJ, Creagh CE et al: Complications of assisted ventilation: a prospective study of 354 consecutive episodes, *Am J Med* 57:161, 1974.

9. Mallampati RS, Gatt SP, Gugino LD et al: A clinical sign to predict difficult tracheal intubation: a prospective study, *Can Anaesth Soc J* 32:429, 1985.

10. Samsoon GLT, Young JRB: Difficult tracheal intubation: a retrospective study, *Anaesthesia* 42:487, 1987.

11. Benumof JL: Management of the difficult airway: with special emphasis on awake tracheal intubation, *Anesthesiology* 75:1087, 1991.

Chapter 14

CONVENTIONAL (LARYNGOSCOPIC) OROTRACHEAL AND NASOTRACHEAL INTUBATION (SINGLE-LUMEN TUBE)

Jonathan L. Benumof

I. CONVENTIONAL (LARYNGOSCOPIC) OROTRACHEAL INTUBATION

The oral route is the easiest and most frequently used approach for tracheal intubation and should be the first technique learned. It is very commonly used for the administration of anesthesia, resuscitative efforts, and other short-term situations requiring airway intubation. Visualization of the glottis is obtained by the introduc- tion of a laryngoscope through the mouth. A tracheal tube is then inserted through the glottis into the trachea under direct vision. The laryngoscope is removed, and the tube is secured to the face or teeth.

A. PRELARYNGOSCOPY MANEUVERS

Box 14-1 lists the basic materials that are to be present and immediately available for conventional orotracheal and nasotracheal intubation. The materials are grouped according to the temporal sequence of intubation events. Whenever there is a choice in size, the size that is thought to be the right one (medium, in Box 14-1), one size larger (large, in Box 14-1), and one size smaller (small, in Box 14-1) should be available. The equipment listed in Box 14-1 is considered basic for either perform- ing tracheal intubation or preventing a major complica- tion, or both.

Box 14-2 lists the proper temporal sequence of essential prelaryngoscopy maneuvers. If the intubation is being performed in an intensive care location, adequate access to the patient's head must be arranged and may include removal of the headboard of the bed. The height of the surface upon which the patient rests (bed,

---

BOX 14-1   Basic equipment for tracheal intubation

Preoxygenation and ventilation

1. Oxygen source should be turned on and attached to a self-inflating ventilation bag
2. Small, medium, and large anesthesia masks must be present
3. Small, medium, and large oropharyngeal and nasopharyngeal airways
4. Tongue depressor

Preparation of the endotracheal tube

5. Small, medium, and large orotracheal tubes
6. Small, medium, and large nasotracheal tubes
7. Malleable stylet
8. Syringe, 10-ml
9. Jelly and ointment, 4% lidocaine (Xylocaine)

Anesthesia

10. Intravenous anesthetics and muscle relaxants
11. Syringes and needles
12. Lidocaine 4% multidose and two ampules of phenylephrine (Neo-Synephrine)
13. Laryngotracheal anesthesia kit, atomizer, and local anesthetic

Laryngoscopy

14. Suction apparatus should be turned on and hard plastic suction catheter attached
15. Magill forceps
16. All sized Miller blades with functioning light source
17. All sized Macintosh blades with functioning light source
18. Towels to put patient's head and neck in "sniff" position

Fixation of the endotracheal tube

19. Tincture of benzoin
20. Adhesive or umbilical tape or both

Determination of endotracheal tube location (see Chapter 27)

21. Stethoscope
22. End-tidal CO_2 monitor
23. Pulse oximeter

BOX 14-2   Prelaryngoscopy maneuvers

1. Have equipment and suction available (Box 14-1).
2. Clear access to patient's head.
3. Place patient's head in sniff position.
4. Preoxygenate.
5. Have adequate help available.

---

who have suffered airway trauma (blood), who have had a cardiac and/or pulmonary arrest (stomach contents and secretions), and who have had a failure in immediate previous intubation attempts (secretions). A curved, clear, hard plastic suction catheter should be used.

The correct head position for laryngoscopy is extremely important. Successful direct laryngoscopy requires aligning the oral, pharyngeal, and laryngeal axes (Fig. 14-1) such that the passageway from the incisor teeth to the glottis is almost a straight line. If the head is simply placed on the resting surface in a neutral position (with no head support), the oral, pharyngeal, and laryngeal axes form a C-shaped curve (Fig. 14-1, *A*). To bring the laryngeal axis in line with the pharyngeal axis, the neck first must be flexed on the chest by 35 degrees[1] by elevating the head about 10 cm with pads under the occiput (shoulders ordinarily remaining on the table) (Fig. 14-1, *B*). To bring the oral axis in line with both the pharyngeal axis and laryngeal axis, the head must also be extended on the neck (extension of the junction of the spine and skull [atlantooccipital joint]) so that the angle between the nose-occiput axis of the head forms an 80- to 85-degree angle with the long axis of the neck and the plane of the face is 15 degrees from the horizontal plane (Fig. 14-1, *C*).[1] This position of the head and neck is commonly called the sniff position.

Placing the patient's head in an optimal head and neck position is the first and perhaps the most important maneuver that can routinely and predictably improve laryngoscopy and intubation outcome. It must be understood that there are two basic components to the sniff position: slight flexion of the neck on the chest and severe extension of the head on the neck at the atlantooccipital joint. Achievement of these head-face-neck-chest axes is best appreciated by a lateral view of the patient. The sniff position may not be achieved in some patients by simply placing the head on some sort of elevated support; for example, in very obese patients it takes a good deal of effort to also elevate and support the scapula, shoulders, and the nape of the neck (which creates room for extension of the head) as well as the head (Fig. 14-2; see later discussion). If optimal head and neck position is not achieved *prior to* the first attempt at laryngoscopy, it may be very difficult to achieve later at the time of crisis. In normal-appearing patients (i.e., the vast majority) the achievement of the sniff position

operating room table, gurney, and so forth) should be adjustable (to the level of the intubationist's midintercostal margin), and the surface should be nonmovable (rolling parts locked). An experienced aide should be in constant attendance to hand items such as suction lines, airways, tubes, drugs, and so on to the intubationist.

Suctioning the pharynx may be necessary at any time in any patient, but it is most likely to be necessary in patients who have eaten recently (stomach contents),

HEAD AND NECK POSITION AND THE
AXES OF THE HEAD AND NECK AND UPPER AIRWAY

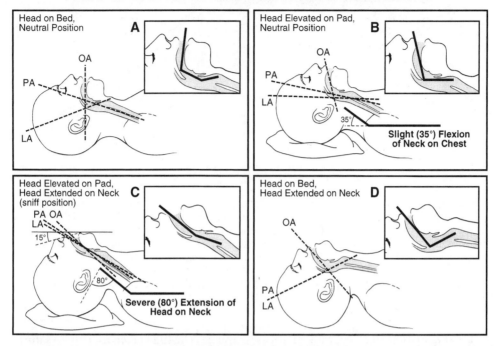

Fig. 14-1. This schematic diagram shows the alignment of the oral axis (OA), pharyngeal axis (PA), and laryngeal axis (LA) in four different head positions. Each head position is accompanied by an inset that magnifies the upper airway (the oral cavity, pharynx, and larynx) and superimposes, as a variously bent bold line, the continuity of these three axes within the upper airway. **A,** The head is in a neutral position with a marked degree of nonalignment of the LA, PA, and OA. **B,** The head is resting on a large pad that flexes the neck on the chest and aligns the LA with the PA. **C,** The head is resting on a pad (which flexes the neck on the chest); concomitant extension of the head on the neck, which brings all three axes into alignment (sniff position), is shown. **D,** Extension of the head on the neck without concomitant elevation of the head on a pad, which results in nonalignment of the PA and LA with the OA.

may be facilitated by placing the patient's head and neck in a commercially made soft (foam-sponge consistency) premolded head and neck piece (American Medical Development Company). The failure to use optimal head and neck position may explain why there is a commonly observed increase in the incidence of failed intubation when general anesthesia is induced after a failed regional anesthetic (Robert Caplan, personal communication, 1993).[2]

Occasionally in obese patients it is necessary to also place towels and blankets under the scapula, shoulders, and nape of the neck, as well as the head, in order to appropriately flex the neck on the chest (Figs. 14-1, *B* and 14-2) and extend the head on the neck (Figs. 14-1, *C* and 14-2); in this instance, the purpose of the scapula, shoulder, and neck support is to give the head room so that it may be extended on the neck. When in doubt, the final assessment of the correctness of the sniff position should be from a lateral view of the patient because only a lateral view enables precise assessment of the chest, neck, face, and head axes (Figs. 14-1, *C* and

14-2). Full extension of the head without elevation of the occiput (Fig. 14-1, *D*) is contraindicated because this position increases the lips-to-glottis distance; rotates the larynx anteriorly, unaligning the oral axis from the pharyngeal and laryngeal axes; and may necessitate subsequent leverage on the maxillary teeth or gums with the laryngoscope blade to expose the larynx.

The upper airway is maximally patent in the sniff position and is the reason that long-distance runners instinctively assume this head position. Thus the same positioning movements that make the airway largest also make the airway straightest.

From the moment a resuscitator begins laryngoscopy to the initiation of positive pressure ventilation via the tracheal tube, a period of time must pass. The duration of this period is directly proportional to the degree of difficulty of exposure of the larynx and inversely proportional to the skill of the intubationist. Since even skilled intubationists may require 30 seconds to 1 minute for this period, preoxygenation with 100% oxygen ventilation via face mask is almost always indicated (see

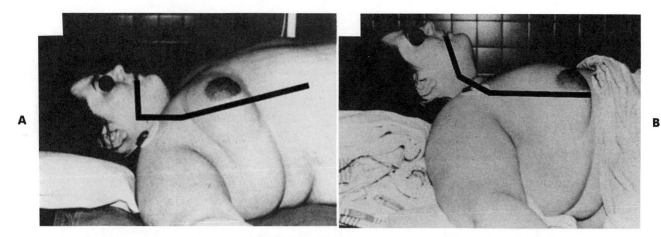

Fig. 14-2. A, In some obese patients, simply placing the head on a pillow does not result in the sniff position; in the obese patient shown, and as illustrated by the overlying heavy bold black line, the oral and laryngeal axes are perpendicular to one another, the neck is not flexed on the chest, and the head is not extended on the neck at the atlantooccipital joint. **B,** In the same patient, placing support (blankets, towels, and the like) under the scapula, shoulders, nape of the neck, and head results in a much better sniff position; the oral, pharyngeal, and laryngeal axes form only a slightly bent curve, the neck is flexed on the chest, and the head is extended on the neck at the atlantooccipital joint.

later discussion). Preoxygenation may be with either positive or negative pressure breathing. If the tidal volume is large and the rate is rapid (i.e., minute ventilation is high), the duration of preoxygenation need only be for 1 minute,[3] whereas if the tidal volume is small and/or the rate is slow (i.e., minute ventilation is low), the duration of preoxygenation should be for 3 to 4 minutes.[4]

Two notes of caution about preoxygenation are necessary. First, even in normal patients, in instances of poor spontaneous or positive pressure ventilation via mask, the PaO_2 may actually decrease during attempts to preoxygenate. Ventilation via mask may be inadequate because of the presence of a large mask leak or airway obstruction or some combination of both (see Chapter 12). Under these circumstances, partial pressure of carbon dioxide in end-tidal gas ($PETCO_2$) from capnography is not accurate and is, by definition, falsely low. The immediate assessment of the adequacy of ventilation under these circumstances in an urgent clinical situation is a matter of experience and medical judgment.

Second, a morbidly obese patient has multiple pulmonary abnormalities, which include decreased vital capacity, expiratory reserve volume, inspiratory capacity, and functional residual capacity (FRC). Furthermore, assumption of the recumbent position for induction of anesthesia in such patients further decreases expiratory reserve volume and FRC and increases the possibility of tidal volume falling within the closing capacity. The diminished FRC results in decreased stores of oxygen to meet the metabolic requirements when the patient is apneic. The time taken for oxygen saturation to decrease to 90% after 5 minutes of preoxygenation or until expired nitrogen concentration was less than 5%, has been found to be 364 ±24 seconds in normal patients (within 20% of their ideal body weight), 247 ±21 seconds in obese patients (more than 20%, but less than 45 kg over ideal body weight) and 163 ±15 seconds in morbidly obese patients (more than 45 kg over ideal body weight).[5] Thus obese patients are at significantly increased risk to develop decreased arterial oxygen tension when apneic.

Pharyngeal insufflation of oxygen can significantly prolong the safe duration of apnea (i.e., prevent arterial desaturation). In a typical apneic adult, approximately 250 ml/min of oxygen are transferred from the lungs into the bloodstream, while only 100 to 200 ml/min of CO_2 enter the lungs from the bloodstream; the remainder of the body's CO_2 production is buffered by red blood cells or dissolved in tissues. This alveolar gas deficit causes alveolar pressure to become slightly subatmospheric; if the airway is patent, there will be a net flow of gas from the pharynx into the alveoli. If following adequate preoxygenation, the pharynx is filled with oxygen, the onset of hypoxia will be delayed, since oxygen, rather than air, would be drawn into the lungs by this mechanism. Pharyngeal insufflation may be conveniently achieved by passing a catheter into the pharynx through a soft indwelling nasopharyngeal airway and oxygen insufflated at 3 L/min.[5] When preoxygenation is followed by pharyngeal insufflation as described previously, in normal but apneic patients (ASA Class I or II with a preapneic pulse oximetry (SpO_2) greater than 98 and the

Opening the Mouth for Laryngoscopy: Extraoral Technique

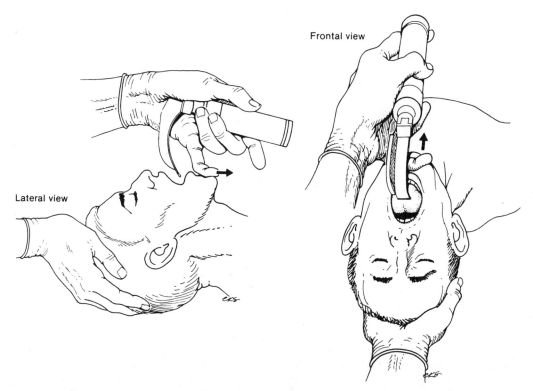

Fig. 14-3. The mouth can be opened wide by concomitantly extending the head on the neck with the right hand while the small finger and medial border of the left hand push the anterior aspect of the mandible in a caudad direction (extraoral technique). As the blade approaches the mouth, it should be directed toward the right side of the mouth. Gloves should be worn during laryngoscopy because the hands may come into contact with patient secretions.

airway kept patent by jaw thrust and the nasopharyngeal airway), the Spo_2 remains 98% or greater for a minimum of 10 minutes (although at the end of 10 minutes the $Paco_2$ may be expected to be approximately 70 to 80 mm Hg).[6]

B. LARYNGOSCOPY

The laryngoscope handle is held in the left hand. There are two ways to open the mouth wide. First, extension of the head on the neck (by the right hand) causes the lips to part and the mouth to open (Fig. 14-3). If the small finger and medial border of the left hand (which also holds the laryngoscope handle) simultaneously push in a caudad direction on the anterior aspect of the mandible, the mouth will open further. Second, the thumb of the right hand can press (caudad direction) on the right lower posterior molar teeth, and the index finger of the right hand can simultaneously press up (cephalad direction) on the right upper posterior molar teeth (Fig. 14-4). The two forces in opposite directions on the upper and lower molar teeth cause the mouth to open widely.

There are two basic types of laryngoscope blades: the curved blade (Macintosh) and the straight blade with curved tip (Miller). Each of these blades has a flange on the left side of the blade for keeping the tongue out of the line of sight (Figs. 14-5 to 14-10, pp. 267-269). The flange of the blade also houses the light source. Each blade has an open right side for visualization of the larynx and for insertion of the endotracheal tube (Figs. 14-5 to 14-10).

Following opening the mouth, and with the laryngoscope held in the left hand, the laryngoscope blade is inserted into the right side of the mouth (Fig. 14-5, *A*). During the insertion of the laryngoscope the patient's right lower lip should be pulled away from the lower incisors (with the right hand or by an assistant) to prevent injury to the lower lip by catching the lower lip between the laryngoscope blade and the incisor teeth. (This complication is avoided in Figs. 14-5, *A*, 14-9, and 14-10). The blade is then simultaneously advanced forward toward the base of the tongue (partly by rotating the left wrist [Fig. 14-5, *B*]) and swept centrally toward the midline so that the tongue is completely pushed over

Opening the Mouth for Laryngoscopy: Intraoral Technique

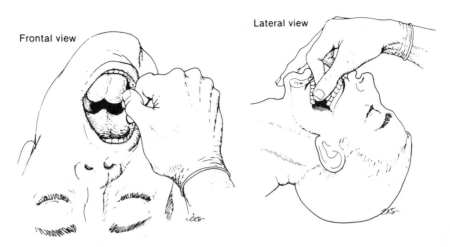

Fig. 14-4. The mouth can be opened wide by pressing the thumb of the right hand on the right lower posterior molar teeth in a caudad direction while the index finger of the right hand simultaneously presses on the right upper posterior molar teeth in a cephalad direction (intraoral technique). Gloves should be worn during laryngoscopy because the hands may come into contact with patient secretions.

to the left side of the mouth by the flange of the laryngoscope blade. After the blade has been applied to the base of the tongue the laryngoscope is lifted to expose the epiglottis (Fig. 14-5, *C*). Hereafter, the left wrist of the operator should remain straight, all lifting being done by the left shoulder and arm. If the laryngoscopist follows a natural inclination to rotate and flex the wrist further, thereby raising the laryngoscope like a lever whose fulcrum is the upper incisor or gum, broken teeth or gum bleeding is likely to result. With the patient in a sniff position, the direction of force necessary to lift the mandible and tongue and thereby expose the glottis is along an approximately 45 degree straight line above an imaginary line from the patient's ear to feet. Careful study of Figs. 14-1, *C* and 14-5 makes this consideration obvious.

Once the epiglottis is visualized, the next step depends on the type of laryngoscope blade being used. If the blade is curved (Macintosh), the tip should be placed in the vallecula (space between the base of the tongue and the pharyngeal surface of the epiglottis) (Fig. 14-5, *D*). Subsequent forward and upward movement of the blade (exerted along the axis of the handle, not by pulling back on the handle) stretches the hyoepiglottic ligament, causing the epiglottis to move upward, exposing first the arytenoid cartilages and then, with favorable anatomy, allowing more and more of the glottic opening and vocal cords to come into view (Fig. 14-5, *D*).

The identification (or failure to identify) the epiglottis and the lifting of the epiglottis anteriorly to reveal progressively more of the glottic aperture, from a progressively posterior (the arytenoid cartilages) to an anterior aspect (the commissure) has led to a convenient

and useful system for grading the laryngoscopic view (see Fig. 6-2).[7-9] Grade I laryngoscopic view consists of visualization of the vocal cords. The percentage of the vocal cords visualized was not specified in the original reports, but obviously it may range from 1% to 100%. Grade II laryngoscopic view is visualization of the posterior portion of the laryngeal aperture (the arytenoid cartilages) but not any portion of the vocal cords. Grade III laryngoscopic view is visualization of just the epiglottis, but not the posterior portion of the laryngeal aperture. Again, the percentage of the epiglottis visualized was not specified in the original reports, but obviously it may range from just the tip to the whole of the epiglottis. Grade IV laryngoscopic view is visualization of just the soft palate, but not the epiglottis.

Insertion of a blade too far into the vallecula, as well as continued rotation of the handle to the vertical, may push the epiglottis down over the glottic opening, resulting in limited exposure of the larynx (Fig. 14-6). If the blade is straight (Jackson, Wisconsin, or Miller), the tip should extend just behind (posterior to) or beneath the laryngeal surface of the epiglottis (Fig. 14-7). As with a curved laryngoscope blade, subsequent forward and upward movement of the straight blade (exerted along the axis of the handle, not by pulling back on the handle) exposes the glottic opening (Fig. 14-7).

With either type of laryngoscope blade (straight or curved) the use of optimal external laryngeal pressure can significantly improve the laryngoscopic view and in some patients is a factor that can make the difference between intubation failure and success. For example, routine use of external laryngeal pressure may reduce

Conventional Laryngoscopy with a Curved Blade

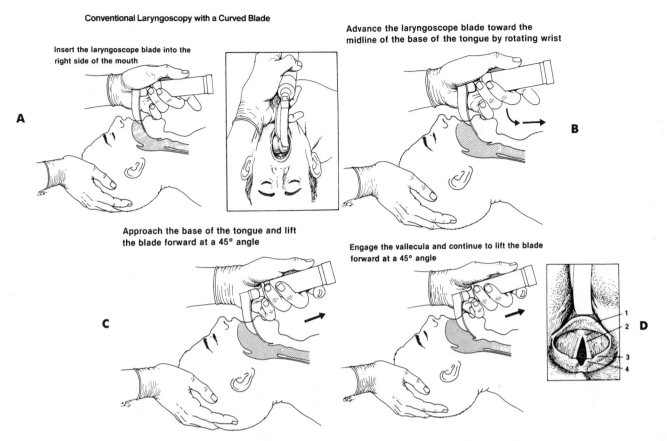

A, Insert the laryngoscope blade into the right side of the mouth

B, Advance the laryngoscope blade toward the midline of the base of the tongue by rotating wrist

C, Approach the base of the tongue and lift the blade forward at a 45° angle

D, Engage the vallecula and continue to lift the blade forward at a 45° angle

Fig. 14-5. This four-part schematic diagram shows how to perform laryngoscopy with a Macintosh blade (curved blade). **A** and **D,** Both lateral and frontal views are shown. **B** and **C,** Lateral views. **A,** The laryngoscope blade is inserted into the right side of the mouth so that the tongue is to the left of the flange. **B,** The blade is advanced around the base of the tongue, in part by rotating the wrist so that the handle of the blade becomes more vertical (*arrows, C*). **C,** The handle of the laryngoscope is lifted at a 45-degree angle (*arrow*) as the tip of the blade approaches the base of the tongue, thereby exposing the epiglottis. **D,** The laryngoscope blade is placed in the vallecula with continued lifting of the laryngoscope handle at a 45-degree angle, resulting in exposure of the laryngeal aperture. *1,* Epiglottis; *2,* vocal cords; *3,* cuneiform part of arytenoid cartilage; and *4,* corniculate part of arytenoid cartilage.

the incidence of Grade III view from 9% to a range from 5.4% to 1.3%.[9] Optimal external laryngeal pressure is probably not cricoid pressure (the cricoid cartilage is 2 cm caudad to the larynx); it may be pressure that is backward, upward, and to the right on the thyroid cartilage,[10] but the best way to determine optimal laryngeal pressure is for the laryngoscopist to determine this with his or her own free right hand (Fig. 14-8).

Curved blades are thought to be less traumatic to the epiglottis for two reasons. First, the tip of a curved blade does not have to touch the epiglottis. Second, the pharyngeal surface of the epiglottis is innervated by the glossopharyngeal nerve, whereas the laryngeal surface of the epiglottis is innervated by the superior laryngeal nerve. Stimulation of the laryngeal surface of the epiglottis is thought to predispose to laryngospasm and bronchospasm more than stimulation of the pharyngeal surface of the epiglottis. Curved blades are also thought

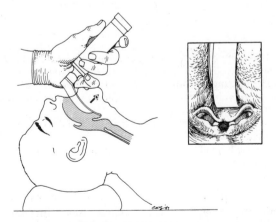

Fig. 14-6. Insertion of the laryngoscope blade too deeply into the vallecula may push the epiglottis down over the laryngeal aperture, diminishing exposure of the vocal cords.

Conventional Laryngoscopy with a Straight Blade

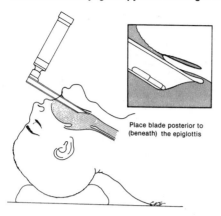

Place blade posterior to (beneath) the epiglottis

Fig. 14-7. Conventional laryngoscopy with a straight blade. A straight laryngoscope blade (Miller) should be passed underneath the laryngeal surface of the epiglottis; then the handle of the laryngoscope should be elevated at a 45-degree angle, similar to the lifting that takes place in the use of a curved laryngoscope blade.

DETERMINING OPTIMAL EXTERNAL LARYNGEAL MANIPULATION WITH FREE (right) HAND

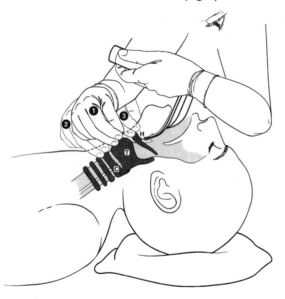

Fig. 14-8. Optimal external laryngeal manipulation to improve the laryngoscopic view is determined by the laryngoscopist by quickly pressing in both the cephalad and posterior direction with the right hand over, *1,* the thyroid (T) (most common), *2,* cricoid (C), and, *3,* hyoid cartilages (H). If the laryngoscopic view is critically improved by this maneuver, the laryngoscopist can use an assistant's hands or fingers as an extension of his or her own right hand to reproduce the optimal external laryngeal manipulation.

to be less traumatic to the teeth and to provide more room for passage of the tracheal tube through the oropharynx. On the other hand, straight blades definitely provide a better view of the glottis in a patient with a long, floppy epiglottis or an anterior larynx. Therefore

Insertion of the Laryngoscope Blade Too Deeply into the Pharynx Elevates the Larynx and Exposes the Esophagus

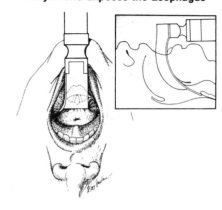

Fig. 14-9. Insertion of the laryngoscope blade too deeply into the pharynx may result in elevation of the entire larynx so that the opening of the esophagus rather than the glottic aperture will be visualized. The esophagus is located just to the right of the midline and posteriorly, and the esophageal opening is round and puckered with no structures around it.

straight blades are the blade of choice in infants, pediatric patients, and patients with an anterior larynx. Use of a long blade (curved or straight) is indicated in very large patients and patients with very long mandibles in the neck.

Four major common problems are encountered in performing laryngoscopy. First, with either laryngoscope blade, inserting the blade too deeply into the pharynx may elevate the entire larynx, so that the opening of the esophagus will be visualized rather than the glottic aperture (Fig. 14-9). The tracheal and esophageal openings are differentiated as follows: the esophagus is located just to the right of the midline and posteriorly, and the esophageal opening is round and puckered, with no structures around it (Fig. 14-9). The glottis is located in the midline, has a triangular shape, and contains the prominent knobs of the arytenoids posteriorly and the pale white vocal cords laterally. The dark cavity of the trachea can be seen beyond the glottis (Figs. 14-5, *D* and 14-10, *A*); when the trachea is illuminated by the light of the laryngoscope blade, the cartilaginous tracheal rings appear as prominent anterior arches or ridges that extend from the 8-o'clock to the 4-o'clock position (Fig. 14-10, *A*).

Second, it is very important to keep the tongue completely to the left side of the mouth with the flange of the laryngoscope blade. Many unsuccessful or difficult intubations result from the tongue flopping over the flange of the blade toward the right side of the mouth, thus establishing a narrow "tunnel" through which the vocal cords must be visualized and the endotracheal tube passed (Fig. 14-10, *B*). Vision is obscured further when part of the narrow tunnel is subsequently occupied by the

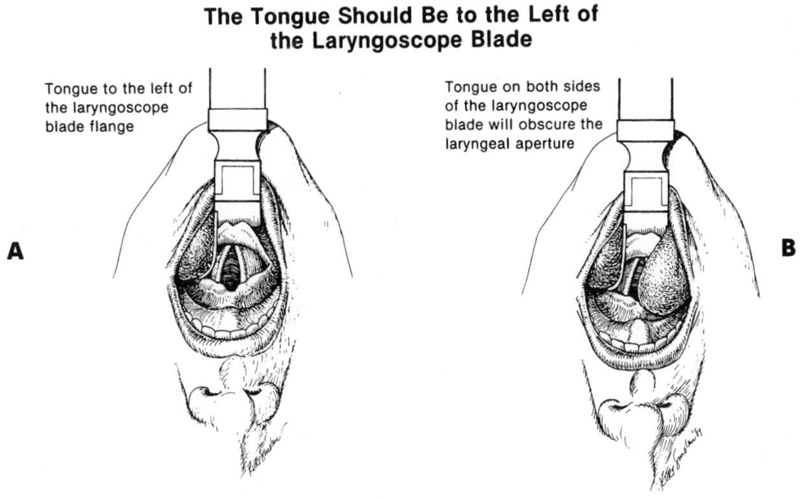

The Tongue Should Be to the Left of the Laryngoscope Blade

Fig. 14-10. The tongue should be to the left of the laryngoscope blade. **A,** The flange on the laryngoscope blade should keep the tongue completely to the left side of the mouth. If this is accomplished, the tongue does not obstruct the view of the vocal cords. The tracheal rings on the anterior aspect of the trachea are evident. **B,** If the tongue slips over the laryngoscope blade and occupies part of the right side of the mouth, the view of the vocal cords is obscured by the part of the tongue that is on the right side of the mouth.

endotracheal tube. Thus with a tunnel view the endoscopist can partially visualize, but not instrument, the larynx. Therefore all of the tongue must be to the left of the blade (Fig. 14-10, *A*).

A third common error in performing laryngoscopy is getting too close to the objects being viewed. In the properly positioned patient with the vocal cords exposed, the mouth is only 6 to 8 inches from the cords. This is barely the distance that most people require to focus their eyes on a close object. Yet the beginner at intubation is often seen with one eye virtually in the patient's mouth, as if taking aim with a shotgun. This close distance compromises vision, which is better at a slightly greater distance, and denies the advantage of depth perception, which depends greatly on the use of both eyes.

Fourth, in barrel-chested and obese patients and large-breasted women, it may be difficult to insert the blade of a laryngoscope correctly into the mouth and avoid interruption of this procedure by anterior chest wall obstruction to movement of the handle of the laryngoscope. In these patients further initial skull-spine extension (atlantooccipital joint) or 90-degree rotation of the laryngoscope to the right permits easier introduction of the blade of the laryngoscope into the mouth and avoids anterior chest wall obstruction to the movement of the handle of the laryngoscope. Finally, one can insert an unattached blade into the right side of the mouth until it is possible to reattach the handle without experiencing chest wall obstruction.

The choice of relaxant is a complicated matter, but it may significantly determine the number of laryn-

goscopies required for intubation as well as the ultimate outcome. If no relaxant is used (perhaps because the first laryngoscopy is used as a diagnostic tool), the attempt may be suboptimal. If succinyldicholine is used and difficulty is encountered, then after several minutes or after a few attempts, muscle tone will return and subsequent laryngoscopy attempts (and mask ventilation) may be compromised (even though an appropriate adjustment, such as institution of optimal head and neck position, external laryngeal pressure, or using a different blade, or a combination of these, has been made). When a nondepolarizing muscle relaxant is used (which removes the highs and lows of muscle relaxation encountered with single or even multiple doses of succinyldicholine), the ability to return to spontaneous ventilation is compromised (although it does not necessarily mean there must be more intubation attempts). It is obvious from the preceding that understanding the advantages and disadvantages of the various muscle relaxants can significantly affect outcome, but the choice of muscle relaxant remains an issue of judgment.

C. TRACHEAL INTUBATION

The actual insertion of the tracheal tube is usually easy once the vocal cords are exposed (and the tongue is out of the way) (Fig. 14-10, *A*). Tracheas in adult women and men readily accept tracheal tubes with internal diameters of 7 to 8 mm and 8 to 9 mm, respectively (see Chapter 29 for pediatric sizes). If it is thought that fiberoptic bronchoscopy will be necessary subsequently for either diagnosis or therapy, the larger size should be used. If it is thought that the space between the upper and lower teeth will be small and the cuff of the tube may come in contact with the teeth, the distal tube and cuff should be lubricated to facilitate the cuff sliding by the teeth. The tip of the endotracheal tube should be introduced into the right corner of the mouth and passed along an axis that intersects the line of the laryngoscope blade at the glottis. In that way the tube does not interrupt the view of the vocal cords. The common error of trying to use the laryngoscope blade as a midline guide, under which the tube is passed, violates this principle, obscures vision, and is a significant source of difficulty for the inexperienced operator. The tube tip is passed through the cords, stopping 2 cm after the tube cuff disappears from sight or when the external markings are at the 21- and 23-cm marks at the incisors in adult women and adult men, respectively; when these external markings are at the lower incisors, the tip of the tube is at the midtrachea.[11] It is of paramount importance that the endoscopist not take his or her eye off the laryngeal aperture until the cuff disappears beyond the vocal cords.

Because the glottic opening can be unexpectedly anterior and therefore unvisualized, a precurved stylet should be placed in the endotracheal tube whenever a curved laryngoscope blade is used. To intubate an unvisualized glottis and trachea, the tube must pass along, but to the right of, the curved route made by the blade (as described earlier), and when the styleted tube reaches the end of the blade, it must dip around the epiglottis (by gentle probing) until it "falls into" the glottic opening (as indicated by a loss of resistance). I always use a stylet because if the larynx is anterior (expectedly or unexpectedly), no time will be lost in locating and then placing a stylet in an endotracheal tube. This is an avoidable delay that can only harm the patient. In general, when intubation speed is important (as in a patient with a full stomach), an endotracheal tube should always be styleted. A stylet should be malleable and lubricated and never extend beyond the end of the lumen of the tube. Occasionally a curved, styleted endotracheal tube impinges on the anterior tracheal wall as it is being inserted. Under these circumstances, while the endotracheal tube is through the vocal cords, the stylet should be withdrawn, which will give the tip of the endotracheal tube its inherent flexibility and permit further passage caudad.

The laryngoscope is removed from the mouth with the left hand. The cuff of the tube is blown up until moderate tension is felt in the pilot balloon to the cuff. The tube should then be connected to a source of ventilation with 100% O_2 and held in place by one hand. The thumb and index finger should hold the tube or the corrugated tubing while the other three fingers are in contact with the cheek. In this way, if the patient's head were to be turned to one side suddenly, the hand and the tube would

---

> **BOX 14-3   Signs of tracheal intubation**
>
> *Non–fail-safe signs*
> 1. Breath sounds over chest
> 2. No breath sounds over stomach
> 3. No gastric distention
> 4. Chest rise and fall
> 5. Intercostal spaces filling out during inspiration
> 6. Large spontaneous exhaled tidal volumes
> 7. Respiratory gas moisture disappearing on inhalation and reappearing on exhalation
> 8. Hearing air exit from the endotracheal tube when the chest is compressed
> 9. Reservoir bag having the appropriate compliance
> 10. Reciprocating pulsed pressures to and from supersternal notch and to and from balloon on the pilot tube of the endotracheal tube
> 11. Progressive arterial desaturation by pulse oximetry
>
> *Near fail-safe signs*
> 1. Carbon dioxide excretion waveform
> 2. Rapid expansion of a tracheal indicator bulb
>
> *Fail-safe signs*
> 1. Endotracheal tube visualized between vocal cords
> 2. Fiberoptic visualization of cartilaginous rings of the tracheal and tracheal carina

follow (rather than the hand remain stationary, which would pull the tube outward).

The next, most important task is to ascertain that the tube has, indeed, been inserted into the tracheobronchial tree rather than the esophagus (Box 14-3). This issue is extensively discussed in Chapter 27, and only a brief summary of the signs of tracheal intubation is given here. Simple but not fail-safe signs of tracheal intubation consist of breath sounds over the chest, lack of breath sounds over the stomach, lack of gastric distention, the rise and fall of the chest, the filling out during inspiration of the intercostal spaces, large spontaneous exhaled tidal volumes, respiratory gas moisture in the endotracheal tube that disappears on inhalation and reappears on exhalation, the sound of air exiting from the endotracheal tube when the chest is compressed, manual squeezing of a reservoir bag that has an appropriate compliance, and pulsing pressure on the suprasternal notch and feeling the pulse transmitted to the pilot balloon of the cuff, or conversely, palpation of a transmitted pulse from the endotracheal tube pilot tube to the cuff to the supersternal notch. A progressive decrease in Sp_{O_2} may indicate failure to intubate the trachea, but it is a late sign of esophageal intubation and it may also indicate bronchospasm, endobronchial intubation, aspiration, kinking of the tube, machine or equipment malfunction, or the like.

Near fail-safe signs of tracheal intubation are the presence of a normal CO_2 waveform and rapid expansion of a large rubber tracheal indicator bulb (see Chapter 27). Cardiac arrest (when no CO_2 is excreted),[12] severe bronchospasm, or kinking or massive plugging of the endotracheal tube may prevent the appearance of CO_2 in the exhaled gas (a false-negative finding), and CO_2 will appear if the tip of the tube is proximal to, but near the larynx (a false-positive finding). The esophageal-tracheal detector bulb has a very high sensitivity and specificity, but it is not perfect and false-negative and false-positive findings can occur.

The only fail-safe, but invasive, methods of definitively determining tracheal intubation are direct observation of the endotracheal tube going through the vocal cords and the use of a fiberoptic bronchoscope. Direct visualization of the tube lying in the glottic opening may be enhanced by pressing the concavity of the tube posteriorly, which may pull the glottic opening posteriorly and into better view. The fiberoptic bronchoscope allows visualization of the cartilaginous rings of the trachea and the tracheal carina. However, the fiberoptic bronchoscope cannot be regarded as a practical method of determining tracheal intubation.

If there is no CO_2 excretion waveform, breath sounds cannot be heard, and/or no chest movement occurs, pull the endotracheal tube out, ventilate the patient with a mask and bag system several times with 100% O_2, and reattempt tracheal intubation again after inspecting the tube for plugs. Changes in the curvature of the endotracheal tube and in the position of the head and neck and the need for anterior tracheal pressure should be considered and coordinated during the period of mask ventilation.

The next task is to ascertain that the tip of the endotracheal tube is above the carina and that ventilation is symmetric. This is done by observing equal expansion of both hemothoraces and by stethoscopic examination for breath sounds throughout both peripheral lung fields. However, hearing uniform breath sounds throughout all lung fields does not guarantee that the tube does not lie in a mainstem bronchus. (If it does, it almost always will be in the right mainstem bronchus.) If there is any question about a mainstem bronchus intubation, one should retract the tube about 1 cm at a time and reexamine the breath sounds. In one study an insertion depth of 21 cm in adult women and 23 cm in adult men resulted in no incidence of mainstem bronchial intubation.[11] Simultaneous palpation of pulsed pressures both in the cuff in the suprasternal notch and the pilot balloon of the cuff (as described earlier) is another simple way of determining the location of the tube in the trachea. Fiberoptic bronchoscopy is another, but complex, way of determining the location of the tube in the trachea. Outside of the operating room, it is always advisable to confirm endotracheal tube position by chest x-ray. Ideally the tip of the tube should be at the clavicular (midtracheal) level.

When the tracheal tube is placed and during taping of the endotracheal tube, the marking of the endotracheal tube at the level of the lower teeth must be noted. This is important for four reasons. First, as discussed earlier, if the tube is inserted to the 21-cm mark in adult women and to the 23-cm mark in adult men, there will be virtually no incidence of mainstem bronchial intubation.[11] Second, during taping of the tube to the face, anxious beginners have a tendency to unwittingly advance the tube further into the trachea. Third, the patient may cough or make bucking or vomiting-like movements after intubation and, unless the tube has been continuously secured, the patient may self-extubate the tracheal tube. Movements of the initial marking outward facilitates this diagnosis. Fourth, following intubation of the trachea and the initiation of positive pressure ventilation, if the left side of the chest suddenly stops moving or no left-side chest breath sounds can be heard, there are two likely causes, which the mark of the tube at the teeth can help to determine: (1) the tube has advanced into the right mainstem bronchus, causing left lung atelectasis and (2) a left pneumothorax, possibly under tension, has developed. If the tube was marked when ventilation was normal bilaterally and this mark subsequently advanced into the patient's mouth, bronchial intubation would be much more likely than pneumothorax, whereas the converse would be true if the mark were stationary. Similar considerations apply to apparent absent ventilation of the right side of the lungs.

D. SECUREMENT OF THE TUBE

After the mark of the tube at the lower teeth level has been noted, the tube should be tightly secured in place. This is important not only to prevent accidental extubation, but also to minimize tube movement within the airway. Taping the tube to the skin with adhesive tape is the most common method of securing the tube. Fig. 14-11 suggests two different ways to tape the tube in place. The securement of the tube in place can be increased by having the lateral ends of the tape (shown in Fig. 14-11) completely encircle the jaw and neck. (Place the tape all the way around the posterior neck over to the contralateral neck and jaw.) Application of tincture of benzoin to the skin before the tape is applied helps provide a stronger bond between the tape and skin. In case of prolonged intubation, changing the tape and reapplying it to a new area on the face every 2 days helps prevent maceration of the skin. In patients with beards or in whom the adhesive tape fails to stick to the skin, the tube can be tied into place with a length of umbilical tape that encircles the tube with a nonslipping knot and then

Securing the Endotracheal Tube with Tape

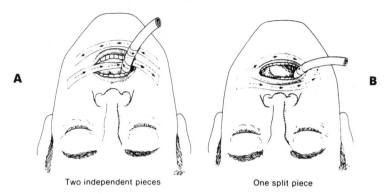

Two independent pieces   One split piece

Fig. 14-11. This schematic diagram depicts two ways of taping an oral endotracheal tube in place. **A,** Thin (½-inch) tape can be brought from one lateral jaw around the tube over the other lateral jaw, both above the upper lip and below the lower lip. Securement of the tube is increased by placing tincture of benzoin over the skin prior to taping and taping all the way around the back of the neck over to the contralateral jaw. **B,** Thick (1-inch) tape can be brought from a lateral jaw to the angle of the mouth, the tape split in half, with the upper half crossing above the upper lip as an anchor to the skin and with the lower half wrapped around the tube and then over to the contralateral jaw, holding the tube in place. The same, but oppositely directed, taping procedure may be done starting from the contralateral jaw with the thick unsplit tape.

encircles the neck with another nonslipping knot. Adhesive tape may be used over the umbilical tape for added security. Another very reliable method of securing an orotracheal tube is to wire the tube to a tooth. One or two layers of adhesive tape are wrapped around the tube at the level of the lower incisor teeth. Stainless steel wire (25 to 28 gauge) is passed around a lower incisor tooth and twisted around the tape on the tube. In anesthetized patients a suture may be passed through the gum and then either around a ring of adhesive tape on the endotracheal tube (as with wire) or through the wall of the endotracheal tube and then tied to the tube. A bite block, rolled gauze, or an oral airway (used in the vast majority of tracheal intubations for anesthesia) should be placed between the teeth to prevent the patient from biting down and occluding the lumen of an oral tube. The mouth and pharynx should be suctioned. The tube cuff then should be deflated so that a gas leak occurs during a positive pressure inspiration and reinflated to a just-seal volume during the next few peak positive pressure inspirations.

II. CONVENTIONAL (LARYNGOSCOPIC) NASOTRACHEAL INTUBATION

Intubation by the nasal route is generally a more difficult procedure than oral intubation. On the other hand, nasal tubes are thought to be better tolerated than oral tubes. Therefore nasal tubes are considered the tube of choice for long-term mechanical ventilation. The tracheal tube is inserted into a nostril and then passed through the nasal cavity and nasopharynx to the oropharynx. Once the tube has been passed into the oropharynx, it can be guided into the glottis with conventional direct laryngoscopic vision and without any special grasping aid, or it can be grasped additionally by a forceps (Magill) and manually directed into the glottis.

A. PRELARYNGOSCOPY MANEUVERS

Prior to insertion of the nasotracheal tube into the nose, the nasal mucosa should be sprayed with a vasoconstrictor drug. Vasoconstriction of blood vessels in the nasal mucosa minimizes bleeding that is due to the trauma of passing nasotracheal tube through the nose, and it increases the diameter of the nasal passages by constricting (shrinking) the nasal mucosa. In addition, softening the tip of the nasotracheal tube by soaking it in a warm saline solution may decrease the incidence of mucosal damage and bleeding. The naris selected should be the one that the patient thinks offers the least resistance to breathing while the other naris is occluded. However, if both nares offer equal resistance, then the left-side naris should be chosen because the bevel of the nasotracheal tube, when introduced through the left-side naris, will face the turbinates, reducing damage to the turbinates (Fig. 14-12). In addition, the left-side naris should be chosen because entry of the tube into the oropharynx from the left side will permit more room for the laryngoscopic blade and Magill forceps on the right side of the oropharynx. In the vast majority of adults, tubes with an internal diameter of 7.0 to 7.5 mm pass through the nares. The other prelaryngoscopy maneuvers described under direct-vision orotracheal intuba-

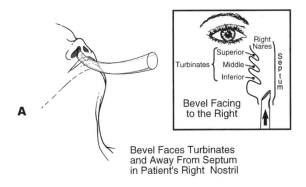

Bevel Faces Turbinates
and Away From Septum
in Patient's Right Nostril

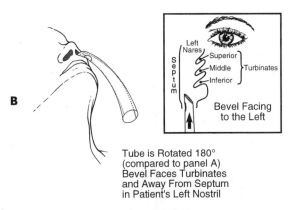

Tube is Rotated 180°
(compared to panel A)
Bevel Faces Turbinates
and Away From Septum
in Patient's Left Nostril

Fig. 14-12. Insertion of a nasotracheal tube into the nares. **A,** When the nasotracheal tube is passed into the right nares, the bevel should be facing to the right toward the turbinates (see inset). In this way the tip of the tube is against the septum and the risks of catching the tip of the tube on a turbinate and tearing or dislocating it are minimized. In this orientation the concavity of the tube is pointing anteriorly. **B,** When the nasotracheal tube is passed into the left nares, the bevel should be facing to the left toward the turbinates (see inset). In this way the tip of the tube is against the septum and the risks of catching the tip of the tube on a turbinate and tearing or dislocating it are minimized. In this orientation the concavity of the tube is pointing posteriorly.

tion (positioning of the head, suctioning, and preoxygenation) should be performed for direct-vision nasal intubation. The nasotracheal tube should be lubricated and passed through the nose in one smooth posterior, caudad, medially directed movement until resistance to forward movement significantly decreases as the tube enters the oropharynx (usually at the 15- to 16-cm mark).

The pathway that the nasotracheal tube takes should be visualized as a ∪ lying on its side. The curve of the tracheal tube should be aligned to facilitate passage along this curved course. As the tube passes through the nose into the nasopharynx, it must turn downward to pass through the pharynx. In making this turn, it may impact against the posterior nasopharyngeal wall and resist any attempt to push it further. The tube should be pulled back a short distance, and the patient's head should be extended further to facilitate attempts to pass

this point smoothly and atraumatically. If this is not done and the tube is forced, the mucosal covering of the posterior nasopharyngeal wall may be torn open and the tube may be passed into the submucosal tissues.

B. LARYNGOSCOPY

The laryngoscopy for nasal intubation is identical to that described for oral intubation.

C. TRACHEAL INTUBATION

Once the tube is in the oropharynx, the tip of the tube must be aligned with the glottic opening. If the tip of the tube is excessively anterior, posterior, or lateral to the glottic opening, it will not enter this orifice. If necessary, the tube must be withdrawn slightly, before any of the corrective measures, described next, are taken (Fig. 14-13).

Lateral tip location, as indicated either by direct vision or by observing bulging soft tissue in the lateral neck, can be corrected in either direction by twirling or rotating the adapter of the tube at the nose. If the bulge is on the right, the proximal end of the tube is rotated in a counterclockwise direction and is advanced again (Fig. 14-13, *A*). If the bulge is on the left, the proximal end of the tube is rotated in a clockwise direction (Fig. 14-13, *B*). Alternatively, this problem can be identified by noting the rotation of a curved adapter, whose curve lies in the same vertical plane as the concave curve of the tube, away from the midline.

Anterior tip location, as indicated by either direct vision or bulging soft tissue under the mandible, can be corrected by flexion of the head or by picking up the larynx and trachea externally (anterior displacement) (Fig. 14-13, *C*). Both of these maneuvers cause the tip of the tube to become more posterior in relation to the glottis. Sometimes sitting the patient up correctly aligns the tip of the tube with the laryngeal aperture (Fig. 14-3, *C* and *D*).

Posterior tip location almost always means esophageal intubation and is indicated either by direct vision or by loss of breath sounds heard or felt from the tube. Posterior tip location can be corrected by extending the patient's head, which causes the tip of the tube to become more anterior in relation to the larynx (Fig. 14-13, *D*). Posterior direction can also be corrected by using a ring tube (Endotrol). A ring tube has a cord that runs from the anterior surface of the tip of the tube up the length of the tube to a ring on the proximal end of the tube. Pulling on the ring causes anterior bending of the tip of the tube. Posterior tip location can be corrected by pushing the larynx down (posterior displacement), which causes the larynx to become more posterior in relation to the tip of the tube (Fig. 14-13, *D*). Both anterior and posterior tip location may also be corrected by sitting the patient upright (Fig. 14-13, *C* and

NASOTRACHEAL INTUBATION:
ALIGNMENT OF TIP OF NASOTRACHEAL TUBE WITH GLOTTIS

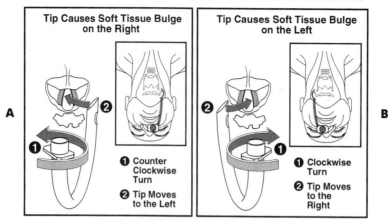

Tip Causes Soft Tissue Bulge on the Right

A

❶ Counter Clockwise Turn

❷ Tip Moves to the Left

Tip Causes Soft Tissue Bulge on the Left

B

❶ Clockwise Turn

❷ Tip Moves to the Right

NASOTRACHEAL INTUBATION:
ALIGNMENT OF TIP OF NASOTRACHEAL TUBE WITH GLOTTIS

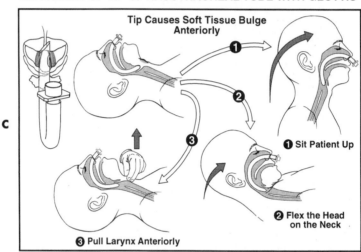

Tip Causes Soft Tissue Bulge Anteriorly

C

❶ Sit Patient Up

❷ Flex the Head on the Neck

❸ Pull Larynx Anteriorly

NASOTRACHEAL INTUBATION:
ALIGNMENT OF TIP OF NASOTRACHEAL TUBE WITH GLOTTIS

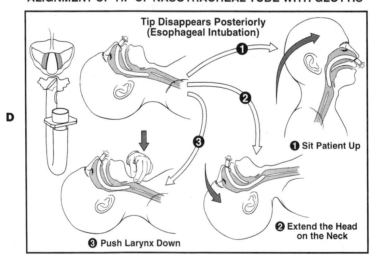

Tip Disappears Posteriorly (Esophageal Intubation)

D

❶ Sit Patient Up

❷ Extend the Head on the Neck

❸ Push Larynx Down

Fig. 14-13. Nasotracheal intubation: alignment of tip of nasotracheal tube with glottis (correcting malalignment of nasotracheal tube with the glottis). **A,** Right lateral malalignment is corrected by counterclockwise rotation of proximal end of endotracheal tube. **B,** Left lateral malalignment is corrected by clockwise rotation of proximal end of nasotracheal tube. **C,** Anterior malalignment is corrected by, *2,* flexion of the head on the neck or by, *3,* pulling the larynx anteriorly, or both. **D,** Posterior malalignment is corrected by, *2,* extension of the head on the neck, by, *3,* pushing the larynx posteriorly, by using a tip-controlled tube (Endotrol), or by a combination of these. **C** and **D,** Correct alignment of the tip of the tube with the glottic opening may result from, *1,* sitting the patient up.

Guiding a Nasotracheal Tube into the Larynx Using a Magill Forceps

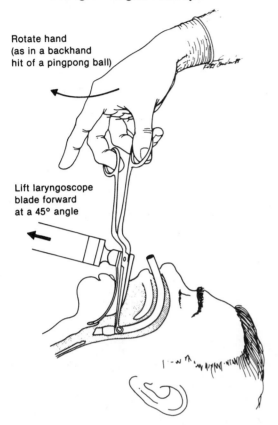

Rotate hand
(as in a backhand
hit of a pingpong ball)

Lift laryngoscope
blade forward
at a 45° angle

Fig. 14-14. A nasotracheal tube can be guided under direct vision (laryngoscopic control) through the laryngeal aperture with a Magill forceps by simply rotating the hand as one would do when using a backhand motion in hitting a Ping-Pong ball. The Magill forceps should grab the nasotracheal tube proximal to the cuff of the endotracheal tube..

D). The procedures described earlier for correction of the anterior, posterior, and lateral malpositions of the tube tip can be performed more precisely under direct vision than with blind attempts and result in success more easily.

Since one hand must hold the laryngoscope and another hand may be necessary for manipulation of the head or larynx, an assistant may be necessary to push the tube into the larynx when the appropriate elements are lined up correctly. In addition, if the tube is in the midline but too posterior and this is not corrected by extension of the head, force on the anterior trachea, or use of the ring on an Endotrol tube, the tube must be grasped in the pharynx with a Magill forceps (avoiding the cuff on the tube) and directed anteriorly through the vocal cords (Fig. 14-14). The advantage of the design of these forceps is that when the grasping ends are parallel

to the long axis of the tracheal tube, the handle is outside of the right side of the mouth and at a right angle to the long axis of the tube. Since the handle is outside the right side of the mouth, it is away from the line of sight. Since the forceps are grasped parallel to the long axis of the tube, a backhand motion of the right hand passes the tube toward the glottic opening (Fig. 14-14). Thus the intubationist can have the larynx exposed by the laryngoscope held in the left hand, the tube in full view, a means (the forceps) of manipulating the alignment of the tube, and a means of advancing the tube. However, it is often desirable to have an assistant advance the proximal end of the tube so that the intubationist is free to simply guide the tube into the larynx without having to pull it along with the Magill forceps.

In some patients, as the tube enters the trachea, the tube's anterior curvature may direct it against the anterior tracheal wall and interfere with passage past this point. To resolve this difficulty, the head must be lifted (flexed) slowly as the tube is advanced. A nasotracheal tube should be advanced until the cuff is 2 cm below the vocal cords or until the external markings are 24 cm for women and 26 cm for men (3 cm more than for oral tubes) at the nares. The tube's correct placement must be verified as in any intubation (see orotracheal intubation), but this is particularly critical with nasal intubations because the relationship to external tube markings and the location of the tube tip is not as firmly established as it is for orotracheal tubes. If nasal bleeding occurs, it is probably wise to leave the tube in place to act as a tamponade. If the bleeding is severe, the tube can be retracted and the cuff inflated to act as a better tamponade.

D. SECUREMENT OF THE TUBE

The nasotracheal tube can be secured with adhesive tape as described for orotracheal tubes. In addition, a nasotracheal tube can be secured by a suture through the nasal septum and then tied, after being tightly wound around an adhesive band on the tube or passed through the wall of the tube by a needle and then tied.

REFERENCES

1. Horton WA, Fahy L, Charters P: Defining a standard intubating position using "angle finder," *Br J Anaesth* 62:6, 1989.
2. Caplan R: Personal Communication, 1993.
3. Gold MI, Durate I, Muravchick S: Arterial oxygenation in conscious patients after 5 minutes and after 30 seconds of oxygen breathing, *Anesth Analg* 60:313, 1981.
4. Gambee AM, Hertzka RE, Fisher DM: Preoxygenation techniques: comparison of three minutes and four breaths, *Anesth Analg* 66:468, 1987.
5. Jense HG, Dubin SA, Silverstein PI et al: Effect of obesity on safe duration of apnea in anesthetized humans, *Anesth Analg* 72:89, 1991.
6. Teller LE, Alexander CM, Frumin MJ et al: Pharyngeal insufflation of oxygen prevents arterial desaturation during apnea, *Anesthesiology* 69:980, 1988.

7. Samsoon GLT, Young JRB: Difficult tracheal intubation: a retrospective study, *Anaesthesia* 42:487, 1987.

8. Cormack RS, Lehane J: Difficult tracheal intubation in obstetrics, *Anaesthesia* 39:1105, 1984.

9. Wilson ME, Spiegelhalter D, Robertson JA et al: Predicting difficult intubation, *Br J Anaesth* 61:211, 1988.

10. Knill RL: Difficult laryngoscopy made easy with a "Burp," *Can J Anaesth* 40:279, 1993.

11. Owen RL, Cheney FW: Endobronchial intubation: a preventable complication, *Anesthesiology* 67:255, 1987.

12. Garnett AR, Ornato JF, Gonzalez ER et al: End-tidal carbon dioxide monitoring during monitoring during cardiopulmonary resuscitation, *JAMA* 257:512, 1987.

Chapter 15

BLIND DIGITAL INTUBATION

Michael F. Murphy
Orlando R. Hung

I. HISTORY

Although probably first described by Herholdt and Rafn[1] in 1796 for the management of drowning victims, blind digital orotracheal intubation had received scant attention in the medical literature until the mid 1980s, when revived by Stewart[2,3] in emergency medicine and prehospital care. Notable publications on the topic over the years have portrayed the technique as an acceptable, if not preferable, alternative to standard laryngoscopic endotracheal intubation, particularly when the standard technique is contraindicated, has failed, or is not possible because of lack of equipment.

In 1880 MacEwen[4] described the technique utilizing a curved metal tube in awake patients, and Sykes[5] recommended the routine use of the digital technique in anesthetic practice in the 1930s. Siddall[6] and Lanham[7] relegated the technique to last-ditch efforts following the failure of conventional intubation methods.[3] The technique has been described in neonatal resuscitation[8] and as an adjunct in blind nasotracheal intubation.[9]

Currently there is widespread variation in awareness, expertise, and application of the technique in anesthesia, emergency medicine, and prehospital care. Although advances in airway management equipment and expertise have made obsolete the routine use of blind digital orotracheal intubation, it remains a valuable skill in some patients, especially in the emergency setting.[3]

II. INDICATIONS

The use of the digital technique is neither aesthetically pleasing, easily accomplished, nor entirely safe. As one might imagine, placing one's fingers far enough down a patient's throat to elevate the epiglottis and guide an endotracheal tube into the trachea has implications related to patient selection and the manual dexterity and anatomic features of the intubator.

The technique has found some popularity in the prehospital care environment where difficult patient position, poor lighting conditions, disrupted anatomy, potential cervical spine instability, and unknown status regarding infectious disease are the norm. Digital intubation is ordinarily used when other maneuvers have failed or are likely to fail, or when alternative equipment is unavailable or inoperative.

Successful digital intubation demands that the patient be unconscious to tolerate the intense oropharyngeal stimulus and prevent bite injuries to the intubator. Neuromuscular blockade facilitates the technique, although it is relatively contraindicated in patients with anatomically difficult or disrupted airways. Digital intubation may be indicated as follows:

   1. When equipment required to undertake alterna-

tive techniques is unavailable or inoperative.

2. When positioning of the patient or the intubator prevents conventional intubation.

3. When other methods have failed or are likely to fail and the skill and experience of the intubator make the digital technique the technique of choice.

4. In the face of potential or actual cervical spine instability the intubator selects the digital technique on the basis of the risk-benefit analysis. While there is no evidence to suggest that the technique of digital intubation will alter the neurologic outcome in a patient, we believe that there is less cervical spine motion during intubation with the digital technique as compared with the conventional laryngoscopic orotracheal intubation without in-line stabilization.

5. When adequate visualization of the airway to allow conventional intubation is not possible because of the absence of adequate suction to clear secretions, blood, or vomitus in the oropharynx or because of traumatic disruption of the upper airway anatomy.

III. TECHNIQUE OF DIGITAL INTUBATION

A. PREPARATION

As with any intubation technique, preparation involves assembling the necessary equipment and personnel, including emergency drugs and adequate suction, to optimize success and preserve ventilation and oxygenation. An appropriate size of endotracheal tube (ET) is selected. The use of a stiff but malleable stylet increases maneuverability during the intubation. Lubrication of the stylet with a water-soluble lubricant ensures easy retraction following the placement of the tip of the ET in the glottic opening. The stylet is inserted into the ET so that the distal end of the stylet is at the level of the Murphy eye. With the stylet in place, bend the distal half of the ET and the stylet (ET-ST) unit to a ∪ configuration (Fig. 15-1). The proximal half of the ET is then bent approximately 90 degrees to the dominant side of the intubator to allow manipulation of the ET-ST by the dominant hand during intubation (Figs. 15-2 and 15-3). The degree of bend should be individualized and depends on the intubator's experience. The tip of the ET should be well lubricated with a water-soluble lubricant. In the uncommon event that the intubation is performed in an awake patient, especially an uncooperative patient, a bite block should be placed between the patient's molars on one side to prevent injury to the intubator's fingers.

B. POSITIONING

The patient should be supine with the head in a slight sniffing position as for laryngoscopic intubation. The intubator stands (or kneels if the patient is on the ground) beside the patient so that the nondominant side

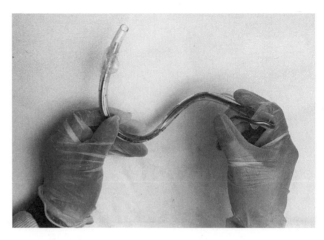

Fig. 15-1. With the stylet in place, the distal half of the tube is bent in a ∪ shape.

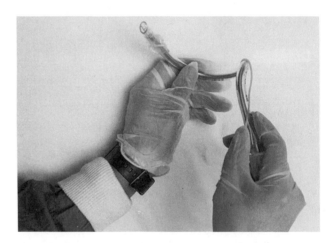

Fig. 15-2. The proximal half of the endotracheal tube is bent 90 degrees toward the dominant side of the intubator.

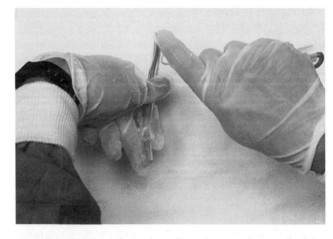

Fig. 15-3. Final configuration allows improved control of the endotracheal tube with both hands. During the intubation the index finger of the dominant hand can help advance the endotracheal tube while the index and middle fingers of the nondominant hand guide the tip of the tube into the glottis.

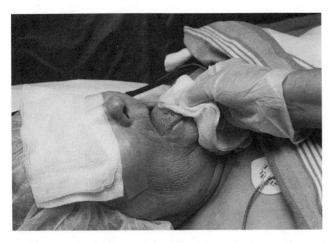

Fig. 15-4. An assistant retracts the tongue using a piece of gauze.

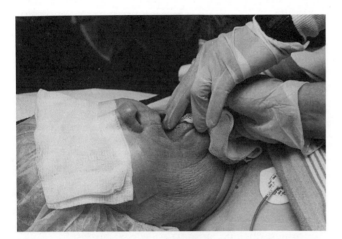

Fig. 15-5. The index and middle fingers of the nondominant hand are inserted into the mouth palm down.

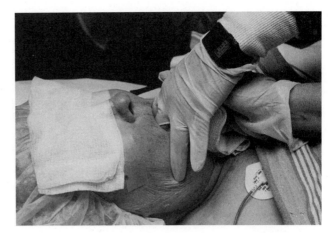

Fig. 15-6. The fingers are advanced to the point where the middle finger is able to palpate the tip of the epiglottis and push it anteriorly.

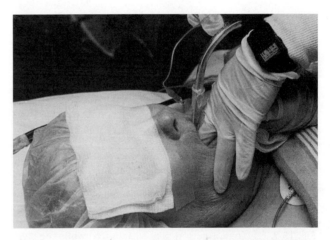

Fig. 15-7. The endotracheal tube and stylet unit (ET-ST) is advanced along the groove between the index and middle fingers, over top of the tongue.

of the intubator is closest to the patient. An assistant facilitates the procedure.

C. TECHNIQUE

It is my experience that retraction of the tongue facilitates palpation of the epiglottis, improving the success rate for digital intubation. The patient's mouth is opened and the tongue grasped gently by the assistant with a gauze sponge. (Fig. 15-4). Traction on the tongue moves the epiglottis slightly cephalad, enhancing its palpability and facilitating the placement of the tip of the ET into the glottic opening. Insert the index and middle fingers of the nondominant hand into the oral cavity, and slide the palm down along the surface of the tongue (Fig. 15-5). The tip of the middle finger contacts the tip of the epiglottis, which is then directed anteriorly (Fig. 15-6). The ease of palpating and lifting the epiglottis depends on the length of the intubator's fingers, the height of the patient, the anatomy of the oropharynx, and the presence or absence of teeth. Once the epiglottis is identified

and directed anteriorly, the ET-ST is inserted through the corner of the mouth (Fig. 15-7). The ET-ST glides along the groove between the middle and index fingers on the palmar surface of the nondominant hand. While firm anterior pressure is maintained against the epiglottis with the middle finger, the ET-ST is advanced slowly into the glottic opening by the dominant hand (Fig. 15-8). The index finger may be used to guide the tip of the ET-ST into the glottic opening. Stabilize the ET while withdrawing the stylet (Fig. 15-9), and advance the ET slowly into the trachea. During the intubation the ET-ST should never be advanced forcefully against resistance. Accurate placement is confirmed by conventional techniques, such as end-tidal carbon dioxide monitoring and auscultation.

Occasionally the tip of the epiglottis cannot be palpated. An upward (cephalad) and backward (poste-

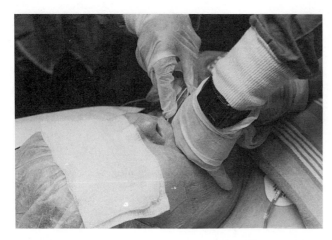

Fig. 15-8. The ET-ST is guided into the glottis, directed by the index finger tip if necessary.

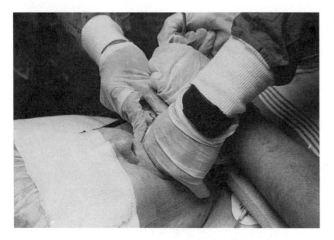

Fig. 15-9. The endotracheal tube is stabilized while the stylet is removed.

rior) pressure applied anteriorly to the larynx by an assistant may be helpful. As an alternative, the index and middle fingers of the nondominant hand may be used to keep the ET-ST in midline while observing tissue movement in the anterior neck during gentle rocking of the ET-ST back and forth in an attempt to locate the glottic opening.

This potentially lifesaving procedure is a relatively simple technique and can be learned easily. The following case history serves to illustrate the role of digital intubation in the emergency airway management of a patient who could not be intubated by the conventional method.

IV. CASE HISTORY

A call was received by the 911 center of a large, urban emergency medical services system (EMS), reporting a "man not breathing" at a downtown hotel. A mobile intensive care unit from the nearest ambulance station was dispatched within 40 seconds of the call having been received.

On arrival 3 minutes later, the EMS team was directed to the top floor of the hotel, where a wedding reception was in progress. On the floor of a small washroom the 120-kg patient was found in cardiac arrest, pulseless, and not breathing. According to the history given by relatives, the patient had chest pain while dancing after a large meal. He went into the washroom and collapsed.

Cardiopulmonary resuscitation (CPR) with bag-mask ventilation was begun immediately. Vomiting ensued, obscuring the view of the paramedic who was attempting orotracheal intubation. Suctioning was attempted using a portable suction unit, but so much vomitus was present that the collecting bottle of the suction unit filled rapidly and further suctioning was not successful in clearing the upper airway. "Quick-look" paddles revealed asystole.

While chest compressions and bag-mask ventilation continued, attempts at intravenous access were successful. Second and third attempts at direct-vision tracheal intubation resulted in esophageal placement, readily recognized by the paramedic team.

It became clear that attempts at direct visualization of the airway would not be successful because of the large amount of vomitus in the oropharynx. Because of this, the decision was made to place the ET using the tactile (digital) method. Using a 7.5-mm ET, a physician carried out a digital intubation through the vomitus and secretions and was successful on the first attempt. Ventilation and suctioning were begun through the in-place ET and the patient's color improved. CPR continued during transport to a local hospital.

V. LIMITATIONS

The more alert the patient is, the less the likelihood that digital intubation will be tolerated or successful. The very setting, by itself, of a patient who is already the victim of multiple failed intubation attempts places limitations on the likelihood of success of the digital technique. Patients with limited mouth opening, carious or prominent dentition, small mouths, and large tongues can be predictably difficult to intubate, no matter what method is employed, including the digital method. With practice, however, digital intubation has been shown to be an effective, alternative method of intubation.[2]

The risk of injury to the intubator by the patient's teeth and body fluids is real. This risk can be minimized by selecting unconscious or paralyzed patients or by placing a bite block between the patient's molars. In our experience double gloving provides a measure of protection against barrier interruption, injury from teeth, and the potential for disease transmission.

As with other techniques of intubation, complications such as trauma to the upper airways can occur during the digital intubation. However, trauma can be minimized by advancing the ET gently during the intubation. Other potential complications of digital intubation, including esophageal intubation, can be avoided by good technique and gentle manipulation.

Digital intubation is a "blind" technique and therefore relatively contraindicated in patients with upper airway compromise resulting from such disorders as infectious diseases, neoplasms, foreign bodies, caustic and thermal burns, and anaphylaxis.

VI. CONCLUSION

Digital intubation is seldom the method of first choice in securing a definitive airway. However, it offers an alternative that, in the event of failure of conventional techniques, may prove lifesaving. Successful digital intubation depends largely on the intubator's preparation, experience, and skill.

REFERENCES

1. Herholdt JD, Rafn CG: *Life-saving measures for drowning persons,* Copenhagen, 1796, H. Tikiob.
2. Stewart RD: Tactile orotracheal intubation, *Ann Emerg Med* 13:175, 1984.
3. Stewart RD: Digital intubation. In Dailey RH, Simon B, Stewart RD et al, editors: *The airway: emergency management,* St Louis, 1992, Mosby.
4. MacEwen W: Clinical observations on the introduction of tracheal tubes by the mouth instead of performing tracheotomy or laryngotomy, *Br Med J* 1:163, 1880.
5. Sykes WS: Oral endotracheal intubation without laryngoscopy: a plea for simplicity, *Curr Res Anesth Analg* 16:133, 1937.
6. Siddall WJW: Tactile orotracheal intubation, *Anaesthesia* 21:221, 1966.
7. Lanham HG: Tactile orotracheal intubation, *JAMA* 236:2288, 1976 (letter).
8. Woody NC, Woody HG: Direct digital intratracheal intubation for neonatal resuscitation, *J Pediatr* 73:903, 1968.
9. Korber TE, Henneman PL: Digital nasotracheal intubation, *J Emerg Med* 7:275, 1989.

Chapter 16

FIBEROPTIC ENDOSCOPY-AIDED TECHNIQUES

Andranik Ovassapian
Melissa Wheeler

1. **Knowing the instrument**
2. **Handling the instrument**
   a. PRACTICE ON A TRACHEOBRONCHIAL
      TREE MODEL
   b. PRACTICE ON THE INTUBATION
      MANNEQUIN
   c. PRACTICE ON PATIENTS
   d. FIBEROPTIC TRACHEAL INTUBATION OF
      THE PATIENT
3. **Additional learning aids**
4. **Assessing proficiency**
5. **Introducing fiberoptic intubation into one's
   own practice**
X. **CONCLUSION**

I. HISTORICAL BACKGROUND

The first recorded fiberoptic nasotracheal intubation was performed in 1967 on a patient with Still's disease, using a flexible fiberoptic choledochoscope.[1] Five years later, a fiberoptic bronchoscope (FOB) was used for nasotracheal intubation in patients with severe rheumatoid arthritis in which conventional endotracheal intubation techniques were not possible.[2,3] The first series of 100 fiberoptic endotracheal intubations was reported by Stiles et al.[4] in 1972. Intubations were performed both orally and nasally; four intubations failed because of copious secretions. Stiles et al. indicated that with experience, fiberoptic intubation can be performed in less than 1 minute.

In 1973 Davis[5] mentioned the use of the FOB to check endotracheal tube (ET) position in relation to the carina. Reports of fiberoptic evaluation of ET position and fiberoptic repositioning of ET intraoperatively soon followed.[6-8] Fiberoptic evaluation of ET position was demonstrated to be as good as chest radiograph evaluation in both adults and children.[9-10]

Raj et al. in 1974 were the first to report the use of the FOB to assist placement and positioning of a left-sided double-lumen endobronchial tube.[11] Other reports of the use of the FOB for positioning single-lumen and double-lumen endobronchial tubes followed.[12,13] Ovassapian and Schrader[14] described a new fiberoptic technique for positioning of right-sided double-lumen tubes in 1987. Benumof et al.[15] published their findings on evaluation of the left and right mainstem bronchi in 1987, demonstrating the high safety margin of the left-sided double-lumen tube and further demonstrating why placement of a right-sided double-lumen tube is not possible in some patients.

The use of the FOB in critically ill pediatric patients to evaluate the upper and lower airway has expanded in recent years.[16-20] Fiberoptic bronchoscopy is a bedside procedure that does not require general anesthesia. It may be performed orally, nasally, or through endotra-

cheal or tracheostomy tubes. The main disadvantage of its use through airway devices is the increased airway resistance encountered, since the fiberscope occupies a significant portion of the endotracheal lumen.

The FOB was not originally developed for the management of the difficult intubation.[21] The value of the FOB, however, in this area was recognized by anesthesiologists from the beginning, and they played an important role in expanding its use in the management of the difficult airway.[1-4,22] The FOB was used for patients with Ludwig's angina,[23] rheumatoid arthritis,[24,25] trauma,[26,27] unstable cervical spine,[28] cut throat (disruption) injuries,[29] acromegaly,[30] Pierre-Robin syndrome,[31,32] and many other difficult airway conditions.[33-40]

The significant role of the FOB in securing the airway in the conscious patient, especially when associated with an increased risk of aspiration, has been demonstrated by several investigators.[33-38] Ovassapian et al.[41] reported the first series of 129 patients at increased risk of aspiration who were subjected to awake fiberoptic intubation, without any evidence of aspiration after successful completion of the technique.

The relative ease of exploring the upper and lower airway with or without the benefit of general anesthesia has expanded the role of the anesthesiologist as a diagnostician in the perioperative period.[42] The many uses of the FOB include evaluation of severe postextubation laryngeal spasm and preoperative or postextubation stridor, and identification of unexpected hypoxemia caused by acute atelectasis or by unintentional endobronchial intubation, ET blockage by secretions, and kinking or cuff herniation, as well as incidental discoveries of laryngeal polyps or other airway lesions.

The continuous improvement and refinement of technique, the development of new FOBs and related ancillary equipment, and recognition of the value of the FOB in airway management have led to the enormous popularity that the FOB enjoys today. Increased publication of papers related to fiberoptic airway management and books and monographs entirely devoted to fiberoptic use in anesthesia attest to the widespread interest of clinicians in this area.[43-45]

The teaching of and training for fiberoptic airway endoscopy have been introduced and expanded in most training programs during the last decade. Most anesthesiologists who had completed their training earlier have had to learn this new skill on their own and by participating in special training workshops organized for this purpose.

A graduate-level training program was developed by Ovassapian et al.[46,47] to teach fiberoptic intubation to anesthesia residents. This program was later incorporated into a workshop format for training clinicians in practice.[48] Since then, a number of new ideas have been

BOX 16-1   Indications for fiberoptic intubation

I. Difficult intubation
   A. Known or anticipated
   B. Unanticipated failed intubation
II. Compromised airway
   A. Intubation in the conscious patient
      1. High risk of aspiration
      2. Movement of neck not desirable
      3. Known difficult mask ventilation
      4. Morbid obesity
      5. Self-positioning
   B. High risk of dental damage
   C. Previous tracheostomy or prolonged intubation
   D. Routine intubation

introduced for the step-by-step, progressive training of the art of fiberoptic intubation.[49-51]

This chapter covers fiberoptic intubation techniques and procedures in adults and children, including ET changing techniques. It explores how one may learn and teach the art of fiberoptic intubation and develop a proficiency in its application. The chapter begins with a brief discussion of the physics of the FOB and its general care and maintenance.

II. THE INSTRUMENT

The first fiberoptic bronchoscope was designed and produced based on specifications provided by Ikeda[21] in 1966. Since then, FOBs in various sizes and lengths have been introduced.[44] These can be used for airway management in adults and premature neonates (Box 16-1). The knowledge of the basic physical principles involved in construction of an FOB is essential for understanding how the FOB functions and how one can avoid damaging the instrument. This knowledge is critical because the FOB is an expensive instrument and special care is required to ensure the expected years of service. Frequent damage to the instrument is not only costly but also means the FOB is unavailable and therefore underused.

Fiberoptic laryngoscopes and bronchoscopes are manufactured by various companies using the same basic principles and design. The FOB has three main components: the handle, the insertion cord, and the universal cord. Each of these is designed to contribute to the overall function of the FOB (Fig. 16-1).

The handle contains the eyepiece for viewing, the lever for controlling the bending section of the tip, the suction button, and the access port to the suction channel. The eyepiece contains a diopter adjustment ring to focus and adjust the eyepiece to fit each viewer's vision. The bending lever is located on the back of the handle and controls movement of the insertion cord

tip in one plane of motion. Handles are designed to be held comfortably by either hand and to allow maneuvering of the bending lever by the thumb and activation of the suction by the index finger. This one-handed operation allows the operator's other hand to be free to advance, withdraw, or manipulate the insertion cord or ET.

The second component of the FOB is the insertion cord. The insertion cord is that portion of the FOB that is inserted into the patient and over which ETs are passed during fiberoptic intubation.

The insertion cord contains the light and image transmission bundles, the suction channel, and the tip bending control wires. These components are held together with a stainless steel mesh and are wrapped with a water-impermeable plastic coating. The outside diameter of the insertion cord is what determines the size of the smallest ET that can be used. The insertion cord is flexible and tolerates gentle bending to accommodate the curves of the airway. Keep in mind, however, that the only portion of the insertion cord that is designed for maximum bending is the distal tip. Vigorous bending of other areas of the insertion cord results in breakage of fiberoptic fibers.

Light is transmitted within the insertion cord through one or two light transmission bundles to the tip of the FOB. The glass fibers of the light transmission bundles extend to the light guide bundle of the universal cord, which is connected to the external light source.

The viewing portion of the FOB incorporates part of the handle (the eyepiece) and parts of the insertion cord (the image transmission bundle and objective lens). All FOBs are "frontal view" instruments; that is, the objective lens is perpendicular to the longitudinal axis of the instrument. Thus the image viewed through the lens is in the same orientation as the actual object. The FOB also has "fixed focus" at the distal tip.

Light reflected off the object is focused by the objective lens onto the distal end of the image transmission bundle. This image is then transmitted to the proximal end of the image transmission bundle near the eyepiece. The glass fibers in the image transmission bundle are placed so that each fiber is in the same relative location on both ends of the bundle to represent the true nature of the object (coherent bundle).

The suction channel extends from the handle of the fiberscope to the tip of the insertion cord and can be used to suction secretions, spray local anesthetics, pass various biopsy and brush instruments, or insufflate oxygen.

The bending of the distal section of the insertion cord is achieved by movement of the bending lever located at the handle. Two wires originating from the bending lever and ending at the tip of the fiberscope provide the mechanism for bending of the distal section of the insertion cord (Fig. 16-2). When the lever is moved

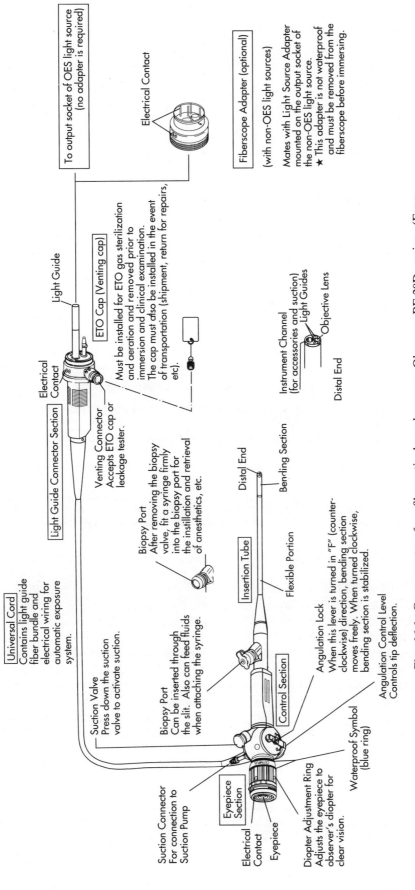

Fig. 16-1. Components of a fiberoptic bronchoscope. Olympus BF-20D series. (From Ovassapian A: *Fiberoptic airway endoscopy in anesthesia and critical care*, New York, 1990, Raven.)

To output socket of OES light source (no adapter is required)

Electrical Contact

Fiberscope Adapter (optional)

(with non-OES light sources)

Mates with Light Source Adapter mounted on the output socket of the non-OES light source.
★ This adapter is not waterproof and must be removed from the fiberscope before immersing.

Light Guide

Electrical Contact

Light Guide Connector Section

ETO Cap (Venting cap)

Must be installed for ETO gas sterilization and aeration and removed prior to immersion and clinical examination. The cap must also be installed in the event of transportation (shipment, return for repairs, etc).

Venting Connector Accepts ETO cap or leakage tester.

Biopsy Port
After removing the biopsy valve, fit a syringe firmly into the biopsy port for the instillation and retrieval of anesthetics, etc.

Instrument Channel (for accessories and suction)
Light Guides
Objective Lens

Distal End

Distal End

Bending Section

Insertion Tube

Flexible Portion

Universal Cord
Contains light guide fiber bundle and electrical wiring for automatic exposure system.

Suction Valve
Press down the suction valve to activate suction.

Biopsy Port
Can be inserted through the slit. Also can feed fluids when attaching the syringe.

Angulation Lock
When this lever is turned in "F" (counterclockwise) direction, bending section moves freely. When turned clockwise, bending section is stabilized.

Angulation Control Level
Controls tip deflection.

Control Section

Waterproof Symbol (blue ring)

Suction Connector
For connection to Suction Pump

Eyepiece Section

Electrical Contact

Eyepiece

Diopter Adjustment Ring
Adjusts the eyepiece to observer's diopter for clear vision.

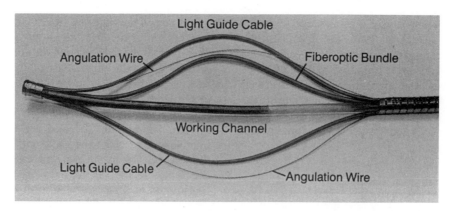

Fig. 16-2. Inside a fiberoptic bronchoscope insertion tube. Two angulation wires control the bending of the tip of the fiberoptic. Two light guide cables contain fiberoptic bundles (incoherent), which bring light to the tip of the fiberscope. The fiberoptic bundle contains the coherent bundle, which transmits images from the objective lens at the tip of the fiberscope to the eyepiece of the fiberscope. The working channel is used for suctioning of secretions, instillation of local anesthetics, and insufflation of oxygen. (From Ovassapian A: *Fiberoptic airway endoscopy in anesthesia and critical care,* New York, 1990, Raven.)

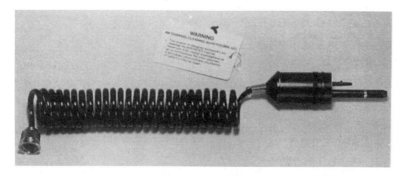

Fig. 16-3. Air leak tester. The cap is attached to the fiberscope venting connector. The adapter is attached to the light source. The air pumped by the light source pressurizes the fiberscope. Any air leak from the fiberscope indicates that the waterproof system is damaged and needs to be repaired before it can be soaked in solution (From Ovassapian A: *Fiberoptic airway endoscopy in anesthesia and critical care,* New York, 1990, Raven.)

downward, the wire that controls the anterior deflection of the tip is tightened and the tip of the fiberscope bends upward or anteriorly. When the lever is moved upward, the tip of the FOB bends downward or posteriorly. Substantial usage and improper handling, such as applying excessive pressure on the lever while the tip of FOB is inside the ET lumen, result in breakage of the delicate wire and loss of bending control.

The universal cord contains the light transmission fiber bundle and electrical wiring for the automatic photography system and ends in a light source connector. The light source connector contains the plug, air vent connector, and electrical contacts for photography. It is plugged into the light source before use of the FOB. The air vent connector is where the ethylene oxide (ETO) sterilization venting cap and leakage tester are placed (Fig. 16-3). When the ETO cap is attached, it provides venting of the FOB interior to equalize internal and external pressures. The ETO

cap must be installed when FOB is subjected to gas sterilization and aeration and during air freight transportation. The ETO cap must be removed before immersion of the FOB into water or disinfectant solution or when the FOB is in use.

The light source is an integral part of the fiberoptic endoscope system. Various light sources are available, which provide adequate illumination not only for viewing but also for taking photographs or videotapes. An intense light is generated and is focused on the proximal end of the light guide cable by a source lens or a spheric reflecting mirror. A heat filter or reflecting mirror is used to reduce the amount of heat focused on the light guide cable.

A. CLEANING AND DISINFECTING THE FIBERSCOPE

Universal precautions are now mandatory in every health-care institution to minimize the risk of transmission of infectious diseases. Cleaning and disinfecting the FOB following each use are a must for safe practice of bronchoscopy.[52,53]

After each use the FOB should be cleaned and disinfected to prevent damage to the FOB and to prevent transmission of disease from patient to patient. Specific recommendations for sterilization or disinfection made by the manufacturer and by each health-care facility should be followed. Most modern FOBs are constructed to withstand complete immersion in disinfectant solution.

The FOB should be washed immediately after each use, and the working channel should be flushed with water to remove secretions before they dry. The use of a cleaning brush may be needed for complete removal of secretions from the working channel. The brush should be inserted through the suction port at the handle downward toward the tip of insertion cord to avoid FOB damage. Retrograde insertion of a wire through the working channel is not recommended because it increases the risk of damage to the internal lining of the suction channel of the FOB. Before being soaked in disinfecting solution, the FOB should be inspected for defects that might allow liquids to penetrate inside the FOB. The rubber covering of the distal portion of the insertion cord should be carefully examined, since frequent use of the FOB may cause tears and defects in this covering. The FOB should be tested for leaks using a leakage tester and pressurized air while the FOB is immersed in water. If an air leak is detected, the instrument should promptly be sent to the manufacturer for appropriate repair.

After initial inspection the suction and biopsy port assembly should be removed and the FOB placed in disinfectant solution. With a syringe the working channel of the FOB should be filled with disinfecting solution. One such solution is 2% alkaline glutaraldehyde. Recommended immersion times after use in noninfected patients vary from 10 minutes for glutaraldehyde to 20 minutes for the iodine-containing solutions. Each solution is potentially caustic to the materials in the FOB; thus the manufacturers' recommendations for disinfectant concentration and maximum soaking time should be carefully observed. The FOB should be washed and the working channel suctioned with water to remove all traces of the disinfectant solution. Suctioning air for 10 to 15 seconds dries the inside of the suction channel.

If the patient has tuberculosis or another transmissible illness, the FOB should be sterilized. Sterilization of the bronchoscope is also critical before use in patients with immune deficiencies. Complete sterilization of the FOB can be accomplished with ETO gas. The ETO cap must be securely attached to the venting connector and must remain in place throughout the sterilization and aeration process. The gas sterilization procedure is

lengthy; it may take as long as 24 hours before the FOB is ready for use.

After cleaning, the FOB should be dried thoroughly and stored for subsequent use. The ideal container allows the insertion cord to remain straight. Carrying cases or small sterilization trays, in which the insertion cord is bent, are less desirable for storage, since the bending ultimately changes the shape and integrity of the insertion cord. The storage location must be clean, dry, well ventilated, and maintained at room temperature. Direct sunlight, high temperature, high humidity, and x-ray exposure may cause damage to the FOB.

III. FIBEROPTIC INTUBATION OF THE ADULT TRACHEA

The value of the FOB in difficult endotracheal intubation is well established.[22-40,44,54] However, the use of an FOB should not be limited to patients in whom endotracheal intubation may be difficult (Table 16-1). Many other patients who might be denied general anesthesia or might receive tracheostomy can be safely intubated with the help of the FOB.

Fiberoptic intubation is accomplished simply, quickly, and easily when certain preparatory steps are taken.

A. PREPARATION FOR FIBEROPTIC INTUBATION

Anesthesiologists must be prepared to manage any kind of airway at any time. The ability to rapidly transport fiberoptic equipment and supplies is critical for effective use of this instrument, especially when emergency conditions exist. Unexpected failed intubations in the operating room may also require the immediate availability of the FOB.

A mobile bronchoscopy cart should be readily available for the emergency situation previously described (Fig. 16-4). The cart should have large wheels for stability and easy transport and be equipped with FOBs, a light source, drugs for application of topical anesthesia, and various other airway supplies such as gauzes, tongue blades, intubating and nasal airways, cotton-tipped swabs, bronchoscopy swivel adapter, lubricant (K-Y jelly or silicone lubricant), and endoscopy masks, which may be needed for fiberoptic intubation. All equipment and supplies for administration of anesthesia, resuscitation, and monitoring should be available in the operating room and should be checked following a standard protocol. In the operating room the fiberoptic cart is placed at the left side of the endoscopist. The FOB is connected to the light source, the light is turned on, and the focus is adjusted by looking at written material until a clear view is obtained. The light is then turned off until the time of intubation. The insertion cord of the FOB and the ET (with cuff checked and cut to an appropriate length)

Table 16-1. Characteristics of fiberoptic bronchoscopes

Instrument	Insertion cord diameter (mm)	Insertion cord length (mm)	Working channel (mm)	Tip bending (degrees)	Field of view (degrees)
Olympus					
LF-2*	4.0	600	1.5	Up 130 Down 130	90
LF-P†	2.2	600	None	Up 120 Down 120	75
LF	1.8	550	None	None	75
BF-3C30	3.6	550	1.2	Up 180 Down 130	120
BF-P30	5.0	550	2.2	Up 180 Down 130	120
Pentax			1.2	Up 130 Down 130	90
FB-10X	3.5	600	1.2	Up 180 Down 130	95
FB-15X	4.9	600	2.2	Up 180 Down 130	100
VB-1530‡	5.5	600	1.2	Up 180 Down 130	120

*Intubation fiberscopes.
†Smallest with directable tip.
‡Video bronchoscope.

are placed in warm water. The necessary supplies are laid out on top of the fiberoptic cart, and the suction catheter is connected to the suction port. Routine preoperative preparation of the patient and routine monitoring are applied to all patients receiving airway endoscopy, whether the procedure is performed in the operating room suite, intensive care unit, or any other location. When everything is ready, anesthesia, intravenous sedation, or application of topical anesthesia is started based on the needs of the patient. Fiberoptic intubation starts as soon as patient preparation is completed.

1. Ancillary equipment

Various intubating airway devices—nasopharyngeal airways, endoscopy masks, and bronchoscopy swivel adapters—have been applied to facilitate fiberoptic ET intubation.[55-63]

a. INTUBATING AIRWAYS

i. Berman II intubating airway. This airway is disposable and is tubular along its entire length[61] (Fig. 16-5). It was originally designed for blind orotracheal intubation. It has also been used for fiberoptic intubation.[44] It has a longitudinal opening on its side, which can be opened wide to disengage it from the ET; then it can be removed from the patient's mouth. The airway is available in different sizes. Because of its length and tubular shape, the FOB cannot be maneuvered by bending its tip once it is placed through the airway.

Therefore, if the distal end of the airway is not in line with the glottic opening, exposure of the cords can be accomplished only by partial withdrawal of the airway.

ii. Ovassapian fiberoptic intubating airway. This airway is designed to provide an open air space in the oropharynx, to protect the FOB from being bitten by the patient, and to be removed from the mouth without disconnecting the ET adapter[57] (Fig. 16-6). This airway has a flat lingual surface on the proximal half, which minimizes its movement. The wide distal half of the airway curves to prevent the tongue and soft tissues of the anterior pharyngeal wall from falling back and obstructing the view of the glottis. This feature also maintains an open space for maneuvering the tip of the fiberscope. This airway accommodates an endotracheal tube up to 8.5 mm ID (inner diameter).

iii. Patil fiberoptic airway. This airway is available in only one size and is made of aluminum.[56] A groove at the middle portion of the distal part of the airway provides room for anterior-posterior maneuvering of the fiberscope. However, an ET will not pass through the airway, and it should be removed before advancement of the ET.

iv. Williams airway intubator. This airway was designed for blind orotracheal intubation, but its use in fiberoptic intubation has been described.[58] The proximal half is cylindric; the distal half has an open lingual surface. The airway is made in two sizes, 90 and 100 mm, which admit ETs up to 8 and 8.5 mm ID, respectively (Fig. 16-7). Because of its design, the tip of the FOB cannot be

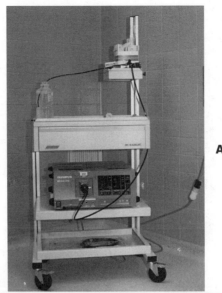

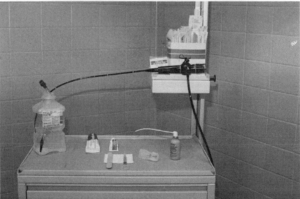

Fig. 16-4. A, A simple fiberoptic cart arrangement. Fiberoptic bronchoscope, after being cleaned and disinfected after each use, is stored on the top of cart covered with towels. All necessary supplies are in drawer. **B,** Close view of the top of the fiberoptic cart showing the equipment and drugs prepared for an awake intubation (warm water bottle with endotracheal tube and fiberoptic bronchoscope placed inside, lubricant, local anesthetic jelly, tongue blade, local anesthetic solution for transtracheal injection, intubating airway, and lidocaine spray).

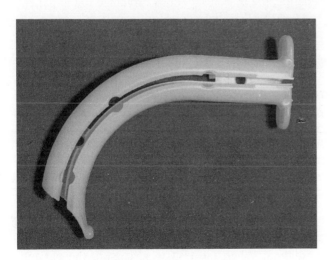

Fig. 16-5. Berman airway.

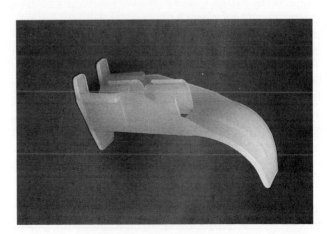

Fig. 16-6. Ovassapian airway.

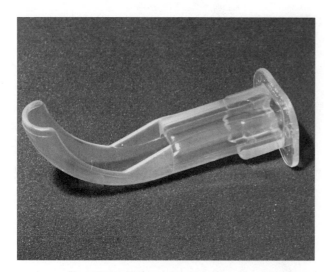

Fig. 16-7. Williams airway.

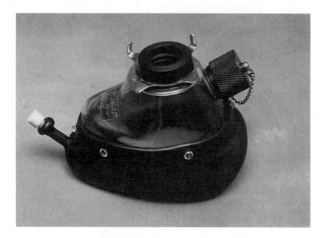

Fig. 16-8. Patil-Syracuse mask.

maneuvered in an anteroposterior or a lateral direction. If the distal end of the airway is not in line with the glottic opening, the exposure of the cords becomes difficult, necessitating partial withdrawal of the airway. The ET adapter should be removed before intubation to allow removal of the airway.

b. ENDOSCOPY MASK

A face mask with an endoscopy port to assist fiberoptic intubation in anesthetized patients was first described by Mallios[55] in 1980 and later by Patil et al.[56] (Fig. 16-8). Modification of oropharyngeal airways and pediatric anesthesia masks to facilitate pediatric fiberoptic intubation is also described.[62,63] The endoscopy mask permits passage of a FOB through the port into the oropharynx in an anesthetized patient being ventilated by face mask. Because a rubber diaphragm covers the port, an air leak is not developed and mask ventilation can be continued throughout the procedure.

More recently, a new mask adapter for fiberoptic intubation of the anesthetized patient has been re-

ported. This adapter consists of two parts: a rotating disk, which possesses a port, and the body of the adapter, which attaches to the face mask.[59]

B. FIBEROPTIC INTUBATION OF THE CONSCIOUS PATIENT

1. General considerations (psychologic and pharmacologic preparation)

When the airway is compromised and difficult intubation is expected, awake intubation with or without conscious sedation is indicated.[44,54] Awake intubation should also be considered in the following circumstances: for patients at high risk of gastric aspiration, for those who have an unstable cervical spine, for the morbidly obese, and for patients in ventilatory failure or who are otherwise seriously ill. Patients with tracheal stenosis or with extrinsic compression of the trachea associated with thoracic aortic aneurysm, substernal thyroid, or mediastinal mass may also benefit from awake intubation. The advantages of fiberoptic intubation for these patients are the maintenance of spontaneous ventilation and the ability to precisely position the tip of the ET beyond the compression site. Fiberoptic intubation is easiest in the awake patient because the tongue does not fall back in the pharynx, and spontaneous ventilation tends to keep the airway open. In addition, by deep breathing the patient can assist the operator in locating the glottis when the airway anatomy is distorted.

Four factors are critical for successful execution of an awake fiberoptic tracheal intubation. These are proper psychologic preparation of the patient, proper pharmacologic preparation of the patient, an expert endoscopist, and a properly functioning FOB (Box 16-2).

Psychologic preparation starts with an informative, reassuring preoperative visit to the patient. A detailed explanation of the technique is provided, and questions are answered. If intubation is to be performed with no sedation, the reason should be explained to the patient, emphasizing that this is done for the patient's safety. The patient's active participation in the process of intubation is asked for. The patient is informed of what he or she can do to assist in a smooth intubation, for example, maintaining the head position, taking deep breaths, or swallowing secretions when requested. A well-informed patient who knows that the technique is chosen to maximize his or her safety appreciates the efforts and helps the physician in the process of intubation. When minimal or no sedation is used, the patient should also be informed that recall of the procedure is expected to minimize psychologic impact for future anesthetics. If the patient's condition permits providing conscious sedation, then the patient should be further assured that it is most likely he or she will not remember the intubation. When the visit is successful, the patient's apprehension is relieved and therefore the need for

---

BOX 16-2   Steps for successful awake intubation

I. Psychologic preparation: informative, reassuring preoperative visit
II. Pharmacologic preparation
   A. Premedication
      1. Light or no sedation for calm patients
      2. Heavy sedation for anxious patients
      3. Narcotics when pain is present
      4. Specific drugs for habitual drug users
      5. Antisialagogue unless contraindicated
   B. Intravenous sedation
      1. No sedation for patients with severely compromised airway
      2. Conscious sedation for most patients
      3. Heavy sedation for uncooperative patients
   C. Topical anesthesia
      1. Oral intubation: oropharynx, laryngotracheal
      2. Nasal intubation: nasal mucosa, laryngotracheal
III. Expert endoscopist
IV. Good, functional fiberoptic bronchoscope

---

sedation is lessened and the patient's cooperation is maximized.

Pharmacologic preparation consists of premedication, conscious sedation at the time of intubation, and application of topical anesthesia. The goal of premedication is twofold. One goal is to provide sedation that will complement the psychologic preparation of the patient. The second is to provide an antisialagogue to reduce secretions. Benzodiazepines are the most commonly prescribed drugs for premedication and sedation. Diazepam (Valium) 5 to 10 mg by mouth or intramuscular (IM) midazolam 1 to 3 mg provide adequate sedation in most patients. Opioids should be considered if the patient is in pain or is a habitual user.

An antisialagogue agent is used to reduce secretions. This is essential for establishing good topical anesthesia.[44,54,64] Glycopyrrolate and atropine are given in doses of 0.2 to 0.4 mg and 0.4 to 0.6 mg IM, respectively. Because glycopyrrolate does not cross the blood-brain barrier and causes less tachycardia, it is considered the anticholinergic agent of choice.

The next phase of pharmacologic preparation is conscious sedation administered intravenously in immediate preparation for intubation. Conscious sedation is desirable to minimize awareness of the procedure and to increase patient acceptance, provided that safety is not compromised. The main goal of conscious sedation is to have an awake, calm, and cooperative patient who can follow verbal commands and maintain adequate oxygenation and ventilation.

Depending on the patient's condition and the indication for awake intubation, an opioid, a sedative, or a combination is used. Opioids produce profound analgesia, are strong depressants of the airway reflexes, and facilitate airway instrumentation while the patient is still capable of following verbal commands. However, patients become more susceptible to aspiration of gastric contents if regurgitation or vomiting does occur. Airway protective reflexes remain more active when a sedative such as diazepam or midazolam is used, but the patient may be less cooperative and react more vigorously to instrumentation of the airway. A combination of fentanyl and midazolam (1.5 µg/kg and 30 µg/kg, respectively) has been used successfully for conscious sedation.

The last phase of pharmacologic preparation is application of topical anesthesia. Instrumentation of the airway without adequate topical anesthesia is uncomfortable and distressing to a conscious patient. Awake airway instrumentation must be made painless and nonstressful, especially in those who may need repeated operations. Good topical anesthesia of the respiratory tract mucous membranes eliminates pharyngeal, laryngeal, and tracheobronchial reflexes. Judicious use of topical anesthetics requires a sound knowledge of their pharmacology and technical skills in its application. Reduction of secretions to provide a dry mucosa is essential to good topical anesthesia. Excess secretions dilute the local anesthetic solution, create a barrier between agent and mucosa, and carry the local anesthetic away from the sight of action.[44,64]

The principles and guidelines for the safe use of topical anesthetics have been summarized by Adriani et al.[65] It is essential to know the optimum effective concentration of each drug, the rapidity of onset of action, the recommended maximum safe dose, and the appropriate techniques for application. The onset time shortens and the duration of anesthesia lengthens as the concentration of drug is increased. However, the maximum effective concentration is not necessarily either safe or recommended. For example, cocaine is maximally effective at 20% concentration, far in excess of the 4% to 10% recommended for clinical use. Combining two local anesthetics at their maximum effective concentrations neither improves nor prolongs the duration of topical anesthesia. However, systemic effects of the two drugs are additive and increase the possibility of systemic toxicity.[66] In a mixture of short- and long-acting drugs, the duration of anesthesia will be that of the longer-acting drug. Benzocaine, with its rapid onset, and tetracaine, with its prolonged action, complement each other.

The rate and amount of topical anesthetic absorbed varies according to the site of application, the dose of the drug, and general condition of the patient.[67-70] Absorption is more rapid from alveoli than from the tracheobronchial tree and more rapid from the tracheobronchial tree than from the pharynx. Vasoconstrictor added to solutions of topical anesthetics neither slows the absorption nor prolongs the duration of topical anesthesia.[65] Plasma levels rise more rapidly after topical application to the respiratory tract than after injection into tissue; therefore recommended doses of topical anesthetics for use within the respiratory tract are approximately half of the doses of the same drug injected into tissue.

The techniques of topical anesthesia application differ for the oral versus the nasal approach and are discussed in the following sections.

2. Orotracheal intubation

With proper preparation and technique a successful orotracheal intubation can be accomplished in almost all patients. In addition to the preparation described earlier, monitoring of blood pressure, electrocardiogram, and oximetry is required. Also, oxygen is provided by nasal cannula at a flow rate of 3 L/min to all patients undergoing awake intubation.

a. TOPICAL ANESTHESIA

Application of topical anesthesia should begin after sedation to minimize patient discomfort.

For the oropharynx, application of a 4% solution or a 10% aerosol preparation of lidocaine spray provides excellent topical anesthesia by abolishing pain sensation and obtunding gag and swallowing reflexes.

For topical anesthesia of the larynx and trachea, 4% lidocaine can be injected translaryngeally or sprayed through the FOB. Translaryngeal injection using a 20-gauge catheter or a 22-gauge needle provides good topical anesthesia of the trachea and larynx. Most patients cough, often for period of 8 to 20 seconds. The main advantage of this technique is that the topical anesthesia is established prior to endoscopy. This feature prevents severe cough and laryngeal spasm that is seen by premature advancement of the FOB when the airway is not anesthetized. In addition, it provides better, more solid topical anesthesia than "spray as you go" technique.[71] Sixty to 90 seconds after translaryngeal injection a local anesthetic jelly, lidocaine 5% or benzocaine 20% (Americaine) is applied to the base of the tongue and to the anterior tonsillar pillars with a tongue blade. This maneuver checks the adequacy of the oropharyngeal topical anesthesia by the lidocaine spray and supplements the block if it is not adequate.

The spray of local anesthetic through the FOB "spray as you go" method is the simplest, preferred way of anesthetizing bronchial mucosa.

The "spray as you go" method involves spraying topical anesthetic through the suction channel of an advancing FOB.[71] The epiglottis and vocal cords are visualized through the FOB and sprayed directly. After 30 to 45 seconds the FOB is advanced into the trachea,

the anterior wall is sprayed, and as the FOB is advanced toward the carina, incremental doses are sprayed on the walls of the tracheobronchial tree. The size of the FOB channel is important with this technique. A small suction channel (0.5 to 1.0 mm) enables the operator to use 0.2 ml of solution at a time and produces a fine stream that reaches the targeted area. Most adult FOBs have larger suction channels (2 to 2.5 mm) that are essential for suctioning, brushing, and using biopsy forceps. With this larger channel, spray of small volumes of local anesthetic becomes difficult, and spread of the solution is less uniform. This problem can be overcome by passing an epidural catheter (internal diameter, 0.5 to 1 mm cut to the length of the insertion cord), through the suction channel and using it for spraying the local anesthetic.[44] Placing a three-way stopcock at the hub of the epidural catheter allows suctioning and spraying intermittently without losing the anesthetic solution during suctioning. The three-way stopcock is closed during suctioning and open during spraying. The "spray as you go" technique provides flexibility for the operator to anesthetize part or all of the respiratory passages. It is ideal for most awake tracheal intubations, especially in patients at high risk of aspirating gastric contents, since the topical anesthetic is applied only *after* the vocal cords are exposed and intubation is achieved without the lower airway being anesthetized.

Anesthesia of the airway may be supplemented with bilateral superior laryngeal and lingual nerve blocks.[54,64] The sensory innervation of the larynx above the level of the vocal cords is supplied by the superior laryngeal nerve. This branch of the vagus nerve is easily blocked bilaterally by injecting 2 to 3 ml of 1% lidocaine by an anterior neck approach. The lingual branch of the glossopharyngeal nerve carries the sensory innervation of the pharynx, tonsils, and posterior third of the tongue. The block of lingual nerve bilaterally depresses the gag reflex during tracheal intubation in the conscious patient. In a small number of patients, if topically applied local anesthetic is not satisfactory, injection of local anesthetic (2 ml of 1% lidocaine on each side) at the palatolingual arch (anterior tonsillar pillar) blocks the lingual branch of the glossopharyngeal nerve.

b. PROCEDURE

After topical anesthesia has been established, the patient head is put into a neutral position for intubation, an airway intubator is placed in the mouth, the oropharynx is suctioned, and the lubricated endotracheal tube is placed 4 to 5 cm inside the intubating airway. The fourth and fifth fingers of the right hand hold the endotracheal tube to prevent premature advancement of the tube, while the index finger and thumb advance the FOB through the ET (Fig. 16-9). As the FOB is advanced toward the oropharynx, the white pharyngeal surface of the airway, soft palate, and uvula will come into view

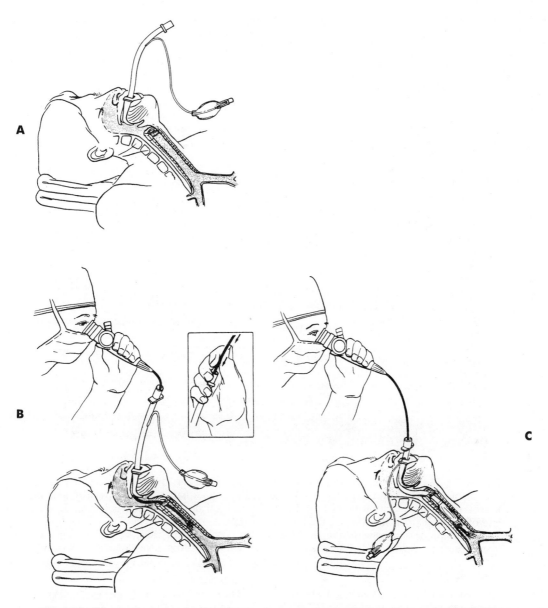

Fig. 16-9. Fiberoptic orotracheal intubation in a conscious patient. **A,** Ovassapian intubating airway and endotracheal tube position. **B,** The bronchoscope is advanced through endotracheal tube into midtrachea. Insert illustrates position of hand for holding tracheal tube and advancing the bronchoscope. **C,** The tube is advanced over the bronchoscope into the trachea (From Ovassapian A: *Fiberoptic airway endoscopy in anesthesia and critical care,* New York, 1990, Raven.)

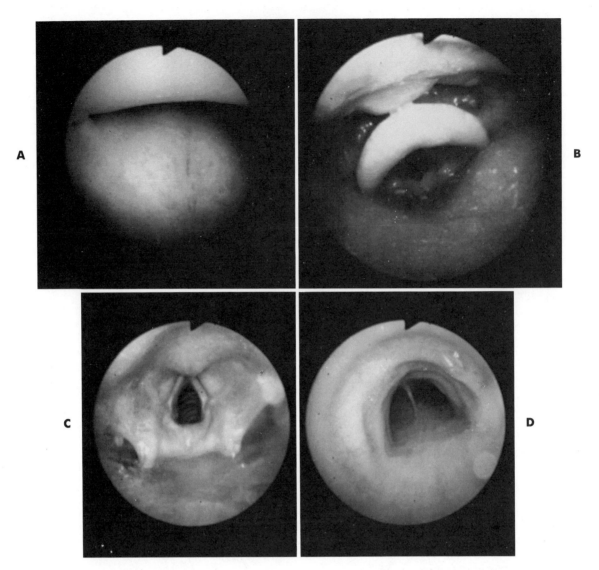

Fig. 16-10. Bronchoscopic views during fiberoptic orotracheal intubation. **A,** Pharyngeal surface of the Ovassapian airway is seen in white in the upper half of the picture. Soft palate is seen in the lower half of the picture. **B,** The tip of bronchoscope is in oropharynx. Distal end of Ovassapian airway covering the base of the tongue. Epiglottis is in view. **C,** The tip of bronchoscope passed beneath the tip of epiglottis. Glottis is in view. **D,** The tip of the bronchoscope in lower third of the trachea. Carina is in view. (From Ovassapian A: *Fiberoptic airway endoscopy in anesthesia and critical care,* New York, 1990, Raven.)

(Fig. 16-10). With farther advancement of the FOB its tip is deflected anteriorly to expose the epiglottis and vocal cords. In the presence of a large, floppy epiglottis the tip of the FOB should be manipulated underneath the tip of the epiglottis to visualize the vocal cords. Extending the head at the atlantooccipital joint and keeping the mouth closed keeps the epiglottis away from posterior pharyngeal wall. On rare occasions, during an awake intubation a jaw thrust or pulling the tongue forward may be necessary to facilitate glottic exposure. After the vocal cords are exposed they are maintained in the center of the field of view by fine rotation of the body of the FOB and manipulations of the tip control lever while the FOB is being advanced. Without such maneuvering the tip of the FOB often ends up in the anterior commissure or against the anterior laryngeal wall. Pulling the FOB back and flexing the tip of the FOB posteriorly brings the laryngeal and tracheal lumen into view. The FOB is then advanced into the midtrachea, and the ET is slipped over the firmly held stationary FOB into the trachea. The FOB is kept stationary to ensure that it is not advanced farther down into the tracheobronchial tree during advancement of the endotracheal tube. The tip of the ET is positioned 3 to 4 cm above the carina.

The oral approach can be somewhat more difficult

than the nasal approach because of the sharp curve leading from the oral cavity into the larynx. In many patients, even though the FOB has entered the trachea, the ET impinges on the epiglottis or on the vocal cords or it lodges in the pyriform sinus and cannot be advanced into the trachea.[44,72] When this happens, the ET is pulled back over the FOB, rotated 45 to 90 degrees, and readvanced during deep inspiration. In some patients this maneuver may have to be repeated two to three times, particularly when a small-size FOB is used for placement of a large-size ET. The larger a gap is between the FOB and ET, the more chance there is that the tube may not have slipped into the trachea.[44] In two patients, when repeated attempts at advancing an 8.5-mm ID tube over a 4-mm FOB failed, the tube was easily advanced when the small FOB was changed to a 6-mm FOB. A more pliable tube decreases this incidence. The main reason for placing the ET in warm water is to make the tube more pliable, thereby increasing its successful passage into the trachea.[44] In a recent publication it was demonstrated that the passage of a spiral-wound (anode) ET is less likely to be impeded by glottic structures.[72] In 19 of 20 patients the anode tube entered the trachea on the first attempt, compared with 7 of 20 successful first attempts with the standard endotracheal tube. When 7 of 20 standard tubes did not enter into the trachea after the third attempt, changing the tube to an anode tube allowed successful passage of the tube in all 7 cases. The authors suggested that these points should be considered in the management of the difficult airway. Laryngospasm resulting from poor topical anesthesia may also prevent ET advancement. In this circumstance, additional topical anesthesia applied through the FOB improves conditions for intubation.

3. Nasotracheal intubation

Fiberoptic nasotracheal intubation is often easier than the oral approach because the FOB is usually pointed straight at the glottis as it enters the oropharynx, there is no sharp turn to negotiate, and the vocal cords are usually visible from a distance.[38,44] For nasotracheal intubation in conscious patients, either the ET is placed in the nostril first and the FOB is passed through it or the ET is mounted over the FOB, which is then passed through the nostril. Placing the tube first avoids the possibility of nasal secretions covering the objective lens and obscuring the view, and a tight nasal passage can be recognized when the FOB is being advanced. Once the FOB has been passed through the ET into the trachea, advancement of the tube over the FOB is easily accomplished. The disadvantages are a higher possibility of causing nasal bleeding and that, in some patients, the tube may not make the bend to enter the oropharynx. The main disadvantage of passing the FOB first is that the adequacy of the nasal passage cannot be judged and insertion of a 4- or 5-mm OD (outside diameter) FOB through the nose does not guarantee the subsequent passage of a 7- or 8-mm ID ET. In the case of a tight nasal passage, if the tube is advanced over the FOB by force, removal of the FOB may be impossible, necessitating removal of the tube and fiberscope together.

a. TOPICAL ANESTHESIA

To anesthetize the mucous membrane of the nose, select the most patent nostril and fill it with 2% lidocaine gel. Then cotton-tipped applicators soaked in 4% to 5% cocaine or a mixture of 3% lidocaine with 0.25% phenylephrine (Neo-Synephrine) (3 ml 4% lidocaine plus 1 ml 1% phenylephrine) can be placed in the nose with minimal patient reaction. These agents provide topical anesthesia and shrinkage of the nasal mucosa. Allow 4 minutes for maximal anesthetic and vasoconstrictive effect. Two ml of agent is adequate for anesthetizing one nostril. Using cotton-tipped applicators is also helpful in evaluating the patency of nasal passages and in predicting the angle for endotracheal tube insertion.

Laryngotracheal anesthesia is achieved by translaryngeal injection as described or by spraying through the fiberscope during the process of intubation. There is no need for application of topical anesthesia to the oropharynx, since the gag reflex is not stimulated by the nasal route.[38,44]

b. PROCEDURE

The softened endotracheal tube is lubricated generously and is introduced gently through the anesthetized nostril until it just enters the posterior oropharynx. If it does not make the bend, it is pulled back, rotated 90 degrees to the right or left, and reintroduced. If this maneuver is unsuccessful, the FOB is used to direct the ET into the oropharynx. After the tube is placed in the oropharynx, the secretions are suctioned through the ET and the lubricated FOB is advanced through it into the oropharynx (Fig. 16-11). In 80% to 85% of patients the epiglottis and vocal cords are seen with minimal or no manipulation of the tip of the FOB.[38] In heavily sedated patients or in elderly, edentulous patients the tongue and pharyngeal tissue may fall back and block the exposure of the larynx and vocal cords. Extending the head, applying jaw thrust, or pulling the tongue forward helps in visualizing the vocal cords. The FOB is advanced into the midtrachea, followed by the ET. With nasotracheal intubation the incidence of the ET meeting resistance and not entering the trachea is low.

C. FIBEROPTIC INTUBATION IN THE ANESTHETIZED PATIENT

Fiberoptic intubation with the patient under general anesthesia is accomplished with the patient either breathing spontaneously or paralyzed and receiving controlled ventilation. The main disadvantages of intu-

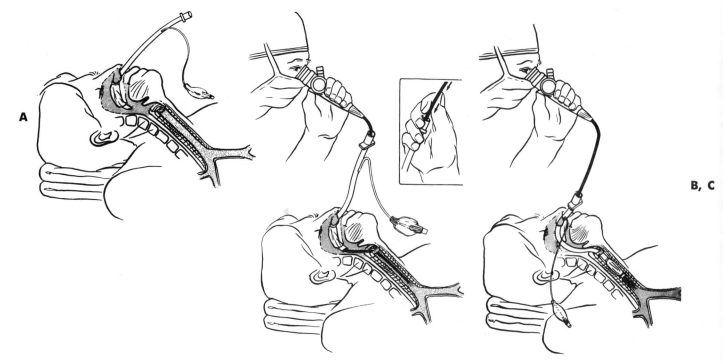

Fig. 16-11. Fiberoptic nasotracheal intubation in conscious patient. **A,** The position of the tip of the nasotracheal tube making the bend into oropharynx. **B,** The fiberscope advanced through the nasotracheal tube into the midtrachea. Insert illustrates position of hand for holding tracheal tube and advancing the fiberscope. **C,** The tracheal tube threaded over the fiberscope into the trachea. (From Ovassapian A: *Fiberoptic airway endoscopy in anesthesia and critical care,* New York, 1990, Raven.)

bation under general anesthesia is that the tongue and pharyngeal tissues lose their tonicity and close down the pharyngeal space, blocking visualization of the larynx. To minimize apnea time and to facilitate laryngeal exposure, an assistant is needed. The assistant is directed to do the following tasks: first, to mount the endotracheal tube on the lubricated FOB and have it ready to hand to the anesthesiologist as soon as the anesthesia mask is removed; second, to apply jaw thrust to maintain an open oropharynx; and, third, to observe the apnea time and monitor the patient. The endoscopy cart is placed at the head of the table on the left side of the patient while the assistant stands on the patient's left side facing the anesthesiologist.

1. Orotracheal intubation

After general anesthesia and muscle relaxation are established, the anesthesia mask is removed, the intubating airway is placed inside the mouth, and the oropharynx is suctioned. Ventilation is resumed by mask and continued for 30 to 60 seconds. The assistant at this time has the FOB ready, with the endotracheal tube mounted on its insertion cord. The anesthesia mask is removed, and the anesthesiologist grasps the body of the FOB with the left hand and the tip of the insertion cord with the right hand. The tip of the insertion cord is placed inside the intubating airway and advanced into the oropharynx. The assistant applies a jaw thrust after handing the FOB to the endoscopist. This maneuver is vital and constitutes the most important step in fiberoptic intubation under general anesthesia.

If an intubating airway is not available, the assistant may pull the patient's tongue forward away from the palate and posterior pharyngeal wall. This maneuver also moves the epiglottis away from the posterior pharyngeal wall, thus assisting exposure of the vocal cords. The assistant may also use both hands to apply jaw thrust, while simultaneously opening the mouth by downward pressure on the chin.[44] Forceful stretch of the tongue over the lower teeth may cause trauma and laceration of the tongue. Lung forceps and mouth gag with tongue holder have been applied to keep the tongue forward.[22,73] Without the intubating airway it is more likely that the FOB will move from the midline position and make exposure of the vocal cords somewhat more difficult.[22] After placement of the FOB in the midtrachea the endotracheal tube is advanced with a rotating motion into the trachea; the tip of the tube is placed 3 cm above the carina. If the endotracheal tube faces resistance and does not enter the trachea, it is pulled back, rotated 90 degrees or more to the right or left, and then advanced while the assistant continues to apply jaw thrust. The FOB is then removed, and the breathing system is attached to the ET. In case of a prolonged intubation time the position of the ET should be checked only after ventilation has been resumed.

2. Nasotracheal intubation

The general preparation for and the technique of intubation are as described for orotracheal intubation, and the assistant performs the same duties. An oropharyngeal airway or an intubating airway is used to retract the tongue from the posterior pharyngeal wall. Application of a vasoconstrictor to the nostril prior to intubation either before or after induction of anesthesia is recommended to minimize the incidence of bleeding. The lubricated ET is mounted on the insertion cord of the FOB, and as soon as the anesthesia mask is removed the operator grasps the FOB as described earlier and inserts its tip into the selected nostril; while looking through the FOB, the operator advances it toward the larynx and trachea. The assistant applies jaw thrust to keep the oropharyngeal space open. After the FOB is placed in the midtrachea, the endotracheal tube is threaded over the FOB into the trachea.

3. Rapid-sequence induction and intubation

The combination of a difficult intubation and full stomach in patients receiving emergency operation presents a special problem. If the patient is uncooperative, is intoxicated, or is a child, awake intubation to secure the airway before induction of general anesthesia may not be a viable option. Under these conditions general anesthesia using rapid-sequence induction and intubation technique is commonly used. Compression of cricoid cartilage to block passive regurgitation of gastric contents into the oropharynx is applied with this induction technique. Failure of endotracheal intubation with rigid laryngoscopy during a rapid-sequence induction leaves the patient's airway vulnerable to aspiration. Fiberoptic intubation while cricoid pressure is maintained is a possibility that should seriously be considered. Advanced experience and confidence in the use of FOB are necessary for successful use of FOB under these circumstances.[74]

The ability to perform rapid fiberoptic intubation in patients at high risk for aspiration may play an important role in diminishing major airway-related catastrophes. Repeated attempts at blind nasal or rigid laryngoscopy for endotracheal intubation traumatize the airway and may change a manageable airway into an unmanageable one. The application of a rapid fiberoptic intubation, before unduly traumatizing the airway, is a lifesaving measure.

Fiberoptic rapid induction and intubation may be applied from the beginning if the patient has history of difficult intubation but mask ventilation is known to be

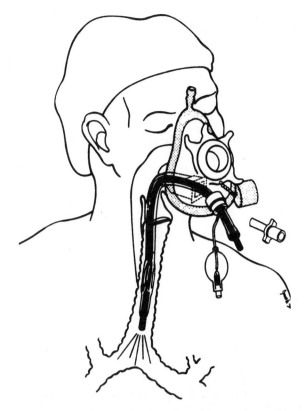

Fig. 16-12. Intubation through endoscopy mask. Schematic diagram showing fiberoptic orotracheal intubation through endoscopy mask in an anesthetized and paralyzed patient. The fiberoptic bronchoscope and endotracheal tube have been introduced through the diaphragm in the endoscopy mask. After intubation, the fiberoptic bronchoscope is removed from within the endotracheal tube and the endoscopy mask is removed over the endotracheal tube. Endotracheal tube adapter is replaced and connected to anesthesia machine breathing system (From Rogers SN, Benumof JL: *Anesthesiology* 59:569, 1983.)

easy in the patient. One assistant applies cricoid pressure, and one passes the FOB to the anesthesiologist and applies jaw thrust.

4. Intubation aided by an endoscopy mask

The technique of combining an intubating airway and anesthesia mask with endoscopy port for fiberoptic orotracheal intubation has been described.[25,43,55] To apply this technique, an assistant who is capable of administering anesthesia and maintaining mask ventilation is essential. Anesthesia is induced and maintained with an endoscopy mask. An intubating airway is placed inside the mouth, the oropharynx is suctioned, and mask ventilation is resumed. The FOB, with the ET (without its adapter) mounted on it, is advanced through the rubber diaphragm of the endoscopy port into the intubating airway and through the vocal cords into the trachea[25] (Fig. 16-12). The ET is threaded over the FOB through the endoscopy port and intubating airway into the trachea. After the FOB is removed, the endoscopy mask is disengaged from the ET and removed. The ET adapter is now replaced and connected to the anesthesia circuit. Caution should be exercised to avoid accidental injury of face or eyes during placement of the endotracheal tube adapter, which must be pushed into the ET securely. The use of an intubating airway is mandatory with this technique.

It is possible to use the endoscopy mask for nasotracheal intubation. However, the length of an uncut endotracheal tube threaded over the FOB may prevent placement of the tip of the FOB in the midtrachea without advancing the ET through the diaphragm of the endoscopy port. As soon as the ET is passed through the diaphragm, it opens the system and positive pressure ventilation cannot be continued. A bronchoscope with an insertion cord length of 60 cm, such as the Olympus LF-2, reaches the midtrachea before the nasotracheal tube reaches the endoscopy port, avoiding the problem mentioned earlier.

5. Modified endoscopy mask technique

Advancing the ET over the FOB, then through the endoscopy port and intubating airway into the trachea is hard on the instrument and may cause instrument damage. In addition, during nasotracheal intubation before the tip of the FOB has reached the midtrachea the ET may often pass through the diaphragm of the endoscopy port, which violates the closed anesthesia circuit system, interfering with assisted or controlled mask ventilation. To avoid both of these shortcomings, a modified technique has been applied.

The ET is prepared with its adapter loosely attached to the tube for later easy disconnection.[44] A bronchoscopy swivel adapter is mounted on the ET adapter. The 15-mm side arm of the swivel adapter is blocked with tape. The prepared ET is lubricated and is passed through the diaphragm of the endoscopy mask port by about 10 cm (Fig. 16-13). Additional lubrication is applied to the distal end of the ET after it has passed through the diaphragm. Anesthesia is induced using a regular anesthesia mask. After achieving surgical depth of anesthesia and complete relaxation, the anesthesia mask is removed, an intubating airway is placed, and the oropharynx is suctioned. The endoscopy mask mounted with the ET is now placed over the face with the distal 2 inches of the ET entering inside the airway. The anesthesia is continued with the new mask in place. With this technique, while the ET is positioned inside the airway the anesthesia breathing system remains closed. The FOB is now advanced through the bronchoscopic port of the swivel adapter, through the ET into the oropharyngeal airway intubator and into the trachea. The ET is advanced over the FOB into the trachea. The FOB and two adapters are removed together, leaving the

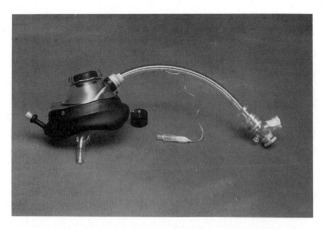

Fig. 16-13. Modified endoscopy mask technique of fiberoptic intubation. Endoscopy mask mounted with endotracheal tube with loosely attached tracheal tube and bronchoscopy swivel adapters. (From Ovassapian A: *Fiberoptic airway endoscopy in anesthesia and critical care,* New York, 1990, Raven.)

ET in place. The endoscopy mask is then disengaged from the ET and removed. The ET adapter is reattached to the ET, completing the intubation process.

For nasotracheal intubation, the ET with loosely attached adapters is mounted over the FOB before intubation. The breathing circuit remains closed when the ET passes through the endoscopy port.

6. Intubation using the nasal airway

In the anesthetized, spontaneously breathing patient anesthesia may be maintained through a nasopharyngeal airway to allow time for unhurried tracheal intubation. For orotracheal intubation a binasal airway is placed in the nostrils and connected to the anesthesia breathing system. An intubating airway is placed, and the FOB mounted with the ET is inserted through the airway to perform the intubation.[43] For nasotracheal intubation a nasopharyngeal airway mounted with an ET adapter is inserted in one nostril.[75,76] The breathing circuit of the anesthesia machine is attached to the nasopharyngeal airway. The fiberscope mounted with the ET is passed through the other nostril to perform tracheal intubation.

With both the oral and the nasal approach, because the patient is breathing spontaneously and the level of anesthesia is maintained, plenty of time is provided for intubation. The FOB provides the option of spraying local anesthetic to the larynx to minimize laryngeal reaction and spasm. This may become necessary when the depth of anesthesia is inadequate for airway manipulation.

7. Combining fiberoptic with other intubation techniques

The FOB can be used in combination with other intubation techniques to overcome many difficult and seemingly impossible airways. The FOB can be used in combination with a rigid laryngoscope, laryngeal mask airway, or a Combitube. It can be used to improve the technique of a retrograde wire intubation or of a blind nasal intubation. The principles of light wand intubation can be applied with an FOB.

a. FIBEROPTIC INTUBATION AIDED BY RIGID LARYNGOSCOPY

In patients with an oropharyngeal mass, upper airway edema, or a posteriorly displaced epiglottis (because of a supraglottic mass or because the epiglottis is large and floppy) the passage of an FOB beneath the epiglottis to expose the glottic opening may be extremely difficult. Combining rigid laryngoscopy with fiberoptic intubation is helpful under these circumstances.[44,77-79]

The epiglottis is exposed using a rigid laryngoscope by a second anesthesiologist. By looking directly inside the mouth (not through the FOB), the first anesthesiologist passes the tip of the FOB under the epiglottis.[44] The tip of the fiberscope can also be guided toward the glottis by the anesthesiologist who performs the rigid laryngoscopy while the first one is looking through the fiberscope.[77,78] If successful, this allows easy exposure of the vocal cords and advancement of the FOB into the trachea to complete the intubation.

The combined use of rigid and fiberoptic laryngoscopes is also useful in changing an existing endotracheal tube in a patient with a history of difficult intubation. Excessive pharyngeal soft tissue, edema of the airway, and a large volume of secretions are common in these patients and interfere with fiberoptic visualization of the larynx. Rigid laryngoscopy helps in exposing the supraglottic area and allows complete suctioning of secretions. In addition, a curved blade lifts the epiglottis, which may be embracing the endotracheal tube, and allows passage of the FOB beneath the epiglottis. This is crucial for exposure of the anterior commissure and passage of the FOB into the trachea alongside an existing tube.[44]

b. FIBEROPTIC INTUBATION THROUGH THE LARYNGEAL MASK AIRWAY

The laryngeal mask airway (LMA) is gaining popularity as a routine airway management tool for the administration of general anesthesia.[80,81] Its ease and speed of insertion without the use of rigid laryngoscopy or muscle relaxants has prompted the anesthesiologist to use the laryngeal mask for management of the difficult airway and failed intubation.[81-92] A number of case reports attest to the value of the LMA in failed intubation and in restoring artificial ventilation when it otherwise could not be achieved by bag and face mask.[82-84] Endotracheal intubation through the LMA has been successfully carried out in awake and anesthetized patients, using blind or fiberoptic-aided techniques.[85-92]

The LMA is placed, and breathing through the LMA is confirmed. An appropriate-size ET (cuffed, 6 mm ID for sizes 3 and 4 LMAs) is passed blindly through the LMA shaft into the trachea.[85] Instead of an ET, a bougie or tube changer could be passed blindly through the LMA into the trachea and then could be used as a guide for tracheal intubation after the LMA is removed.[86-88]

To avoid blind passage of the tube or bougie into the trachea and improve the success rate of intubation through the LMA, the FOB has been used (Fig. 16-14). A well-lubricated 4-mm FOB loaded with 6.5-mm ID tube is advanced through a size 4 LMA.[89] A 6.5-mm ID ET passes through the shaft of a size 4 LMA, but it is tight and requires some manipulation to pass it through. The larynx is exposed, and the FOB is advanced into the trachea. The ET is threaded over the FOB into the trachea, and the cuff of the ET is inflated. The FOB is removed, and ventilation is carried out through the endotracheal tube. At the conclusion of anesthesia the ET is removed first, allowing the patient to breath through the LMA until protective airway reflexes return. Then the LMA can be removed.

The shortcoming of the LMA is the limitation imposed on the size of the ET that can be placed. A 6-mm ET is inadequate for prolonged general endotracheal anesthesia and mechanical ventilation. Another potential problem is the length of the 6-mm ET and the possibility of intralaryngeal placement of the tube cuff. The 6-mm cuffed ET is 28 cm in length. The length of a size 4 LMA is 19 cm, and the distance from the LMA grille to the vocal cords is 3.5 cm. This allows only 5 cm of the ET to go beyond the vocal cords.[93] As a result, the cuff of the ET may be inflated in the larynx rather than the trachea and this may cause recurrent laryngeal nerve palsy. Removing the adapter of the LMA before intubation shortens the length of the LMA by 18 mm, which leads to deeper placement of the ET inside the trachea and, it is hoped, prevents this problem.

If a larger ET is desired, the 6-mm tube may be changed to a larger-size tube with the help of a tube changer or the FOB.

Hasham et al.[91] used the FOB to place a guide tube into the trachea through the LMA. An 8.5-mm ET was then railroaded over the guide tube into the trachea.

In an attempt to overcome the limitation of the 6.5-mm tube for LMA tracheal intubation a longitudinally split, size 3 LMA has been recommended. Through this LMA a larger-size ET can be advanced into the trachea over the fiberscope.[92] The cuff of the split LMA is sealed with silicone, and the LMA shaft bound with micropore tape. The split, taped LMA is inserted, and its cuff fully inflated. The FOB mounted with the ET is passed through the LMA into the trachea. The LMA is then deflated. The tape is removed from the LMA, and the ET threaded over the FOB through the LMA into the trachea.

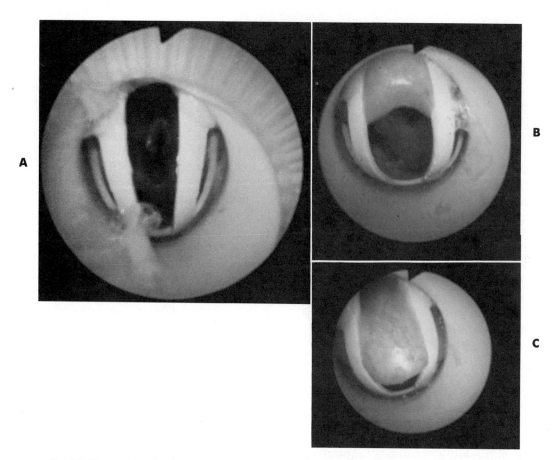

Fig. 16-14. Endoscopic view through laryngeal mask airway (LMA). The fiberoptic broncho-scope is placed inside the LMA with the tip 2 cm away from the inside bars of the LMA. **A,** Perfect positioning of LMA. The epiglottis is out of view. Blind intubation through LMA is highly likely but still may fail, depending on the position of the tip of the tube in relations to glottic anatomy. Fiberoptic intubation would be successful. **B,** The tip of epiglottis blocking half of the LMA distal opening. Blind tracheal intubation may be successful; however, the chance of failure is great. Fiberoptic intubation would be successful. **C,** The epiglottis blocking more than 90% of the distal opening of the LMA. Blind tracheal intubation through LMA not possible. Fiberoptic intubation is likely.

Another approach for avoiding the use of a small-size tube is to pass a bougie or a tube changer under fiberoptic observation through the LMA into the tra-chea.[94] The tube changer is advanced and manipulated toward the glottis and trachea. The LMA cuff is then deflated, and the LMA is pulled up over the insertion cord of the FOB. The FOB is then removed, leaving the bougie inside the trachea. A 7- to 8-mm ID ET is then advanced over the bougie into the trachea.

c. FIBEROPTIC TRACHEAL INTUBATION WITH A COMBITUBE IN PLACE

When tracheal intubation has failed and mask venti-lation is impossible, other approaches may be taken to establish ventilation to avoid anoxic brain damage. Esophageal-tracheal double-lumen tube (Combitube) is one such device that is recommended for rapid estab-lishment of ventilation.[95] The Combitube provides ventilation whether it is placed in the esophagus (common) or in the trachea (uncommon). The Com-bitube is placed blindly, and more than 90% of the time it enters the esophagus. Ventilation is achieved through the pharyngeal lumen of the airway while the esophageal cuff blocks the air entry into the esophagus and the pharyngeal cuff seals the upper airway. With the Combitube in the esophagus, suctioning of the trachea is not possible. The Combitube is also not recommended for prolonged mechanical ventilation. Replacement of the Combitube with an ET is necessary to avoid possible complications, to provide a more secure airway, and to have access to the trachea for suctioning.

In a series of 14 patients fiberoptic intubation of the trachea was attempted in the presence of a Combitube.[96] Tracheal intubation was successful in 12 patients. In one patient the fiberoptic intubation failed because of poor relaxation, and in the other the Combitube was removed before intubation was completed. The tongue became engorged in eight patients and remained so until the Combitube oropharyngeal cuff was deflated. The peak airway pressure during controlled ventilation through the Combitube averaged 6 cm H_2O higher, compared with mechanical ventilation through the endotracheal tube. Oxygenation and ventilation was achieved with ease in all patients.

The Combitube often elevates the epiglottis, making fiberoptic exposure of the vocal cords easy. However, because of the large tube size of the Combitube, manipulation of the FOB can be difficult. Combination of blind placement of the Combitube followed by fiberoptic endotracheal intubation may be an effective means of emergency airway management.

d. FIBEROPTIC-ASSISTED BLIND NASAL INTUBATION

The FOB can be used in two different ways to assist in completion of a difficult or failed blind nasotracheal intubation.

When the size of the nasal passage prohibits passage of the FOB through the nasotracheal tube, the FOB may be introduced through the contralateral nostril to visualize the position of the tip of the tube and assist in its passage through the vocal cords.[39] Under visual observation the nasotracheal tube and the patient's head are manipulated to direct the nasotracheal tube toward the larynx.

In some patients with a distorted and compromised airway, blind nasotracheal intubation and fiberoptic exposure of the glottis may independently fail. A combination of blind nasal and fiberoptic intubation techniques may prove successful. The nasotracheal tube is advanced blindly, gently, and slowly while the practitioner is listening to the breath sounds of the spontaneously breathing patient. The advancement of the tube is stopped when the breath sounds are the loudest. At this position the tip of the tube is a short distance from the glottic opening, and the tube has passed beyond the distorted obstructed airway. Passage of a lubricated FOB through the nasotracheal tube brings the tip of the FOB close to the glottis. The epiglottis and the glottic opening are easily identified. The FOB is advanced into the trachea and followed by the nasotracheal tube to complete intubation.

e. FIBEROPTIC-ASSISTED RETROGRADE GUIDEWIRE INTUBATION

A guidewire introduced through the cricothyroid membrane may be used to direct the fiberscope toward the glottis and trachea when attempts at conventional retrograde technique of intubation have failed. Two different principles have been applied for completion of retrograde intubation with the FOB. First, the ET that cannot be advanced over the guidewire into the larynx is left in place. The FOB is inserted into the ET and is advanced alongside the guidewire past the end of the ET and is advanced beyond the entrance of the guidewire into the trachea. When the position of the FOB is ensured in the lower trachea, the guidewire is removed and the ET is threaded over the FOB into the trachea.[97]

The second approach is to pass the guidewire in a retrograde fashion through the suction channel of an FOB that is mounted with an ET. The FOB is guided and advanced over the guidewire into the trachea. The wire is removed, and the ET is threaded over the FOB into the trachea.[98]

Gerrish and Weston[99] applied the same principle under a different circumstance. When an FOB mounted with the ET was advanced into the trachea with great difficulty, the ET could not be advanced into the trachea because of unexpected tracheal stenosis as a result of previous tracheostomy. Before the FOB was removed, a guidewire was advanced through the suction channel into the trachea. The FOB was removed, the ET was changed to a smaller tube, and the fiberscope mounted with a smaller tube was threaded over the guidewire into the trachea, followed by the ET.

f. USE OF THE FIBERSCOPE AS A LIGHTWAND

The lightwand is a lighted stylet with a bright light on its tip and is applied for blind tracheal intubation. The lightwand is loaded with the ET and is advanced blindly toward the trachea. Strong transillumination of the anterior neck confirms its entrance into the trachea, at which time the ET is railroaded over the stylet into the trachea. If the lightwand is not advanced enough to reach the larynx or if it enters the esophagus, the light is not transmitted through the anterior neck. When the lightwand is off center, the light is detected on the lateral aspect of the larynx in the lateral neck.

The FOB has a strong light and can be used as a lightwand to enter the trachea by observing the distribution of the light on the anterior neck. This approach may prevent failure of fiberoptic intubation when copious secretions or blood interferes with visualization of the airway anatomy. We have used this approach on a few occasions and it has also been described by others.[100] The FOB loaded with the ET is passed through the intubating airway toward the larynx. While jaw thrust is applied, the FOB is advanced, first keeping its distal tip straight to facilitate its passage beneath the epiglottis and then deflecting it anteriorly to enter the larynx. The position of the transilluminated light on the neck dictates the maneuvers necessary to enter the trachea.

IV. FIBEROPTIC INTUBATION IN CHILDREN AND INFANTS

The technique of fiberoptic endoscopy for airway management in the adult patient is well established. Less frequently discussed are the uses of fiberoptic endoscopy for the management of the pediatric airway. This is

---

BOX 16-3   Acquired disease associated with difficult airway

Infection: epiglottitis, upper airway abscess
Obesity
Trauma and burns
Tumors and masses: upper and lower airways

---

unfortunate because the difficult pediatric airway can be a frightening and challenging experience for any anesthesiologist, and any technique that can be added to our airway management skills should be understood and used. In particular, with the introduction of ultrathin fiberoptic endoscopes that have directable tips even neonates requiring tubes as small as 2.5 mm ID are not excluded from the option of a fiberoptic approach to airway management.

All indications for fiberoptic endoscopic airway management in adult patients can also be applied to pediatric patients. However, conditions that are more frequently or are exclusively found in the pediatric population warrant special mention. Conditions that are unique to or more common in children and are associated with difficult airway fall into the following broad categories: (1) acquired pathology and (2) congenital syndromes and hereditary diseases (Boxes 16-3 and 16-4).

Although airway management is potentially adversely affected in any of these syndromes, some generalizations can be made about the type of problem each may present. In syndromes associated with macroglossia or with midface hypoplasia mask airways tend to be challenging, but intubations are usually not difficult. In syndromes associated with limited temporomandibular motion or limited mouth opening, intubations tend to be difficult but mask airways may or may not be difficult. In syndromes associated with obstructing masses, distorted facial features, or enlarged or abnormal mandible or syndromes with micrognathia, mask airways and difficult intubations may both be challenging. A fiberoptic approach to airway management must be considered in children who have syndromes associated with an anomaly that may cause a potentially difficult intubation.

Patients with potential cervical instability or immobility are particularly good candidates for fiberoptic endoscopy airway management because this can be undertaken without the need for neck manipulation, which rigid laryngoscopy often requires.

Fiberoptic endoscopic airway management for some of these conditions have been described in the literature* (Table 16-2).

*References 27, 31, 32, 39, 40, 101-110.

A. SELECTION OF TECHNIQUE AND PREPARATION OF THE PEDIATRIC PATIENT

A challenge of pediatric anesthesia is the great variety in both patient age and size. The skill this challenge requires is nowhere more evident than when faced with a child who has a potential airway problem. The choice of technique must be both age appropriate and airway appropriate. For example, conscious sedation might be the best choice for a 13-year-old with high-level thoracic myelomeningocele who is obese and barrel-chested and is known to have had a difficult mask airway and difficult rigid laryngoscopy, but a 5-year-old with Down syndrome and documented cervical instability may require a full general anesthetic before fiberoptic endoscopy.

B. SEDATION IN CHILDREN: SPECIAL CONSIDERATIONS

Traditionally the approach to the anticipated difficult airway in adults is to place the endotracheal tube and secure the airway while the patient is awake but with topical anesthesia and conscious sedation. Commonly applied in adults, the benzodiazepine and narcotic combination for conscious sedation is also quite effective for adolescents and mature preteens. This type of sedation, which helps an older patient comply with the safe securing of the airway, may only serve to disinhibit an already frightened young child. "Enough" sedation to ensure compliance of a 2-year-old child with fiberoptic endoscopy may be "too much" to preserve adequate spontaneous ventilation. There are, however, safe and effective alternatives to the benzodiazepine-narcotic combinations (Box 16-5).

Ketamine is a potent hypnotic and analgesic agent that produces a "dissociative" anesthetic.[111] In most circumstances ketamine preserves adequate spontaneous ventilation while providing adequate anesthesia to prevent reaction to airway manipulation. These characteristics make it an ideal anesthetic for the infant, the young child, or the mentally delayed older child or adolescent. It may be used alone or in conjunction with midazolam. Another attractive feature of ketamine is that it has many routes for administration. If an intravenous line is difficult or impossible to obtain, a small intramuscular, intranasal, oral, or rectal dose can be effectively used for heavy sedation. An intravenous line can then be secured, and further sedation, if necessary, may be given intravenously.

Ketamine has not been widely used in adult anesthesia because of its high incidence of psychomimetic emergence reactions.[111] However, these reactions are less common in children,[112] particularly if ketamine is combined with midazolam.[113] Also, ketamine can produce increased upper airway secretions, which might interfere with fiberoptic airway management. However,

---

BOX 16-4   Congenital syndromes and hereditary diseases associated with difficult airway

Micrognathia and mandibular hypoplasia

Carpenter's syndrome
Christ-Siemens-Touraine syndrome
Cri du chat syndrome
DiGeorge syndrome
Edwards' syndrome (trisomy 18)
Goldenhar's syndrome
King-Denborough syndrome
Letterer-Sewe disease
Meckel's syndrome
Möbius' syndrome
Noonan's syndrome
Osteochondrodystrophies (dwarfism)
Patau syndrome (trisomy 13)
Pierre Robin syndrome
Smith-Lemli-Opitz syndrome
Treacher Collins syndrome
Turner's syndrome

Macroglossia

Beckwith-Wiedemann syndrome
Down syndrome (trisomy 21)
Farber's disease
Hurler's syndrome (mucopolysaccharidosis, type I)
Pompe's disease (glycogen storage disease, type II)

Cervical instability or limited cervical mobility

Arnold-Chiari malformation
Down syndrome (see Macroglossia)
Hurler's syndrome (see Macroglossia)
Klippel-Feil syndrome
Larsen's syndrome
Marfan syndrome
Maroteaux-Lamy syndrome (mucopolysaccharidosis, type VI)
Morquio's syndrome (mucopolysaccharidosis, type IV)
Osteochondrodystrophies (dwarfism)

Syndromes affecting temporomandibular joint and limited mouth opening

Arthrogryposis
Behçet's syndrome
Cockayne-Touraino syndrome (dystrophic epidermolysis bullae)
CREST syndrome
Epidermolysis bullosum
Freeman-Sheldon syndrome (whistling face)
Juvenile rheumatoid arthritis (Still's disease)
Myositis ossificans
Scleroderma
Treacher Collins syndrome

Midface hypoplasia and prominent or abnormal mandible

Andersen's syndrome
Apert's syndrome
Crouzon syndrome
Hallermann-Streiff syndrome
Oral-facial-digital syndrome
Pfeiffer's syndrome
Rieger's syndrome

Obstructing mass

Cherubism (tumors)
Encephalocele
Farber's disease (tumors of larynx; see Macroglossia)
Kasabach-Merritt syndrome (hemangioma)
Letterer-Siwe disease (laryngeal fibrosis; see Micrognathia)
Neurofibromatosis (fibroma)
Stevens-Johnson syndrome (bullae)
Sturge-Weber syndrome (hemangioma)

Enlarged mandible or distortion of facial features

Gaucher disease
Maroteaux-Lamy syndrome
Morquio's syndrome
Pyle's disease
Saethre-Chotzen syndrome
Sanfilippo's syndrome (mucopolysaccharidosis, type III)
Sotos' syndrome (cerebral gigantism)

---

a preoperative antisialogogue, in conjunction with preendoscopy suctioning of the airway, alleviates this problem. There are anecdotal reports of "hyperreactive" airway reflexes when ketamine is used. However, adequate ketamine or ketamine-midazolam doses combined with good suctioning and skilled endoscopy techniques are the best defense against airway reactivity. In fact, ketamine is a commonly described anesthetic agent for fiberoptic airway management in children with difficult airways, and no problems with increased airway reactivity have been noted.

Propofol infusion titrated to provide a more profound degree of sedation but maintain spontaneous ventilation is another anesthetic option.[114] The technique is tricky, however, and advanced experience is required because of the risk of oversedation and apnea. But propofol has the advantage of quick awakening after the infusion is discontinued, unlike titrated doses of ketamine. Propofol is useful in patients for whom conscious sedation is not an option.

As an alternative, for patients in whom conscious sedation is not an option, a careful inhalation induction

Table 16-2. Fiberoptic endoscopy for pediatric airway management: case reports

Author(s)	Reference no.	Patient age(s)	Precipitating disease(s)	Indication for intubation	Complications
Alfery et al., 1979	39	Newborn*	Fusion of the jaws	Examination of the jaws	None
Rucker et al. 1979	27	18 mo to 16 yr (22 children)	Trauma, asthma, seizures, Reye's syndrome, croup, pneumonia, epiglottitis, encephalitis	Ventilatory failure or impending ventilatory failure	None
Rucker et al., 1979	27	9 yr	Marfan's syndrome	Mitral valve replacement	None
Berthelsen et al., 1985	101	6 mo†	History of difficult intubation	Intraocular surgery	None
Kleeman et al., 1987	31	30 mo	Ankylosis of temporomandibular joint (congenital)	Plastic surgery	None
Kleeman et al., 1987	31	18 mo	Ankylosis of temporomandibular joint (congenital)	Plastic surgery	None
Kleeman et al., 1987	31	3 mo	Pierre Robin syndrome	Plastic surgery	None
Gouverneur et al., 1987	102	2 weeks*	Klippel-Feil syndrome	Ventriculoperitoneal shunt	None
Baines et al., 1989	103	6 yr	Swollen tongue	Airway obstruction	None
Wilder and Belanti, 1990	104	12 yr	Hurler's syndrome	Incarcerated umbilical hernia	Pulmonary edema
Tassony et al., 1990	105	4 to 9 yr (four children)	Noma (gangrenous stomatitis)	Various surgical procedures	
Audenaert et al., 1991	106	20 children‡: 1 day to 17 yr	Amyoplasia; cerebral palsy; congenital anomalies; arthrogryposis with Klippel-Feil, Hurler's, Hallermann-Streiff, Pierre Robin, Schwartz-Jampel syndromes; C_{1-2} subluxation, Still's disease	Various surgical procedures	20 intubations: one had epistaxis; two had O_2 desaturation levels below 90%
Montgomery et al., 1991	107	13 yr	Goldenhar's syndrome	Harrington rod instrumentation	None
Monrigal and Granry, 1991	40	9 days to 6 mo (10 infants)	Four patients with history of difficult intubation, six with "facial abnormalities"	Various surgical procedures	None
Scheller and Schulman, 1991	32	1 mo†	Pierre Robin syndrome	Pyloromyotomy	None
Finer and Muzyka, 1992	108	31.5 to 60 weeks post gestation (23 neonates)	Goldenhar's, Pierre Robin, Larsen's micrognathia; stridor, failed intubation, hydrocephalus	Respiratory failure, various surgical procedures	Transient desaturation
Asada et al., 1994	109	8 yr	Farber's disease	Excision of airway granulomas	None
Roth et al., 1994	110	1 to 24 mo (20 infants)	Healthy children (prospective study)	Various surgical procedures	Two patients had barky cough 24 hours after intubation

*Intubation under fiberoptic observation.
†Three-stage technique.
‡Retrograde-assisted technique.

> **BOX 16-5   Sedation for fiberoptic intubation in pediatrics**
>
> Ketamine 0.5 mg/kg, intravenous (IV) in incremental doses
> Midazolam 10 µg/kg, IV in incremental doses
> Fentanyl 0.5 µg/kg, IV in incremental doses
> Propofol 1 to 2 mg/kg, IV bolus; 150 to 300 µg/kg/minute, IV infusion

Table 16-3. Lidocaine nebulizer: suggested doses for pediatrics

Patient weight (kg)	4% Lidocaine (ml)	Normal saline (%)
10 to 14	0.5	2
15 to 19	1.0	2
20 to 24	1.5	3
25 to 29	2.0	4
30 to 34	2.5	—
35 to 39	3.0	—
40 to 44	3.5	—
45 and up	4.0	—

with halothane may be undertaken. Controlled ventilation is gradually assumed, and this ensures that the child's airway can be managed by mask. If mask ventilation is easily performed, a muscle relaxant can be given and fiberoptic intubation begun. This approach obviates any risk of laryngospasm or of sudden patient movement, which can occur with sedation or light anesthesia, with preserved spontaneous ventilation. However, time for each fiberoptic attempt for intubation is decreased because of the patient's apnea. If the use of a muscle relaxant is unadvisable and maintaining spontaneous ventilation increases patient safety, 4% lidocaine should be sprayed on the vocal cords to prevent or minimize the incidence and severity of laryngospasm before advancement of the fiberscope into the trachea.

C. TOPICAL ANESTHESIA: SPECIAL CONSIDERATIONS

For tracheal intubation under sedation and general anesthesia with spontaneous ventilation, topical anesthesia of the airway improves patient acceptance, prevents laryngospasm, and increases the success rate by decreasing airway reflexes.

In general, all techniques that are used in adults may be used in children, with a few caveats. Keep in mind the smaller size of the patient and the subsequent restrictions on the volumes and amount of local anesthetic that can be used. Also, Cetacaine spray and Americaine ointment, because they contain the ingredient benzocaine, may cause methemoglobinemia in infants; it is best to avoid using them.[115] Translaryngeal injection is technically difficult in infants less than 6 months of age and therefore should be avoided in these children.

Nebulized lidocaine has been used successfully in adults.[116] We have used nebulized lidocaine in children as well. This technique seems ideal for young children. Children seem to get a better anesthetic effect from this technique than do adults. Also, many children have used nebulizers in the treatment of asthma or bronchospastic disease and therefore readily accept the lidocaine nebulizer.[116] A suggested dosing schedule for nebulized lidocaine is presented in Table 16-3.

D. PEDIATRIC FIBEROPTIC INTUBATION

All fiberoptic techniques will be more successful if a preoperative antisialagogue is administered either intramuscularly or intravenously before proceeding with the fiberoptic intubation. Except for intubation of the older child or adolescent under conscious sedation, an assistant is necessary to aid in the safe monitoring of the patient and to provide jaw thrust. Jaw thrust is necessary to elevate the tongue off the posterior pharynx and facilitate visualization of the vocal cords.

Ancillary equipment to facilitate fiberoptic tracheal intubation is more limited for the pediatric population. At present, the various intubation airways designed to facilitate orotracheal intubation are available only for the adult-size patient. Modification of oropharyngeal airways and pediatric anesthesia masks to facilitate fiberoptic intubation in pediatrics has been described.[62,63] A new mask adapter consisting of a rotating disk with a port and the body of adapter that attaches to the face mask can also be applied in pediatric patients.[59] In addition, the LMA can be useful as a guide for fiberoptic intubation.[90]

1. Single-stage intubation

The single-stage intubation or routine technique is the traditional adult technique as described previously in this chapter. This is the method of choice if a small, directable-tip FOB is available. For example, the Olympus LFP directable-tip FOB, which has an external diameter of 1.8 to 2.2 ml, may be used in ETs as small as 2.5 mm ID.

Preparation for fiberoptic intubation should include checking the FOB, light source, and related supplies, as well as preparation of rigid laryngoscopy equipment, masks, circuit, appropriate drugs, ETs, and stylets. When a small FOB with no suction channel is used, the regular suction catheter is applied to clear the oropharyngeal secretions. The part of the suction catheter is blocked by tape to make it suitable for one-hand operation.

A method for delivering supplemental oxygen should

also be available. The type of supplemental oxygen used depends on the technique. For patients who are breathing spontaneously. (Supplemental oxygen is provided using the blow-by from the circuit technique or delivered through an insufflation catheter placed inside the mouth or through a nasal cannula.) For patients who are paralyzed, an endoscopy mask or an LMA may be used in conjunction with the FOB to provide oxygen and ventilation if required.

The patient should be positioned in an appropriate fashion to ensure the greatest possibility of success. The body should be positioned with the arms tucked on either side. A strap should be placed over the legs. For infants, a papoosing technique is useful. This technique keeps arms restrained but maintains a free excursion of the chest and abdomen. Head position should be neutral or extended rather than sniffing, since the neutral or extended position ensures a better angle for visualization of the larynx with the FOB.

When beginning fiberoptic intubation after the patient has been properly prepared, the assistant should provide jaw thrust. This brings the tongue up off the posterior pharynx and provides an unobstructed view of the larynx. The mouth should then be suctioned. It is important to place the FOB into the mouth in a midline position. This is done by looking directly at the FOB (not through the FOB) while it is being placed into the mouth. Midline position is especially critical in small infants and neonates because it is easy to become confused about anatomic features if the initial central position is not ensured. A good method to maintain this midline position is to rest the right hand on the patient's face and hold the insertion cord of the FOB in the midline position. The FOB is advanced using the fingers of the right hand, while directing the FOB tip with the thumb of the left hand. When needed, the body of the FOB may be rotated to change the orientation of the tip of the FOB. If the view through the FOB is a pink mass, pull back the FOB: recognizable structures usually come into view. The most common mistake is to advance the FOB too deep, thus entering the esophagus, particularly if one is used to adult airways.

Keep in mind several anatomic differences between adults and children, which affect the fiberoptic technique. The airway distances are much shorter in neonates, infants, and young children than in adults. Therefore laryngeal structures come into view very quickly; hence the importance of strict midline placement and of advancing the FOB only when you see recognizable landmarks. Remember also that neonates and infants have a larynx that is more cephalad, vocal cords that are angled more anteriorly, and an epiglottis that is more angulated, long, and stiff.[117] These differences make it critical that the larynx be approached with

the FOB in the midline position, not from the sides of the mouth. If the approach is not midline, the insertion cord may not pass easily through the glottis.

Also, recall that the cricoid cartilage in children as opposed to the glottic opening in adults, is the narrowest portion of the airway. For this reason uncuffed ETs are used in children. This presents a problem unique to children: an inability to effectively ventilate or protect the airway after ET placement because the inserted tube is too small! One solution is to use a tube changer to switch to an ET a half-size larger. The FOB can then be used to help confirm the correct placement of the new ET.

As an alternative, the FOB can be loaded with the new ET and the tip directed to the larynx. An assistant can then withdraw the old tube as the FOB is directed through the glottis. The new ET is then advanced into the trachea, and the fiberscope removed as usual.

The single-stage or routine technique of fiberoptic intubation may also be used with a nasal rather than an oral approach, but be aware of the possibility of sheared adenoid tissue, particularly in children between 2 and 6 years of age, when adenoid tissue can be hypertrophied. In general, there is no clear advantage to the nasal approach. The oral approach with good jaw thrust is easily performed, and the potential problems of shearing adenoid tissue and of creating a nasal bleed are avoided. If a nasal approach is used in young children, phenylephrine drops may be used to vasoconstrict the nasal passages. This may ease placement and decrease the possibility of bleeding.

2. Two-stage intubation

The two-stage intubation technique is used in infants and small children when the FOBs that are available are too large to pass through the appropriate-size ET. In the original technique described by Stiles[118] a standard cardiac catheter and guidewire with the proximal connector removed were used. An FOB with a working channel is required for this technique. The cardiac catheter guidewire is passed through the working channel of the FOB to within 1 inch of its distal portion. The FOB is then introduced into the mouth and positioned at the top of the vocal cords. The guidewire is then advanced under direct observation through the glottis into the trachea. The FOB is removed, leaving the guidewire in place. The patient then receives mask ventilation while an assistant passes the cardiac catheter over the guidewire. The cardiac catheter is used to stiffen the guidewire, to facilitate passing the ET over the guidewire and catheter into the trachea. The catheter-guidewire combination is then removed, leaving the ET in the trachea. This technique has been used for the intubation of an infant with the Pierre Robin syndrome.[32] However, those authors found that threading of the cardiac catheter over the guidewire was an unnecessary step and that the 3.5-mm ID ET could be passed directly over the guidewire into the trachea without difficulty. Modification of this technique when the FOB has no working channel has also been described.[119] In that report the authors used a no. 8 French red rubber catheter attached by waterproof tape to the insertion cord of the FOB. The larynx was visualized in the usual fashion, then a cardiac catheter guidewire was threaded through the rubber catheter into the trachea. With the guidewire in position the FOB was then withdrawn, and an ET was passed into the trachea over the guidewire.

3. Three-stage intubation

A three-stage fiberoptic intubation technique for infants has been described.[101] For this technique an ET that is larger than the larynx of the infant is advanced over the FOB and positioned on top of the vocal cords. The FOB is then removed, and a tube changer or catheter is advanced into the trachea through the endotracheal tube. The larger tube is then removed and the appropriate-size ET is threaded over the tube changer or catheter into the trachea. This approach is another alternative that can be used when the FOB is too large and lacks a working channel. This technique was used successfully in a 6-month-old infant whose operation had been previously canceled because of failure to intubate.[101]

4. Intubation under fiberoptic observation

This technique is an alternative that can be used for nasotracheal intubation when the FOB is too large to pass through the appropriate-size ET. In this technique the FOB is introduced through one naris while the ET is passed through the second naris. The tube is manipulated into the glottis while the glottis and the tip of the tube are observed through the FOB.[39] As an alternative, if the observed ET is not easily passed into the glottis, a small catheter may be more easily manipulated into the glottic entry and then used as a stylet to pass the ET into the trachea.[102] A disadvantage of these techniques is that a minimum of two people, and ideally a third person, are needed to perform the manipulations. One person would perform the fiberoptic laryngoscopy to expose the larynx and ET, a second person would hold and manipulate the head of the patient, and the third person would manipulate the tube or catheter into the larynx followed by the endotracheal tube. These techniques were used successfully in two neonates; one had congenital fusion of the jaws, and the other had Dandy-Walker syndrome associated with Klippel-Feil syndrome, micrognathia, hypoplasia of the soft palate, and anteversion of the uvula.[39,102]

> **BOX 16-6   Indications for changing endotracheal tube**
>
> Inability to ventilate through the tube
>   Blockade of the tube
>   Major cuff leak
>   Tube too short (laryngeal placement)
>   Broken cuff
> Tube too small for bronchoscopy or major surgery
> Sinusitis complicating nasal intubation
> Change orotracheal tube to nasotracheal tube for patient comfort
> Changing single-lumen tube to double-lumen tube for thoracotomy
> Changing double-lumen tube to single-lumen tube for postoperative ventilatory support

V. FIBEROPTIC CHANGING OF THE ENDOTRACHEAL TUBE

It may be necessary to replace an ET for a variety of reasons[44,120] (Box 16-6). Replacement of a small tube with a larger tube may be necessary if a small tube is placed for rigid laryngoscopy and biopsy before a major head and neck surgery. After the laryngoscopy procedure the small tube should be replaced with a larger one for a lengthy major operation. Changing a single-lumen tube to a double-lumen endobronchial tube at the beginning of a thoracotomy and replacing the double-lumen tube with a single-lumen tube at the conclusion of a thoracotomy are often necessary (Box 16-6).

Emergency intubation during cardiopulmonary resuscitation or ventilatory failure is usually accomplished by the oral route. When prolonged mechanical ventilatory support is required, a change to nasotracheal intubation may be preferred for patient comfort and to provide a better-secured tube. Sinusitis caused by prolonged nasotracheal intubation may necessitate a change back to an orotracheal tube.

Before changing an ET three basic steps should be followed. First, the patient should be evaluated to verify the need for changing the tube. Second, the route of intubation should be decided. Third, all necessary equipment should be secured and an assistant enlisted before beginning the procedure (Box 16-7). The route of intubation (oral or nasal) is often optional but may be mandated by the patient's condition and the reason for tube change.[120]

Three different techniques may be applied for changing an endotracheal tube: a tube changer, rigid laryngoscopy, and fiberoptic laryngoscopy[44,120] (see Chapter 39). The tube changer may be used when the route of intubation remains the same. After preparing the patient and suctioning the trachea, the appropriate-size tube changer is introduced and advanced until it passes

BOX 16-7   Steps and techniques for changing an endotracheal tube

1. Evaluation and verification of the need for tube change
    Immediate (emergent)
    Urgent
    Nonurgent
2. Determination of the route of intubation
    Unchanged
    Changed from oral to nasal route or vice versa
3. Determination of the technique for tube changing
    Direct rigid laryngoscopy
    Use of tube changer
    Fiberoptic technique

BOX 16-8   Indications for fiberoptic tube changing

Initial difficult intubation
Unstable cervical spine
Gastric pull-up operation (postsurgical patient)
High positive end-expiratory pressure required for oxygenation

beyond the tip of the ET. The depth of insertion is predetermined by noticing the length of the ET at nose or mouth level. The tube changer is held firmly while the existing ET is being removed. The new tube is then advanced over the tube changer into the trachea.

Both the rigid laryngoscope and the FOB can be applied for tube changing that maintains the same route or when the route of intubation is changed. The most common technique applied for tube changing is the rigid laryngoscope. It is easy to use, and all anesthesiologists are familiar and experienced with it.[120]

When the use of rigid laryngoscope is difficult or may be hazardous, the fiberoptic option should be considered. In four groups of patients fiberoptic tube change may be advantageous (Box 16-8). Patients with acute ventilatory failure who require high positive end-expiratory pressure (PEEP) (10 to 20 cm H_2O) to maintain a minimum acceptable Pao_2 will decompensate very quickly when mechanical ventilation and high PEEP are disrupted. Mask ventilation with 100% oxygen is usually ineffective to maintain or improve the Pao_2 in these patients. The removal of the existing ET, followed by a failure to immediately reintubate, may be extremely dangerous. Fiberoptic tube change is also preferred when accidental esophageal intubation must be avoided, for example, in patients who have undergone esophagectomy with a gastric pull-up to prevent potential trauma at the site of the anastomosis. Although use of the fiberscope does not guarantee avoidance of inadvertent esophageal intubation, it minimizes the incidence of such occurrences. Two other groups of patients who may benefit from fiberoptic tube change are patients with a known difficult intubation and patients with unstable cervical spine.

A. FIBEROPTIC CHANGE OF AN ORAL TO A NASAL TUBE

The first use of FOB to change an ET was reported in 1981.[121] If the patient is conscious, the procedure is explained and patient cooperation is secured. An antisialagogue is administered intravenously or intramuscularly 15 to 30 minutes before tube change to minimize secretions. A narcotic is included with intravenous sedation to assist in suppression of the pharyngeal and laryngeal reflexes. The nasal mucosa is anesthetized with 4% cocaine or mixture of lidocaine and phenylephrine as previously described. The softened ET is lubricated with a clear, water-soluble lubricant, inserted into the nose, and advanced into the oropharynx. The tracheal tube cuff is rechecked to ensure that the integrity of the cuff is not violated. The pharynx is thoroughly suctioned, and the FOB is advanced through the nasal tube into the pharynx. All secretions are suctioned, and 4 to 5 ml of 4% lidocaine is sprayed over the larynx to provide topical anesthesia of the larynx. After 2 to 3 minutes the airway is suctioned. An assistant applies jaw thrust or helps pull the tongue forward. The goals are to advance the FOB alongside the existing tube into the trachea and position the tip of the FOB just above the carina. Positioning the tip of the FOB next to the carina prevents accidental extubation of the FOB during removal of the existing ET.

The ET occupies the posterior half of the larynx and lies against the arytenoids and interarytenoid muscle, leaving the anterior portion of the glottis open. The FOB is maneuvered so that its tip will be placed anterior to the existing ET to bring the anterior commissure of the larynx into view[44] (Fig. 16-15). With some maneuvering the FOB is advanced into the larynx and trachea until ET cuff is identified. The cuff of the orotracheal tube is deflated, and the FOB is advanced beyond the endotracheal tube cuff 2 to 3 cm above the carina. The tape is removed from the existing tube and, while the operator is looking through the FOB to ensure that the FOB tip stays close to the carina, the assistant pulls out the existing tube. As soon as the tube is out of the larynx, the new tube is threaded over the FOB into the trachea. The FOB is removed, and ventilation is resumed.

If the FOB could not be advanced into the trachea, a second approach to tube changing would be to position the FOB on top of the vocal cords.[44] For complete clearance of secretions the cuff of the existing orotracheal tube is deflated and one or two positive-pressure ventilation breaths are given to move secretions accumulated above the cuff into the oropharynx. The cuff is

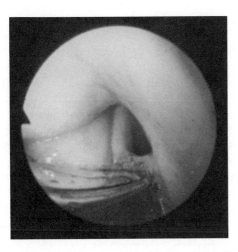

Fig. 16-15. Endoscopic view of the existing orotracheal tube. The anterior commissure is free. The tip of the fiberoptic bronchoscope, which is rotated to the left 90 degrees, is positioned above the orotracheal tube and is ready to enter the larynx.

BOX 16-9   Advantages of fiberoptic intubation

Related to the instrument

Flexible instrument adaptable to airway anatomy
Applied orally or nasally
Applicable to all age-groups
Excellent visualization of the airway
Ability to apply topical anesthesia and insufflate oxygen
   during intubation
Ability to use video system

Related to intubation

High success rate in difficult intubation
Prevention of unrecognized esophageal and endobronchial intubation
Definitive check of tube position
Provides evaluation of the airway before intubation
Less traumatic than rigid laryngoscopic intubation
Less cardiovascular response during awake intubation
   than with rigid laryngoscopic intubation
Excellent patient acceptance of awake intubation

---

reinflated, and all secretions are suctioned again. The cuff is then deflated, and the tube is pulled out while jaw thrust is maintained. As soon as the tube leaves the larynx, the FOB is advanced into the trachea followed by the ET. The shortcoming and the danger of this approach are that after extubation secretions and soft tissue may block the laryngeal view and delay or cause failure of tracheal intubation. This necessitates mask ventilation before a second attempt at intubation. The failure rate with this technique is high.[44,121-123] Combining rigid laryngoscopy with fiberoptic intubation increases the success rate of tube changing under difficult conditions. Published reports on this particular approach for tube changing are few and describe a limited number of cases. More work is needed to establish its value under specific conditions.

B. FIBEROPTIC CHANGE OF A NASAL TO AN ORAL TUBE

Most of the considerations described earlier for change from an oral to a nasal tube also apply to fiberoptic change of a nasal to an oral tube. The nasal tube lies against the posterior pharyngeal wall and therefore interferes less with advancement and manipulation of the fiberscope. However, there is less restriction in selection of the size of an oral tube, and there is much less of a possibility of accidental damage to the tube cuff. The technique for advancement of the fiberscope alongside the existing nasotracheal tube, removal of the existing tube, and advancement of the orotracheal tube is similar to the technique described for fiberoptic change of an oral and a nasal tube.

VI. ADVANTAGES OF FIBEROPTIC INTUBATION

The primary advantage of fiberoptic intubation is its effectiveness in the management of both difficult and failed conventional tracheal intubation (Box 16-9). The FOB is flexible and can be used orally or nasally and for all age groups. Whenever the movement of the head and neck is not possible or is undesirable and the opening of the mouth is restricted, the FOB provides the most successful and an easy approach for securing the airway.

Another major advantage of fiberoptic intubation is placement of the ET under visual observation and therefore avoidance of esophageal or endobronchial intubation. In a patient with abnormal airway anatomy and in the presence of secretions it is possible that the FOB may be advanced into the esophagus instead of the trachea. The lumen of the esophagus is usually flat, but on occasion the lumen of the esophagus is open and tubular and may be mistaken for the trachea, especially in the presence of secretions and poor visualization. When tracheal rings are not satisfactorily identified, the FOB should be advanced farther to expose the carina. The presence of tracheal bifurcation excludes the possibility of esophageal intubation.

Fiberoptic intubation of the trachea in conscious patients is well tolerated, less stressful, and associated with a lesser degree of hypertension and tachycardia compared to rigid laryngoscopy.[124-126] However, cardiovascular response to fiberoptic intubation under general anesthesia has not been shown to be more favorable when compared with rigid laryngoscopy.[127,128]

Another advantage of this technique is the excellent visualization of the airway, which allows evaluation of the larynx and trachea before intubation. This may provide critical information in patients with compromised airway. The FOB makes precise placement of the ET beyond the tracheal compression possible in patients with anterior mediastinal mass.[44,129] This is a critical

---

BOX 16-10   Disadvantages of fiberoptic intubation

Instrument

Instrument is delicate, balky, and expensive.
Separate light source is required.
Instrument is difficult to clean and disinfect.
Vision is obscured easily by secretions.
Small fiberoptic bronchoscopes lack suction channel and tip control mechanism.

Technique

Different skill is required than in rigid laryngoscopy.
Lack of expertise is a disadvantage if the practitioner is not taught during training.
Most of the lumen of the endotracheal tube is blocked by fiberscope.
Passage of the tube through the vocal cords is blind.
Advancement of the endotracheal tube into the trachea may pull the fiberoptic bronchoscope out of trachea.
Resistance during advancement of endotracheal tube into the trachea is common.

---

factor in avoiding airway disasters such as those reported during anesthetic management of patients with anterior mediastinal mass.[129-132]

After completion of intubation, the distance from the tip of the tube to carina is measured and the length of the tube at teeth level is recorded. This information is useful for subsequent repositioning or retaping of the tube in critically ill patients to avoid bronchial intubation and to obviate the need for chest radiographic confirmation.

Fiberoptic intubation can easily be applied with the patient in the supine, sitting, lateral, or even prone position. The FOB provides the only hope for securing the airway and providing general anesthesia to patients in whom access to the anterior neck is not possible because of severe cervical flexion deformity.[35] Other advantages include less trauma and avoidance of tooth damage, which is a common complication and the most common cause of malpractice suits against anesthesiologists.[133,134]

The ability to apply topical anesthesia and insufflate oxygen through the working channel of FOB and the option of using a videocamera system are additional advantages of this technique.

VII. DISADVANTAGES AND COMPLICATIONS OF FIBEROPTIC INTUBATION

The two major disadvantages of the FOB itself are the high cost of the instrument and its size (Box 16-10). Bronchoscopes are delicate instruments and need a separate light source for proper illumination during endoscopy; therefore they occupy a larger space and need their own cart and setup. Cleaning, sterilization, and storage consume more time and resources. Another major disadvantage of the FOB is that a small amount of secretions and blood may completely obscure the view and interfere with airway evaluation and tracheal intubation. As the FOB is advanced through the tracheal tube, the effective lumen left for air exchange is compromised and airway resistance increases greatly when compared with the rigid bronchoscope, which provides a large lumen for air exchange. Many small-size FOBs used for neonates lack the tip control mechanism or suction channel, which limits the value and maneuverability of the instruments.

With fiberoptic intubation the passage of the endotracheal tube through the vocal cords is done blindly, and the depth of tracheal tube cuff placement inside the trachea is unknown. Blind passage of the ET through the vocal cords may result in intralaryngeal placement of the ET cuff with the potential of causing recurrent laryngeal nerve injury and vocal cord palsy. Resistance to advancement of the tube into the trachea is common, especially when a small FOB is used to advance an 8-mm ID or a larger ET. The free lumen of the endotracheal tube predisposes the tube to move away from the insertion cord of the FOB and catch the laryngeal structures, therefore interfering with smooth entrance of the tube into the trachea.[44] Pulling the tube up and rotating the tube while readvancing often overcomes this problem. Forceful advancement of the tube should be avoided because it may traumatize the larynx.

A poorly lubricated FOB with a tight fit may cause intussusception of the outer cover of the FOB, complete obstruction of the tube, and failure to withdraw the FOB.[135] Passing the FOB through the Murphy eye, or side opening, of the ET can cause failure of intubation and inability to remove the FOB.[136] Foreign body aspiration during fiberoptic intubation aided with endoscopy mask has also been reported.[137-139]

Positioning of the FOB into the trachea also does not guarantee tracheal placement of the ET. While the FOB is in the trachea, the ET may enter the esophagus, pulling the FOB out of the trachea. This is most likely to happen when a small-size FOB is used for passage of a large ET.[44] In addition, a correctly placed ET may inadvertently be withdrawn from the trachea during taping of the tube and patient positioning. Checking tube position and its relation to the carina with the FOB after completion of intubation and taping ensures the correct placement of the tube.

The commonly applied clinical evaluations for checking the tube position should also be used (see Chapter 27). Observation of symmetric bilateral movement of the upper chest wall, auscultation of apical and midaxillary area, and auscultation of the epigastrium during ventilation should be performed after each intubation. Measuring exhaled tidal volume and noting the characteristic feel of the reservoir bag and its refilling during exhalation are helpful in confirming correct tube placement. Other techniques have also been applied for confirming correct tube placement.[140] The most reliable technique is measurement of end-tidal volume of carbon dioxide, provided the equipment is functioning properly. Easily identifiable carbon dioxide curves are obtained with ventilation through the tracheal tube.[141,142]

Because fiberoptic airway management training is a recent introduction in residency training programs, a large number of anesthesiologists and other physicians involved in airway management lack the necessary expertise for its effective use. This has resulted in underuse of FOB in anesthesia and critical care.

The hemodynamic response to tracheal intubation during awake fiberoptic intubation has been shown to be less severe when compared with the response with rigid laryngoscopic intubation.[124-126] This advantage of fiberoptic intubation has not been shown to be true when intubation has been performed in anesthetized patients.[127,128,143] In one such study the fiberoptic intubation was associated with a greater increase in systolic blood pressure and heart rate as compared with rigid laryngoscopic intubation. Fiberoptic intubations were performed by holding the tongue and pulling it forward, which could be painful. Prolonged intubation time and retraction of the tongue may have contributed to this exaggerated response.[127] In another study no differences were demonstrated in systolic blood pressure; however, the increase in pulse rate was higher in the fiberoptic group than in the rigid laryngoscopy group.[143] In a more recent publication Schaefer et al.[50] demonstrated no difference in hemodynamic response to tracheal intubation with fiberoptic bronchoscopic or rigid laryngoscopic techniques. More studies are needed to clarify the differences reported by various investigators. Schaefer et al.[50] also reported that the incidence of postoperative sore throat, dysphagia, and hoarseness after fiberoptic intubation was similar to that with rigid laryngoscopic intubation, despite a longer period of airway manipulation and lack of visual control of tracheal tube insertion in the fiberoptic group.

Of 111 pediatric fiberoptic intubations in 15 reports, six complications were noted.* Of 20 patients who required fiberoptic intubation for a variety of illnesses, oxygen saturation levels of 86% and 89% were noted in two patients.[106] However, no supplemental oxygen was being used in these patients, and saturation levels rapidly returned to normal with administration of supplemental oxygen. In another study of 20 patients intubated by FOB, two patients were noted by the parents to have a barky cough 24 hours after intubation. These coughs resolved without consequence.[110] It should be noted that

*References 27, 31, 32, 39, 40, 101, 102, 104, 106-110.

> **BOX 16-11   Causes of failure of fiberoptic intubation**
>
> Lack of expertise
> Presence of secretions and blood
> Fogging of the objective and focusing lenses
> Poor topical anesthesia
> Decreased space between epiglottis and the posterior pharyngeal wall
> Distorted airway anatomy
> Passage of bronchoscope through the Murphy eye
> Inadequate lubrication of a tight-fit bronchoscope

in a control group of children who had traditional intubation, two of 20 also had a barky cough at 24 hours after surgery and that these children also resolved their cough without consequence.[110] In a report of 20 intubations in four children with gangrenous stomatitis, one episode of epistaxis was reported.[105]

The most dramatic complication associated with the fiberoptic intubation is a case report of postobstructive pulmonary edema in a 12-year-old child with Hurler's syndrome.[104] Hurler's syndrome is a mucopolysaccharidase deficiency that results in deposition of mucopolysaccharides in tissues, causing facial and airway deformities. Postobstructive pulmonary edema has been described in normal children because of acute airway obstruction associated with forceful respiratory attempts after extubation.[144] The technique of intubation does not contribute to the development of this complication.

VIII. CAUSES OF FAILURE OF FIBEROPTIC INTUBATION

A large, floppy epiglottis or the presence of secretions or blood contributes to a difficult fiberoptic intubation. The objective lens at the tip of the FOB is easily covered with secretions and blood, which interfere with the visualization of laryngeal structures[44] (Box 16-11). Administration of an adequate dose of an antisialagogue and proper suctioning of secretions before intubation are important preliminary steps in avoiding this problem. In case of unexpected difficult rigid laryngoscopy and tracheal intubation, fiberoptic intubation should be instituted as soon as possible and before causing trauma and bleeding. The conscious patient can be asked to swallow or breathe deeply to clear secretions. Secretions can also be suctioned through the working channel of the FOB. Insufflation of oxygen through the suction channel helps keep secretions away and improves exposure, but one should be aware of the possibility of barotrauma to lungs if the FOB is advanced through a narrowed airway, limiting the oxygen escape from the lungs. If all intubation attempts are unsuccessful, the FOB should be removed, the tip cleaned, and the

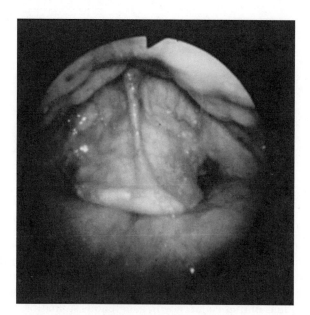

Fig. 16-16. Large, floppy epiglottis blocks the view of the glottis. Jaw thrust or pulling the tongue forward will move the tip of the epiglottis away from the posterior pharyngeal wall, making exposure of the glottis possible. (From Ovassapian A: *Fiberoptic airway endoscopy in anesthesia and critical care,* New York, 1990, Raven.)

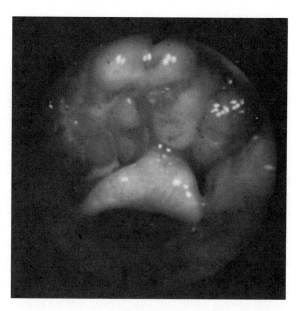

Fig. 16-17. A large, benign lymphoid mass at the base of the tongue compressing the epiglottis. This condition makes fiberoptic exposure of the glottis opening difficult and may interfere with smooth passage of the endotracheal tube over the fiberoptic bronchoscope into the trachea.

oropharynx thoroughly suctioned before the next attempt at laryngoscopy.

Fogging of objective and ocular lenses also interferes with exposure of the laryngeal structures. Insertion of the tip of the insertion cord in warm water solves the problem of objective lens fogging. Exit of exhaled air from the upper border of the operator's protective face mask causes fogging of the ocular lens in a cold operating room. Applying the face mask tightly to the nose and keeping the lower part of it loose directs exhaled air downward, avoiding fogging of the ocular lens. In case of inadequate topical anesthesia, instrumentation of the oropharynx increases secretions and causes coughing, swallowing, and vomiting. Swallowing or coughing moves the laryngeal structures out of the visual field. Laryngospasm is likely if poorly anesthetized vocal cords are touched with the FOB. Even if the FOB can be passed through the vocal cords, it may be impossible to pass the ET.

In many patients the tip of the epiglottis may be next to the posterior pharyngeal wall, which interferes with navigating the FOB beneath the epiglottis. In the presence of a large, floppy epiglottis application of jaw thrust or pulling the tongue moves the epiglottis away from the posterior pharyngeal wall and corrects the problem (Fig. 16-16). If difficulty is experienced because of a supraepiglottic mass or inflammation and edema of the upper airway, simple jaw thrust may not solve the problem. Under these circumstances, even if the FOB is

advanced into the trachea, threading the ET over the FOB into the trachea may fail (Fig. 16-17). Anterior displacement of the base of the tongue with a rigid laryngoscope may be necessary to assist the passage of the ET. With severe flexion deformity of the cervical spine the entire larynx is pushed backward against the posterior pharyngeal wall, making fiberoptic intubation quite difficult[44] (Fig. 16-18).

Distorted anatomy that is due to previous surgery, a mass, edema, or soft tissue contracture may contribute to the difficult vocal cord exposure (Fig. 16-19). For nasotracheal intubation the nostril toward which the larynx is deviated is selected for intubation. This may make the exposure of the glottis easy. For orotracheal intubation the tip of the FOB should be directed toward the side to which the larynx is deviated.

A deviated nasal septum may direct a nasotracheal tube away from the glottis, and in severe cases, even though the FOB may enter the trachea, the ET may not follow it.

Difficulty in advancing the ET into the trachea is a common phenomenon during orotracheal intubation. Pulling the ET back up the FOB, rotating it 45 to 90 degrees, and readvancing it often solve the problem. If still unsuccessful, the following maneuvers may be helpful: an assistant can apply a jaw thrust or pull the tongue forward, the awake patient may be asked to take a deep breath while one advances the tube, and the base of the tongue and epiglottis may be elevated with a tongue retractor or rigid laryngoscope to assist the passage of the tube into the trachea. Difficulty in

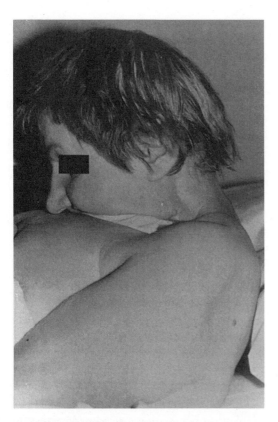

Fig. 16-18. Lateral view of a patient with severe degree of cervical spine flexion deformity resulting from advanced rheumatoid arthritis and pathologic fracture of cervical vertebrae due to fall. Fiberoptic exposure of the vocal cords was extremely difficult because posterior displacement of the entire larynx was pushing the tip of epiglottis against posterior pharyngeal wall. (From Ovassapian A: *Fiberoptic airway endoscopy in anesthesia and critical care,* New York, 1990, Raven.)

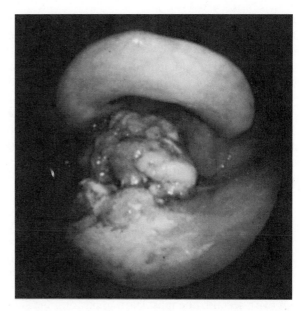

Fig. 16-19. Large malignant mass of larynx originating from left piriform sinus. The tip of epiglottis is in view with large fungating mass beneath it. The glottic opening can not be seen. A 6-mm internal diameter (ID) tube was passed atraumatically into the trachea using Olympus LF-1 fiberoptic intubation scope. The fiberoptic scope was passed from the 1 o'clock position to the back of the mass where glottic opening with normal vocal cords could be seen. Moderately difficult fiberoptic intubation.

advancing the tube into the trachea is less common with nasotracheal intubation.

Advancement of the tracheal tube may also be difficult when the FOB is passed through the Murphy eye rather than the distal opening of the ET.[136] When the FOB is passed through the Murphy eye of the endotracheal tube, withdrawal of the FOB may be difficult or impossible without damaging the instrument. In this instance the FOB and ET should be withdrawn together as a unit, the FOB disengaged, and the procedure repeated. It may also be difficult to remove an unlubricated FOB that has a tight fit. If the FOB has a loose plastic cover and the ET is a tight fit, intussusception can result, leading to difficulty in removing the instrument from the ET.[135]

The single most common cause of failure of fiberoptic intubation is lack of training and experience. In the absence of bloody field or distorted anatomy there is no reason that a fiberoptic intubation should fail.[44]

IX. LEARNING FIBEROPTIC INTUBATION*

The flexible fiberoptic choledochoscope was the first of the new generation of flexible instruments to be used for difficult tracheal intubation.[1] Shortly after the introduction of the FOB into clinical bronchology practice, its use was applied to difficult tracheal intubation by anesthesiologists.[2-4,21] Despite the early recognition by some anesthesiologists of the value of flexible fiberoptic instruments in airway management and their early introduction into clinical anesthesia practice, widespread introduction of the instrument into clinical practice has been slow. This has remained so, despite newer, modern instrument design and equipment and their efficacy in a wide range of clinical circumstances of importance to the anesthesiologist.

In recent years there has been a significant interest in and increase in learning this valuable skill by many disciplines of medicine involved in airway management, especially by anesthesiologists. This view is supported by the large number of regional and national scientific meetings devoted entirely or in part to the role of the FOB in airway management and by the increased number of publications about fiberoptic airway management.

*See Chapters 41 and 42.

Our "hands-on" workshop teaching the use of the FOB in airway management was started in 1984. Over the past 5 years the number of workshops devoted to airway management and fiberoptic intubation has escalated. This is in keeping with the findings of a 1985 survey of academic department chairpersons, members of the Society for Education in Anesthesia, and private-practice anesthesiologists, who were asked which procedural skills should be learned by anesthesia residents: fiberoptic intubation received one of the highest priorities.[145]

A. METHODS OF LEARNING

Fiberoptic tracheal intubation is a psychomotor skill completely different from conventional techniques. There are three components to learning the art of fiberoptic intubation. First, one must understand the instrument, its application, and the skills required (cognitive); second, one must learn to perform the skills (psychomotor); and third, one must be able to apply the new skills in clinical practice.

1. Knowing the instrument

Understanding the physical characteristics of the bronchoscope, the manner in which it functions, and how to avoid damaging it are critical for its successful use. Demonstration of the FOB and in-service training for the physicians, nurses, and technicians who use and take care of the bronchoscope are essential to avoid unnecessary breakage, which contributes to underuse of the instrument.

The endoscopist should have a clear understanding of what the instrument can do, its limitations, and how it can be used most beneficially. Viewing of various videotapes that demonstrate the clinical application of the instrument, its characteristics, and handling is a basic step in learning its use.[46]

2. Handling the instrument

The handling and maneuvering of the FOB can be learned by working on models, patients, or both. It seems logical that the early phase of exercise for getting acquainted with the instrument and developing the dexterity that is essential for successful use of this instrument be done on models. Working on the model is easy and avoids the stress of the operating room. Exercise can be done at any time, and valuable operating room time will not be consumed for this purpose. The most important advantage is becoming dexterous and learning what to do when the technique will be applied to the patient.

The selection of patients for the first few fiberoptic intubations is also critical. Patients with normal airway anatomy provide the opportunity to train the eye to the airway anatomy, manage problems created by secretions, and learn to keep the larynx in visual field during patient movement and swallowing. Only then does the management of a complicated, difficult airway with FOB with low incidence of failure become practical. The following steps are suggested for learning proper maneuvering of the FOB.

a. PRACTICE ON A TRACHEOBRONCHIAL TREE MODEL

"Hands-on" work is necessary to educate the trainee to maneuver the fiberscope and develop the eye-motor coordination and optic recognition essential to its use. Manipulation of the instrument should be natural and spontaneous and can easily be achieved by working on a tracheobronchial model.[46-48,51]

The practitioner should have access to the instrument and the model for unlimited practice. Practice on a tracheobronchial model is critical for learning effective and proper manipulation of the fiberscope. Practice should continue until the operator can quickly and predictably maneuver the instrument in a given direction to expose various segments of the lung model. An acceptable level of dexterity is achieved with 3 to 4 hours of independent practice.

b. PRACTICE ON THE INTUBATION MANNEQUIN

An intubation mannequin is used to demonstrate the steps of fiberoptic intubation that are performed in awake and anesthetized patients. ET position is checked by measuring the distance between the tip of the ET and carina. Fiberoptic tube changing techniques are also practiced. Each procedure is practiced several times to become familiar with the steps of intubation.[46-51]

c. PRACTICE ON PATIENTS

The main requirement for successful fiberoptic intubation is the ability to locate the epiglottis and the glottic opening and to recognize the problems created by secretions. This goal was initially achieved by performing, in patients who gave prior consent, fiberoptic nasopharyngolaryngoscopy during recovery from general anesthesia in the post anesthesia care unit.[46]

More recently, Smith et al.[51] have applied the same training principle by allowing trainees to expose the laryngeal structures in anesthetized and intubated patients. This approach is more practical, since fiberoptic intubation is now considered a routine procedure and the trainee has greater access to the FOB and the patient. In our institution this exercise is applied in training the resident in the technique of fiberoptic endotracheal tube changing.

Exposure of the vocal cords in the anesthetized, paralyzed, and intubated patient is more difficult and requires more maneuvering of the fiberscope than in the awake or anesthetized but not intubated patient. In addition, a jaw-thrust maneuver performed by an assistant to lift up the relaxed pharyngeal structures is often necessary.

d. FIBEROPTIC TRACHEAL INTUBATION OF THE PATIENT

The final stage of learning flexible fiberoptic intubation involves performing intubations in awake and anesthetized patients. The early recommendation of performing only awake fiberoptic nasotracheal intubation was based on an overwhelming preference for nasotracheal intubation.[46,47] Today fiberoptic orotracheal intubation is a daily procedure, and one can learn the technique without waiting for opportunities to perform the much less common nasotracheal intubation. Intubations performed orally or nasally with the patient either sedated or anesthetized and paralyzed have all been suggested.[46-51,146]

A sedated patient in stable condition with good topical anesthesia provides an unrushed opportunity for the inexperienced endoscopist to try his or her first fiberoptic intubation. The important contribution of the safe use of conscious sedation, combined with topical anesthesia of the airway, toward completion of successful flexible fiberoptic intubation should be kept in mind. Because patients present new challenges, such as airway secretions, blood, fogging, and inadequate topical anesthesia with airway reactivity and movement, the endoscopist gains confidence in handling these occurrences with successful routine experience. Because overall patient acceptance of awake or sedated fiberoptic intubations is excellent, more liberal use of awake intubations should be encouraged.[44]

Teaching fiberoptic orotracheal intubation with the patient under general anesthesia is an alternative method with its own advantages (see Chapter 41). The number of patients available for teaching is not limited, and the anxiety of performing a new technique in a conscious patient is avoided.[50] Fiberoptic orotracheal intubations are performed routinely in less than 60 seconds; therefore time is not usually a factor.

Initial intubations by the inexperienced endoscopist should be limited to patients with normal upper airway anatomy who are scheduled for routine surgical procedures.[46-51] The instructor who is teaching the technique should emphasize the role of an assistant in performing the maneuvers that support the relaxed oropharyngeal structures in the anesthetized patient. With experience, intubation of patients with abnormal airway anatomy and patients in whom rigid laryngoscopy has failed becomes an easier task to perform.

Regularly performed nasal intubations using the FOB in patients undergoing oral surgery were reported in a large series by Davies.[147] These were performed with patient under general anesthesia, breathing spontaneously, after the application of topical anesthesia to the nose and larynx.

3. Additional learning aids

In addition to the tracheobronchial model and intubation mannequin, other equipment is helpful in teaching fiberoptic intubation. The fiberoptic teaching attachment makes it possible for the instructor and trainee to simultaneously observe and demonstrate the intubation procedure. A video camera and television screen can be used to demonstrate the techniques for tracheal intubation, airway evaluation, or the positioning of endobronchial tubes. Smith et al.[51] have demonstrated that the use of a video system was more effective in teaching the step-by-step technique of fiberoptic intubation than other methods.

4. Assessing proficiency

Proficiency in fiberoptic intubation technique cannot simply be based on the number of performances attempted. Trainees who have learned the use and proper manipulation of the FOB by practicing on a tracheobronchial tree model and have used the FOB to expose laryngeal structures can be successful in more than 85% of their first six attempts at nasotracheal intubation in patients with normal airway anatomy.[47]

Johnson and Roberts[146] reported that an acceptable level of technical expertise in fiberoptic intubation can be obtained by performing 10 intubations in anesthetized patients. This finding is based on the performance of four anesthesia residents with at least 8 months of training and with no previous experience in fiberoptic intubation. Each resident had a 15-minute practice session on a teaching mannequin with an instructor before attempting orotracheal intubation in anesthetized patients.

If intubation was not achieved within 3 minutes, ventilation in the patient was performed before a second attempt was made. The duration of the intubation procedure was measured from the last mask ventilation to the first breath via the ET, minus the time during which a second mask ventilation was performed. In the first five intubations, the success rate for first attempt at fiberoptic intubation was 50%; the rate improved to 90% in the next five patients and to 100% in the following five patients.[146]

The authors concluded that an acceptable level of technical expertise in fiberoptic intubation is achieved within 10 intubations and that the time needed for intubation remains stable after the tenth intubation at an average level of 1.2 to 1.5 minutes. Their findings were similar to the experience of Delaney and Hessler,[148] who reported their clinical experiences in the use of the FOB in emergency room nasotracheal intubations; they found a significant decrease in the time needed for intubation after their ninth to tenth cases.

Although the level of proficiency cannot be based only on the number of intubations performed by the individual, in our experience most trainees, after practicing on tracheobronchial and intubation models, learn to use the FOB effectively in awake patients with normal airway anatomy after 15 to 20 such intubations. The same number of intubations with patients under general anesthesia seems to be adequate to give the trainee the necessary skill and experience for independent use of the FOB. However, the amount of training or experience necessary for safe, effective use of the FOB in patients with compromised airways is not known and needs to be studied. Based on the observations of a few of our anesthesia fellows and staff, who have used the FOB for considerable lengths of time, expert mastery of the FOB requires significant experience of 100 cases or more. A varied exposure to multiple airway evaluations, tracheal intubations, endotracheal tube changes, and double-lumen tube placement may be needed to gain the necessary experience for independent, successful use of the FOB in patients with compromised airways.

Minimal competency standards for cognitive and technical skills to perform fiberoptic tracheal intubation, placement, and positioning of double-lumen tubes and limited bronchoscopy should be established. A selected minimum number of fiberoptic intubation performances should be only one of the criteria used to judge competency. Each trainee must be evaluated individually regarding overall performance.

If instruction in flexible fiberoptic laryngoscopy is initiated early in the anesthesia training program, there will be ample time and opportunity for every trainee to become proficient in the use of the FOB. Successful teaching of a psychomotor skill requires an instructor who is knowledgeable and proficient in the skill and displays a positive attitude toward the clinical applications and effectiveness of the technique.[48]

5. Introducing fiberoptic intubation into one's own practice

Anesthesiologists who have not been trained to perform fiberoptic intubation during their residency training program face a special challenge in introducing this new technique into their daily practice. The following steps are suggested to assist with the smooth introduction of the technique.

The first step requires gaining the necessary cognitive skills concerning the instrument and its clinical application by referring to the published literature. The second step requires organizing a fiberoptic cart that is reliably maintained with all necessary required equipment and supplies, along with a system for the routine care and cleaning of the FOB. The learning of basic technique by participating in fiberoptic workshops, along with practice on tracheobronchial and intubation models, is the third step before fiberoptic intubation in patients is attempted.[48]

When the basic knowledge and handling of the FOB is learned and an organized, well-functioning fiberoptic cart assembled, an assistant who can be present during intubation should be enlisted for assistance. Attempts at laryngeal exposure in the anesthetized patient tend to proceed smoothly and to have a relatively high success rate. The well-prepared anesthesiologist does not appear to be clumsy or leave a negative impression on the surgeon or other personnel in the operating room. Initial failure of a technique, particularly when it is new, is an acceptable and familiar circumstance to most individuals who work in the operating room environment. However, attempting a technique without any preparation is unacceptable and leaves a bad impression.

The goal of the first few attempts at fiberoptic intubation should be limited to laryngeal exposure only. The importance of jaw thrust in the anesthetized patient, the role of the assistant, and difficulties created by secretions will all be appreciated. Very soon, laryngeal exposure time will be minimized, and time will be available to complete the process of intubation. A colleague, nurse, or technician should provide the necessary assistance for performing intubation with the patient under general anesthesia.

X. CONCLUSION

The maintenance of a patent airway is one of the fundamental responsibilities of every anesthesiologist. Unexpected difficult intubations associated with difficult mask ventilation are responsible for a large proportion of anesthetic-related complications that result in permanent disability or death. When an airway problem is encountered, one should use the technique that one is most familiar or experienced with, to gain control of the situation. However, this should not be used as an excuse to avoid learning new techniques that may be superior or more successful under those difficult circumstances. Two recent editorials have emphasized the value of fiberoptic intubation technique and the importance of developing training programs to teach every anesthesia trainee.[149,150]

Fiberoptic intubation has proven itself to be the technique of choice for the management of securing the difficult airway. The appropriate selection and use of the FOB minimize disastrous outcomes and increase the safety of airway management. Fiberoptic tracheal intubation is critical in airway management and should be mastered by all physicians involved in airway management.

REFERENCES

1. Murphy P: A fibre-optic endoscope used for nasal intubation, *Anaesthesia* 22:489, 1967.
2. Taylor PA, Towey RM: The broncho-FB as an aid to intubation, *Br J Anaesth* 44:611, 1972.
3. Conyers AB, Wallace DH, Mulder DS: Use of the fiberoptic bronchoscope for nasotracheal intubation: a case report, *Can Anaesth Soc J* 19:654, 1972.
4. Stiles CM, Stiles QR, Denson JS: A flexible fiberoptic laryngoscope, *JAMA* 221:1246, 1972.
5. Davis NJ: A new fiberoptic laryngoscope for nasal intubation, *Anesth Analg* 52:807, 1973.
6. Whitehouse AC, Klock LE: Evaluation of endotracheal tube position with the fiberoptic intubation laryngoscope, *Chest* 68:848, 1975 (letter).
7. Vigneswaran R, Whitfield JM: The use of a new ultra-thin fiberoptic bronchoscope to determine endotracheal tube position in the sick newborn infant, *Chest* 80:174, 1981.
8. Moyers J, Gregory GA: Use of fiberoptic bronchoscopy to reposition an endotracheal tube intraoperatively, *Anesthesiology* 43:685, 1975.
9. O'Brien D, Curran J, Conroy J et al: Fiber-optic assessment of tracheal tube position: a comparison of tracheal tube position as estimated by fiber-optic bronchoscopy and chest X-ray, *Anaesthesia* 40:73, 1985.
10. Dietrich KA, Strauss RH, Cabalka AK et al: Use of flexible fiberoptic endoscopy for determination of endotracheal tube position in the pediatric patient, *Crit Care Med* 16:884, 1988.
11. Raj PP, Forestner J, Watson TD et al: Technics for fiberoptic laryngoscopy in anesthesia, *Anesth Analg* 53:708, 1974.
12. Aps C, Towy RM: Experiences with fiber-optic bronchoscopic positioning of single-lumen endobroncheal tubes, *Anaesthesia* 36:415, 1981.
13. Shinnick JP, Freedman AP: Bronchofiberoscopic placement of a double-lumen endotracheal tube, *Crit Care Med* 10:544, 1982.
14. Ovassapian A, Schrader SC: Fiber-optic aided bronchial intubation, *Semin Anesthesia* 6:133, 1987.
15. Benumof JL, Partridge BL, Salvatirra C et al: Margin of safety in positioning modern double-lumen endobroncheal tubes, *Anesthesiology* 67:729, 1987.
16. Fitzpatrick SB, Marsh B, Stokes D et al: Indications for flexible fiberoptic bronchoscopy in pediatric patients, *Am J Dis Child* 137:595, 1983.
17. Fan L, Flynn JW: Laryngoscopy in neonates and infants: experience with the flexible fiberoptic bronchoscope, *Laryngoscope* 91:451, 1981.
18. Wood RE: Spelunking in the pediatric airways: explorations with the flexible bronchoscope, *Pediatr Clin North Am* 31:785, 1984.
19. Shinwell ES, Higgins RD, Auten RL et al: Fiberoptic bronchoscopy in the treatment of intubated neonates, *Am J Dis Child* 143:1064, 1989.
20. Fan LL, Sparks LM, Dulinski JP: Applications of an ultra-thin flexible bronchoscope for neonatal and pediatric airway problems, *Chest* 89:673, 1986.
21. Ikeda S: *Atlas of flexible bronchofiberoscopy,* Baltimore, 1974, University Park.
22. Ovassapian A, Dykes MHM: The role of fiberoptic endoscopy in airway management, *Semin Anesthesia* 6:93, 1987.
23. Schwartz HC, Bauer RA, Davis J et al: Ludwig's angina: use of fiberoptic laryngoscopy to avoid tracheostomy, *J Oral Surg* 32:608, 1974.
24. Messeter KH, Petersson KI: Endotrachea intubation with the fiberoptic bronchoscope, *Anaesthesia* 35:294, 1980.
25. Rogers SN, Benumof JL: New and easy techniques for fiberoptic endoscopy-aided tracheal intubation, *Anesthesiology* 59:569, 1983.
26. Mulder DS, Wallace DH, Woolhouse FM: The use of the fiberoptic bronchoscope to facilitate endotracheal intubation following head and neck trauma, *J Trauma* 15:638, 1975.
27. Rucker RW, Silva WJ, Worcester CC: Fiberoptic bronchoscopic nasotracheal intubation in children, *Chest* 76:56, 1979.
28. Sidhu VS, Whitehead EM, Ainsworth QP et al: A technique of awake fiberoptic intubation: experience in patients with cervical spine disease, *Anaesthesia* 48:910, 1993.
29. Davies JR: The fiberoptic laryngoscope in the management of cut throat injuries, *Br J Anaesth* 50:511, 1978.
30. Ovassapian A, Doka JC, Romsa DE: Acromegaly: use of fiberoptic laryngoscope to avoid tracheostomy, *Anesthesiology* 54:429, 1981.
31. Kleeman PP, Jantzen JP, Bonfils P: The ultra-thin bronchoscope in management of the difficult paediatric airway, *Can J Anaesth* 34:606, 1987.
32. Scheller JG, Schulman SR: Fiberoptic bronchoscopic guidance for intubating a neonate with Pierre Robin syndrome, *J Clin Anesth* 3:45, 1991.
33. Wang JF, Reves JG, Corssen G: Use of the fiberoptic laryngoscope for difficult tracheal intubation, *Ala Med* 13:247, 1976.
34. Edens ET, Sia RL: Flexible fiberoptic endoscopy in difficult intubations, *Ann Otol Rhinol Laryngol* 90:307, 1981.
35. Ovassapian A, Land P, Schafer MF et al: Anesthetic management for surgical correction of severe flexion deformity of the cervical spine, *Anesthesiology* 58:262, 1987.
36. Nakayama M, Kataoka N, Usui Y et al: Techniques of nasotracheal intubation with the fiberoptic bronchoscope, *J Emerg Med* 10:729, 1992.
37. Keenan MA, Stiles CM, Kaufman RL: Acquired laryngeal deviation associated with cervical spine disease in erosive, poliarticular arthritis: use of the fiberoptic bronchoscope in rheumatoid arthritis, *Anesthesiology* 58:441, 1983.
38. Ovassapian A, Yelich SJ, Dykes HM et al: Fiberoptic nasotracheal intubation: incidence and causes of failure, *Anesth Analg* 62:692, 1983.
39. Alfrey DD, Ward CF, Harwood IR et al: Airway management for a neonate with congenital fusion of the jaws, *Anesthesiology* 51:340, 1979.
40. Monrigal JP, Granry JC, Le Rolle T et al: Difficult intubation in newborns and infants using an ultra-thin fiberoptic bronchoscope, *Anesthesiology* 75:A1044, 1991.
41. Ovassapian A, Krejcie TC, Yelich SJ et al: Awake fiberoptic intubation of the patient at high risk of aspiration, *Br J Anaesth* 62:13, 1989.
42. Ovassapian A: Fiberoptic airway endoscopy in critical care. In Ovassapian, A, editor: *Fiberoptic airway endoscopy in anesthesia and critical care,* New York, 1990, Raven.
43. Patil V, Stehling LC, Zauder HL: Fiberoptic endoscopy in anesthesia, St Louis, 1983, Mosby.
44. Ovassapian A: *Fiberoptic airway endoscopy in anestheisa and critical care,* New York, 1990, Raven.
45. Roberts JT: Fiberoptics in anesthesia, *Anesth Clin North Am* 9:1, 1991.
46. Ovassapian A, Dykes MHM, Golmon ME: A training programme for fiberoptic nasotracheal intubation. Use of model and live patients. *Anaesthesia* 38:795, 1983.
47. Ovassapian A, Yelich SH, Dykes MHM et al: Learning fiberoptic intubation: use of simulators V. traditional teaching, *Br J Anaesth* 61:217, 1988.
48. Dyked MHM, Ovassapian A: Dissemination of fiberoptic airway endoscopy skills by means of a workshop utilizing models, *Br J Anaesth* 63:595, 1989.
49. Coe PA, King TA, Towey RM: Teaching guided fiberoptic nasotracheal intubation: an assessment of an anaesthetic technique to aid training, *Anaesthesia* 43:410, 1988.

50. Schaefer HG, Marsch SCU, Keller HL et al: Teaching fiberoptic intubation in anaesthetized patients, *Anaesthesia* 49:331, 1994.

51. Smith JE, Fenner SG, King MJ: Teaching fiberoptic nasotracheal intubation with and without closed circuit television, *Br J Anaesth* 71:206, 1993.

52. Hanson PJV, Meah S, Tipler D et al: Infection control in endoscopy units: does it cost more to be clean? *Br Med J* 298:866, 1989.

53. Hanson PJV, Collins JV: AIDS, aprons, and elbow grease: preventing nosocomial spread of human immunodeficiency virus and associated organisms, *Thorax* 44:778, 1989.

54. Benumof JL: Management of the difficult adult airway, *Anesthesiology* 75:1087, 1991.

55. Mallios C: A modification of the Laerdal mask for nasotracheal intubation with the fiberoptic laryngoscope, *Anaesthesia* 35:599, 1980.

56. Patil V, Stehling LC, Zauder HL et al: Mechanical aids for fiberoptic endoscopy, *Anesthesiology* 57:69, 1982.

57. Ovassapian A: A new fiberoptic intubating airway, *Anesth Analg* 66:S132, 1987.

58. Williams RT, Harrison RE: Prone tracheal intubation simplified using an airway intubator, *Can Anaesth Soc J* 28:288, 1981.

59. Imai M, Kemmotsu Q: A new adapter for fiberoptic endotracheal intubation for anesthetized patients, *Anesthesiology* 70:374, 1989 (letter).

60. Davis K: Alterations to the Patil-Syracuse mask for fiberoptic intubation, *Anesth Analg* 74:472, 1992 (letter).

61. Berman RA: A method for blind oral intubation of the trachea or esophagus, *Anesth Analg* 56:866, 1977.

62. Frei FJ: A special mask for teaching fiber-optic intubation in pediatric patients, *Anesth Analg* 76:458, 1993 (letter).

63. Wilton NCT: Aids for fiberoptically guided intubation in children, *Anesthesiology* 75:549, 1991.

64. Reed AP, Han DG: Preparation of the patient for awake fiberoptic intubation, *Anesthes Clin North Am* 9:69, 1991.

65. Adriani J, Zepernick R, Arens J et al: The comparative potency and effectiveness of topical anesthetics in man, *Clin Pharmacol Ther* 5:49, 1964.

66. Campbell D, Adriani J: Absorption of local anesthetics, *JAMA* 168:873, 1958.

67. Bourke DL, Katz J, Tonneson A: Nebulized anesthesia for awake endotracheal intubation, *Anesthesiology* 63:690, 1985.

68. Chinn WM, Zavala DC, Ambre J: Plasma levels of lidocaine following nebulized aerosol administration, *Chest* 71:346, 1977.

69. Patterson JR, Blaschke TF, Hunt KK et al: Lidocaine blood concentrations during fiberoptic bronchoscopy, *Am Rev Respir Dis* 112:53, 1975.

70. Chu SS, Rah KH, Brannan MD et al: Plasma concentration of lidocaine after endotracheal spray, *Anesth Analg* 54:438, 1975.

71. Webb AR, Fermando SSD, Dalton HR et al: Local anesthesia for fiberoptic bronchoscopy: transcricoid injection or the "spray as you go" technique? *Thorax* 45:474, 1990.

72. Brull SJ, Wiklund R, Ferris C et al: Facilitation of fiberoptic orotracheal intubation with a flexible tracheal tube, *Anesth Analg* 78:746, 1994.

73. Pelimon A, Simunovic Z: Mouth gag and tongue holder for fiberoptic laryngoscopy, *Anaesthesia* 40:386, 1985 (letter).

74. Ovassapian A, Krejcie TC, Joshi CW: Fiberoptic vs. rigid laryngoscopy for rapid sequence intubation of the trachea, *Anesth Analg* 74:S229, 1992.

75. Wangler MA, Weaver JM: A method to facilitate fiberoptic laryngoscopy, *Anesthesiology* 61:111, 1984.

76. Lu GP, Frost EAM, Goldiner PL: Another approach to the problem airway, *Anesthesiology* 65:101, 1986.

77. Johnson C, Hunter J, Ho E et al: Fiberoptic intubation facilitated by a rigid laryngoscope, *Anesth Analg* 72:714, 1991 (letter).

78. Couter P, Perreault C, Girard D: Fiberoptic bronchoscopic intubation after induction of general anesthesia: another approach, *Can J Anaesth* 39:99, 1992.

79. Russell SH, Hirsch NP: Simultaneous use of two laryngoscopes, *Anaesthesia* 48:918, 1993.

80. Brain AIJ: The laryngeal mask: a new concept in airway management, *Br J Anaesth* 55:801, 1983.

81. Pennant JH, White PF: The laryngeal mask airway: its uses in anesthesiology, *Anesthesiology* 79:144, 1963.

82. Brain AIJ: Three cases of difficult intubation by the laryngeal mask airway, *Anaesthesia* 40:353, 1985.

83. Calder I, Ordman AJ, Jackowski A et al: The Brain laryngeal mask airway: an alternative to emergency tracheal intubation, *Anaesthesia* 45:137, 1990.

84. Nath G, Major V: The laryngeal mask in the management of a paediatric difficult airway, *Anaesth Intensive Care* 20:518, 1992.

85. Heath ML, Allagain J: Intubation through the laryngeal mask: a technique for unexpected difficult intubation, *Anaesthesia* 46:545, 1991.

86. Chadd GD, Ackers JW, Bailey PM: Difficult intubation aided by the laryngeal mask airway, *Anaesthesia* 45:1015, 1990.

87. McCrirricka, Pracilio A: Awake intubation: a new technique, *Anaesthesia* 46:661, 1991.

88. Brimacombe J, Berry A: Placement of a Cook airway exchange catheter via the laryngeal mask airway, *Anaesthesia* 48:351, 1993.

89. Benumof JL: Use of the laryngeal mask airway to facilitate fiberscope-aided tracheal intubation, *Anesth Analg* 74:313, 1992.

90. Johnson CM, Sims C: Awake fiberoptic intubation via a laryngeal mask in an infant with Goldenhar's syndrome, *Anaesth Intensive Care* 22:194, 1994.

91. Hasham F, Kumar CM, Lawler PGP: The use of laryngeal mask airway to assist fiberoptic orotracheal intubation, *Anaesthesia* 46:891, 1991.

92. Darling JR, Keohane M, Murray JM: A split laryngeal mask as an aid to training in fiberoptic tracheal intubation: a comparison with the Berman II intubating airway, *Anaesthesia* 48:1079, 1993.

93. Asai T, Latto IP, Vaughan RS: The distance between the grille of the laryngeal mask airway and the vocal cords, *Anaesthesia* 48:667, 1993.

94. Allison A, McCrory J: Tracheal placement of a gum elastic bougie using the laryngeal mask airway, *Anaesthesia* 45:419, 1990.

95. Frass M, Frenzer R, Rauscha F et al: Evaluation of esophageal tracheal Combitube in cardiopulmonary resuscitation, *Crit Care Med* 15:609, 1986.

96. Ovassapian A, Liu S, Krejcie TC: Fiberoptic tracheal intubation with Combitube in place, *Anesth Analg* 75:S315, 1993.

97. Barriot P, Riou B: Retrograde technique for tracheal intubation in trauma patients, *Crit Care Med* 16:712, 1988.

98. Lechman MJ, Donahoo JS, MacVaugh HIII: Endotracheal intubation using percutaneous retrograde guide wire insertion followed by antegrade fiberoptic bronchoscopy, *Crit Care Med* 14:589, 1986.

99. Gerrish SP, Weston GA: The use of a biopsy brush wire as a bronchoscope guide, *Anaesthesia* 41:444, 1986.

100. Whitlock JE, Calder I: Transillumination in fiberoptic intubation, *Anaesthesia* 42:570, 1987.

101. Berthelsen P, Prytz S, Jacobsen E: Two-stage fiberoptic nasotracheal intubation in infants: a new approach to difficult pediatric intubation, *Anesthesiology* 63:457, 1985.

102. Gouverneur JM, Veyckemans F, Licker M et al: Using an ureteral catheter as a guide in difficult neonatal fiberoptic intubation, *Anesthesiology* 66:436, 1987.

103. Baines DB, Goodrick MA, Beckenham EJ et al: Fiberoptically guided endotracheal intubation in a child, *Anaesth Intensive Care* 17:354, 1989.

104. Wilder RT, Belani KG: Fiberoptic intubation complicated by

pulmonary edema in a 12-year-old child with Hurler syndrome, *Anesthesiology* 72:205, 1990.

105. Tassony E, Lehman C, Gunning K et al: Fiberoptically guided intubation in children with gangrenous stomatitis (Noma), *Anesthesiology* 73:348, 1990.

106. Audenaert SM, Montgomery CL, Stone B et al: Retrograde-assisted fiberoptic tracheal intubation in children with difficult airways, *Anesth Analg* 73:660, 1991.

107. Montgomery G, Dueringer J, Johnsoon C: Nasal endotracheal tube change with an intubating stylette after fiberoptic intubation, *Anesth Analg* 72:713, 1991 (letter).

108. Finer NN, Muzyka D: Flexible endoscopic intubation of the neonate, *Pediatr Pulmonol* 12:48, 1992.

109. Asada A, Tatekawa S, Terai T et al: The anesthetic implications of a patient with Farber's lipogranulomatosis, *Anesthesiology* 80:206, 1994.

110. Roth AG, Wheeler M, Stevenson GW et al: Comparison of the use of a rigid laryngoscope with the ultrathin fiberoptic laryngoscope for intubation of infants, *Can J Anaesth* 41:1069, 1994.

111. White, PE: Ketamine update: its clinical uses in anesthesia, *Semin Anesth* 7:113, 1988.

112. Hollister GR, Burn JMB: Side effects of ketamine in pediatric anesthesia, *Anesth Analg* 53:264, 1974.

113. Cartwright PD, Pingel SM: Midazolam and diazepam in ketamine anesthesia, *Anaesthesia* 39:439, 1984.

114. Marsh B, White M, Morton N et al: Pharmacokinetic model driven infusion of propofol in children, *Br J Anaesth* 67:41, 1991.

115. Hughes JR: Infantile methemoglobinemia due to benzocaine suppository, *J Pediatr* 66:797, 1965.

116. Bourke Dl, Katz J, Tonneson A: Nebulized anesthesia for awake endotracheal intubation, *Anesthesiology* 63:690, 1985.

117. Eckenhoff JE: Some anatomic considerations of the infant larynx influencing endotracheal anesthesia, *Anesthesiology* 12:401, 1951.

118. Stiles CM: A flexible fiberoptic bronchoscope for endotracheal intubation of infants, *Anesth Analg* 53:1017, 1974.

119. Ford RWJ: Adaptation of the fiberoptic laryngoscope for tracheal intubation with small diameter tubes, *Can Anaesth Soc J* 28:479, 1981.

120. Alfery DD: Changing an endotracheal tube. In Benumof JL, editor: *Procedures in anesthesia and intensive care*, Philadelphia, 1991, Lippincott.

121. Rosenbaum SH, Rosenbaum LH, Cole RP et al: Use of the flexible fiberoptic bronchoscope to change endotracheal tube in critically ill patients, *Anesthesiology* 54:169, 1981.

122. Watson CB: Fiberoptic bronchoscopy for anesthesia, *Anesthesiology Rev* 9:17, 1982.

123. Halebian P, Shires T: A method for replacement of the endotrachial tube with continuous control of the airway, *Surg Gynecol Obstet* 161:285-286, 1985.

124. Southerland AD, Sale JP: Fiberoptic awake intubation: a method of topical anaesthesia and orotracheal intubation, *Can Anaesth Soc J* 33:502, 1986.

125. Ovassapian A, Yelich SJ, Dykes MHM et al: Blood pressure and heart rate changes during awake fiberoptic nasotracheal intubation, *Anesth Analg* 62:951, 1983.

126. Schrader S, Ovassapian A, Dykes MHM et al: Cardiovascular changes during awake rigid and fiberoptic laryngoscopy, *Anesthesiology* 67:A28, 1987.

127. Smith JE: Heart rate and arterial pressure changes during fiberoptic tracheal intubation under general anesthesia, *Anaesthesia* 43:629, 1988.

128. Smith M, Calder I, Dobst ChB et al: Oxygen saturation and cardiovascular changes during fiberoptic intubation under general anaesthesia, *Anaesthesia* 47:158, 1992.

129. Prakash UBS, Abel MD, Hubmayr RD: Mediastinal mass and tracheal obstruction during general anesthesia, *Mayo Clin Proc* 63:1004, 1988.

130. Piro AH, Weiss DR, Hellman S: Mediastinal Hodgkin's disease: a probable danger for intubation anesthesia, *Int J Radiol Oncol Biol Phys* 1:415, 1976.

131. Keon TP: Death on induction of anesthesia for cervical node biopsy, *Anesthesiology* 55:471, 1981.

132. Price SL, Hecker BR: Pulmonary edema following airway obstruction in a patient with Hodgkin's disease, *Br J Anaesth* 59:518, 1987.

133. Wright RB, Manfield FFV: Damage to teeth during the administration of general anesthesia, *Anesth Analg* 53:405, 1974.

134. Burton JF, Baker AB: Dental damage during anaesthesia and surgery, *Anaesth Intensive Care* 15:262, 1987.

135. Siegal M, Coleprate P: Complications of fiberoptic bronchoscope, *Anesthesiology* 61:214, 1984.

136. Ovassapian A: Failure to withdraw flexible fiberoptic laryngoscope after nasotracheal intubation, *Anesthesiology* 63:124, 1985.

137. Zornow MH, Mitchell MM: Foreign body aspiration during fiberoptic assisted intubation, *Anesthesiology* 64:303, 1986.

138. Williams L, Teague PD, Nagia AH: Foreign body from a Patil-Syracuse mask, *Anesth Analg* 73:359, 1991.

139. Patil VU: Concerning the complications of the Patil-Syracuse mask, *Anesth Analg* 76:1165, 1993 (letter).

140. Wee MYK: The esophageal detecter device, *Anaesthesia* 43:27, 1988.

141. Murray IP, Modell JH: Early detection of endotracheal tube accidents by monitoring carbon dioxide concentration in respiratory gas, *Anesthesiology* 59:344, 1983.

142. Birmingham PK, Cheney FW, Ward RJ: Esophageal intubation: a review of detection techniques, *Anesth Analg* 65:886, 1986.

143. Finfer SR, MacKenzie SIP, Saddler JM et al: Cardiovascular responses to tracheal intubation: a comparison of direct laryngoscopy and fibreoptic intubation, *Anaesth Intensive Care* 17:44, 1989.

144. Ondjhane K, Bowen AD, Oh KS et al: Pulmondary edema complicating upper airway obstruction in infants and children, *Can Assoc Radiol J* 43:278, 1992.

145. Spielman FJ, Levin KJ, Matherly LA et al: Which procedural skills should be learned by anesthesiology residents? *Anesthesiology* 69:A798, 1988.

146. Johnson C, Roberts JT: Clinical competence in the performance of fiberoptic laryngoscopy and endotracheal intubation: a study of resident instruction, *J Clin Anesth* 1:344, 1989.

147. Davies NJ: A new fiberoptic laryngoscope for nasal intubation, *Anesth Analg* 52:807, 1978.

148. Delaney KA, Hessler R: Emergency flexible nasotracheal intubation: a report of 60 cases, *Ann Emerg Med* 17:919, 1988.

149. Mason RA: Learning fiberoptic intubation: fundamental problems, *Anaesthesia* 47:729, 1992.

150. Vaughan RS: Training in fiberoptic laryngoscopy *Br J Anaesth* 66:538, 1991 (editorial).

Chapter 17

RETROGRADE INTUBATION TECHNIQUE

Antonio Sanchez
Vincente Pallares

I. HISTORY

The first reported case of retrograde intubation (RI) was by Butler and Cirillo in 1960.[1] The technique involved passing a red rubber catheter cephalad through the patient's previously existing tracheostomy. Once the catheter exited the oral cavity it was tied to the endotracheal tube (ET), allowing it to be pulled into the trachea.

The first person to perform RI as presently practiced was Waters, a British anesthesiologist in Nigeria.[2] In 1963 he reported treating patients who had cancrum oris, an invasive gangrene that deforms the oral cavity, severely limiting mouth opening. His technique involved passing a standard Tuohy needle through the cricothyroid membrane (CTM) and feeding an epidural catheter cephalad into the nasopharynx. He "fished" the catheter out of the nasopharynx through the nares, using a hook he devised. The epidural catheter was then used as a stylet to guide the ET through the nares and into the trachea.

Over the ensuing years RI did not gain clinical acceptance because of its invasiveness and the potential for complications from the CTM puncture. After 1964, when fiberoptic technology became available, RI was irregularly but occasionally discussed in the literature.[1-102] In 1993, RI was designated as part of the anesthesiologist's armamentarium by the ASA Difficult Airway Task Force.[102]

The name "retrograde intubation," used by Butler and Cirillo, is a misnomer.[14] The technique is actually a translaryngeal guided intubation, but for historical reasons we will continue using the name "retrograde intubation."

BOX 17-1   Number of retrograde intubations in the literature (383 patients and 117 cadavers)

Oral cavity

Calncrum oris, 27
Mandibular or maxillary fracture, 31
Perimandibular abscess, 1
Ankylosis of temporomandibular joint, 5
Microstomia, 1
Macroglossia, 1
Cancer of tongue, 8
Oral myxoma, 1

Cervical

Spinal cord injury, 66
Ankylosing spondylitis, 11
Rheumatoid arthritis, 32

Pharynx and larynx

Laryngeal cancer, 70
Pharyngeal abscess, 1
Epiglottitis, 1
Pharyngeal edema, 1
Laryngeal edema after burn, 2

Others

Pediatric anomalies, 24
Obesity, 11
Coronary artery bypass grafting (failure to intubate), 28
Tracheostomy stoma, 16
Trauma (failure to intubate), 33
Disease not specified (failure to intubate), 12
Cadaver studies, 117

From UCI Department of Anesthesia: *Teaching aids.*

BOX 17-2   Characteristics of retrograde intubations in the literature

1. Number of adult patients (RI): 357
2. Number of pediatric patients (RI): 26
3. Age range: (1 day old; weight, 2.9 kg) to 84 years
4. Average time for technique: 2.5 min (range, 0.5 to 15 min)
5. Elective cases: 113 patients
6. Failed attempts using RI: 5 patients

From UCI Department of Anesthesia: *Teaching aids.*

injury) and its use has been reported in facial trauma. It has been employed in both adults and pediatric patients with success (Box 17-2).

Not all reported cases have described the amount of time required to perform the technique, but in one study involving emergency medical service personnel (paramedics and registered nurses) using training mannequins the average time was 71 seconds (range, 42 to 129 seconds).[103] Barriot and Riou[4] described 13 patients with maxillofacial trauma who could not be intubated "in the field" using direct laryngoscopy (six attempts: average time, 18 minutes). Intubation was subsequently performed in the patients on the first RI attempt in an average time of less than 5 minutes. An additional six patients were intubated in less than 5 minutes when RI was used as the initial method of choice. The investigators concluded that the RI technique was a rapid, efficacious method for intratracheal intubation of trauma patients, especially patients with maxillofacial trauma.

Historical indications for RI are the following:
1. Failed attempts at laryngoscopy and/or fiberoptic intubation
2. Emergent establishment of an airway where visualization of the vocal cords is prevented by blood, secretions, or anatomic derangement
3. Elective use when deemed necessary in clinical situations such as unstable cervical spine, maxillofacial trauma, or anatomic anomaly

III. CONTRAINDICATIONS

Contraindications to RI have been cited, often anecdotally (Box 17-3). Most are relative contraindications and can be divided into four categories: unfavorable anatomy, laryngotracheal disease, coagulopathy, and infection.

A. UNFAVORABLE ANATOMY

Since in most cases retrograde intubation is performed above or below the cricoid cartilage, the absolute lack of access to this region, as in severe flexion deformity of the neck, is a contraindication if not an

II. INDICATIONS

The RI technique has been used both in the hospital setting and in prehospital mobile units (in the field).[4,33] It has been employed with the anticipated[2,4,28,49,63] and unanticipated* difficult airway, following failure to intubate using conventional means (direct laryngoscopy,[8,33,49] blind nasal intubation,[6,8] bougie,[9,81] and fiberoptic laryngoscopy).[18,22,23,25] It has been employed in both humans and animals.[51,98] In the literature, as well as in the author's experience, there have been approximately 500 reported cases using RI (383 patients and 117 cadavers). Although in the majority of cases RI has been used to place a single-lumen ET, one case report described placement of a double-lumen ET via RI.[63]

Airway disease necessitating RI has been of a wide variety (Box 17-1). Retrograde intubation has been most frequently associated with limited range of motion of the neck (153 trauma victims with potential cervical spine

---

*References 2, 4, 6, 8, 9, 18, 19, 23, 27, 31, 33, 37, 47, 53.

BOX 17-3   Contraindications to retrograde intubation and examples

Unfavorable anatomy

Lack of access to cricothyroid muscle (severe flexion deformity of the neck)
Poor anatomic landmarks (obesity)
Pretracheal mass (thyroid goiter)

Laryngotracheal disease

Malignancy
Stenosis

Coagulopathy

Infection (pretracheal abscess)

From UCI Department of Anesthesia: *Teaching aids.*

impossibility.[104,105] For the same reason, the patient with nonpalpable landmarks,[5,16,26] obesity,[101] overlying malignancy,[5] or large thyroid goiter[5] should be approached cautiously. Shantha[80] reported a case of RI in a patient with a large thyroid goiter. After failure of conventional intubating methods (including fiberoptic) the surgeons dissected down to the cricothyroid membrane (CTM) and subsequently passed the catheter cephalad. Eleven cases of RI have been reported in the obese without major complications.[23,47,100,101]

B. LARYNGOTRACHEAL DISEASE

Theoretically, laryngotracheal stenosis[2,16] may contraindicate RI, since narrowing of the trachea or larynx could be made worse by either the needle puncture or the catheter.[2,16] However, RI has been used in patients with laryngeal cancer,[36] epiglottitis,[32] and laryngeal edema resulting from burn injuries.[19,25] It should not be used when there is laryngeal tracheal stenosis directly under the intended puncture site.

C. COAGULOPATHY*

Preexisting bleeding diathesis should be considered a relative contraindication. Although there is a potential for bleeding, the CTM is considered a relatively avascular plane (see Anatomy). A small, self-limited hematoma[49] was reported in a patient who underwent coronary artery bypass graft with intraoperative heparin and postoperative disseminated intravascular coagulation.

D. INFECTION

RI in the presence of preexisting infection over the puncture site or in the path of the puncture, as in pretracheal abscess, could result in transmittal of bacterial flora into the trachea and should be avoided. This, again,

*References 5, 16, 50, 70, 93, 106-108.

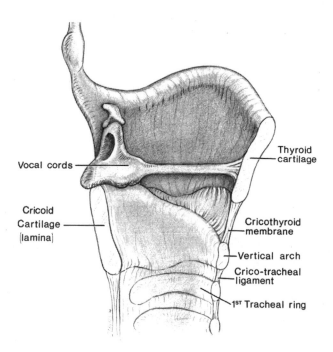

Fig. 17-1. Anatomy of the cricoid cartilage. Midsagittal view of the larynx and trachea. (From Sanchez AF: *The retrograde cookbook*, 1993, University of California-Irvine Department of Anesthesia.)

should be considered a relative contraindication, since transtracheal aspiration is performed for sputum sample in patients with pneumonia, despite the possibility of pretracheal abscess (see Complications).[5,16,108-111]

IV. ANATOMY

The performance of RI requires basic anatomic knowledge of the cricoid cartilage (Fig. 17-1) and the structures above and below it, to minimize complications and failure. Indeed, regardless of the intubation technique planned, the cricoid cartilage and CTM should be identified preoperatively in every patient.[99] Cartilage and membrane, vascular structures, and the thyroid gland are relevant anatomy.

A. CARTILAGE AND MEMBRANE

The cricoid cartilage is in the shape of signet ring (Fig. 17-1). It consists of a broad, flat, posterior plate called the lamina and a narrow, convex, anterior structure called the arch.[112,113] In most cases the cartilage can be easily palpated by identifying the thyroid notch and running a finger down the midline in a caudad direction until a rigid rounded structure is encountered. The vertical height (Fig. 17-2) of the arch is 0.5 to 0.7 cm.[113] The CTM connects the superior border of the arch to the inferior border of the thyroid cartilage and measures approximately 1 cm in height[112] and 2 cm in width.[114] The lateral borders are the paired cricothyroid muscles.[111] The cricotracheal ligament connects the

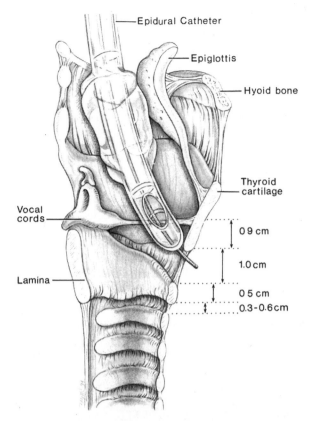

Fig. 17-2. Midsagittal view of the larynx and trachea showing the distance between the vocal cords and the upper border of the first tracheal ring. Only a small portion of the endotracheal (ET) Murphy eye is below the vocal cords. (From Sanchez AF: *The retrograde cookbook,* 1993, University of California-Irvine Department of Anesthesia.)

inferior border of the arch to the upper border of the first tracheal ring and measures 0.3 to 0.6 cm in height.[52] The distance between the inferior border of the thyroid cartilage and the vocal cords varies with gender but is approximately 0.9 cm.[115]

B. VASCULAR STRUCTURES

There are paired major blood vessels above and below the cricoid cartilage: the cricothyroid artery and the superior thyroid artery (Fig. 17-3).

The cricothyroid artery,[113-117] a branch of the superior thyroid artery, runs along the anterior surface of the CTM, usually close to the inferior border of the thyroid cartilage. In some cases the cricothyroid arteries anastomose in the midline and give rise to a descending branch that feeds the middle lobe of the thyroid gland when present. Based on dissections on cadavers performed by the author, the cricothyroid artery becomes insignificant in size as it approaches the midline. No mention of a major venous plexus could be found in the literature or in dissections by the author.

The anterior branch of the superior thyroid artery[113,115-117] runs along the upper border of the thyroid isthmus to anastomose with its counterpart from the opposite side. The inferior thyroid artery also anastomoses with the superior thyroid artery at the level of the isthmus. The arteries are remarkable for their large size and frequent anastomoses. In less than 10% of the population an unpaired thyroid ima artery ascends ventral to the trachea (from either the aortic arch or brachiocephalic artery) to anastomose at the level of the

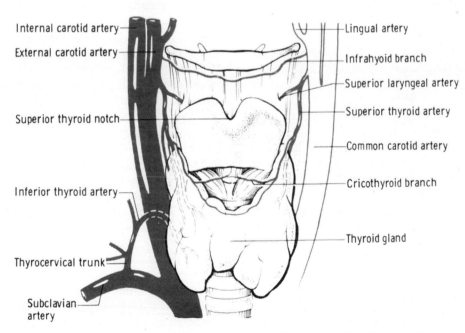

Fig. 17-3. Vascular anatomy above and below the cricoid cartilage. (Modified from Naumann H, editor: *Head and neck surgery,* Philadelphia, 1984, WB Saunders.)

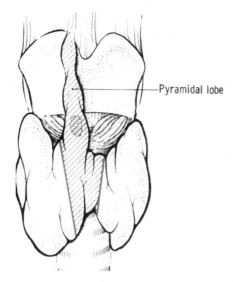

Fig. 17-4. Pyramidal lobe of the isthmus. (Modified from Naumann H, editor: *Head and neck surgery,* vol 4, Philadelphia, 1984, WB Saunders.)

isthmus. It is usually small but may be very large. A rich venous plexus is formed in and around the isthmus.

C. THYROID GLAND (ISTHMUS, PYRAMIDAL LOBE)

The isthmus of the thyroid gland (Fig. 17-3) is rarely absent and generally lies anterior to the trachea between the first and the fourth tracheal rings (usually between the second and third), although there are many variations. Its size and vertical height vary; the average vertical height and depth are 1.25 cm. Extending from the isthmus, the highly vascular pyramidal lobe (Fig. 17-4) is well developed in one third of the population. It is found more frequently on the left of the midline and may extend up to the hyoid bone. (The upper continuation is usually thyromuscular.) [51,112,113,116,117]

V. PHYSIOLOGY

Sympathetic stress response (increased heart rate, blood pressure, intraocular pressure, and intracranial pressure and elevated catecholamine levels) has been reported with laryngoscopy, endotracheal intubation, coughing, translaryngeal local anesthesia, laryngotracheal anesthesia, and fiberoptic intubation. Therefore concern is appropriate when performing RI in patients with coronary artery disease, elevated intraocular pressure, and elevated intracranial pressure. [104,105,118-125] It is reasonable to argue, however, that RI, performed skillfully, need not be more stimulating than any other technique for managing the airway.

No apparent significant changes in hemodynamics were reported in multiple case reports of patients with cardiac disease (congenital anomalies, ischemic coronary artery disease, valvular disease, pericarditis, and congestive heart failure) who underwent RI, both awake

Table 17-1. Hemodynamic effects of retrograde intubation

	Laryngoscopy	Retrograde intubation
HR	Increase	No change from baseline
MAP	Increase	No change from baseline
CI	Decrease	No change from baseline
PCWP	Increase	No change from baseline
ECG	3-mm ST depression	No change from baseline

Modified from Casthely PA et al: *Can Anaesth Soc J* 32:661, 1985. HR, heart rate; MAP, mean arterial pressure; CI, cardiac index; PCWP, pulmonary capillary wedge pressure; ECG, electrocardiogram (ST segment changes in lead V_5)

with topical anesthesia and under general anesthesia.* Casthely[49] reported 25 patients with difficult airway because of rheumatoid arthritis who came for open heart surgery (coronary artery bypass graft and valvular replacement). The patients had invasive monitors placed (Swan-Ganz catheters and peripheral arterial lines) preoperatively. The initial 24 patients underwent a cardiac induction of anesthesia (diazepam 10 mg, fentanyl 25 to 30 µg/kg and pancuronium 0.1 mg/kg) before rigid laryngoscopy followed by retrograde intubation. Comparison of hemodynamic responses to rigid laryngoscopy (Macintosh and Miller blades) versus RI demonstrated that the former was more stressful (Table 17-1). Patient no. 25 underwent RI before induction of anesthesia after application of topical anesthesia with no significant hemodynamic response.

Two case reports[27,28] documented patients with previous history of difficult airway and intracranial disease (pseudotumor cerebri and intracranial tumor with elevated intracranial pressure) who underwent elective, awake RI after topical anesthesia with no evidence of further increase in intracranial pressure.

The author, unmedicated except for topical lidocaine, underwent awake RI with no significant hemodynamic changes.[99]

VI. TECHNIQUES
A. PREPARATION
1. Positioning

The ideal position for RI is in the supine sniffing position with the neck hyperextended.[41,42] In this position the cervical vertebrae push the trachea and cricoid cartilage anteriorly and displace the strap muscles of the neck laterally. As a result, the cricoid cartilage and the structures above and below it are easier to palpate. Retrograde intubation can also be performed with the patient in a sitting position,[99] which may be the only position in which some patients can breathe comfortably. Potential cervical spine injury or limited range of motion of the cervical spine may necessitate RI with the neck in

*References 8, 18, 31, 32, 35, 43, 48, 49, 55, 66, 126.

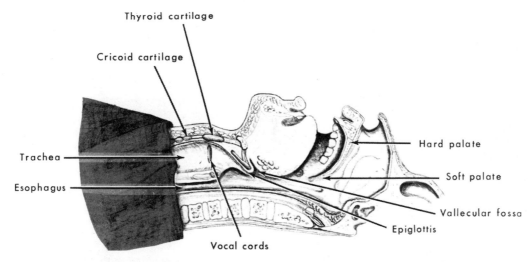

Fig. 17-5. Midsagittal view of the head and neck. (From Sanchez AF: *The retrograde cookbook,* 1993, University of California-Irvine Department of Anesthesia.)

a neutral position, which is a well-documented practice (Box 17-1).

2. Skin preparation

Although most documented retrograde intubations have not been elective, every effort should be made to perform RI using aseptic technique.

3. Anesthesia

If time permits, the airway should be anesthetized to prevent sympathetic stimulation, laryngospasm, and discomfort. In the literature many different combinations of techniques have been described as follows:

1. Translaryngeal anesthesia during intravenous sedation or general anesthesia*
2. Translaryngeal anesthesia with superior laryngeal nerve block[4,33,39]
3. Translaryngeal anesthesia with topicalization of the pharynx (aerosolized or sprayed)[10,27,63,127]
4. Glossopharyngeal nerve block and superior laryngeal nerve block with nebulized local anesthetic[31]

Refer to Chapter 9 for a detailed description of neural blockade of the airway.

In the author's experience[99] an awake RI can be performed with translaryngeal anesthesia (4 ml 2% lidocaine) supplemented with topicalization (nebulized or sprayed local anesthetics) of the pharynx and hypopharynx. Special caution should be exercised when performing the translaryngeal anesthesia, since coughing, grunting, sneezing, or swallowing causes the cricoid cartilage to travel cephalad with the potential for breaking the needle in the trachea.[128,129] To avoid this, one can insert a 20-gauge angiocatheter and remove the needle before injecting the local anesthetic.

*References 2, 6, 13, 19, 23, 28, 49.

4. Entry site

The transtracheal puncture for RI can be made either above or below the cricoid cartilage. The CTM is relatively avascular and has less potential for bleeding (see Anatomy). The disadvantage of the CTM is that initially only 1 cm of ET is actually placed below the vocal cords and the angle of entry of the ET into the trachea is more acute. A cricotracheal ligament puncture site allows a longer initial length of ET below the vocal cords. The disadvantage is that this site has more potential for bleeding (although none has been reported). Both entry sites have been used successfully. In cadaver studies[38,79] the success rate for RI was higher with less vocal cord trauma when the cricotracheal ligament rather than the CTM was used. Vocal cord trauma has not been reported in living patients.

B. CLASSIC TECHNIQUE

Classically and simply the retrograde intubation is performed percutaneously using a standard 17-gauge Tuohy needle and epidural catheter.

After positioning (Fig. 17-5), skin preparation, and anesthesia, a right-hand dominant person should stand on the right side of a supine patient. The left hand is used to stabilize the trachea by placing the thumb and third digit on either side of the thyroid cartilage. The index finger of the left hand is used to identify the midline of the CTM and the upper border of the cricoid cartilage.

Since the Tuohy needle is blunt, a small incision through the skin and subcutaneous tissue with a no. 11 scalpel blade is recommended. Because of the significant force required to perforate the skin and the CTM, there is a risk of perforating the posterior tracheal wall as well. This has been verified in cadaver studies using a fiberoptic bronchoscope (FOB).[101]

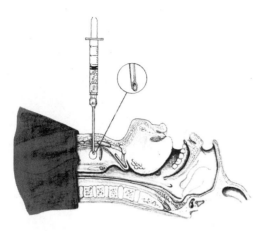

Fig. 17-6. Standard no. 17 Tuohy needle (with saline-filled syringe) is advanced (with bevel pointing cephalad) through the cricothyroid membrane (CTM) at a 90-degree angle (trying to stay as close as possible to the upper border of the cricoid cartilage). Entrance into the trachea is verified by aspiration of air. (From Sanchez AF: *The retrograde cookbook,* 1993, University of California-Irvine Department of Anesthesia.)

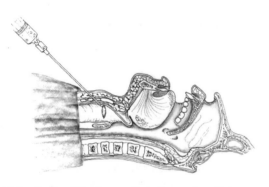

Fig. 17-7. Angle of Tuohy needle is changed to 45 degrees with bevel pointing cephalad (again verifying position by aspirating air). (From Sanchez AF: *The retrograde cookbook,* 1993, University of California-Irvine Department of Anesthesia.)

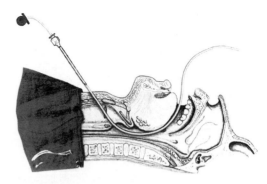

Fig. 17-8. Epidural catheter is advanced through the vocal cords and into the pharynx. During this time the patient is asked to stick tongue out, or tongue can be pulled out manually. Most of the time the epidural catheter comes out of the mouth on its own. Tuohy needle is then withdrawn to the caudal end of epidural catheter. (From Sanchez AF: *The retrograde cookbook,* 1993, University of California-Irvine Department of Anesthesia.)

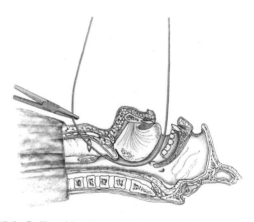

Fig. 17-9. Pull epidural catheter out of the mouth to an appropriate length; then clamp a hemostat flush with the skin. (From Sanchez AF: *The retrograde cookbook,* 1993, University of California-Irvine Department of Anesthesia.)

The right hand then grasps the Tuohy needle and saline syringe like a pencil (using the fifth digit to brace the right hand on the patient's lower neck) and performs the puncture, aspirating to confirm placement in the lumen of the airway (Figs. 17-6 and 17-7).

Once the Tuohy needle is in place, the epidural catheter is advanced into the trachea (Fig. 17-8). When advancing the epidural catheter, it is important to have the tongue pulled anteriorly to prevent the catheter from coiling up in the oropharynx. The catheter usually exits on its own from either the oral (Fig. 17-9) or nasal cavity. A hemostat should be clamped to the catheter at the neck skin line to prevent further movement of the epidural catheter. If the catheter has to be retrieved from the oropharynx, the author's preferred instrument is a nerve hook (V. Mueller NL2490, Baxter, Deerfield, Ill.). Magill forceps have been used, but these were designed to grasp large structures like an ET and may not grip the relatively small catheter (the distal tips of

the forceps do not completely occlude) and, in addition, may traumatize the pharynx.

Originally the catheter was threaded through the main distal lumen (beveled portion) of the ET. Bourke and Levesque[7] modified the technique by threading the catheter through the Murphy eye (Fig. 17-10), reasoning that this would allow an additional 1 cm of ET to pass through the cords. Lleu et al.[38,79] in cadaver studies showed that using the cricotracheal ligament as the puncture site in combination with threading the epidural catheter through the Murphy eye enhanced success over the original technique.

When the ET is being advanced over the epidural catheter (Figs. 17-11 to 17-13), a moderate amount of tension should be employed.[9,70] Excessive tension pulls the ET anteriorly, making it more likely to get caught up against the epiglottis, vallecula, or anterior commissure of the vocal cords. If there is difficulty in passing the opening of the glottis, the ET can be rotated 90 degrees

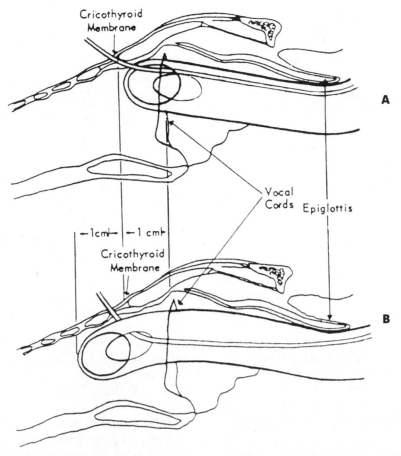

Fig. 17-10. Cross-section of larynx and trachea with ET and catheter guide passing through the CTM. **A,** Catheter passes through end of ET, and 1 cm of ET passes the cords. **B,** The catheter exits the side hole, allowing 2 cm of ET to pass beyond the vocal cords.

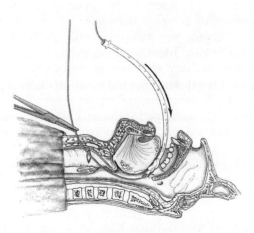

Fig. 17-11. Thread a well-lubricated endotracheal tube (ET) over the epidural catheter. Maintain a moderate amount of tension on the epidural catheter as you advance the ET *(arrow)* forward: you will feel a small click as ET travels through the vocal cords. (From Sanchez AF: *The retrograde cookbook,* 1993, University of California-Irvine Department of Anesthesia.)

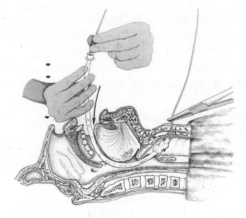

Fig. 17-12. When the ET reaches the CTM, it is important to maintain pressure *(small arrows)*, forcing the ET into the oropharynx *(large arrow)* to cause continuing pressure against the CTM with the tip of the ET. (*Note:* You are still maintaining moderate tension on the epidural catheter.) (From Sanchez AF: *The retrograde cookbook,* 1993, University of California-Irvine Department of Anesthesia.)

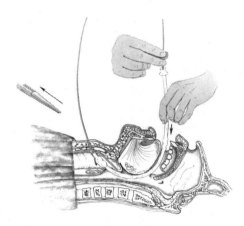

Fig. 17-13. Have an assistant remove hemostat *(large arrow)* while pressure is maintained *(small arrow)* to push the ET up against the CTM. (The epidural catheter may be cut flush with the hemostat before hemostat is removed.) (From Sanchez AF: *The retrograde cookbook,* 1993, University of California-Irvine Department of Anesthesia.)

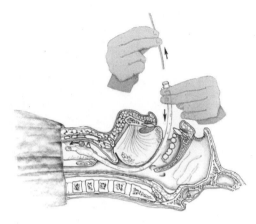

Fig. 17-14. Simultaneously *(straight arrows)* remove epidural catheter as you advance the ET. The tip of the ET will drop from its position up against the CTM to midtrachea *(curved arrow).* Advance ET to desired depth. (From Sanchez AF: *The retrograde cookbook,* 1993, University of California-Irvine Department of Anesthesia.)

counterclockwise[9,62,101] or exchanged for a smaller tube.[101]

Ideally, one would like to verify that the ET is below the vocal cords *before* removing the epidural catheter (Figs. 17-13 and 17-14). The methods are the following:

1. By direct vision, using the fiberoptic bronchoscope (see Fiberoptic Technique)
2. If the patient is breathing spontaneously, by listening to breath sounds through the endotracheal tube
3. By capnography, using a fiberoptic elbow adapter connected to a capnograph[62]

C. GUIDEWIRE TECHNIQUE

The modified technique using a guidewire* developed because the flexible epidural catheter is prone to kinking.[9,22,51] Equipment consists of an 18-gauge angiocatheter, a J-tip guidewire (0.038-inch outer diameter and 110 to 120 cm in length), and a guide catheter (Fig. 17-15).

Use of a guidewire offers the following advantages:

1. The J tip tends to be less traumatic to the airway.[15,25,50,127]
2. Retrieval of the guidewire from the oral or nasal cavity is easier.[15,26,127]
3. The guidewire is less prone to kinking.[3]
4. The guidewire can be used with the FOB (see Fiberoptic Technique).
5. The guidewire is easy to handle.[5,15,39]
6. The technique takes less time to perform than the classic technique.[26,103]

Discrepancy between the external diameter of the guidewire and the internal diameter of the ET allows a railroading effect to occur, with the tip of the ET

*References 5, 9, 11, 13-16, 18, 21, 22, 25-27, 32, 39, 50, 51, 53-56, 58, 63, 64, 67, 119-122, 127.

catching peripherally on the arytenoids or vocal cords instead of going straight through the cords. Sliding the guide catheter over the guidewire from above (antegrade) once it has exited the mouth or nose increases the external diameter of the guidewire,[62] and use of the guide catheter in combination with a smaller-diameter ET allows the ET to enter the glottis in a more centralized position with respect to the glottic opening.

Various types of antegrade guide catheters have been used: fiberoptic bronchoscopes (see next section), nasogastric tubes,[87,101] suction catheters,[17,101] plastic sheaths from Swan-Ganz catheters,[58] Eschmann's stylets[9] and tube changers.[21,25] The Cook Critical Care retrograde guidewire kit (Cook Incorporated, Bloomington, IN) contains a tapered antegrade guide catheter, which is the author's choice of antegrade guide catheters (Fig. 17-15) and is used to describe the basic guidewire and antegrade guide catheter technique.

The guidewire and antegrade guide catheter technique is as follows: Identify the trachea in Figs. 17-16 to 17-18 with the syringe and 18-gauge angiocatheter. The J wire is then fed through the intratracheal catheter (Fig. 17-19) until it passes out the mouth (Fig. 17-20). The guidewire is then clamped at the neck skin line, and the tapered antegrade guide catheter fed over the guidewire (Fig. 17-21) until the antegrade guide catheter reaches the CTM (Fig. 17-22). The ET is then fed over antegrade guide catheter (Figs. 17-23 and 17-24, p. 331) and the antegrade guide catheter is then removed (Fig. 17-25, p. 331).

Two other modifications have been reported using guide catheters. First, remove the guidewire once the guide catheter abuts against the CTM (Fig. 17-21). The guide catheter alone is then advanced further into the trachea and used as a stylet for the ET.[13,21,58] Second, perform a RI with the bare guidewire (or

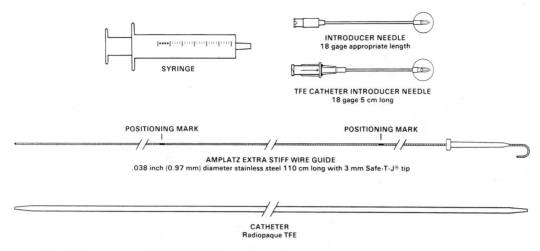

Fig. 17-15. Retrograde kit TFE (Teflon guide catheter). (From Cook Inc., Bloomington, Ind.)

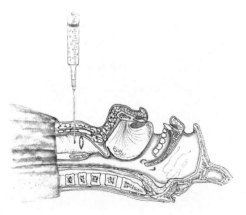

Fig. 17-16. 18-gauge Angiocatheter (18-gauge) placed at 90-degree angle to the CTM, aspirating for air to confirm position. (From Sanchez AF: *The retrograde cookbook,* 1993, University of California-Irvine Department of Anesthesia.)

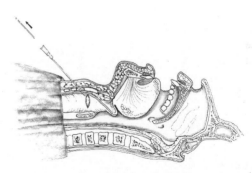

Fig. 17-18. Advance sheath of angiocatheter cephalad, and remove needle. (From Sanchez AF: *The retrograde cookbook,* 1993, University of California-Irvine Department of Anesthesia.)

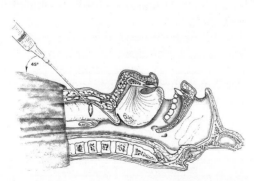

Fig. 17-17. Angle is changed to 45 degrees (again aspirating air to confirm position). (From Sanchez AF: *The retrograde cookbook,* 1993, University of California-Irvine Department of Anesthesia.)

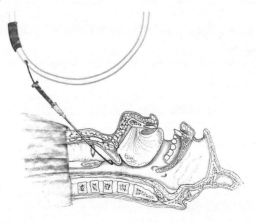

Fig. 17-19. Advance J-tip guidewire through angiocatheter sheath. (From Sanchez AF: *The retrograde cookbook,* 1993, University of California-Irvine Department of Anesthesia.)

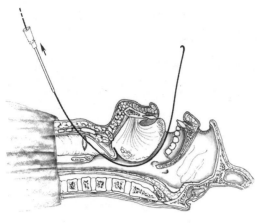

Fig. 17-20. Retrieve end of guidewire from mouth as in classic technique. Remove angiocatheter *(small arrow)*. (From Sanchez AF: *The retrograde cookbook,* 1993, University of California-Irvine Department of Anesthesia.)

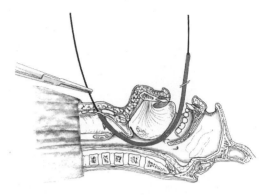

Fig. 17-22. Advance guide catheter to CTM. (From Sanchez AF: *The retrograde cookbook,* 1993, University of California-Irvine Department of Anesthesia.)

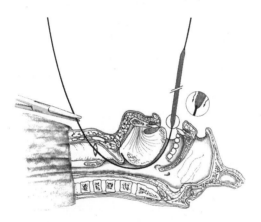

Fig. 17-21. Clamp hemostat flush with neck skin, and advance tapered tip of guide catheter *(inset)* over guidewire into mouth. (From Sanchez AF: *The retrograde cookbook,* 1993, University of California-Irvine Department of Anesthesia.)

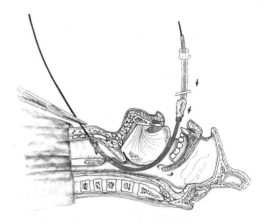

Fig. 17-23. Advance ET over entire structure *(arrows)*. Use an ET that has 6 7 mm internal diameter. Size of the ET is dictated by the external diameter of the guide catheter. (From Sanchez AF: *The retrograde cookbook,* 1993, University of California-Irvine Department of Anesthesia.)

epidural catheter) alone. Once the ET abuts the CTM, the guide catheter is advanced through the ET from above (antegrade), passing distally to the carina.[8] The guidewire is then removed and the guide catheter is again used as a stylet for the ET. In the author's opinion the best results from a blind RI would be to use the cricotracheal ligament as a puncture site and use the guide catheter over the guidewire technique.

D. FIBEROPTIC TECHNIQUE

The FOB is a versatile tool for the anesthesiologist,[117] but the FOB, like RI, has its limitations. In some cases the combination of two techniques when both alone have failed* allows achievement of tracheal intubation. The combination of RI with direct laryngoscopy[32] and RI using FOB[18,27,39,53,55] can improve the chance of successful intubation.

*References 18, 27, 32, 39, 53, 55, 62, 101.

The advantages of passing a FOB antegrade over a guidewire placed by RI are as follows:

1. The outer diameter of the guidewire and the internal diameter of the suction port of the FOB form a tight fit that prevents railroading between both cylinders, allowing the FOB to follow a straight path through the vocal cords without getting caught on anatomic structures.
2. The FOB acts as a large antegrade guide catheter (see Guidewire Technique) and prevents railroading of the ET.
3. Once the FOB has passed over the wire through the vocal cords, it can be advanced freely beyond the puncture site to the carina, which eliminates the problem of distance between vocal cords and puncture site.
4. Use of the FOB allows placement of the ET under direct vision.

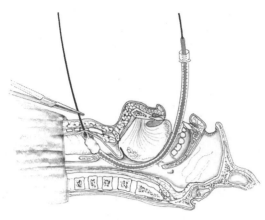

Fig. 17-24. Advance ET through vocal cords and up against the CTM. (From Sanchez AF: *The retrograde cookbook,* 1993, University of California-Irvine Department of Anesthesia.)

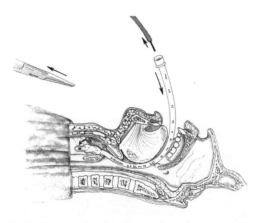

Fig. 17-25. Removal of wire and catheter as in classic technique, except the guidewire and guide catheter are removed simultaneously. (From Sanchez AF: *The retrograde cookbook,* 1993, University of California-Irvine Department of Anesthesia.)

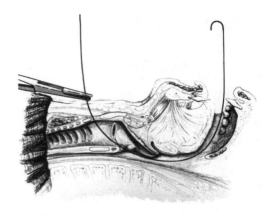

Fig. 17-26. Guidewire placed as in guidewire technique and pulled out to appropriate length to accommodate fiberoptic bronchoscope (FOB) (hemostat in place). (From Sanchez AF: *The retrograde cookbook,* 1993, University of California-Irvine Department of Anesthesia.)

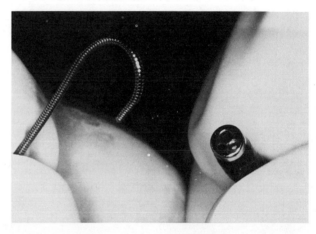

Fig. 17-27. Close-up view of J tip of guidewire and distal tip of FOB. (From Sanchez AF: *The retrograde cookbook,* 1993, University of California-Irvine Department of Anesthesia.)

5. The FOB can be used by the less experienced operator.
6. Oxygen can be delivered continuously through the FOB with the guidewire still in place (see Pediatrics).

Preparation of the FOB should be completed before RI is initiated. The rubber casing from the proximal portion of the suction port must be removed (to allow the guidewire to exit from the FOB handle), and the FOB should be armed with the appropriate ET. The RI is performed using the guidewire technique (Fig. 17-26), and the FOB then passed antegrade over the guidewire like a guide catheter (Figs. 17-27 to 17-30). Once the tip of the FOB abuts the CTM (Fig. 17-31), there are the following options:

1. Remove the guidewire distally (Fig. 17-32) or proximally (through the fiberoptic handle) and, after advancing under direct vision to the carina, intubate (Figs. 17-33 and 17-34). Removal of guidewire distally is less likely to dislodge the FOB from the trachea, but anecdote suggests that removal proximally should decrease the incidence of infection from oral contaminants.[61]
2. Instead of removing the guidewire, allow it to relax caudad into the trachea, advance the FOB below the cricoid cartilage, and then remove the guidewire. This allows for a greater length of the FOB in the trachea before the guidewire is removed.
3. Remove the guidewire proximally only until it is seen through the FOB to have popped out of the CTM and into the trachea; then advance it through the FOB to the carina. The FOB can then be advanced antegrade over the guidewire to the carina. (Caution: Be sure both ends of the guidewire are floppy.)
4. Tobias[53] used a fiberoptic technique that did not

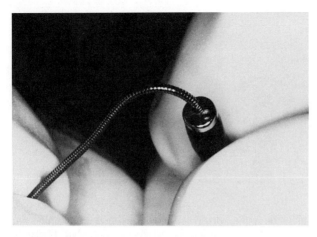

Fig. 17-28. Close-up view of J tip being fed into suction port of FOB. (From Sanchez AF: *The retrograde cookbook,* 1993, University of California-Irvine Department of Anesthesia.)

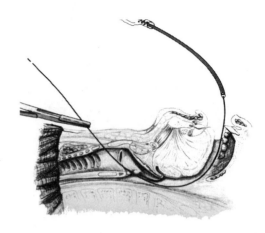

Fig. 17-30. Begin advancing the FOB (armed with the ET) over the guidewire. (From Sanchez AF: *The retrograde cookbook,* 1993, University of California-Irvine Department of Anesthesia.)

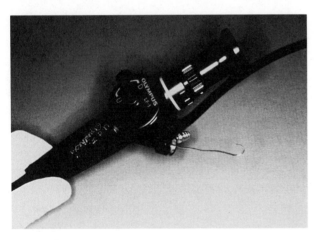

Fig. 17-29. J tip exiting from FOB handle. (From Sanchez AF: *The retrograde cookbook,* 1993, University of California-Irvine Department of Anesthesia.)

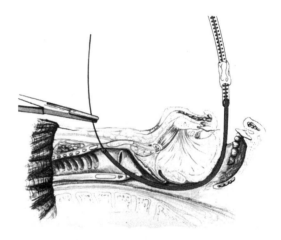

Fig. 17-31. Advance FOB to the CTM. (From Sanchez AF: *The retrograde cookbook,* 1993, University of California-Irvine Department of Anesthesia.)

make use of the suction port of the FOB. He performed a standard retrograde intubation, feeding the guidewire or epidural catheter, first, through the main lumen (bevel) of the ET and immediately exiting out of the Murphy eye. The ET was then advanced to the level of the CTM (Fig. 17-35). At this time the FOB was advanced proximally through the ET to the level of the carina. The retrograde guidewire was then removed, and a standard fiberoptic intubation was performed.

The author prefers the third option.

The combination of FOB and RI is the easiest to perform of all the RI techniques. The disadvantages are that it requires more equipment (not readily available in cases of emergency) and more preparation time and may not be suitable in certain conditions (airway with large amounts of blood or secretions).

E. SILK PULL-THROUGH TECHNIQUE

Various pull-through techniques have been described using epidural catheters,[50,90] CVP catheters,[126] monofilament sutures[10] and Fogarty catheters[89]: the silk technique is also a pull-through technique.[99-101] The basic principle involves advancing the epidural catheter retrograde as in the classic technique, attaching it to a length of silk, attaching the length of silk to the tip of the ET, and then using the catheter-silk combination to pull the ET into the trachea. The silk technique offers the following advantages:

1. Equipment is readily available in the operating room.
2. The silk is intimately attached to the ET, eliminating railroading.
3. Multiple attempts at intubation are allowed.
4. Oxygen can be delivered via the ET using a standard anesthesia circle system, and in-line

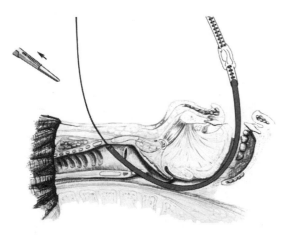

Fig. 17-32. Have assistant remove hemostat *(arrow)*. (From Sanchez AF: *The retrograde cookbook,* 1993, University of California-Irvine Department of Anesthesia.)

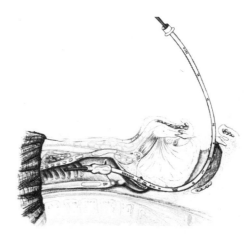

Fig. 17-34. Continue as you would in a standard fiberoptic intubation. (From Sanchez AF: *The retrograde cookbook,* 1993, University of California-Irvine Department of Anesthesia.)

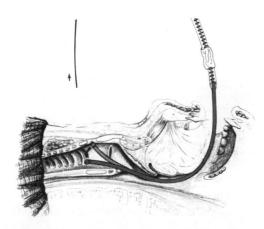

Fig. 17-33. Remove guidewire from the CTM *(straight arrow).* The tip of the FOB will then drop into midtracheal position *(curved arrow).* (From Sanchez AF: *The retrograde cookbook,* 1993, University of California-Irvine Department of Anesthesia.)

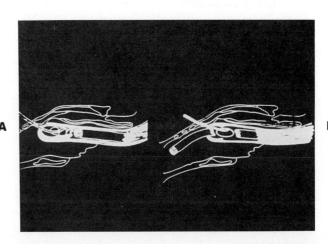

Fig. 17-35. A, Midsagittal view of the larynx with the ET tip at the level of the CTM. The FOB is advanced through the main lumen of the ET. **B,** The FOB is advanced to the level of the carina, *before* the guidewire is removed. (Modified from Tobias R: *Anesth Analg* 62:366, 1983.)

capnography can be used to verify placement of the ET.
5. If necessary, postoperative reintubation can be accomplished using the silk, which is left in place until time of discharge from the recovery room.

The silk technique employs the principles and equipment of the classic technique, with the addition of a length of silk suture (3.0 nylon monofilament may also be used). Once the epidural catheter (which is used only to place the silk) is out of the oral or nasal cavity (Fig. 17-36), the silk suture is tied to the cephalad end of the catheter (Fig. 17-36) and the silk is pulled antegrade through the CTM (Fig. 17-37). The epidural catheter is cut off and discarded (Fig. 17-37), and the cephalad end of the silk is tied to the Murphy eye (Fig. 17-38). The silk suture is then used to gently pull the ET into the trachea

(Figs. 17-38 and 17-39). When a floppy epiglottis causes obstruction, one can deliberately intubate the esophagus: as the ET is being gently withdrawn from the esophagus, tension applied simultaneously to the distal end of the silk pops the tip of the ET anteriorly, lifts up the epiglottis, and allows the ET to enter the larynx. Once the ET abuts up against the CTM, the tension on the silk suture is released (Fig. 17-40) and the ET passed further enter the trachea (Fig. 17-40).

If a nasal intubation is required, a urologic catheter can be used to cause the epidural catheter to exit the nasal rather than the oral cavity (Figs. 17-41 to 17-44).

In practice, my residents have found it difficult to suture the silk onto the epidural catheter. A small "learning curve" is required to not allow any slack on the silk until the cricothyroid membrane is reached and to

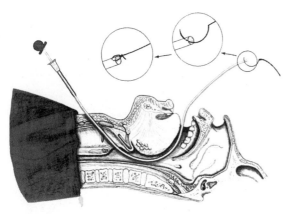

Fig. 17-36. After proceeding as in classic technique, when the epidural catheter has exited the oral cavity, it is tied to a 3.0 noncutting silk suture (30-inch length), as shown in the insets. (From Sanchez AF: *The retrograde cookbook,* 1993, University of California-Irvine Department of Anesthesia.)

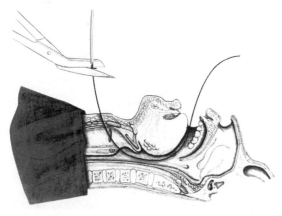

Fig. 17-37. Pull the epidural catheter caudad until the silk suture exits the skin above the CTM; then cut off the epidural catheter. (From Sanchez AF: *The retrograde cookbook,* 1993, University of California-Irvine Department of Anesthesia.)

properly gauge the fine balance between pulling on the silk and simultaneously advancing the ET. The technique is easy, and because the silk can be left in place with no discomfort for the duration of the anesthetic and after extubation, emergent reintubation can be accomplished. The author has had two occasions to reintubate in the recovery room using this technique: both patients had suffered maxillofacial trauma, had initially been intubated awake using retrograde silk technique, and had arch bars placed in the operating room.

VII. PEDIATRICS

In pediatric patients the physician is faced with the formidable problems of small anatomic structures that are difficult to palpate, immature anatomic structures such as anterior larynx and narrow cricoid cartilage, congenital anomalies, and pathologic disorders that

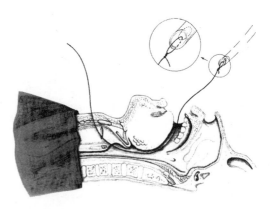

Fig. 17-38. Tie the suture to the Murphy eye as shown. Have assistant pull patient's tongue forward. Begin pulling the suture with one hand while the opposite hand holds the ET steady and in midline. At all times maintain tension on the suture while advancing the ET. (From Sanchez AF: *The retrograde cookbook,* 1993, University of California-Irvine Department of Anesthesia.)

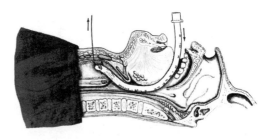

Fig. 17-39. Simultaneously pull the silk caudad *(arrow)* as you advance the ET *(arrow)* with the opposite hand. Advance ET to the CTM. (From Sanchez AF: *The retrograde cookbook,* 1993, University of California-Irvine Department of Anesthesia.)

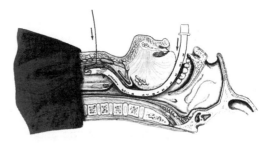

Fig. 17-40. Release the suture, and with the opposite hand advance the ET to desired depth. The suture will partially retract *(arrow)* into the trachea as the ET is advanced *(arrow)* past the CTM. The remaining suture is secured to the neck with transparent dressing. On extubation the silk is left in place as a precaution, should reintubation be required. The suture is removed in the recovery room upon patient discharge by cutting it flush with the skin and pulling it out of the oral cavity. (From Sanchez AF: *The retrograde cookbook,* 1993, University of California-Irvine Department of Anesthesia.)

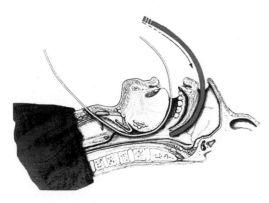

Fig. 17-41. With the epidural catheter already in place, a 16-French red rubber urologic catheter is advanced *(arrow)* through the nose. (From Sanchez AF: *The retrograde cookbook,* 1993, University of California-Irvine Department of Anesthesia.)

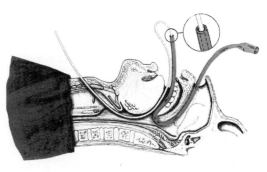

Fig. 17-43. The epidural catheter is fed into the urologic catheter *(inset)* and may be tied together. (From Sanchez AF: *The retrograde cookbook,* 1993, University of California-Irvine Department of Anesthesia.)

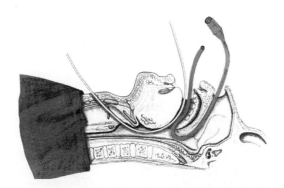

Fig. 17-42. The tip of the urologic catheter is retrieved from the oral cavity. (From Sanchez AF: *The retrograde cookbook,* 1993, University of California-Irvine Department of Anesthesia.)

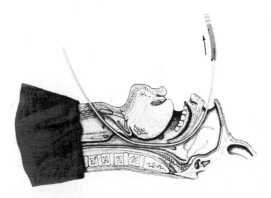

Fig. 17-44. Urologic catheter is removed *(arrow),* with the epidural catheter now exiting the nose. The epidural catheter can now be used as a nasotracheal guide. (From Sanchez AF: *The retrograde cookbook,* 1993, University of California-Irvine Department of Anesthesia.)

intimately affect the airway (e.g., acute epiglottitis). Because the pediatric airway is different, concerns have been raised as to whether RI is indicated or contraindicated in infants.[41,42,44,127] Some have claimed RI to be outright dangerous[44] without citing any clinical supportive evidence. The number of articles and case reports in the medical literature on the subject of RI in the pediatric population is limited.*

Retrograde intubation has been used in the anticipated and the unanticipated difficult pediatric airway, primarily after failure of conventional intubating techniques (blind nasal intubation, direct laryngoscopy, or fiberoptic intubation). The technique used is the same as in the adult, but a higher incidence of difficulties has been reported, including problems in cannulating the ET and the inability to pass the ET through the glottic opening.[8,39,46]

In some cases, combined techniques have offered more success than blind RI. In one case report of a 16-year-old with acute epiglottitis, intubation was ac-

complished only by RI combined with rigid laryngoscopy; the retrograde catheter marked a path through an otherwise completely distorted anatomy.[32] The largest pediatric series with the highest success rate was reported by Audenaert et al.[39]; in that series RI was performed in 20 pediatric patients, aged 1 day to 17 years, with difficult airways primarily resulting from congenital anomalies (Table 17-2). The authors' preferred approach, a combination of fiberoptic with retrograde guidewire intubation, offered the following:

1. Higher success rate
2. Faster intubation
3. Ability to insufflate oxygen through the suction port of the FOB with the guidewire in place (Table 17-3)
4. No hanging up of the ET in the glottis
5. No need to rely on anatomic landmarks to guide the FOB into the trachea
6. Less requirement for experience to manage the FOB

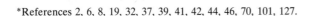

*References 2, 6, 8, 19, 32, 37, 39, 41, 42, 44, 46, 70, 101, 127.

Table 17-2. Summary of clinical approaches to pediatric patients with airways difficult to manage clinically

Case no.	Age	Weight (kg)	Primary/surgical diagnosis	Airway problems	Scope	Tube	Rationale or failed means of tracheal intubation
1	1 day	2.9	Congenital anomalies/omphalocele	Micrognathia, nonvisualization	AUR-8	3.0	A,D
2	6 mo	4.5	Congenital anomalies/bilateral radial club hand	Nonvisualization	AUR-8	3.0	D
3	7 mo	5.7	Amyoplasia/congenital hip dislocation	Micrognathia, nonvisualization, limited mouth opening	AUR-8	4.0	A,D,F*
4	8 mo	6.8	Amyoplasia/clubfoot	Micrognathia, limited mouth opening, nonvisualization	AUR-8	4.0	A,D
5	10 mo	4.9	Pierre Robin syndrome/cleft palate	Micrognathia, nonvisualization	AUR-8	3.5	A,D
6	11 mo	7.8	Arthrogryposis/clubfoot	Klippel-Feil, micrognathia	AUR-8	4.0	A
7	15 mo	8.0	Undiagnosed congenital anomalies/congenital hip dislocation	Nonvisualization	AUR-8	4.0	D
8	24 mo	13.2	Hurler's syndrome/bone marrow transplant	Short neck, large tongue, limited neck motion, nonvisualization	AUR-8	4.0	A,D
9	26 mo	11.4	Camptomelic dysplasia/cervical fusion	Cervical spine abnormalities and instability, limited motion of neck, mouth	AUR-8	3.0	A,C
10	3 yr	11.2	Hallermann-Streiff syndrome/ophthalmologic procedures	Narrowed trachea, micrognathia, malar hypoplasia, microstomia, nonvisualization	AUR-8	4.5	A,D
11	5 yr (6 yr)	15.1 (16.9)	Escobar syndrome (multiple pterygium)/orthopedic and plastic procedures	Klippel-Feil, brevicollis, limited mouth and neck motion, nonvisualization	LF-1	5.0	A,D
12	6 yr	11.3	Multiple congenital anomalies/infantile scoliosis	Micrognathia, cervical hemivertebra, limited mouth opening, nonvisualization	LF-1	5.0	H,A, D,R,F*
13	7 yr	17.1	Spondyloepiphyseal dysplasia congenital/C1-2 subluxation	C-spine abnormalities	LF-1	5.5	C
14	7 yr (7 yr)	15.9 (17.1)	Schwartz-Jampel syndrome/C2-3 subluxation	Microstomia, limited neck, mouth motion, C-spine abnormalities	LF-1	5.0	A,C
15	9 yr	14	Cerebral palsy/congenital hip dislocation	Nonvisualization	AUR-8	5.5	D
16	12 yr	22	Escobar syndrome (multiple pterygium)/scoliosis	Klippel-Feil, brevicollis, limited mouth, neck motion, micrognathia nonvisualization	LF-1	5.5	A,D,L
17	12 yr	15.2	Undiagnosed congenital progressive neuromuscular disease/extreme cervicothoracolumbar fixed lordosis for release and fusion	Extreme fixed cervicothoracic lordosis, micrognathia nonvisualization	AUR-8	5.0	A,D
18	14 yr	51	Juvenile rheumatoid arthritis/joint fusion	Limited motion, neck and mouth	LF-1	5.5	H,A
19	15 yr	71	Juvenile rheumatoid arthritis/phalangeal replacements	Limited motion, neck and mouth	LF-1	6.0	H,A
20	17 yr	74	Trauma/cervical spine and facial fractures	Facial fractures, in cervical traction, unstable cervical spine	LF-1	7.5	C

From Audenaert SM et al: *Anesth Analg* 73:660, 1991.

*Use of a Bullard rigid fiberoptic laryngoscope afforded an excellent view of the vocal cords, but owing to limited mouth opening the endotracheal tube could not be properly positioned.

Case numbers have been assigned for reference and convenience only. The tracheas of patients 11 and 14 have each been intubated twice with retrograde-assisted fiberoptic technique. Under "airway problems," nonvisualization refers to failure to expose the cords or arytenoid cartilages with direct laryngoscopy. On all occasions where the AUR-8 scope was used, the 22-gauge catheter and 0.018-in wire (see text) were also used. Likewise, where the LF-1 scope was used, the 20-gauge catheter and 0.025-in wire (see text) were used. "Tube" refers to the endotracheal tube's internal diameter in millimeters. The "rationale or failed means of tracheal intubation" column reveals a few patients where this technique was used primarily, usually for cervical spine consideration (C) or when the airway was known to be extremely difficult by history/previous experience (H), or by preoperative assessment (A). Direct laryngoscopy (D), fiberoptic laryngoscopy (F), lightwand (L), and retrograde alone (R) techniques were attempted unsuccessfully where so noted.

Table 17-3. Flow measurement of various fiberscopes

Scope (mfg)	Outer scope diameter (mm)	Inner lumen diameter (mm)	Working length (cm)	Maximum tip flexion (°)	Scope configuration	Maximum O_2 flow (L/min)
AUR-8 (Circon ACMI)	2.7	0.8	37	140	Straight	9.4 ± 0.1
					90° curve and 90° tip flexion	9.4 ± 0.0
					90° curve with 0.018-in wire in place	4.37 ± 0.01
LF-1 (Olympus)	3.8	1.2	60	120	Straight	18.1 ± 0.2
					90° curve and 90° tip flexion	17.9 ± 0.1
					90° curve with 0.025-in wire in place	12.4 ± 0.1
BF-1 (Olympus)	5.9	2.8	55	100	Straight	159 ± 5
					90° curve and 90° tip flexion	152 ± 1
					90° curve with 0.035-in wire in place	145 ± 1

From Audenaert SM et al: *Anesth Analg* 73:660, 1991.
Flow measurements represent mean ± SD.
Mfg, manufacturer.

No major complications were reported, and the technique was considered a valuable addition to pediatric airway management.

VIII. COMPLICATIONS AND CAUTIONS

Although it has been demonstrated that transtracheal needle puncture is safe and is associated with only minor complications (Box 17-4), numerous potential complications of RI have been cited in the literature (Box 17-5). Documented complications from RI are relatively few, and most were self-limited (Box 17-6). The most common complications were bleeding* and subcutaneous emphysema.[3,33,37]

A. BLEEDING

With RI one can expect insignificant bleeding (four to five drops of blood) with CTM puncture.[3,70] Even a patient who received heparin intraoperatively and had postoperative disseminated intravascular coagulation had only a small, self-limited hematoma.[49] Controversy exists with respect to making the puncture below the cricoid cartilage because of a greater potential for bleeding.[2,50,79] Three studies[33,37,50] involving 57 patients who underwent RI with punctures at the cricotracheal ligament or between the second and third tracheal ring showed no evidence of major bleeding. There are, however, scattered reports of severe hemoptysis following transtracheal needle puncture with resultant hypoxia, cardiorespiratory arrest, dysrhythmias, and death.[106,107,130-132] Two patients had epistaxis[51,70] after nasal intubation. (No vasoconstricting agent was used.) The following measures have been suggested to decrease the potential for bleeding:

1. Avoid RI in patients with bleeding diathesis.
2. Apply pressure to the puncture site for 5 minutes.

*References 3, 4, 16, 33, 36, 49, 50, 70.

BOX 17-4   Translaryngeal anesthesia (complications)

17,500 reported cases

2 broken needles
2 laryngospasms
4 soft tissue infections

Modified from Gold MI, Buechel DR: *Anesthesiology* 20:181, 1959.

BOX 17-5   Potential complications of retrograde intubation

Esophageal perforation
Hemoptysis
Intratracheal submucosal hematoma with distal obstruction
Laryngeal edema
Laryngospasm
Pretracheal infection
Tracheal fistula
Tracheitis
Vocal cord damage

From UCI Department of Anesthesia: *Teaching aids.*

---

3. Apply pressure dressing to the puncture site for 24 hours.
4. Maintain patient in the supine position for 3 to 4 hours after puncture.

B. SUBCUTANEOUS EMPHYSEMA*

Subcutaneous emphysema localized to the area of a transtracheal needle puncture site is common but self-limited. In severe cases air may track through the fascial planes of the neck, leading to tracheal compres-

*References 3, 33, 37, 93, 104, 105, 129, 132-136.

BOX 17-6   Reported complications of retrograde intubation

Self-limited

Bleeding
    Puncture site, 8
    Peritracheal hematoma, 1
    Epistaxis, 2
Subcutaneous emphysema, 4
Pneumomediastinum, 1
Breath holding, 1
Catheter traveling caudad,[1] 2

Not self-limited

Trigeminal n. trauma, 1
Pneumothorax, 1
Loss of hook,[2] 2

From UCI Department of Anesthesia: *Teaching aids.*
[1]Refers to catheter traveling in a caudad direction toward the lungs instead of cephalad towards the oral cavity.
[2]Refers to Dr. Waters' technique of retrieving catheter from nasopharynx using a self-made hook. From Waters DJ: *Anaesthesia* 18:158, 1963.

sion with airway compromise, pneumomediastinum, and pneumothorax.* Accumulation of air occurs gradually[93,134] in 1 to 6 hours after a transtracheal puncture. Severe subcutaneous emphysema has been attributed to use of a large-bore needle and exposure of the puncture site to persistent elevated intratracheal pressure (coughing, grunting, or sneezing). In addition, pneumomediastinum has been reported in patients who underwent transtracheal puncture with a needle and was attributed to elevated endotracheal pressure (paroxysmal coughing and sneezing).[93,106,108] Once the patient has been intubated via the retrograde technique, elevated peak inspiratory and/or end-expiratory pressures (PIP and PEEP, respectively) should not increase the likelihood of these complications intraoperatively, since the puncture site would be located above the ET cuff. The result is that the area of the initial puncture site would not be exposed to high pressure. Lee et al.[35] reported a patient (history of noncardiogenic pulmonary edema and atelectasis) who, after RI, received 7.5 cm of water with PEEP (PIP values were not reported) with no complications.

C. OTHER COMPLICATIONS

Other reported self-limited complications were breath holding[70] and the catheter (a straight, flexible guidewire) traveling caudally.[37,67]

Complications that were not self-limited were as follows:

*References 68, 93, 104, 105, 107, 128, 134, 135.

1. Trigeminal nerve trauma,[47] which the author suspects was due to multiple laryngoscopies
2. Guidewire fracture, in which wire had to be surgically removed[48]
3. Loss of hook (the type that was originally used by Waters and is no longer used)[2,46,70]
4. Pneumothorax, which necessitated a chest tube[93]

IX. CONCLUSION

The anesthesiologist is charged with the responsibility for securing the airway. In the vast majority of cases this can be accomplished using conventional techniques, but in a small number of cases these techniques cannot be successfully applied to the clinical problem at hand. No method, including RI, offers 100% success; therefore it is wise to have multiple available options and to be facile with alternative techniques for intubation.

Retrograde intubation has been a particularly useful alternative in difficult intubations after multiple manipulations have caused bleeding, in facial injuries where bleeding is already present, and in patients with limited neck movement and mouth opening. The technique is easy to learn, requires little equipment, and in practiced hands is a rapid, safe, and effective method for intubating the trachea.

In the author's opinion, RI is a valuable additional airway management technique and should be included as part of the armamentarium of physicians involved in the care of seriously injured or ill patients.

ACKNOWLEDGMENTS

Dedicated to my daughter Danielle. With special thanks to Dr. Debra E. Morrison for her long hours at the editing table, Tay McClellan for her outstanding medical illustration, Mr. Seath Eaker for his research assistance, and Doreen Hasson for her renowned secretarial work.

REFERENCES

1. Butler FS, Cirillo AA: Retrograde tracheal intubation, *Anesth Analg* 39:333, 1960.
2. Waters DJ: Guided blind endotracheal intubation: for patients with deformities of the upper airway, *Anaesthesia* 18:158, 1963.
3. Powell WF, Ozdil T: A translaryngeal guide for tracheal intubation, *Anesth Analg* 46:231, 1967.
4. Barriot P, Riou B: Retrograde technique for tracheal intubation in trauma patients, *Crit Care Med* 16:712, 1988.
5. McNamara RM: Retrograde intubation of the trachea, *Ann Emerg Med* 16:680, 1987.
6. Borland LM, Swan DV: Difficult pediatric endotracheal intubation: a new approach to the retrograde technique, *Anesthesiology* 55:577, 1981.
7. Bourke D, Levesque PR: Modification of retrograde guide for endotracheal intubation, *Anesth Analg* 53:1013, 1974.
8. Cooper CMS, Murray-Wilson A: Retrograde intubation: management of a 4.8 kg. 5-month infant, *Anaesthesia* 42:1197, 1988.
9. Freund PR, Rooke A, Schwid H: Retrograde intubation with a modified Eschmann stylet, *Anesth Analg* 67:596, 1988 (letter).

10. Harrison CA, Wise CC: Retrograde intubation *Anaesthesia* 43:609, 1988 (letter).

11. Yealy DM, Paris PM: Recent advances in airway management, *Emerg Med Clin North Am* 7:83, 1989.

12. Cossham PS: Difficult intubation, *Br J Anaesth* 57:239, 1985.

13. King HK, Wang LF, Khan AK: Translaryngeal guided intubation for difficult intubation, *Crit Care Med* 15:869, 1987.

14. King HK, Wang LF, Wooten DJ: Endotracheal intubation using translaryngeal guided intubation vs percutaneous retrograde guidewire insertion, *Crit Care Med* 15:183, 1987 (letter).

15. Gerenstein RI, Arria-Devoe G: J-wire and translaryngeal guided intubation, *Crit Care Med* 17:486, 1989 (letter).

16. Guggenberger H, Lenz G: Training in retrograde intubation, *Anesthesiology* 69:292, 1980 (letter).

17. Harmer M, Vaughan R: Guided blind oral intubation, *Anaesthesia* 35:921, 1986 (letter).

18. Lechman MJ, Donahoo JS, Macvaugh H: Endotracheal intubation using percutaneous retrograde guidewire insertion followed by antegrade fiberoptic bronchoscopy, *Crit Care Med* 14:589, 1986.

19. Manchester GH, Mani MM, Master FW: A simple method for emergency orotracheal intubation, *Plast Reconstr Surg* 49:312, 1972.

20. Payne KA: Difficult tracheal intubation, *Anaesth Intensive Care* 8:84, 1980.

21. King KK et al: Antegrade vs retrograde insertion introducer for guided intubation in needle laryngostomized patient, *Can J Anaesth* 68:823, 1989.

22. Heller EM, Schneider K, Saven B: Percutaneous retrograde intubation, *Laryngoscope* 99:555, 1989.

23. Rossini L: The tunneling technique: an approach to difficult intubations, *J Am Assoc Nurse Anesth* 52:189, April, 1984.

24. Gordon RA: Anesthetic management of patients with airway problems, *Int Anesthesiol Clin* 10:37, 1972.

25. Hines MH, Meredith JW: Modified retrograde intubation technique for rapid airway access, *Am J Surg* 159:597, 1990.

26. Stern Y, Spitzer T: Retrograde intubation of the trachea, *J Laryngol Otol* 105:746, 1991.

27. Gupta B, McDonald JS, Brooks HJ: Oral fiberoptic intubation over a retrograde guidewire, *Anesth Analg* 68:517, 1989.

28. Amanor-Boadu SD: Translaryngeal guided intubation in a patient with raised intracranial pressure, *Afr J Med Med Sci* 21:65, 1992.

29. Talyshkhanov KK: Retrograde intubation of the trachea, *Anesteziol Reanimatol*, 5,6:58, 1992.

30. Yoneda I, Nakamura M, Satoh T: A simple method of retrograde intubation, *Masui (Jpn J Anesthesiol)* 40:124, 1991.

31. Pintanel T, Font M, Aguilar JL et al: Intubation orotracheal retrograde (Cartas al director), *Rev Esp Anestesiol Reanim* 35:344, 1988.

32. Heslet L, Christensen KS, Sanchez R et al: Facilitated blind intubation using a transtracheal guide wire, *Dan Med Bull* 32:275, 1985.

33. Mahiou, Bouvet FR, Korach JM: Proceedings of the thirty-first Congress De Intubation Tracheal, July 14, 1983 Intubation retrograde (abstract R26) Paris.

34. Stordahl A, Syrovy G: Blind endotracheal intubation over retrograde, *Tidsskr Nor Laegeforen* 106:1590, 1986.

35. Lee YW, Lee YS, Kim JR: Retrograde tracheal intubation, *Yonsei Med J* 28:228, 1987.

36. Guggenberger H, Lenz G, Heumann H: Success rate and complications of a modified guided blind technique for intubation in 36 patients, *Anaesthesist* 36:703, 1987.

37. VanNiekerk JV, Smalhout B: Retrograde endotracheal intubation using a catheter, *Ned Tijdschr Geneeskd*, 131:1663, 1987.

38. Lleu JC, Forrler M, Forrler C et al: L'intubation oro-tracheale par void retrograde, *Ann Fr Anesth Reanim* 8:632, 1989.

39. Audenaert SM, Montgomery CL, Stone B: Retrograde-assisted fiberoptic tracheal intubation in children with difficult airways, *Anesth Analg* 73:660, 1991.

40. Scurr C: A complication of guided blind intubation, *Anaesthesia* 30:411, 1975 (letter).

41. France NK, Beste DJ: Anesthesia for pediatric ear, nose and throat surgery. In Gregory GA, editor: *Pediatric anesthesia,* ed 2, New York, 1989, Churchill Livingstone.

42. Gregory GA: Induction of anesthesia. In Gregory GA, editor: *Pediatric anesthesia,* ed 2, New York, 1989, Churchill Livingstone.

43. Schmidt SI, Hasewinkel JV: Retrograde catheter-guided direct laryngoscopy, *Anesthesiology Rev* 16:6, 1989.

44. Levin RM: Anesthesia for cleft lip and cleft palate, *Anesthesiology Rev* 6:25, 1979.

45. Lopez G, James NR: Mechanical problems of the airway, *J Clin Anesth* 36:8, 118-122, 1984.

46. Akinyemi OO, John A: A complication of guided blind intubation, *Anaesthesia* 29:733, 1974.

47. Faithfull NS: Injury to terminal branches of the trigeminal nerve following tracheal intubation, *Br J Anaesth* 57:535, 1985.

48. Contrucci RB, Gottlieb JS: A complication of retrograde endotracheal intubation, *Ear Nose Throat J* 69:776, 1989.

49. Casthely PA, Landesman S, Fynaman PN: Retrograde intubation in patients undergoing open heart surgery, *Can Anaesth Soc J* 32:661, 1985.

50. Abou-Madi MN, Trop D: Pulling versus guiding: a modification of retrograde guided intubation, *Can J Anaesth* 36:336, 1989.

51. Corleta O, Habazettl H, Kreimeier U: Modified orotracheal intubation technique for airway access in rabbits, *Eur Surg Res* 24:129, 1992.

52. Shantha TR: Retrograde intubation using the subcricoid region, *Br J Anaesth* 68:109, 1992.

53. Tobias R: Increased success with retrograde guide for endotracheal intubation, *Anesth Analg* 62:366, 1983 (letter).

54. Roberts KW: New use for Swan-Ganz introducer wire, *Anesth Analg* 60:67, 1981 (letter).

55. Carlson CA, Perkins HM: Solving a difficult intubation, *Anesthesiology* 64:537, 1986.

56. Dhara SS: Retrograde intubation: a facilitated approach, *Br J Anaesth* 69:631, 1992.

57. King KH, Wang LF, Khan AK: Soft and firm introducers for translaryngeal guided intubation, *Anesth Analg* 68:826, 1989 (letter).

58. King HK: Translaryngeal guided intubation using a sheath stylet, *Anesthesiology* 63:567, 1985.

59. King HK: Translaryngeal guided intubation, *Anesth Analg* 64:650, 1985 (letter).

60. Poradowska-Jeszke M, Falkiewicz H: Intubation retrograde chez un nourrisson atteint de maladie de Pierre Robin, *Cah Anesthesiol* 37:605, 1989.

61. Rizzi F, Ambroselli V, Mezzetti MG: Sull'impiego dell'intubazione retrograda in emergenza, *Minerva Anestesiol* 57:1705, 1991.

62. Benumof JL: Management of the difficult adult airway, *Anesthesiology* 75:1087, 1991.

63. Alfery DD: Double-lumen endobronchial tube intubation using retrograde wire technique, *Anesth Analg* 76:1374, 1993 (letter).

64. Gerenstein RI: J-wire facilitates translaryngeal guided intubation, *Anesthesiology* 76:1059, 1992 (letter).

65. Benumof JL: Retrograde intubation, *Anesthesiology* 76:1060, 1992 (letter).

66. Maestro CM, Andujar MJJ, Sancho CJ et al: Intubacion retrograda en un paciente con una malformacion epiglotica (Cartas al director), *Rev Esp Anestesiol Reanim* 35:344, 1988.

67. Criado A, Planas A: Intubacion orotraqueal retrograda (Cartas al director), *Rev Esp Anestesiol Reanim* 35:344, 1988.

68. Van Der Laan KT, Bllast B, Wouters B: Retrograde endotracheale intubatie met behulp van een catheter, *Ned Tijdschr Geneeskd* 131:2324, 1987.

69. Williamson R: Pediatric intubation: retrograde or blind? *Anaesthesia* 42:802, 1988 (letter).

70. Akinyemi OO: Complications of guided blind endotracheal intubation, *Anaesthesia* 34:590, 1979.

71. King HK, Khan AK, Wooten DJ: Translaryngeal guided intubation solved a critical airway problem, *J Clin Anesth* 1:112, 1988.

72. King HK: Translaryngeal guided intubation: a lifesaving technique. A review and case report, *Anesth Sinica* 22:279, 1984.

73. Faithfull NS: Retrograde intubation. Summary of papers presented at the sixth European Congress, *Anaesthesia* (suppl 22)1:458, 1982.

74. Latto IP, Rosen M, editors: *Management of difficult intubation: difficulties in tracheal intubation,* 1984, Balliere Tindall.

75. Dhara SS: Guided blind endotracheal intubation, *Anaesthesia* 35:81, 1980 (letter).

76. Graham WP III, Kilgore ES III: Endotracheal intubation in complicated cases, *Hosp Physicians* 3:60, 1987.

77. Mclean D: Guided blind oral intubation, *Anaesthesia* 37:605, 1982 (letter).

78. Ward CF, Salvatierra: Special intubation techniques for the adult patient. *Clinical procedures in anesthesia and intensive care,* New York, 1992, JB Lippincott.

79. Lleu JC, Forrler M, Pottecher T: Retrograde intubation using the subcricoid region, *Br J Anaesth* 55:855, 1983 (letter).

80. Shantha TR: Retrograde intubation, *Br J Anaesth* 55:855, 1983 (letter).

81. Dennison PH: Four experiences in intubation of one patient with Still's disease, *Br J Anaesth* 50:636, 1978.

82. Greaves JD: Endotracheal intubation in Still's disease, *Br J Anaesth* 51:75, 1979.

83. Salem MR, Mathrubhutham M, Bennett EJ et al: Difficult intubation: medical intelligence current concepts, *N Engl J Med* 295:879, 1976.

84. Linscott MS, Horton WC: Management of upper airway obstruction, *Otolaryngol Clin North Am* 12:351, 1979.

85. Roberts JR: *Clinical procedures in emergency medicine,* Philadelphia, 1985, WB Saunders.

86. Miller RD: Endotracheal intubation. In *Anesthesia,* ed 3, New York, 1986, Churchill Livingstone.

87. Luhrs R, Fuller E: A case study: the use of trans-tracheal guide for a patient with a large protruding oral myxoma, *J Am Assoc Nurse Anesth* 55:81, 1987.

88. Layman PR: An alternative to blind intubation, *Anaesthesia* 38:165, 1983.

89. Carlson RR, Sadove MS: Guided non-visualized nasal endotracheal intubation using a transtracheal Fogarty catheter, *Illinois Med J* 143:364, 1973.

90. Kubo K, Takahashi S, Oka M: A modified technique of guided blind intubation in oral surgery, *J Maxillofac Surg* 8:135, 1980.

91. Ramsay MAE, Salyer KE: The management of a child with a major airway abnormality, *Plast Reconstr Surg* 67:668, 1981.

92. Reynaud J, Lacour M, Diop L et al: Intubation tracheale guidee a bouche fermee (technic de D.J. Waters), *Bull Soc Med Afr Noire Lang Fr* 12:774, 1967.

93. Poon YK: Case history number 89: A life-threatening complication of cricothyroid membrane puncture, *Anesth Analg* 55:298, 1976.

94. Riou B: Intubation difficile. In *Conference d'actualisation, 1990, Societe Francaise d'Anesthesie Reanimation,* Paris, July 3, 1990, Masson.

95. Faithfull NS, Erdmann W, Groenland THN: Alternatieve intubatie routes, *Ned Tijdschr voor Anaesthesie-medewerkers* 25:8, 1985.

96. Finucane BT, Santora AH: *Principles of airway management,* Philadelphia, 1988, FA Davis.

97. Yonfa AE et al: Retrograde approach to nasotracheal in a child with severe Pierre Robin syndrome, *Anesthesiol Rev,* 10:28, 1983.

98. Sanchez AS: Retrograde intubation in the llama. Presented at the American Association of Zoological Veterinarians, annual meeting, St Louis, Nov. 3, 1993.

99. Sanchez AS: ASA airway safety video. II. Cricothyroid membrane. 1992.

100. Sanchez AF: Preventing the difficult from becoming the impossible airway: retrograde intubation. Presented at the annual meeting of the American Society of Anesthesiologist, Las Vegas, Oct. 16, 1990.

101. Sanchez AS: The retrograde cookbook. Presented at the first international symposium on the difficult airway Newport Beach, California 1993.

102. ASA Difficult Airway Task Force: Practice guidelines for management of the difficult airway, *Anesthesiology* 78:597-602, 1993.

103. Van Stralen DW, Rogers M, Perkin RM et al: Retrograde intubation training using mannequin. Presented at the eighth annual conference of the National Association of EMS Physicians, June 16, 1992 (abstract).

104. Ovassapian A: Topical anesthesia. In *Fiberoptic airway endoscopy in anesthesia and critical care,* New York, 1990, Raven.

105. Ovassapian A: Fiberoptic tracheal intubation. In *Fiberoptic airway endoscopy in anesthesia and critical care,* ed 3, New York, 1990, Raven.

106. Kalinske RW, Parker RH, Brandt D: Diagnostic usefulness and safety of transtracheal aspiration, *N Engl J Med* 276:604, 1967.

107. Unger KM, Moser KM: Fatal complication of transtracheal aspiration: a report of two cases, *Arch Intern Med* 132:437, 1973.

108. Ries K, Levison ME, Kaye D et al: Transtracheal aspiration in pulmonary infection, *Arch Intern Med* 133:453, 1974.

109. Green DC, Strait GB: A complication of transtracheal anesthesia: nocardia cellulitis, *Ann Thorac Surg* 8:561, 1969.

110. Yoshikawa TT, Chow AW, Montgomerie JZ et al: Paratracheal abscess: an unusual complication of transtracheal aspiration, *Chest* 65:105, 1974.

111. Deresinski SC, Stevens DA: Anterior cervical infections: complications of transtracheal aspirations, *Am Rev Respir Dis* 110:354, 1974.

112. Caparosa RJ, Zavatsky AR: Practical aspects of the cricothyroid space, *Laryngoscope* 67:577, 1957.

113. Clemente C: *Gray's anatomy,* ed 13, 1985, Lea & Febiger.

114. Kress TD, Balasubramaniam S: Cricothyroidotomy, *Ann Emerg Med* 11:197, 1982.

115. Naumann H: *Head and neck surgery,* Philadelphia, 1984, WB Saunders.

116. Bergman R, Thompson S, Afifi AK et al: *Compendium of human anatomic variation: text, atlas, and world literature,* Baltimore, Munich, 1988, Urban & Schwarzenberg.

117. Anson BJ: *Morris human anatomy: a complete system treatise,* ed 12, New York, 1966, McGraw-Hill.

118. Kaplan JA: Postoperative respiratory care. In *Thoracic anesthesia* New York, 1983, Churchill Livingstone.

119. Miller RD: *Anesthesia,* ed 3, vol 2, New York, 1990, Churchill Livingstone. Shapiro HM and Drummond JC: Neurosurgical "Anesthesia and Intracranial Hypertension," pg 1737-89, 1990.

120. Stone DJ, Gal TJ: Airway management. In Miller RD, editor: *Anesthesia,* ed 3, vol 2, New York, 1990, Churchill Livingstone.

121. Wedel DJ, Brown DL: Nerve blocks. In Miller RD, editor: *Anesthesia,* ed 3, vol 2, New York, 1990, Churchill Livingstone.

122. Shapiro HM, Drummond JC: Neurosurgical anesthesia and intracranial hypertension. In Miller RD, editor: *Anesthesia,* ed 3, vol 2, New York, 1990, Churchill Livingstone.

123. Barash PG, Cullen BF, Stoelting RK, editors: *Clinical anesthesia,* Philadelphia, 1989, JB Lippincott.
124. Cuchiara RF, Black S, Steinkeler JA: Anesthesia for intracranial procedures. In Barash PG, Cullen BF, Stoelting RK, editors: *Clinical anesthesia,* Philadelphia, 1989, JB Lippincott.
125. Stehling SC: Management of the airway. In Barash PG, Cullen BF, Stoelting RK, editors: *Clinical anesthesia,* Philadelphia, 1989, JB Lippincott.
126. Raza S, Levinsky L, Lajos TZ: Transtracheal intubation: useful adjunct in cardiac surgical anesthesia, *J Thorac Cardiovasc Surg* 76:721, 1978.
127. Dailey RD, Simon B: Retrograde tracheal intubation. In Purcell T, editor: *The airway emergency management,* St Louis, 1992, Mosby.
128. Willson JKV: Cricothyroid bronchography with a polyethylene catheter: description of a new technique, *Am J Roentgenol* 81:305, 1959.
129. Newman J, Schultz S, Langevin RE: Bronchography by cricothyroid catheterization, *Laryngoscope* 75:774, 1965.
130. Spencer CD, Beaty HN: Complications of transtracheal aspiration, *N Engl J Med* 286:304, 1972.
131. Schillaci RF, Iacovoni VE, Conte RS et al: Transtracheal aspiration complicated by fatal endotracheal hemorrhage, *N Engl J Med* 295:9, 488, 1976.
132. Hemley SD, Arida EJ, Diggs AM et al: Percutaneous cricothyroid membrane bronchography, *Radiology* 76:763, 1961.
133. Hahn HH, Beaty HN: Transtracheal aspiration in the evaluation of patients with pneumonia, *Ann Intern Med* 72:183, 1970.
134. Massey JY: Complications of transtracheal aspiration: a case report, *J Arkansas Med Soc* 67:254, 1971.
135. Won KH, Rowland DW, Croteau JR et al: Massive subcutaneous emphysema complicating transcricothyroid bronchography, *Am J Roentgenol Radium Ther Nucl Med* 101:953, 1967.
136. Radigan LR, King RD: A technique for the prevention of postoperative atelectasis, *Surgery* 47:184, 1960.

Chapter 18

ILLUMINATING STYLET (LIGHTWAND)

Orlando R. Hung
Ronald D. Stewart

I. INTRODUCTION

Although a prompt, accurate placement of an endotracheal tube (ET) is one of the most important aspects of modern airway management, the concept of placing an ET is almost 1000 years old. The procedure was first performed on pigs by the Arab Avicenna between 980 and 1037,[1,2] but it was not until 1796 that Herholdt and Rafn[3] described the blind tactile digital intubation in a resuscitation protocol for drowning victims.[3] MacEwen[4] later reported the placement of a curved metal tube into the trachea orally by tactile means in awake patients in 1880. However, modern methods of tracheal intubation did not emerge until early in the 20th century following the introduction of a flexible metal tube by Kuhn and a laryngoscope by Jackson.[5]

Over the years laryngoscopic intubation has been shown to be an effective, safe, and relatively easy technique. In fact, it has become the standard method of tracheal intubation in the operating room, intensive care unit, and emergency department. Even in the hands of experienced laryngoscopists, however, accurate and prompt placement of the ET remains a significant challenge in some patients. This is particularly true in "unprepared" patients, that is, patients requiring emergency intubation. Visualization of the glottis directly can be difficult in the presence of an anatomic abnormality such as a receding mandible, prominent upper incisors, a restricted mouth opening, or a limited movement of the cervical spine. It has been estimated that between 1% and 3% of surgical patients have "difficult" airways, making laryngoscopic intubation difficult and sometimes impossible.[6] In obstetric patients the incidence of failed laryngoscopic intubation has been reported to be between 0.05% and 0.35%.[7] Many predictors of difficult laryngoscopic intubation have been suggested in the literature over the past few decades.[8,9] However, there is no single predictor that is reliable in predicting difficult laryngoscopic intubating.[10] Because of these difficulties, alternative intubation techniques have been developed over the past several decades, such as fiberoptic intubation. Although this technique is effective and reliable, it requires expensive equipment and its operation requires special skill and training. Furthermore, this technique is difficult to use in emergency situations with "unprepared" and uncooperative patients or in patients with copious secretions or blood in the oropharynx.

Because of the difficulties posed by direct-vision laryngoscopic intubation, particularly in emergency situations, the search for other techniques has led to the development of blind techniques using a variety of devices. Over the past few decades, light-guided intubation using the principle of transillumination has proven itself to be an effective, safe, and simple technique. The objectives of this chapter are to briefly review the concept of transillumination, to introduce a new lighted stylet (lightwand), and to describe the technique of intubation using this new device (Trachlight, Laerdal Medical Corp., Long Beach, Calif.).

Although many versions of the lighted stylet have been commercially available for many years, the authors have considerably more experience with the newly developed Trachlight device. Hence the lightwand discussion refers specifically to the use of the Trachlight. It should be emphasized, however, that the concepts and techniques of light-guided intubation are applicable to other lightwand devices.

II. HISTORY OF THE LIGHTWAND AND THE PRINCIPLE OF TRANSILLUMINATION

In 1958 Macintosh and Richards[11] reported the use of a lighted introducer to assist the placement of an ET into the trachea under direct vision using a laryngoscope. However, they did not describe the technique of transillumination of the soft tissues of the neck. The technique of transillumination was probably first described by Yamamura et al.[12] in 1959 when they reported the use of a lighted stylet for nasotracheal intubation.

A lighted stylet uses the principle of transillumination of the soft tissues of the anterior neck to guide the tip of the ET into the trachea. It also takes advantage of the anterior (superficial) location of the trachea relative to the esophagus. When the tip of the lighted ET enters the glottic opening as seen under fluoroscopy (Fig. 18-1), a well-defined, circumscribed glow slightly below the thyroid prominence can readily be seen in the anterior neck (Fig. 18-1, *inset*). However, if the tip of the tube is in the esophagus (Fig. 18-2), the transmitted glow is diffuse and cannot be detected easily under ambient lighting conditions (Fig. 18-2, *inset*). If the tip of the ET is placed in the vallecula above the epiglottis as shown in Fig. 18-3, the light glow is diffuse and is slightly above the thyroid prominence (Fig. 18-3, *inset*). Using this principle, the lighted stylet can guide the tip of the ET easily and safely into the trachea without the use of a laryngoscope.

Despite its potential clinical application, intubation using the lighted stylet did not receive widespread popularity until a commercial product became available. During the past decade, several versions of lighted stylet have been introduced, including the Fiberoptic Lighted-Intubation Stilette (Benson Medical Industries, Inc.,

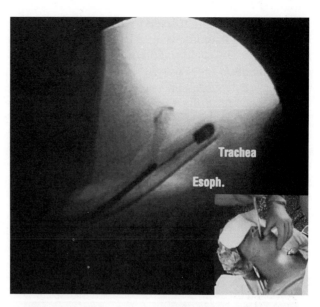

Fig. 18-1. When the tip of the endotracheal tube is placed at the glottic opening under fluoroscopy, there is a well-defined circumscribed glow *(arrow)* in the anterior neck just below the thyroid prominence *(inset)*. *Esoph,* Esophagus.

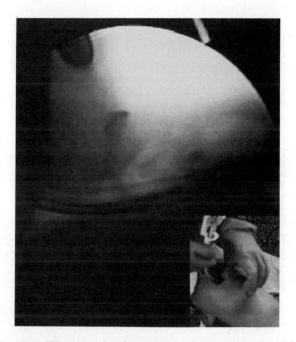

Fig. 18-2. When the tip of the endotracheal tube is placed in the esophagus under fluoroscopy, transillumination is poor and the transmitted glow is diffuse in the anterior neck and cannot be seen easily under ambient lighting condition *(inset)*.

Markham, Ontario, Canada), Flexilum (Concept Corporation, Clearwater, Fla.), Tubestat (Concept Corporation), and Fiberoptic Lighted Stylet (Fiberoptic Medical Products, Inc., Allentown, Penn.) (Fig. 18-4). After more than a decade of experience, these devices have proven to be effective and safe in placing the ET both orally and nasally.[13-16]

In 1985 Vollmer et al.[13] reported an 88% success rate in 24 field intubations using the Flexilum, with three failures. The average duration of the intubation procedure (intubation time) was 20 seconds. In 1986 Ellis et al.[14] reported successful intubations in 50 elective surgical patients using the Tubestat with an average intubation time of 37 seconds. Most of the patients (72%) were intubated following one attempt; in 22% two attempts were required, and in 6% three attempts. In a larger study with 200 patients, Ainsworth and Howells[15] accomplished successful intubation in all patients using

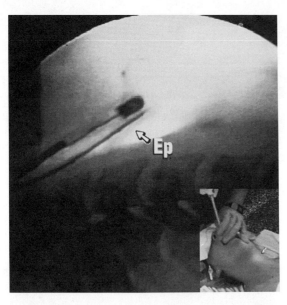

Fig. 18-3. When the tip of the endotracheal tube is placed above the epiglottis (Ep) under fluoroscopy, the light glow *(arrow)* is diffuse and is slightly above the thyroid prominence *(inset).*

the Tubestat within 60 seconds. However, the authors commented that "satisfactory conditions are met only when a darkened environment can be obtained and [that] transillumination in daylight may not be a reliable indicator of successful intubation." Weis and Hatton[16] also reported successful intubations in 250 patients using the lightwand, with three failures in patients who had gross obesity.

Despite the favorable and successful results, there were some difficulties with the lightwand devices, largely resulting from the following design-related shortcomings:

1. The intensity and beam direction of the lightbulb were insufficient to produce adequate transillumination under ambient light. Successful intubation with previous versions of lighted stylets required a darkened environment for optimal transillumination. This can be inconvenient at times and even impossible in a "field environment" or in the ambulance. In addition, a darkened environment can be dangerous for patients with a high risk of reflux, since regurgitation may not be easily detected during intubation.

2. The design of the older versions of the lighted stylet permits the light source to shine only forward without lateral projection. As shown in Fig. 18-5, the light beam shines only forward from the three older versions of lighted stylets. In these, visualization of the transilluminated light is adequate only if the tip of the stylet is pointing toward the skin surface. However, this is not always possible, since during intubation the tip of the stylet may sometimes be pointing down the trachea. A wider angle of light beam projected from the tip of the

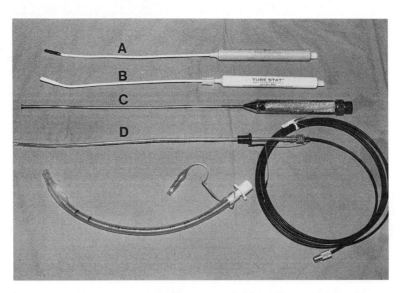

Fig. 18-4. Commercially available lighted stylets. **A,** Flexilum; **B,** Tubestat; **C,** Fiberoptic Lighted-Intubation Stilette; and **D,** Fiberoptic Lighted Stylet.

lighted stylet provides better illumination of the soft tissues of the neck.

3. The length of some of the stylets, such as Flexilum and Tubestat, was inadequate, which restricted their use to short or cut (25-cm) ETs.

4. A device (clamp or connector) to secure the ET onto the lightwand was not incorporated in some of the designs, such as Flexilum and Fiberoptic Lighted-Intubation Stilette, making it necessary in some cases to tape the ET to the devices.

5. The light switch was placed awkwardly at the proximal end of the devices. This necessitates the use of two hands to operate the lighted stylets during intubation.

6. Because of the rigidity of the wand portion of the device, the ET was occasionally dislodged from the glottic opening when the lightwand was withdrawn from the ET following intubation. In addition, after the withdrawal of the stylet from the ET it is impossible to detect the location of the tip of the ET. This may lead to an inadvertent esophageal intubation. The rigidity of the lighted stylets also hampers the use of these devices for nasotracheal intubation.

7. The Flexilum and Tubestat were designed for a single use (disposable unit), which has substantially increased the cost of intubation.

Because of the shortcomings of the existing lighted stylets, a new lighted stylet (Trachlight) has been developed. It has an improved light source and a more flexible wand portion of the device. This added flexibility broadens the utility of the device for both oral and nasal intubation, improves the ease of intubation, and permits the evaluation of the position of the tip of the ET following the intubation.

III. A NEW LIGHTWAND (TRACHLIGHT)

The Trachlight consists of three parts: a reusable handle, a flexible wand, and a stiff, retractable stylet (Fig. 18-6). The power-control circuitry and batteries are encased within the handle. The Trachlight requires three AAA alkaline batteries, which are readily changed as necessary. A locking clamp located on the front of the handle accepts and secures a standard ET connector. The wand consists of a durable, flexible plastic shaft with a bright lightbulb affixed at the distal end. With the improved bulb technology, the light emitted by the Trachlight is extremely bright, with minimal heat production (a maximum surface temperature of approximately 60° C). In addition to a forward projection as with most of the lighted stylets, the light of the Trachlight also projects laterally at a much wider angle (Fig. 18-5). This additional feature further improves transillumination of the soft tissues of the neck. The improved light source of the Trachlight permits intubation to be performed under ambient lighting conditions, making it unnecessary to dim the room light in most cases. After 30 seconds of illumination the lightbulb blinks to minimize heat production. Since the tip of the lightbulb is encased within the ET, it is extremely unlikely that the bulb would cause any thermal injury during intubation.

Affixed to the other end of the wand is a rigid plastic connector with a release arm, allowing its connection to the grooves in the wand handle. This connector allows adjustment of the wand along the handle by depressing the release arm and gliding it along the handle to

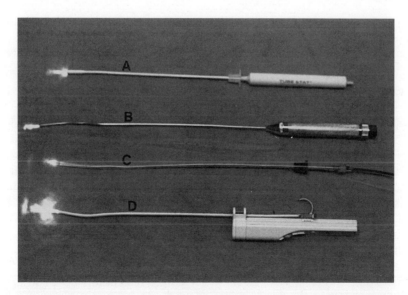

Fig. 18-5. The light beam shines only forward from the tip of the three older versions of lightwands: **A,** Tubestat; **B,** Fiberoptic Lighted-Intubation Stilette; and **C,** Fiberoptic Lighted Stylet. The light beam of, **D,** the Trachlight shines forward and laterally with a wider angle.

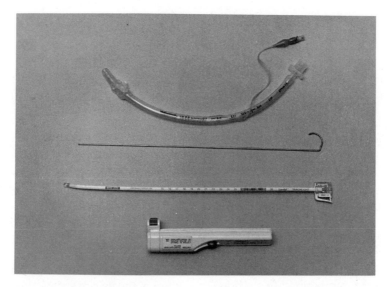

Fig. 18-6. The Trachlight consists of 3 parts: a handle, a flexible wand, and a stiff internal stylet.

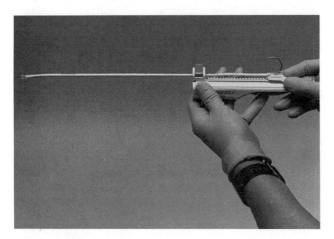

Fig. 18-7. The length of the wand can be adjusted by depressing the release arm of the wand and gliding it along the handle of the Trachlight.

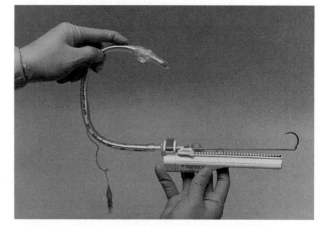

Fig. 18-8. After retraction of the stiff internal stylet the distal part of the wand and endotracheal tube becomes pliable, facilitating the entry of the tube into the trachea.

accommodate ETs of varying lengths (Fig. 18-7). Enclosed within the wand is a stiff but malleable, retractable stylet. With the stylet retracted the wand becomes pliable, permitting the endotracheal tube to advance easily into the trachea (Fig. 18-8). In essence, this is the most important feature of this lightwand device, significantly improving its ease of use.

The stiff, retractable stylet gives sufficient stiffness to the device to allow one to shape the wand in a "field hockey stick" configuration (Fig. 18-9). This configuration directs the bright light of the lighted stylet against the anterior wall of the larynx and trachea. In addition, the "hockey stick" configuration also enhances maneuverability during intubation and facilitates the placement of the ET into the glottic opening. Once through the glottis, however, the "field hockey stick" configuration

impedes further advancement of the tube into the trachea. Retraction of the stiff stylet produces a pliable ET-Trachlight unit (ET-TL) that allows advancement into the trachea (Fig. 18-8). This flexibility also allows accurate placement of the tip of the ET. Once the internal stiff stylet is retracted, the pliable ET-TL can be advanced into the trachea until the tip reaches the sternal notch. At the sternal notch the tip of the endotracheal tube is about halfway between the vocal cords and the carina.[17]

IV. TECHNIQUE OF LIGHTWAND INTUBATION

Since the authors have had significant involvement in the development of the Trachlight, the following intubation technique is a reflection of our experience and bias with the Trachlight. However, the concept of

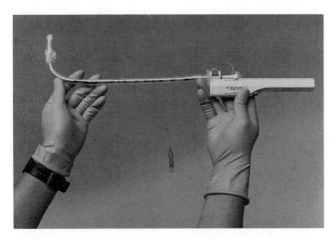

Fig. 18-9. After the insertion of the wand of the Trachlight into the endotracheal tube, a 90-degree bend is made at the distal end of the tube to form the "field hockey stick" configuration.

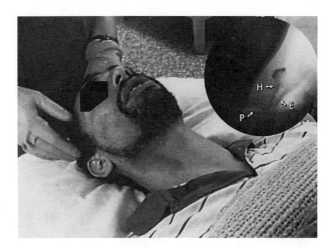

Fig. 18-10. When the head is in a sniffing position, the epiglottis (E) is almost in contact with the posterior pharyngeal wall (P), making it difficult for the lighted stylet to go underneath the epiglottis. *H,* hyoid bone.

intubation using transillumination is applicable to other types of lighted stylets. Undoubtedly, successful intubation using a lighted stylet, including the Trachlight, depends in part on the intubator's experience and skill. In other words, as with any intubation technique, regular use of and practice with the Trachlight will improve performance and may also reduce the likelihood of complications.

A. PREPARATION

Lubrication of the stiff internal stylet of the wand using silicone fluid ensures its easy retraction during intubation. With the stiff internal stylet in place, the wand is attached to the handle. The internal wall of the ET should be well lubricated with a water-soluble lubricant to facilitate retraction of the wand following the ET placement. Insert the wand into the ET, ensuring that the tube is firmly attached to the handle. The length of the wand is adjusted by sliding the wand along the handle (Fig. 18-7), placing the lightbulb close to, but not protruding beyond, the tip of the ET. With the Trachlight (TL) in place, bend the ET-TL unit at a 90-degree angle just proximal to the cuff of the tube in the shape of a field hockey stick (Fig. 18-9). Although the degree of bend should be individualized, a right-angle bend generally makes the intubation considerably easier. When the tip of the ET is in the glottic opening, a right-angle bend allows the maximum light intensity pointing to the surface of the skin with a well-defined circumscribed glow. However, the maximum light intensity will be pointing down the trachea if the Trachlight bends to 45 degrees. In other words, a 90-degree bend generally provides better transillumination, making the light-guided intubation much easier. Although the wider angle of light projection from the lightbulb of the Trachlight enhances transillumination substantially, it is

our preference to keep a "tight" 90-degree bend for most intubations. For obese patients or patients with short necks a more acute bend (greater than a 90-degree bend) provides better transillumination. To facilitate the tip of the ET to "slip" into trachea during intubation, the tip of the tube should also be lubricated with a water-soluble lubricant.

B. POSITIONING

The intubator usually stands at the head of the table (bed). It is possible to use the device from the front or side of the patient, which enhances the utility of the device in the prehospital environment. Although the height of intubators may vary considerably, it is advisable to lower the table to allow maximal visualization of the anterior neck of the patient during intubation. A footstool may be extremely helpful when it is not possible to lower the table or bed, such as in the emergency department. In contrast to the sniffing position for laryngoscopic intubation, the patient's head and neck should be in a neutral or relatively extended position. The epiglottis is almost in contact with the posterior pharyngeal wall when the head is in the sniffing position (Fig. 18-10), making it difficult for the Trachlight to go underneath the epiglottis. However, the epiglottis is lifted off the posterior pharyngeal wall when the head is extended (Fig. 18-11). This facilitates the entrance of the ET into the glottic opening. In addition, the extended neck position also allows maximal exposure of the anterior neck. Therefore it is generally recommended that the patient's head and neck be placed in a slightly extended position in the absence of potential cervical spine instability. In obese patients or patients with extremely short necks, placing a pillow under the

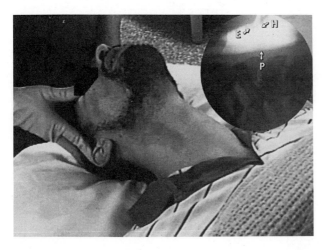

Fig. 18-11. When the head and neck are in extension, the epiglottis (E) is lifted off the posterior pharyngeal wall (P). *H,* hyoid bone.

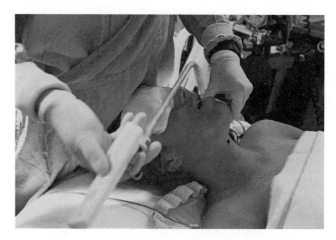

Fig. 18-12. The jaw is grasped by the nondominant hand and lifted upward to elevate the tongue and epiglottis. The nondominant hand must be kept close to the corner of the mouth to ensure an unobstructed path in the midline for the lightwand. The endotracheal tube–Trachlight unit (ET-TL) is inserted into the oropharynx using the dominant hand.

shoulders and neck further extends the neck, which makes the lightwand intubation substantially easier.

C. CONTROL OF THE AMBIENT LIGHT

With the improved bulb technology the light emitted by the Trachlight is extremely bright. This enhances transillumination of the neck soft tissues. In most cases patients can be intubated easily under ambient lighting conditions. In particularly thin patients the lightbulb is so bright that it is possible to mistakenly interpret an esophageal intubation as an intratracheal placement. Therefore it is recommended that all tracheal intubations using the Trachlight be carried out under ambient light. Room lights should be dimmed only when absolutely necessary, such as for obese patients or patients with thick necks, when transillumination may be less than ideal. In the emergency department or prehospital setting, when controlling the ambient lighting is not possible, shading the neck with a towel or hand may be helpful.

D. TECHNIQUE

1. Oral intubation

As with other intubating techniques, proper oxygenation of the patient should precede the light-guided intubation. With the patient lying supine, the jaw is grasped and lifted upward using the thumb and index finger of the nondominant hand (Fig. 18-12). This lifts the tongue and epiglottis away from the posterior pharyngeal wall to facilitate placement of the tip of the ET into the glottic opening. The nondominant hand must be kept close to the corner of the mouth to ensure an unobstructed path in the midline for the lightwand. The Trachlight is switched on, and the ET-TL inserted into the midline of the oropharynx using the dominant hand. The midline position of the ET-TL is maintained

while the device is advanced gently in a rocking motion along an imaginary arc. The ET-TL should always be advanced gently. When resistance is felt, the ET-TL should be "rocked" backward (cephalad) and the tip redirected toward the laryngeal prominence, using the glow of the light as a guide. A faint glow seen above the thyroid prominence indicates that the tip of the ET-TL is located in the vallecula (Fig. 18-3). A jaw-lift maneuver helps to elevate the epiglottis and enhance the passage of the ET-TL under the epiglottis. When the tip of ET-TL enters the glottic opening, a well-defined circumscribed glow can be seen in the anterior neck slightly below the thyroid prominence (Fig. 18-13). However, the ET-TL cannot be advanced into the trachea because of the "hockey stick" configuration of the Trachlight. Retracting the stiff inner stylet approximately 10 cm makes the ET-TL more pliable, which allows advancement into the trachea with reduced risk of trauma (Fig. 18-14). The ET-TL is then advanced until the glow begins to disappear at the sternal notch (Fig. 18-15), which indicates that the tip of the ET is approximately halfway between the vocal cords and the carina.[17] After release of the locking clamp the Trachlight can be removed from the ET.

Occasionally the circumscribed glow cannot be readily seen in the anterior neck because of anatomic features such as morbid obesity or short necks. Neck extension as described earlier may be helpful. Retraction of the breast or chest wall tissues, together with indentation of the tissues around the trachea by an assistant, enhances transillumination of the soft tissues in the anterior neck. Dimming the lights is required only rarely.

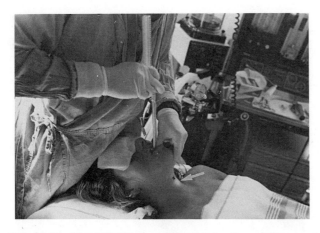

Fig. 18-13. The ET-TL is positioned in the midline and advanced gently in a rocking motion along an imaginary arc. A bright, well-defined, circumscribed glow *(arrow)* is seen below the thyroid prominence (marked *X*) when the ET-TL enters the glottic opening.

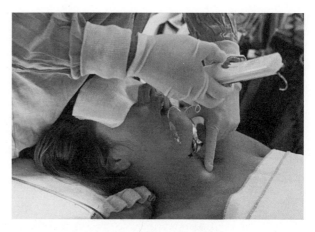

Fig. 18-15. Following retraction of the stiff internal stylet, the ET-TL becomes pliable, permitting the ET to be advanced further into the trachea. The ET is advanced until the glow is at the sternal notch.

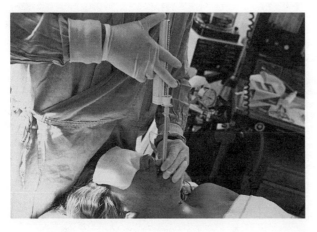

Fig. 18-14. When the ET-TL is at the glottic opening, the stiff internal stylet is retracted while holding the ET close to the lips with the nondominant hand.

After the retraction of the stiff stylet the tip of the tube and lightwand can sometimes be caught at the vestibular folds of the cords (hung up) and cannot be advanced into the trachea readily because the tip of the ET is pointing toward the anterior wall of the larynx. While maintaining contact with the laryngeal wall, the ET-TL should be rotated sideways 90 degrees or more to the right or left side of the head. The tip of the ET will then be pointing sideways or downward, which enhances the entrance of the ET into the trachea. As an alternative, grasping the anterior larynx with the nondominant hand with an upward lift helps the tip of the ET to come off the vestibular folds.

2. Nasal intubation

Although nasotracheal intubation is used only infrequently by anesthesiologists for oral procedures, it remains a useful alternative technique for many situations, particularly in emergency conditions. Light-guided nasotracheal intubation using the Trachlight is particularly useful when blind nasal intubation is indicated, such as in emergency airways for patients with a limited mouth opening and/or cervical spine instability.

Removal of the stiff internal stylet before the insertion of the Trachlight into the ET makes the ET-TL pliable and permits nasotracheal intubation (Fig. 18-16). Application of a vasoconstrictor nasal spray to the nostril before intubation minimizes mucosal bleeding. Immersing the ET-TL in a bottle of warm sterile water or saline solution softens the ET and further minimizes the potential for mucosal damage during the nasal intubation. Water-soluble lubricant is applied to the nostril to facilitate entry of the ET-TL through the nose. As with oral intubation, the jaw is grasped and lifted upward, elevating the tongue and epiglottis away from the posterior wall of the pharynx and facilitating the placement of the tip of the ET into the glottic opening (Fig. 18-17). The Trachlight is switched on once the tip of the ET-TL has advanced into the oropharynx. The ET-TL is positioned in the midline and advanced, using the light glow as a guide. The ET-TL must advance gently. When resistance is felt, the ET-TL should be withdrawn slightly and the tip redirected toward the thyroid prominence, using the glow of the light as a guide. A faint glow seen above the thyroid prominence indicates that the tip of the ET-TL is located in the vallecula. A jaw-lift maneuver helps to elevate the epiglottis and enhance the passage of the ET-TL under it. As an alternative, the neck of the patient can be flexed while advancing the tip of ET-TL slowly. When the ET-TL enters the glottic opening, a well-defined circumscribed glow is seen in the anterior neck just below the thyroid prominence (Fig. 18-18). To ensure that the tip of the ET-TL is located at the optimal position within the

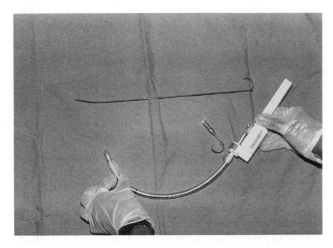

Fig. 18-16. Following the removal of the stiff internal stylet from the wand, the ET-TL becomes pliable and flexible, permitting light-guided blind nasal tracheal intubation.

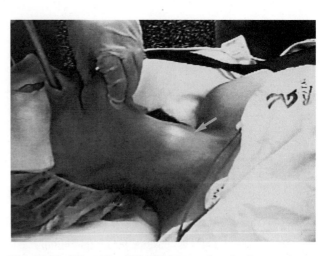

Fig. 18-18. When the ET-TL enters the glottic opening, a well-defined circumscribed glow *(arrow)* is seen in the anterior neck just below the thyroid prominence.

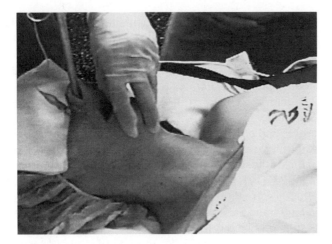

Fig. 18-17. The jaw is grasped and lifted upward by the nondominant hand. This elevates the tongue and epiglottis away from the posterior wall of the pharynx to facilitate the placement of the tip of the ET into the glottic opening. The ET-TL is positioned in the midline and advanced gently into the glottic opening using the light glow as a guide.

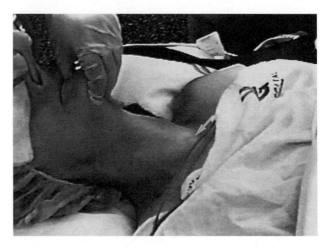

Fig. 18-19. To ensure that the tip of the ET-TL is located at the optimal position within the trachea, the tip of the ET is advanced until the glow begins to disappear at the sternal notch *(arrow)*.

trachea, the tip of the ET is advanced until the glow begins to disappear at the sternal notch (Fig. 18-19). Following the release of the locking clamp the Trachlight is withdrawn from the ET. The correct tube placement is confirmed by means of the end-tidal carbon dioxide or auscultation, or both.

V. CLINICAL APPLICATIONS OF THE TRACHLIGHT

The authors conducted a study involving 950 elective surgical patients that compared the effectiveness and safety of oral intubation using the Trachlight with standard laryngoscopic intubation.[18] The Trachlight has significant advantages compared with standard laryngoscopic intubation (Table 18-1). Although there is a statistically significant difference in the total intubation time between the groups (15.9 seconds for the Trachlight versus 19.9 seconds for laryngoscopy), the small difference probably has no clinical significance. However, it compares favorably with the conventional intubation technique with regard to its effectiveness and failure rate. Furthermore, there were fewer patients with complications and sore throats following the intubation using the Trachlight as compared with laryngoscopy. The ease of intubation using the Trachlight, in contrast to laryngoscopy, does not appear to be influenced by the anatomic variabilities of the upper airways, which suggests that the device may be a useful alternative for patients with "difficult" airways.

Recent evidence suggests that intubation using the light-guided intubation technique is associated with fewer hemodynamic changes as compared with the conventional technique using a laryngoscope.[19] In a study of 450 elective surgical patients the increase in

Table 18-1. Results of orotracheal intubation using either the Trachlight or laryngoscope

	Trachlight	Laryngoscopy
No. of patients	479	471
Total time-to-intubate (sec)	15.7 ± 10.8	19.6 ± 23.7*
No. of patients intubated with one attempt	442	422†
No. of patients requiring two or more attempts	37	49†
No. of failures	5	13†
No. of patients with sore throat	82	119*
No. of patients with hoarseness	2	5†
No. of patients with trauma	10	37*

*Statistically significant difference between the groups.
†No statistically significant difference between the groups.

mean arterial pressure and heart rate following intubation was significantly less with use of the Trachlight than with laryngoscopy.[19]

Fewer failures and complications as compared with the conventional technique using laryngoscopy and the ease of intubation irrespective of patients' upper airway anatomy led to speculation that the Trachlight might be useful in intubation of patients with difficult airways. In an ongoing study we investigated 186 patients with difficult airways (84 with documented previous difficult intubation, 58 with cervical spine instability, 32 with stiff temporomandibular joints, 8 with morbid obesity, and 4 with miscellaneous syndromes) and 49 patients with unanticipated failed laryngoscopic intubation.[20] All but two patients (a morbidly obese patient weighing 220 kg and a patient with severe flexion deformity of the cervical spine) were successfully intubated using the Trachlight. The tracheas of three patients were intubated awake with topical anesthesia, and the remaining 232 patients were intubated under general anesthesia. Eighteen patients had nasal intubation, and the remainder had oral intubation. The mean (±sd) intubation time was 24.2 seconds (range, 5 to 130 seconds) using the Trachlight. A majority of the patients were intubated following one attempt, 38 required two attempts, and 8 required three attempts. Apart from minor mucosal bleeding, no complications occurred in any of these patients. The results of this study indicated that the Trachlight is a useful, effective alternative technique for placement of ET both nasally and orally in patients with difficult airways. The brighter light source allowed intubation under ambient light, and the retractable stylet markedly improved the success rate of the intubation compared with the older versions of the lightwand. The following case history serves to highlight the role of the Trachlight and other lighted stylets in airway management in patients with difficult airways.

VI. CASE HISTORY

A healthy 23-year-old man was scheduled to have cervical laminectomy for cervical radiculopathy. Preoperative examination showed that he had a restricted mouth opening and discomfort with neck extension. Under general anesthesia, only the tip of the epiglottis could be seen when using a laryngoscope. The patient had adequate ventilation with the use of a no. 4 laryngeal mask airway (LMA). Manipulation of a fiberoptic bronchoscope through the LMA was found to be difficult because of the acute angle of the glottis relative to the epiglottis. An attending staff anesthesiologist who was experienced with the Trachlight was called to assist the placement of the ET. After proper preparation, intubation was successfully performed using the Trachlight in less than 8 seconds. The position of the tube was confirmed using the end-tidal carbon dioxide and auscultation.

VII. LIMITATIONS

Although the lightwand has been demonstrated to be an effective, safe device for intubation, the technique requires transillumination of the soft tissues of the anterior neck without visualization of the laryngeal structure. Therefore, the lightwand should be avoided in patients with known abnormalities of the upper airway, such as tumors, polyps, infection (e.g., epiglottis and retropharyngeal abscess), and trauma of the upper airway, or if there is a foreign body in the upper airway. In these cases other alternatives using direct vision, such as fiberoptic intubation, should be considered. The lightwand should also be used with caution in patients in whom transillumination of the anterior neck may not be adequate, such as patients who are grossly obese or patients with limited neck extension. However, these contraindications and precautions may become irrelevant when a patient's airway is compromised and urgent intubation is indicated. Furthermore, this light-guided technique should not be attempted with an uncooperative awake patient unless a bite block is used to prevent damage to the device or injury to the intubator.

VIII. CONCLUSION

Occasional difficult laryngoscopic intubation has led to the development of many alternative intubating techniques. Transillumination of the soft tissues of the neck using a lighted stylet has been shown to be an effective intubation technique for decades. While many versions of lighted stylets are available, a newly developed lighted stylet (Trachlight) has incorporated many design modifications to facilitate both oral and nasal intubation in both awake and anesthetized patients. It has been demonstrated as an effective, safe intubating device in a large number of surgical patients and patients with documented difficult airways. However, it should be avoided in patients with anatomic abnormalities of the upper airways. As with any intubation technique, regular use of and practice with the lightwand will improve its performance and may also reduce the likelihood of complications.

REFERENCES

1. Frostad AB: Tracheostomy in acute obstructive laryngitis, *J Laryngol Otol* 87:1101, 1973.
2. Mihic D, Binkert E, Novoselac M: The first endotracheal intubation, *Anesthesiology* 52:523, 1980 (letter).
3. Herholdt JD, Rafn CG: *Life-saving measures for drowning persons,* Copenhagen, H Tikiob, 1796, pp 52-53.
4. MacEwen W: Clinical observations on the introduction of tracheal tubes by the mouth instead of performing tracheostomy or laryngotomy, *Br Med J* 122:163, 1880.
5. Jackson C: The technique of insertion of intratracheal insufflation tubes, *Surg Gynecol Obstet* 17:507, 1913.
6. Latto IP: Management of difficult intubation. In Latto IP, Rosen M, editors: *Difficulties in tracheal intubation,* London, 1987, Bailliere Tindall.
7. Davies JM, Weeks S, Crone LA et al: Difficult intubation in parturients, *Can J Anaesth* 36:668, 1989.
8. Mallampatti SR, Gatt SP, Gugino LD et al: A clinical sign to predict difficult tracheal intubation: a prospective study, *Can Anaesth Soc J* 32:427, 1985.
9. Wilson ME, Speiglhalter D, Robertson JA et al: Predicting difficult intubation, *Br J Anaesth* 61:211, 1988.
10. Oates JDL, Oates PD, Pearsall RJ et al: Comparison of two methods for predicting difficult intubation, *Br J Anaesth* 66:305, 1991.
11. Macintosh R, Richards H: Illuminated introducer for endotracheal tubes, *Anaesthesia* 12:223, 1957.
12. Yamamura H, Yamamoto T, Kamiyama M: Device for blind nasal intubation, *Anesthesiology* 20:221, 1959.
13. Vollmer TP, Stewart RD, Paris PM et al: Use of a lighted stylet for guided orotracheal intubation in the prehospital setting, *Ann Emerg Med* 14:324, 1985.
14. Ellis GE, Jakymec A, Kaplan RM et al: Guided orotracheal intubation in the operating room using a lighted stylet: a comparison with direct laryngoscopic technique, *Anesthesiology* 64:823, 1986.
15. Ainsworth QP, Howells TH: Transilluminated tracheal intubation, *Br J Anaesth* 62:494, 1989.
16. Weis FR, Hatton MN: Intubation by use of the lightwand: experience in 253 patients, *J Oral Maxillofac Surg* 47:577, 1989.
17. Stewart RD, Larosee A, Kaplan RM et al: Correct positioning of an endotracheal tube using a flexible lighted stylet, *Crit Care Med* 18:97, 1990.
18. Hung OR, Pytka S, Murphy MF et al: Clinical trial of a new lightwand to intubate the trachea, *Anesthesiology* 1995.
19. Hung OR, Pytka S, Murphy MF et al: Comparative hemodynamic changes following laryngoscopic or lightwand intubation, *Anesthesiology* 79(suppl 3A):A497, 1993.
20. Hung OR, Stevens SC, Pytka S et al: Clinical trial of a new lightwand device for intubation in patients with difficult airways, *Anesthesiology* 79(suppl 3A):A498, 1993.

Chapter 19

LARYNGEAL MASK AIRWAY

Girish P. Joshi
Ian Smith
Paul F. White

I. INTRODUCTION

The laryngeal mask airway (LMA) is an innovative device designed for upper-airway management. It was originally described by Dr. A.I.J. Brain primarily as an alternative to the face mask and the endotracheal tube.[1]

It has been described as the missing link between those devices.[2] Compared to the face mask, the LMA maintains a better airway, frees the hands and reduces fatigue of the anesthesiologist, and does not require neuromuscular blockade or laryngoscopy for placement. In addition, its insertion is associated with minimal pressor response and minimal increase in the intraoccular pressure compared to the endotracheal tube. Furthermore, it is well tolerated at the time of recovery and provides a clear airway in the postoperative period.[3]

In the short period following its introduction in the early 1980s, the LMA has gained widespread popularity and is now extensively used during general anesthesia and in situations of difficult or failed intubations.[3,4] Extensive correspondence, several review articles, and editorials have been published relating to its use. The device is a useful advance in airway management and is easy to use. However, few well-designed randomized studies have been performed. Also, its inappropriate and/or incorrect use can lead to mishaps and serious complications. It is important to have adequate knowledge of the indications and contraindications of using the LMA in order to optimize its use.[5,6]

II. HISTORICAL PERSPECTIVE

The LMA was invented and developed by Dr. A.I.J. Brain, a British anesthesiologist, at the London Hospital in 1981. The use of a prototype was first described in 1983.[1,7] Although a number of airway devices similar to the LMA were described previously, none gained the popularity of the LMA. One such device was a "pharyngeal bulb gasway," described in 1937 by Dr. B.C. Leech of Regina, Saskatchewan.[8,9] The "Leech Gasway" consisted of a detachable soft rubber bulb fitted to a modified metal oropharyngeal airway. In contrast to the LMA, which forms a seal around the perimeter of the larynx, the "Leech Gasway" formed a seal around the perimeter of the pharynx.

On examination of postmortem specimens of the larynx, Brain noted that an airtight seal could be achieved around the laryngeal inlet by an inflated cuff in the hypopharynx. Plaster-of-Paris molds of cadaveric pharynx showed that the space around and posterior to the glottis was boat shaped, with the sharp end facing caudad.[7] Similarities between the pharyngeal casts and the cuff of the Goldman dental nasal mask led to the construction of a prototype LMA. The flanges of the cuff were joined together and a diagonally cut endotracheal tube incorporated onto the base of the mask. The elliptical cuff was attached to the distal end of a pilot tube, with a nonreturn valve making it inflatable. When inflated the cuff formed an airtight seal around the laryngeal inlet.

In the summer of 1981, the prototype LMA was used for the first time, successfully and without any complications, in a male patient undergoing hernia repair.[7] Although a pilot study was highly encouraging, a number of shortcomings became apparent.[1,10] It was noticed that inadequate size of the mask caused laryngeal obstruction and leaks. In addition, occasional folding down of the epiglottis caused partial or complete obstruction of the glottis. A stainless-steel introducer attached to the front of the mask was used to facilitate insertion and to draw the epiglottis into the normal position during the device's removal.

While developments in the design of the LMA continued, it was being used in approximately 1000 patients a year. In February 1983, the LMA prototype was used successfully in a case of failed intubation.[11] In an attempt to provide easy escape to regurgitated gastric

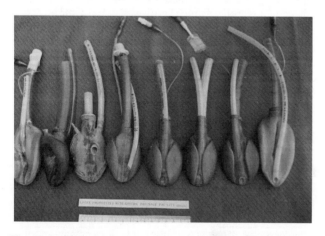

Fig. 19-1. Some prototype laryngeal mask (From Brain AIJ: *Eur J Anaesthesiol Suppl* 4:5, 1991.)

contents and thus prevent pulmonary aspiration, prototypes were designed to provide access to both the trachea and the stomach. In 1985, silicone-mask prototypes were made, featuring a silicone cuff with a double bar at the aperture to prevent the epiglottis from folding down and blocking the aperture (Fig. 19-1).

The new silicone mask was superior to previous prototypes, allowing a smoother insertion and discontinuation of the introducer tool. While further developments of the LMA continued, an independent clinical trial confirmed that a clear and unobstructed airway could be achieved in 98% of the patients.[2] Subsequently, the LMA was used in children and infants with success. A nasal prototype was also developed. The LMA design was finalized in January 1988, and three more sizes were constructed based on the dimensions of the silicone or latex prototypes.

The LMA was first marketed in the United Kingdom in mid-1988. It was used in 500 United Kingdom hospitals within 1 year; in only 2 years, every hospital where surgery was performed had purchased the LMA.[4] Following the approval of the LMA by the United States Food and Drug Administration in 1991, increasing interest has developed in the United States.[3] It is presently sold in more than 60 countries. The LMA has become available, and has gained widespread popularity, in most of Europe, Australia, North America, and Japan.

III. DESCRIPTION OF THE LMA

The current commercially available LMA is manufactured from medical-grade silicone and consists of an obliquely cut tube mounted into the concave central part of an oval mask (Fig. 19-2). The angle between the tube and inflated mask is 30 degrees. A pilot tube with a balloon is attached to the inflatable cuffed rim of the mask. The proximal end of the tube consists of a standard 15-mm tapered connector that fits a breathing circuit. Two vertically placed bars at the junction of the tube and the mask are designed to prevent the epiglottis from obstructing the lumen of the tube. A black line runs through the posterior length of the tube to provide orientation and to prevent twisting of the mask. The LMA is now available in five sizes, developed for use in neonates and adults (Fig. 19-2). A size 5 LMA has recently been introduced in the United Kingdom and is used for large adults. The differences in the various sizes of the LMA are described in Table 19-1.

IV. ANATOMIC CONSIDERATIONS

The LMA was designed to allow an end-to-end connection between the anatomical airway and the external breathing circuit.[7] The LMA achieves this by surrounding the opening of the larynx as it enters obliquely into the hypopharynx. The space occupied by the LMA is well adapted to the presence of foreign bodies (in the form of food), so it is not surprising that the presence of an inflated cuff is better tolerated in the hypopharynx than in the trachea. In addition, the posterior aspect of this space is firm (being supported by the anterior surfaces of the upper cervical vertebrae), so that the cuff of the LMA can press against the posterior wall and form a seal around the larynx.

When the LMA is correctly positioned, its anterior margin lies at the base of the hypopharynx, with the tip

at the opening of the esophagus against the upper esophageal sphincter. The lateral portions of the cuff lie in the piriform fossae, while the upper border of the cuff lies at the base of the tongue, below the level of the tonsils. Because the cuff is soft, it can conform to the contours of the larynx, thereby forming a relatively good seal.

When optimally inserted, the deflated wedge-shaped leading edge of the LMA cuff passes between the tip of the epiglottis and the posterior pharyngeal wall, so that the epiglottis retains its usual location following cuff inflation (Fig. 19-3). However, in many cases the epiglottis may be folded down by passage of the LMA. In the worst cases, this may deflect its tip onto the vocal cords, inducing coughing and laryngospasm.[12] The folded-down epiglottis may also cause airway obstruction. Complete obstruction is rare, partly because the two bars over the opening of the LMA tube help prevent the epiglottis from totally occluding the aperture. Radiologic studies in adults[13] and children[14] have demonstrated that downward displacement of the epiglottis is very common, although this does not necessarily result in clinical evidence of airway obstruction. However, it may cause problems when trying to intubate or view the larynx with a fiberoptic scope through the LMA. The likelihood of folding down the epiglottis can be reduced by avoiding incorrect insertion technique (Fig. 19-4).[12]

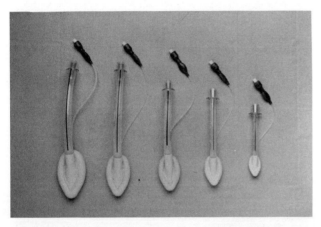

Fig. 19-2. Five different sizes of laryngeal mask airways (from right to left, sizes 1, 2, 2.5, 3, 4). (From Gensia Inc., San Diego, CA.)

Table 19-1. Description of different sizes of laryngeal mask airway devices

Mask size	Patient weight (kg)	Internal diameter (ID. mm)	Length (cm)	Cuff volume (ml)	Largest ET (ID. mm)	FOB size (mm)	Type of FOB that will pass through
1	<6.5	5.25	10.0	2-4	3.5	2.7	Olympus PF-27M ENF-P2 BF-N20 Pentax FB-10H FI-10P
2	6.5-20	7.0	11.5	10	4.5	3.5	Olympus ENF-P3 BF-3C20 Pentax FNL-15S
2.5	20-30	8.4	12.5	15	5.0	4.0	Olympus LF-1
3	30-60	10.0	19.0	20	6.0 cuffed	5.0	Olympus BF-2TR BF-P20D
4	>60	10.0	19.0	30	6.5 cuffed	5.0	Pentax FB-19H FB-19H3

ET = endotracheal tube; FOB = fiberoptic bronchoscope
Modified from Pennant JH, White PF: The laryngeal mask airway: its uses in anesthesiology, *Anesthesiology* 79:144, 1993.

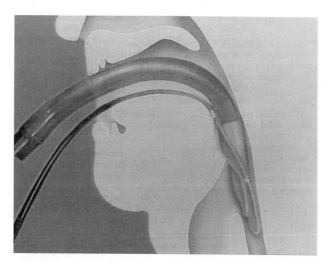

Fig. 19-3. Correct insertion avoids both the epiglottis and the glottis, with the mask tip reaching into the base of the hypopharynx. (From Brain AIJ: The Intravent laryngeal mask instruction manual, Berkshire, U.K., 1992, *Brain Medical.*)

V. PRACTICAL CONSIDERATIONS

A. PREPARATION FOR PLACEMENT

Because the LMA is a reusable, sterilizable device, it should be inspected and tested before every use. The anesthesiologist should confirm that the LMA has been adequately sterilized, and examine the device for cracks and other defects. Checking that the cuff can remain both fully inflated and deflated tests the integrity of the cuff and inflation-tube valve. The cuff should be inflated with a volume of air 50% greater than the recommended maximum volume and checked for herniations and/or thinning of the cuff wall. The LMA should be discarded if it is discolored or if the tube kinks when it is flexed to 180 degrees.

The classic insertion technique requires that the cuff should be deflated so that the tip forms a flat leading edge.[12] This is best accomplished by pressing the concave surface of the LMA against a clean surface while aspirating all of the air from the cuff. The cuff should deflate to form a flat disk, with the rim facing away from the LMA aperture (Fig. 19-5). The rear (convex) surface of the LMA should then be carefully lubricated using a water-soluble jelly. This should not be done until immediately before the LMA is to be inserted, to prevent drying of the lubricant. Lubricating the concave surface of the LMA does not help insertion, and may lead to aspiration of lubricant, causing coughing and/or laryngospasm. Compared to K-Y jelly, the use of 2% lidocaine jelly/ointment as a lubricant is reported to reduce the incidence of coughing during emergence.[15] However, the use of local anesthetic containing lubricants is controversial.

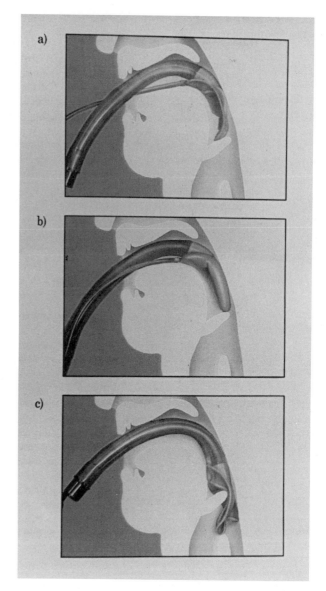

Fig. 19-4. If the mask is deflected forward as in **A,** or inadequately deflated as in **B,** it may either push the epiglottis down or penetrate the glottis as in **C.** (From Brain AIJ: The Intravent laryngeal mask instruction manual, Berkshire, U.K., 1992, *Brain Medical.*)

B. INDUCTION OF ANESTHESIA

Although the LMA can be inserted under topical anesthesia (e.g., to facilitate fiberoptic bronchoscopy), it is normally used as part of a general anesthetic technique. Correct insertion requires an adequate level of anesthesia to obtund pharyngeal reflexes. However, in contrast to a tracheal tube, muscle-relaxant drugs are unnecessary. Of the available intravenous induction agents, propofol appears to yield the best conditions for insertion of the LMA, which is possible within 30 seconds of administering propofol, 2.0-2.5 mg·kg^{-1} IV.[7]

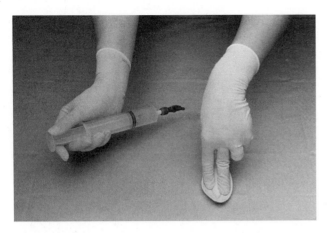

Fig. 19-5. Deflate mask as completely as possible so there are no folds near the tip. Always deflate so rim faces away from mask aperture. (From Brain AIJ: The Intravent laryngeal mask instruction manual, Berkshire, U.K., 1992, *Brain Medical.*)

Other intravenous induction drugs (e.g., thiopental) do not produce as satisfactory conditions,[16,17] and it is necessary to either give a dose that exceeds the usual induction dose or to "deepen" anesthesia with a volatile agent. The LMA can also be easily inserted following an inhalation induction.[18]

C. TECHNIQUES OF INSERTION

Insertion of the LMA can be achieved in a high proportion of patients with little practice. However, careful attention to the details of the insertion technique is necessary to ensure optimal placement of the LMA and an unobstructed airway. Partial obstruction is often caused by folding down of the epiglottis. While this may cause little functional impairment during brief procedures, it can impair the efficiency of ventilation, and is particularly undesirable when the LMA is being used as a conduit for fiberoptic bronchoscopy. A poor insertion technique may also cause misplacement of the LMA, resulting in coughing, straining, and even loss of the airway.

The standard insertion technique is described in the LMA instruction manual[12] and summarized in Box 19-1. Following adequate induction of anesthesia (i.e., sufficiently deep as to ensure jaw relaxation), place the patient into the "sniffing the morning air" position, with neck flexed and head extended. Place the deflated and lubricated LMA into the open mouth, and press it back against the hard palate so that the LMA is seen to flatten (Fig. 19-6). It is especially important to check that the rim of the LMA does not become folded back on itself at this stage, which will inevitably prevent correct insertion (Figs. 19-7 and 19-8). From this point, slide the LMA behind the tongue and into the pharynx (Figs. 19-9 and 19-10). Smooth passage is aided by the use of

BOX 19-1   Guidelines for insertion of the LMA after induction of anesthesia

- Deflate cuff while pressing bowl of the LMA against a clean, flat surface.
- Lubricate rear (convex) surface of the LMA with water-based lubricant.
- Induce adequate depth of anesthesia (e.g., propofol 2-2.5 mg·kg^{-1}).
- Push on back of patient's head to extend the head and flex the neck.
- Insert the LMA into patient's mouth, pressing back against the palate.
- LMA should be seen to flatten out against the palate.
- Push the LMA into oral cavity, while continuing to press against roof of mouth.
- Once past the tongue, the LMA will move easily into position.
- Stop insertion when resistance is met (LMA is at the esophageal sphincter).
- If insertion fails, consider deepening anesthetic or partially inflating LMA cuff.
- Inflate cuff (the LMA will protrude slightly).
- Connect breathing circuit, insert (soft) bite block, and secure with tape.

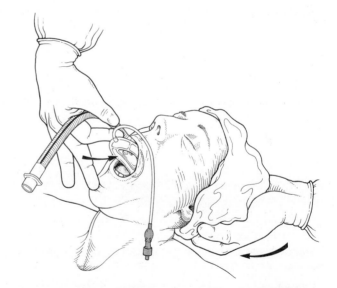

Fig. 19-6. Following stabilization of occiput with the left hand, place deflated and lubricated LMA into the open mouth. It should be pressed against the hard palate so the LMA is seen to flatten. (From Brain AIJ: The Intravent laryngeal mask instruction manual, Berkshire, U.K., 1992, *Brain Medical.*)

lubricant, which should not be allowed to dry out before insertion. A definite resistance is felt when the LMA reaches its final location. Inflate the cuff at this stage, during which the LMA should be free to move and will invariably center itself over the laryngeal opening (Fig. 19-11). The LMA should be secured with tape, taking care to ensure that the tube does not become twisted, which can cause the LMA to rotate away from the larynx. A black line is printed along the posterior surface of the LMA tube, which gives a visual confirmation of correct orientation. Insert a soft gauze bite block to protect the tube from the patient's teeth.

A variety of alternative insertion techniques have also been described, including insertion with the cuff partially inflated,[19] and insertion with the opening of the LMA facing posteriorly, followed by rotation through 180 degrees (as for a Guedel airway).[20] A comparative study has demonstrated that the conventional technique results in the highest rate of correct LMA placements in adults (as judged by fiberoptic inspection).[21] However, the alternative methods may prove effective in children and when insertion by the usual technique has failed.[20] With adequate anesthesia and appropriate choice of

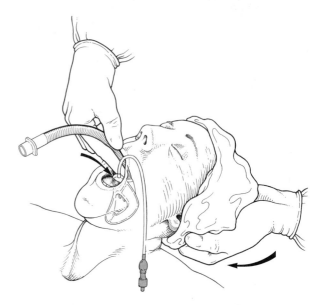

Fig. 19-9. With patient's neck flexed and head extended, slide the LMA behind the tongue and into the pharynx using the index finger of the right hand. (From Brain AIJ: The Intravent laryngeal mask instruction manual, Berkshire, U.K., 1992, *Brain Medical.*)

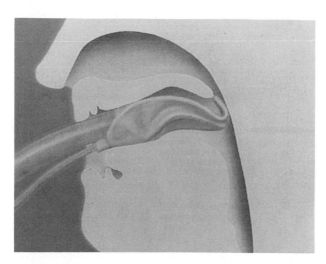

Fig. 19-7. Failure to press deflated mask against the hard palate, or inadequate lubrication or deflation, can cause the mask tip to fold back on itself; this causes it to jam against the posterior pharyngeal wall. (From Brain AIJ: The Intravent laryngeal mask instruction manual, Berkshire, U.K., 1992, *Brain Medical.*)

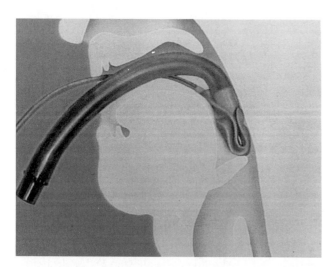

Fig. 19-8. Once mask tip has started to fold over it may continue to do so, pushing the epiglottis into a folded-down position and causing obstruction. (From Brain AIJ: The Intravent laryngeal mask instruction manual, Berkshire, U.K., 1992, *Brain Medical.*)

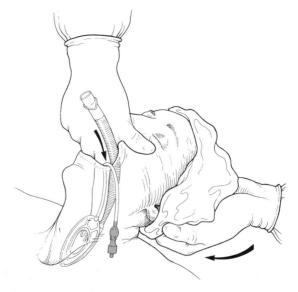

Fig. 19-10. Continue pushing with the ball of the index finger to guide the mask into position. (From Brain AIJ: The Intravent laryngeal mask instruction manual, Berkshire, U.K., 1992, *Brain Medical.*)

LMA size, it should rarely prove necessary to use a laryngoscope or other form of introducer. Although muscle relaxants are not required for LMA insertion, they may be used when it is desirable to use an intermittent positive pressure ventilation (IPPV) technique (or following failed intubation). The use of muscle relaxants does not interfere with LMA placement.

D. VENTILATION THROUGH THE LMA

For the majority of patients and procedures, spontaneous ventilation through the LMA is satisfactory, even for prolonged procedures lasting several hours. IPPV can also be applied, although it is strongly recommended

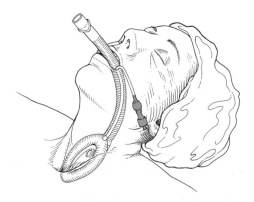

Fig. 19-11. When mask is inflated with the recommended volume of air (without the tube being held), the LMA may protrude slightly. (From Brain AIJ: The Intravent laryngeal mask instruction manual, Berkshire, U.K., 1992, *Brain Medical.*)

that the novice first gain considerable experience using the LMA with spontaneous ventilation. The two main problems in applying IPPV with the LMA are the comparatively low pressure seal and the variable relationship of the esophagus to the LMA opening. The seal between the LMA and the larynx will leak at pressures of 15 to 20 cm H_2O (often lower when the LMA is first inserted), and a minor (clinically insignificant) leak may be present at lower pressures. At 15 cm H_2O, the leak fraction was 13% (Fig. 19-12). However, this increased to 21% at 20 cm H_2O and 25% at 25 cm H_2O.[22] This means that ventilation will only be satisfactory if the lungs are reasonably compliant. Any subsequent change in compliance will alter the ventilatory pattern. Therefore, a sudden increase in leakage usually signals the need for additional muscle relaxant rather than displacement of the LMA.

Because the opening of the esophagus often lies within the bowl of the LMA, gastric distention is a possibility during prolonged IPPV, especially at high inflation pressures. Gastroesophageal insufflation occurred in less than 10% of patients ventilated through an LMA at pressures of 20 cm H_2O and below, although this increased to 20% or more at pressures above 25 cm H_2O (Fig. 19-13).[22] The use of a nasogastric tube has previously been recommended when performing IPPV through the LMA,[23] although more recent evidence suggests that clinically significant gastric insufflation is no more common during IPPV with the LMA than with an endotracheal tube, provided inflation pressures remain below 20 cm H_2O.[24] Gastric inflation is more

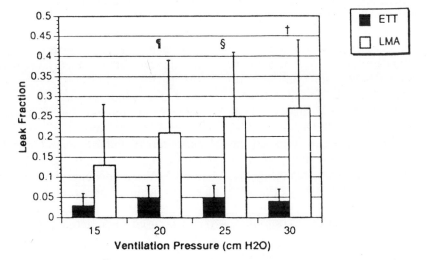

Fig. 19-12. Leak (mean ± SD), expressed as a fraction of inspired volume, with laryngeal mask airway (LMA) and endotracheal tube (ET) at different ventilation pressures. There is a significant interaction between airway device and ventilation pressure (P < 0.0001), with a diverging pattern of leak fraction with increasing ventilation pressure. The difference in leak fraction between ventilation pressures of 15 and 20 cm H_2O (P < 0.0001), 20 and 25 cm H_2O (P < 0.005), and 25 and 30 cm H_2O (P < 0.05) were statistically significant. (From Devitt JH, Wenstone R, Noel AG, O'Donnell MP: *Anesthesiology* 80:550, 1994.)

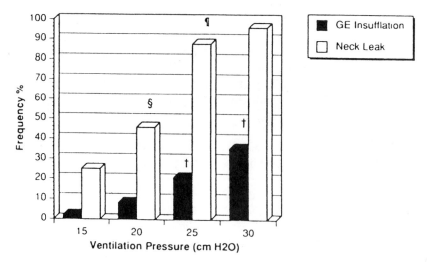

Fig. 19-13. Frequency of gastroesophageal insufflation and neck leak at different ventilation pressures. There was a significant increase in the frequency of neck leak at ventilation pressures from 15 to 20 cm H_2O (P < 0.005), and 20 to 25 cm H_2O (P < 0.0001). There was also a significant increase in the frequency of gastroesophageal insufflation at ventilation pressure from 20 to 25 cm H_2O (P < 0.0001) and 25 and 30 cm H_2O (P < 0.05). (From Devitt JH, Wenstone R, Noel AG, O'Donnell MP: *Anesthesiology* 80:550, 1994.)

likely if inadequate anesthesia or muscle relaxation allow closure of the vocal cords, which forces ventilator-driven gas into the stomach.[25]

E. REMOVAL OF THE LMA

The LMA is well tolerated even at light levels of anesthesia[26] and can be left in situ while the patient emerges from anesthesia. The patient will frequently remove the LMA themselves, and secretions that have accumulated above the mask can be withdrawn with the LMA, or swallowed. Leaving the LMA in place until return of consciousness ensures a clear airway until normal protective reflexes have returned; it is a practice recommended by the manufacturers.[12] The LMA can also be removed while the patient is still anesthetized, although the airway will then need to be supported by jaw lifting (and possibly even an oral airway). This technique appears to offer little advantage in adults, although the incidence of coughing is reduced in children by removing the LMA while they are still anesthetized.[27] It is important to avoid removing the LMA during light planes of general anesthesia because this may cause airway obstruction as a result of partial displacement of the LMA. Accumulated secretions may also induce laryngospasm.

Once the LMA is removed, it should be washed with warm, soapy water, using a bottle brush to clean the inside of the tube. It can be immersed in an 8.4% solution of bicarbonate to dissolve secretions before washing. The air should be removed from the cuff and the LMA should then be sterilized by autoclaving at a temperature of no higher than 134°C. Chemical disinfectants or ethylene oxide should not be used because they may damage the device.

VI. SPECIFIC USES OF THE LMA

A. SUPERFICIAL PROCEDURES

Body-surface surgery generally requires little (if any) muscle relaxation. While a face mask can provide for acceptable anesthetic conditions, use of the LMA ensures a clearer airway with improved hemoglobin oxygen saturation, and reduces fatigue in the anesthesiologist.[28] A further advantage is that the anesthesiologist's hands are free for record keeping, drug administration, and other tasks. Examples of the superficial surgical procedures that are frequently performed using the LMA include excision biopsies (e.g., lipomas, sebaceous cysts, tumors), varicose vein surgery, peripheral orthopedic procedures (e.g., carpal tunnel, halux valgus procedures) and peripheral plastic surgery. Inguinal herniorrhaphy can also be satisfactorily managed with the LMA. An adequate degree of muscle relaxation is usually achieved using a volatile anesthetic and spontaneous ventilation. However, muscle relaxants and IPPV may be used when necessary.

B. AMBULATORY SURGICAL PROCEDURES

Many of the surgical procedures for which the LMA has particular advantages are usually performed on ambulatory patients. In addition, use of the LMA provides additional benefits for outpatients by avoiding some of the adverse effects of endotracheal intubation.[29]

Side effects that would be considered minor in another context may be especially troublesome to outpatients. Muscle pains caused by succinylcholine are reported to be more common in patients who ambulate early than in patients who are hospitalized following surgery.[30] Although it has been alleged that myalgias can be attenuated by pretreatment with nondepolarizing muscle relaxants, well-controlled studies have failed to verify this clinical impression. In addition, this pretreatment may cause unpleasant effects such as diplopia, weakness, and, occasionally, difficulty in breathing immediately prior to induction of anesthesia. Since the LMA can easily be inserted without the use of muscle relaxants (unlike an endotracheal tube), it avoids succinylcholine-induced myalgia. Nondepolarizing muscle relaxants can also be avoided by using the LMA, which can usually be used satisfactorily with spontaneous ventilation. While not producing myalgias, the nondepolarizing relaxants increase the risk of intraoperative awareness and may result in residual weakness (and respiratory insufficiency) if their effects are inadequately reversed at the end of surgery. Furthermore, there is also evidence to suggest that the use of reversal agents (e.g., neostigmine/glycopyrrolate) may increase the incidence of postoperative nausea and vomiting.[31]

A common source of morbidity following endotracheal intubation is sore throat, which can persist for 24 hours. In one comparative study, endotracheal intubation was associated with a 49% incidence of sore throats, which was reduced to only 7% by use of the LMA.[32] Other reports have placed the incidence of postoperative sore throat with the LMA at up to 19%.[2,28,33,34] Endotracheal intubation is also associated with postoperative changes in the voice that persist for up to 24 hours. In contrast, the LMA causes fewer vocal changes[35] and is less likely to cause laryngeal damage,[36] making it the technique of choice in professional singers undergoing ambulatory surgery.

A further source of morbidity results from teeth and crowns being damaged by metal laryngoscope blades or by patients biting the oral airway during the emergence phase. Such damage may be both expensive and inconvenient, and there is also the risk that small tooth fragments may be aspirated into the airway. These sources of morbidity may be avoided by the use of the LMA and a folded gauze bite block.[37]

C. OPHTHALMIC SURGICAL PROCEDURES

While the LMA provides a useful method of securing the airway during extraocular procedures (e.g., strabismus correction), its use during intraocular operations is more controversial. The anesthetic technique for open-eye surgery should ideally avoid increases in intraocular pressure (IOP) before surgery, and should aim to

eliminate coughing and straining in the immediate postoperative period. It is essential that IOP also remain low (and reasonably constant) while the eye is open, to avoid the possibility of loss of intraocular contents.

The reduced pressor response caused by the LMA may offer advantages over an endotracheal tube for intraocular surgery. IOP decreased following induction of anesthesia and LMA insertion, whereas it increased following endotracheal intubation in a similar group of patients undergoing elective intraocular surgery. Furthermore, IOP increased again when the trachea was extubated, though no increase was observed following removal of the LMA.[38] These findings were confirmed in a follow-up investigation in which the LMA was associated with significantly smaller increases in IOP than an endotracheal tube, both on insertion and removal.[39] An additional advantage of the LMA is that its use for intraocular surgery results in a much lower incidence of coughing in the postoperative period compared to the use of an endotracheal tube.[33,39] Coughing is undesirable following eye surgery because it may elevate IOP by as much as 50 mm Hg.[39] These potential advantages of the LMA are also observed in patients with glaucoma, who are at a greater risk of vision loss if IOP rises excessively. Induction of anesthesia with propofol, followed by LMA insertion, resulted in a 40% reduction in IOP from the awake level.[40] In contrast, IOP exceeded baseline values following endotracheal intubation in patients receiving an identical anesthesia-induction regimen (Fig. 19-14). The LMA may also be preferable to an endotracheal tube when anesthesia is required for the measurement of IOP (e.g., "examinations under anesthesia" in children).[41]

Although investigations to date have generally been associated with satisfactory intraoperative conditions, concern has been expressed about the safety of using the LMA during open-globe procedures. The intraocular contents could be put at risk if misplacement of the LMA caused an increase in IOP secondary to coughing or airway obstruction. Although such misplacement of the LMA has been reported,[42] no serious adverse events appear to have occurred. In one series of more than 400 intraocular procedures, the LMA was used without the occurrence of any adverse event.[43] In another series of 593 uses, the LMA was incorrectly located in one patient and became displaced in another, giving an overall complication rate of 0.3%. This contrasted with a 1.6% incidence of serious problems occurring with endotracheal tubes over a similar period, including cases of laryngospasm, difficult intubation, and pulmonary edema.[42] Clearly, the results of even larger series are needed before declaring the LMA safe for routine intraocular surgery. However, careful attention to the insertion technique and the maintenance of an adequate

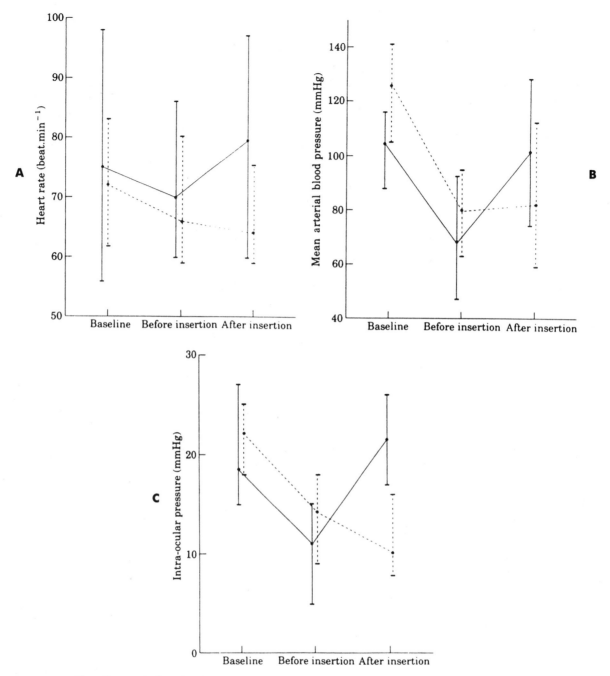

Fig. 19-14. Median (95% confidence interval) heart rate (**A**), arterial pressure (**B**), and intraocular pressure (**C**) before induction of anesthesia (baseline), after induction of anesthesia (before insertion), and after insertion of either a laryngeal mask (--●--) or an endotracheal tube (–●–) (after insertion). (From Barclay K, Wall T, Wareham K, Asai T: *Anaesthesia* 49:159, 1994.)

degree of anesthesia and muscle relaxation should reduce the likelihood of serious complications.[44]

D. ORAL AND ENT SURGICAL PROCEDURES

Anesthesia for oral and ENT surgery requires that the need for unrestricted surgical access to balanced against maintenance and protection of the airway. A variety of techniques, including insufflation and nasal masks, have been used in the past, although endotracheal intubation is most commonly employed. A further alternative is the LMA, which occupies most of the hypopharynx, reducing the space that requires packing and providing excellent protection of the larynx from blood and other debris.[1] When methylene blue was introduced into the pharynx above an LMA, subsequent inspection of the larynx and trachea with a fiberoptic bronchoscope failed to detect any staining with the dye.[45] In a large series of patients undergoing dental extraction, the laryngeal (inside) surface of the LMA was bloodstained in only 3% of cases.[18] Compared to a nasal mask for simple dental extraction in children, the LMA provided a greatly superior airway, and allowed the placement of a more effective throat pack.[18,46,47]

There is also increasing experience in the use of the LMA for adenotonsillectomy. One early problem that was encountered was compression of the soft LMA tube by the Boyle-Davis gag, leading to partial airway obstruction. A reinforced LMA (RLMA), which incorporates a wire spiral, has been developed to eliminate this problem.[48] However, the tube of the RLMA is more flexible than the standard LMA, which can make its insertion more difficult. The use of a gum elastic bougie to stiffen the tube during insertion has been recommended.[49] In one randomized comparison, surgical access when using the RLMA was indistinguishable from access when using an endotracheal tube. In addition, the RLMA appeared to offer better protection of the trachea from blood contamination compared to a noncuffed endotracheal tube in small children.[50] However, it is important to ensure an adequate level of anesthesia during surgery to prevent laryngospasm in response to surgical stimuli.[51] Following adenotonsillectomy with the RLMA, recovery appears to be "smoother," with a lower incidence of stridor, laryngospasm, and oxygen desaturation compared with endotracheal intubation.[4,50,51]

Laser surgery of the upper airway is becoming increasingly common, and presents problems in the prevention of airway fires. Preliminary studies suggest that the LMA may be comparatively resistant to perforation by laser equipment.[52] However, other investigators have failed to confirm this observation, and advocate shielding the LMA tube and protecting the cuff with wet gauze swabs.[53]

E. ENDOSCOPIC PROCEDURES

Simple endoscopic procedures such as cystoscopy and arthroscopy are frequently performed under general anesthesia. These procedures rarely require muscle relaxation, but they are of sufficient duration (about 1 hour) to make the use of a face mask inconvenient. The LMA is an ideal solution; during arthroscopic surgery it provided a superior airway compared to a face mask.[28]

The LMA can also serve as a conduit for fiberoptic bronchoscopy, improving the speed of access to the larynx while avoiding the trauma of nasal insertion or endotracheal intubation.[54] By avoiding endotracheal intubation, a larger area of the airway is available for ventilation, which may be particularly advantageous in

children.[54-56] In addition, since the LMA may be placed without muscle relaxants, a dynamic view of vocal cord movements can be obtained.[54,55,57]

The use of the LMA for laparoscopic procedures is considerably more controversial.[58] The combination of intraperitoneal gas insufflation and the Trendelenburg position are said to increase the risk of regurgitation and also to compromise spontaneous ventilation, leading to carbon dioxide retention. However, it has been shown that lower-esophageal sphincter tone rises in response to raised intraabdominal pressure,[59] so that gastroesophageal "barrier" pressure actually increases. Furthermore, no aspiration occurred in a large series of approximately 5000 patients undergoing pelvic laparoscopy while breathing spontaneously via a face mask.[60] In addition, several investigators have found similar arterial or $ETCO_2$ values with either spontaneous or assisted ventilation during short laparoscopic procedures.[61,62]

Goodwin and colleagues studied 40 women who underwent laparoscopy while spontaneously breathing through an LMA.[63] Anesthesia was maintained either by a propofol infusion or enflurane with nitrous oxide, 70% in oxygen. Neither technique produced significant adverse respiratory or cardiac effects, and no episode of aspiration was recorded. In a comparison with endotracheal intubation for gynecological laparoscopy, similar intraoperative conditions were obtained with either technique. The use of the LMA was associated with a higher incidence of nausea in the early postoperative period, which may have been due to gastric insufflation caused by the use of assisted ventilation during the period of pneumoperitoneum.[64]

Although no cases of aspiration have been reported in connection with the use of the LMA for laparoscopy, relatively little experience of this technique has been described in the peer-reviewed literature. However, Malins and Cooper have used the LMA (with controlled ventilation) for more than 3000 gynecologic laparoscopies over a six-year period. Two patients regurgitated, although neither aspirated. However, in a similar period one patient for whom endotracheal intubation was planned regurgitated and aspirated following induction of anesthesia. These authors stress that the use of large volumes of insufflating gas, steep head-down tilt (e.g., >90 degrees), prolonged surgery, and obesity all increase the risk of aspiration during the use of the LMA for laparoscopy, and should be considered contraindications.[65] Although the LMA appears to be safe, its role in laparoscopic surgery will remain uncertain until the results of even larger series of patients are available.

F. PEDIATRIC SURGICAL PROCEDURES

The smaller size (1 to 2.5) LMA devices have been developed for use in children. Despite being scaled-down versions of the adult LMA (which was carefully developed with reference to anatomical specimens), airway complications and difficulties in LMA placement are similar in children.[4] Compared to a face mask, use of the LMA in children improves oxygen saturation and surgical conditions.[66] The pattern of use of the LMA in children is principally influenced by the different range of procedures being performed. For example, sedation-type anesthesia is often required to ensure cooperation and immobility during diagnostic, imaging, and radiotherapy procedures, which rarely require monitored anesthesia care in adults. Many of these procedures can satisfactorily be managed using the LMA.[14,67,68] The RLMA may provide advantages when imaging or radiotherapy require that the child be placed in awkward positions, with the risk of kinking the LMA tube.[49] The metal spiral precludes the use of the RLMA during magnetic resonance imaging, although the standard LMA is safe, provided that a special nonmetallic valve is fitted to the pilot tube.

In children, insertion of the LMA may be more successful on the first attempt if the cuff is partially inflated to remove all folds and indentations.[15] Alternatively, insertion of the LMA with the opening facing posteriorly, followed by rotation through 180 degrees (similar to a Guedel airway) has been reported to overcome some cases of difficult insertion.[20] Removal of the LMA under "deep" anesthesia can reduce the incidence of coughing compared to removal from awake children.[27]

G. OBSTETRIC ANESTHESIA

The increased risk of pulmonary aspiration in obstetric patients, resulting from the effects of pregnancy on gastric emptying, contraindicate the routine use of the LMA. However, the LMA may have a place in the emergency management of the airway following failed endotracheal intubation. One case has been reported in which adequate oxygenation could not be achieved using a bag and face mask, but which responded to insertion of the LMA.[69] Manual ventilation via the LMA restored oxygen saturation and then permitted anesthesia to be maintained during the subsequent cesarean section, which was urgently required for persistent fetal bradycardia.

It is anticipated that even the emergency use of the LMA in pregnant patients will be limited. The accepted management of failed intubation in obstetric practice is to allow the patient to wake up, unless the planned operation is extremely urgent. In this event, oxygenation and anesthesia should be supplied by face mask. The LMA should not routinely be used, since attempts to pass it may precipitate vomiting. However, as described, the LMA may be lifesaving when an adequate airway cannot be achieved with a face mask.

H. DIFFICULT INTUBATION (VENTILATION AND/OR INTUBATION THROUGH THE LMA)

The LMA may have a role in cases involving both anticipated and unanticipated difficult endotracheal intubation (see also Chapter 16). For example, the LMA was successfully placed in a patient with a severe fixed flexion deformity of the neck and limited mouth opening as a result of facial burns.[70] Similarly, Brain described the trouble-free passage of a prototype LMA in a patient known to have been previously difficult to intubate. Indeed, successful insertion of the LMA may actually be easier in patients with some anatomical causes of difficult intubation.[11] Insertion of the LMA with the neck in the neutral position (as in cervical spine injury) appears to be almost as successful as the conventional technique.[71] Although elective use of the fiberoptic laryngoscope is often considered to be the technique of choice in cases of anticipated difficulty in intubation, the LMA may be the only practical option when the presence of blood or pulmonary edema make fiberoptic intubation virtually impossible.[72]

If the anesthesiologist can secure the difficult airway with the LMA, several choices for subsequent management are available (Box 19-2). At worst, the LMA will allow adequate oxygenation while definitive management is planned, or the patient is allowed to awaken. Awake endotracheal intubation may then be performed. In some situations the LMA may represent a satisfactory alternative to the planned anesthetic technique, in which case surgery can be allowed to proceed. Rarely, a combination of unusual circumstances may necessitate the use of the LMA to provide anesthesia for procedures normally requiring endotracheal intubation (e.g., cardiac surgery).[73] However, in most cases (especially emergency cases), the risk of pulmonary aspiration will require the airway to be secured with an endotracheal tube or tracheostomy while using the LMA as a conduit or a temporary airway.

In adults, a 6-mm internal-diameter endotracheal tube can be passed through the tube of size 3 and 4 LMAs (Box 19-3). Provided that the LMA is correctly located, a well-lubricated, uncut 6-mm endotracheal tube can be blindly advanced through the aperture of the LMA and into the larynx. Rotation of the endotracheal tube 90 degrees to the left can prevent the bevel of the tube catching on the bars of the LMA aperture.[74] Tracheal intubation by this method was found to be possible in 90% of cases, with most failures being due to an inability to correctly insert the LMA.[75] Passage of the endotracheal tube through the larynx may be aided by the use of deep anesthesia or muscle relaxants. Extending the atlantooccipital joint may assist intubation when it proves difficult to pass the tube with the patient in the classic "sniffing" position. The type of endotracheal tube

<table>
</table>

BOX 19-2   Management of "difficult intubation" once an LMA has been inserted and is functioning satisfactorily

Abandon surgery

- Use LMA to permit oxygenation while patient awakens; operation subsequently performed using local or regional anesthesia or by first performing awake endotracheal intubation, then inducing general anesthesia.

Use LMA for anesthesia

- Continue surgery while maintaining anesthesia via LMA using either spontaneous or controlled ventilation.

Intubate trachea using LMA as a conduit

- Pass uncut 6-mm ID endotracheal tube directly through LMA.
- Pass gum-elastic bougie via LMA into trachea; remove LMA, railroad endotracheal tube.
- Pass fiberoptic bronchoscope (with premounted endotracheal tube) via LMA into larynx; cut LMA longitudinally and peel away from fiberoptic scope; advance endotracheal tube into trachea.

Maintain oxygenation via LMA while securing airway by alternative means

- Perform surgical tracheostomy.
- Perform cricothyroid puncture and pass catheter retrograde into mouth.
- Pass nasal catheter and retrieve from mouth; pass catheter into trachea via LMA; remove LMA, sew catheters together, and use as guide to blind nasal intubation.

BOX 19-3   Techniques of direct endotracheal intubation through the LMA

Preparation

- Prepare uncut 6-mm ID endotracheal tube with connector firmly inserted.
- Lubricate outside surface of endotracheal tube with water-based lubricant.

Technique

- Place size 3 or 4 LMA, strictly following the preferred insertion technique (to prevent folding down of epiglottis).
- Inflate cuff with 10 to 15 ml air (low volumes make intubation easier).
- Ensure correct position of LMA by adequate ventilatory pattern.
- Administer muscle relaxant or ensure deep anesthesia to prevent laryngospasm on intubation.
- Insert endotracheal tube through tube of LMA.
- Rotate endotracheal tube through 90 degrees to the left so that bevel faces anteriorly.
- Once tube passes bars of LMA, (about 20 cm), allow it to rotate back (90 degrees) to normal position.
- Advance endotracheal tube gently until fully inserted (connector touches that of the LMA).
- Confirm correct position by capnography or esophageal detector device.
- Inflate endotracheal tube cuff (will require large volume) and secure both tube and LMA.
- Assisted ventilation is preferable (except for brief cases) because of the small tube diameter.

If trachea is not entered

- Alter relative positions of patient's head and neck.
- Adjust volume of air in LMA cuff.
- Try different make of endotracheal tube (Portex nasal and Mallinckrodt reinforced are associated with a high success rate).
- In emergencies, try transiently releasing cricoid pressure (after other methods have failed).

---

can also influence the success of endotracheal intubation through the LMA.[76] Once the endotracheal tube has been fully advanced, its position can be confirmed by capnography or the esophageal detector device.[77] There is little experience of the use of the LMA to permit intubation of pediatric patients. However, a 4-kg, 1-day-old neonate with the Pierre Robin syndrome was successfully intubated by the blind passage of a 3-mm endotracheal tube through a size 1 LMA following failed direct laryngoscopy.[78]

Although direct intubation through the LMA is often effective, it is limited by the inability to pass a tube larger than 6 mm. Furthermore, the anesthesiologist has little control over the final location of the endotracheal tube, which in some cases may not be long enough to allow the endotracheal tube cuff to be positioned below the level of the cords.[79] Brain has described a prototype LMA that permits the passage of larger sizes of endotracheal tube.[11] Until the larger intubating LMA is routinely

available, the LMA must be removed after passage of an intubating guide in order to insert a larger (>6 mm) endotracheal tube. For example, a gum-elastic bougie can be passed through the LMA and into the larynx; after removal of the LMA, an endotracheal tube is passed over this guide.[80] Passage of the bougie is facilitated by angulation of the tip anteriorly until the aperture of the LMA is passed, followed by rotation of the tip through 180 degrees to guide it into the larynx. Preliminary trials produced successful endotracheal intubation in 84% of patients, with failure being most commonly associated with poor positioning of the LMA.[81] A variant of this technique that permits nasal intubation has also been described.[82]

If a fiberoptic laryngoscope or bronchoscope is available, a suitable endotracheal tube (cuffed 6-mm ID) can be mounted at the top of the fiberscope before it is passed through the LMA (see also Chapter 16). This technique allows the larynx to be located even when the position of the LMA prevents blind intubation. It appears that the larynx can be visualized in virtually all patients in whom a LMA can be placed.[83] Once the fiberoptic laryngoscope is passed into the larynx, the cuffed 6-mm ID is passed over the fiberscope into the trachea until the adapter of the 6-mm ID endotracheal tube is flush with the adapter of the LMA. The LMA will have to be removed before a larger endotracheal tube can be slid into place. With care, the LMA tube can be slit longitudinally and peeled away from the fiberoptic endoscope. If difficulty has been anticipated in advance, it is possible to use a presplit LMA, which can subsequently be reused. The open ends of the cuff of the split LMA can be sealed with vulcanized silicone, which preserves normal function and withstands repeated autoclaving.[84] In rare situations, none of these methods may be applicable or effective, in which case the airway may have to be secured by alternative means (e.g., tracheostomy, retrograde intubation) while the LMA serves as a method of maintaining oxygenation.

In the management of an unanticipated (or failed) intubation in a nonfasting patient, it is essential that cricoid pressure be maintained in order to prevent regurgitation and aspiration of stomach contents. Several investigators have examined the effect of cricoid pressure on the success of LMA insertion and subsequent intubation through the LMA. Asai et al. attempted to simulate unexpected failed intubation after administration of muscle relaxants to nonfasting patients. After placement of the LMA, satisfactory ventilation was achieved in only 50% of patients receiving two-handed cricoid pressure, compared to 95% of a control group without cricoid pressure. Furthermore, when a fiberoptic bronchoscope was passed through the LMA, the position of the airway was judged to be "correct" in only 10% of patients with cricoid pressure, and endotracheal intubation (guided by the bronchoscope) was possible in only 15%. Transient release of the cricoid pressure increased the number of patients who could be successfully intubated, but the total was still only 34%.[85]

In contrast, a second study involving simulated failed intubation found that the application of single-handed cricoid pressure only reduced successful insertion with the LMA (judged by fiberoptic evaluation and ability to ventilate the lungs) from 98% to 90%.[86] However, no attempt was made to intubate the trachea in this study. Differences between these results may be due to the use of one versus two hands to apply cricoid pressure, and the position of the patient's neck (flexed versus ex-

tended). Application of cricoid pressure with the patient's neck extended is known to compress most of the hypopharynx, and would be expected to impede correct LMA placement. While application of cricoid pressure with the neck flexed may make LMA insertion more successful, it is not known if this will effectively prevent regurgitation.[87] Until this issue is resolved, it would seem prudent to avoid the use of LMA when cricoid pressure is required unless it is impossible to manage the airway in any other way. If it becomes necessary to insert an LMA, cricoid pressure should be maintained until the patient is awake or the trachea is intubated. Cricoid pressure should only be released to aid insertion of the LMA if this is considered to be a lifesaving maneuver. Strang has demonstrated in cadavers that once the LMA is correctly positioned, cricoid pressure is effective in preventing regurgitation of barium inserted into the esophagus with pressures which are encountered clinically.[88]

I. EMERGENCY AIRWAY MANAGEMENT (USE IN RESUSCITATION)

The LMA may be a useful alternative to reintubation of the trachea for management of postoperative problems following elective surgery (e.g., inadequate reversal of muscle relaxants, upper-airway obstruction),[89] though intubation of the trachea remains the "gold standard" for the management of the airway in emergency situations (e.g., cardiac arrest, major trauma). Nevertheless, skilled medical personnel may not be immediately available, and there have been increasing efforts to train paramedical staff to intubate the trachea. It is well recognized that adequate training is time-consuming, and that the skills need to be practiced regularly if they are to be retained. Several investigators have studied the ease with which paramedical staff can be trained to use the LMA. One group of inexperienced medical trainees were given instruction in LMA and endotracheal-tube insertion techniques using a video instruction program, a mannequin for practice, and a live demonstration. Following this training period, the trainees successfully inserted the LMA in 94% of cases, compared to a 51% success rate in achieving endotracheal intubation within 40 seconds. More importantly, the trainees inadvertently intubated the esophagus in 13% of cases.[90] In a second study involving medical and paramedical students, the LMA was inserted significantly sooner compared to endotracheal intubation (39 versus 88 seconds). Five students were unable to intubate the trachea after three attempts, yet all inserted an LMA into the same patient on their first attempt.[91]

For personnel who have not received instruction in endotracheal intubation, the use of a bag and face mask may be the only method available for resuscitation. Following a brief period of training, volunteers were able to insert an LMA and maintain adequate ventilation in 87% of patients, compared to a 43% success rate using a bag, mask, and Guedel airway.[92] Also following minimal training, nurses were able to achieve significantly more effective ventilation in patients when using the LMA than when using a face mask.[93]

The LMA has also successfully been used for prehospital resuscitation of unconscious victims of motor-vehicle accidents in whom entrapment within the vehicle wreckage made endotracheal intubation impossible.[94] The LMA acted as a temporary method for airway management, with definitive control being established once the victim was freed.

Although the need to provide oxygenation without aspiration requires that endotracheal intubation remain an essential component of all resuscitation protocols, the LMA may provide better airway management than the use of a face mask or attempts at intubation by inadequately trained persons. The reduced period of training required for LMA insertion would allow a higher proportion of paramedical staff to have sufficient airway-management skills to prevent hypoxia until more experienced personnel are available to provide definitive care.

VII. ADVANTAGES

Compared to face-mask and endotracheal intubation, the LMA is associated with relatively few complications. The LMA can be placed easily, and an adequate airway can be established in the majority of patients. It provides a superior airway (e.g., less hemoglobin desaturation) compared to a face mask with an oral airway.[28] In addition, use of the LMA eliminates fatigue seen in the anesthesiologist managing the airway with a face mask and allows the anesthesiologist to perform other tasks such as drug administration and record keeping.[28]

Placement of the LMA does not require muscle relaxation and laryngoscopy and thus may prevent the associated problems (e.g., muscle pains, damage to teeth and crowns). The LMA offers advantages over the endotracheal tube with respect to hemodynamic and intraocular pressure stability. Hemodynamic responses following the placement of the LMA are reduced compared to laryngoscopy and endotracheal intubation, and are similar to those associated with insertion of the Guedel airway.[38,40,95-97] Similarly, the pressor response during the patient's emergence from general anesthesia with the LMA in situ was significantly lower than that with the endotracheal tube in place.[98] The insertion of the LMA leads to a smaller increase in the IOP values than laryngoscopy and endotracheal intubation in patients with normal IOP and in those with glaucoma.[38,40]

Because the LMA is tolerated at a lighter depth of anesthesia than an endotracheal tube, its use may permit more rapid awakening and earlier discharge after ambulatory surgery.[26] In the postoperative period, the LMA is well tolerated and can be left in situ to provide an unobstructed airway and adequate oxygenation until return of consciousness ensures a clear airway. The incidence of sore throat following the use of the LMA is reported to be between 7% and 12%.[28,32,34,99] The incidence of throat soreness is lower than following endotracheal intubation, and comparable to that seen with oral airways.[28,32] Because of the absence of contact with the vocal cords, the LMA may decrease morbidity in professional singers.[36]

The LMA can serve as a conduit for fiberoptic bronchoscopy and allow a dynamic view of vocal-cord movements. It has proved useful in situations involving unanticipated difficult endotracheal intubation. Its use has been incorporated into the protocol for difficult intubation. In addition, the LMA may be useful in prehospital resuscitation of trauma victims because it is easy to use and also avoids the risk of esophageal or endobronchial intubation.[91]

Both in vitro and in vivo studies demonstrate that the resistance and work of breathing through the LMA is significantly lower than that through an endotracheal tube.[100,101] This may be important in patients with pulmonary disease breathing spontaneously through the LMA.

Although the LMA is reusable, it is expensive ($200) compared to the endotracheal tube ($1.50). It is estimated that the LMA can be reused 40 to 100 times.[4,6] Analysis of all direct and indirect costs suggest that the use of the LMA device can prove cost effective for surgical procedures that do not require the use of muscle relaxants.[102]

VIII. DISADVANTAGES

One of the major limitations of the LMA is that it does not guarantee a seal against pulmonary aspiration of gastric contents and other secretions. In 10% to 15% of patients, the esophagus is ensnared within the cuff of the LMA, which may lead to gastric distention during positive pressure ventilation.[103-105] In addition, inadequate depth of anesthesia may cause the patient to swallow air during spontaneous ventilation through the LMA, which may cause gastric distention.[106] Furthermore, compared with the lower esophageal sphincter tone in anesthetized patients breathing spontaneously through a face mask and Guedel airway, the tone in patients breathing through the LMA is significantly lower.[107] Rabey et al. suggest that distention of the hypopharyngeal space by the LMA may result in reflex relaxation of the lower esophageal sphincter. However, the upper esophageal sphincter remains competent during the use of the LMA and the face mask, but becomes incompetent following the use of muscle relaxants for endotracheal intubation.[108]

Following the introduction of the LMA, aspiration was reported in several patients for whom there were contraindications to its use (e.g., emergency surgery, recent trauma). Of more concern were the sporadic reports of regurgitation occurring in adequately fasting, elective-surgery patients with no apparent evidence of a full stomach. Regurgitation usually provided little warning, with the first indication being the appearance of gastric secretions in the tube of the LMA. Some of the reported episodes were triggered by moving the patient, while others occurred during recovery from anesthesia.[109-112] It is likely that abdominal contraction and attempted inspiration against a closed glottis—in response to surgical stimulation during inadequate anesthesia, or muscle relaxation in the case of IPPV—may trigger regurgitation.[25] Fortunately, most of the reported cases have resulted in favorable outcomes because the regurgitated material was not aspirated, or the aspiration was relatively mild. The ability of the vocal cords to contract beneath the LMA may offer some protection against serious aspiration.

In one series (n = 56) in which patients swallowed a capsule of methylene blue dye before anesthesia, the incidence of gastric regurgitation in those patients breathing spontaneously via the LMA was reported to be 25%, whereas there was no regurgitation in patients breathing through the face mask and Guedel airway.[113] However, another similar study (n = 60) using methylene blue as a marker reported no regurgitation in patients breathing either through the LMA or the face mask and Guedel airway.[114] In a study comparing the incidence of regurgitation and aspiration between spontaneously breathing patients and those undergoing mechanical ventilation through the LMA, 1 out of 25 patients (4%) in each group regurgitated methylene blue dye.[115] However, in the patient who was ventilated mechanically, the dye was also present in the trachea and bronchi.

A recent preliminary study (n = 55) describing the use of esophageal pH electrodes reported a significantly higher incidence of gastroesophageal reflux with the use of the LMA compared with the use of a face mask.[116] In contrast, another study using a similar technique could not demonstrate gastric regurgitation in anesthetized patients breathing spontaneously through either the LMA or the endotracheal tube.[117] The inconsistent results between these two studies emphasizes the importance of further research on this topic.

The incidence of silent regurgitation during general anesthesia is between 5% and 20%.[118-121] The incidence of clinically significant pulmonary aspiration reported by large surveys is between 0.01% and 0.8%.[122-124] Because the incidence of pulmonary aspiration is very small, a large, prospective, randomized trial comparing pulmonary aspiration when the endotracheal tube, LMA, and face mask are used will be necessary to avoid a type II statistical error.

Except for case reports, there are no large studies comparing the incidence of pulmonary aspiration when the endotracheal tube, LMA, and face mask are used. The reporting of critical incidents is notoriously unreliable, so that the overall incidence of aspiration with the LMA is unknown. In those series that have been published, the incidence appears to range from 1 in 3500 to 1 in 4300, which is comparable to the overall incidence of aspiration in elective surgery using face masks and tracheal tubes.[42,122-125] It has been suggested that IPPV via the LMA may increase the incidence of regurgitation (due to gastric distention). The maintenance of adequate depth of anesthesia and muscle relaxation appears to be especially important during IPPV through the LMA.[25] The incidence of aspiration associated with the LMA, according to a metaanalysis of randomized studies and case reports, is 2 in 10,000 patients.[126] However, the issue would be more easily resolved if the results of the enormous amount of clinical experience with the LMA to date were available for analysis.

The management of a patient who regurgitates or vomits during general anesthesia via the LMA is controversial. One of the recommendations is that upon suctioning of the hypopharynx, the LMA be removed immediately and replaced with the endotracheal tube.[3,127] In contrast, Brain recommends leaving the LMA in situ, placing the patient in the Trendelenburg position, increasing the FiO_2 to 1, and then suctioning through the LMA tube once the oxygenation is satisfactory.[128] Following this, tracheal intubation and fiberoptic bronchoscopy can be performed. Furthermore, he suggests that regurgitation or vomiting may be detected earlier with the LMA in position compared with a face mask because the gastric contents can be noticed earlier coming through the transparent tube of the LMA. It is suggested that patients who aspirate gastric contents be observed for at least two hours after surgery because those who develop symptoms within two hours of aspiration are likely to have respiratory complications.[122]

There is a small incidence (1% to 5%) of failed placement of the LMA, although this decreases with increasing experience of the anesthesiologist.[129] In addition, selection of the right LMA size, adherence to correct insertion technique, and maintenance of adequate depth of anesthesia during insertion are important factors for successful placement of the LMA.

The LMA cuff is permeable to nitrous oxide and carbon dioxide, which results in significant increases in cuff pressures and volume during anesthesia.[130,131] Although these changes did not increase the pressure exerted upon the pharyngeal mucosa, it may be an important consideration when prolonged or repeated LMA use is anticipated.[131] In addition, airway obstruction may occur from overinflation caused by diffusion of nitrous oxide into the cuff.[132] It is possible that the increased intracuff pressures may increase the incidence of postoperative sore throats or cause transient dysarthria. A pressure-relief valve fitted to the cuff of the LMA[130] and inflating the cuff with volumes not exceeding its residual volumes[131] may decrease diffusional overinflation. Although the manufacturers recommend intracuff pressure monitoring, they do not suggest an acceptable pressure.

Edema of the epiglottis resulting from its entrapment in the bars at the distal aperture of the LMA may lead to airway obstruction.[133] Swelling of the uvula and trauma to the posterior pharyngeal wall have also been reported.[134-136] Bacteremia following the placement of the LMA may be of concern in immunocompromised patients.[137,138] With repeated use, the cuff or the tube of the LMA may fracture or leak, although this should usually be detected during testing prior to use.[139,140] Other problems with the LMA include dislodgment and kinking and the presence of foreign bodies in the tube of the LMA, leading to airway obstruction.[141] Accidental (inadvertent) disposal of this reusable device can also be a costly problem. Fortunately, this problem can be minimized with proper in-service education of the operating-room staff.

IX. CONTRAINDICATIONS

Although the LMA has advantages in many clinical situations, it is not suitable for all patients and procedures. With increasing experience there are increasing reports of mishaps with the use of the LMA. Interestingly, most of the complications reported may have been prevented if the contraindications to the use of the LMA had been followed.[5,6,142]

The LMA instruction manual suggests that the LMA should only be used in "fasting" patients.[12] Because the LMA does not protect against aspiration of gastric contents and may increase the incidence of aspiration by preferentially directing regurgitated material into the airway, it is contraindicated in patients at risk of regurgitation. The use of the LMA is contraindicated in obese patients, patients with hiatus hernias, pregnant patients, and those with a history of gastric regurgitation, heartburn, ileus, and "full stomach."

The LMA is relatively contraindicated in patients with low pulmonary compliance or high pulmonary resistance who may require inflation pressures of more than 20 cm H_2O to ventilate through the LMA. Because the LMA seal pop-off pressure is 15 to 20 cm H_2O, high inflation pressures may lead to inadequate ventilation and gastric distention, which may increase the incidence of gastric regurgitation.

Because the LMA may be dislodged, its use is relatively contraindicated whenever access to the patient's airway is difficult or endotracheal intubation cannot be readily accomplished (e.g., operations when the patient is in prone, lateral, and jackknife position, or when the operating table is turned away from the anesthesiologist).[5,192] Of interest, the LMA has been safely used when the patient is in the prone position.[49,143]

Although the LMA may have a role in unanticipated or failed endotracheal intubation, it is relatively contraindicated in patients with known history of difficult endotracheal intubation or signs suggesting the possibility of difficult intubation. Thus it should not be used as a substitute for endotracheal intubation in such patients. In addition, it is contraindicated in patients with pathology in the pharynx, such as abscess, hematoma, edema, tissue disruption, or tumor. Furthermore, upper airway obstruction due to laryngeal pathology is also a contraindication for the use of the LMA.

X. FUTURE OF THE LMA

The LMA was originally marketed in four different sizes. Since then, a size 2.5 has been added, which bridges the considerable difference in size between 2 and 3 masks. More recently, wire-reinforced LMAs have been introduced (in the same five sizes), for use in situations where kinking of the LMA tube is a concern. It is now possible to choose a suitable-size LMA for most patients and situations in which the technique is appropriate. The biggest disadvantage of the current LMA is that it does not seal the trachea against aspiration. While efforts continue to develop the ultimate LMA (which would offer this protection), it may still be necessary to intubate the trachea even after the airway has been established using the LMA (e.g., failed intubation). While direct passage of an endotracheal tube through the LMA is less successful than fiberoptic intubation, it is invariably quicker, requires no special (or expensive) equipment, and does not require any interruption in ventilation during intubation. However, the size of the endotracheal tube is currently limited to a maximum internal diameter of 6 mm, and the position of the endotracheal-tube cuff is dependent upon the length of the LMA tube. A prototype "intubating LMA" was described as long ago as 1985,[11] but a commercial version has not been released. The prototype comprised a standard LMA bowl attached to a wide-bore tube, which would permit the passage of endotracheal tubes up to 9 mm in internal diameter. The ideal intubating LMA would also have a shorter tube, to permit greater control of the depth of endotracheal-tube insertion (ST-LMA).

The ultimate LMA would protect the trachea against aspiration.[7] A variety of prototype designs have been evaluated that incorporate tubes or grooves to drain the esophagus.[7,144] Unfortunately, these modifications increase the complexity (and cost) of the device, and also make insertion more difficult. A hybrid device, comprising a hollow esophageal obturator attached to the convex surface of the LMA, has been evaluated with a small number of patients. Although the prototype appeared to be effective in separating the trachea and esophagus, insertion appeared to be more difficult and was associated with a higher incidence of complications.[145] In addition, it would seem unlikely that such a device could be reliably inserted in the presence of cricoid pressure. Until the ultimate LMA device is developed, a better solution would appear to be insertion of a separate gastroesophageal tube after placing the LMA.[144]

Based on the enormous experience gained by the inventor of the LMA in its development, a variety of more-specialized LMAs are under development. One of the more interesting variants is the "nasal LMA," which would comprise a detachable tube. After placing the LMA conventionally, the tube would be detached and removed from the mouth, to be inserted through the nose and reattached to the bowl.[7] However, in the absence of specific indications for such a device, it is unlikely that it will become available for clinical use. A novel version of the LMA has been developed that incorporates an oximeter probe to permit measurement of hemoglobin oxygen saturation from the pharyngeal mucosa.

XI. CONCLUSION

The LMA is easy to use and provides a clear airway, in both adults and children, in a wide variety of clinical situations. The LMA combines several advantages and prevents the morbidity associated with both the endotracheal tube and face masks. It may also be more cost-effective than the endotracheal tube in surgical procedures performed on outpatients. The LMA has proved to be useful in the management of unanticipated difficult endotracheal intubation and in fiberoptic visualization of the upper and lower airway. In addition, it may have a role in securing the airway for emergency use in or out of the hospital. However, it is important to recognize the limitations of the LMA and to adhere to the contraindications for its use. Proper selection of patients and learning the correct insertion technique are necessary before use. Maintenance of adequate depth of anesthesia should prevent most common problems associated with the LMA, namely difficulty in its placement, difficult ventilation, gastric distention, coughing, and laryngospasm. Monitoring for gastric distention may help in preventing regurgitation of gastric contents. The LMA has a great potential in the modern anesthetic practice. With availability of results of well-designed trials, the role of the LMA may expand in the future.

ACKNOWLEDGMENTS

The authors would like to thank Dr. A.I.J. Brain for sharing his views on the future of the laryngeal mask airway.

REFERENCES

1. Brain AIJ: The laryngeal mask: a new concept in airway management, *Br J Anaesth* 55:801, 1983.
2. Brodrick PM, Webster NR, Nunn JF: The laryngeal mask airway: a study of 100 patients during spontaneous breathing, *Anaesthesia* 44:238, 1989.
3. Pennant JH, White PF: The laryngeal mask airway: its uses in anesthesiology, *Anesthesiology* 79:144, 1993 (review).
4. Leach AB, Alexander CA: The laryngeal mask: an overview, *Eur J Anaesthesiol* 4:19, 1991 (review).
5. Benumof JL: Laryngeal mask airway: indications and contraindications, *Anesthesiology* 77:843, 1992 (editorial).
6. Asai T, Vaughan RS: Misuse of the laryngeal mask airway, *Anaesthesia* 49:467, 1994 (editorial).
7. Brain AI: The development of the laryngeal mask: a brief history of the invention, early clinical studies and experimental work from which the laryngeal mask evolved, *Eur J Anaesthesiol* 4:5, 1991.
8. Leech BC: Pharyngeal bulb gasway: a new aid in cyclopropane anesthesia. *Anesth Analg* 16:22, 1937.
9. Bodman R: Deja vu, *Br J Anaesth* 64:406, 1990 (letter).
10. Brain AIJ, McGhee TD, McAteer EJ et al: The laryngeal mask airway: development and preliminary trials of a new type of airway, *Anaesthesia* 40: 356, 1985.
11. Brain AIJ: Three cases of difficult intubation overcome by the laryngeal mask airway, *Anaesthesia* 40:353, 1985.
12. Brain AIJ: *The Intravent laryngeal mask instruction manual,* ed 2, Berkshire, U.K., 1992, Brain Medical.
13. Nandi PR, Nunn JF, Charlesworth CH et al: Radiological study of the laryngeal mask, *Eur J Anaesthesiol* 4:33, 1991.
14. Goudsouzian NG, Denman W, Cleveland R et al: Radiologic localization of the laryngeal mask airway in children. *Anesthesiology* 77:1085, 1992.
15. O'Neill B, Templeton JJ, Caramico L et al: The laryngeal mask airway in pediatric patients: factors affecting ease of use during insertion and emergence. *Anesth Analg* 78:659, 1994.
16. Scanlon P, Carey M, Power M et al: Patient response to laryngeal mask insertion after induction of anaesthesia with propofol or thiopentone, *Can J Anaesth* 40:816, 1993, (erratum appears on p 1006).
17. Brown GW, Patel N, Ellis FR: Comparison of propofol and thiopentone for laryngeal mask insertion, *Anaesthesia* 46:771, 1991.
18. Young TM: The laryngeal mask in dental anaesthesia, *Eur J Anaesthesiol* 4:53, 1991.
19. Newman PTF: Insertion of partially inflated laryngeal mask airway, *Anaesthesia* 46:235, 1991 (letter).
20. Chow BF, Lewis M, Jones SE: Laryngeal mask airway in children: insertion technique, *Anaesthesia* 46:590, 1991 (letter).
21. Brimacombe J, Berry A: Insertion of the laryngeal mask airway: a prospective study of four techniques, *Anaesth Intensive Care* 21:89, 1993.
22. Devitt JH, Wenstone R, Noel AG et al: The laryngeal mask airway and positive-pressure ventilation, *Anesthesiology* 80:550, 1994.
23. Brain AIJ: Further developments of the laryngeal mask, *Anaesthesia* 44:530, 1989 (letter).
24. Graziotti PJ: Intermittent positive pressure ventilation through a laryngeal mask airway: is a nasogastric tube useful? *Anaesthesia* 47:1088, 1992.

25. Brain AIJ: Risk of aspiration with the laryngeal mask, *Br J Anaesth* 73:278, 1994 (letter).
26. Wilkins CJ, Cramp PG, Staples J et al: Comparison of the anesthetic requirement for tolerance of laryngeal mask airway and endotracheal tube, *Anesth Analg* 75:794, 1992.
27. Varughese A, McCulloch D, Lewis M et al: Removal of the laryngeal mask airway (LMA) in children: awake or deep? *Anesthesiology* 81:A1321, 1994 (abstract).
28. Smith I, White PF: Use of the laryngeal mask airway as an alternative to a face mask during outpatient arthroscopy, *Anesthesiology* 77:850, 1992.
29. Smith I, Joshi G: The laryngeal mask airway for outpatient anesthesia, *J Clin Anesth* 5 (suppl):22S, 1993 (review).
30. Churchill-Davidson HC: Suxamethonium (succinylcholine) chloride and muscle pains, *BMJ* 1:74, 1954.
31. Ding Y, Fredman B, White PF: Use of mivacurium during laparoscopic surgery: effect of reversal drugs on postoperative recovery, *Anesth Analg* 78:450, 1994.
32. Alexander CA, Leach AB: Incidence of sore throats with the laryngeal mask, *Anaesthesia* 44:791, 1989 (letter).
33. Akhtar TM, McMurray P, Kerr WJ et al: A comparison of laryngeal mask airway with tracheal tube for intra-ocular ophthalmic surgery, *Anaesthesia* 47:668, 1992.
34. Sarma VJ: The use of a laryngeal mask airway in spontaneously breathing patients, *Acta Anesthesiol Scand* 34:669, 1990.
35. Lee SK, Hong KH, Choe H et al: Comparison of the effects of the laryngeal mask airway and endotracheal intubation on vocal function, *Br J Anaesth* 71:648, 1993.
36. Harris TM, Johnston DF, Collins SRC et al: A new general anesthetic technique for use in singers: the Brain laryngeal mask airway versus endotracheal tube, *J Voice* 4:81, 1990.
37. Brain AIJ: The laryngeal mask in patients with chronic respiratory disease, *Anaesthesia* 44:790, 1989 (letter).
38. Lamb K, James MF, Janicki PK: The laryngeal mask airway for intraocular surgery: effects on intraocular pressure and stress responses, *Br J Anaesth* 69:143, 1992.
39. Holden R, Morsman CD, Butler J et al: Intra-ocular pressure changes using the laryngeal mask airway and tracheal tube, *Anaesthesia* 46:922, 1991.
40. Barclay K, Wall T, Wareham K et al: Intra-ocular pressure changes in patients with glaucoma: comparison between the laryngeal mask airway and tracheal tube, *Anaesthesia* 49:159, 1994.
41. Watcha MF, White PF, Tychsen L et al: Comparative effects of laryngeal mask airway and endotracheal tube insertion on intraocular pressure in children, *Anesth Analg* 75:355, 1992.
42. Haden RM, Pinnock CA, Campbell RL: The laryngeal mask for intraocular surgery, *Br J Anaesth* 71:772, 1993 (letter).
43. Holden R, Morsman D, Butler J et al: The laryngeal mask airway and intraocular surgery: a reply, *Anaesthesia* 47:446, 1992 (letter).
44. Brain AIJ: The laryngeal mask for intraocular surgery, *Br J Anaesth* 71:772, 1993 (letter).
45. John RE, Hill S, Hughes TJ: Airway protection by the laryngeal mask: a barrier to dye placed in the pharynx, *Anaesthesia* 46:366, 1991.
46. Bailie R, Barnett MB, Fraser JF: The Brain laryngeal mask: a comparative study with the nasal mask in paediatric dental outpatient anaesthesia, *Anaesthesia* 46:358, 1991.
47. Noble H, Wooler DJ: Laryngeal masks and chair dental anaesthesia, *Anaesthesia* 46:591, 1991 (letter).
48. Alexander CA: A modified Intravent laryngeal mask for ENT and dental anaesthesia, *Anaesthesia* 45:892, 1990 (letter).
49. Moylan SL, Luce MA: The reinforced laryngeal mask airway in paediatric radiotherapy, *Br J Anaesth* 71:172, 1993 (letter).
50. Williams PJ, Bailey PM: Comparison of the reinforced laryngeal mask airway and tracheal intubation for adenotonsillectomy, *Br J Anaesth* 70:30, 1993.
51. Webster AC, Morley FP, Dain S et al: Anaesthesia for adenotonsillectomy: a comparison between tracheal intubation and the armoured laryngeal mask airway, *Can J Anaesth* 40:1171, 1993.
52. Brimacombe J, Sher M, Laing D: Incendiary characteristics of the laryngeal and re-inforced laryngeal mask airway, *Anaesthesia* 49:171, 1994 (letter).
53. Pennant JH, Gajraj NM: Lasers and the laryngeal mask airway, *Anaesthesia* 49:448, 1994 (letter).
54. Maekawa H, Mikawa K, Tanaka O et al: The laryngeal mask may be a useful device for fiberoptic airway endoscopy in pediatric anesthesia, *Anesthesiology* 75:169, 1991 (letter).
55. Rowbottom SJ, Morton CP: Diagnostic fibreoptic bronchoscopy using the laryngeal mask, *Anaesthesia* 46:161, 1991 (letter).
56. Walker RW, Murrell D: Yet another use for the laryngeal mask airway, *Anaesthesia* 46:591, 1991 (letter).
57. Lawson R, Lloyd TA: Three diagnostic conundrums solved using the laryngeal mask airway, *Anaesthesia* 48:790, 1993.
58. Smith I, White PF: Anesthetic considerations for laparoscopic surgery. In Cuschieri A, MacFadyen BV, editors: Seminars in laparoscopic surgery, Philadelphia, 1994, WB Saunders.
59. Jones MJ, Mitchell RW, Hindocha N: Effect of increased intra-abdominal pressure during laparoscopy on lower esophageal sphincter, *Anesth Analg* 68:63, 1989.
60. Scott DB: Regurgitation during laparoscopy, *Br J Anaesth* 52:559, 1980 (letter).
61. Harris MNE, Plantevin OM, Crowther A: Cardiac arrhythmias during anaesthesia for laparoscopy, *Br J Anaesth* 56:1213, 1984.
62. Kenefick JP, Leader A, Maltby JR et al: Laparoscopy: blood gas values and minor sequelae associated with three techniques based on isoflurane, *Br J Anaesth* 59:189, 1987.
63. Goodwin AP, Rowe WL, Ogg TW: Day case laparoscopy: a comparison of two anaesthetic techniques using the laryngeal mask during spontaneous breathing, *Anaesthesia* 47:892, 1992.
64. Swann DG, Spens H, Edwards SA et al: Anaesthesia for gynaecological laparoscopy: a comparison between the laryngeal mask airway and tracheal intubation, *Anaesthesia* 48:431, 1993.
65. Malins AF, Cooper GM: Laparoscopy and the laryngeal mask airway, *Br J Anaesth* 73:121, 1994 (letter).
66. Johnston DF, Wrigley SR, Robb PJ et al: The laryngeal mask airway in paediatric anaesthesia, *Anaesthesia* 45:924, 1990.
67. Waite K, Filshie J: The use of a laryngeal mask airway for CT radiotherapy planning and daily radiotherapy, *Anaesthesia* 45:894, 1990 (letter).
68. Grebenik CR, Ferguson C, White A: The laryngeal mask airway in pediatric radiotherapy, *Anesthesiology* 72:474, 1990.
69. McClune S, Regan M, Moore J: Laryngeal mask airway for caesarean section, *Anaesthesia* 45:227-8, 1990.
70. Thomson KD, Ordman AJ, Parkhouse N et al: Use of the Brain laryngeal mask airway in anticipation of difficult tracheal intubation, *Br J Plasti Surg* 42:478, 1989.
71. Brimacombe J, Berry A: Laryngeal mask airway insertion: a comparison of the standard versus neutral position in normal patients with a view to its use in cervical spine instability, *Anaesthesia* 48:670, 1993.
72. Calder I, Ordman AJ, Jackowski A et al: The Brain laryngeal mask airway: an alternative to emergency tracheal intubation, *Anaesthesia* 45:137, 1990.
73. White A, Sinclair M, Pillai R: Laryngeal mask airway for coronary artery bypass grafting, *Anaesthesia* 46:234, 1991 (letter).
74. Heath ML: Endotracheal intubation through the laryngeal mask: helpful when laryngoscopy is difficult or dangerous, *Eur J Anaesthesiol* 4:41, 1991.
75. Heath ML, Allagain J: Intubation through the laryngeal mask: a

technique for unexpected difficult intubation, *Anaesthesia* 46: 545-8, 1991.

76. Lim SL, Tay DH, Thomas E: A comparison of three types of tracheal tube for use in laryngeal mask assisted blind orotracheal intubation, *Anaesthesia* 49:255, 1994.

77. Wee MYK: The oesophageal detector device: assessment of a new method to distinguish oesophageal from tracheal intubation, *Anaesthesia* 43:27-29, 1988.

78. Wheatley RS, Stainthrop SF: Intubation of one-day-old baby with Pierre-Robin syndrome via a laryngeal mask, *Anaesthesia* 49:733, 1994 (letter).

79. Asai T, Latto IP, Vaughan RS: The distance between the grille of the laryngeal mask airway and the vocal cords: is conventional intubation through the laryngeal mask safe? *Anaesthesia* 48:667, 1993.

80. Chadd GD, Ackers JW, Bailey PM: Difficult intubation aided by the laryngeal mask airway, *Anaesthesia* 44:1015, 1989 (letter).

81. Allison A, McCrory J: Tracheal placement of a gum elastic bougie using the laryngeal mask airways, *Anaesthesia* 45:419, 1990 (letter).

82. Thomson KD: A blind nasal intubation using a laryngeal mask airway, *Anaesthesia* 48:785, 1993.

83. Silk JM, Hill HM, Calder I: Difficult intubation and the laryngeal mask, *Eur J Anaesthesiol* 4:47, 1991.

84. Darling JR, D'Arcy JT, Murray JM: Split laryngeal mask airway as an aid to fibreoptic intubation, *Anaesthesia* 48:79, 1993 (letter).

85. Asai T, Barclay K, Power I et al: Cricoid pressure impedes placement of the laryngeal mask airway and subsequent tracheal intubation through the mask, *Br J Anaesth* 72:47, 1994.

86. Brimacombe J, White A, Berry A: Effect of cricoid pressure on ease of insertion of the laryngeal mask airway, *Br J Anaesth* 71:800, 1993.

87. Asai T, Barclay K, Power I et al: Single- compared with double-handed cricoid pressure for insertion of an LMA, *Br J Anaesth* 72:733, 1994 (letter).

88. Strang TI: Does the laryngeal mask airway compromise cricoid pressure? *Anaesthesia* 47:829, 1992.

89. Kumar CM: Laryngeal mask airway for inadequate reversal, *Anaesthesia* 45:792, 1990 (letter).

90. Davies PR, Tighe SQ, Greenslade GL et al: Laryngeal mask airway and tracheal tube insertion by unskilled personnel, *Lancet* 336:977, 1990.

91. Pennant JH, Walker MB: Comparison of the endotracheal tube and laryngeal mask in airway management by paramedical personnel, *Anesth Analg* 74:531, 1992.

92. Alexander R, Hodgson P, Lomax D et al: A comparison of the laryngeal mask airway and Guedel airway, bag and facemask for manual ventilation following formal training, *Anaesthesia* 48:231, 1993.

93. Martin PD, Cyna AM, Hunter WA et al: Training nursing staff in airway management for resuscitation: a clinical comparison of the facemask and laryngeal mask, *Anaesthesia* 48:33, 1993.

94. Greene MK, Roden R, Hinchley G: The laryngeal mask airway: two cases of prehospital trauma care. *Anaesthesia* 47:688, 1992.

95. Braude N, Clements EA, Hodges UM et al: The pressor response and laryngeal mask insertion: a comparison with tracheal intubation, *Anaesthesia* 44:551, 1989.

96. Wilson IG, Fell D, Robinson SL et al: Cardiovascular responses to insertion of the laryngeal mask, *Anaesthesia* 47:300, 1992.

97. Hickey S, Cameron AE, Asbury AJ: Cardiovascular response to insertion of Brain's laryngeal mask, *Anaesthesia* 45:629, 1990.

98. Joshi GP, Morrison SG, Gajraj NM et al: Hemodynamic changes during emergence from anesthesia: use of the laryngeal mask airway vs endotracheal tube, *Anesth Analg* 78(suppl):185, 1994 (abstract).

99. Maltby Jr, Loken RG, Watson NC: The laryngeal mask airway: clinical appraisal in 250 patients, *Can J Anaesth* 37:509, 1990.

100. Bhatt SB, Kendall AP, Lin ES et al: Resistance and additional inspiratory work imposed by the laryngeal mask airway: a comparison with tracheal tubes, *Anaesthesia* 47:343, 1992.

101. Joshi GP, Morrison SG, Miciotto CJ et al: Evaluation of work of breathing during anesthesia: use of laryngeal mask airway versus tracheal tube, *Anesthesiology* 81:A1449, 1994 (abstract).

102. Joshi GP, Smith I, Watcha M et al: A model for studying the cost effectiveness of airway devices: laryngeal mask airway versus tracheal tube, *Anesth Analg* (Suppl):219, 1995.

103. Fullekrug B, Pothmann W, Werner C et al: The laryngeal mask airway: anesthetic gas leakage and fiberoptic control or positioning, *J Clin Anesth* 5:357, 1993.

104. Payne J, Edwards J: The use of the fibreoptic laryngoscope to confirm the position of the laryngeal mask, *Anaesthesia* 44:865, 1989 (letter).

105. Wittmann PH, Wittmann FW: Laryngeal mask and gastric dilatation, *Anaesthesia* 46:1083, 1991 (letter).

106. Brimacombe JR: Laryngeal mask anaesthesia and recurrent swallowing, *Anaesth Intensive Care* 19:275, 1991.

107. Rabey PG, Murphy PJ, Langton JA et al: Effect of the laryngeal mask airway on lower oesophageal sphincter pressure in patients during general anaesthesia, *Br J Anaesth* 69:346, 1992.

108. Vanner RG, Pryle BJ, O'Dwyer JP et al: Upper oesophageal sphincter pressure during inhalational anaesthesia, *Anaesthesia* 47:950, 1992.

109. Alexander R, Arrowsmith JE, Frossard RJ: The laryngeal mask airway: safe in the X-ray department? *Anaesthesia* 48:734, 1993 (letter).

110. Lack A: Regurgitation using a laryngeal mask, *Anaesthesia* 48:734, 1993 (letter).

111. Campbell JR: The laryngeal mask: cautionary tales, *Anaesthesia* 45:167, 1990 (letter).

112. Criswell J, John R: The laryngeal mask: cautionary tales, *Anaesthesia* 45:168, 1990 (letter).

113. Barker P, Langton JA, Murphy PJ et al: Regurgitation of gastric contents during general anaesthesia using the laryngeal mask airway, *Br J Anaesth* 69:314, 1992.

114. El Milkatti N, Luthra AD, Healy TE et al: Gastric regurgitation during general anaesthesia in the supine position with the laryngeal and face mask airways, *Br J Anaesth* 69: 529, 1992 (abstract).

115. Akhtar TM, Street MK: Risk of aspiration with the laryngeal mask, *Br J Anaesth* 72:447, 1994.

116. Owens T, Robertson P, Twomey K et al: Incidence of gastroesophageal reflux with the laryngeal mask, *Anesthesiology* 79:1053, 1993 (abstract).

117. Joshi GP, Morrison SG, Okonkwo N et al: Continuous hypopharyngeal pH monitoring: use of laryngeal mask airway versus tracheal tube, *Anesthesiology* 81:A1281, 1994 (abstract).

118. Illing L, Duncan PG, Yip R: Gastro-esophageal reflux during anesthesia, *Can J Anaesth* 39:466, 1992.

119. Carlsson C, Islander G: "Silent" gastropharyngeal regurgitation during general anesthesia, *Anesth Analg* 60:655, 1981.

120. Turndof H, Rodis ID, Clark TS: Silent regurgitation during general anesthesia, *Anesth Analg* 53:700, 1974.

121. Blitt CD, Guttman HL, Cohen D et al: "Silent" regurgitation and aspiration during general anesthesia, *Anesth Analg* 49:707, 1970.

122. Warner MA, Warner ME, Weber JG: Clinical significance of pulmonary aspiration during the perioperative period, *Anesthesiology* 78:56, 1993.

123. Olsson GL, Hallen B, Hambraeus-Jonzon K: Aspiration during anesthesia: a computer-aided study of 185,358 anesthetics, *Acta Anesthesiol Scand* 30:84, 1986.

124. Cohen MM, Duncan PG, Pope WDB et al: A survey of 112,000

anaesthetics at one teaching hospital, *Can Anaesth Soc J* 33:22, 1986.

125. Brimacombe J, Berry A: Incidence of aspiration with the laryngeal mask airway, *Br J Anaesth* 72:495, 1994 (letter).

126. Brimacombe JR, Berry A: The incidence of aspiration associated with the laryngeal mask airway: a meta-analysis of published literature, *J Clin Anesth* 1995.

127. Nanji GM, Maltby JR: Vomiting and aspiration pneumonitis with the laryngeal mask airway, *Can J Anaesth* 39:69, 1992.

128. Brain AIJ: The laryngeal mask and the oesophagus, *Anaesthesia* 46:701, 1991 (letter).

129. Verghese C, Smith TG, Young E: Prospective survey of the use of the laryngeal mask airway in 2359 patients, *Anaesthesia* 48:58, 1993.

130. Lumb AB, Wrigley MW: The effect of nitrous oxide on laryngeal mask cuff pressure: in vitro and in vivo studies, *Anaesthesia* 47:320, 1992.

131. Marjot R: Pressure exerted by the laryngeal mask airway cuff upon the pharyngeal mucosa, *Br J Anaesth* 70:25, 1993 (erratum on p 711).

132. Collier C: A hazard with the laryngeal mask airway, *Anaesth Intensive Care* 19:301, 1991 (letter).

133. Miller AC, Bickler P: The laryngeal mask airway: an unusual complication, *Anaesthesia* 46:659, 1991.

134. Lee JJ: Laryngeal mask and trauma to uvula, *Anaesthesia* 44:1014, 1989 (letter).

135. Brain AIJ: Laryngeal mask and trauma to the uvula: a reply, *Anaesthesia* 44:1015, 1989 (letter).

136. Marjot R: Trauma to the posterior pharyngeal wall caused by a laryngeal mask airway, *Anaesthesia* 46:589, 1991 (letter).

137. Stone JM, Karalliedde LD, Carter ML et al: Bacteraemia and insertion of laryngeal mask airways, *Anaesthesia* 47:77, 1992 (letter).

138. Brimacombe J, Shorney N, Swainston R et al: The incidence of bacteraemia following laryngeal mask insertion, *Anaesth Intensive Care* 20:484, 1992.

139. Crawford M, Davidson G: A problem with a laryngeal mask airway, *Anaesthesia* 47:76, 1992 (letter).

140. Squires SJ: Fragmented laryngeal mask airway, *Anaesthesia* 47:274, 1992 (letter).

141. Conacher ID: Foreign body in a laryngeal mask airway, *Anaesthesia* 46:164, 1991 (letter).

142. Fisher JA, Ananthanarayan C, Edelist G: Role of the laryngeal mask in airway management, *Can J Anaesth* 39:1, 1992 (editorial).

143. Ngan Kee WD: Laryngeal mask airway for radiotherapy in the prone position, *Anaesthesia* 47:446, 1992.

144. Brain AIJ: The oesophageal vent–laryngeal mask, *Br J Anaesth* 72:727, 1994 (letter).

145. Akhtar TM: Oesophageal vent–laryngeal mask to prevent aspiration of gastric contents, *Br J Anaesth* 72:52, 1994.

Chapter 20

THE EVOLUTION OF UPPER-AIRWAY RETRACTION: NEW AND OLD LARYNGOSCOPY BLADES

Sheila D. Cooper

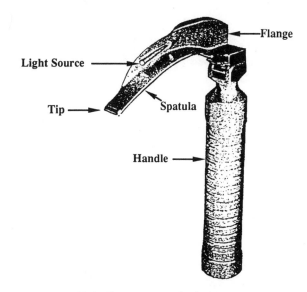

Fig. 20-1. Components of a laryngoscope.

I. INTRODUCTION: LARYNGOSCOPE AND BLADE BASICS

A. COMPONENTS OF A LARYNGOSCOPE

The basic components of a laryngoscope are the handle, blade, and light source (Fig. 20-1). The two main categories of handles are the L type and the U type. The U type, introduced by Jackson (see later section), has been abandoned in favor of the L type, which is lighter and less bulky. Most handles lie at a right angle to the blade. But several modifications of the blade angle have been made to facilitate entry of the blade into the oropharynx in specific clinical situations (i.e., Polio blade to intubate patients in an iron-lung machine) that diminish the tendency of the endoscopist to use the patient's upper incisors as a fulcrum during direct laryngoscopy. The handle can be further classified based on the method of attachment to the blade. There are permanently attached blades (rarely found today) and "hook-on" folding blades. This hook-on or hinged folding mechanism not only facilitates attachment of the blade to the handle but contains an automated switch to provide illumination from the light source when the blade is lifted into the working position.

The earliest laryngoscope used proximal lighting — that is, the light sources came from a point between the laryngoscopist and the laryngoscope. Examples of commonly used proximal light sources included head mirrors, headlamps, and electric lights directed into the oropharynx by a prism or mirror. The invention of the electric lightbulb carrier by Einhorn in 1902 led to the introduction of distal lighting in 1907 by Jackson, which provided illumination to the blade tip. In 1913 Janeway incorporated the battery into the handle to power the light source, a system that has become a standard for laryngoscopes used by anesthesiologists.[1] Morch's laryngoscope incorporated the light source in the handle so that blades of any design could be attached to the handle.[2]

The blade itself is composed of the spatula, flange, and tip. The spatula is designed to compress and manipulate the soft tissues of the lower jaw to facilitate a direct line of vision past the upper incisors and around the bulk of the tongue to get a view of the larynx during direct laryngoscopy. The long axis of the spatula is either straight or curved in all or part of its length. The flange projects off the side of the spatula to deflect tissues out of the line of vision during laryngoscopy. The flange is a component of the cross-sectional shape of the blade, which varies from blade to blade: from no flange, so that the blade resembles a straight or curved tongue depressor (e.g., the double-angle blade), to a completely closed tube or O-shaped blade. Intermediate cross-sectional curves include a C, a flattened C, a U turned on its side, or a Z in reverse (i.e., "Ƨ"). The vertical height of the cross-sectional shape of a blade is occasionally referred to as the "step."

The blade tip is designed to elevate the epiglottis either directly or indirectly to facilitate a view of the larynx. The tip of straight blades is of multiple designs; it has been ridged, curved, slotted, and hooked in an effort to lift the epiglottis more directly and effectively. Solutions to aid in indirect elevation of the epiglottis have included various curved and angled blades to blades that have bifid tips that straddle the hyoepiglottic ligament in the vallecula. The blade tip or "beak" is blunt and thickened to prevent trauma to the oropharyngeal tissues and is either flat, curved or slightly uplifted (see Fig. 20-1).

B. ORIGINAL DIRECT-VISION LARYNGOSCOPES

More than 50 descriptions of laryngoscope blade designs have been published since William MacEwan, a distinguished surgeon of the Glasgow Royal Infirmary,

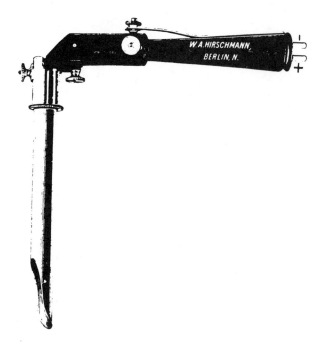

Fig. 20-2. Kirstein's original autoscope. (From Hirsch NP, Smith GB, Hirsch PO: *Anaesthesia* 41:42, 1986.)

first passed a tube through the mouth into the trachea using his fingers as the guide in 1878. This method of intubation by palpation continued for several decades. But even in experienced hands, it was an uncertain and often traumatic event. Although indirect laryngoscopy using a mirror antedated MacEwan's experience (a method originally used by Manuel Garcia in 1854 and then Turck and Czermak[3]), many clinicians thought it would be impossible to visualize the vocal cords directly while passing an endotracheal tube (ET) due the geometric relationship between the mouth and the vocal cords. This notion was erased by the introduction of the first direct-vision laryngoscope by Alfred Kirstein in Berlin in 1895.

Kirstein's device was the forerunner to the modern-day laryngoscope. It was developed after Kirstein's colleague Rosenheim informed him that an esophageal scope had accidentally slipped into the trachea, giving rise to a perfect view of the bronchial bifurcation. From this information, Kirstein devised a reproducible method of viewing the larynx directly. His initial device consisted of a 25-cm esophagoscope attached to an electroscope (an electric hand lamp) that was used as the handle (Fig. 20-2).[4] He termed this combination electroscope-esophagoscope the "autoscope." Due to concern about the pressure the autoscope placed on the upper incisors and the marked neck extension necessary for direct laryngoscopy, he modified the original autoscope by replacing the cylindrical esophagoscope with one of two different designs of semicircular blades (Fig. 20-3),

which are strikingly similar to those described in the 1940s by Drs. Macintosh[5] and Miller.[6] Kirstein's other claim to fame was his appreciation of proper positioning of the patient's head; he was most certainly the first to describe what is now referred to as the "sniff" or Magill position.

Gustav Killian, a pupil of Kirstein, enthusiastically supported his concepts and used this autoscope or laryngoscope. He was not only the first to introduce a tube into the trachea but also used the Kirstein laryngoscope to aid in the first successful extraction of a foreign body from the right mainstem bronchus via the translaryngeal route on March 30, 1897. He subsequently performed other successful foreign body translaryngeal extractions using a suspension laryngoscope. He is commonly referred to as the father of bronchoscopy.[7] The Kirstein direct-vision laryngoscope initially had no light attached to it and was used in conjunction with an electric light that was reflected down the lumen by a prism. Electrical wires trailed from the laryngoscope to a separate battery box; eventually the cord was passed through the hollow handle of the instrument. This arrangement continued until 1913 when the battery itself was housed in the handle, making the entire apparatus self-contained and much easier to maneuver.[8]

The development of the ordinary hand laryngoscope can be attributed to multiple individuals, most notably Chevalier Jackson in 1907. His straight-bladed laryngoscope with the O-shaped flange had a U-type handle that looked like three sides of a square with the lifting handgrip parallel to the blade. This facilitated exposure of the larynx without applying direct pressure to the upper teeth (Fig. 20-4).[9] The Jackson laryngoscope became a standard instrument for laryngeal examinations and was used to directly inspect the vocal cords prior to intubation, a technique advocated by Charles Elsberg, a New York surgeon, in 1912. Jackson pointed out that the use of a gag (e.g., a suspension laryngoscope), commonly used by other laryngoscopists of the day, should be abandoned because a sufficiently anesthetized patient should not need one and wide gagging defeats exposure of the larynx by jamming the mandible. He wrote that "the most important thing of all is the position of the patient, and next to that comes recognition of the epiglottis, and then the application of a proper lifting motion of the hyoid bone which all aid in exposing the larynx."[9]

The use of the straight O-shaped Jackson blade continued for many years despite the introduction of a slightly curved O-shaped blade attached to an L-type handle by Henry Janeway, another American surgeon, in 1913.[10,11] His instrument was notable as the first laryngoscope to have an internal light source powered by batteries contained in the handle. The use of O-shaped tubelike blades was a carryover from the esophagoscopes

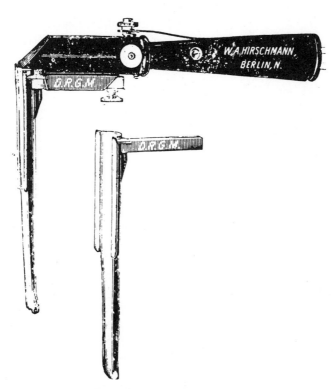

Fig. 20-3. Kirstein's modified autoscope. Standard blade is attached to handle. Intralaryngeal blade is shown separately, *bottom.* (From Hirsch NP, Smith GB, Hirsch PO: *Anaesthesia* 41:42, 1986.)

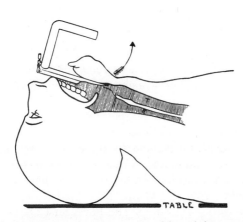

Fig. 20-4. Jackson laryngoscope positioned in oropharynx. Arrow illustrates direction of motion that should be imparted on laryngoscope blade to assist in exposure of the larynx and insertion of endotracheal tube (ET). (From Jackson C: *Surg Gynecol Obstet* 17:507, 1913.)

used in the late 19th century. This closed tube was either slotted or segmented to facilitate its removal after the introduction of a bronchoscope. As the laryngoscope became more commonly used for orotracheal intubation, the lateral segment was removed completely (usually from the right side) so that the blade became C shaped.

The best known examples of the original C-shaped straight blades are the Magill (1920) and Flagg (1928)

laryngoscopes. In an effort to decrease the amount of volume the blade occupied in the oropharynx, the C shape was flattened in the upper portion (i.e., the flat C shape) (Elam [1935], Murphy [ca. 1940], Miller [1941]), Wis-Foregger [ca. 1940]) and in the upper and lower curves (i.e., to produce a lateral U shape) (Bruening [1909], Guedel [1927], Waters-Hipple [ca. 1940]). Other changes in the shape of the flange cross-sectional area included a reversed Z shape ("Ƨ") (Seldon [1938], Macintosh [1943]) and a shallow upside-down and reversed L ("⌐") (Bennett (1943]). Despite the many modifications of laryngoscopes, particularly the blade shape, only the Macintosh and Miller laryngoscope blades introduced in the 1940s have achieved lasting popularity.

C. MILLER LARYNGOSCOPE BLADE

By 1941 Miller recognized that existing laryngoscopes were too thick at the base, thereby increasing the risk of trauma to the teeth. He additionally noted that the blade tips did not have the proper shape to lift the epiglottis, the blades were often too short, the curve of the blades was too distal, and the flat bottom tended to push the tongue against the floor of the mouth, thereby inhibiting adequate exposure in "difficult" patients (i.e., those with a deep throat, thick tongue, or prominent upper incisors).[6] To overcome these deficiencies, Miller de-

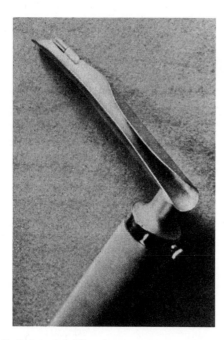

Fig. 20-5. Original Miller laryngoscope blade. Note long, narrow shape. (From Miller RA: A new laryngoscope, *Anesthesiology* 2:317, 1941.)

Table 20-1. Comparison of Miller blade with other blades in the early 1940s

Other blades	Miller blade
High base	Shallow
Flat bottom	Round
Wide end	Narrow
Curve at the tip	Curve 2 inches back
Large and medium sizes	One size (useful in all patients and infants)

signed a laryngoscope that was longer, rounded on the bottom, smaller at the tip, and had a shallower base and an extra curve beginning 2 inches from the distal tip (Fig. 20-5). These changes resulted in less required mouth opening and allowed for freer anterior movement of the mandible so that when the small, round end of the blade pressed up against the tongue and the distal tip entrapped the epiglottis, a channel was created through which the larynx was exposed. Miller noted that although the epiglottic entrapment technique of intubation was used (see Chapter 14), the decrease in required mouth opening limited the area for tube manipulation, so that oftentimes it was necessary to use a stylet to pass a larger ET. Since its introduction, the Miller blade has become the standard to which other subsequently developed laryngoscope blades are compared. Table 20-1 compares the advantages of the Miller blade to other laryngoscope blades available in the early 1940s.

D. MACINTOSH LARYNGOSCOPE BLADE

Although his original laryngoscope blade was fashioned after a Boyle-Davis gag, Sir Robert Macintosh recognized the limitations of a suspension laryngoscope and in 1943 introduced his sharply curved blade specifically designed not to entrap the epiglottis (Fig. 20-6). Human had advised that in some cases the blade of the laryngoscope should be passed only until the epiglottis comes into view and then the ET should be guided behind the epiglottis into the trachea.[12] The Macintosh

laryngoscope blade is introduced into the right side of the mouth by pushing the tongue to the left and is advanced until the distal tip of the short, curved blade rests in the glossoepiglottic fold (vallecula) (Fig. 20-7). Upward traction is exerted on the base of the tongue by lifting the laryngoscope to elevate the epiglottis upward, facilitating exposure of the larynx (Fig. 20-8). If the tongue is not adequately retracted to the left and bulges over the blade, the view of the larynx is obscured. Due to the diminished blade contact with the extensively innervated epiglottis, Macintosh claimed it could be used under a lighter plane of anesthesia. He also claimed that his blade design resulted in less risk of damage to the teeth, owing to its completely open top section. He further explained that the shape of the blade did not matter much provided it did not go beyond or make contact with the epiglottis and that the degree of curvature accommodated the natural curve of a Magill-type ET. He, in fact, used blades ranging from those with a well-marked curve to those that were perfectly straight (Fig. 20-9).[13] Many refinements followed from different inventors. A hinge was incorporated between the blade and handle by the Welch-Allyn Company so that the blade could be folded against the handle to allow for easy transportation.[14] An automated switch was later incorporated into the hinge mechanism to provide illumination from the light source when the blade was lifted into the working position. The Foregger Company was given the right to copy the Macintosh laryngoscope blade for the North American market in 1943. The inventors (Macintosh and a Mr. Salt, the senior chief technician of the Nuffield Department of Anaesthetics) sent a prototype to Foregger expecting their engineers to refine it, only to discover later that the blade had been marketed in its original form.

From the primary three laryngoscope blade types—straight blade (Jackson), curved tip (Miller), and curved (Macintosh)—many modifications were proposed because even in the most experienced hands, there were still occasional patients in whom intubation was found to be difficult or impossible with existing techniques. Most of these modifications were attempts to overcome

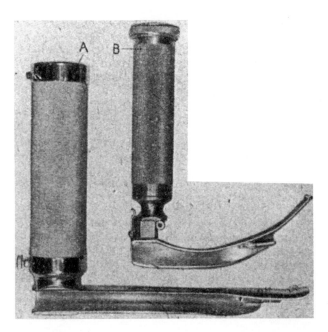

Fig. 20-6. A, Standard Miller long, straight laryngoscope blade. **B,** Macintosh short, curved blade. (From Macintosh RR: A new laryngoscope, *Lancet* 1:205, 1943.)

specific anatomic variations of the mouth or pharynx that contributed to intubation difficulties. A broad categorization of these variations includes: an anterior larynx, limited mouth opening, decreased size of the infraoral cavity, immobile or unstable cervical spine, large or protruding sternal region,[15] pediatric patients, and excess secretions or blood obstructing the line of vision. To emphasize clinical function, this chapter organizes the more effective laryngoscope blades developed over the past 50 years into these categories. Although they are placed in specific categories based on the primary anatomic variations they were designed to overcome, there is considerable overlap. Many of the blades might fit in multiple categories; where appropriate, this is elaborated on in the following sections. Schematics of intubation techniques as well as peer-reviewed clinical experiences are presented for the most promising of the recently introduced laryngoscope blades.

II. MODIFICATIONS OF LARYNGOSCOPE BLADES BASED ON SPECIFIC ANATOMIC VARIATIONS

A. ANTERIOR LARYNX

1. Cassels laryngoscope blade

Shortly after the introduction of the Miller laryngoscope blade in 1941, Cassels wrote that tradition in medicine "has obscured the advantages of modifications in technic and design."[16] He was referring to the fact that the laryngoscopes of that day still had a C-shaped cross section rather than open edges that came out straight. This was a carryover from the bronchoscopist's instrument that had a sliding piece completing a circle, fitting in the gap through which long, straight instruments were passed. He further pointed out that insertion of a curved, flexible ET was markedly different from the insertion of a rigid, straight bronchoscope. This, he believed, mandated a different device to expose the larynx. Because the amount of mouth opening limits the upward angulation that can be applied on the laryngoscope without applying pressure on the upper teeth, only the posterior part of the larynx is exposed with a straight blade (Fig. 20-10). Curving the distal tip of the blade as Miller did facilitated anterior exposure without necessitating an increase in mouth opening or interfering with the anesthetist's view. Cassels's support of the curved-tip Miller blade for facilitating exposure of an anterior larynx has been echoed by multiple anesthesiologists over the many years since its introduction.[17]

2. Siker laryngoscope blade

a. DESCRIPTION

In addition to assisting with exposure of an anterior larynx, the Siker blade (1959) was developed to overcome other anatomical variations such as a recessed mandible, prominent and/or overriding upper incisors (buck teeth), and an increased tongue size, all of which contributed to intubation difficulty.[18] Siker incorporated a mirror onto the blade, which was positioned 3 inches from the distal tip (Fig. 20-11). The blade distal to the mirror makes an angle of 135 degrees to the 2.5 inch proximal portion. The mirror is attached to the blade via a copper jacket, which facilitates conduction of the patient's heat to minimize fogging of the mirror during exhalation.

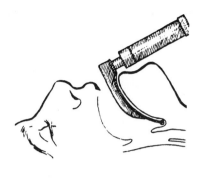

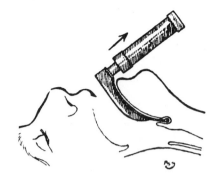

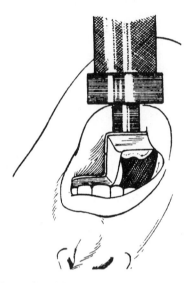

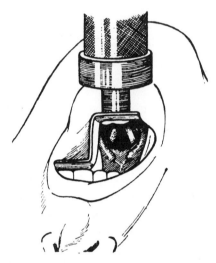

Fig. 20-7. Correct positioning and view obtained prior to lifting Macintosh laryngoscope blade. (From Macintosh RR: A new laryngoscope, *Lancet* 1:205, 1943.)

Fig. 20-8. Direction of motion applied to Macintosh laryngoscope blade and view obtained of larynx. (From Macintosh RR: A new laryngoscope, *Lancet* 1:205, 1943.)

b. TECHNIQUE

The original description of the technique for using this laryngoscope cautioned the operator to condition himself to viewing and working with inverted structures since the mirror reflected an inverted image. Keeping this in mind, the operator inserts the blade in the usual manner, pushing the tongue to the left side and looking through the proximal mirror to view the structures at the distal end of the blade. Once the oropharyngeal curve is negotiated, the epiglottis appears in the lower portion of the mirror and is then elevated with the tip of the blade. When a view of the vocal cords is obtained, an ET is inserted with the aid of the stylet to help direct it around the curvature of the laryngoscope blade. As the ET is passed through the laryngeal inlet, the reflected image in the mirror will appear as though the tube is moving in a posterocaudad direction. When the tip of the ET passes through the cords, the laryngoscope is removed and intubation is completed by threading the ET off the stylet and into the trachea.

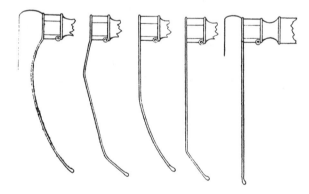

Fig. 20-9. Range of blade curvatures Sir Robert Macintosh experimented with in developing final version of Macintosh blade (on far left). (From Macintosh RR: Laryngoscope blades, *Lancet* 1:485, 1944.)

c. CLINICAL EXPERIENCE

Siker's initial experience with his blade was extremely favorable. Out of 100 randomly selected patients who required endotracheal intubation, laryngoscopy was successfully performed in all but one. This one failure

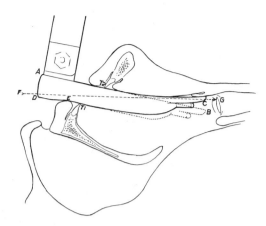

Fig. 20-10. Illustration by Cassels depicting advantages of a curved laryngoscope blade. Limited mouth opening (T_1 to T_2) limits amount of upward angulation that can be applied on laryngoscope blade without damaging teeth. With a straight blade (A-B), only the posterior portion of the larynx is exposed if T_1-T_2 is small, but curving the tip (A-C) faciliates a more anterior view from point D looking along line F-G without an increase in T_1-T_2. Flaring the proximal end along E-D might facilitate an even better laryngeal view. (From Cassels WH: Advantages of a curved laryngoscope, *Anesthesiology* 3:580, 1942.)

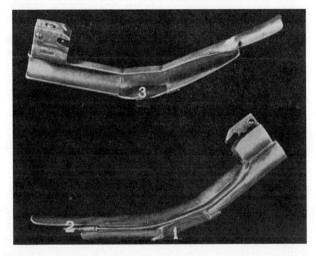

Fig. 20-11. Siker mirror laryngoscope. **1,** Copper jacket. **2,** Light source. **3,** Stainless steel mirror. (From Siker ES: A mirror laryngoscope, *Anesthesiology* 17:38, 1956.)

was attributed to the large size of the blade; the distal tip was in the larynx prior to the mirror entering the oral cavity. Furthermore, Siker cited three cases in which laryngoscopy and intubation were easily accomplished with his blade where the "classical" (Miller) and Macintosh laryngoscope blades had failed.[18] The primary disadvantage of this instrument is that extensive practice is required to become adept at its use, thereby necessitating a committed period of learning even in the hands of experienced laryngoscopists. The Siker laryngoscope blade is rarely used today.

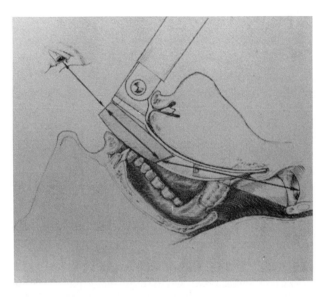

Fig. 20-12. Huffman prism laryngoscope. With Macintosh laryngoscope in proper position, prism allows a 30-degree refraction in the direction of the larynx. (From Huffman JP, Elam JO: Prisms and fiber optics for laryngoscopy, *Anesth Analg* 50:64, 1971.)

3. Huffman laryngoscope blade

The introduction of prisms for indirect laryngoscopy dates back to MacKenzie (1865) and Janeway (1913), but Huffman was the first to apply a prism to the curved Macintosh laryngoscope.[10,19-21] The idea of indirect laryngoscopy arose from experience with a small percentage of the adult population in whom direct laryngoscopy with a curved or straight standard laryngoscope blade was either impossible or extremely traumatic. The anatomic variations contributing to intubation difficulty and subsequent development of this laryngoscope blade included obesity, macroglossia, micrognathia, postirradiation distortion, acute edematous conditions, and an anteriorly situated larynx.

Huffman fitted a standard Macintosh no. 3 laryngoscope with a Plexiglas prism that fastened onto the blade with a steel clip, allowing for 30-degree refraction in the direction of the larynx (Fig. 20-12). For markedly limited head extension, Huffman also designed a prism pharyngolaryngoscope. This instrument consists of two prisms fitted onto a pharyngoscope and resembles a conventional Fink no. 3 oral airway with a vallecular extension (Fig. 20-13).[22] These prisms result in a combined angle of refraction measuring 80 degrees. Illumination is provided by means of a plastic fiberoptic light guide positioned on the left side of the blade. Both of these blades fit onto standard laryngoscope handles. Because of the refraction curvatures with the two blades (30 degrees and 80 degrees), it is necessary to elevate the tip of the tube to achieve successful intubation. The original investigations with these blades used them as inspection

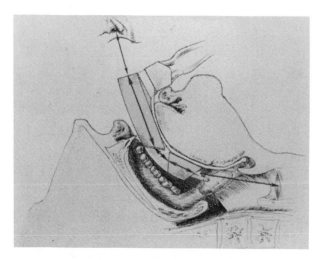

Fig. 20-13. Huffman prism pharyngolaryngoscope. With proper positioning, 80 degrees of refraction is possible in the direction of the larynx, minimizing head extension. (From Huffman JP, Elam JO: Prisms and fiber optics for laryngoscopy, *Anesth Analg* 50:64, 1971.)

devices of the hypopharynx and larynx during inhalation anesthesia and not necessarily as intubation devices for difficult airways. The concept of using a prism to assist with laryngeal exposure was later elaborated on with the introduction of the Belscope by Dr. Bellhouse (see section 5).

4. Grant laryngoscope blade

The Grant laryngoscope blade is another variation of the Macintosh laryngoscope blade. It incorporates a spring-loaded lever on the front of the handle to facilitate endotracheal intubation in situations where an introducing stylet would be required to guide the ET anteriorly.[23] When pressure is applied on the lever, it is transmitted to a second lever on the blade (the blade lever) that moves the blade lever upward (Fig. 20-14). To use the laryngoscope, the blade lever is closed by squeezing the handle lever and the blade is then inserted into the mouth (Fig. 20-15). The distal tip is placed in the vallecula. Before the tongue and epiglottis are lifted, pressure on the handle lever is released, allowing the blade lever to fall into the oropharyngeal cavity. The ET is then introduced into the mouth and positioned close to the blade. If the tip of the tube needs to be lifted to facilitate intubation, the handle lever is squeezed and the blade lever lifts the tube tip to the desired position (Fig. 20-16). Once the ET is advanced between the cords, the blade is carefully removed, closing the lever upon withdrawal. The author-inventor wrote that field evaluations were being conducted at the time of the original report in the United Kingdom, Australia, and

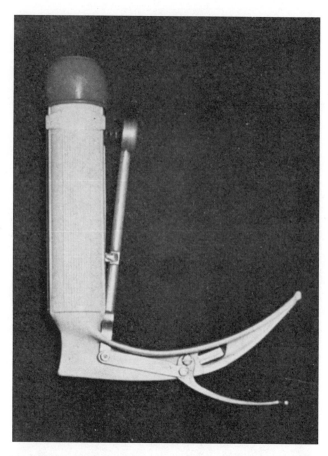

Fig. 20-14. Grant laryngoscope with its manipulating mechanism. (From Grant GC: A new laryngoscope, *Anaesth Intens Care* 5:263, 1977.)

New Zealand, but no clinical studies have appeared in the literature.

5. Belscope
a. DESCRIPTION

The Belscope is an angulated, straight-bladed laryngoscope bent forward 45 degrees at the midpoint. It is available in three lengths (6.7, 8, and 9 cm, from tip to angle) (Fig. 20-17).[24] It was designed to combine the attractive features of both straight and curved laryngoscope blades and is similar conceptually to the Siker blade; a prism mechanism provides an indirect view of the larynx to assist with difficult intubations. When the angle of the blade blocks a view of the larynx, the prism is used to "see" around this corner and provide an indirect view of the glottic opening. This may be easier to conceptualize than the inverted image obtained by looking in the mirror with the Siker blade. In contrast to the Siker blade, it is less bulky and has an inverted L-shaped cross section (vs. the C-shaped cross section of the Siker blade) so that in the majority of laryngoscopies a direct view of the larynx is obtained, making it useful

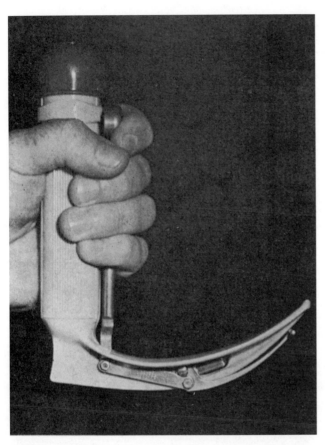

Fig. 20-15. Blade lever is closed prior to insertion of the blade. (From Grant GC: A new laryngoscope, *Anaesth Intens Care* 5:263, 1977.)

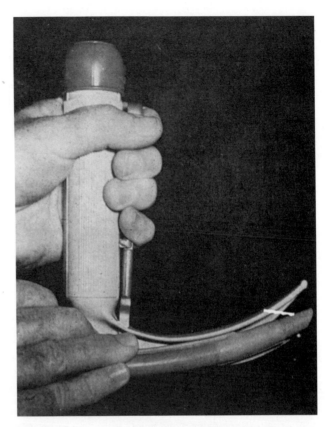

Fig. 20-16. If tip of the ET needs to be lifted, the handle lever is squeezed, allowing the blade lever to lift ET to desired position for insertion between vocal cords. (From Grant GC: A new laryngoscope, *Anaesth Intens Care* 5:263, 1977.)

for routine intubations as well. Compared to the Macintosh blade, the Belscope has a significantly smaller step with a shorter vertical component; this, in combination with the inverted L-shaped cross section, leaves more room to manipulate an ET in the oropharynx.

b. TECHNIQUE

i. Without prism. For the majority of laryngoscopies, the Belscope is used much like a conventional straight laryngoscope blade (see Chapter 14). The tip of the blade traps the epiglottis so that the view is obtained by looking along the straight part of the distal end of the flange (Fig. 20-18).

ii. With prism. If the laryngoscope blade has been optimally placed and the view is still impaired (patients with limited atlantooccipital extension, a short mandible, or a large tongue), the prism is used. When viewed through the proximal end (Fig. 20-19), it provides an indirect view of the larynx. The prism rotates the image of the larynx by 34 degrees, which often necessitates the use of a curved stylet to direct the tip of the ET anteriorly. When the prism is used, it is important to prevent fogging either by using a commercial antifog

preparation or by warming the prism in a towel prior to attaching it to the blade.

c. CLINICAL EXPERIENCE

Dr. Bellhouse's clinical experience in more than 4000 intubations has been favorable; he has been successful with both routine as well as known difficult intubations in patients with major anatomic abnormalities such as poor neck extension, short mandible, and large tongues. The longest blade was used in 80% of cases, the medium blade in 20% of cases, and the shortest blade in 0.5% of cases (5 per 1000). This angulated laryngoscope was designed for the prism but is advantageous for routine intubations without the prism as well. In fact, the prism has been found to be necessary in only 0.3% of cases (3 times per 1000). Experience from other evaluators has also been favorable, but comparison studies with other similar laryngoscope blades are lacking.[25] An important caveat mentioned by all users is that the angulated blade feels different than other blades and therefore practice is essential. In fact, Bellhouse himself recommends that 50 intubations should be performed without the prism and then another 20 or 30 with the prism before the user can be expected to be comfortable with the blade.

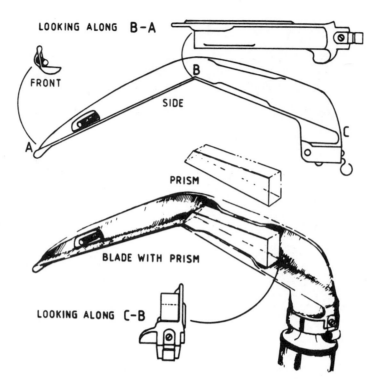

Fig. 20-17. Scale drawings of the Belscope angulated laryngoscope. Top diagram shows view obtained looking forward from the angle along the distal part of blade in direction B-A. Bottom diagram shows prism in position on blade. When prism is used, view of larynx is obtained by looking along line C-B through prism. (From Bellhouse CP: An angulated laryngoscope for routine and difficult tracheal intubation, *Anesthesiology* 69:126, 1988.)

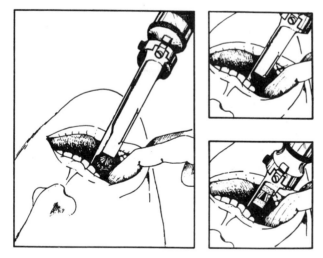

Fig. 20-18. *Left,* angulated laryngoscope in oropharynx, facilitating direct view of larynx. *Top right,* uncommon situation where oropharyngeal tissues push laryngoscope angle back into pharynx, obscuring view of larynx. *Bottom right,* attachment of prism affords indirect view of larynx. (From Bellhouse CP: An angulated laryngoscope for routine and difficult tracheal intubation, *Anesthesiology* 69:126, 1988.)

6. Neustein laryngoscope blade

The Neustein laryngoscope is a small, angulated, hollow, rigid guide channel attached to a mirror (Fig. 20-20).[26] The guide on this device accepts a soft catheter, which is directed through the vocal cords while they are visualized indirectly in the mirror. The Neustein laryngoscope is used in conjunction with a Macintosh laryngoscope blade. Once the Macintosh blade is correctly positioned, the guide is then placed cephalad and posterior to the epiglottis, with the distal end of the rigid tube on the posterior aspect of the guide directed under the epiglottis. The light source from the Macintosh blade illuminates the mirror to provide an indirect view of the larynx. Once the vocal cords are visualized, an assistant is necessary to pass a catheter through the guide and into the trachea. The device is then removed and the catheter is used as a guide over which an ET is blindly passed. Recognized limitations of this laryngoscope by the inventor include the lack of a catheter that is rigid enough and specifically designed for use with the guide to direct an ET into the trachea. Other limitations include the requirement of an assistant (the operator is holding the two laryngoscopes) and the fact that the guide channel location behind the mirror may preclude visualization beneath the epiglottis by limiting the

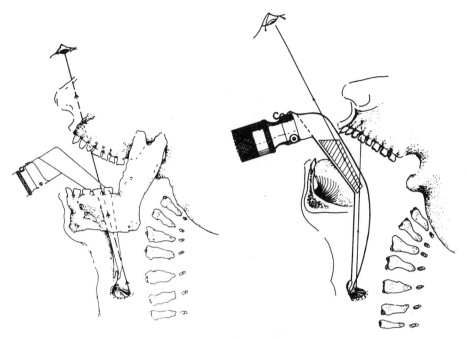

Fig. 20-19. *Left,* in the majority of laryngoscopies with the Belscope, a view of posterior commissure (and usually much more) is seen when the lip is pulled upward and outward by looking along the right side of the maxilla. *Right,* in difficult laryngoscopies when the laryngoscope angle cannot be pulled forward sufficiently for direct viewing of the larynx, attachment of prism will provide an indirect view. (From Bellhouse CP: An angulated laryngoscope for routine and difficult tracheal intubation, *Anesthesiology* 69:126, 1988.)

amount of space posterior to the epiglottis for positioning of the mirror. There have been no clinical studies with the Neustein laryngoscope and it is not yet commercially available on a widespread basis.

B. LIMITED MOUTH OPENING

1. Soper laryngoscope blade

The Soper blade was introduced in 1947. Although quoted as the first true derivative of the Macintosh laryngoscope, its shape is similar to the Miller blade. This blade was developed as a result of the perceived disadvantages of the Macintosh laryngoscope; elevating the epiglottis indirectly did not always result in exposure of the cords, especially when there was a large "flabby" epiglottis to contend with. It was also found that although the laryngeal opening was visualized, it was often necessary to use a stiffener inside the ET to manipulate it around the curvature of the blade.[27]

The Soper laryngoscope (Fig. 20-21), like the Macintosh, has a Z-shaped section on the flange instead of the older C-shaped section. However, the blade portion is straight and similar in length to the Miller. It is designed to elevate the epiglottis in the usual way and has a slot built into the tip, which is intended to prevent the epiglottis from slipping off the blade. Two sizes, adult and child, were available from the Longworth Scientific

Instrument Company, Oxford, England. This laryngoscope was never very popular and now serves only as a point of historical interest.

2. Parrott laryngoscope blade

Although the first modification of the Macintosh blade was the Soper laryngoscope blade, the Parrott laryngoscope was the first to address changes in the blade's curvature, a feature that Macintosh did not consider of primary importance.[28] This laryngoscope was designed to facilitate intubation in patients with prominent teeth and receding jaws. It is 2.5 cm longer than the original Macintosh laryngoscope with a less-pronounced curvature (Fig. 20-22). This lessened curvature presumably facilitated easier passage of an ET, and the additional length was useful in larger patients. This laryngoscope blade originally incorporated a removable lamp carrier, but this was later abandoned.

3. Gould laryngoscope blade

To reduce damage to the upper teeth, Gould modified the Soper blade by flattening the proximal end from the standard Z shape to a "spatulate appearance" with a rubber lining.[29] He also replaced the sharp, ratchetlike distal end with a blunt edge (Fig. 20-23). Apparently similar modifications were made to the Macintosh blade, but neither Gould blade gained widespread recognition.

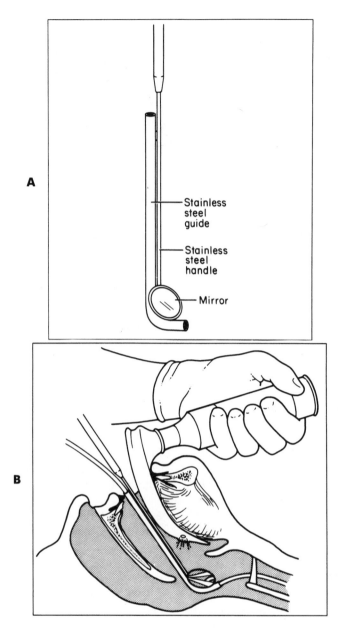

Fig. 20-20. A, Neustein laryngoscope. **B,** Macintosh laryngoscope is used to lift tongue and illuminate the mirror of the Neustein laryngoscope. Indirect view of larynx is seen in mirror; the guide is used to position catheter in trachea. (From Neustein SM: The Neustein laryngoscope: a new solution to the difficult intubation, *Anesth Review* XIX:54, 1992.)

4. Bowen-Jackson laryngoscope blade

According to Ronald Bowen and Ian Jackson, laryngoscopy and endotracheal intubation are easily accomplished in most patients, and that skill is more important than the type of blade used provided the anesthetist places the patient in the amended Chevalier Jackson position—that is, flexion of the neck with extension of the head.[30] These investigators reviewed both straight and curved blades and found that each type of laryngoscope had advantages and disadvantages that varied with the anatomy of the specific patient. They thought that a compromise between a straight and curved blade might

facilitate intubation in all patients. After experimenting with five different blade shapes, they introduced the Bowen-Jackson (B-J) blade (Fig. 20-24). The B-J blade has a bifid distal end that straddles the glossoepiglottic fold in the recesses of the vallecula (also see Augustine guide). The major portion of the blade is straight with a marked distal curvature that is intended to create greater space for manipulation of an ET. The length is adequate to accommodate even the largest patient. The step of the blade (the vertical portion of the flange) is used to control the tongue and is similar to that on the Macintosh laryngoscope. But the depth of the step is very

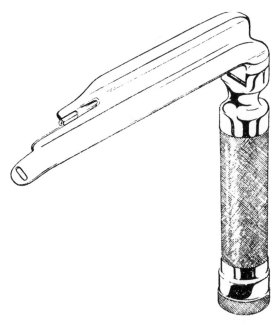

Fig. 20-21. Soper laryngoscope. (From Soper RL: A new laryngoscope for anaesthestists, *Br Med J* 1:265, 1947.)

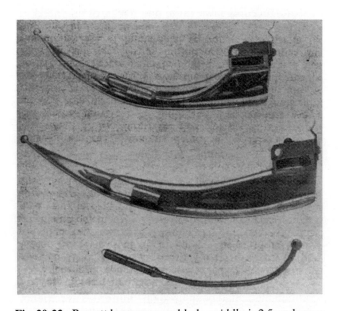

Fig. 20-22. Parrott laryngoscope blade, *middle,* is 2.5 cm longer than the Macintosh blade, *bottom,* and has a separate bulb assembly that facilitates cleaning, *top.* (From Parrott CM: Modification of Macintosh's curved laryngoscope, *Br Med J* 2:1031, 1951.)

shallow, providing more space between large or protruding teeth. The maximum depth of the step is in the middle of the blade to control the main bulk of the tongue in the faucial region. An additional feature is that the handle is set back so that it forms an approximate 100-degree angle with the blade to help avoid contact of the handle with the chest. The blade was recommended

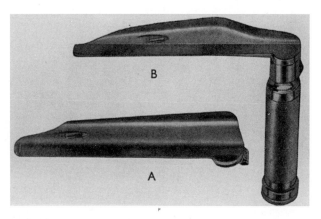

Fig. 20-23. Gould laryngoscope blade, **B,** is a modified version of Soper blade. **A,** Proximal end of Gould blade has been flattened to reduce risk of damage to teeth. It is also slightly longer than Soper blade. (From Gould RB: Modified laryngoscope blade, *Anaesthesia* 9:125, 1954.)

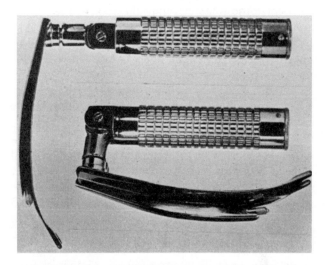

Fig. 20-24. Bowen-Jackson (B-J) laryngoscope. (From Bowen RA, Jackson I: A new laryngoscope, *Anaesthesia* 7:254, 1952.)

for use in patients aged 4 years and older and attained a limited following.

5. Gabuya-Orkin laryngoscope blade

Drs. Gabuya and Orkin faulted the Macintosh laryngoscope on several points: (1) it lacked flexibility for manipulation without imposing trauma to the teeth; (2) it interfered with binocular vision; and (3) it was a suboptimal device for intubation in infants and children.[31] Their modifications of the Macintosh laryngoscope blade resulted in less required mouth opening for exposure of the laryngeal inlet and consisted of the following: The distal two thirds of the blade forms an S curve starting 2.5 cm from the proximal end, which raises the base of the tongue during laryngoscopy (Fig. 20-25). The tip of the blade is curved transversely much like the Miller blade that, in the proper position, pulls on the

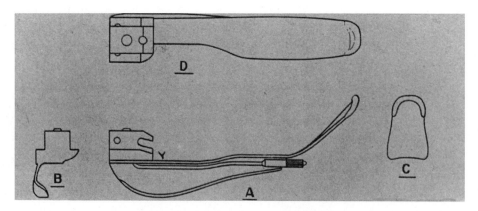

Fig. 20-25. A schematic of the Gabuya-Orkin laryngoscope blade. **A,** View of right side. **B,** View of top. **C,** End view of distal tip. **D,** End view of joint section. **Y,** Center of the radius of blade. (From Gabuya R, Orkin LR: Design and utility of a new curved laryngoscope blade, *Anesth Analg* 38:364, 1959.)

glossoepiglottic folds elevating the root of the tongue anteriorly. The flat portion of the blade is malleable so that individual adjustments can be made, but it is reportedly strong enough to hold its shape during laryngoscopy. The vertical height is limited to 1.8 cm and is slanted sideward to facilitate binocular vision.

This laryngoscope blade was compared to a similarly sized Macintosh laryngoscope blade in 100 patients undergoing electroconvulsive therapy (ECT). After induction of general anesthesia and elicitation of mild convulsions for ECT, laryngoscopy was performed by a single individual, who made the following observations: (1) the new blade allowed for greater exposure (2 to 5 mm) in grade II or greater laryngoscopic views; (2) exposure was better with a lateral versus midline approach for both blades; (3) the most effective angle for the distal tip to facilitate exposure was 35 degrees from the horizontal; (4) the use of binocular vision was more apparent with the new blade than with the Macintosh blade; and (5) pressure was exerted more frequently on the upper teeth with the flange of the Macintosh blade. Furthermore, the flexible blade angle was thought to be an additional advantage in patients with unusual anatomic variations of the oropharynx, although this was never investigated.[31] Gabuya and Orkin had planned to develop a mirror clip accessory to facilitate indirect laryngoscopy, but no formal reports of this modification have been reported in the literature and no further clinical studies have been performed.

6. Bizzarri-Giuffrida laryngoscope blade

The first radical change in the shape of the Macintosh laryngoscope was proposed by Drs. Bizzarri and Giuffrida in 1958.[32] They modified the shape based on the frequent contact the vertical flange on the original Macintosh made with the upper incisors during laryn-

goscopy, especially in patients with limited mobility of the mandible. In an effort to overcome this problem, they eliminated the vertical component entirely (Fig. 20-26). Their experience in more than 200 patients found this blade particularly useful in patients with protruding incisors, receding jaws, large bull necks, or an anteriorly positioned larynx. Other than their initial report, little other clinical evaluation is available on this blade.

7. Onkst laryngoscope blade

Dr. Onkst also recognized the problem of the immobile vertical flange on the Macintosh laryngoscope that often made contact with the upper teeth, resulting in injury and hampering maneuverability. His effort to overcome this limitation included cutting the flange from the bulb to the base of the flange and interposing a hinge (Fig. 20-27).[33] A coiled spring holds the flange at a right angle to the blade so that any pressure on the flange causes it to fold toward the midline up to a maximum 90 degree arc until it lies parallel to the blade (Fig. 20-28). The flange is prevented from folding away from the midline and into the laryngoscopist's line of vision by a metal piece incorporated into the flange itself. Onkst's modified blade had been used on "hundreds of patients" prior to its first appearance in the literature and apparently "satisfaction" was achieved by all who used it.[33] No formal clinical trials have been reported.

8. Orr laryngoscope blade

The Orr U-shaped laryngoscope blade was designed to eliminate contact with the upper incisor teeth, particularly useful in patients with protruding upper incisors and receding lower jaws.[34] The blade has two right-angle bends (Fig. 20-29) so that when the functional portion of the blade is properly positioned in the oropharynx, the proximal portion is not in contact with

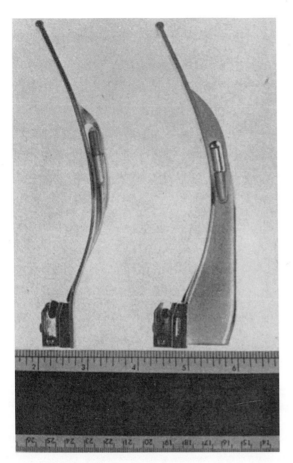

Fig. 20-26. Bizzarri-Giuffrida laryngoscope blade, *left,* compared to Macintosh laryngoscope blade, *right.* Bizzarri-Giuffrida blade is substantially thinner with essentially no vertical component, dramatically reducing potential damage to teeth. (From Bizzarri DV, Giuffrida JG: Improved laryngoscope blade designed for ease of manipulation and reduction of trauma, *Anesth Analg* 37:231, 1958.)

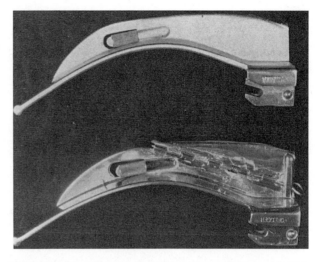

Fig. 20-27. *Top,* a lateral view of the standard Macintosh blade, and *bottom,* modified Onkst blade with hinged flange. (From Onkst HR: Modified laryngoscope blade, *Anesthesiology* 22: 846, 1961.)

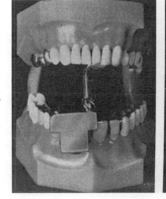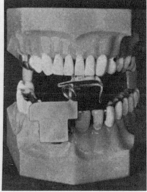

Fig. 20-28. A, Onkst blade in place with no pressure on flange. **B,** With pressure on the flange, it folds to the lowest position. Vertical dimension is dramatically decreased. In addition, the entire broad, flat surface of flange contacts upper incisors, distributing pressure over a wide surface area. (From Onkst HR: Modified laryngoscope blade, *Anesthesiology* 22:846, 1961.)

the teeth, thereby shifting the fulcrum away from the teeth to a point lower in the pharynx. It is used much like a straight blade, elevating the epiglottis with the distal blade tip to expose the larynx. Once the vocal cords are visualized, the ET is inserted from the right side of the mouth.

A small clinical trial was performed by Dr. Orr on 12 patients with known difficult airways. He was successful in intubating the trachea of all patients including two in whom the vocal cords could not be visualized with any existing available blade at the time. In addition, there are anecdotal reports of less damage to the teeth.

The Orr laryngoscope blade is available in two sizes. The shorter version is used when the distal tip enters the esophagus since even partial withdrawal would result in impingement of the upper incisor teeth on the vertical portion. The Foregger Company originally manufactured this blade, which is rarely used today.

9. Phillips laryngoscope blade

The Phillips laryngoscope blade combines features of both the Jackson and Miller blades: the shaft of the Jackson and the curved tip of the Miller, with the light bulb on the left side of the blade.[35] The curved tip of the Phillips blade lifts the hyoid and attached structures, affording good visualization of the glottis; the rounded shaft offers a conduit for passage of the ET.

Clinical experience with the Phillips laryngoscope included its use by a variety of anesthesia personnel (residents, nurse anesthetists, student nurses, and anesthesia faculty at the University of Pittsburgh) in 1038

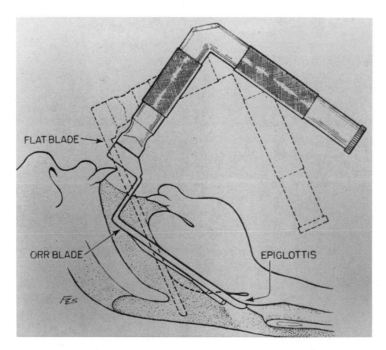

Fig. 20-29. Orr blade in position. (From Orr RB: A new laryngoscope blade designed to facilitate difficult endotracheal intubation, *Anesthesiology* 31:377, 1969.)

patients, ranging in age from 6 weeks to adulthood.[35] Multiple attempts were necessary in 16% of all intubations; a stylet was used in 17% of the cases. Although the study was poorly controlled, the number of attempts and the need for a stylet to facilitate intubation was reportedly higher when using either a Miller or Macintosh blade as compared to the Phillips blade. However, most personnel chose the blade most familiar to them when they were confronted with difficult intubation situations. Since the original report, no further clinical comparison studies have been done with this laryngoscope blade. But as Dr. Schapira commented in a guest editorial, the Phillips blade is close to the "perfect laryngoscopy blade," permitting visualization of the vocal cords during difficult intubations as well as routine intubations and thus enabling the laryngoscopist to become thoroughly comfortable with its use.[36] He further pointed out that the problem with specialty blades (such as the Siker[18] or Orr[34] blades) was that they were not intended for daily use and were only for use in difficult situations. This is obviously doomed to failure since the laryngoscopist is likely to be unfamiliar with their use. Interestingly, Schapira developed his own modified version of the straight blade that same year.

10. Schapira laryngoscope blade

The Schapira blade is a modified version of the Wis-Foregger laryngoscope blade; the vertical component was eliminated and it has a slightly different curvature (Fig. 20-30).[37] These changes were thought to

afford easier insertion without risking damage to the teeth while providing excellent visualization of the glottis and the cords.

11. Improved-vision Macintosh laryngoscope blade

When Sir Robert Macintosh first presented his laryngoscope blade in 1943, it was curved with a markedly flattened midportion. Since the device's inception, the flattened midportion disappeared and the blade has assumed a curved shape, which was retained largely due to manufacturing considerations.[14] Unfortunately, the curve in the midportion often inhibits visualization of the larynx, especially in patients with prominent teeth, receding jaws, or poor cervical-spine mobility. The improved-vision (IV) Macintosh laryngoscope sought to correct this perceived disadvantage by replacing the convex curvature with a concave midportion curvature while maintaining the outer-edge curved appearance (Fig. 20-31).[38] Limited clinical experience has demonstrated improved visibility, although no formal clinical trials have been performed. This laryngoscope blade is manufactured by and available from Anesthesia Medical Specialties (Santa Fe Springs, California).

12. Callender-Thomas laryngoscope blade

Another modification of the Macintosh blade was proposed by Callender and Thomas, who reduced the height of the flange to make insertion in patients with limited mouth opening much easier (Fig. 20-32).[39] In addition, the decreased flange height resulted in less risk

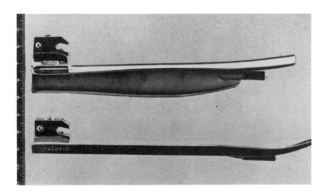

Fig. 20-30. Lateral view of Wis-Foregger, *top,* and Schapira, *bottom,* blades. Note larger vertical component of Wisconsin blade. (From Schapira M: A modified straight laryngoscope blade designed to facilitate endotracheal intubation, *Anesth Analg* 52:553, 1973.)

of damage to the teeth, especially in patients with prominent upper incisors. Apparently, this laryngoscope blade is manufactured in England, but little other information is available.

13. Pressure-sensitive laryngoscope blade

Injury to the teeth is a common complication from direct laryngoscopy and is most often a result of pressure on the upper teeth from the laryngoscope.[40] Preventive solutions to this problem include using rubber or plastic guards, tape, and blades of varying design.[41] Racz and Allen designed a new adult laryngoscope blade to reduce the potential for dental injury by incorporating a flexible hinged proximal portion on a straight blade that displaces laterally when pressure is applied (similar conceptually to the Onkst laryngoscope blade) (Fig. 20-33).[42] The hinged portion is concave along its entire length, and the convexity of the main portion of the blade is slightly greater than a standard Miller blade so that vision is not impeded with maximum displacement of the hinged portion. The spring tension is set below the lowest mastication pressure so that the hinged portion starts to bend at only 0.68 kg of pressure to a maximum displacement at 1.8 kg of pressure. Although this laryngoscope blade is available, no clinical studies have been performed on it.

14. Kawahara laryngoscope blade

In response to the difficulty experienced in performing endotracheal intubation in patients with fractured mandibles, ankylosis of the jaw, tumors of the neck, and malformation of the orofacial region, Kawahara et al. evaluated a laryngoscope equipped with fiberoptics as an alternative to their usual intubating techniques in these clinical situations (e.g., awake blind nasal intubation, retrograde intubation, or intubation using a flexible fiberoptic bronchoscope).[43] The flexible fiberoptic bronchoscope was considered their method of choice. But the

skilled use of it, as the authors correctly pointed out, required extensive training and practice. This laryngoscope was composed of a curved blade, slightly more curved than a standard Macintosh blade, with an attached fiberoptic eyepiece at the proximal end (Fig. 20-34).

To use this fiberoptic laryngoscope, the lens is first defogged and focused, and then the blade is inserted into the oropharynx in the standard fashion. It is advanced until the epiglottis comes into view through the eyepiece. The glottis is then visualized by elevating the epiglottis slightly with the distal blade tip. Once the glottic opening comes into focus, the ET is advanced through the vocal cords. Because the glottis is viewed indirectly, it is initially cumbersome and spatially difficult to advance the ET through the vocal cords, but with practice it is reported to become easier. The reported advantage of this blade is that neither extensive mouth opening nor extreme hyperextension of the neck are necessary for successful intubation. No clinical comparison studies have been performed.

15. Double-Angle laryngoscope blade

The Double-Angle blade (prototype made by Anesthesia Medical Specialties, Santa Fe Springs, California, U.S. patent pending) was designed by Dr. Choi in an effort to combine the advantageous features of the Miller and Macintosh laryngoscope blades while eliminating their disadvantages.[44] This blade incorporates two incremental curves, 20 degrees and 30 degrees, which allow for visualization of an anteriorly situated larynx without having to tilt the laryngoscope posteriorly. The vertical flange was eliminated entirely to reduce the risk of tooth damage and create more room for intubation. The blade tip is also wider and flatter, which allows for easier manipulation of a large tongue or floppy epiglottis (Fig. 20-35).

The blade is introduced into the oropharynx in the standard fashion, and visualization of the glottis is achieved either directly by lifting the epiglottis or indirectly by placing the blade tip in the vallecula. Elimination of the flange is thought to decrease damage to the upper incisors while maintaining the ability to displace the tongue out of the line of vision (Fig. 20-36 on p. 394). The simplicity of this blade is its most attractive feature, but it needs to be tested clinically prior to widespread recommended use.

16. Levering laryngoscope blade

Certain oropharyngeal anatomic peculiarities allow for exposure of the epiglottis but preclude elevation of it; these abnormalities include decreased mouth opening, a large tongue, and prominent or bucked upper teeth. The natural inclination in these situations is to lever the laryngoscope backward in an attempt to entrap

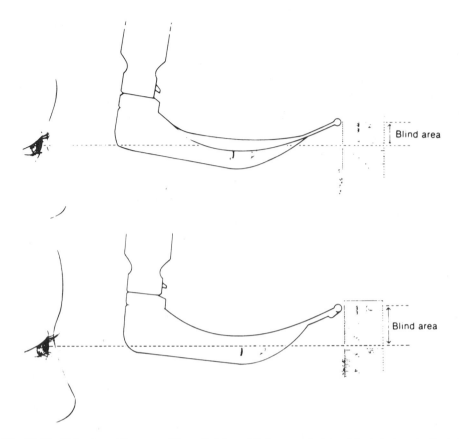

Fig. 20-31. Side view of improved line of vision with improved-vision Macintosh as indicated on the ruler, *top,* compared with standard Macintosh laryngoscope, *bottom.* (From Racz GB: Improved vision modification of the Macintosh laryngoscope. Letter-to-the-Editor, *Anaesthesia* 39:1249, 1984.)

and lift the epiglottis, often resulting in damage to the upper teeth. The levering laryngoscope is a modification of the standard Macintosh curved laryngoscope that eliminates contact with the upper incisors while maintaining the fulcrum at a lower point in the pharynx.[45] It differs from the Macintosh in that it has a hinged tip, a lever at the proximal end, a spring-loaded drum, and a connecting shaft that links the spring-loaded drum to the hinged tip (Fig. 20-37). The blade fits onto a standard laryngoscope handle. The intubation technique is similar to that in using a Macintosh laryngoscope; it is inserted into the oropharynx, and the distal tip of the blade is positioned in the vallecula. Compression of the lever toward the handle results in elevation of the hinged tip approximately 70 degrees upward, which exerts traction on the hyoepiglottic ligament, elevating the epiglottis and exposing the larynx. Intubation of the trachea is accomplished in the usual manner. Then the lever is released, allowing the tip of the blade to assume its normal, resting position (Fig. 20-37). Although the inventors found that the amount of force necessary for visualization of the larynx was decreased with this blade, no clinical comparison studies have been performed. However, there have been several anecdotal

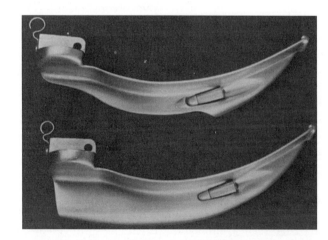

Fig. 20-32. Callender-Thomas modification of the Macintosh laryngoscope, *top,* consists of a reduction of the height of flange at the hilt of blade without an alteration in the position of the light source, compared with the standard Macintosh laryngoscope, *bottom.* (From Callander CC, Thomas J: Modification of Macintosh laryngoscope for difficult intubation. Letter-to-the-Editor, *Anaesthesia* 42:671, 1987.)

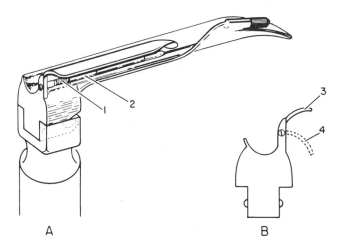

Fig. 20-33. Illustration of side (**A**) and back (**B**) views of pressure-sensitive laryngoscope blade: *1,* spring; *2,* threaded screw; *3,* normal position; *4,* full displacement of flexible portion. (From Racz GB, Allen FB: A new pressure-sensitive laryngoscope, *Anesthesiology* 62:356, 1985.)

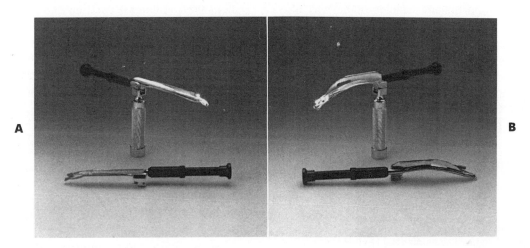

Fig. 20-34. Kawahara laryngoscope with fiberoptics. **A,** Miller. **B,** Macintosh. (From Kawahara M, Takeshita T, Akitu S: A new model of laryngoscope equipped with fiberoptics, *Anesth Prog* 36:70, 1989.)

reports that it has been advantageous in cases of difficult intubations.[46-49]

C. SMALL INFRAORAL CAVITY

1. Snow laryngoscope blade

Dr. Snow was a strong advocate of straight blades to facilitate intubation but found fault with both the Wis-Foregger and Miller blades; the Wis-Foregger did not predictably lift the epiglottis, and there was occasionally lack of space with the Miller laryngoscope blade to pass the ET, although the vocal cords were clearly visualized.[50] He therefore combined features of both of these blades to overcome the perceived limitations of each. His blade is curved 1 inch from the rounded distal tip and is specifically designed for raising the epiglottis. It also contains a semicircular groove with a concavity to the right, which not only provides a pathway for visualizing the larynx but allows easier passage of an ET

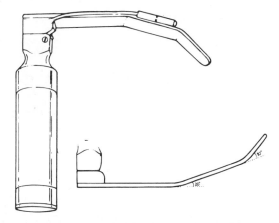

Fig. 20-35. Double-Angle blade with 20-degree and 30-degree incremental curvatures . (From Choi JJ: A new Double-Angle blade for direct laryngoscopy, *Anesthesiology* 72:576, 1990.)

while it holds the tongue to the left side of the mouth (Fig. 20-38). Snow found that "intubation is easier and more successful with this blade . . . than with any other blade."[50] Despite his enthusiasm, little else is written about the Snow laryngoscope blade.

2. DeCiutiis laryngoscope blade

Dr. DeCiutiis modified the Macintosh laryngoscope for the specific purpose of facilitating intubation in patients with thick, heavy tongues and in edentulous patients with small mouths.[51] His modification included widening the blade while maintaining the "essential" curvature (remembering of course that Macintosh himself thought that the shape of the curvature was inconsequential). These changes were thought to facilitate support of a large, beefy tongue and to hold the cheek at a distance from the viewing edge of the blade so that little right-to-left motion was necessary to view the larynx. A proportionally smaller blade was also

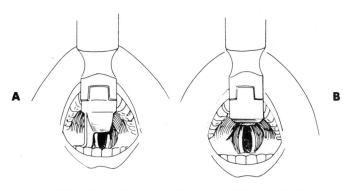

Fig. 20-36. Schematic comparison of the Macintosh, **A,** and Double-Angle, **B,** blades. The nonflanged Double-Angle blade improves vision, provides more room for passage of an ET, and should reduce risk of tooth damage. (From Choi JJ: A new Double-Angle blade for direct laryngoscopy, *Anesthesiology* 72:576, 1990.)

available for infants but neither gained widespread acceptance.

3. McWhinnie laryngoscope blade

McWhinnie's modification of the Macintosh blade involved widening the flange where the bulk of the tongue sits to hold the tongue and endotracheal tube out of the way and provide room for intubation as well as manipulation of other devices, including Magill forceps, which were often used to assist with nasogastric-tube insertion (Fig. 20-39).[52] This idea was originally proposed by Campbell and Millar,[53] but because of its limited applicability for routine use, neither laryngoscope blade has gained much attention.

4. Left-handed laryngoscopes

The first left-handed Macintosh laryngoscope blade was designed by E.S. Pope as an aid to intubation in a patient with unilateral swelling of the upper jaw. He thought that in addition to this particular case, this instrument would be useful in a variety of other situations such as with patients with dental lesions on the upper right jaw or with injuries to the right side of the face resulting in scarring and immobility, or as a uniquely suited tool for left-handed beginning laryngoscopists.[54] Various left-handed versions of both the Macintosh and Miller laryngoscope blades are still available today.[55] The ridge of the curve is on the right side of the blade so that when it is inserted on the left side of the mouth, the tongue is pushed to the right. When a patient has extensive right hemifacial lesions, these blades are thought to facilitate better laryngeal exposure.

5. Bainton pharyngolaryngoscope

a. DESCRIPTION

In 1987 Dr. Bainton introduced a new laryngoscope blade to the anesthesia community that he designed

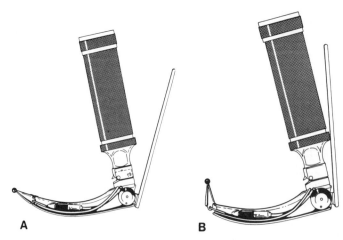

Fig. 20-37. Illustration of levering laryngoscope blade attached to standard handle in normal position (**A**) and with the distal tip elevated (**B**). (From McCoy ED, Mirakhur RK: The levering laryngoscope, *Anaesthesia* 48:516, 1993.)

specifically for use in patients with pharyngeal obstructions.[56] The etiology of acute upper-airway obstruction includes laryngopharyngeal neoplasms, infections, neck trauma, surgery, and other conditions that can lead to life-threatening swelling and edema. In these situations, a standard nontubular laryngoscope blade is unable to create sufficient viewing space since the mucosa and/or scar tissue envelopes the blade, obliterating both the viewing space and the light source on direct laryngoscopy. Several ENT tubular laryngoscopes (Jackson, Holinger, Jako, and Dedo-Pilling, Pilling Co., Washington, Pennsylvania) exist that create space within the pharynx and have an intraluminal light source that prevents the edematous tissue from obstructing the illumination. The problems with these laryngoscope blades is that they are too long to facilitate easy passage of an ET, and as the ET is inserted, the view is obstructed, making stabilization of the ET's position during removal of the laryngoscope difficult. Therefore Bainton developed a pharyngolaryngoscope that achieved the following objectives: (1) created pharyngeal space using a tubular design; (2) optimized the passing of endotracheal tubes through or around the blade into the larynx using the tubular structure; and (3) fit onto existing, standardized light handles.

The Bainton pharyngolaryngoscope (model 52-2220, Pilling Instruments, Fort Washington, Pennsylvania) resembles a standard, straight blade with a 7-cm tube incorporated onto the distal portion. A dual fiberoptic light source is recessed within the lumen to protect it from secretions and obstruction by surrounding oropharyngeal tissue (Fig. 20-40). The distal tip of the blade is beveled at a 60-degree angle, creating an oval opening. An 8.0 ID or smaller ET is easily accommodated through the tubular lumen without significantly obstructing the view.

b. TECHNIQUE

The intubation technique is similar to any straight blade. It is inserted in the right side of the mouth, pushing the tongue to the left and advanced until the distal tip entraps the epiglottis. Once the glottic opening is visualized, an ET is placed through the tubular lumen

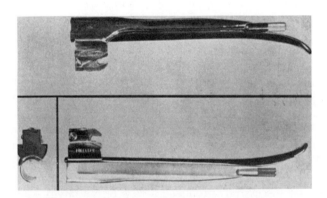

Fig. 20-38. Snow laryngoscope blade. Blade is curved 1 inch from distal tip and has a semicircular groove with the concavity to the right, which permits visualization of larynx and easy passage of an ET while preventing obstruction of the view by surrounding edematous tissues or protruding teeth. (From Snow JC: Modification of laryngoscope blade, *Anesthesiology* 23:294, 1962.)

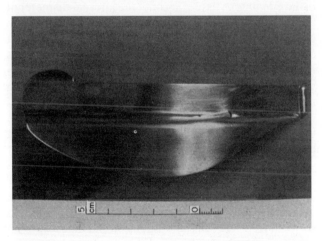

Fig. 20-39. McWhinnie modification of standard Macintosh blade, with markedly widened flange. (From McWhinnie F: Modification of laryngoscope for nasogastric intubation. Letter-to-the-Editor, *Anaesthesia* 41:218, 1986.)

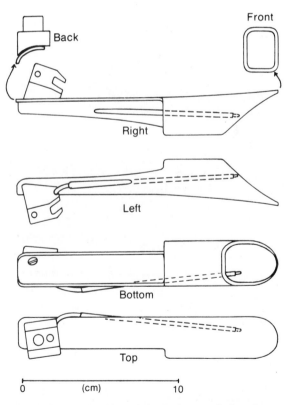

Fig. 20-40. Scale drawings of the Bainton tubular pharyngo-laryngoscope. (From Bainton CR: A new laryngoscope blade to overcome pharyngeal obstruction, *Anesthesiology* 67:767, 1987.)

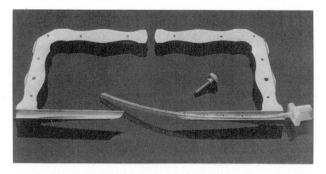

Fig. 20-42. Two-piece tubular pediatric laryngoscope. The two handle-blades are held together by a knurled screw during orotracheal intubation. (From Diaz JH, Guarisco JL, LeJeune FE: A modified tubular pharyngolaryngoscope for difficult pediatric laryngoscopy, *Anesthesiology* 73:357, 1990.)

and passed through the vocal cords. The device is then divided in half along the long axis of the scope and the two halves are removed around the ET (Fig. 20-41).

c. CLINICAL EXPERIENCE

This laryngoscope blade was first tested in a dog that was injected with a saline solution in the pharyngeal submucosa and the base of the tongue to simulate an edematous pharynx. Visualization of the larynx was easily accomplished with the new blade whereas both the Guedel and Macintosh laryngoscope blades failed to produce an adequate view. Other clinical experience by Bainton included 12 patients with edematous pharynges and one with a bleeding pharyngeal tumor in whom this blade successfully produced a view of the larynx while other blades failed. Bainton's experience has not been repeated in any formal clinical trials but his patient trials have emphasized three important features of the pharyngolaryngoscope. First, the tubular portion of the blade must extend to the tip so that the tip remains in the visual field during insertion; otherwise it will get lost in the edematous tissue. Second, the internal diameter of the tubular portion should be approximately 20 mm to create sufficient viewing space as well as to prevent obstruction of the laryngeal view when the ET is inserted. And third, the length of the tubular portion should be limited to the pharynx; longer tubes extending into the mouth are more difficult to manage.

A pediatric version was proposed by shortening the length of the blade and decreasing the outer diameter, but it has not been developed. However, in subsequent years a modified two-piece pharyngolaryngoscope was developed for pediatric use (Fig. 20-42).[57] Two handle-blades are held together by a screw, and each blade contains a dual fiberoptic light source. Once the glottis is visualized via direct suspension laryngoscopy, an appropriately sized ET is passed through the lumen and into the glottic opening. As the patient's trachea is intubated, the laryngeal view is temporarily obstructed. Another minor disadvantage is the difficulty in stabiliz-

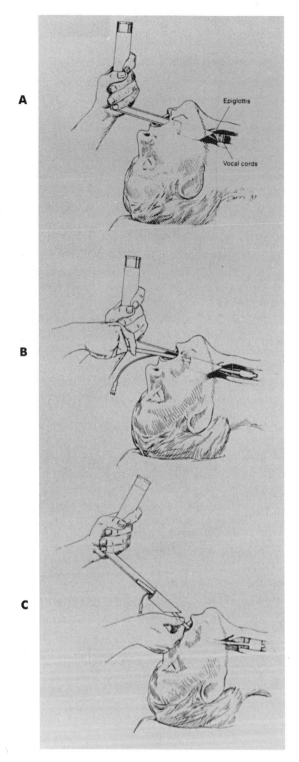

Fig. 20-41. Schematic of intubation technique with Bainton tubular pharyngolaryngoscope. **A,** Tubular portion, pictured in cutaway, fits within the pharyngeal space. Tip of blade elevates epiglottis to permit a view of larynx. **B,** ET without an adapter (stylet optional) is inserted into tubular portion of blade and advanced into larynx. ET cuff is inflated. **C,** syringe and stylet are removed from ET and pharyngolaryngoscope is withdrawn from mouth. Right hand of operator stabilizes ET as blade is elevated over proximal end of ET and cuff pilot tube. (From Bainton CR: A new laryngoscope blade to overcome pharyngeal obstruction, *Anesthesiology* 67:767, 1987.)

ing the ET as the blade is dismantled and removed from the oropharynx. The authors have found this device to be useful in patients with acquired pediatric microsomia and intraoral cystic hygroma because of its unique ability to create viewing space within the oropharynx by gently compressing surrounding edematous tissue, masses, or scars.[57] In addition, this device, like the Bainton blade, may have a distinct advantage over flexible fiberoptic intubation techniques because this instrument prevents blood, secretions, and/or edematous tissues from obscuring the view and the illumination source. The disadvantages of this blade and the Bainton pharyngolaryngoscope are similar to the disadvantages of all straight blades; they may not work well for the "anterior" larynx. As with any new device, they are initially bulky and awkward to manipulate; both require practice to become skilled at their use. Although there is little clinical research in support of either blade, some anesthesiologists have found the Bainton pharyngolaryngoscope useful in obstetrics, particularly for the occasional preeclamptic parturient requiring an urgent anesthetic with a rapid-sequence intubation.

D. IMMOBILE/UNSTABLE CERVICAL SPINES

Direct laryngoscopy is the easiest, quickest, and surest method of endotracheal intubation, but it requires flexion of the cervical spine and altantooccipital extension for alignment of the oral, pharyngeal, and laryngeal axes to create a direct line of vision from the mouth to the vocal cords. There are situations when such patient positioning is impossible or contraindicated, such as in a patient with a fused cervical spine or with cervical-spine instability following injury. In elective situations, fiberoptic bronchoscopy is probably the preferred method of intubation. In an emergency setting, a rapid sequence induction with in-line manual axial traction has been recommended as a stabilization maneuver but, as emphasized by Hastings and Mark in a subsequent study, the potential for neck movement does exist with this approach, although neurologic sequelae are infrequent.[58-59] Several new laryngoscopes address this concern.

1. Bullard laryngoscope

a. DESCRIPTION

The Bullard laryngoscope (BL) (Circon, ACMI, Stamford, Connecticut) is one of these new intubating devices. This rigid instrument functions as an indirect fiberoptic laryngoscope; the blade portion is designed to match the anatomical airway. This feature negates the need for manipulation of the patient's head and neck to visualize the larynx, an obvious advantage in patients with cervical-spine pathology. Specifications of this blade include: length, 13.2 cm; width, 1.3 cm; radius of curvature, 3.4 cm; and blade thickness, 0.64 cm. The fiberoptic bundle is positioned along the posterior aspect of the blade and the distal end of the fiber comes to within 26 mm of the distal tip of the blade, placing the endoscopist's view in the posterior pharynx. This facilitates excellent visualization of the larynx. Other features include a bifurcated 3.7-mm channel incorporated into the laryngoscope at its proximal end. One port of the bifurcation is equipped with a Luer-lock fitting for attachment of a three-way stopcock to provide suction or insufflation of oxygen or installation of local anesthetics. The other port of the bifurcation accepts the proximal end of a new, dedicated, nonmalleable intubating stylet, the newest device to aid in intubation (Fig. 20-43). The original intubating mechanisms included: (1) a styleted ET shaped to mimic the curve of the Bullard blade; (2) an ET with a directional tip (e.g., Endotrol, Mallinckrodt Critical Care, Glens Falls, New York); and (3) use of the Bullard intubating forceps, a thumb lever–activated device that allows the operator to advance the intubating forceps into the larynx and release the ET once it is through the vocal cords. The intubating forceps have recently been abandoned in favor of the nonmalleable intubating stylet.

b. TECHNIQUE

To use the intubating stylet, the ET must be preloaded prior to attaching the stylet onto the laryngoscope. First the stylet is well lubricated. After removal of the ET adapter, the ET is positioned on the stylet so that the distal end of the stylet projects through the Murphy eye of the ET. The ET can then be either advanced proximally over the length of the stylet if there is limited mouth opening or left in position near the distal tip of the blade. The stylet clips onto a designated port on the BL, so that when it is correctly attached, the stylet-ET apparatus lies along the right side of the posterior spine of the blade. Since the new intubating stylet hugs the posterior surface of the blade, the BL must be used like a modified Miller blade; the epiglottis is retracted against the posterior part of the tongue. If the epiglottis is not retracted, the ET will impact the vallecula as it is advanced off the stylet.

The technique of intubation with the BL is in the following manner (Fig. 20-44): The BL, held in the left hand, is inserted into the mouth in the horizontal plane. Once it clears the tongue, the blade is rotated to a vertical plane by allowing it to slide around the midline of the tongue. The laryngoscope is then momentarily dropped into the posterior pharynx. With a scooping motion, gentle traction is applied in the vertical plane to lift the blade against the posterior surface of the tongue. Either the epiglottis or the vocal cords will come into view. If the epiglottis is the only structure visualized with initial blade insertion, the blade is dropped back into the posterior pharynx followed by the application of a more-pronounced scooping motion on the blade in an

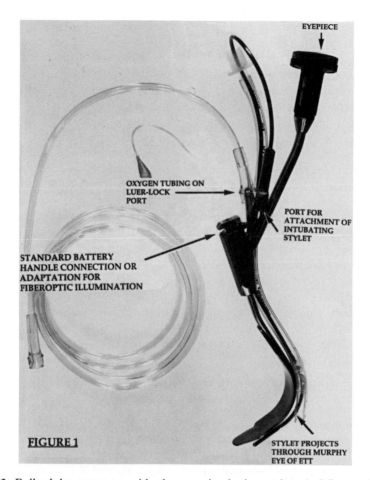

Fig. 20-43. Bullard laryngoscope with the new intubating stylet. A 3.7-mm channel is incorporated into the laryngoscope, which is bifurcated at its proximal end. One port is equipped with a Luer-lock fitting for attachment of a three-way stopcock to provide suction, insufflation of oxygen, or the application of local anesthetics. The other port of the bifurcation accepts the proximal end of the dedicated, nonmalleable intubating stylet. ET is positioned on the well-lubricated stylet so that the distal end of the stylet projects through the Murphy eye of ET. Removal of ET adapter enables proximal positioning of ET on stylet, thereby reducing amount of mouth opening required for blade insertion. Stylet then clips onto its designated port so stylet-ET apparatus hugs right side of the posterior surface of blade when stylet is correctly attached. (From Cooper SD, Benumof JL, Ozaki GT: Evaluation of the Bullard laryngoscope using the new intubating stylet: comparison with conventional laryngoscopy, *Anesth Analg* 79:965, 1994.)

attempt to position the laryngoscope under the epiglottis and obtain a clear, unobstructed view of the glottic opening and vocal cords. With the stylet pointed directly at the glottic opening, the ET is advanced off the stylet with the right hand and through the laryngeal aperture until the cuff passes just beyond the vocal cords under direct vision. The BL is then removed in the opposite way from that by which it was inserted; the right hand stabilizes the ET and the left hand rotates the blade from a vertical to a horizontal plane, taking care that the stylet remains in close contact with the blade to avoid injury to the teeth or face.

c. CLINICAL EXPERIENCE

Several authors have described their experiences with the BL. Bjoraker detailed the characteristics of the BL and described the three original intubating techniques recommended by the manufacturer mentioned previously.[60] He concluded that, although the BL affords excellent visualization of the glottis, serious commitment and training are necessary to become skillful at intubation with any one of these techniques. Dyson et al. compared the learning curves of first-year anesthesia residents using both the fiberoptic bronchoscope and the BL in a mannequin modified to make intubation difficult.[61] They found that the time course for proficiency using either device was similar, but passage of the ET through the laryngeal aperture took longer with the BL (using one of the three originally described intubation techniques). Borland and Casselbrant used the pediatric BL in 93 patients (ages 1 day to 10.7 years), 64

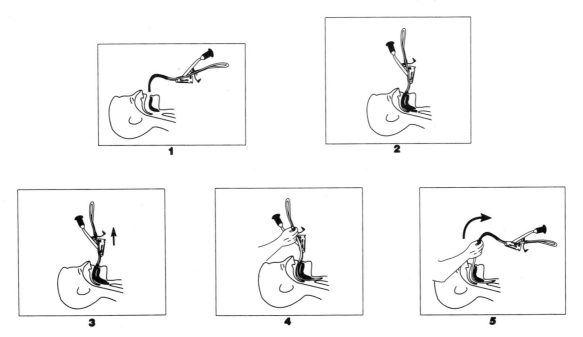

Fig. 20-44. Panels illustrate intubation technique with new intubating stylet. *1,* Bullard laryngoscope (BL) with a preloaded, attached intubating stylet is inserted into mouth in horizontal plane; less than 6 mm of opening between teeth is required when ET is positioned on the proximal end of the stylet. *2,* handle is rotated to the vertical plane, allowing the blade to slide around tongue. Blade is then allowed to drop momentarily into the posterior pharynx. *3,* Blade is elevated against tongue's dorsal surface with upward pressure on handle so that epiglottis is trapped by the blade, exposing glottic opening. *4,* ET is advanced off the stylet through glottic opening and into trachea. Placement is initially visually confirmed. *5,* with ET secured at proximal end, BL and intubating stylet are removed by rotating unit forward and then back to horizontal plane, and gently lifting it out of mouth. (From Cooper SD, Benumof JL, Ozaki GT: Evaluation of the Bullard laryngoscope using the new intubating stylet: comparison with conventional laryngoscopy, *Anesth Analg* 79:965, 1994.)

with normal airway anatomy and 29 with known abnormal upper-airway anatomy.[62] Intubation was successful in 97% of the cases (intubation technique not mentioned). Difficulty occurred in two patients with excessive secretions. In a third patient, intubation failed because of a small mouth that did not allow adequate space to direct and insert the endotracheal tube. Saunders and Giesecke reported the use of the BL in a variety of circumstances including patients with uncomplicated airways (n = 40), cervical-spine instability (n = 5), rapid-sequence intubations (n = 10), and awake patients (n = 3).[63] In the first three patient groups there was an 88% intubation success rate in under 24 seconds by passing a styleted ET freehand. For unexplained reasons, three intubations failed in the group with uncomplicated airways; they were intubated by other, unspecified means. All three awake intubation attempts (5% of all study patients) failed secondary to poor visualization. In these patients, intubation was accomplished by, again, other unspecified means. Gorback presented five case reports of successful intubation with the BL in which a styleted ET was passed freehand in adults with unusual airway anatomy (grade III and IV airways, limited temporomandibular joint mobility, and limited cervical spine mobility).[64] He concluded that, although there might be a steep learning curve, the BL is a worthwhile addition to any anesthesiologist's armamentarium in approaching a potentially difficult airway.

Most recently Cooper et al. determined that the optimal intubating mechanism with the BL was the new dedicated intubating stylet; fewer attempts were required and it took less time to achieve successful endotracheal intubation compared with the original three intubating mechanisms.[65] Their results also suggested that time to successful intubation with the BL using the intubating stylet was not affected by the conventional laryngoscopic grade; it was just as easy (and difficult) to intubate a conventional grade I laryngoscopic-view patient (full glottic view) as it was to intubate a conventional grade III laryngoscopic-view patient (visualization of just the epiglottis) with the BL. There were two failed intubations with the BL (3%) due to an inability to trap the epiglottis. Based on these results and the results of other investigators, the BL may be uniquely useful in trauma patients with uncleared cervical spines and in other patients with whom the head and neck cannot be manipulated.[65] Of interest, Hastings et al. recently found that some, albeit minimal, neck

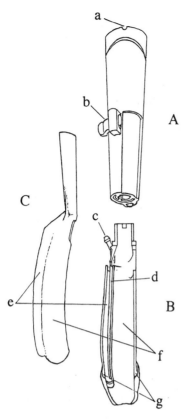

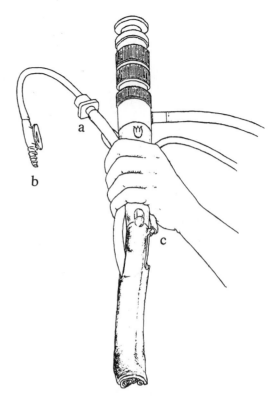

Fig. 20-45. Schematic representation of components of WuScope system: **A,** handle, **B,** main blade, and **C,** bivalve element; *a,* locator on handle that aligns with locator on the fiberscope; *b,* latch for proximal interlocking mechanism; *c,* oxygen port; *d,* oxygen channel; *e,* fibercord passageway; *f,* ET passageway; and *g,* slits for distal interlocking mechanism. (From Wu T, Chou H: A new laryngoscope: the combination intubating device, *Anesthesiology* 81(4):1085, 1994.)

Fig. 20-46. WuScope system with rigid and flexible portions fitted together and properly assembled with *a,* ET in ET passageway, *b,* suction catheter in ET lumen, and *c,* oxygen tubing connected to oxygen port. (From Wu T, Chou H: A new laryngoscope: the combination intubating device, *Anesthesiology* 81(4):1085, 1994.)

movement does occur when using the BL for intubation.[66] Whether or not this results in any neurologic sequelae is not yet known, but preliminary results show this blade to be quite favorable in patients with cervical-spine pathology.

2. WuScope system

a. DESCRIPTION

The WuScope system (Achi Corp., Dublin, California) is similar to both the tubular pharyngolaryngoscope and the Bullard laryngoscope. This system consists of a rigid blade portion and a separate flexible fiberoptic portion (Olympus fiberscope LF-1, LF-2, or rhinolaryngoscope ENF-P3 are recommended) (Figs. 20-45 and 20-46). When assembled, the laryngoscope is essentially a tubular, curved, bivalved rigid blade with an incorporated flexible fiberscope as its optical guide. The assembly is somewhat complex for the beginner, but after a few trial-and-error sessions, is readily accomplished. A detailed description of the assembly is nicely outlined in

the instruction manual available from the manufacturer. Two adult sizes are available.

b. TECHNIQUE

The WuScope system is suitable for endotracheal intubations in awake or anesthetized patients, through the oral or nasal routes. The technique for orotracheal intubation is strikingly similar to that for the Bullard laryngoscope. Maintaining the patient's head in the neutral position, the device is introduced into the patient's mouth at the midline with the help of a tongue depressor, much like inserting an oral airway. With the handle in the operator's left hand, it is gradually rotated around the contour of the tongue until the handle reaches a vertical position (Fig. 20-47). It is recommended that the user look through the eyepiece as soon as the tip of the blade enters the oropharynx to follow the progress as the blade is rotated. Experience has revealed that maintaining a midline position with proper orientation of the airway structures as the blade is advanced greatly facilitates laryngeal inlet exposure. Once the vocal cords come into view, the ET and distal blade are aligned with the glottis and the ET is advanced through the tubular main blade until the cuff is observed to pass through the vocal cords. The inventors report that first

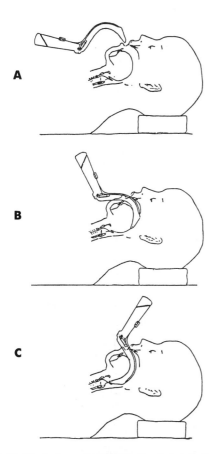

Fig. 20-47. Technique for orotracheal intubation with the WuScope system. **A,** With patient's head in neutral position, device is introduced into patient's mouth in the horizontal axis at the midline. Tongue depressor is often used to aid with insertion. **B,** Blade is maintained in a midline position and rotated around tongue until handle reaches vertical position. **C,** Once glottis is in view, ET and distal blade are aligned with glottic opening and ET is advanced through tubular blade until cuff is observed to pass through vocal cords. (From Wu T, Chou H: A new laryngoscope: the combination intubating device, *Anesthesiology* 81(4):1085, 1994.)

passing a suction catheter through the vocal cords may serve as a reliable conduit to aid in alignment of the ET with the glottis. The WuScope blade is then disassembled and carefully removed from the patient's mouth while the ET is held firmly in place. Once the usual steps have been taken to confirm the intratracheal location of the ET, it is secured.

The shape of the blade and its fiberoptic viewing ability preclude the need for alignment of the upper oral airway to visualize the larynx. This feature is advantageous when head and neck manipulation are contraindicated (i.e., suspected or known unstable cervical-spine injuries). The tubular aspect of the main blade helps create viewing space when tumors, trauma, edema, or inflammation obscure the posterior pharynx. This tubular portion also contains the fiberoptic bronchoscope

and protects the optics from being obscured by blood, secretions, or soft oropharyngeal tissues.

c. CLINICAL EXPERIENCE

The inventors (Drs. Wu and Chou) have extensive experience with this intubating system, having achieved great success in their clinical trials. They have found it useful in awake or anesthetized patients in routine as well as difficult intubations.[67] Theoretically, unexpected difficult intubation will not exist if the WuScope system is used routinely. Limitations for its use include: limited mouth opening (temporomandibular joint dysfunction, rheumatoid arthritis) and extreme fixed-flexion neck deformity. Reported complications are similar to those with the use of other rigid laryngoscopes; sore throat, chipped teeth, and mucosal injury. Other than the inventors' clinical experience, there is no published data on the use of the WuScope system. Obviously, more experience is necessary before it can be recommended for widespread clinical use.

3. Augustine guide

a. DESCRIPTION

Another intubation device that is rapidly gaining in popularity is the Augustine guide (AG; Augustine Medical Inc., Eden Prairie, Minnesota), originally designed for blind orotracheal intubation. The AG is a two-piece device that is constructed of medical-grade plastic and consists of an intubation guide and stylet (Fig. 20-48). The intubation guide is curved in shape and is designed to follow around the back of the tongue and fit into the vallecula. The distal edge has a midline indentation and two lateral bulbous protrusions. When the leading or distal edge is properly seated in the vallecula, the midline indentation straddles the hyoepiglottic ligament and the lateral bulbous protrusions lock into the recesses of the vallecula, sitting beneath the hyoid bone. Proper positioning is verified by palpating lateral movements of the hyoid bone when the intubation guide is moved from side to side. A hollow guide channel runs along the interior and underside of the intubation guide. When properly oriented, the guide channel is positioned directly opposite the glottic opening. The stylet has an S-shaped molded tip with six aspiration holes (three on each side) and is connected to a 35-ml syringe. It is used as an esophageal detector device (see Chapter 27) and as a guide to facilitate easy passage of the ET.

b. TECHNIQUE

Prior to blade insertion into the oropharynx, the well-lubricated intubating stylet is placed through a 7.0-mm, 7.5-mm, or 8.0-mm ID ET. The S-shaped molded portion of the stylet is then advanced to the edge of the open tip of the ET and the ET and stylet are inserted into the guide channel of the AG (Fig. 20-49). A special bite block is included with the AG to facilitate introduction of the device into the mouth.

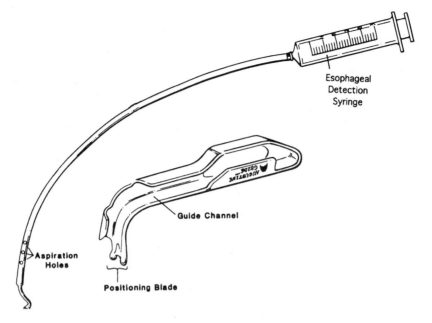

Fig. 20-48. Components of Augustine guide: Augustine stylet, *top,* and intubation guide, *bottom.* (From Carr RJ, Belani KGB: Clinical assessment of the Augustine guide for endotracheal intubation, *Anesth Analg* 78:983, 1994.)

The intubation technique involves opening the mouth and inserting the bite block between the molars on the right to ensure that the mouth remains open. Once the bite block is properly positioned, a 4 × 4 gauze is used to pull the tongue out of the patient's mouth. The preloaded AG is then inserted into the oropharynx. The leading edge is advanced toward the vallecula by rotating the guide handle from a horizontal to a vertical position until it is at 90 degrees to the plane of the face (similar to positioning the BL and WuScope system). To ensure proper placement of the AG in the vallecula, the hyoid bone is palpated and the guide handle is gently moved from side to side. The hyoid bone will move if the guide is correctly seated in the glossoepiglottic fold (Fig. 20-50). The stylet is then gently advanced into the larynx until the syringe contacts the ET connector. If an obstruction is met, gentle probing may be necessary until the stylet advances easily. The plunger of the syringe is then aspirated to its full volume. Free and easy return of air confirms successful placement of the stylet in the trachea (see Chapter 27) (Fig. 20-51). Any resistance to aspiration or recoil with release of the plunger implies that the soft muscular walls of the esophagus are being sucked over the perforations in the stylet, creating a vacuum.

Once the intratracheal position of the stylet is verified, the right hand grasps the AG handle while the left hand disengages the ET from the guide channel and advances it over the stylet into the trachea (Fig. 20-52). Rotation of the AG may be necessary if resistance is

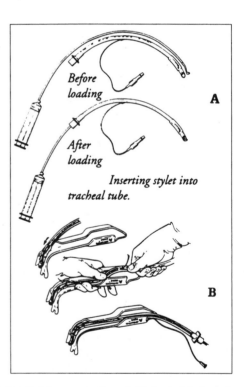

Fig. 20-49. Guide preparation. **A,** Stylet is lubricated well and placed through a 7.0-mm, 7.5-mm, or 8.0-mm ID ET. **B,** S-shaped molded portion of stylet is then advanced to edge of open tip of ET. ET and stylet are inserted into guide channel of Augustine guide. (Courtesy of Augustine Medical Inc. From Kovac AL: *Anesthesiology Review* 1:25, 1993.)

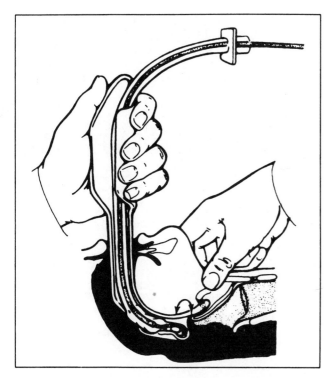

Fig. 20-50. Guide inserted into vallecula. Palpable movement of hyoid bone with gentle side-to-side motion of guide indicates guide is properly engaged in vallecula around hyoepiglottic ligament. (Courtesy of Augustine Medical Inc. From Kovac AL: *Anesthesiology Review* 1:25, 1993.)

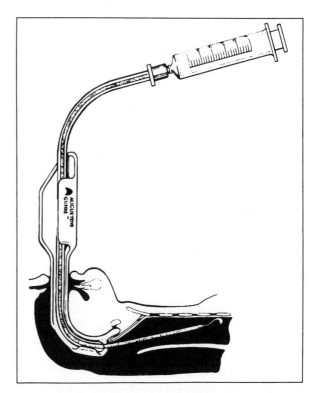

Fig. 20-51. Stylet is used to locate trachea. Free return of air with syringe aspiration with no vacuum-like resistance indicates intratracheal location. (Courtesy of Augustine Medical Inc. From Kovac AL: *Anesthesiology Review* 1:25, 1993.)

encountered. The intubation guide and stylet are carefully removed and verification of proper ET placement is accomplished using conventional criteria.

c. CLINICAL EXPERIENCE

The AG has been shown to facilitate rapid, blind, orotracheal intubation in adults (no pediatric version is available).[68,69] A recent report described the successful use of the AG in patients with normal airways who had operations under general anesthesia.[70] They found that the AG was a safe and effective device in achieving rapid, blind, orotracheal intubation in 94% of patients studied. Since this is a blind intubating device, blood, vomitus, and secretions in the oropharynx that would obscure direct vision with conventional laryngoscopy or fiberoptic bronchoscopy do not pose a problem. In addition, head and neck manipulation are not required to achieve successful intubation with this device. This makes this device uniquely useful in patients with known or suspected cervical-spine injury.[71] It has also been found to be useful in intubating the trachea of an adult with Treacher Collins syndrome.[72]

The primary disadvantage is that it is a blind technique. However, the reliability of correct placement with the esophageal detector device (the stylet) has been established.[68] In addition, Dr. Augustine has recently

developed a prototype that incorporates fiberoptic viewing capability onto the standard AG. It is currently undergoing clinical trials (Fig. 20-53). In addition, many anesthesiologists have evolved a technique wherein a flexible fiberoptic bronchoscope (FOB) is independently passed down the ET in a correctly positioned AG, converting the blind technique to a fiberoptic one; the ET is advanced over the FOB into the trachea under direct vision.[73] The AG appears to be a promising new tool to add to the anesthesiologist's armamentarium for managing difficult airway problems.

E. ENLARGED STERNAL REGION

The curved Macintosh laryngoscope is at a right angle to the blade.[5] It is the most widely used instrument for direct viewing of the larynx in a variety of patients, including obstetrical patients. However, parturients requiring general anesthesia present problems that affect the ease of intubation, including the risk of aspiration, airway edema, and engorged and enlarged breasts. To prevent aspiration a rapid sequence induction with the application of cricoid pressure (Sellick's maneuver) is employed. The combination of an assistant's hand on the cricoid cartilage and the patient's enlarged breasts may make insertion of the laryngoscope blade difficult. Many

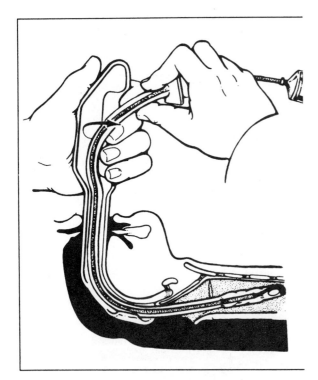

Fig. 20-52. ET is firmly grasped to stabilize it while it is detached from guide. (Courtesy of Augustine Medical Inc. From Kovac AL: *Anesthesiology Review* 1:25, 1993.)

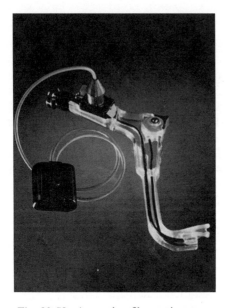

Fig. 20-53. Augustine fiberoptic scope.

solutions to overcome this problem have been proposed including: (1) remove the blade from the handle and reconnecting it after it is inserted into the oropharynx,[74] (2) use a short laryngoscope handle,[75] (3) insert the blade into the corner of the patient's mouth with the

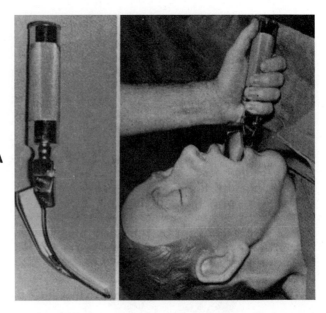

Fig. 20-54. A, Polio blade, **B,** inserted into patient's mouth. (From Weeks DB: A new use for an old blade, *Anesthesiology* 40:200, 1974.)

handle parallel to the patient's shoulder and then rotate it to the correct position,[76-78]) and (4) alter the angle the blade makes with the handle. These techniques have not only been used in the obstetrical population but also for obese patients, patients with kyphosis and with severe barrel-chest deformity, and patients with short necks.

1. Polio laryngoscope blade

The use of a Polio blade, originally designed for intubating the tracheas of patients in iron-lung machines, has been one option in overcoming these problems (Fig. 20-54).[79-81] However, the very obtuse angle it forms with the handle makes it difficult to apply pressure to the tongue in the correct direction to facilitate a view of the glottic opening. It is therefore not easy to use.

2. Kessel laryngoscope blade

Dr. Kessel took a standard Macintosh laryngoscope blade and varied the fitting so that it came off the handle at approximately 110 degrees (Fig. 20-55).[82] In his experience it felt no different than the standard Macintosh and achieved the goal of avoiding impingement on both the chest wall and the assistant's hand applying cricoid pressure upon insertion. It is manufactured by Pen Medic Ltd. in New Zealand and apparently is distributed by HI Clements Pty., Ltd., in Australia.

3. Jellicoe and Harris adapter

Jellicoe and Harris further modified the standard Macintosh arrangement by interposing an adapter between the laryngoscope handle and the blade. This

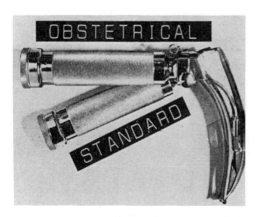

Fig. 20-55. Comparison of angles of obstetrical and standard laryngoscope handles with superimposed blades. (From Kessel J: A laryngoscope for obstetrical use: an obstetrical laryngoscope, *Anaesth Intens Care* 5:265, 1977.)

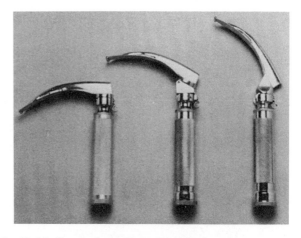

Fig. 20-56. Comparison of standard Macintosh arrangement, *left,* standard laryngoscope with adapter in place *middle,* and Polio blade, *right.* (From Jellicoe JA, Harris NR: A modification of a standard laryngoscope for difficult tracheal intubation in obstetric cases, *Anaesthesia* 39:800, 1984.)

adapter tilts the angle between the blade tip and handle to 90 degrees, a marked increase over the 58-degree angle between the blade tip and handle of the standard Macintosh laryngoscope (Fig. 20-56).[83] This enables introduction of the blade tip in the vertical plane while maintaining the handle in the horizontal plane, easily clearing the patient's chest and the assistant's hand on the cricoid cartilage. This adapter will fit onto any standard laryngoscope handle and is widely used in the obstetric population in England.

4. Patil and Stehling laryngoscope handle

An extension of this idea is the adjustable laryngoscope handle, which allows positioning of the Macintosh blade at four different angles to the handle: 180 degrees, 135 degrees, 90 degrees, and 45 degrees (Fig. 20-57).[84] If the handle contacts the patient's chest upon initial insertion of the blade into the mouth, the lock on the handle (see arrow, Fig. 20-57) is released until the blade position lies parallel to the handle (180-degree angle). After it is inserted into the patient's mouth, the blade-handle angle is readjusted to 90 degrees and standard laryngoscopic technique follows.

5. Yentis laryngoscope blade

The solution proposed by Yentis was the development of a laryngoscope adapter that maintains the normal angle between the handle and blade but allows lateral rotation of the laryngoscope handle (Fig. 20-58).[85] The adapter is a 2.5 × 2.5 × 2.5–cm block that fits between a standard screw-fit Penlon laryngoscope handle and the Macintosh blade. When the blade is inserted into the patient's mouth, the handle is pointing 90 degrees to the right, avoiding contact with the patient's chest and/or an assistant's hand (Fig. 20-59). The handle is then swiveled back to its normal position and laryngoscopy is performed in the standard fashion.

This device might also be uniquely advantageous for intubating patients in the left lateral decubitus position.

6. Dhara and Cheong adapter

Another adjustable multiple-angle laryngoscope adapter was developed by Dhara and Cheong.[86] Their adapter also fits onto a standard laryngoscope handle and unlike the Patil adapter, allows the operator to choose from a wider variety of clinically useful angles, (180, 150, 130, 110, 90, and 65 degrees) single-handedly (Fig. 20-60). The adapter hooks onto a standard laryngoscope handle on one end; another similar arrangement is on the opposite end for attachment of a Macintosh laryngoscope blade. The rotating mechanism is operated by a push rod connected to a spring-loaded pin in the middle of the adapter (Fig. 20-61 on p. 408). The laryngoscope is held and used in the standard fashion with the operator's left hypothenar eminence positioned near the push rod. If the clinical situation dictates, pressure from the hypothenar area toward the handle will release the rotating mechanism. When the blade reaches the desired angle, the blade is locked in position by releasing the push rod. The inventors have found this device to be "convenient and easy to use in difficult clinical situations,"[86] but no other formal clinical experience has appeared in the literature.

F. PEDIATRIC LARYNGOSCOPES

The usual method of laryngoscopy using a standard straight blade involves lifting the epiglottis with the distal tip of the laryngoscope blade. Because the infant epiglottis differs from that of an adult—it is longer, floppier, U or Omega shaped, sits higher, and projects backward in the pharynx—this is not always easily accomplished. Use of a standard Macintosh laryngo-

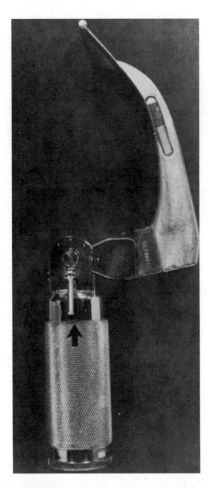

Fig. 20-57. Adjustable laryngoscope handle. Blade lock *(arrow)* allows positioning of blade at 180, 135, 90, or 45 degrees to handle. (From Patil VU, Stehling LC, Zauder HL: An adjustable laryngoscope handle for difficult intubations. Letter-to-the-Editor, *Anesthesiology* 60:609, 1984.)

scope blade is similarly inadequate because its use is based on the principle of lifting the base of the tongue and with it the epiglottis. This would seem to overcome the problem of trapping and lifting the abnormally shaped pediatric epiglottis, but often the smaller blades were too curved to adequately move the epiglottis out of the line of vision. As a result of these observations, many investigators modified the standard straight blade for use in infants and children.

1. Seward laryngoscope blade

Although a child-sized version of the Soper and Miller laryngoscope blades had been previously introduced, E.H. Seward was the first to design a blade specifically for children, the Seward laryngoscope.[87] The straight blade portion is 10.5 cm long and the bulb is the same as those on an adult laryngoscope (Fig. 20-62). The smaller handle was found to be more convenient in the pediatric population. The blade is intended for use in children less than 5 years old, and interestingly was originally designed for anesthesiologists who "do not

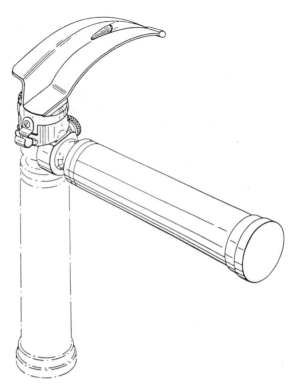

Fig. 20-58. Laryngoscope and adapter assembled illustrating lateral pivoting ability. (From Yentis SM: A laryngoscope adaptor for difficult intubation, *Anaesthesia* 42:764, 1987.)

often use a laryngoscope."[87] Although no formal clinical studies have been performed with the Seward laryngoscope blade, it is still commonly found and used in many pediatric anesthesia departments.

2. Bryce-Smith laryngoscope blade

Drs. Bryce and Smith, in conjunction with the now infamous Richard Salt (of Macintosh fame), also developed a laryngoscope blade designed for use in children, from newborn to age 3 (Fig. 20-63).[88] Their blade is essentially straight with a slight, 2.5-cm distal curvature. It has a three-quarter-circle cross section throughout most of its length, and tapers from a maximum width of 1.8 cm at the proximal end to a 1-cm width at the distal tip. The right side is open and the left side is guarded, which facilitates retraction of the tongue. The broad overhang on the open side helps prevent the lips from obscuring the view. A satisfactory view of the cords is obtained whether it is positioned anterior or posterior to the epiglottis and whether the head is extended or flexed. The introduction of both this laryngoscope blade and the Seward laryngoscope blade paved the way for the development of many more pediatric laryngoscope blades.

3. Mark infant laryngoscope blade

The Mark infant laryngoscope was designed by F.L. Robertshaw, who published his design in 1962.[89] The

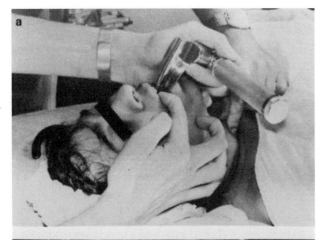

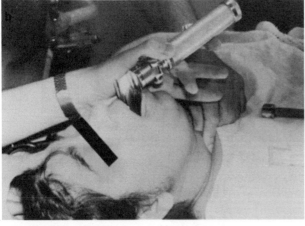

Fig. 20-59. Pivoting adapter in use. **A,** Insertion of blade into patient's mouth. **B,** Handle in normal position. (From Yentis SM: A laryngoscope adaptor for difficult intubation, *Anaesthesia* 42:764, 1987.)

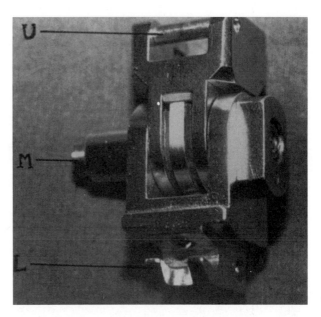

Fig. 20-60. Adapter. A hook-on arrangement fits onto a standard laryngoscope handle, *L.* Push rod in middle section, *M,* operates spring-loaded pin that engages or disengages rotating mechanism. On top, a bar arrangement, *U,* engages hook-on type of laryngoscope blade. (From Dhara SF, Cheong TW: An adjustable multiple angle laryngoscope adaptor, *Anaesth Intens Care* 19:243, 1991.)

Mark-1 was fashioned after the baby Soper blade[27] but with a slightly curved tip rolled at the end. It was found to be useful in newborns and children up to 5 years old. The original Mark-1 blades were made of brass with chromium plating. They were subsequently fashioned out of stainless steel in an effort to increase production and decrease cost. The lateral wall was also removed, facilitating a view of the glottic opening with both eyes on direct laryngoscopy (Fig. 20-64). The edges of the newer Mark-2 blade are more rounded to minimize potential trauma to the oropharynx should the blade slip out of position. Although no clinical studies have been done with these laryngoscope blades, they are still occasionally found in pediatric anesthesia departments.

4. Jones laryngoscope blade

Since the advent of the original pediatric laryngoscope blades (Miller, Seward, Bryce-Smith, and Mark), many subtle changes have been suggested in the design of the straight Miller blade to facilitate pediatric laryngoscopy and provide for oxygen supplementation during endoscopy and intubation. These modifications have included, but are not limited to, widening the distal portion of the blade, decreasing the width of the C-shaped flange, adhering a strip of rough adhesive tape to the blade's lingual surface, increasing the angle between the blade and handle, and adapting blades for insufflation of oxygen by taping, threading, or soldering an insufflation channel along the blade.[90-97]

Jones's modification included shortening the Welch-Allyn Miller-1 blade by removing the distal 13 mm to decrease the working length to 67 mm, compared with the original 80-mm length.[98] This positioned the lamp closer to the larynx, which greatly improved illumination on direct laryngoscopy for patients less than 5 months old. There were no perceived disadvantages of this laryngoscope blade in the inventor's experience. No clinical comparison studies with this blade or any other pediatric laryngoscope blade have appeared in literature. Therefore the anesthesiologist is left to decide which pediatric laryngoscope blade to use on an entirely subjective basis.

G. LARYNGOSCOPE BLADES WITH SPECIAL ACCESSORIES

1. Suction integrated laryngoscope blade

Instead of modifying the shape of the standard Macintosh and Miller laryngoscope blades, various inventors attached devices to these blades to facilitate ease of laryngoscopy. One modification consists of an integrated stainless steel tube on the lingual surface of

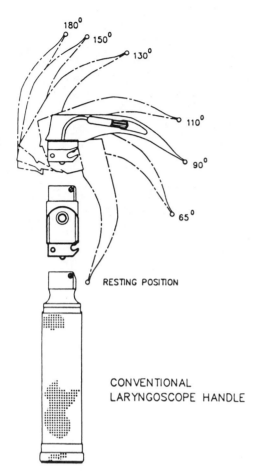

Fig. 20-61. Adapter illustrating available angles. (From Dhara SF, Cheong TW: An adjustable multiple angle laryngoscope adaptor, *Anaesth Intens Care* 19:243, 1991.)

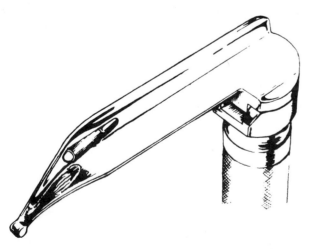

Fig. 20-62. Seward laryngoscope blade for pediatrics. (From Seward EH: Laryngoscope for resuscitation of the newborn, *Lancet* 2:1041, 1957.)

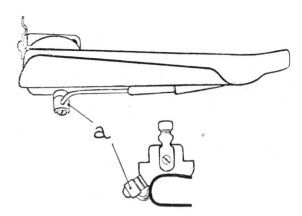

Fig. 20-63. Bryce-Smith infant laryngoscope blade; *a* represents light carrier. (From Bryce-Smith R: A laryngoscope blade for infants, *Br Med J* 1:217, 1952.)

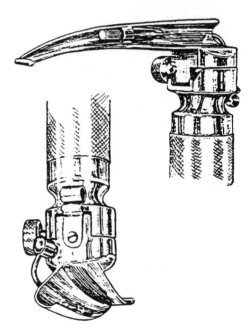

Fig. 20-64. Mark-1 infant laryngoscope blade, two views. (From Robertshaw FL: A new laryngoscope for infants and children, *Lancet* 2:1034, 1962.)

a standard Macintosh laryngoscope blade that opens into a slot positioned at the distal blade tip (Fig. 20-65).[99] The proximal end of the tube can then be attached to a vacuum source to remove blood and secretions during laryngoscopy. The suction conduit itself does not interfere with a direct view of the glottis on laryngoscopy since the channel is incorporated onto the blade itself, limiting any increase in bulk. In addition to providing suctioning capability, fresh gas flow can be insufflated through this channel to augment oxygen delivery or to add an anesthetic gas mixture during prolonged laryngoscopy. The potential usefulness of this laryngoscope blade has yet to be formally evaluated.

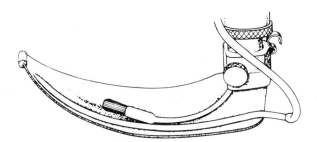

Fig. 20-65. Suction integrated laryngoscope blade. Plastic tubing attached to end of suction conduit leads to a vacuum source via a Y connector taped to laryngoscope handle. (From Gabrielczyk MR: A new integrated suction laryngoscope. Letter-to-the-Editor, *Anaesthesia* 41:970, 1986.)

2. Fishelev laryngoscope blade

The integrated suction idea was further elaborated upon by Fishelev et al., who welded either metal rings (adult version) or a metallic tube (infant version) onto the left side of a standard Macintosh blade.[100] These conduits were designed to accommodate wide-bore suction catheters (Fig. 20-66). The distal end of a suction catheter is placed through the rings or the tube and is then positioned just beyond the tip of the laryngoscope blade. This facilitates easy and efficient suctioning of oropharyngeal secretions. The inventors found that in rapid-sequence intubation situations with the application of cricoid pressure, the suctioning capability helped to decrease the incidence of aspiration of gastric contents. Similar modifications, to provide either suctioning capability or the application of fresh gas flow and anesthetic through channels or tubes incorporated onto standard laryngoscope blades, have subsequently been suggested by other authors.[101]

3. Khan laryngoscope blade

One of these inventors was Khan, who was the first to incorporate a suction tube on a standard straight Miller blade.[102] The tube (2.5 mm, with an ID of 1.75 mm) has a hub on the proximal end that can readily be occluded by the operator's thumb, allowing for control of suctioning once it is attached to a vacuum apparatus. As with the previously discussed laryngoscope blades, this blade allows for continuous suctioning during uninterrupted intubation attempts.

III. CONCLUSION

Most patients can be intubated with one of the three primary laryngoscope blade types: the straight blade (Jackson), the curved tip (Miller), or the curved blade (Macintosh). However, despite careful preinduction assessment of the airway, there are still occasional patients in whom intubation is difficult or impossible with these conventional laryngoscope blades. When this situation occurs, many options exist including using one

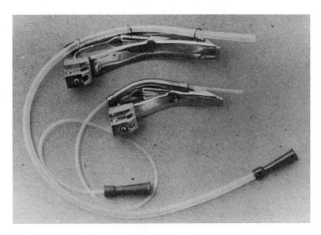

Fig. 20-66. Modified Macintosh laryngoscopes with added suction catheters placed through metallic rings (*top,* adult version) or a welded tube (*bottom,* infant version). (From Fishelev W, Vatashsky E, Aronson HB: Suction catheter attached to laryngoscope, *Anaesthesia* 39:188, 1984.)

or more of the other blades discussed. The best choice enables the laryngoscopist to obtain the best view possible without putting pressure on the teeth or stressing the temporomandibular joint. The basis of design of new laryngoscope blades ranges from individual clinical experience to x-ray[22,31] and anatomical studies, as well as the use of an animal model;[56] overall, the evolution of laryngoscopes has been a relatively arbitrary process. In fact, Sikes aptly stated, "Accessories for endotracheal anaesthesia are without end. There is no living anaesthetist who holds the distinction of not having designed one or more devices."[103]

Scientific evaluation of the performance of any particular laryngoscope blade is rare; critical analysis or comparison with other blades is essentially nonexistent. Marks et al. have recently proposed a theoretical method for blade analysis based on a previous investigative x-ray laryngoscopy study of normal patients where a single "ease of intubation" angle was found to correlate with intubation difficulty.[104] This angle is the connection of three points: from the internal midpoint of the symphysis menti to the tip of the upper incisors and from there to a point just behind the thyroid cartilage. The measurement of this angle is representative of the space available behind the mandible into which the tongue is compressed during laryngoscopy to permit laryngeal exposure.[105] The Marks' study measured two characteristics of the Macintosh sizes 3 and 4, Miller size 3, and the Soper size 3 laryngoscope blades: the amount of space that the blade occupies behind the mandible and the amount of deviation from the ideal line of vision during laryngoscopy.[104] They found that the Macintosh sizes 3 and 4 curved blades were distinctly better in forward space enhancement and provided higher eye-line deviation (e.g., better approximation of the ideal line of vision) on laryngoscopy compared to the Miller or Soper blades. In addition, the Macintosh blades and the Miller size 3 blade were found to be superior to the Soper size 3 blade on both characteristics.[104] They believe that their study establishes a theoretically reproducible method for performance analysis in contrast to simple comparative clinical trials, which can be faulted for multiple reasons, the major one being variation in skills that can influence the incidence of critical events, trauma, and mortality.[106]

This theoretical analysis of laryngoscope blades by Marks et al. is a rational beginning to the selection of a particular laryngoscope blade to manage a specific clinical situation rather than simply choosing a blade based solely on familiarity with its use. Gaining experience with several different laryngoscope blades designed to address specific anatomic variations that contribute to intubation difficulties should begin in anesthesia training. At the University of California, San Diego, Cooper and Benumof have pioneered a dedicated 1-month specialty rotation into the clinical anesthesia–2 year specifically designed to create nonurgent, nonstressful clinical situations that facilitate learning various airway-management techniques, including the use of multiple laryngoscope blades.[107] Their concepts are further elaborated on in Chapter 42.

REFERENCES

1. Collins VJ: *Endotracheal anesthesia: basic considerations in principles of anesthesiology,* ed 2, Philadelphia, 1976, Lea & Febiger.
2. Gillespie NA: *Equipment and apparatus in endotracheal anesthesia,* Madison, 1963, University of Wisconsin Press.
3. Fink BR: *The human larynx: a functional study,* New York, 1975, Raven Press.
4. Hirsch NP, Smith GB, Hirsch PO: Alfred Kirstein, pioneer of direct laryngoscopy, *Anaesth* 41:42, 1986.
5. Macintosh RR: A new laryngoscope, *Lancet* 1:205, 1943.
6. Miller RA: A new laryngoscope, *Anesthesiology* 2:317, 1941.
7. Zollner F: Gustav Killian, father of bronchoscopy, *Arch Otolaryngol Head Neck Surg,* 82:656, 1965.
8. Sykes WS: The Cheerful Centenarian, or the Founder of Laryngoscopy. In Sykes WS: *Essays on the first hundred years of anaesthesia,* vol 2, Huntington, NY, 1972, Robert E. Kreiger Publishing Co.
9. Jackson C: The technique of insertion of intratracheal insufflation tubes, *Surg Gynecol Obstet* 17:507, 1913.
10. Janeway HH: Intratracheal anesthesia from the standpoint of the nose, throat and oral surgeon with a description of a new instrument for catheterizing the trachea, *Laryngoscope* 23:1082, Nov 1913.
11. Calverly RK: Intubation in anaesthesia. In Atkinson RS, Boulton TB, editors: *The history of anesthesia,* Royal Society of Medical International Congress and Symposium, series 134, Park Ridge, NJ, 1989, Parthenon.
12. Human JU: Blind intubation and the signs of anaesthesia, London, 1941,
13. Macintosh RR: Laryngoscope blades, *Lancet* 1:485, 1944.
14. Jephcott A: The Macintosh laryngoscope: a historical note on its clinical and commercial development, *Anaesth* 39:474, 1984.
15. McIntyre JNR: Laryngoscope design and the difficult adult tracheal intubation, *Can J Anaesth* 36:94, 1989.
16. Cassels WH: Advantages of a curved laryngoscope, *Anesthesiology* 3:580, Sept 1942.
17. Wiggin SC: A new modification of the conventional laryngoscope and technic for laryngoscopy, *Anesthesiology* 5:61, 1944.
18. Siker ES: A mirror laryngoscope, *Anesthesiology* 17:38, 1956.
19. MacKenzie MI: The use of the laryngoscope in diseases of the throat, Philadelphia, 1865, Lindsay and Blackstone.
20. Huffman JP: The application of prisms to curved laryngoscopes: a preliminary study, *AANA J* 36:138, 1968.
21. Huffman JP, Elam JO: Prisms and fiber optics for laryngoscopy, *Anesth Analg* 50:64, 1971.
22. Fink BR: Roentgenographic studies of the oropharyngeal airway, *Anesthesiology* 18:711, 1957.
23. Grant GC: A new laryngoscope, *Anaesth Intensive Care* 5:263, 1977.
24. Bellhouse CP: An angulated laryngoscope for routine and difficult tracheal intubation, *Anesthesiology* 69:126, 1988.
25. Mayall RM: The Belscope for management of the difficult airway, *Anesthesiology* 76:1059, 1992.
26. Neustein SM: The Neustein laryngoscope: a new solution to the difficult intubation, *Anesthesiology Review* 19:54, 1992.
27. Soper RL: A new laryngoscope for anaesthestists, *Br Med J* 1:265, 1947.
28. Parrott CM: Modification of Macintosh's curved laryngoscope, *Br Med J* 2:1031, 1951.
29. Gould RB: Modified laryngoscope blade, *Anaesth* 9:125, 1954.
30. Bowen RA, Jackson I: A new laryngoscope, *Anaesth* 7:254, 1952.
31. Gabuya R, Orkin LR: Design and utility of a new curved laryngoscope blade, *Anesth Analg* 38:364, 1959.
32. Bizzarri DV, Giuffrida JG: Improved laryngoscope blade designed for ease of manipulation and reduction of trauma, *Anesth Analg* 37:231-232, 1958.
33. Onkst HR: Modified laryngoscope blade, *Anesthesiology* 22:846, 1961.
34. Orr RB: A new laryngoscope blade designed to facilitate difficult endotracheal intubation, *Anesthesiology* 31:377, 1969.
35. Phillips OC, Duerksen RL: Endotracheal intubation: a new blade for direct laryngoscopy, *Anesth Analg* 52:691, 1973.
36. Schapira M: Guest discussion on: a new blade for direct laryngoscopy, *Anesth Analg* 52:698, 1973.
37. Schapira M: A modified straight laryngoscope blade designed to facilitate endotracheal intubation, *Anesth Analg* 52:553, 1973.
38. Racz GB: Improved vision modification of the Macintosh laryngoscope, *Anaesth* 39:1249, 1984 (letter).
39. Callender OC, Thomas J: Modification of Macintosh laryngoscope for difficult intubation, *Anaesth* 42:671, 1987 (letter).
40. Wright RB, Manfield FFV: Damage to teeth during the administration of general anesthesia, *Anesth Analg* 53:405, 1974.
41. Evers W, Racz GB, Glazer J et al: Orahesive as a protection for the teeth during general anesthesia and endoscopy, *Can Anaesth Soc J* 14:123, 1967.
42. Racz GB, Allen FB: A new pressure-sensitive laryngoscope, *Anesthesiology* 62:356, 1985.
43. Kawahara M, Takeshita T, Akitu S: A new model of laryngoscope equipped with fiberoptics, *Anesth Prog* 36:70, 1989.
44. Choi JJ: A new Double-Angle blade for direct laryngoscopy, *Anesthesiology* 72:576, 1990.
45. McCoy ED, Mirakhur RK: The levering laryngoscope, *Anaesth* 48:516, 1993.
46. Marks R: The levering laryngoscope, *Anaesth* 48:1008, 1993.
47. Ward M: The McCoy levering laryngoscope blade, *Anaesth* 49:357, 1993.
48. Farlings PA: The McCoy levering laryngoscope blade, *Anaesth* 49:358, 1993.
49. Johnston HML, Rao U: The McCoy levering laryngoscope blade, *Anaesth* 49:358, 1993.

50. Snow JC: Modification of laryngoscope blade, *Anesthesiology* 23:294, 1962.

51. DeCiutiis VL: Modification of Macintosh [sic] laryngoscope, *Anesthesiology* 20:115, 1959.

52. McWhinnie F: Modification of laryngoscope for nasogastric intubation, *Anaesth* 41:218, 1986 (letter).

53. Campbell BB, Millar R: Modification of laryngoscope for nasogastric intubation, *Anaesth* 40:703, 1985.

54. Pope ES: Left handed laryngoscope, *Anaesth* 15:326, 1960.

55. Lagade MRG, Poppers PJ: Use of left-entry laryngoscope blade in patients with right-sided oro-facial lesions, *Anesthesiology* 58:300, 1983.

56. Bainton CR: A new laryngoscope blade to overcome pharyngeal obstruction, *Anesthesiology* 67:767, 1987.

57. Diaz JH, Guarisco JL, LeJeune FE: A modified tubular pharyngolaryngoscope for difficult pediatric laryngoscopy, *Anesthesiology* 73:357, 1990.

58. Grande CM, Barton CR, Stene JK: Appropriate techniques for airway management of emergency patients with suspected spinal cord injury, *Anesth Analg* 67:714, 1988.

59. Hastings RH, Mark JD: Airway management for trauma patients with potential cervical spine injuries, *Anesth Analg* 73:471, 1991.

60. Bjoraker DG: The Bullard intubating laryngoscopes, *Anesthesiology Review* 17(5):64, 1990.

61. Dyson A, Harris J, Bhatta K: Rapidity and accuracy of tracheal intubation in a mannequin: comparison of the fiberoptic with the Bullard laryngoscope, *Br J Anaesth* 65:268, 1990.

62. Borland LM, Casselbrant M: The Bullard laryngoscope: a new indirect oral laryngoscope (pediatric version), *Anesth Analg* 70:105, 1990.

63. Saunders PR, Giesecke AH: Clinical assessment of the adult Bullard laryngoscope, *Can J Anaesth* 36:518, 1989 (abstract).

64. Gorback MS: Management of the challenging airway with the Bullard laryngoscope, *J Clin Anesth* 3:473, 1991.

65. Cooper SD, Benumof JL, Ozaki GT: Evaluation of the Bullard laryngoscope using the new intubating stylet: comparison with conventional laryngoscopy, *Anesth Analg* 79:965, 1994.

66. Hastings RH, Vigil CC, Hanna R et al: Cervical spine movement during laryngoscopy with the Bullard, Macintosh and Miller laryngoscopes, *Anesthesiology* (in press).

67. Wu T, Chou H: A new laryngoscope: the combination intubating device, *Anesthesiology* 81(4):1085, 1994.

68. Kovac AL: The Augustine guide: a new device for blind orotracheal intubation, *Anesthesiology Review* 1:25, 1993.

69. Krafft P, Fitzgerald R, Pernarstorfer T et al: A new device for blind oral intubation in routine and difficult airway management, *Eur Anaesth* 11:207, 1994.

70. Carr RJ, Belani KGB: Clinical assessment of the Augustine guide for endotracheal intubation, *Anesth Analg* 78:983, 1994.

71. Cicala RS, Grande CM, Stene JK et al: *Emergency and elective airway management for trauma patients: textbook of trauma anesthesia and critical care,* Baltimore, 1993, Mosby–Year Book.

72. Kovac AL: Use of the Augustine stylet anticipating difficult tracheal intubation in Treacher-Collins syndrome, *J Clin Anesth* 4:409, 1992.

73. LaTourette P, Patil VU: The Augustine guide as a fiberoptic bronchoscopic guide, *Anesth Analg* 76:1164, 1993.

74. Bourke DL, Lawrence J: Another way to insert a Macintosh blade, *Anesthesiology* 39:80, 1983.

75. Datta S, Briwa J: Modified laryngoscope for endotracheal intubation of obese patients, *Anesth Analg* 60:120, 1981.

76. Kubota Y: Mammomegaly and intubation, *Anaesth* 37:779, 1982.

77. Kay NH: Mammomegaly and intubation, *Anaesth* 37:221, 1982.

78. Jephcott A: Mammomegaly and intubation: the polio blade, *Anaesth* 37:780, 1982.

79. Wilson J, Kerr M: *Operative obstetrics,* ed 10, London, 1982, Balliere-Tindall.

80. Lagade MRG, Poppers PJ: Revival of the Polio laryngoscope blade, *Anesthesiology* 57:545, 1982.

81. Weeks DB: A new use for an old blade, *Anesthesiology* 40:200, 1974.

82. Kessel J: A laryngoscope for obstetrical use: an obstetrical laryngoscope, *Anaesth Intensive Care* 5:265, 1977.

83. Jellicoe JA, Harris NR: A modification of a standard laryngoscope for difficult tracheal intubation in obstetric cases, *Anaesth* 39:800, 1984.

84. Patil VU, Stehling LC, Zauder HL: An adjustable laryngoscope handle for difficult intubations, *Anesthesiology* 60:609, 1984 (letter).

85. Yentis SM: A laryngoscope adaptor for difficult intubation, *Anaesth* 42:764, 1987.

86. Dhara SF, Cheong TW: An adjustable multiple angle laryngoscope adaptor, *Anaesth Intensive Care* 19:243, 1991.

87. Seward EH: Laryngoscope for resuscitation of the newborn, *Lancet* 2:1041, 1957.

88. Bryce-Smith R: A laryngoscope blade for infants, *Brit Med J* 1:217, 1952.

89. Robertshaw FL: A new laryngoscope for infants and children, *Lancet* 2:1034, 1962.

90. Buekes HvZ, Mostert JW: A new anatomic laryngoscope, *Anesthesiology* 57:552, 1982.

91. Matsuki A: New pediatric laryngoscope, *Anesthesiology* 57:556, 1982.

92. Rokowski WJ, Gurmarnik S: Laryngoscope blades modified for neonates and infants, *Anesth Analg* 62:241, 1983.

93. Moynihan P: Modification of pediatric laryngoscope, *Anesthesiology* 56:330, 1982.

94. Wung J, Stork R, Indyk L et al: Oxygen supplement during endotracheal intubation of the infant, *Pediatrics* 59:1046, 1977.

95. Cork RC, Woods W, Vaughan RW et al: Oxygen supplementation during endotracheal intubation of infants, *Anesthesiology* 51:186, 1979.

96. Hencz P: Modified laryngoscope for endotracheal intubation of neonates, *Anesthesiology* 53:84, 1980.

97. Diaz JH: Further modifications of the Miller blade for difficult pediatric laryngoscopy, *Anesthesiology* 60:612, 1984.

98. Jones RDM: Lamp placement and the Miller-1 laryngoscope blade, *Anesthesiology* 62:207, 1985.

99. Gabrielczyk MR: A new integrated suction laryngoscope, *Anaesth* 41:970, 1986 (letter).

100. Fishelev W, Vatashsky E, Aronson HB: Suction catheter attached to laryngoscope, *Anaesth* 39:188, 1984.

101. Loeser EA: Oxygen and suction-equipped laryngoscope blade, *Anesthesiology* 62:376, 1985.

102. Khan AK: A controllable suctioning laryngoscope, *Anesth Analg* 71:200, 1990.

103. Sykes WS: The Cheerful Centenarian, or the Founder of Laryngoscopy. In Sykes WS: *Essays on the first hundred years of anesthesia,* vol 2, Huntington, NY, 1972, Robert E. Kreiger Publishing Co.

104. Marks RD, Hancock R, Charters P: An analysis of laryngoscope blade shape and design: new criteria for laryngoscope evaluation, *Can J Anaesth* 40(3):262, 1993.

105. Horton WA, Fahy L, Charters P: Factor analysis in difficult tracheal intubation: laryngoscopy induced airway obstruction, *Br J Anaesth* 65:801, 1990.

106. MacIntyre JWR: Tracheal intubation and laryngoscope design, *Can J Anaesth* 40(3):193, 1993 (editorial).

107. Cooper SD, Benumof JL: Teaching the management of the difficult airway: the UCSD airway rotation, *Anesthesiology,* 81(3A):A1241, 1994.

Chapter 21

SEPARATION OF THE TWO LUNGS (DOUBLE-LUMEN TUBES, BRONCHIAL-BLOCKERS, AND ENDOBRONCHIAL SINGLE-LUMEN TUBES)

Jonathan L. Benumof

5. **Methods to obtain a just-seal volume in the bronchial-blocker cuff**
6. **Firm clinical indications for use of the Univent bronchial-blocker system**
   B. BRONCHIAL BLOCKERS THAT ARE INDEPENDENT OF A SINGLE-LUMEN TUBE
V. ENDOBRONCHIAL INTUBATION WITH SINGLE-LUMEN TUBES
VI. CONCLUSION

I. INTRODUCTION

The complete functional separation of the two lungs is often the most important consideration in inducing anesthesia in patients undergoing thoracic surgery. The procedure can occasionally be lifesaving and frequently facilitate greatly the conduct of surgery. Newly introduced disposable, plastic double-lumen tubes (DLTs) which are relatively nontraumatic and easy to insert, and the advent of fiberoptic bronchoscopy, which makes location of a DLT under direct vision possible and therefore a precise, repeatable, low-risk maneuver, have greatly increased the efficacy and use of DLTs. In addition, the new Univent bronchial-blocker tube makes the use of a bronchial blocker much easier and simpler by coupling the insertion of the main single-lumen tube with the insertion of the bronchial blocker. Since the single-lumen tube and bronchial blocker are inserted together, the only new skill required is in pushing, under fiberoptic guidance and during continuous ventilation, the bronchial blocker into the desired mainstem bronchus.

This chapter sequentially discusses the indications for separation of the two lungs, conventional techniques of DLT insertion, and determination of precise DLT position by fiberoptic bronchoscopy. It then considers how to position the bronchial blocker of the Univent tube properly. It ends with a brief discussion of endobronchial intubation with a single-lumen tube.

II. INDICATIONS FOR SEPARATION OF THE TWO LUNGS

There are several absolute and relative indications for separation of the two lungs during thoracic operations or procedures (Box 21-1).

A. ABSOLUTE INDICATIONS

Separation of the two lungs for any of the absolute indications discussed here should be considered a lifesaving maneuver because failure to separate the two lungs under any of these conditions could result in a life-threatening complication or situation. There are three absolute indications for separating the two lungs (Box 21-1). First, separation of one lung from the other

---

> **BOX 21-1 Indications for separation of the two lungs (double-lumen tube intubation) and/or one-lung ventilation**
>
> I. Absolute
>   1. Isolation of one lung from the other to avoid spillage or contamination
>   A. Infection
>   B. Massive hemorrhage
>   2. Control of the distribution of ventilation
>   A. Bronchopleural fistula
>   B. Bronchopleural cutaneous fistula
>   C. Surgical opening of a major conducting airway
>   D. Giant unilateral lung cyst or bulla
>   E. Tracheobronchial-tree disruption
>   F. Life-threatening hypoxemia due to unilateral lung disease
>   3. Unilateral bronchopulmonary lavage
>   A. Pulmonary alveolar proteinosis
> II. Relative
>   1. Surgical exposure — high priority
>   A. Thoracic aortic aneurysm
>   B. Pneumonectomy
>   C. Thoracoscopy
>   D. Upper lobectomy
>   E. Mediastinal exposure
>   2. Surgical exposure — medium (lower) priority
>   A. Middle and lower lobectomies and subsegmental resections
>   B. Esophageal resection
>   C. Procedures on the thoracic spine
>   3. Postcardiopulmonary bypass pulmonary edema/hemorrhage after removal of totally occluding unilateral chronic pulmonary emboli
>   4. Severe hypoxemia due to unilateral lung disease

---

is absolutely necessary to prevent spillage of pus or blood from an infected (abscessed) lung or bleeding lung, respectively, to a noninvolved lung. Acute contamination of a lung with either blood or pus from the other lung usually results in severe massive (bilateral) atelectasis, pneumonia, and sepsis. Second, a number of unilateral lung problems can prevent adequate ventilation of the noninvolved side. A large bronchopleural or bronchopleural cutaneous fistula, or a surgically opened conducting airway, may have such a low resistance to gas flow that a tidal inspiration delivered by positive pressure will exit via the low-resistance pathway, making the adequate ventilation of the other, more normal, lung impossible. A giant, unilateral bulla or cyst may rupture if exposed to positive-pressure ventilation and result in a tension pneumothorax or pneumomediastinum. Very severe or life-threatening hypoxemia due to unilateral lung disease may require differential lung ventilation and positive end-expiratory pressure (PEEP).[1] Finally, positive-pressure ventilation of a lung with a tracheobronchial-tree disruption can result in dissection of gas into the pulmonary interstitial space or mediastinum, resulting in a tension pneumomediastinum. Third, separation of the two lungs is absolutely necessary to perform unilateral bronchopulmonary lavage in patients with pulmonary alveolar proteinosis (and rarely, asthma and cystic fibrosis).

B. RELATIVE INDICATIONS

There are many relative indications for separation of the two lungs, and they are all for the purpose of facilitating surgical exposure by collapsing the lung in the operative hemithorax. These indications can be divided into categories of high priority and medium (lower) priority (Box 21-1). Of the relative indications, repair of a thoracic aortic aneurysm is usually the highest priority because it requires exposure of the thoracic aorta as it runs the entire length of the left hemithorax. A pneumonectomy, especially if performed through a median sternotomy,[2] is greatly aided by the wide exposure of the lung hilum that is afforded by collapse of the operative lung. Similarly, an upper lobectomy (technically the most difficult lobectomy) and many mediastinal exposures may be made much easier by eliminating ventilation to the lung on the side of the procedure. Examination of the pleural space (thoracoscopy) and pulmonary resections through a thoracoscope is considerably aided by collapse of the ipsilateral lung.

The surgical items in the medium- (lower-) priority category do not routinely require collapse of the lung on the operative side but still significantly aid surgical exposure and eliminate the need for the surgeon to handle (retract, compress, pack away) the operative lung. Severe intraoperative retraction of the lung on the operated side can traumatize the operative lung and impair gas exchange both intraoperatively[3,4] and postoperatively.[5,6] The lower-priority items consist of middle and lower lobectomies, less-extensive pulmonary resections, thoracic spinal procedures that are approached anteriorly through the chest,[7] and esophageal surgery. However, even relatively small operations such as wedge and segmental resections benefit by DLT insertion because of the ability to alternate easily and quickly between lung collapse and inflation, which is sometimes required to better visualize lung morphology and to facilitate identification and separation of important planes and fissures.

Finally, the separation of the lungs following removal of totally occluding and predominantly unilateral chronic pulmonary emboli (postcardiopulmonary bypass) can be very helpful if significant transudation of hemorrhagic fluid across the alveolar capillary membrane in the region of the lung supplied by the previously occluded vessel occurs postcardiopulmonary bypass (reperfusion of a previously and chronically nonperfused vascular bed). Should significant and predominantly unilateral postthromboembolectomy/postcardiopulmonary-bypass pulmonary edema occur, the patient should be returned to cardiopulmonary bypass, and a double-lumen endotracheal tube should be inserted so that differential lung ventilation may be used. Also, significant hypoxemia due to unilateral lung disease may more easily be treated by differential lung ventilation and PEEP.[1]

III. DOUBLE-LUMEN TUBE INTUBATION

Double-lumen endotracheal intubation has become the lung-separation technique of choice in the majority of thoracic surgery cases. Bronchial blockade with the Univent tube in adults is also greatly increasing. DLTs are favored over bronchial blockers and endobronchial tubes for lung separation primarily because they are more versatile. The most important double-lumen function not available with a bronchial blocker is independent bilateral suctioning. In addition, it is easier to apply continuous positive airway pressure (CPAP) to the nonventilated operative lung with a DLT than with a bronchial blocker. Endobronchial tubes are very limited in function and allow only one-lung ventilation.

There are two firm disadvantages or contraindications to the use of a DLT compared with a bronchial blocker. First, very distorted tracheobronchial-tree anatomy, including exophytic and stenotic lesions, as well as tortuosity, may preclude successful positioning of a DLT. Second, changing from a double-lumen tube to a single-lumen tube during or at the end of a case can be a difficult or risky procedure. Examples of a requirement for a change from a double-lumen tube to a single-lumen tube during the operative period are turning the patient from the supine to the prone position (45% of cases involving an anterior approach to surgery on the vertebral bodies[7]) and at the end of the case for postoperative ventilation in the ICU. There are many known anatomical causes of difficult laryngoscopy and intubation,[8] but the most important intraoperative/postoperative risk factor for making them difficult is the infusion of massive amounts of blood and fluids (i.e., the upper airway becomes edematous).

DLTs have two relatively minor in-situ disadvantages, which are related to the fact that the lumens of a DLT may be narrow. First, suctioning may be more difficult down a narrow lumen, though this is usually not a problem with the new disposable Robertshaw-type DLTs, which have nonadhering suction catheters that slide easily down the lumens of the double-lumen tube. Second, airway resistance may be increased with a narrow lumen, but this can easily be overcome by positive-pressure ventilation.[9]

DLTs are essentially two catheters bonded together; each lumen is intended to ventilate one of the two lungs.

Double-Lumen Tubes

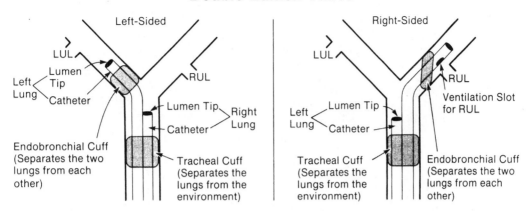

Fig. 21-1. Essential features and parts of left-sided and right-sided double-lumen tubes. *RUL,* right upper lobe; *LUL,* left upper lobe. (From Benumof JL: *Anesthesia for thoracic surgery,* Philadelphia, 1987, W.B. Saunders Co.)

DLTs are made as left- and right-sided tubes. A left-sided tube means that the left-lung catheter is placed into the left mainstem bronchus, whereas the right-lung catheter ends in the trachea; therefore, for a left-sided tube, the left-lung catheter is longer than the right-lung catheter (Fig. 21-1). A right-sided tube means that the right-lung catheter is placed into the right mainstem bronchus, whereas the left-lung catheter ends in the trachea; therefore, for a right-sided tube, the right-lung catheter is longer than the left-lung catheter (Fig. 21-1). All the DLTs have a proximal cuff for the trachea and a distal cuff for a mainstem bronchus; the endobronchial cuff causes separation and sealing off of the two lungs from each other, and the tracheal cuff causes separation and sealing off of the lungs from the environment. The part of the right-lung catheter of the right-sided DLT that is in the right mainstem bronchus must be slotted to allow for ventilation of the right upper lobe (Fig. 21-1) because the right mainstem bronchus is too short to accommodate both the right lumen tip and the right endobronchial cuff. All the double-lumen endotracheal tubes have two curves that lie in planes approximately 90° apart. The distal curve is designed to facilitate placement of the distal catheter tip into the appropriate mainstem bronchus and the proximal curve is designed to approximate the oropharyngolaryngeal curve.

The original Robertshaw DLT, introduced in 1962, was made as a reusable, red rubber tube. This tube was designed to provide the largest possible lumen to decrease airway resistance and to facilitate removal of secretions. The lumens are D shaped and lie side by side. As with the other double-lumen endotracheal tubes, it has two curves (in planes 90° apart) that facilitate intubation and proper endobronchial placement. The Robertshaw-type tube is now made of a clear, nontoxic

tissue-implantable plastic (denoted by the marking "Z-79") and is disposable (Fig. 21-2). The tubes are made in sizes 41, 39, 37, 35, 28, and 26 French gauge (internal diameter [ID] of each lumen is approximately 7.4, 7.0, 6.5, 6.0, 4.5, and 4.0 mm, respectively). These tubes are relatively easy to insert compared with other lung separation tubes, and have appropriate end-of-lumen and cuff arrangements that minimize lobar obstruction. Each lumen is color coded (bronchial is blue and tracheal is clear colorless) and labeled. The endobronchial cuff is colored brilliant blue, an important feature for recognition when using a fiberoptic broncho-scope. The ends of both lumens have a black radiopaque line, an essential recognition marker when viewing a chest x-ray film. The tubes have high volume–low pressure tracheal and endobronchial cuffs; the usual just-seal volume and intracuff pressure relationship of the endobronchial cuff is approximately 1-2 ml and 15 to 30 cm H_2O (see section III G). Mucosal perfusion is probably maintained, since the actual pressure transmitted to the bronchial wall is only approximately 10% to 20% of the measured intracuff pressure (the difference between measured intracuff pressure and the pressure applied to the bronchial wall is the pressure required simply to distend and maintain the inflation of the cuff itself).[10-13] The slanted, doughnut-shaped endobronchial cuff on the Mallinckrodt right-sided DLT allows the right uper lobe ventilation slot to ride off of (away from) the orifice of the right upper lobe, which minimizes the chance of obstruction of the right upper lobe by the tube. The clear, see-through color-coded tubing is helpful because it permits continuous observation of the tidal movement of respiratory moisture as well as observation of secretions from each lung. When the polyvinylchloride material heats to body temperature, the tube shape changes to approximate more closely the

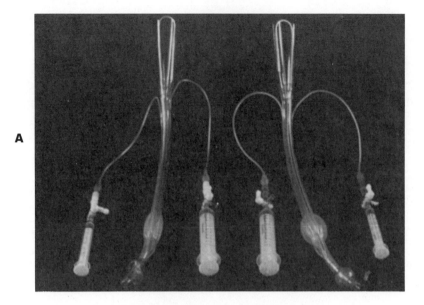

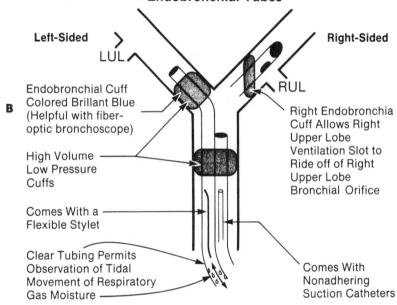

**The Advantages of the Modern
Plastic Disposable Robertshaw Double-Lumen
Endobronchial Tubes**

Left-Sided

LUL

Right-Sided

RUL

B

Endobronchial Cuff
Colored Brillant Blue
(Helpful with fiber-
optic bronchoscope)

High Volume
Low Pressure
Cuffs

Comes With a
Flexible Stylet

Clear Tubing Permits
Observation of Tidal
Movement of Respiratory
Gas Moisture

Right Endobronchia
Cuff Allows Right
Upper Lobe
Ventilation Slot to
Ride off of Right
Upper Lobe
Bronchial Orifice

Comes With
Nonadhering
Suction Catheters

Fig. 21-2. A, Left- and right-sided disposable Robertshaw double-lumen tubes. **B,** Advantages
of left- and right-sided modern Robertshaw double-lumen endobronchial tubes, which are
plastic and disposable. Both lumens of the left-sided double-lumen tube are shown, whereas
only the distal endobronchial lumen of the right-sided double-lumen tube is shown. (From
Benumof JL: *Anesthesia for thoracic surgery,* Philadelphia, 1987, W.B. Saunders Co.)

shape of the airway. The tubes are packaged with
malleable stylets and are relatively easy to insert and to
position. These tubes have large internal-to-external
diameter ratios and gentle curvatures and therefore
allow suctioning to be done relatively easily, and they
have a low resistance to air flow. They are packaged with
their own nonadhering suction catheters. For these
reasons the Robertshaw-type tubes are now considered
by far the double-lumen endotracheal tube of choice by
most anesthesiologists. As expected, several manufac-

turers make these DLTs (Mallinckrodt, Sheridan,
Rusch, Portex).

A. THE CONVENTIONAL (NONFIBEROPTIC) DOUBLE-LUMEN TUBE INTUBATION PROCEDURE

1. Choice of left- versus right-sided double-lumen tube

It has been recommended that the nonoperated
mainstem bronchus be routinely intubated, since intubation of the operative mainstem bronchus may interfere

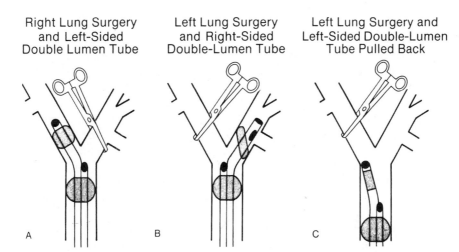

Right Lung Surgery
and Left-Sided
Double Lumen Tube

Left Lung Surgery
and Right-Sided
Double-Lumen Tube

Left Lung Surgery and
Left-Sided Double-Lumen
Tube Pulled Back

A   B   C

Fig. 21-3. Use of left-sided and right-sided double-lumen tubes for left- and right-lung surgery (as indicated by clamp). When surgery is going to be performed on right lung, a left-sided double-lumen tube should be used **(A).** When surgery is going to be performed on left lung, a right-sided double-lumen tube may be used **(B).** However, because of uncertainty as to alignment of right upper–lobe ventilation slot to the right upper–lobe orifice, a left-sided double-lumen tube can also be used for left-lung surgery **(C).** If left-lung surgery requires a clamp to be placed high on left mainstem bronchus, the left endobronchial cuff should be deflated, the left-sided double-lumen tube pulled back into the trachea, and the right lung ventilated through both lumens (use double-lumen tube as a single-lumen tube). (From Benumof JL: *Anesthesia for thoracic surgery,* Philadelphia, 1987, W.B. Saunders Co.)

with surgery. Consequently, there is no controversy regarding using a left-sided double-lumen endotracheal tube for right thoracotomies requiring collapse of the right lung and ventilation of the left lung (Fig. 21-3). However, there is controversy regarding using a right-sided DLT for left-lung surgery. For this reason, either a left- or right-sided tube may be used for left thoracotomies requiring collapse of the left lung and ventilation of the right lung (Fig. 21-3). However, since the right upper lobe ventilation slot of a right-sided tube has to be closely apposed to the right upper lobe orifice for unobstructed right upper lobe ventilation to occur and since there is considerable anatomic variation in the exact position of the right upper lobe orifice and, therefore, length of the right mainstem bronchus. (In fact, it is well known that an anomalous right upper lobe can take off from the trachea; the incidence is 1:250 in normal patients and 1:50 in patients who have some other congenital defect.) Use of a right-sided tube for left-lung collapse introduces the risk of inadequate ventilation of the right upper lobe. For this reason, a left-sided tube is preferable for most patients requiring one-lung ventilation. If clamping of the left mainstem bronchus is necessary, the tube can be withdrawn at that time into the trachea and then used in the same manner as a single-lumen endotracheal tube (ventilate the right lung with both lumens with the endobronchial cuff deflated; Fig. 21-3). If after withdrawal the tracheal cuff is supraglottic, then the bronchial cuff should be inflated and the patient ventilated through the bronchial lumen.

A contraindication to the use of a left-sided double-lumen tube is proximal left mainstem bronchial lesions that could be traumatized by the passage of a left-sided tube. These lesions include strictures, endoluminal tumors, tracheobronchial disruptions, and compression of the airway by an external mass (including a thoracic aortic aneurysm).[13] In addition, tumors of the left lower lobe and left upper lobe may push and pull, respectively, the left mainstem bronchus off the trachea at a very acute angle. This distortion of the tracheobronchial tree may make it impossible to cannulate the left mainstem bronchus, even over a fiberoptic bronchoscope (FOB). Finally, sleeve resection of the proximal left mainstem bronchus contraindicates the presence of an endobronchial catheter in the surgical field. The largest-sized tube that can comfortably pass the glottis should be used, since a relatively small DLT may require excessive cuff volume for an endobronchial cuff seal to be obtained (see the discussion of endobronchial cuff problems in section III A3c and Fig. 21-12); may be inadvertently inserted too deeply; may not protect against transbronchial spread of pus, blood, or necrotic tumor if the endobronchial cuff is deflated during two-lung ventilation (larger space around small lumen);[14] and may cause difficulty with suctioning secretions.

2. Choice of size of double-lumen tube

The appropriate DLT size is one that results in a just-seal volume for the endobronchial cuff that is greater than 1 ml but less than 3 ml. If the endobronchial just-seal cuff volume is less than 1 ml, then the outside diameter of the bronchial lumen and the risk of bronchial-wall damage is increased especially if the DLT is inserted too deeply. If the endobronchial just-seal cuff volume is greater than 3 ml, then the outside diameter of the endobronchial tube is too small in relation to the bronchial lumen and the intracuff pressures will be excessive (the bronchial cuff will behave as a high-pressure cuff)[15] and the risk of bronchial wall damage will be increased, especially if nitrous oxide is used; other considerations for the size of the DLT are listed in the previous paragraph.

In general, as height and weight increase, the appropriate DLT size tube (as defined in the previous paragraph) increases, although height is much more important than weight.[16,17] Since women are usually shorter than men, sizes 35 French and 37 French are ordinarily appropriate for women, whereas sizes 39 French and 41 French are appropriate for men. However, choice of a DLT by height, irrespective of gender, makes more sense.[16,17]

3. The double-lumen tube intubation procedure

a. PREINTUBATION PROCEDURES

Prior to intubation with a double-lumen endotracheal tube, both cuffs and lumen connections are checked. A 3-ml syringe should be placed on the end of the bronchial-cuff pilot tube, and a 5- or 10-ml syringe should be placed on the tracheal-cuff pilot tube. Both cuffs should be tested for leaks. Since the high volume–low pressure cuffs can be easily torn by teeth, the distal tube is coated with a lubricating ointment (preferably containing a local anesthetic) to minimize this possibility. If a less-than-optimal view of the larynx is anticipated, the stylet that comes packaged with the tube is lubricated, inserted into the endobronchial (in this case, the left) lumen, and appropriately curved. The patient is then anesthetized and paralyzed.

b. THE INTUBATION

A curved open-phalanged blade (Macintosh) is usually preferred for laryngoscopy, since it approximates the curvature of the tube and therefore provides the largest possible area through which to pass the tube. However, a straight (Miller) blade may be a better choice in patients with overriding teeth or an excessively anterior larynx.

Double-lumen endotracheal tubes with carinal hooks are first inserted through the vocal cords with the distal curve concave anteriorly (just like a single-lumen tube) and the hook facing posteriorly. When the tip of the tube has passed the vocal cords, the tube is rotated 180 degrees, so that the hook passes anteriorly through the glottis. After the tube tip and the hook pass the larynx, the tube is rotated 90 degrees so that the tip is curved toward and enters the appropriate bronchus and the hook engages the carina.

The Robertshaw double-lumen tube (without carinal hook) is passed with the distal curvature initially concave anteriorly, as with a single-lumen tube (Fig. 21-4, *A*). After the tube tip passes the larynx and while anterior force on the laryngoscope is continued, the stylet (if used) is removed and the tube is carefully rotated 90 degrees (so that the distal curve is now concave toward the appropriate side and the proximal curve is concave anteriorly) to allow endobronchial intubation on the appropriate side (Fig. 21-4, *B*). Continued anterior force by the laryngoscope during tube rotation prevents hypopharyngeal structures from falling in around the tube and interfering with a free 90-degree rotation of the tip of the distal tube. Failure to obtain close to a 90-degree rotation of the tip of the distal tube, while the proximal end does rotate 90 degrees, will cause either a kink or twist in the shaft of the tube and/or prevent the distal end of the lumen from lying free in the mainstem bronchus (i.e., not against the bronchial wall). After rotation, the tube is advanced until most of it is inserted, (28 to 30 cm) (Fig. 21-4, *C*).[17]

When the proper depth of insertion is defined as the cephalad surface of the bronchial cuff immediately below the carinal bifurcation, the average depth of insertion for both male and female patients 170 cm tall is 29 cm, and for each 10-cm increase or decrease in height, average placement depth is increased or decreased 1 cm.[17] The correlation between depth of insertion and height is highly significant ($P < .0001$) for both male and female patients. Nevertheless, it should be understood that the depth of DLT insertion at any given height is still normally distributed and correct DLT position should always be confirmed fiberoptically after initial placement.

If the proximal end of the common or two-lumen binding mold is near or at the level of the teeth (i.e., at a depth of 32 to 33 cm) in a normal-sized person and/or moderate resistance to further passage is encountered, it usually means that the tube has been pushed in too far and the tube has been firmly seated in a distal bronchus. Double-lumen endotracheal tubes may also be passed successfully via tracheostomy, although it should be remembered that the tracheal cuff may be at the tracheal stoma or lie partly outside the trachea in this situation.[18,19] A special DLT has been designed for use with tracheostomies.[20]

c. ROUTINE CHECKING OF POSITION OF DOUBLE-LUMEN TUBE

Once the tube tip is thought to be in an endobronchial position, the following directions are carried out to ensure proper functioning of the tube. Inflate the tracheal and endobronchial cuffs until moderate tension is palpated in the external pilot balloons. The endobronchial cuff should not require more than 2 to 3 ml of air; if it does, the cuff may be herniating out of the mainstem

Passage of Left-Sided Double-Lumen Tube

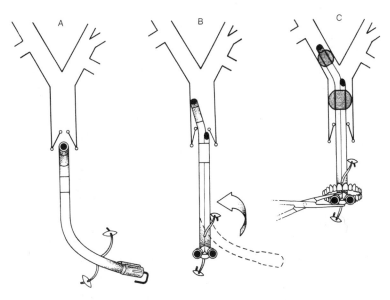

Fig. 21-4. Passage of the left-sided double-lumen tube in a supine patient. **A,** Tube is held with distal curvature concave anteriorly and proximal curve concave to the right and in a plane parallel to floor. Tube is then inserted through vocal cords until left cuff passes vocal cords. Stylet is then removed. **B,** Tube is rotated 90 degrees counterclockwise so that distal curvature is concave to the left and in a plane parallel to the floor and proximal curvature is concave anteriorly. **C,** Tube is inserted until either 30-cm mark is at incisors, a moderate resistance to further passage is encountered, or end of common molding of two lumens is at teeth. Both cuffs are then inflated, and both lungs are ventilated. Finally, one side is clamped while other side is ventilated, and vice versa (see text for further explanation). (From Benumof JL: *Anesthesia for thoracic surgery,* Philadelphia, 1987, W.B. Saunders Co.)

bronchus (which is, by far, the most likely possibility) or the mainstem bronchus is malotic, or the size of the DLT is inappropriately small. Later, after one has completed fiberoptic confirmation of proper position of the DLT, the tracheal lumen can be clamped and the endobronchial cuff deflated. Then, while ventilating through only the endobronchial lumen, its cuff can be slowly inflated until the minimum amount of air needed to prevent an air leak is determined (the "just-seal" volume of air). Other, more quantitative methods of determining the just-seal volume of cuff air are the positive-pressure ventilation–air bubble under water technique (see section III F), negative circle system pressure/collapse of reservoir bag, and use of capnography (see Figs. 21-18 to 21-20).[21-23] Determination of an air leak when the cuff is deflated is important because it rules out the possibility that the DLT is too tightly impacted in the bronchus.

Several positive-pressure ventilations should be delivered and the chest auscultated and observed bilaterally to determine that the trachea, rather than the esophagus, has been intubated and that both lungs are being ventilated (Fig. 21-4,*C*). In addition to seeing the tube go through the vocal cords, the intubationist should check the correct intubation position by feeling and

observing the anesthesia reservoir bag to make sure it has the appropriate compliance and movement, maintaining normal pulse oximetry and end-tidal CO_2 values, and perhaps palpating the tracheal cuff in the neck. If only unilateral breath sounds or chest movements are present, it is likely that both of the lumens of the tube have entered a mainstem bronchus. (If both of the lumens enter the left mainstem bronchus, the findings may mimic an esophageal intubation and vice versa). In this situation, quickly deflate the cuffs, withdraw the tube 1 to 2 cm at a time, inflate the cuffs, and reassess ventilation until bilateral breath sounds are heard. If bilateral breath sounds are not heard and the tube has been withdrawn a significant amount, the entire procedure must be repeated, beginning with establishing the airway and oxygen ventilation via mask, laryngoscopy, and reinsertion of the DLT through the vocal cords. If bilateral breath sounds are present, then one side is clamped, and breath sounds and chest movement should disappear on the ipsilateral side and remain on the contralateral side. Next, the clamped side should be unclamped and the breath sounds and chest movement should reappear on that side. During unilateral clamping the breath sounds on the ventilated side should be compared with and calibrated against unilateral chest-

Correct Position of Double-Lumen Tube and Unilateral Clamping

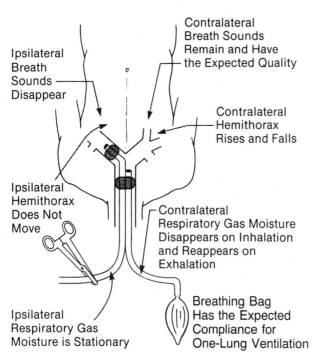

Fig. 21-5. Results of unilateral clamping when double-lumen tube is in correct position. (From Benumof JL: *Anesthesia for thoracic surgery,* Philadelphia, 1987, W.B. Saunders Co.)

wall movements and the inspiratory disappearance and expiratory appearance of respiratory-gas moisture in the clear tubing of the ventilated side (Fig. 21-5). In addition, the compliance of the lung should be gauged by using hand ventilation. The unilateral clamping and unclamping should then be repeated on the opposite side to assure adequate lung separation and cuff seal.

In summary, when the position of the double-lumen endotracheal tube is correct, the breath sounds are normal and follow the expected unilateral pattern with unilateral clamping, the chest rises and falls in accordance with the breath sounds, the ventilated lung feels reasonably compliant, no leaks are present, and respiratory-gas moisture appears and disappears with each tidal ventilation (Fig. 21-5). When comparing both lumens during two-lung ventilation and when changing from two-lung ventilation to one-lung ventilation with a known constant tidal volume, the exhaled tidal volume should not decrease by more than 15%, expiratory flow rate from either lung should not slow markedly, peak airway pressure should not increase by more than 60%, and there should be no obvious difference in the rate of appearance of the fog in the two lumens during exhalation. However, it should be realized that in the presence of advanced lung disease, loss of lung tissue, or

atelectasis, more exaggerated changes in the above-mentioned variables are expected when switching from two-lung ventilation to diseased-lung ventilation. It should be noted that the auscultation findings with a DLT whose endobronchial cuff has gone past an upper-lobe orifice, but that still allows the upper lobe to be ventilated by the tracheal lumen, may closely mimic the findings expected for a properly positioned DLT during two-lung ventilation.[24,25] Conversely, when the double-lumen endotracheal tube is malpositioned, any or all of the following may occur: the breath sounds are poor and correlate poorly with unilateral clamping; the chest movements do not follow the expected pattern; the ventilated lung feels noncompliant; leaks are present; or the respiratory-gas moisture in the clear tubing is relatively stationary. It is important to realize, however, that even if the DLT is thought to be properly positioned based on clinical signs, subsequent fiberoptic bronchoscopy will reveal a 40% to 48% incidence of malpositioning.[26,27] (see section III D). Obviously, the auscultation and fiberoptic findings can always be supplemented by direct observation of the operative lung and mediastinum when the chest is open.

Whether the endobronchial cuff should be left inflated or deflated after confirmation of proper position of the DLT is controversial (see section III B). On the one hand, deflation of the cuff during two-lung ventilation during the initial stages of surgery (preparing the chest, draping, opening the chest wall, etc.) minimizes the chance of pressure damage to the bronchial mucosa. On the other hand, leaving the cuff inflated (after readjustment to a just-seal volume) prevents trans–mainstem-bronchial spread of secretions (pus, blood) and necrotic tumor. In cases where migration of material from the nondependent to the dependent lung is a possibility, adjustment of the cuff to a just-seal volume would seem to minimize risk and maximize benefit.

d. AUSCULTATION AND UNILATERAL CLAMPING MANEUVERS TO DIAGNOSE MALPOSITION OF DOUBLE-LUMEN TUBE

When it is believed that the double-lumen endotracheal tube is malpositioned based on clinical signs, it is theoretically possible to diagnose the malposition of the tube more precisely by a combination of several unilateral clampings, chest auscultation, and left endobronchial-cuff inflation-deflation maneuvers (Fig. 21-6). With reference to a left-sided double-lumen endotracheal tube, there are three possible gross malpositions: in too far on the left (both lumens in the left mainstem bronchus), out too far (both lumens in the trachea), and in or down the right mainstem bronchus (at least the left lumen is in the right mainstem bronchus). When the right (tracheal) side is clamped and the tube is in too far on the left side, breath sounds will be heard only on the

Double-Lumen Tube Malpositions

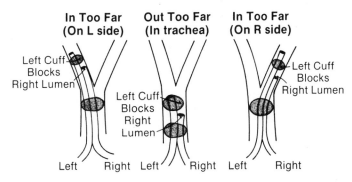

Procedure	Breath Sounds Heard		
Clamp Right Lumen Both Cuffs Inflated	Left	Left and Right	Right
Clamp Left Lumen Both Cuffs Inflated	None or Very ↓↓	None or Very ↓↓	None or Very ↓↓
Clamp Left Lumen Deflate Left Cuff	Left	Left and Right	Right

Fig. 21-6. There are three major (involving a whole lung) malpositions of a left-sided double-lumen endotracheal tube. The tube can be in too far on the left (both lumens are in the left mainstem bronchus), out too far (both lumens are in the trachea), or down the right mainstem bronchus (at least the left lumen is in the right mainstem bronchus). In each of these three malpositions, the left cuff, when fully inflated, can completely block the right lumen. Inflation and deflation of the left cuff while the left lumen is clamped creates a breath-sound differential diagnosis of tube malposition. See text for full explanation. (*L*, left; *R*, right; ↓, decreased). (From Benumof JL: *Anesthesia for thoracic surgery,* Philadelphia, 1987, W.B. Saunders Co.)

left side. When the tube is out too far and the right side is clamped, breath sounds will be heard bilaterally (the tube needs to be advanced further). When the tube is in or down the right side and the right lumen is clamped, breath sounds will be heard only on the right side (the tube needs to be pulled back, rerotated, and readvanced). When the left side is clamped and the left endobronchial cuff is inflated, the right lumen is blocked by the left cuff in all three malpositions. Consequently, with the left side clamped and the left cuff inflated, no or very diminished breath sounds will be heard bilaterally in all three malpositions and there will be marked resistance to air flow (the right lumen opens between two inflated cuffs). When the left side is clamped and the left cuff is deflated so that the right lumen is no longer blocked by the left cuff, breath sounds will be heard only on the left side when the tube is in too far on the left (the tube needs to be pulled back), breath sounds will be heard bilaterally if the tube is out too far (the tube needs to be advanced), and breath sounds will be heard only on the right side when the tube is in the right side (the tube needs to be pulled back, rerotated, and readvanced). The left cuff inflation-deflation findings provide the key diagnostic data because they essentially define the

position of the right tracheal lumen by blocking and unblocking it with the left cuff. Another possible diagnostic sequence is presented in Figure 21-7.[28]

There are, however, several situations in which unilateral clamping, auscultation, and cuff inflation and deflation maneuvers for determining the integrity of lung separation are either unreliable or impossible. First and most importantly, when the patient is in the lateral decubitus position, has had a skin preparation, and is draped, access to the chest wall is impossible, and the anesthesiologist cannot listen to the chest. Second, the presence of unilateral or bilateral lung disease, which either preexisted before anesthesia and surgery or was induced by anesthesia, may markedly obscure the crispness of the chest auscultation end points. Third, the diagnosis of exactly where the double-lumen endotracheal tube has located may be confused when the tube is just slightly malpositioned. Fourth, the tube may have moved because of some event such as coughing, turning into the lateral decubitus position, and tracheal manipulation and hilar retraction by the surgeon. Finally, some combination of the above circumstances may culminate in uncertainty as to where the double-lumen tube has located. The solution to any uncertainty as to the exact

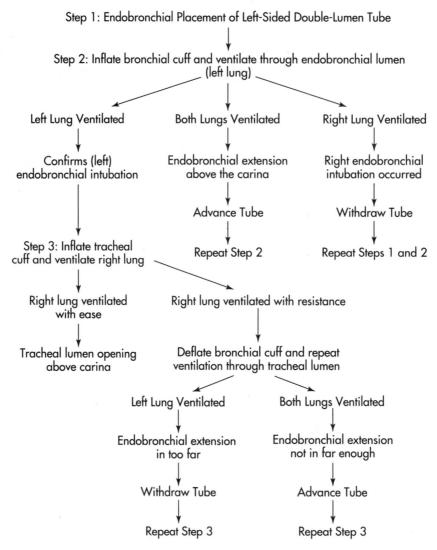

Fig. 21-7. Decision tree outlining a sequence of cuff inflation and positive-pressure ventilation through a left-sided double-lumen tube that will ensure proper functioning of the tube. (From Katz JA, Fairley HB: Pulmonary surgery. In Marshall BE, Longnecker DF, Fairley HB, editors: *Anesthesia for thoracic procedures,* Boston, 1988, Blackwell Scientific.)

position of the double-lumen tube is to determine the position by use of fiberoptic bronchoscopy (see section III C).

B. USE OF FIBEROPTIC BRONCHOSCOPE TO INSERT THE BRONCHIAL LUMEN OF A DOUBLE-LUMEN TUBE INTO A MAINSTEM BRONCHUS

The insertion of the bronchial lumen of a double-lumen tube into the appropriate mainstem bronchus may be aided by the use of a fiberoptic bronchoscope (Fig. 21-8). The procedure is indicated whenever the endobronchial lumen will not locate in the appropriate mainstem bronchus by blind insertion (e.g., ventilation through only the endobronchial lumen results in breath sounds over the wrong lung field or side); when the endobronchial lumen needs to be maneuvered past some sort of pathology (e.g., stenosis in left mainstem bronchus due to thoracic aortic aneurysm)[13]; or when intubation is known to be difficult and intubation of an awake (or anesthetized) patient with a DLT over a fiberoptic bronchoscope (FOB) is indicated[29,30] (as it would be for a single-lumen tube; of course, the awake patient requires topical and nerve-block anesthetic).[29]

The DLT is usually first placed in the trachea in a conventional manner (laryngoscopy or manual tube insertion) (unless the patient is awake and the fiberscope is used from the outset) until the tracheal cuff just passes

**Use of Fiberoptic Bronchoscope to
Insert Left-Sided Double-Lumen Tube**

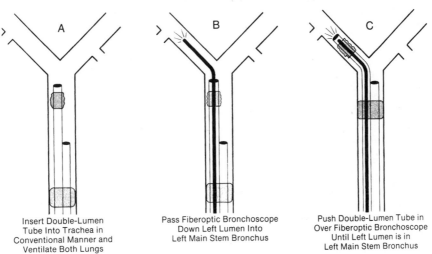

Insert Double-Lumen
Tube Into Trachea in
Conventional Manner and
Ventilate Both Lungs

Pass Fiberoptic Bronchoscope
Down Left Lumen Into
Left Main Stem Bronchus

Push Double-Lumen Tube in
Over Fiberoptic Bronchoscope
Until Left Lumen is in
Left Main Stem Bronchus

Fig. 21-8. Double-lumen tube can be put into trachea in a conventional manner, and both lungs can be ventilated by both lumens (**A**). Fiberoptic bronchoscope may be inserted into left lumen of double-lumen tube through a self-sealing diaphragm in the elbow connector to the left lumen; this allows continued positive pressure ventilation of both lungs through right lumen without creating a leak. After fiberoptic bronchoscope has been passed into the left mainstem bronchus (**B**), it is used as a stylet for left lumen (**C**), fiberoptic bronchoscope is then withdrawn. Final precise positioning of double-lumen tube is performed with fiberoptic bronchoscope in right lumen (see Fig. 21-9 and 21-10). (From Benumof JL: *Anesthesia for thoracic surgery,* Philadelphia, 1987, W.B. Saunders Co.)

the vocal cords. The tracheal cuff is then inflated, and both lungs are ventilated with both lumens (the double-lumen tube is used as if it were a single-lumen tube). A pediatric fiberoptic bronchoscope can then be inserted into the bronchial lumen through a self-sealing diaphragm in the elbow connector to the bronchial lumen, which permits continued positive-pressure ventilation through that lumen around the fiberoptic bronchoscope, and passed into the appropriate mainstem bronchus.[29,31] The tracheal cuff is then deflated and the bronchial lumen is passed over the FOB stylet into the appropriate mainstem bronchus. With respect to placing a right-sided DLT correctly (i.e., getting the right upper lobe ventilation slot opposite the right upper lobe bronchial orifice), the right upper lobe bronchial orifice may first be identified fiberoptically. Then, while the FOB is held steady, the endobronchial lumen is passed over the FOB into the right mainstem bronchus (the tip of the FOB must be returned to a neutral position during passage of the DLT over the tip of the FOB until the tip of the FOB can be used to look through the right upper lobe ventilation slot into the right upper lobe bronchial orifice (see Fig. 21-13, *B* on p. 428). The fiberoptic bronchoscope is then withdrawn from the bronchial lumen to determine the precise DLT position (see section III C).

Alternatively, once the DLT is in the trachea, the fiberoptic bronchoscope can be inserted into the tra-

cheal lumen through a self-sealing diaphragm in the elbow connector to the tracheal lumen, which permits continued positive-pressure ventilation through that lumen around the FOB, and passed just proximally to the tracheal carina.[32] While the carina and the two mainstem bronchial orifices are in view, the DLT can be advanced and the degree of lateral rotation adjusted so that the left lumen enters the left mainstem bronchus. Final precise positioning (see the section III C) can be done with the FOB remaining in the tracheal lumen.

C. USE OF FIBEROPTIC BRONCHOSCOPE TO DETERMINE PRECISE POSITION OF DOUBLE-LUMEN TUBE

The deleterious consequences of a malpositioned DLT can be great, even life threatening. With almost all DLT malpositions, gas exchange can be significantly or profoundly impaired, the nonoperative lung can be difficult or impossible to ventilate, and the operative lung may not collapse on the initiation of one-lung ventilation. In addition, failure to separate the lungs in some specific situations may result in such additional catastrophes as a tension pneumothorax and flooding both lungs with blood, pus, or lavage fluid.

There is a very high incidence of malpositioned DLTs, as determined by using an FOB, when the DLT is inserted "blindly" (i.e., without an FOB). In one study, 48% of all DLTs were found to be malpositioned.[33] In another study, 83% of disposable right-sided DLTs were malpositioned.[34] In a third study, fiberoptic bronchoscopy after auscultation (which led the physician to believe the DLT was in optimal position) resulted in repositioning of 78% of left-sided DLTs and 83% of right-sided DLTs.[35] In a fourth study, 38% of all DLTs were malpositioned.[36] In a fifth study, 44% of disposable tubes required readjustment using the fiberoptic bronchoscope during the initial intubation and 30% required readjustment using the fiberoptic bronchoscope during the operation.[37] The authors of the last three studies concluded that "auscultation is an unreliable method of confirming the position of DLTs and should be followed by fiberoptic bronchoscopy,"[35] "because auscultation for tube position is unreliable, bronchoscopic assessment of final position should be performed in every instance"[36] and that "in certain situations the fiberoptic bronchoscope may have been life-saving."[37]

Given the high incidence of malpositioned DLTs when DLT position is determined by only auscultation (i.e., blindly) and the potentially serious consequences associated with a malpositioned DLT, it is only a matter of common sense to use an FOB routinely to determine easily, quickly, and precisely the position of the DLT. In the studies quoted above, it is open to conjecture and speculation as to what would have happened if the position of the DLT was not corrected with the aid of an FOB. However, one study has shown that when the position of the DLT is checked only by clinical signs, 25% of the time there will be intraoperative problems with either deflating the nondependent lung, ventilating the dependent lung, or completely separating the two lungs.[38]

If one accepts the premise that the position of a DLT should be confirmed by an FOB, then I also contend that it should be done first in the supine position, again after the patient has been turned into the lateral decubitus position, and again during the case whenever there is a question about the position of a DLT (in conjunction with other maneuvers such as palpation of the lumen tips by the surgeon and observation of the operative lung, mediastinum, etc.). There are several reasons for repeating fiberoptic bronchoscopy. First, when the patient is supine, access to the patient's head and DLT is optimal, the orientation of the patient and FOB most certain, and it is easiest to correlate the auscultatory findings (by whatever unilateral clamping and auscultation technique one prefers)[28,39-41] with the FOB findings. The main value of fiberoptic bronchoscopy at this time (supine position), given that all auscultation algorithms can rule in/out cannulation of the wrong mainstem bronchus or failure to cannulate either mainstem bronchus, is to rule in/out upper-lobe obstruction by deter-

mining endobronchial-cuff position or by visualizing the upper-lobe bronchial orifice. I do not believe one can accurately diagnose upper-lobe obstruction by auscultation alone because breath sounds are transmitted from the ipsilateral lower lobe and across the mediastinum from the contralateral lung. Second, if the DLT is properly positioned in the supine position with certainty (i.e., with FOB confirmation), then the second and more important confirmation of DLT position after the patient is in the lateral position is greatly facilitated by the first look in the supine position. In addition, events that take place between the supine and lateral decubitus position may affect the functioning of the DLT. For example, placement of the axillary roll has caused almost complete obstruction of the right mainstem bronchus in a 10-year-old child.[42] Similarly, third and further intraoperative views are facilitated by the second view in the lateral position. This series/cascade of FOB views of DLT position interact and overlap to give the anesthesiologist much tighter control of vital respiratory functions throughout the administration of anesthetic, with very little risk.

The exact position of a left-sided double-lumen endotracheal tube can be ascertained at any time, in less than a minute, by simply passing a pediatric FOB through the tracheal lumen of the DLT. It is rarely necessary also to have to pass the FOB down the left endobronchial lumen. With reference to a left-sided DLT, looking down the right tracheal lumen the endoscopist should see a clear, straight-ahead view of the tracheal carina (the tracheal lumen should be approximately 2 cm above the carina), the left lumen going off to the left, and the upper surface of the left endobronchial balloon just below the tracheal carina (Fig. 21-9 and 21-10).

The margin of safety in positioning a left-sided DLT is the difference between the length of the left mainstem bronchus (approximately 50 mm) and the length of tube between the proximal margin of the left endobronchial cuff and the left lumen tip (approximately 30 to 35 mm).[43] If the proximal margin of the left endobronchial cuff can be seen just below the carina then it is not possible for the left upper lobe to be obstructed because of the relatively large margin of safety in positioning left-sided DLTs. The average margin of safety in positioning left-sided DLTs ranges from 16 to 19 mm.[44] These considerations emphasize the importance of not allowing the head to be severely flexed or extended at any time after the DLT has been appropriately positioned (Fig. 21-11 on p. 427).[43]

DLTs with a carinal hook have the hook placed approximately 10 mm proximal to the proximal surface of the endobronchial cuff. Consequently, the tip of the left lumen of a left-sided DLT with a carinal hook enters the left mainstem bronchus 10 mm deeper than a tube

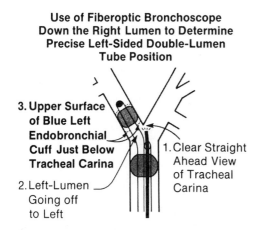

Use of Fiberoptic Bronchoscope Down the Right Lumen to Determine Precise Left-Sided Double-Lumen Tube Position

3. Upper Surface of Blue Left Endobronchial Cuff Just Below Tracheal Carina

1. Clear Straight Ahead View of Tracheal Carina

2. Left-Lumen Going off to Left

Fig. 21-9. Use of fiberoptic bronchoscope down the right lumen to determine precise position of left-sided double-lumen tube. The endoscopist should see a clear straight-ahead view of the tracheal carina, the left lumen going off into the left mainstem bronchus and, most importantly (in bold print), the upper surface of the blue left endobronchial cuff just below the tracheal carina. (From Benumof JL: *Anesthesia for thoracic surgery*, Philadelphia, 1987, W.B. Saunders Co.)

without a carinal hook[45] and the margin of safety is reduced by approximately 10 mm.

It is important that the volume of air used to fill the left endobronchial cuff does not cause the cuff to herniate over the tracheal carina or cause the carina to deviate to the right (Fig. 21-10 and 21-12); both cuff herniation and carinal deviation can be readily appreciated looking down the tracheal lumen. The endoscopist may see a very slight narrowing of the left lumen (because of endobronchial-cuff pressure) as well as the bronchial carina distal to the end of the tube when looking down the left lumen (sometimes done when inserting a left-sided DLT with an FOB [see section III B] and in all cases of bronchopulmonary lavage in which perfect tube position and tight cuff seal are extremely critical) (Fig. 21-10). The endoscopist should not see excessive left-luminal narrowing (because of excessive left-cuff pressure) (Fig. 21-12). Thus, aside from gross malposition, important undesirable findings on endoscopy are related to excessive left-cuff inflation and pressure and consist of cuff herniation over the tracheal carina, carinal deviation to the right (both of which may block the right mainstem bronchial orifice and impair right-lung ventilation), and excessive left-lumen constriction (invagination), which may impair left-lung ventilation (Fig. 21-12).[46] In addition, when an inappropriately undersized tube is used, the volume of the large endobronchial cuff required for cuff seal tends to force the entire DLT cephalad, making a functional bronchial seal more difficult.[47]

With reference to a right-sided DLT, looking down the left (tracheal) lumen the endoscopist should see a clear, straight-ahead view of the tracheal carina, with the right lumen going off to the right (Fig. 21-13, *A* on p. 428). The upper surface of the right endobronchial balloon may not be visible below the tracheal carina depending on the depth of insertion and the design of the right endobronchial cuff (i.e., the shape of the right endobronchial cuff is a function of the manufacturer). Looking down the right lumen, the endoscopist should see the bronchial carina of the right middle-lower lobe distal to the end of the tube. Most importantly, the endoscopist should locate the ventilation slot of the right upper lobe and be able to look directly into the orifice of the right upper lobe through the ventilation slot by simply flexing the tip of the FOB laterally and superiorly (Fig. 21-13, *B*). There should be no overriding of the ventilation slot on the bronchial mucosa, and the bronchial mucosa should not be covering any of the ventilation slot.

The fact that there is little room for error in aligning the slot with the orifice in the right upper lobe means that the positioning margin of safety of right-sided double-lumen tubes is small compared to left-sided double-lumen tubes.[44]

The margin of safety in positioning right-sided tubes is 1 to 10 mm.[44] Obviously with a small margin of safety, head movement is less well tolerated than with left-sided tubes (Fig. 21-11). The Leyland right-sided double-lumen tube has a greater margin of safety than the Rusch (or Mallinckrodt) right-sided double-lumen tube because it has a long (21 mm) ventilation slot for the right upper lobe. However, it should be remembered that the unique, slanted-doughnut shape of the Mallinckrodt right endobronchial cuff of the right-sided double-lumen tube allows the ventilation slot to ride off of the orifice of the right upper lobe, thereby increasing (from 1 mm) to an unknown extent the margin of safety in positioning this particular right-sided tube. The margin of safety in positioning right-sided double-lumen tubes may be negative if the right mainstem bronchus is less than 10 mm (1:6 normal patients)[48] or if the right upper lobe takes off from the trachea (1:250 in normal patients[48] and 1:50 patients with congenital heart disease[49]).

The ventilation slot of the right upper lobe may be easily located by first finding the bronchial lumen radiopaque marker. The radiopaque marker appears as either a white or black line on the inside of the bronchial lumen, which ends at the proximal end of the ventilation slot. If one simply follows the radiopaque line, it will lead the endoscopist to the ventilation slot.

In the author's experience the clinical signs (breath sounds, chest movements, compliance of the lung[s], movement of respiratory-gas moisture) in 8 out of 10 cases indicate that the lungs are clearly and without doubt completely separated when the DLT is first inserted with the patient in the supine position. However, in view of the finding by many authors[33-37] that between 40% and 50% of DLTs are malpositioned to

Use of Fiberoptic Bronchoscope to Determine Precise Left-Sided Double-Lumen Tube Position

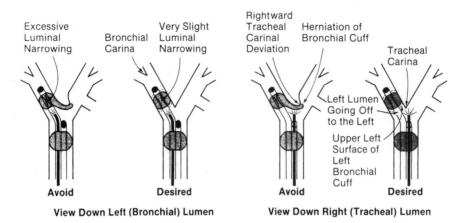

Excessive Luminal Narrowing

Bronchial Carina

Very Slight Luminal Narrowing

Rightward Tracheal Carinal Deviation

Herniation of Bronchial Cuff

Tracheal Carina

Left Lumen Going Off to the Left

Upper Left Surface of Left Bronchial Cuff

Avoid   **Desired**   **Avoid**   **Desired**

View Down Left (Bronchial) Lumen   **View Down Right (Tracheal) Lumen**

Fig. 21-10. Complete fiberoptic bronchoscopy picture of left-sided double-lumen tubes (both desired view and view to be avoided from both lumens). When bronchoscope is passed down the right lumen of the left-sided tube, the endoscopist should see a clear, straight-ahead view of the tracheal carina, the left lumen going off into the left mainstem bronchus and the upper surface of the blue left endobronchial cuff just below the tracheal carina. Excessive pressure in the endobronchial cuff, as manifested by tracheal carinal deviation to right and herniation of endobronchial cuff over carina, should be avoided. When bronchoscope is passed down left lumen of left-sided tube, endoscopist should see a very slight left-luminal narrowing and a clear, straight-ahead view of bronchial carina in the distance. Excessive left-luminal narrowing should be avoided. (From Benumof JL: *Anesthesia for thoracic surgery,* Philadelphia, 1987, W.B. Saunders Co.)

some extent in the supine position, even though the clinical signs may indicate there is no problem it is strongly advisable to check the position of the tube with an FOB when the patient is in the supine position (especially considering that the procedure takes less than a minute). Even if no problem is identified, the procedure still allows the endoscopist to become familiar with the patient's anatomy and facilitates the more important endoscopy performed after turning the patient into the lateral decubitus position. In approximately 2 out of 10 cases there is doubt about tube location in the supine position. In these patients the fiberoptic bronchoscope is always used to correct the DLT malposition. The FOB is always used to determine DLT position after the patient has been turned into the lateral decubitus position. Of course, a determined effort is made to prevent dislodgment of the tube during turning by holding onto the tube at the level of the incisors and by keeping the patient's head absolutely immobile in a neutral or slightly flexed position. Head extension can cause cephalad movement of the tube, which may result in bronchial decannulation; head flexion can cause caudad movement of the tube, which may result in an upper-lobe obstruction or in both lumens being in a mainstem bronchus (see the next section).[43,50] Finally, the FOB is used anytime during the

procedure when there is a question about DLT position. This is not an infrequent occurrence and is usually caused by surgical manipulation and traction on either the hilum, carina, or trachea.

There are a few risks to the routine use of the FOB to determine DLT position. First, depending on the relative sizes of the FOB and the DLT, the use of a self-sealing diaphragm in the elbow connector, and the position of DLT, ventilation may (need to) be interrupted during use of the FOB. Second, if the FOB is inserted through a self-sealing diaphragm in the elbow connector to the side being visualized, one needs to be cognizant of the continuous presence and status of the self-sealing diaphragm (i.e., that a torn fragment is not carried or pushed into the tracheobronchial tree). Third, poor FOB technique may injure the mucosa of the tracheobronchial tree. Fourth, with poor cleaning technique, cross infection or direct mucosal injury (e.g., by Cidex) is possible. Finally, erroneous interpretation of the view is always possible. However, all of these complications are avoidable with proper education, forethought, protocols, and experience. Use of the FOB, especially while the patient is being ventilated or has been hyperventilated on 100% oxygen, should be no more distracting than inserting a central venous line or nasogastric tube, and should also be no more time-

Left Double Lumen Tube Position and
Head Flexion and Extension

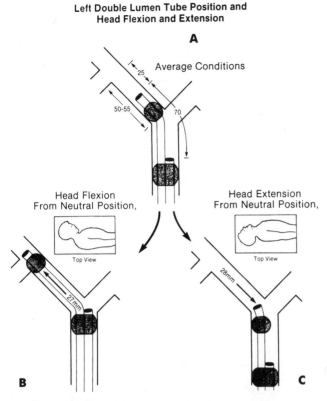

Fig. 21-11. Head flexion moves an endotracheal tube inward, whereas head extension moves outward. **A,** Correct position of left-sided double-lumen tube along with average values (in mm) for left mainstem bronchus, right to left lumen tip and left lumen tip to left upper-lobe lengths; latter length is margin of safety. When left cuff is just below tracheal carina, margin of safety is 25 mm. **B,** Extreme head flexion can cause left upper-lobe obstruction. **C,** Extreme head extension can cause left mainstem bronchial decannulation. (From Benumof JL: *Anesthesia for thoracic surgery,* Philadelphia, 1987, W.B. Saunders Co.)

consuming than the multiple, and often confusing, unilateral clamping and declamping/auscultation periods that are usually required when the DLT is not in the right position.

1. Relationship of size of fiberoptic bronchoscope to size of double-lumen tube

Right- and left-sided double-lumen endotracheal tubes that are clear, plastic, and disposable are manufactured in six sizes: 26, 28, 35, 37, 39, and 41 French. A 5.6-mm outside-diameter diagnostic FOB will not pass down the lumens of any size of DLT. A 4.9-mm external-diameter FOB passes easily through the lumens of the 41-French tube, passes moderately easily with lubrication through the 39-French tube, causes a tight fit that needs a liberal amount of lubrication and a strong pushing force to pass through the 37-French tube, and does not pass through the lumen of the 35-French tube. A silicon-based fluid (such as that made by the American

Excessive Left Cuff Inflation: Problems

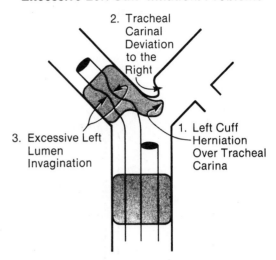

Fig. 21-12. Excessive inflation of left cuff of a left-sided double-lumen tube can cause impaired ventilation of both right and left lungs. Right-lung ventilation may be impaired by left-cuff herniation over tracheal carina (because of excessive left-cuff volume) and by tracheal carinal deviation to the right (because of excessive left-cuff pressure). Left-lung ventilation may be impaired by invagination of the left lumen caused by excessive left-cuff pressure. (From Benumof JL: *Anesthesia for thoracic surgery,* Philadelphia, 1987, W.B. Saunders Co.)

Cystoscope Co.) is the best lubricant for an FOB because it does not dry out or crust and does not interfere with the view even if it coats the tip of the bronchoscope. Fortunately, from the point of view of using a 4.9-mm outside-diameter FOB, a 37-French tube or larger can be used in almost all adult females and 39-French tube or larger can be used in almost all adult males. A 3.6- to 4.2-mm outside-diameter (pediatric) FOB passes easily through the lumens of all adult-sized (35-French or larger) double-lumen endotracheal tubes and, because the bronchoscope has an increased amount of space, the maneuverability of the tip of the bronchoscope is greatly increased. Therefore, the 3.6- to 4.2-mm outside-diameter bronchoscope is obviously the bronchoscope of choice for DLTs for adults. Special neonatal fiberscopes are necessary for use with 28- and 26-French DLTs. Table 21-1 summarizes these FOB-DLT relationships. Several companies (Olympus, Machida, Pentax) presently manufacture 4.9-mm and 3.6- to 4.2-mm outside-diameter FOBs that are of adequate length and have suction channels.

D. USE OF CHEST X-RAY TO DETERMINE POSITION OF DOUBLE-LUMEN TUBE

The chest roentgenogram can be used to determine DLT position. The usefulness of a chest roentgenogram may be greater than conventional unilateral auscultation and clamping in some patients, but it is always less

Use of Fiberoptic Bronchoscope to Determine Precise Right-Sided Double-Lumen Tube Position

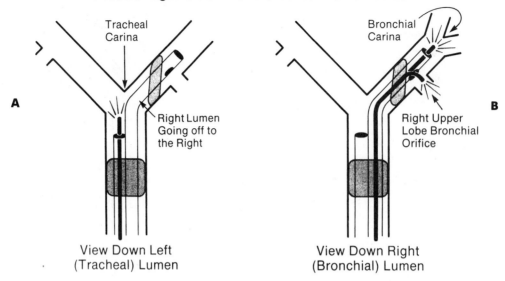

Fig. 21-13. This schematic diagram portrays use of a fiberoptic bronchoscope to determine precise position of right-sided double-lumen tube. **A,** When fiberoptic bronchoscope is passed down left (tracheal) lumen, endoscopist should see a clear, straight-ahead view of the tracheal carina and right lumen going off into right mainstem bronchus. **B,** When fiberoptic bronchoscope is passed down right (bronchial) lumen, endoscopist should see bronchial carina in the distance; when fiberoptic bronchoscope is flexed laterally and cephalad and passed through the ventilation slot of the right upper lobe, the bronchial orifice of the right upper lobe should be visualized. (From Benumof JL: *Anesthesia for thoracic surgery,* Philadelphia, 1987, W.B. Saunders Co.)

Table 21-1. Relationship of FOB* size to DLT* size

FOB size, outside diameter (mm)	DLT size (French)	Fit of FOB inside DLT
5.6	All sizes	Does not fit
4.9	41	Easy passage
	39	Moderately easy passage
	37	Tight fit, needs lubricant,† hand push
	35	Does not fit
3.6-4.2	All sizes	Easy passage
Approximately 2.0	All sizes	Most ORs will need special arrangements to obtain this size FOB

*FOB, fiberoptic bronchoscope; *DLT,* double-lumen tube
†Lubricant recommended is a silicon-based fluid made by the American Cystoscope Co.

precise than fiberoptic bronchoscopy. In order to use the chest roentgenogram, the DLT must have radiopaque markers at the ends of the right and left lumens.

The key to discerning DLT position on the chest roentgenogram is seeing where the marker at the end of the tracheal lumen is in relation to the tracheal carina and whether the endobronchial lumen is located in the correct mainstem bronchus. The end of the tracheal lumen marker must be above the tracheal carina; however, this does not guarantee correct position

because this technique may not reveal a subtle obstruction of an upper lobe. If the tracheal carina cannot be seen, which is often the case with a portable anterior-posterior film, then the chest roentgenogram method of determining DLT position is not usable. Furthermore, the chest roentgenographic method is time-consuming (for film transport, film development), costly, and awkward to perform and may dislodge the tube (the cassettes are often difficult to place under the operating room table and may require moving the patient). Instillation of

Air Bubble Method for Detection of Cuff Seal/Leak

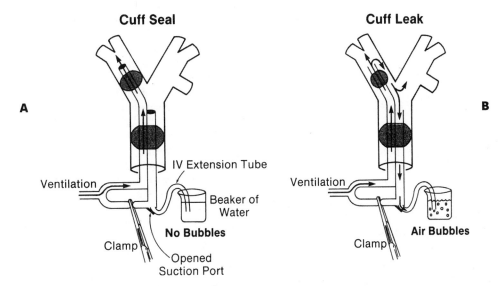

Fig. 21-14. Air-bubble detection method for checking adequacy of the seal of the left endobronchial cuff of a left-sided double-lumen tube. When left lung is selectively ventilated or exposed to any desired distending pressure, and left cuff is adequately sealed, no air will escape around left cuff and out the open right suction port and, thus, no bubbles will be observed passing through beaker of water (**A**). When left lung is ventilated or exposed to any desired distending pressure and left endobronchial cuff is not adequately sealed, air will escape around left cuff and out the open right suction port, and, thus, air bubbles will be observed passing through the beaker of water (**B**). (From Benumof JL: *Anesthesia for thoracic surgery,* Philadelphia, 1987, W.B. Saunders Co.)

1 ml of a radiopaque marker into the endobronchial cuff (renografin 60 is water soluble and is easy to inject, but can be irritating to the bronchial mucosa if it were to leak from a cuff) could enhance the utility of using the chest x-ray to determine DLT position.

E. OTHER METHODS TO DETERMINE POSITION OF DOUBLE-LUMEN TUBE

Three other methods may help to determine the position of a DLT. First, comparison of capnography (waveform and $P_{ET}CO_2$ value) from each lumen may reveal a marked discrepancy. All other conditions being equal, one lung may be very poorly ventilated in relation to the other lung (high $P_{ET}CO_2$) indicating obstruction to that lung. Or one lung may be very overventilated in relation to the other lung (low $P_{ET}CO_2$) indicating, perhaps, just ventilation of a lobe of that lung. Or the capnogram from a given lung may have a much steeper slope to the alveolar plateau, indicating exhalatory obstruction.[51,52] Second, continuous spirometric data (Datex Capnomac Ultima) from both lungs and each individual lung, such as pressure-volume or flow-volume loops, may be displayed and compared to a control loop that is stored in memory.[53] Third, the surgeon may be able to palpate the position of the DLT from within the chest and may be able to redirect or assist in changing the

position of the DLT by, for example, deflecting the DLT away from the wrong lung.[54]

F. QUANTITATIVE DETERMINATION OF CUFF-SEAL PRESSURE HOLD

The use of fiberoptic bronchoscopy to determine DLT position does not provide evidence or a guarantee that the two lungs are functionally separated (i.e., against a fluid and/or air-pressure gradient). There are times, such as during the performance of unilateral pulmonary lavage, when the anesthesiologist must be absolutely certain that functional separation has been achieved. Complete separation of the two lungs by the left endobronchial cuff can be demonstrated in a left-sided tube by clamping the connecting tube to the right lung proximal to the right suction port and attaching a small tube (i.e., intravenous extension tubing) to the open right suction port (by appropriate adapters) (Fig. 21-14). The free end of this tube is submerged in a beaker of water. When the left lung is statically inflated to any pressure considered necessary, and the left endobronchial cuff is not sealed, air will enter the left lung as well as escape out from around the unsealed left cuff, up the right lumen to the small connecting tube and bubble through the beaker of water (Fig. 21-14, *B*). If the left endobronchial cuff is sealed, no bubbles should be

---

BOX 21-2   Complications of double-lumen tubes

1. Malpositioning
2. Tracheobronchial-tree disruption
3. Traumatic laryngitis
4. Suturing of double-lumen tube to intrathoracic structure

BOX 21-3   Endobronchial-cuff considerations to minimize tracheobronchial wall damage (disruption)

1. Be particularly cautious in patients with bronchial-wall abnormalities.
2. Pick an appropriately sized tube.
3. Be certain tube is not malpositioned.* Use fiberoptic bronchoscopy to confirm the position of the double-lumen tube (especially if N_2O is introduced into the inspired gases).
4. Avoid overinflation of endobronchial cuff.*
5. Deflate endobronchial cuff during turning of patient.
6. Inflate endobronchial cuff slowly.
7. Inflate endobronchial cuff with inspired gases.
8. Do not allow tube to move during turning.*

*Most important considerations.

---

observed passing through the beaker of water (Fig. 21-14, *A*). Following demonstration of functional lung separation, the right connecting tube is unclamped, the right suction port is closed, and ventilation to both lungs is resumed. To test for lung separation with the pressure gradient across the endobronchial balloon reversed, the left airway connecting tube is clamped proximal to the left suction port, the left suction port is opened to the beaker of water via the small tube, the right lung is statically inflated to any desired pressure, and the absence or presence of air bubbles in the beaker of water is noted. It should be remembered that even though the left endobronchial cuff may be adequately sealed, it is possible that during these maneuvers compression of the nonventilated lung by the ventilated lung may initially cause some small amount of bubbling in the beaker, which will cease with repeated inflation of the ventilated lung (no bubbles should be seen following several inflations).[46,47] The absence of air flow from the nonventilated-lung suction port is a very simple but sensitive indicator of functional separation of the two lungs. It is possible that a new capnographic method for determining the seal of a bronchial-blocker cuff (see section IV A5) will prove to also be useful for determining endobronchial-cuff seal.

G. COMPLICATIONS OF DOUBLE-LUMEN ENDOTRACHEAL TUBES

In addition to an impediment to arterial oxygenation that is inherent in the use of double-lumen endotracheal tubes for one-lung anesthesia, the tubes themselves are occasionally the cause of other serious complications (Box 21-2). Many of the complications reported in the literature involved the use of the Carlen's tube, which reflects, in part, the long history of the clinical use of this tube. However, as experience with the new disposable polyvinylchloride DLTs increases, so do the number and type of complications associated with this tube, especially tracheobronchial-tree disruption.

In a group of 200 patients in whom the Carlen's tube was used, a 1.5% incidence of traumatic laryngitis occurred, which was probably due to malposition of the carinal hook at the time of intubation.[55] Incorrect intraoperative positioning of the tube was encountered

in at least six patients in this prefiberoptic bronchoscopy series and was felt to be responsible for one intraoperative death. Another death that occurred during the use of a Carlen's tube during pneumonectomy was caused by the inadvertent suturing of a pulmonary vessel to the tube.[56] The possibility of a suture through the endotracheal tube should be considered whenever excessive resistance to extubation is encountered; the consideration of this complication may warrant reexploration of the chest. The possibility of this complication occurring during pneumonectomy should be minimized if an opposite-sided double-lumen endotracheal tube is used or if the double-lumen endotracheal tube is withdrawn into the trachea just before the bronchus is clamped.

The most frequent serious complication is disruption of the tracheobronchial tree, which most often occurs in the posterior membranous wall. The vast majority of significant airway injuries usually present at operation with subcutaneous emphysema, pneumomediastinum and pneumothorax, and perhaps, cardiovascular instability and hemoptysis. They may also occur shortly after the trachea is extubated, with the additional symptoms of dyspnea, tachycardia, persistent cough, and hemoptysis. There are reports of patients showing symptoms up to 24 hours after their tracheal injury.

In a series of approximately 2700 thoracic procedures in which a red rubber Carlen's tube was used, five cases of traumatic tracheobronchial rupture were discovered.[57] In three cases the rupture was noted intraoperatively and in the other two it was discovered early in the postoperative period. All patients underwent successful direct repair of the injuries. The authors suggested that factors leading to this injury included the use of inappropriately sized DLTs, tube malpositioning, and rapid and excessive inflation of tube cuffs (Box 21-3).

These reports emphasize that postoperative bronchoscopy should be performed to rule out the diagnosis of tracheobronchial rupture when an unexplained serious pneumothorax or pneumomediastinum persists after thoracotomy.

Bronchial rupture has also occurred with the use of the red rubber Robertshaw double-lumen endotracheal tube. An intraoperative diagnosis of bronchial rupture was made by the detection of mediastinal bubbles and subsequent direct inspection of the left bronchus; intraoperative repair resulted in an uneventful recovery.[58] The authors suggest that this complication can be avoided by proper selection of tube size, deflation of the endobronchial cuff prior to turning the patient to the lateral decubitus position, and checking the integrity of the previously intubated bronchus at the time of testing the bronchial stump for leaks (Box 21-3). Obviously, great care must be taken when moving the patient from the supine to the lateral decubitus position to prevent tube movement, which can cause not only tube malposition but also tracheobronchial-tree damage (Box 21-3).

Bronchial rupture has also occurred with the use of the red rubber White DLT.[59] In this case of right mainstem bronchial rupture, nitrous oxide diffusion into the right endobronchial cuff causing excessive cuff volumes was believed to be the cause. The authors, therefore, recommend that the cuffs be inflated with a sample of the inspired mixture of gases rather than room air, or that cuff pressures be monitored so that variation in cuff pressure can be observed and corrected (Box 21-3). As a simple method of monitoring cuff pressures and dealing with excessive cuff volumes and pressure, the tension in the pilot balloons to the cuffs can be periodically palpated and gas removed from the cuffs if the tension appears to be increasing (same standard of practice as with single-lumen tubes) (Box 21-3). The authors also noted that bronchial rupture is more likely to occur in patients with congenital abnormalities of the bronchus, weakness of the bronchial wall caused by infiltration of tumor, infection, poor-quality tissue (sepsis, alcoholism, drug abuse), or distortion of the bronchial tree by enlarged mediastinal lymph glands or extrabronchial tumors (Box 21-3). In addition, the authors said they believed that the bevel of the tube or carinal hook could potentially dissect underneath the mucosa. Finally, they correctly warned of the dangers of advancing the stylet beyond the vocal cords and of using force to further advance the tube whenever resistance was encountered.

A common thought in these reports is that excessive air volume and pressure in the bronchial balloon may be a major factor in the genesis of tracheobronchial-tree tears following DLT insertion. Consequently, this complication was the logical inspiration for the development of clear plastic, tissue implantable double-lumen tubes

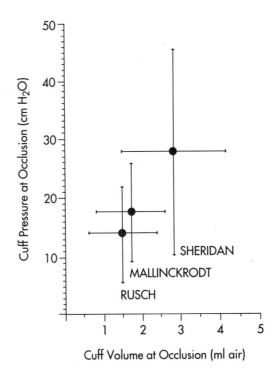

Fig. 21-15. Mean ± SD intracuff volume and pressure during bronchial seal for one-lung ventilation in 48 patients for various brands of double-lumen tubes. (From Slinger P, Chripko D: *Anesthesiology* 77:1233, 1992 [abstract]).

with high volume-low pressure cuffs (as it was the earlier inspiration for single-lumen tubes). The mean ± SD intracuff volume and pressure for the Sheridan, Mallinckrodt, and Rusch left-sided DLTs during clinical one-lung ventilation (n = 48 patients) at peak inspiratory pressures of 35 to 40 cm H_2O are 2.8 ± 1.3 ml and 27.9 ± 17.7 cm H_2O, 1.7 ± 0.9 ml and 17.6 ± 8.5 cm H_2O and 1.5 ± 0.9 ml and 14.1 ± 8.6 cm H_2O, respectively (see Fig. 21-15).[60] These pressures are less than levels associated with mucosal ischemia.[61] Thus, when the tracheobronchial tree is inspected with an FOB after DLT insertion, much less mucosal damage is caused by the tissue-implantable, low-pressure cuffed tubes than with the red rubber, high-pressure cuffed tubes.[62] However, in spite of these expected findings, there have been at least four reports of tracheobronchial-tree disruption following the use of the tissue-implantable, low-pressure cuffed DLTs,[63-66] and the precautions listed in Box 21-3 must be considered even with the modern DLTs. One of the reasons the cuffs of the polyvinylchloride DLTs cause tracheobronchial-tree damage is that the low-pressure cuff assumes the high-pressure characteristics of red rubber, cuffed tubes with volumes greater than 3 ml.[10,66] Of course, as with all medical instruments, manufacturing defects may always be unexpectedly encountered.[67]

Two other relevant predisposing conditions for tracheobronchial-tree damage are possible. First, esoph-

UNIVENT BRONCHIAL BLOCKER TUBE

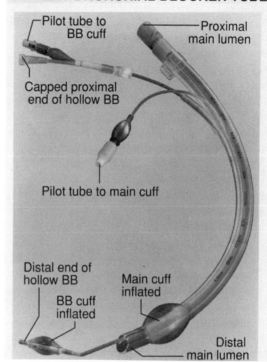

Fig. 21-16. Univent single-lumen tube and bronchial-blocker system.

ageal surgery may cause a specific hazard of tracheobronchial-tree damage by a DLT in that dissection of the upper and cervical esophagus away from the posterior membranous trachea, when it contains an inflated cuff, increases the risk of tracheal tears. This increased risk may be secondary to undermining the support and vascular supply of the membranous trachea during dissection.[68] Second, chronic obstructive airway disease has been suggested as a possible risk factor in tracheal trauma. Emphysema causes the tracheal rings to open and the trachea itself to enlarge. This results in an increase in the size of the membranous portion of the tracheal wall. This is inevitably the portion damaged during intubation. The increase in surface area, along with attenuation of this already vulnerable area, could explain its increased propensity for damage.

H. RELATIVE CONTRAINDICATIONS TO USE OF DOUBLE-LUMEN ENDOTRACHEAL TUBES

There are several types of patients in whom lung separation by a DLT may be relatively contraindicated because insertion of the DLT is either difficult or dangerous (Box 21-4). These include patients who have a full stomach and in whom DLT intubation might be considered time-consuming (risk of aspiration); patients who have a lesion (airway stricture[69,70] or endoluminal tumor) present somewhere along the pathway of the DLT that prevents proper positioning and/or could be traumatized; small patients in whom a 35-French tube is too large to fit comfortably through the larynx and for whom a 28-French tube is considered too small; patients whose upper-airway anatomy precludes either safe insertion of the tube or indicates that a required intraoperative change from a double-lumen tube to a single-lumen tube may be difficult (large tongue, recessed jaw, prominent teeth, bull neck, restricted head and neck motion, or anterior larynx); extremely critically ill patients who have a single-lumen tube already in place and will not tolerate being taken off mechanical ventilation and PEEP (even for the short period of time of one minute); and patients having some combination of all these problems. Under these circumstances, it is still possible to separate the lungs safely and adequately by using a single-lumen tube and fiberoptic bronchoscopic placement of a bronchial blocker or by fiberoptic bronchoscopic placement of a single-lumen tube in a mainstem bronchus.

IV. BRONCHIAL BLOCKERS (WITH SINGLE-LUMEN ENDOTRACHEAL TUBES)

Lung separation can be effectively achieved with the use of a single-lumen tube (SLT) and a fiberoptically placed bronchial blocker (see Figs. 21-16 through 21-23 on pp. 432 to 437). This is often necessary in children, since double-lumen endotracheal tubes are too large to be used in these patients. The smallest DLT available is a 26 French and may be potentially used in patients in the range of 9 to 11 years and weighing 25 to 35 kg. The bronchial blocker most widely used for adults is the movable bronchial blocker that is contained in and is an integral part of the Univent SLT system (Fuji Systems Corp., Tokyo, Japan) (Fig. 21-16).[71-77] The physiology of one-lung ventilation produced by bronchial blockade is

Insertion and Positioning of Univent Bronchial Blocker (BB) System

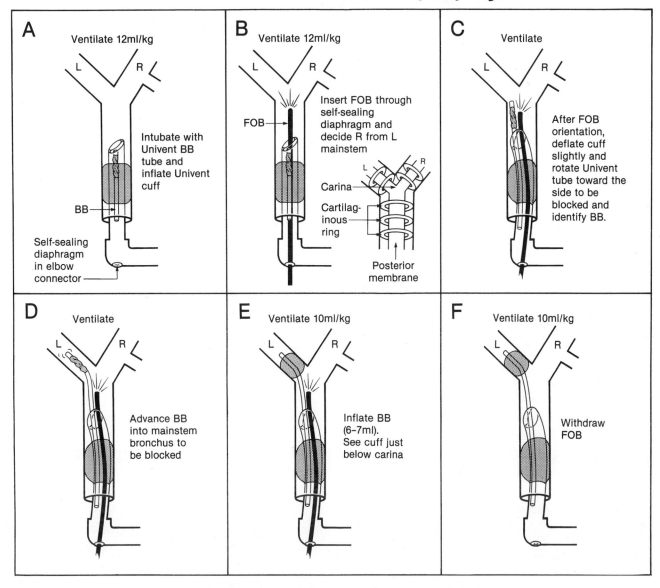

Fig. 21-17. The sequential steps of the fiberoptic-aided method of inserting and positioning the Univent bronchial blocker in the left mainstem bronchus is illustrated. See text for full explanation. One- and two-lung ventilation is achieved by simply inflating and deflating, respectively, the bronchial-blocker balloon. (*L,* left; *R,* right; *FOB,* fiberoptic bronchoscope.) (From Benumof JL: *Anesthesia for thoracic surgery,* Philadelphia, 1987, W.B. Saunders Co.)

identical to that produced by clamping one of the lumens of a DLT.

A. THE UNIVENT BRONCHIAL-BLOCKER (BB) TUBE

1. Description of the Univent bronchial-blocker tube

The Univent bronchial-blocker tube is a Silastic SLT (6 to 9 mm ID, 31 to 37 French) of normal configuration that has a separate, small lumen along the internal anterior concave wall (i.e., at the 12 o'clock position when the tube is held with the natural concavity facing anteriorly) (Figs. 21-16 and 21-17,*A*). The small lumen on the anterior concave side of the tube, in turn, contains a small, hollow lumen catheter (2 mm ID, approximately 17 gauge) that has a cuff at the end of it; this secondary movable (by 8 cm beyond the tip of the SLT), retractable,

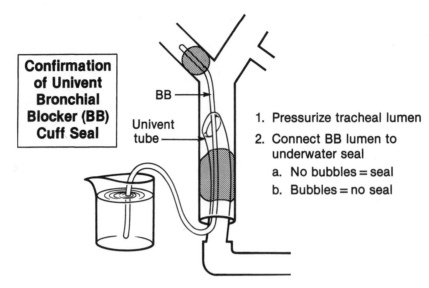

Fig. 21-18. Positive pressure ventilation–air bubble underwater method for determining just-seal volume of bronchial-blocker cuff is the same as for an endobronchial cuff on a double-lumen tube (compare with Fig. 21-14).

catheter serves as a bronchial blocker when the cuff is inflated (and, of course, allows two-lung ventilation when the cuff is deflated). The extra bronchial-blocker channel adds significantly to the anterior-posterior outside diameter so that for a given inside diameter, the outside diameter of the Univent tube is greater than an equivalent internal-diameter SLT and the anterior-posterior diameter is greater than the lateral diameter (Table 21-2 on p. 437). The cuff of the bronchial blocker has a natural volume of 2 ml that creates a spherical or ellipsoid shape with a midcuff diameter of 5 mm; intracuff volume greater than 2 ml converts the cuff from a low-pressure cuff to high-pressure cuff (see section IV A3). However, at the time of this writing, the natural volume of the cuff was being increased to 3 ml.[78]

2. Insertion of the Univent tube and positioning of the bronchial blocker

The tube is inserted in the following manner. First, the SLT along with the bronchial blocker (in the fully retracted position) is inserted as a unit into the trachea (Fig. 21-17, *A*). The cuff on the main endotracheal tube lumen is inflated and the patient is ventilated and oxygenated (Fig. 21-17, *A*). An FOB is inserted through a self-sealing diaphragm in the elbow connector to the SLT while ventilation is maintained around the FOB (but within the SLT) (Fig. 21-17, *B*). The right and left mainstem bronchi are identified (by noting the relationship of the mainstem bronchi to the posterior membrane and the anterior cartilaginous rings [Fig. 21-17, *B*]), the tip of the bronchial blocker is located (by moving the bronchial blocker in and out just beyond the end of its own and the main lumen of the Univent tube [Fig. 21-17,

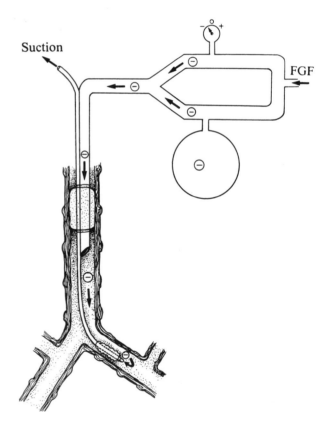

Fig. 21-19. When the bronchial cuff is deflated, negative pressure applied at proximal end of the lumen of the blocker is freely transmitted to reservoir bag of breathing system. *FGF,* fresh gas flow. (From Hannallah M: *Anesthesiology* 75:165, 1991, *and* Hannallah MS, Benumof JL: *Anesth Analg* 75:784, 1992.)

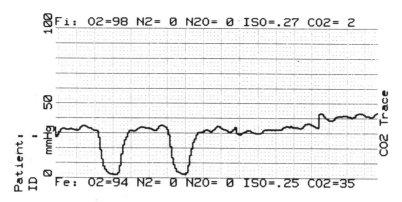

Fig. 21-20. Capnograph tracing showing normal respiratory waveform changing to a straight line as bronchial seal occurs. (From Essig K, Freeman JA: *Anesthesiology* 76:478, 1992.)

A.   Lung Separation With Single Lumen Tube and Left Lung Bronchial Blocker Inside of Single Lumen Tube

B.   Lung Separation With Single Lumen Tube and Right Lung Bronchial Blocker Inside of Single Lumen Tube

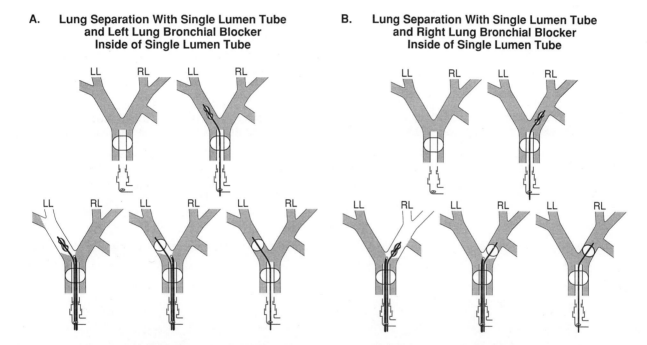

Fig. 21-21. Sequence for lung separation with single-lumen tube and bronchial blocker within the single-lumen tube. **A,** Left-lung bronchial blocker. **B,** Right-lung bronchial blocker. The bronchial blocker (Fogarty embolectomy catheter) is placed in the correct mainstem bronchus under fiberoptic vision. (From Benumof JL: *Anesthesia for thoracic surgery,* Philadelphia, 1987, W.B. Saunders Co.)

C]). The bronchial-blocker cuff is colored blue and is easy to see. It will be seen that the bronchial blocker will almost always enter the right mainstem bronchus if it is simply pushed in (and the main SLT is not turned). If the left mainstem bronchus is to be blocked, the bronchial blocker should be laterally rotated at its distal end (because of the small angle bend at the tip of the bronchial blocker, the tip will flip from side to side or right to left and vice versa) by twirling the proximal end in the fingers. Additionally, the main SLT can be turned

90 degrees to the left (counterclockwise) so that the concavity of the tube is facing toward the left side (Fig. 21-17, *C*), and vise versa for the right side, if necessary. The bronchial blocker is then advanced into the mainstem bronchus under direct vision (Fig. 21-17, *D*). Attempting to advance the bronchial blocker blindly into the appropriate mainstem bronchus (particularly the left) will be unsuccessful 87% of the time and repeated attempts may cause excoriation of the tracheal mucosa.[73] In fact, blindly pushing the somewhat stiff bronchial

blocker may result in perforation of the tracheobronchial tree and tension pneumothorax.[74] The balloon is inflated so that the cephalad surface of the balloon is just below the tracheal carina (Fig. 21-17, *E*) (so that the upper lobe of the blocked lung may also distend if CPAP is applied to the blocked lung) and the FOB is then withdrawn (Fig. 21-17, *F*).

3. Advantages/noteworthy positive attributes of the Univent bronchial-blocker tube system

The Univent bronchial-blocker tube has six important attributes that require special mention (Box 21-5). First, and foremost, the degree of difficulty in inserting the Univent tube is equivalent to a standard SLT and therefore in many instances will be an easier and quicker way to separate the lungs to obtain simple one-lung ventilation (compared to a DLT).[75,77] The Univent tube may thus be preferable, for example, when difficult intubation is anticipated and for a patient who is being given anticoagulants. Second, the patient can be continuously ventilated while the bronchial blocker is being placed into a mainstem bronchus, and the bronchial blocker can be placed into a mainstem bronchus just as easily when the patient is in the lateral decubitus position as in the supine position. Third, the Univent tube may be left in situ for postoperative mechanical ventilation and therefore the risk of a potentially difficult tube change (e.g., from a DLT to an SLT) avoided, provided the postanesthesia care unit and the intensive care unit personnel are instructed in the design and function of the Univent tube, particularly the ventilatory consequence of inflating the bronchial-blocker cuff when the cuff is just distal to the main lumen (i.e., the main lumen will be obstructed).[79] Fourth, and similarly, the Univent tube may be left in situ if a patient is turned from the supine to the prone position midway through a surgical procedure (a common occurrence with surgery on the thoracic spine). Fifth, the unique characteristic of a movable endobronchial blocker permits the Univent endotracheal tube to create selective, partial (a lobe), or total collapse of the targeted lung.[80] The capability of selectively blocking lung segments is extremely impor-

A. **Lung Separation With Single Lumen Tube and Left Lung Bronchial Blocker Outside of Single Lumen Tube**

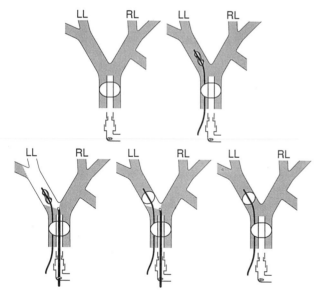

B. **Lung Separation With Single Lumen Tube and Right Lung Bronchial Blocker Outside of Single Lumen Tube**

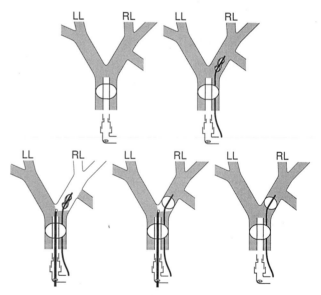

Fig. 21-22. How to separate two lungs with a single-lumen tube, fiberoptic bronchoscope, and a left-lung (**A**) and a right-lung (**B**) bronchial blocker that is outside of the single-lumen tube. Sequence of events is as follows: Single-lumen tube is inserted, and patient is ventilated (upper left diagram, **A** and **B**). Bronchial blocker is passed alongside the indwelling endotracheal tube (upper right diagram, **A** and **B**). Fiberoptic bronchoscope is passed through a self-sealing diaphragm in elbow connector to the endotracheal tube and is used to place bronchial blocker into the appropriate mainstem bronchus under direct vision (lower left diagram, **A** and **B**). Balloon on the bronchial blocker is also inflated under direct vision and is positioned just below the tracheal carina (lower middle diagram, **A** and **B**). During the lower panel sequence (insertion and use of fiberoptic bronchoscope), the self-sealing diaphragm allows patient to continue to be ventilated with positive-pressure ventilation (around the fiberoptic bronchoscope but within the lumens of the endotracheal tube). *LL,* left lung; *RL,* right lung. (From Benumof JL: *Anesthesia for thoracic surgery,* Philadelphia, 1987, W.B. Saunders Co.)

tant in cases of isolated pulmonary hemorrhage. "Partial" versus "total" one-lung ventilation may allow for an improvement in Pao$_2$ in cases of intraoperative hypoxemia during thoracic operations. Finally, it should be noted that it is possible to apply CPAP to the nonventilated operative lung (see Chapter 11) through the lumen of the bronchial blocker;[81] therefore, the Univent tube provides the same best solution to hypoxemia during one-lung ventilation as does a DLT. In fact, except for independent unilateral intermittent positive pressure ventilation and suctioning, all selective differential lung functions possible with a DLT are possible with a Univent bronchial-blocker tube.

4. Potential limitations of the Univent bronchial-blocker tube system and solutions to the limitations

There are several distinct limitations to the Univent bronchial-blocker tube system but fortunately all have relatively simple remedies (Table 21-3). First, the small lumen of the bronchial blocker results in slow inflation of the lung if gases are just insufflated (e.g., at a flow rate

of 10 L/min a lung will require at least 20 seconds to reach total lung capacity) or pushed through the lumen by conventional positive pressure. The operative lung may be made to expand rapidly if the bronchial-blocker cuff is deflated (the operative lung will expand with one positive pressure breath from the main single lumen) or one very short (e.g., <0.5 seconds) wall oxygen-powered 20- to 30-psi jet ventilation (reduced from 50 psi) is administered. However, connection of the bronchial-blocker lumen to a jet ventilator is potentially dangerous (i.e., may cause barotrauma) because the lung can expand extremely rapidly. It is of paramount importance that the anesthesiologist directly observe the lung and that the ventilation be very short or the psi limited to 20 to 30 psi by an additional in-line regulator.

Second, and also because the bronchial-blocker lumen is small, the lung will deflate slowly when blocked. This is easily remedied by deflating the bronchial-blocker cuff (which reestablishes continuity between the operative lung and the main single lumen), disconnecting the patient from the ventilator, and leaving the endotracheal tube open to air while the surgeon gently compresses the lung to evacuate air from the operative lung through the main single lumen. After the lung is thus fully collapsed, the blocker balloon is inflated and ventilation resumed.[75,76] Alternatively, the lumen of the

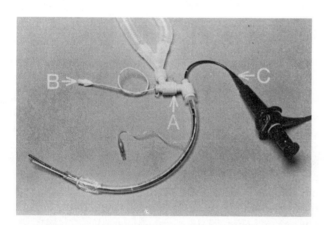

Fig. 21-23. Two elbow connectors *(A)* are shown interposed between anesthesia circuit and endotracheal tube with Fogarty catheter *(B)* inserted through one self-sealing diaphragm and fiberoptic bronchoscope *(C)* inserted through the other self-sealing diaphragm. (From Larson CE, Gaisor TA: *Anesth Analg* 71:311, 1990.)

BOX 21-5 Advantages/noteworthy positive attributes of the Univent bronchial-blocker tube (relative to a double-lumen tube and other bronchial blockers)

1. Easier to insert and properly position
2. Can properly position during continuous ventilation and when patient is in the lateral decubitus position
3. Do not need to change tube for postoperative mechanical ventilation
4. Do not need to change tube intraoperatively when turning patient from supine to prone position
5. Selective blockade of some lobes of each lung
6. Can apply nonventilated operative lung CPAP

Table 21-2. Comparative tube sizes

Univent ID, mm	Univent FG of single main lumen (marked on tube)	Univent OD, mm lateral/AP	Equivalent SLT OD, mm	Equivalent DLT, FG
7.5	31	11.0/12.0	9.6	35
8.0	33	11.5/13.0	10.9	37
8.5	35	12.0/13.5	11.6	39
9.0	37	12.5/14.0	12.2	41

DLT, double-lumen tube, Bronchocath; *SLT,* single-lumen tube, Shiley; *AP,* anteroposterior; *ID,* internal diameter; *OD,* outside diameter; *FG,* French gauge. FG = OD in mm × 3. The AP diameter is greater than the lateral diameter due to the presence of bronchial-blocker lumen. (Data from MacGillvray RG: *Anaesthesia* 43:687, 1988 and Slinger P: *J Cardiothorac Vasc Anesth* 7:18, 1993.)

Table 21-3. Limitations to the use of the Univent bronchial-blocker tube and solutions to the limitations

Limitation	Solution
1. Slow inflation time	1. (a) Deflate bronchial-blocker cuff and administer a positive-pressure breath through the main single lumen; (b) carefully administer one short high-pressure (20-30 psi) jet ventilation.
2. Slow deflation time	2. (a) Deflate bronchial-blocker cuff and compress and evacuate the lung through the main single lumen; (b) apply suction to bronchial-blocker lumen.
3. Blockage of bronchial-blocker lumen by blood or pus	3. Suction, wire stylet, and then suction.
4. High-pressure cuff	4. Use just-seal volume of air.
5. Intraoperative leak in bronchial-blocker cuff	5. Make sure bronchial blocker cuff is subcarinal, increase inflation volume, and rearrange surgical field.

bronchial blocker may be connected to the suction apparatus while the cuff is inflated; a normal amount of wall suction greatly facilitates lung collapse.

Third, and also because the bronchial-blocker lumen is small, the lumen is relatively easily blocked by blood and/or pus. High suction will usually clear the lumen of these materials and total blockage by inspissated secretions can be broken up by a wire stylet.

Fourth, the Univent bronchial blocker behaves as a high-pressure cuff when intracuff volume is less than 2 ml (the resting volume of the cuff). Also, it may be expected to have an intracuff pressure between 150 and 250 mm Hg and a transmural pressure (intracuff pressure within the airway minus intracuff pressure outside of the airway [free in the room]) between 50 and 60 mm Hg when intracuff volumes of 4 to 6 ml are used to seal airways of 12- to 18-mm diameter against the usual proximal airway pressures.[82,83] Thus, the order of usual bronchial-cuff pressures are left-sided polyvinylchloride DLT less than right-sided polyvinylchloride DLT less than Univent bronchial-blocker cuff less than red rubber DLT.[84] These findings underscore the need to inflate the bronchial-blocker cuff with a just-seal volume of air (see next section for three alternative methods to obtain a just-seal volume).

Fifth, the Univent bronchial blocker has been reported to have a minor leak during surgery on occasion (25% in one series).[73] This is not understandable in view of experiments that show that the Univent bronchial-blocker cuff seals within normal-sized mainstem bronchi against proximal airway pressures as great as 100 cm H_2O with inflation volumes that are within the manufacturer's recommendation.[83] Consequently, if (1) less than a 6- to 7-ml intracuff volume has been used, (2) the bronchial-blocker cuff is completely subcarinal (determined by fiberoptic bronchoscopy) and intact, and (3) an intraoperative leak is present, then the intracuff volume should be increased. If (1) an adequate cuff inflation volume has been used (the bronchial blocker can be seen fiberoptically to fill the mainstem bronchus in question), (2) the bronchial-blocker cuff is completely subcarinal (determined fiberoptically) and intact, and (3) an intraoperative leak develops, then the relationship between the mainstem bronchus and the bronchial-blocker cuff may no longer be a simple matter of a sphere or ellipsoid shape being inflated within a cylinder. Under these circumstances the surgeon may need to rearrange the surgical field so that the mainstem bronchus and bronchial-blocker cuff are less distorted. Finally, the addition of the lumen for the bronchial blocker results in an endotracheal tube that has a large outside anterior-posterior diameter relative to its inside diameter.

5. Methods to obtain a just-seal volume in the bronchial-blocker cuff

There are three methods to obtain a just-seal volume of air in the bronchial-blocker cuff. The first method is the same as the one that has already been described for obtaining a just-seal volume of air in the endobronchial cuff of a DLT and consists of pressurizing the main single lumen until air ceases to escape from the bronchial-blocker lumen (detected by connecting the bronchial-blocker lumen to a catheter that is submerged beneath the surface of a beaker of water; when air bubbles cease to come out, the bronchial-blocker cuff has sealed) (Fig. 21-18, compare with Fig. 21-14).

The second method is opposite in concept and uses the negative pressure of the suction apparatus.[21,22] After correct placement of the tube in the trachea and the blocker in the bronchus, the tracheal cuff is inflated in the usual manner, and the patient's lungs are ventilated with 100% oxygen. Ventilation then is discontinued and a fresh gas flow of 5 to 6 L/min is delivered to the system. The reservoir bag will then fully distend (the airway pressure relief valve may need adjustment to distend the bag). Using appropriate connections, negative pressure is applied to the proximal end of the lumen of the blocker. With the bronchial cuff deflated, the distal end of the lumen of the blocker will be freely connected with the trachea and the circle system, the volume of oxygen suctioned out of the system will be more than the volume delivered to it, and the reservoir bag will then begin to deflate (Fig. 21-19). At this point, the bronchial cuff is inflated slowly with 1-ml increments of air, and the breathing bag is watched carefully until it ceases to deflate. This will indicate that there is no longer any communication between the tip of the blocker, where the negative pressure is being applied, and the rest of the breathing system. Complete sealing of the bronchus will have been accomplished at this point. This is confirmed by auscultation of the breath sounds initially and later by observation of the lung's actual collapse, with continued suction, when the chest is opened. Comparison of the first two methods in the same patient show that they yield nearly identical results.[21,22]

The third method appears promising and uses capnography.[23] End-tidal CO_2 analyzers draw gas samples from the anesthesia breathing circuit via tubing terminating distally in a standard Luer-lock male connector that inserts into a female port in the breathing circuit. The male connector also attaches to the female port at the proximal end of the Univent's bronchial blocker. The tracing from a gas analyzer, connected to the blocker with its cuff deflated, shows a typical respiratory waveform. As the blocker's cuff is steadily inflated, a point is reached at which the respiratory waveform abruptly ceases and a straight line is seen, indicating that lung isolation has occurred (Fig. 21-20). CO_2 concentration remains near its end-tidal value until the blocked lung has collapsed, and then rapidly decreases. The strengths of this method include simplicity, repeatability, and ability to ventilate the unblocked lung continuously throughout the procedure.

6. Firm clinical indications for use of the Univent bronchial-blocker system

There are several clinical situations in which the use of the Univent bronchial-blocker tube is relatively indicated. First, whenever it is anticipated that postoperative ventilation will be necessary (e.g., poor pulmonary function preoperatively, anticipated lung damage or massive fluid or blood infusion intraoperatively, anticipated long case), use of the Univent bronchial-blocker tube for lung separation may avoid a risky postoperative DLT-to-SLT change. Second, and similarly, use of the Univent bronchial-blocker tube will avoid a potentially dangerous DLT-to-SLT change in cases of surgery on the thoracic spine where a thoracotomy on a patient in a supine or lateral decubitus position is followed by surgery in the prone position. Third, a very severely distorted airway may prevent successful placement of a DLT, whereas such distortion may have much less of an effect on the proper placement of the Univent tube. Finally, but least predictable and compelling, are situations in which both lungs may need to be blocked (e.g., bilateral operations, trauma cases where a need for a thoracotomy and lung separation and/or one-lung ventilation may arise, indecisive surgeon).

B. BRONCHIAL BLOCKERS THAT ARE INDEPENDENT OF A SINGLE-LUMEN TUBE

Bronchial blockers may also be passed independently of the SLT. Independent bronchial blockers that are balloon-tipped luminal catheters (e.g., Fogarty embolectomy, Foley, and pulmonary-artery catheters) have the advantage of allowing suctioning and injection of oxygen down the central lumen (as with the Univent bronchial-blocker tube). However, most independent bronchial blockers have the disadvantage of sometimes requiring rigid bronchoscopy for placement, and, because they have high-pressure spherically inflating balloons, there is a tendency for them to back out of the bronchus into the trachea.

The independent bronchial blocker most often used for adults is a Fogarty occlusion embolectomy catheter with a 3-ml balloon.[85] The Fogarty embolectomy catheter comes with a stylet in place so that it is possible to place a curvature at the distal tip to facilitate entry into the larynx and either mainstem bronchus by twirling the proximal end. If no endotracheal tube is in place, the operator exposes the larynx and places an SLT with a high-volume cuff in the trachea. The Fogarty catheter is then placed either inside[86,87] or alongside the SLT (Figs. 21-21 and 21-22). Placement of the Fogarty catheter inside the SLT can be greatly facilitated by use of two elbow connectors with self-sealing diaphragms that are connected in series with the anesthesia circuit attached to the proximal end of the proximal elbow connector (Fig. 21-23).[86] The distal end of the distal elbow connector is connected to the patient's single-lumen endotracheal tube. The Fogarty catheter can be easily introduced through the diaphragm of one of the elbow connectors while the other diaphragm allows insertion of an FOB that is used to verify correct placement of the catheter in the mainstem bronchus. In either case (bronchial blocker inside or outside the SLT), a fiberoptic bronchoscope is passed down to the end of the SLT through a self-sealing diaphragm in the elbow connector (which permits continued positive-pressure ventilation around the FOB), and the Fogarty catheter is visualized below the tip of the single-lumen tube. The proximal end of the bronchial blocker is then twirled in the fingertips until the distal tip locates in the desired mainstem bronchus. The catheter balloon is then inflated under direct visualization, and the FOB is withdrawn through the self-sealing diaphragm. The self-sealing diaphragm in the elbow connector containing the bronchial blocker should be made airtight. The bronchial blocker within the SLT technique may be used with a tracheostomy.[87]

For bronchial blockade in very small children (10 kg or less), a Fogarty embolectomy catheter with a balloon capacity of 0.5 ml or a Swan-Ganz catheter (1-ml balloon) should be used.[88] Of course these catheters

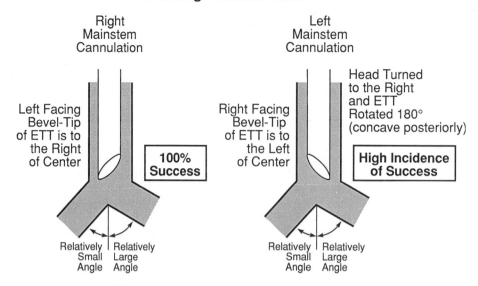

**Cannulation of a Mainstem Bronchus
with a Single Lumen Tube**

Fig. 21-24. Turning face of bevel of endotracheal tube to the side opposite mainstem bronchus to be cannulated places the tip of tracheal tube off center toward the side to be cannulated.[45] In addition, rotation of endotracheal tube 180 degrees so that natural concavity of tube faces posteriorly and turning face/head to right results in cannulation of left mainstem bronchus a high percentage of the time (92%).[43]

have to be positioned under direct vision; a FOB method, as depicted in Figure 21-22, is perfectly acceptable except the FOB outside diameter must be approximately 2 mm to fit inside the endotracheal tube. Otherwise, the bronchial blocker must be situated with a rigid bronchoscope. Pediatric patients of intermediate size will require intermediately sized occlusion catheters and a judgment on the mode of placement (i.e., rigid versus fiberoptic bronchoscope).

Disadvantages of the independent bronchial blockers compared with double-lumen endotracheal tube lung separation include the inability to suction extensively and/or to ventilate the lung distal to the blocker, increased placement time (as well as compared to the Univent tube), and the definite need for a fiberoptic or rigid bronchoscope. In addition, if a mainstem bronchial blocker backs out into the trachea, the seal between the two lungs will be lost, and two catastrophic complications may occur. First, if the bronchial blocker was being used to seal off a fluid (blood or pus) in one lung, then both lungs may become contaminated with the fluid. Second, the trachea will be at least partially obstructed by the blocker, and ventilation will be greatly impaired. Therefore, bronchial blockage requires that the anesthesiologist continuously and intensively monitor the compliance and breath sounds of the ventilated lung.

V. ENDOBRONCHIAL INTUBATION WITH SINGLE-LUMEN TUBES

An SLT may be electively placed in a mainstem bronchus, thereby blocking off the contralateral lung and permitting ventilation of just the ipsilateral lung. If the SLT has to be pushed in blindly, it will enter nearly 100% of the time the right mainstem bronchus when the concavity of the SLT points anteriorly (i.e., the way it is usually held) and the patient's head is in a normal straight-ahead midposition. The SLT will enter the left mainstem bronchus 92% of the time when the tube's concavity is facing posteriorly (180-degree rotation from the usual way it is held) and the head is turned to the right.[89] The reason the SLT enters the right and left mainstem bronchi when the concavity of the tube is anterior or posterior facing, respectively, is because the bevel is left and right facing, respectively (i.e., left-facing bevel enters the right mainstem bronchus and a right-facing bevel enters the left mainstem bronchus) (Fig. 21-24).[90] Unfortunately, blindly placing an SLT into a mainstem bronchus incurs a high risk of blocking the upper lobe of the intubated lung and causing hypoxemia.[91,92] However, if the SLT can be placed proximal to either the right or left upper lobe either with bronchoscopic vision or by surgical manipulation, then the resulting one-lung ventilation gas exchange will be the same as expected for one-lung ventilation with a DLT or with an appropriately placed bronchial blocker.[91,92]

In adults with symptoms including hemoptysis, endobronchial intubation with an SLT is often the easiest, quickest way of effectively separating the two lungs, especially if the left lung is bleeding. If the left lung is bleeding, one can simply take an uncut single-lumen endotracheal tube and advance it inward until moderate resistance is felt (Fig. 21-25, *A*). In the vast majority of

Single Lumen Tube: Lung Bleeding

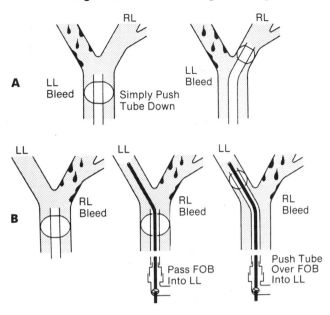

Fig. 21-25. How to separate two lungs with single-lumen tube in presence of massive lung bleeding. When left lung is bleeding **(A)**, an uncut single-lumen tube may simply be inserted its full length, and, in vast majority of cases, will enter right mainstem bronchus, thereby effectively sealing right lung from left lung. However, one can expect that cuff of single-lumen tube will obstruct right upper lobe. When the right lung is bleeding **(B)**, a fiberoptic bronchoscope, which is jacketed on its proximal end with an endotracheal tube, can be passed through a self-sealing diaphragm in elbow connector to endotracheal tube (which allows continued positive-pressure breathing) and, if a moment's view of the tracheal carina can be obtained, passed into left mainstem bronchus. Using fiberoptic bronchoscope as a stylet, endoscopist can pass endotracheal tube over fiberoptic bronchoscope into left mainstem bronchus. Fiberoptic bronchoscope is then withdrawn. *LL,* left lung; *RL,* right lung; *FOB,* fiberoptic bronchoscope. (Reproduced from Benumof JL: *Anesthesia for thoracic surgery,* Philadelphia, 1987, W.B. Saunders Co.)

suctioning through the FOB (through the SLT) may be required in order to visualize the tracheal carina (Fig. 21-25, *B*). The SLT can then be passed over the FOB into the left mainstem bronchus, thereby sealing off the bleeding right lung and allowing for selective ventilation of the left lung. Passing the FOB through a self-sealing diaphragm allows for the continuance of positive-pressure ventilation and PEEP around the bronchoscope. However, it should be realized that visualization of the carina may not be possible when the bleeding is copious and that the only hope for the patient may lie in rapid thoracotomy and control of bleeding from within the chest. In addition, under these very adverse conditions conventional passage of a DLT may more rapidly and effectively separate the two lungs than trying to visualize anatomy with an FOB.

VI. CONCLUSION

In summary, double-lumen endotracheal tubes are the method of choice for separating the lungs in most adult patients. If there is any question, the precise location of a double-lumen tube can be determined by fiberoptic bronchoscopy at any time. There are a number of situations in which insertion of a double-lumen tube may be difficult and/or dangerous. Under these circumstances consideration should be given to separating the lungs with a single-lumen tube alone or in combination with a bronchial blocker (e.g., the Univent tube). However, when using a single-lumen tube in a mainstem bronchus or when using a bronchial blocker, ability to suction the operative site and control ventilation is limited. In addition, placement of the single-lumen tube into one or the other mainstem bronchi and the proper placement of a bronchial blocker require fiberoptic bronchoscopy. Therefore, no matter which method of separating the lungs is chosen, there is a real need for the immediate availability of a small-diameter fiberoptic bronchoscope (for checking the position of the double-lumen tube, placing a single-lumen tube in the left mainstem bronchus, and placing a bronchial blocker) that has a suction port (in order to clear secretions and blood from the airway).

patients the SLT will locate in the right mainstem bronchus, thereby blocking off the bleeding left lung and allowing for selective ventilation of just the right lung. Under these circumstances it is very possible that the right upper lobe bronchus will be blocked off as well, resulting in ventilation of just the right middle and lower lobes. Ventilation of just a soiled right lung or ventilation of just the right middle and lower lobes (even if they are unsoiled) incurs the risk of serious hypoxemia due to the very large transpulmonary shunt that is necessarily created by the single lung (and perhaps bilobar) endobronchial intubation/ventilation.

If the right lung is bleeding, an FOB can be passed through a self-sealing diaphragm in the SLT elbow connector and directed into the left mainstem bronchus. Persistent large soft catheter suctioning of the carinal area through the SLT prior to use of the FOB and

REFERENCES

1. Kvetan V, Carlon GC, Howland WS: Acute pulmonary failure in asymmetric lung disease: approach to management, *Crit Care Med* 10:114, 1982.
2. Urschel HC Jr, Razzuk MA: Median sternotomy as a standard approach for pulmonary resection, *Ann Thorac Surg* 41:130, 1986.
3. Anderson HW, Benumof JL: Intrapulmonary shunting during one-lung ventilation and surgical manipulation, *Anesthesiology* 55:377, 1981 (abstract).
4. Thomson DF, Campbell D: Changes in arterial oxygen tension during one-lung anesthesia, *Br J Anaesth* 45:611, 1973.
5. Boysen PG: Pulmonary resection and postoperative pulmonary function, *Chest* 77:718, 1980.
6. Boysen PG, Block AG, Moulder PV: Relationship between

preoperative pulmonary function tests and complications after thoracotomy, *Surg Gynecol Obstet* 152:813, 1981.

7. Westfall SH, Akbarnia BA, Merenda JT et al: Exposure of the anterior spine: technique, complications and results in 85 patients, *Am J Surg* 154:700, 1987.

8. Benumof JL: Management of the difficult airway: with special emphasis on awake tracheal intubation, *Anesthesiology* 75:1087, 1991.

9. Lack JA: Endobronchial tube resistances, *Br J Anaesth* 46:461, 1974.

10. Neto PPR: Bronchial cuff pressure of endobronchial double-lumen tubes, *Anesth Analg* 71:209, 1990.

11. Brodsky JB, Adkins MO, Gaba DM: Bronchial cuff pressures of double-lumen tubes, *Anesth Analg* 69:608, 1989.

12. Magee PT: Endobronchial cuff pressures of double-lumen tubes, *Anesth Analg* 72:265, 1991.

13. Cohen JA, Denisco RA, Richards TS et al: Hazardous placement of a Robertshaw-type endobronchial tube, *Anesth Analg* 65:100, 1986.

14. Maquire DP, Spiro AW: Bronchial obstruction and hypoxia during one-lung ventilation, *Anesthesiology* 66:830, 1987.

15. Hansen TB, Watson CB: Tracheobronchial trauma secondary to a Carlens tube, presented at the Society of Cardiovascular Anesthesiologists fifth annual meeting, 1983 (abstract).

16. Benumof JL, Partridge BL, Salvatierra C, et al: Margin of safety in positioning modern double-lumen endotracheal tubes, *Anesthesiology* 67:729, 1987.

17. Brodsky JB, Benumof JL, Ehrenwerth J, et al: Depth of placement of left double-lumen endobronchial tubes, *Anesth Analg* 73:570, 1991.

18. Simpson PM: Tracheal intubation with a Robertshaw tube via a tracheostomy, *Br J Anaesth* 48:373, 1976.

19. Seed RF, Wedley JR: Tracheal intubation with a Robertshaw tube via a tracheostomy, *Br J Anaesth* 49:639, 1977 (letter).

20. Brodsky JB, Tobler HG, Mark JBD: A double-lumen endobronchial tube for tracheostomies, *Anesthesiology* 74:387, 1991.

21. Hannallah MS: The Univent tube: bronchial cuff inflation, *Anesthesiology* 75:165, 1991.

22. Hannallah MS, Benumof JL: Comparison of two techniques to inflate the bronchial cuff of the Univent tube, *Anesth Analg* 75:784, 1992.

23. Essig K, Freeman JA: Alternative bronchial cuff inflation technique for the Univent tube, *Anesthesiology* 76:478, 1992.

24. Brodsky JB, Shulman MS, Mark JBD: Malposition of left-sided double-lumen endobronchial tubes, *Anesthesiology* 62:667, 1985.

25. Burk WJ III: Should a fiberoptic bronchoscope be routinely used to position a double-lumen tube? *Anesthesiology* 68:826, 1988.

26. Benumof JL: The position of a double-lumen tube should be routinely determined by fiberoptic bronchoscopy, *J Cardiothorac Vasc Anesth* 7:513, 1993 (editorial).

27. Cohen E, Goldofsky S, Neustein S, et al: Fiberoptic evaluation of endobronchial tube position: red rubber vs polyvinychloride, *Anesth Analg* 68(suppl):54, 1989.

28. Katz JA, Fairley HB: Pulmonary surgery. In Marshall BE, Longnecker DF, Fairley HB, editors: *Anesthesia for thoracic procedures,* Boston, 1988, Blackwell Scientific.

29. Patane PS, Sell BA, Mahle ME: Awake fiberoptic endobronchial intubation, *J Cardiothorac Vasc Anesth* 4:229, 1990.

30. Shulman MS, Brodsky JB, Levesque PR: Fiberoptic bronchoscopy for tracheal and endobronchial intubation with a double-lumen tube, *Can J Anaesth* 34:172, 1987.

31. Ovassapian A, Schrader SC: Fiberoptic-aided bronchial intubation, *Seminars in Anesthesia* 6:133, 1987.

32. Matthew EB, Hirschmann RA: Placing double-lumen tubes with a fiberoptic bronchoscope, *Anesthesiology* 65:118, 1986.

33. Smith GB, Hirsch NP, Ehrenwerth J: Placement of double-lumen endobronchial tubes, *Br J Anaesth* 58:1317, 1986.

34. McKenna MJ, Wilson RS, Bothelho RJ: Right upper lobe obstruction with right-sided double-lumen endobronchial tubes: a comparison of two types, *J Cardiothorac Vasc Anesth* 2:734, 1988.

35. Alliaume B, Coddens J, Deloof T: Reliability of auscultation in positioning of double-lumen endobronchial tubes, *Can J Anaesth* 39:687, 1992.

36. Lewis JW, Serwin JP, Gabriel FS et al: The utility of a double-lumen tube for one-lung ventilation in a variety of noncardiac thoracic surgical procedures, *J Cardiothorac Vasc Anesth* 5:705, 1992.

37. Hurford WE, Alfille PH: A quality improvement study of the placement and complications of double-lumen endobronchial tubes, *J Cardiothorac Vasc Anesth* 7:517-520, 1993.

38. Read RC, Friday CD, Eason CN: Prospective study of the Robertshaw endobronchial catheter in thoracic surgery, *Ann Thorac Surg* 24:156, 1977.

39. Brodsky JB, Shulman MS, Mark JBD: Malposition of left-sided double-lumen endobronchial tubes, *Anesthesiology* 62:667, 1985.

40. Wilson RS: Endobronchial intubation. In Kaplan JA, editor: *Thoracic anesthesia,* ed 2, New York, 1991, Churchill-Livingstone.

41. Hurford WE: Fiberoptic endobronchial intubation, *Anesth Clin N Amer* 9:97, 1991.

42. Benumof JL, Harwood I, Pendleton S: Major obstruction of the right mainstem bronchus caused by placement of a right axillary roll, *J Cardiothorac Vasc Anesth* 7:200, 1993.

43. Saito S, Dohi S, Naito H: Alteration of double-lumen endobronchial tube position by flexion and extension of the neck, *Anesthesiology* 52:696, 1985.

44. Benumof JL, Partridge BL, Salvatierra C et al: Margin of safety in positioning modern double-lumen endotracheal tubes, *Anesthesiology* 67:729, 1987.

45. Komatsu K, Arai T, Hatano Y: A modified double-lumen tube, *Anaesthesia* 43:1064, 1988.

46. Alfery DD, Benumof JL, Spragg RG: Anesthesia for bronchopulmonary lavage. In Kaplan JA, editor: *Thoracic anesthesia,* New York, 1982, Churchill-Livingstone.

47. Spragg RG, Benumof JL, Alfery DD: New methods for performance of unilateral lung lavage, *Anesthesiology* 57:535, 1982.

48. Atwell SW: Major anomalies of the tracheobronchial tree, *Chest* 52:611, 1967.

49. Bloor CM, Liebow AA: *The pulmonary and bronchial circulations in congenital heart disease,* New York, 1980, Plenum Medical.

50. Conrady PA, Goodman LR, Cainge R et al: Alteration of endotracheal tube position: flexion and extension of the neck, *Crit Care Med* 4:8, 1976.

51. Shankar KB, Mosely HSL, Kumar AY: Dual end-tidal CO_2 monitoring and double-lumen tubes, *Can J Anaesth* 39:100, 1991.

52. Shafieha MJ, Sit J, Kartha R et al: End-tidal CO_2 analyzers in proper positioning of the double-lumen tubes, *Anesthesiology* 64:844, 1986.

53. Simon BA, Hurford WE, Alfille PH et al: An aid in the diagnosis of malpositioned double-lumen tubes, *Anesthesiology* 76:862, 1992.

54. Cohen E, Kirschner PA, Goldofsky S: Intraoperative manipulation for positioning of double-lumen tubes, *Anesthesiology* 68:170, 1988.

55. Newman RW, Finer GE, Downs JE: Routine use of the Carlens double-lumen endobronchial catheter: an experimental and clinical study, *J Thorac Cardiovasc Surg* 42:327, 1961.

56. Dryden GE: Circulatory collapse after pneumonectomy (an unusual complication from the use of a Carlens catheter): case report, *Anesth Analg* 56:451, 1977.

57. Guernelli N, Bragaglia RB, Briccoli A et al: Tracheobronchial ruptures due to cuffed Carlens tubes, *Ann Thorac Surg* 28:66, 1979.

58. Heiser M, Steinberg JJ, MacVaugh H et al: Bronchial rupture: a

complication of use of the Robertshaw double-lumen tube, *Anesthesiology* 51:88, 1979.

59. Foster JNG, Lau OJ, Alimo EB: Ruptured bronchus following endobronchial intubation, *Br J Anaesth* 55:687, 1983.

60. Slinger P, Chripko D: A clinical comparison of bronchial cuff pressure in disposable left double-lumen tubes, *Anesthesiology* 77:1233, 1992 (abstract).

61. Knowlson GT, Bassett HF: The pressures exerted on the trachea by endotracheal inflatable cuffs, *Br J Anaesth* 42:834, 1970.

62. Bryce-Smith R, Salt R: A right-sided double-lumen endobronchial tube, *Br J Anaesth* 32:230, 1960.

63. Wagner DL, Gammage GW, Wong ML: Tracheal rupture following the insertion of a disposable double-lumen endotracheal tube, *Anesthesiology* 63:698, 1955.

64. Burton NA, Fall SM, Lyons T et al: Rupture of the left main-stem bronchus with a polyvinylchloride double-lumen tube, *Chest* 83:928, 1983.

65. Hannallah M, Gomes M: Bronchial rupture associated with the use of a double-lumen tube in a small adult, *Anesthesiology* 71:457, 1989.

66. Hasan A, Low DE, Ganado AL et al: Tracheal rupture with disposable polyvinylchloride double-lumen endotracheal tubes, *J Cardiothorac Vasc Anesth* 6:208, 1992.

67. Campbell C, Viswanathan S, Riopelle JM et al: Manufacturing defect in a double-lumen tube, *Anesth Analg* 73:824, 1991.

68. Smith BAC, Hopkinson RB: Tracheal rupture during anesthesia, *Anaesthesia* 39:894, 1984.

69. Cohen JA, Denisco RA, Richard TS et al: Hazardous placement of a Robertshaw-types endobronchial tube, *Anesth Analg* 65:100, 1986.

70. Saito S, Dohi S, Tajima K: Failure of double-lumen endobronchial tube placement: congenital tracheal stenosis in an adult, *Anesthesiology* 66:83, 1987.

71. Inoue H, Shohtsu A, Ogawa J et al: New device for one lung anesthesia: endotracheal tube with moveable blocker, *J Thorac Cardiovasc Surg* 83:940, 1982.

72. Kamaya H, Krishna PR: New endotracheal tube (Univent tube) for selective blockade of one lung, *Anesthesiology* 63:342, 1985.

73. MacGillivray RG: Evaluation of a new tracheal tube with a movable bronchus blocker, *Anaesthesia* 43:687, 1988.

74. Schwartz DE, Yost CS, Larson MD: Pneumothorax complication in the use of a Univent endotracheal tube, *Anesth Analg* 76:443, 1993.

75. Hultgren BL, Krishna PR, Kamava H: A new tube for one lung ventilation: experience with Univent tube *Anesthesiology* 65:481, 1986 (abstract).

76. Karwande SV: A new tube for single lung ventilation, *Chest* 92:761, 1987.

77. Herenstein R, Russo JR, Moonka N et al: Management of one-lung anesthesia in an anticoagulated patient, *Anesth Analg* 67:1120, 1988.

78. Fuji Corp: Personal communication, June, 1994.

79. Hannallah M: Complication of the Univent bronchial blocker tube in the ICU, *Anesthesiology* 77:835, 1992 (letter).

80. Gayes JM: The Univent tube is the best technique for providing one-lung ventilation, pro: one-lung ventilation is best accomplished with the Univent endotracheal tube, *J Cardiothorac Vasc Anesth* 7:103, 1993.

81. Benumof JL, Gaughan S, Ozaki GT: Operative lung constant positive airway pressure with the Univent bronchial blocker tube, *Anesth Analg* 74:406, 1992.

82. Kelley JG, Gaba DM, Brodsky JB: Bronchial cuff pressures of two tubes used in thoracic surgery, *J Cardiothorac Vasc Anesth* 6:190, 1992.

83. Benumof JL, Gaughan SD, Ozaki GT: The relationship among bronchial blocker cuff inflation volume, proximal airway pressure, and seal of the bronchial blocker cuff, *J Cardiothorac Vasc Anesth* 6:404, 1992.

84. Slinger P: The Univent tube is the best technique for providing one-lung ventilation, con: the Univent tube is not the best method of providing one-lung ventilation, *J Cardiothorac Vasc Anesth* 7:108, 1993.

85. Ginsberg RJ: New technique for one lung anesthesia using an endobronchial blocker, *J Thorac Cardiovasc Surg* 82:542, 1981.

86. Larson CE, Gaisor TA: A device for endobronchial blocker placement during one-lung anaesthesia, *Anesth Analg* 71:311, 1990.

87. Zilberstein M, Katz RI, Levy A et al: An improved method for introducing an endobronchial blocker, *J Cardiothorac Vasc Anesth* 4:481, 1990.

88. Veil R: Selective bronchial blocking in a small child, *Br J Anaesth* 41:453, 1969.

89. Kubota H, Kubota Y, Toyoda Y et al: Selective blind endobronchial intubation in children and adults, *Anesthesiology* 67:587, 1987.

90. Baraka A, Akel S, Muallem M et al: Bronchial intubation in children: does the tube bevel determine the side of intubation? *Anesthesiology* 67:869, 1987.

91. El-Baz N, Faber LP, Kittle F et al: Single-lumen tube for two-lung and one-lung ventilation during thoracic surger, *Anesth Analg* 72(suppl):64, 1991.

92. El-Baz N, Faber LP, Kittle F et al: Bronchoscopic endobronchial intubation with a single-lumen tube for one-lung anesthesia, *Anesthesiology* 65:480, 1986 (abstract).

Chapter 22

THE COMBITUBE: ESOPHAGEAL/TRACHEAL DOUBLE-LUMEN AIRWAY

Michael Frass

I. HISTORY AND DEVELOPMENT OF THE COMBITUBE

A. ROLE OF THE ENDOTRACHEAL AIRWAY FOR INTUBATION AND VENTILATION

Rapid establishment of a patent airway to facilitate adequate ventilation during cardiopulmonary resuscitation (CPR) is the primary task of the rescuer. Mouth-to-mouth ventilation carries the disadvantages of possible gastric insufflation and a danger of aspiration. Endotracheal intubation remains the gold standard in airway maintenance. However, this skill is only acquired after intensive training and requires constant practice. Often the people performing a resuscitation are untrained in intubation. In addition, endotracheal intubation is difficult[1] or impossible even for skilled personnel on many occasions, since endotracheal intubation requires good exposure of the patient's airway, a skilled endoscopist, and instruments or facilities for intubation. Therefore, the need arises for a simple and efficient alternative.

B. DEVELOPMENT AND DESCRIPTION OF THE ESOPHAGEAL OBTURATOR AIRWAY AS AN ADJUNCT ALTERNATIVE AIRWAY

The esophageal obturator airway was constructed by Don Michael and Gordon as an alternative to the endotracheal airway during emergency intubation.[2] The esophageal obturator airway is a 34-cm-long tube with a balloon at its distal tip (Fig. 22-1). The balloon should lie below the tracheal bifurcation after insertion. The distal end is blocked. Proximal to the balloon are 16 holes, which are positioned in the region of the hypopharynx after positioning of the airway. At the proximal end, a face mask is connected to the airway, sealing mouth and nose during ventilation.

The esophageal obturator airway is inserted by first grasping the back of the patient's tongue and the lower jaw with thumb and index finger and then guiding the airway gently into the esophagus. The distal balloon is inflated to occlude the esophagus while the mask is pressed against the patient's face. Air enters the proximal end and then enters the hypopharynx through perforations, since the distal end is blocked. From there, air is forced over the open epiglottis into the trachea, since mouth and nose are sealed by the mask and the esophagus by the balloon (Fig. 22-1).

C. STUDIES WITH THE ESOPHAGEAL OBTURATOR AIRWAY

Subsequent physiologic testing and field trials of the esophageal obturator airway were carried out. Schofferman et al.[3] evaluated the airway in 18 patients suffering from cardiac arrest. Resuscitation was performed by paramedics, and arterial blood-gas analysis was obtained during ventilation with the esophageal obturator airway and subsequently with the endotracheal airway. There was little or no improvement in oxygenation after endotracheal intubation, implying that the failures to oxygenate in some patients were not due to the esophageal obturator airway. Shea et al.[4] compared two similar groups of patients during cardiopulmonary arrest with ventricular fibrillation: 296 patients were intubated with either the endotracheal airway or the esophageal obturator airway. Survival rates and neurological sequelae of survivors showed no statistically significant difference between the two groups. Hammargren et al.[5] compared both devices after standardizing the method of oxygen delivery and assuring true sampling of arterial blood. In 48 victims of prehospital cardiac arrest, blood gases were drawn during ventilation with the esophageal obturator airway and subsequent ventilation with the endotracheal airway. There was no statistical significant difference in the Pao_2 or $Paco_2$ between the two devices. The authors

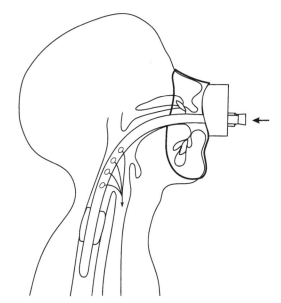

Fig. 22-1. Esophageal obturator airway. Air is blown through proximal port and travels through perforations into hypopharynx (small arrows) and trachea, since mouth and nose are sealed by the mask and esophagus by the balloon.

concluded that the esophageal obturator airway was an effective means of airway management, with the ventilation achieved equal to that of an endotracheal airway.

Nevertheless, it soon became apparent from studies in the controlled environment of the operating room that considerable technical difficulties were associated with the esophageal obturator airway.[6]

D. DISADVANTAGES OF THE ESOPHAGEAL OBTURATOR AIRWAY

The esophageal obturator airway is discussed controversially in the literature because of the following possible complications:

1. There are significant difficulties in obtaining a tight face-mask seal and maintaining the seal during transportation. Effective use requires at least two hands to seal the mask. Complaints are related to significant difficulty obtaining an adequate mask fit particularly in edentulous or bearded patients.[5,6]
2. Inadvertent or unrecognized tracheal intubation.[7] In this case, the patient's airways are completely obstructed, and attempts at repositioning are usually unsuccessful.
3. Esophageal or gastric ruptures.[8-10] Ruptures of the esophagus or the stomach may be due to its length. Since many cardiac-arrest patients exhibit left atrial dilatation with subsequent lateral deviation of the lower half of the esophagus, the esophageal obturator airway may be forced into a left lateral direction in addition to the sagittal curved direction, which might lead to ruptures.

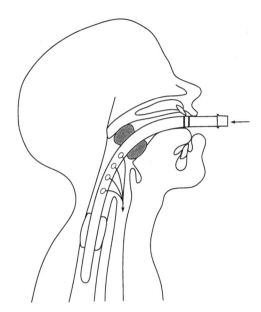

Fig. 22-2. Modified esophageal obturator airway. Mask is replaced by oropharyngeal balloon sealing cavities of mouth and nose.

E. DEVELOPMENT OF THE COMBITUBE ESOPHAGEAL/TRACHEAL DOUBLE-LUMEN AIRWAY

The above disadvantages led to the development of the Combitube. It was devised by the author in cooperation with Reinhard Frenzer and Jonas Zahler, Moedling and Vienna, Austria.[11] Initially, the mask of the esophageal obturator airway was replaced by a special elastic oropharyngeal latex balloon. This balloon fits exactly to the human anatomy and seals the oral and nasal cavity. After inflation, the balloon is pressed against the base of the tongue in a ventrocaudal direction, and closes the soft palate in a dorsocranial direction (Fig. 22-2). In the final position, the ventral part of the balloon reaches the posterior part of the hard palate, thereby anchoring the device during ventilation and transportation without any further need for fixation. The air is blown through the perforations into the hypopharynx. The air cannot escape through mouth or nose because of sealing by the balloon, and thus is forced past the epiglottis into the trachea and lungs.

However, the danger of inadvertent tracheal intubation cannot be prevented by this airway. Therefore, we constructed the Combitube, which has an additional tracheal lumen, to deal effectively with this circumstance.

II. DESCRIPTION OF THE COMBITUBE
A. TECHNICAL DESCRIPTION OF THE COMBITUBE

The Combitube (Kendall Sheridan Catheter Corp., Argyle, New York) is a new device for emergency intubation that combines the functions of an esophageal obturator airway and a conventional endotracheal air-

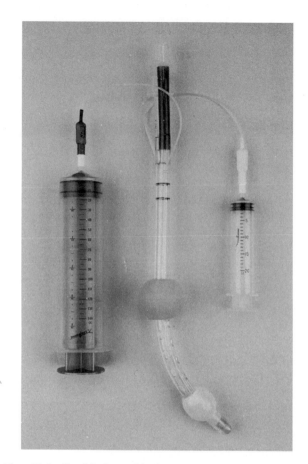

Fig. 22-3. Combitube, with large syringe for inflation of oropharyngeal balloon and small syringe for inflation of distal cuff.

way (Fig. 22-3). The Combitube can be positioned into either the esophagus or the trachea. It is a double-lumen tube (Fig. 22-4): the so-called esophageal lumen has an open upper end and a blocked distal end, with perforations at the pharyngeal level, and the so-called tracheal lumen has an open distal end. The lumens are separated by a partition wall. They are linked by short tubes with connectors. The previously described oropharyngeal balloon is positioned proximal to the pharyngeal perforations. This balloon seals the oral and nasal cavity after inflation. Printed ring marks proximal to the oropharyngeal balloon indicate depth of insertion. At the lower end, a conventional cuff seals either the esophagus or the trachea.

B. DESCRIPTION OF INTRODUCTION

The lower jaw and tongue are lifted by one hand and the tube inserted in a downward curved movement until the printed ring marks lie between the teeth, or the alveolar ridges in edentulous patients (Fig. 22-5, *A*). Next, the oropharyngeal balloon is inflated with 100 ml of air through port no. 1 with the blue pilot balloon using the large syringe (Fig. 22-5, *B*). During inflation, the tube may move slightly out of the patient's mouth.

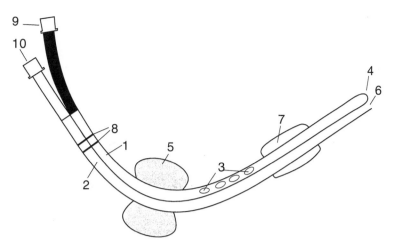

Fig. 22-4. Cross-sectional view of Combitube. *1,* "Esophageal" lumen (longer tube with blocked distal end); *2,* "Tracheal" lumen (shorter tube with open distal end); *3,* Perforations of esophageal lumen 1 at pharyngeal section; *4,* Blocked distal end of esophageal lumen 1; *5,* Oropharyngeal balloon; *6,* Open distal end of tracheal lumen 2; *7,* Distal cuff for obturating either esophagus or trachea; *8,* Printed ring marks for indicating depth of insertion between the teeth or alveolar ridges; *9,* Connector for (blue) tube leading to esophageal lumen 1; *10,* Connector for (clear) tube leading to tracheal lumen 2.

Then, the distal balloon is inflated with 5 to 15 ml of air through port no. 2 with the white pilot balloon using the small syringe. With blind insertion, there is a high probability that the tube will be placed into the esophagus. Therefore, test ventilation is recommended through the longer blue tube no. 1 leading to the esophageal lumen (Fig. 22-5, *C*). Air passes into the pharynx and from there over the epiglottis into the trachea, since the mouth, nose, and esophagus are blocked by the balloons. Auscultation of breath sounds in the absence of gastric insufflation confirm adequate ventilation when the Combitube is in the esophagus. Ventilation is then continued through this lumen. In this position, gastric contents can be suctioned through the other unused tracheal lumen with the help of a small suction catheter included in the kit.

If no breath sounds are heard over the lungs in the presence of gastric insufflation, the Combitube has been placed into the trachea (Fig. 22-5, *D*). Without changing the position of the Combitube, ventilation is changed to the shorter clear tube no. 2, leading to the tracheal lumen, and position is again confirmed by auscultation. Now, air flows directly into the trachea. The oropharyngeal balloon may now be deflated in case of regurgitation. Otherwise, the balloon should remain inflated to stabilize the Combitube.

The Combitube may be inserted blindly. However, the use of a laryngoscope is recommended, if advisable, when for example endotracheal intubation under laryngoscopical view fails and the laryngoscope is still in place.

The anatomical relationships of the oropharyngeal balloon were shown with the help of x-rays. It was demonstrated that the balloon protruded in an oral direction after overinflation so it did not close the epiglottis. Therefore, if sufficient sealing of the mouth and nose cannot be accomplished, the oropharyngeal balloon may be filled with an additional 50 ml of air.[12]

Figure 22-6 shows an MRI image with a cross-sectional view of the Combitube in esophageal position. It displays an anterior movement of the larynx, a situation that can often be observed clinically. Knowledge of this may facilitate subsequent location of the larynx for endotracheal intubation.

III. INDICATIONS FOR USE OF THE COMBITUBE
A. EMERGENCY INTUBATION IN AND OUT OF HOSPITAL

The Combitube is especially suited for emergency intubation in and out of the hospital whenever endotracheal intubation is not immediately possible. It may be used in the following situations: (1) in patients with difficult anatomy (e.g., bull neck, lockjaw; see Box 22-1); (2) under difficult circumstances with respect to space (e.g., difficult access to a patient's head when the patient lies on the floor in a small room, when the patient is lying with his head close to the wall in the general ward or in the ICU with many lines at the side impeding quick access to the head, or with patients trapped in a car after an accident) (3) and under difficult illumination (e.g., bright light might inhibit direct laryngoscopy). In patients with massive bleeding or regurgitation, inability to visualize the vocal cords is no longer an obstacle to intubation. The Combitube prevents aspiration, which might occur with repeated suction maneuvers.

B. ELECTIVE SURGERY

Use of the Combitube is indicated in routine surgery on patients for whom conventional intubation is difficult

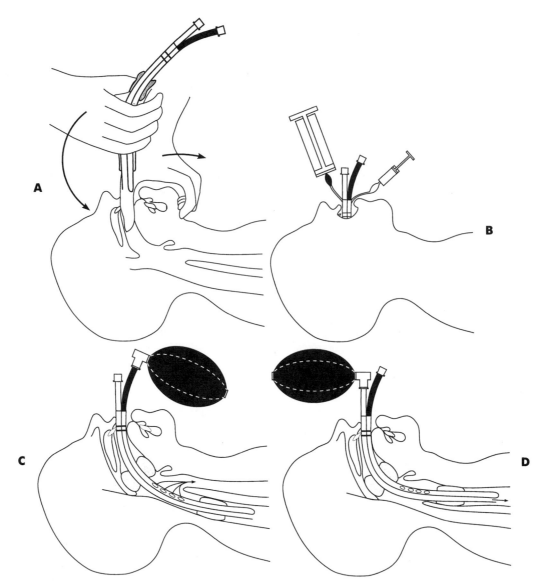

Fig. 22-5. Guidelines for introduction of the Combitube. **A,** Insertion of Combitube: Lifting of chin and lower jaw, introducing of Combitube in downward curved movement. **B,** Inflation of oropharyngeal balloon with 100 ml of air, then distal cuff with 5 to 15 ml of air. **C,** Combitube in esophageal position: Ventilation is performed via longer blue tube no. 1. Air flows through holes into pharynx and from there into trachea. **D,** Combitube in tracheal position: Ventilation is performed via shorter clear tube no. 2. Air flows directly into trachea.

or may be contraindicated: singers and actors, who may be afraid of damage of the vocal cords by endotracheal intubation or rheumatoid arthritis patients with atlanto-axial subluxation. Similar to emergency intubation, it is especially suitable in patients with difficult anatomical situations. Whenever endotracheal intubation cannot be performed immediately, the Combitube might be a helpful alternative (Box 22-1).

There are some special considerations for the use of the Combitube by anesthesiologists who are expert in endotracheal intubation. First, the patient's head does not have to be placed in the traditional "sniffing position" as recommended for conventional endotra-

cheal intubation. The patient's head should remain in a neutral position, which allows free movement of the lower jaw. Depending on the situation, the chin may be lifted toward the patient's chest. Some clinicians prefer to extend the head. However, in patients with cervical spine injury, the head should remain in a neutral position. Second, the position of the operator (Fig. 22-7) may be (1) behind the patient, especially when a laryngoscope is used (Fig. 22-7, *A*); (2) to the side of the patient's head (Fig. 22-7, *B*); or (3) face to face—the operator may stand beside the patient's thorax facing the patient (Fig. 22-7, *C*). In all three positions, it is necessary to insert the Combitube with a curved downward

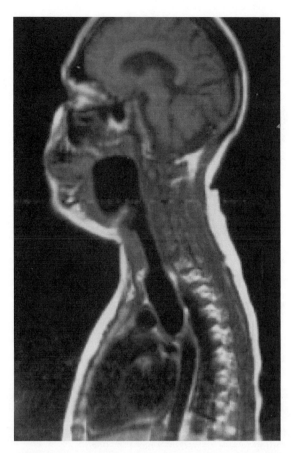

Fig. 22-6. MRI imaging: Cross-sectional view of a patient intubated with Combitube in esophageal position. (Courtesy of Dr. B. Panning, Department of Anesthesiology II, and Dr. C. Ehrenheim, Department of Nuclear Medicine and Special Biophysics, Hannover School of Medicine, Hannover, Germany.)

BOX 22-1   List of suggested indications for use
of the Combitube in anesthesia

  I. Face abnormalities
      A. Congenital (micrognathia, macroglossia, etc.)
      B. Facial trauma
      C. Lockjaw
 II. Cervical-spine abnormalities
      A. Bull neck
      B. Bechterew's disease
      C. Klippel-Feil syndrome
      D. Fractures and luxations
      E. Rheumatoid arthritis with subluxation of the
          atlantoaxial joint
III. Further indications
      A. Preoperative evaluation indications
          1. Previous difficult intubation
          2. Oropharyngeal classification III, IV
          3. Laryngoscopic grade III, IV
      B. Emergency situation
          1. Accidental extubation in patients undergoing
             surgery in prone or sitting position
          2. Cervical hematoma following inadvertent
             puncture of the carotid artery
          3. Unexpected upper-airway bleeding or contin-
             ued vomiting
          4. Cesarean section
          5. Intubation under limited circumstances with
             respect to space
 IV. Main indication: BACK-UP DEVICE

---

movement. Third, during elective surgery it is almost always necessary not only to sedate but also to paralyze the patient to avoid reflexes that impede the insertion of the Combitube. However, grasping and elevating the epiglottis with the fingers during insertion might reduce the need for relaxation. Relaxation may be unnecessary with the use of propofol. Fourth, replacement of the Combitube in esophageal position by an endotracheal airway should be performed as follows: Deflate the oropharyngeal balloon with the Combitube remaining in the esophagus, then insert the endotracheal airway. When insertion of an endotracheal airway is successful, deflate the lower cuff of the Combitube and remove it, so danger of aspiration is prevented. If insertion of the endotracheal airway is not possible, reinflate the oropharyngeal balloon and continue ventilating via the Combitube until the next endotracheal intubation attempt or a surgical airway is established. Fifth, extubation after surgery in the nearly awake patient is possible, and the patient will not show signs of significant distress.

Extubation should be performed after recovery of protective reflexes.

C. ADVANTAGES

The Combitube has a wide range of applications and advantages (Box 22-2). Those benefiting from its use include physicians working in emergency departments, paramedics, medical staff in the military, and physicians in private practice (e.g., when faced with anaphylactic reactions). Cardiac arrests usually do not occur under ideal circumstances, and often, CPR is performed in awkward locations, poorly lit areas, and with difficult access to the patient's head. Since the Combitube can be inserted without a laryngoscope, establishment of a patent airway is not hampered by either adverse environmental factors or staff unskilled in endotracheal intubation.[13] There is no need for additional fixation of the Combitube after inflation of the oropharyngeal balloon.

D. DISADVANTAGES

A potential disadvantage of the Combitube is that suctioning of tracheal secretions is impossible in the esophageal position. However, studies of use of the

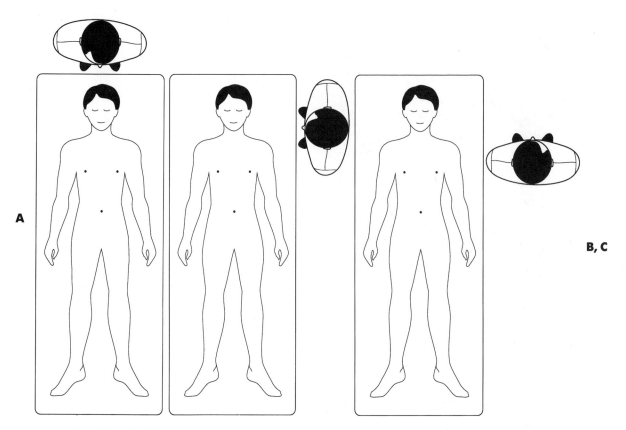

Fig. 22-7. Position of operator during insertion of Combitube. **A,** Behind the patient, especially with use of a laryngoscope. **B,** Operator standing to side of patient's head. **C,** Face to face—operator standing beside patient's thorax.

---

esophageal obturator airway in cardiac-arrest patients[4,5] show that the outcome of those cases is not statistically different when compared with cases in which endotracheal intubation is used. The Combitube is designed to bridge the relatively short gap between the prehospital setting and admission of the patient to the emergency department. If prolonged ventilation is required, the administration of glycopyrronium bromide may be used to suppress tracheal secretions (e.g., during surgery).

E. CONTRAINDICATIONS

The Combitube is contraindicated in the following circumstances:

- Patients with intact gag reflexes, irrespective of their level of consciousness
- Patients under 5 feet with the standard Combitube and under 4 feet with the Combitube SA (small adult, female version)
- Central-airway obstruction
- Patients who have ingested caustic substances
- Patients with known esophageal pathology

F. COMPLICATIONS

Until now, severe complications have not been reported in the literature. Superficial lacerations of the

---

BOX 22-2   Advantages of the Combitube

- Noninvasive as compared to cricothyrotomy
- No preparations necessary; tube and syringes are ready to use
- Blind insertion technique
- Neck flexion unnecessary
- Minimized risk of aspiration
- Simultaneous fixation after inflation of oropharyngeal balloon
- Use of controlled mechanical ventilation possible at higher ventilation pressures
- Independent of power supply (e.g., batteries of laryngoscope)
- Well suited for obese patients
- May be used in paralyzed patients who cannot be intubated or mask ventilated
- Helpful under difficult circumstances with respect to space and illumination
- Works in either tracheal or esophageal position

esophagus could be found in autopsies of patients ventilated with the Combitube. As outlined in the instructions, the Combitube should not be advanced with the use of force. Ovassapian[14] (personal communication) observed livid discoloration of the tongue during ventilation with the Combitube in a few patients without further sequelae.

In a few cases ventilation may be impossible unless the Combitube is pulled about 3 cm out of the patient's mouth with the balloons inflated and then fixed in this position. We suggest that this situation may be caused by closure of the epiglottis.

IV. STUDIES
A. ANESTHESIOLOGIC STUDIES
1. General anesthesia

Function and effectiveness of the Combitube were first tested in animal experiments[15] and subsequently in humans.[16] The effectiveness of ventilation with the Combitube was compared to ventilation with conventional endotracheal airways during routine surgery in a crossover study.[17] Twenty-three patients were ventilated first with the Combitube and then with a conventional endotracheal airway (group 1). In group 2, application of the tubes was performed in a reversed order in eight patients. After 20 minutes of ventilation with each airway, arterial-blood samples were analyzed. In all cases, patients were ventilated with the Combitube without problems. It was demonstrated that ventilation with the Combitube was comparable to ventilation with an endotracheal airway. In addition, arterial-oxygen pressure was higher during ventilation with the Combitube (142 ± 43 mm Hg with the Combitube vs. 119 ± 40 mm Hg with the endotracheal airway in group 1, $P < .001$; 117 ± 16 mm Hg with the endotracheal airway vs. 146 ± 13 mm Hg with the Combitube in group 2, $P < .001$), whereas the differences in arterial–carbon dioxide tension and pH were not significant.

The reasons for increased oxygen tension during ventilation with the Combitube were investigated in another study.[18] In 12 patients undergoing general anesthesia during routine surgery, a thin catheter was placed with its tip 10 cm below the vocal cords. Patients were then ventilated by mask, by the Combitube in esophageal position, and by an endotracheal airway in randomized sequence. Pressures were recorded in the trachea and at the airway openings. Blood gases again showed a higher arterial-oxygen tension with the Combitube when compared to endotracheal airway (151 ± 37 mm Hg vs. 125 ± 32 mm Hg, $P < .05$) and a higher arterial–carbon dioxide tension (36 ± 4 mm Hg vs. 33 ± 4 mm Hg, $P < .05$). This slightly higher carbon dioxide tension with the Combitube might be partly due to the integration of the hypopharynx into the physiologic

dead space. Compared to mask ventilation, carbon dioxide tension was lower with the Combitube.

The following differences in intratracheal pressures were found. The rising pressure during inspiration was highest with the endotracheal airway (19 ± 6 mm Hg/second with the endotracheal airway vs. 14 ± 6 mm Hg/second with the Combitube, $P < .05$). The smaller rising pressure with the Combitube may lead to a more favorable distribution of ventilation. Expiratory flow time was prolonged during ventilation with the Combitube (2.0 ± 1.0 second vs. 1.3 ± 0.6 second with the endotracheal airway). This effect is probably due to an increase in expiratory resistance because of the double-lumen design and might favor the formation of a small positive end-expiratory pressure (PEEP). Auto-PEEP might also be caused by integration of the vocal cords into the airway with the Combitube, while they are bypassed by the endotracheal airway. The auto-PEEP does not exceed 2 mm Hg and therefore does not influence cerebral perfusion during CPR. The smaller rising pressure, prolonged expiratory-flow time, and auto-PEEP together improve conditions for alveolar-arterial–gas exchange.

While peak pressures at the airway openings may be high due to the resistance of the double-lumen airway, intratracheal pressures were comparable between the two tubes (peak endotracheal pressure: 10 ± 4 mm Hg with the Combitube vs. 12 ± 6 mm Hg with the endotracheal airway, $P = $ ns; endotracheal-plateau pressure: 8 ± 2 mm Hg with the Combitube vs. 8 ± 4 mm Hg with the endotracheal airway, $P = $ ns).

The Combitube may also be used for prolonged ventilation.[19] In seven patients in the intensive care unit, the Combitube was used over a period of two to eight hours during mechanical ventilation. Results showed adequate ventilation compared with subsequent endotracheal-airway ventilation.

2. Obstetric anesthesia

Wissler has used the Combitube in obstetric anesthesia.[20] He states that the Combitube is most easily and atraumatically inserted into the esophagus under direct vision using a laryngoscope. In his practice of obstetric anesthesia, the Combitube is his first choice for the anesthetized parturient who cannot be intubated or mask ventilated with cricoid pressure. His reasoning is that it provides a better barrier against regurgitation and aspiration than the laryngeal mask airway (LMA).[20] In addition, ideal insertion conditions for the LMA include lubrication and a special method of cuff deflation, whereas the Combitube is ready to use in its package. In an obstetric patient with increased oxygen consumption, decreased functional residual capacity, and airway obstruction, these differences in preparation time may be clinically important.

B. CARDIAC-ARREST STUDIES

1. In-hospital studies

The application of the Combitube during CPR has been investigated.[21,22] The first paper[21] describes a study consisting of two parts: in the first part, blood-gas analyses of 19 patients after 15 minutes of ventilation with the Combitube are shown. In the second part, a sample of 12 patients, blood-gas analyses during ventilation with the Combitube are compared to subsequent ventilation with a conventional endotracheal airway. Blood-gas analyses again showed higher arterial-oxygen pressures (124 ± 33 mm Hg with the Combitube vs. 103 ± 30 mm Hg with endotracheal airway, P <.001) and a slightly decreased pH during ventilation with the Combitube (7.36 ± 0.08 with the Combitube vs. 7.41 ± 0.05 with the endotracheal airway, P <.02). Carbon dioxide pressure was not significantly different. The second paper[22] reports on the use of the Combitube during in-hospital CPR. In randomized sequence, either the Combitube or a conventional endotracheal airway was used in 43 patients. After stabilization of the patients, each tube was replaced with the other type of tube. Blood-gas analyses again showed the phenomenon of increased oxygen tensions. Intubation time was shorter with the Combitube, which might improve success rates of CPR.

A recent study evaluates the safety and effectiveness of the Combitube as used by ICU nurses under medical supervision compared with endotracheal airway established by ICU physicians during CPR.[23] Intubation time was shorter for the Combitube. Blood gases for each device showed comparable results. The arterial-oxygen tension was slightly higher during ventilation with the Combitube. The study suggests that the Combitube as used by ICU nurses is as effective as the endotracheal airway as used by ICU physicians during CPR.

2. Out-of-hospital studies

Atherton and Johnson investigated the ability of paramedics in a nonurban emergency medical services to use the Combitube in prehospital cardiac-arrest patients.[24] This prospective, controlled study included the evaluation of the difficulty and complications of insertion, recognition of esophageal versus tracheal placement, skill, and skill retention. The ability to use the device in cases of failed endotracheal intubation also was scrutinized. Fifty-two cases of prehospital Combitube insertion by paramedics were examined, and 11 paramedics were evaluated for skill retention. Combitube insertion was attempted on 52 prehospital patients in cardiac arrest, 69% of whom were intubated successfully. Paramedics recognized esophageal versus tracheal placement in 100% of the cases. The Combitube was inserted successfully into 64% of the patients who could not be intubated by the conventional visualized method.

The Combitube was inserted successfully 71% of the time when used as a first-line airway adjunct. A follow-up study on 11 randomly selected paramedics involved in the field study was conducted 15 months later. Nine of 11 paramedics demonstrated inadequate skill retention in the follow-up study (improper insertion angle resulting in resistance and inability to insert the tube, inappropriate inflation of the balloons, insertion too deeply or not deeply enough). Following this reevaluation, the success rate rose to almost 100%.[25] These results demonstrate the necessity of reevaluation of skills a short time after the first training.

D. Lefrançois[26] is performing an ongoing study investigating the Combitube in patients with cardiorespiratory arrest in Montérégie region, Québec. He initiated a semiautomatic defibrillator program in 1992 and added the intubation project using the Combitube in August 1993. Lefrançois is working with 400 basic emergency medical technicians (EMTs) responding to 60,000 calls per year. After exclusion of cases in which intubation by Combitube was unjustified or impossible as evaluated by medical direction of the project, 258 indicated cases were evaluated. The Combitube could be inserted successfully in 98.1% of the cases. In 97.2% of the verified intubations the EMTs had chosen the right lumen for ventilation at the first attempt.

V. GUIDELINES AND REFERENCES REGARDING THE COMBITUBE

The Combitube has gained worldwide interest[27-29] and is now considered to be an adjunct to standard airway equipment in many anesthesiology departments and ambulance services. The Combitube has been recommended in the difficult airway algorithm of the "Practice Guidelines for Management of the Difficult Airway" of the American Society of Anesthesiologists[30] for use when an anesthetized patient can be neither intubated nor mask ventilated. It is also included in the "Guidelines for Cardiopulmonary Resuscitation and Emergency Cardiac Care" of the American Heart Association. In the section "Adult Advanced Cardiac Life Support," the Combitube is described as a valuable tool for emergency intubation.[31]

The Combitube is cited in a review article[29] as an alternative method for artificial ventilation and is recommended for patients with massive regurgitation or airway hemorrhage when visualization of the vocal cords may be impossible.[28]

VI. COMPARISON OF THE COMBITUBE WITH OTHER ALTERNATIVE AIRWAY TECHNIQUES, AND CASE REPORTS

Comparisons among the Combitube, esophageal obturator airway, esophageal gastric tube airway, laryngeal mask airway, and pharyngotracheal lumen airway are

Table 22-1. Comparisons of emergency airway equipment

Description	Esophageal tracheal Combitube	Laryngeal mask airway	Esophageal obturator airway	Esophageal gastric tube airway	Pharyngotracheal lumen airway
Provides barrier to minimize regurgitation of gastric contents	Yes	No	Yes	Yes	Yes
Allows buildup in esophagus of pressure and gastric contents during use	No	No	Yes	No	No
Functions when blindly passed into esophagus	Yes	NA	Yes	Yes	Yes
Functions when blindly passed into trachea	Yes	NA	No	No	Yes
Requires effective mask fit on face	No	No	Yes	Yes	No
Available in pediatric sizes	No	Yes	No	No	No

NA, not applicable
From Wissler RN: The esophageal-tracheal Combitube, *Anesth Review* 20:147, 1993.

shown in Table 22-1.[20] The design of the Combitube has several advantages over the esophageal obturator airway, including an open distal tip that allows decompression and suctioning of the esophagus and stomach in the esophageal position and ventilation in the tracheal position. Also, the Combitube is shorter than the esophageal obturator airway, thereby minimizing the risk of serious complications present with the esophageal obturator airway, including esophageal/gastric rupture. The design of the Combitube prevents airway occlusion with tracheal placement, and postremoval regurgitation and aspiration. In contrast to the Combitube, the esophageal obturator airway as well as the esophageal gastric tube airway require an adequate face-mask seal for effective ventilation. When compared to the laryngeal mask airway, the Combitube provides a decompression barrier (the tracheal lumen) to minimize regurgitation of gastric contents[20] and allows controlled mechanical ventilation with ventilation pressures higher than 20 cm H_2O.

In several unusual cases, the Combitube has proven superior to conventional endotracheal intubation. The Combitube proved to be useful in the case of neck impalement with a large wooden splinter entering at the left angle of the mandible, traversing the pharynx and soft palate and entering the right maxillary cavity below the floor of the orbit;[32] with a bullnecked patient when movement of the neck and opening of the mouth was impossible;[33,34] and in the case of rapidly enlarging cervical hematomas, which caused upper-airway obstruction and thus required immediate intubation after

endotracheal intubation had failed because the epiglottis could not be visualized with a laryngoscope.[35]

VII. FUTURE ASPECTS

The studies demonstrate that the Combitube is an effective alternative to traditional intubation techniques. It has been shown to be as effective as an endotracheal tube in emergency situations. Further studies, especially with respect to management of difficult airways, are needed to elucidate this device fully. The wide range of applications and ease of insertion make it a valuable piece of equipment in the wards, in operating theaters, and in prehospital conditions.

REFERENCES

1. Benumof JL: Management of the difficult adult airway, *Anesthesiology* 75:1087, 1991.
2. Don Michael TA, Lambert EH, Mehran A: Mouth-to-lung airway for cardiac resuscitation, *Lancet* 2:1329, 1968.
3. Schofferman J, Oill P, Lewis AJ: The esophageal obturator airway: a clinical evaluation, *Chest* 69:67, 1976.
4. Shea SR, MacDonald JR, Gruzinski G: Prehospital endotracheal tube airway or esophageal gastric tube airway: a critical comparison, *Ann Emerg Med* 14:102, 1985.
5. Hammargren Y, Clinton JE, Ruiz E: A standard comparison of esophageal obturator airway and endotracheal tube ventilation in cardiac arrest, *Ann Emerg Med* 14:953, 1985.
6. Bryson TK, Benumof JL, Ward CF: The esophageal obturator airway: a clinical comparison of ventilation with a mask and oropharyngeal airway, *Chest* 74:537, 1978.
7. Gertler et al: The esophageal obturator airway: obturator or obtundator? *J Trauma* 25:424, 1985.
8. Scholl DG, Tsai SH: Esophageal perforation following the use of the esophageal obturator airway, *Radiology* 122:315, 1977.

9. Johnson KR, Genovesi MG, Lassar KH: Esophageal obturator airway: use and complications, *JACEP* 5:36, 1976.

10. Crippen D, Olvey S, Graffis R: Gastric rupture: an esophageal obturator airway complication, *Ann Emerg Med* 10:370, 1981.

11. Frass M, Frenzer R, Zahler J: *Respiratory tube or airway,* U.S. patent no. 4,688,568.

12. Frass M et al: Esophageal tracheal Combitube (ETC) for emergency intubation: anatomical evaluation of ETC placement by radiography, *Resuscitation* 18:95, 1989.

13. Johnson JC, Atherton GL: The esophageal tracheal Combitube: an alternate route to airway management, *JEMS* 29, May 1991.

14. Ovassapian A: Personal communication, 1994.

15. Frass M et al: Esophageal tracheal Combitube (ETC): experimental studies with a new airway in emergency cardiopulmonary resuscitation, *Anasthesiol Intensivther Notfallmed Schmerzther* 22: 142, 1987.

16. Frass M et al: First experimental studies with a new device for emergency intubation (esophageal tracheal Combitube), *Intensivmed Notfallmed* 24:390, 1987.

17. Frass M et al: The esophageal tracheal Combitube: preliminary results with a new airway for CPR, *Ann Emerg Med* 16:768, 1987.

18. Frass M et al: Esophageal tracheal Combitube, endotracheal airway and mask: comparison of ventilatory pressure curves, *J Trauma* 29:1476, 1989.

19. Frass M et al: Mechanical ventilation with the esophageal tracheal Combitube (ETC) in the intensive care unit, *Arch Emerg Med* 4:219, 1987.

20. Wissler RN: The esophageal-tracheal Combitube, *Anesth Review* 20:147, 1993.

21. Frass M et al: Evaluation of esophageal tracheal Combitube in cardiopulmonary resuscitation, *Crit Care Med* 15:609, 1987.

22. Frass M et al: Ventilation with the esophageal tracheal Combitube in cardiopulmonary resuscitation: promptness and effectiveness, *Chest* 93:781, 1988.

23. Staudinger et al: Emergency intubation with the Combitube: comparison with the endotracheal airway, *Ann Emerg Med* 22:1573, 1993.

24. Atherton GL, Johnson JC: Ability of paramedics to use the Combitube in prehospital cardiac arrest, *Ann Emerg Med* 22:1263, 1993.

25. Johnson JC: Personal communication, 1995.

26. Lefrançois D: Personal communication, 1994.

27. Clinton JE, Ruiz E: Emergency airway management procedures. In Roberts JR, Hedges JR, editors: *Clinical procedures in emergency medicine,* ed 2, Philadelphia, 1991, W.B. Saunders.

28. Cozine K, Stone G: The take-back patient in ear, nose, and throat surgery. In Benumof JL, editor: *Anesthesiology clinics of North America,* vol 11, no 3, Philadelphia, 1993, W.B. Saunders.

29. Niemann JT: Cardiopulmonary resuscitation: current concepts, *N Engl J Med* 327:1075, 1992.

30. American Society of Anesthesiologists' Task Force on Management of the Difficult Airway: Practice guidelines for management of the difficult airway, *Anesthesiology* 78:597, 1993.

31. American Heart Association: Combination esophageal-tracheal tube. In Guidelines for cardiopulmonary resuscitation and emergency cardiac care: recommendations of the 1992 National Conference of the American Heart Association, *JAMA* 268:2203, 1992.

32. Eichinger S et al: Airway management in a case of neck impalement: use of the oesophageal tracheal Combitube airway, *Br J Anaesth* 68:534, 1992.

33. Frass M et al: Ventilation via the esophageal tracheal Combitube in a case of difficult intubation, *J Cardiothorac Anesth* 1:565, 1987.

34. Banyai M et al: Emergency intubation with the Combitube in a grossly obese patient with bull neck, *Resuscitation* 26:271, 1993.

35. Bigenzahn W, Pesau B, Frass M: Emergency ventilation using the Combitube in cases of difficult intubation, *Eur Arch Otorhinolaryngol* 248:129, 1991.

Chapter 23

TRANSTRACHEAL JET VENTILATION VIA PERCUTANEOUS CATHETER AND HIGH-PRESSURE SOURCE

Jonathan L. Benumof

I. INTRODUCTION

When a patient cannot be intubated or ventilated via a mask and there is no immediately available alternative plan, then death is inevitable.[1] For the purpose of this chapter, *cannot ventilate by mask* means that a reasonably experienced practitioner of medicine cannot cause a life-sustaining amount of gas exchange with a conventional anesthesia mask despite the use of anterior jaw thrust and oropharyngeal and nasopharyngeal airways. In addition, cannot ventilate by mask also means that a laryngeal mask airway does not cause a life-sustaining amount of gas exchange. *Cannot intubate* means that the same medical practitioner cannot pass an endotracheal tube through the vocal cords within a life-sustaining period of time. The incidence of the cannot-ventilate, cannot-intubate situation has ranged from 0.01 to 2.0/10,000 anesthetics (see Chapter 6).[1-6] "Immediately available" transtracheal jet ventilation means that there is a dedicated high-pressure oxygen source and the necessary preassembled noncompliant materials to connect the source to the hub of a transtracheal catheter are already physically present or very close in time (seconds) to being physically present at the bedside.

There is widespread agreement in the literature that percutaneous transtracheal jet ventilation (TTJV) using a large intravenous catheter placed through the crico-

Table 23-1. Minute ventilation (L/min) at $I:E = 1:1$

| | | $C_{set} = 50$ ml/cm H_2O | | | | $C_{set} = 30$ ml/cm H_2O | | | |
| | | Ohmeda | | Dräger | | Ohmeda | | Dräger | |
Test catheter		II	II Plus	2	2A	II	II Plus	2	2A
IV catheter gauge	14	42.0	7.2	39.6	26.4	36.6	4.0	33.6	19.8
	16	31.8	3.6	24.0	13.8	25.8	1.8	22.2	10.8
	18	20.4	1.2	18.6	7.8	15.6	0.0	16.2	4.8
Jet-stylet size	Large	31.8	4.8	28.8	19.2	27.6	3.0	25.2	19.2
	Medium	30.0	1.8	24.0	12.6	25.2	0.6	20.4	9.0
	Small	15.6	0.0	14.4	3.0	13.8	0.0	14.4	1.8

IV, intravenous; *I:E,* inspiratory-to-expiratory ratio, unit of time equal to 1 second; *C_{set},* set compliance of mechanical-lung model.

thyroid membrane is a simple, relatively safe, and extremely effective treatment for the desperate cannot-ventilate-by-mask, cannot-intubate situation.[7-11] Compared to cricothyrotomy and tracheostomy, establishment of percutaneous TTJV (with a high-pressure oxygen source and noncompliant tubing) is ordinarily quicker, simpler, and therefore more efficacious for most anesthesiologists.

Effective TTJV using a 50 psi (pounds per square inch) oxygen source, noncompliant tubing, and a 16-gauge needle was first demonstrated in dogs in 1971. The oxygen flow was great enough so that adequate ventilation occurred without air entrapment.[12] Shortly thereafter, the technique was used in a series of more than 50 patients suffering respiratory distress or cardiopulmonary arrest for the immediate restoration of an adequate airway[13,14] and in many patients undergoing surgical procedures of the upper airway.[15,16] However, it was also recognized that patients who are in respiratory distress with an obstructive lesion of the larynx may have difficulty exhaling gas, which may lead to the stacking of tidal volumes and result in hyperexpansion and barotrauma. It was emphasized that a dangerously high pressure may also occur with a prolonged inspiratory phase of high-pressure oxygen administration.[14-16]

A. MECHANISM OF ACTION AND PROOF OF EFFICACY

TTJV through a suitable cannula (16- or 14-gauge catheter) can potentially provide oxygen for exchange in the alveoli by two mechanisms. The first and most important is by bulk flow of oxygen through the cannula. The second is by translaryngeal entrainment of room air via the Venturi effect, depending on the degree of airway patency above the jet. Studies in experimental models that simulate normal airways (normal airway diameter) and lungs (normal lung compliance) and in normal experimental animals using a driving pressure of 50 psi have demonstrated that the gas flows through 20-, 16-, and 14-gauge cannulas using a driving pressure of 50 psi

are approximately 400 ml/sec,[17] 500 ml/sec,[12] and 1600, ml/sec, respectively.[17] Since the one-second tidal volume with a 14-gauge catheter is equal to 1600 ml, the inspiratory time should be limited to less than one second (e.g., 0.5 second) and the I:E (inspiratory-to-expiratory) ratio should be approximately 1:3 to allow adequate time for exhalation and thereby avoid air trapping and barotrauma. Not surprisingly, as lung compliance decreases and airway resistance increases, the one-second jet-ventilation tidal volume decreases.[17] See Figures 23-13 and 23-14 and Table 23-1 for other typical 14-gauge cannula 50-psi flow rates (as produced by the fresh-gas outlet of an anesthesia machine by activating the flush valve) and the effect of changes in compliance on these flow rates.

In the mechanical model simulating normal tracheo-bronchial-tree dimensions and lung compliance, approximately 50% of the tidal volume is entrained room air.[17] Even in the absence of additional translaryngeal gas entrainment via the Venturi effect, the flow rates with a 14-gauge catheter clearly are adequate to provide excellent ventilation and oxygenation. This is evidenced by numerous animal studies[18-20] as well as human studies and case reports documenting normocarbia or hypocarbia and hyperoxia both in patients undergoing elective surgery and in patients with upper-airway obstruction managed with TTJV for varying periods of time.[21-23]

In the presence of a completely patent glottis, gas entrainment via the Venturi effect may significantly contribute to total tracheal gas flow, adding as much as 40% to 50% more gas to that delivered from the TTJV cannula alone.[12,17,24] However, as the diameter of the tracheobronchial tree decreases, the tidal volume decreases, the amount of room air entrained decreases, and the Fio_2 increases.[17] Indeed, in patients managed with TTJV it appears that translaryngeal entrainment (of room air) has made a negligible contribution to total tracheal gas flow. This contention is supported by two observations. First, arterial blood-gas data in animals as well as healthy patients without lung disease who are managed with TTJV demonstrate PaO_2 values consistent with ventilation with 100% oxygen (no entrainment of room air).[18,19,21] Second, it is likely that negative airway pressure cephalad to the TTJV cannula causes the glottic or periglottic structures to collapse into the glottic aperture on inspiration, thereby further or completely obstructing a partially obstructed or compromised airway and preventing translaryngeal entrainment of room air on inspiration.[12]

Peak inspiratory airway pressures during TTJV will depend upon the cross-sectional area of the trachea; driving pressure; diameter, length, and cross-sectional area of the orifice(s) of the cannula; degree of outflow obstruction; compliance of the lungs and chest wall; and inspiratory time. In animal studies (normal dogs) in which distal airway pressure was measured during TTJV through a 16-gauge needle, it was demonstrated that low-frequency ventilatory rates — that is, less than 30 breaths/min — produced peak airway pressures between 20 and 50 cm H_2O.[12] These peak airway pressures varied linearly with driving pressure when inspiratory time was held constant. Tidal volume also varied linearly with driving pressure. In addition, the tidal volumes and peak inspiratory pressures observed during TTJV were similar to those observed with conventional positive-pressure ventilation via an endotracheal tube.

II. INDICATIONS

A. EMERGENCY SITUATIONS

1. Cannot-ventilate-by-mask, cannot-intubate situation

Acute upper-airway obstructions that cannot be remedied in less than a few minutes by use of a face mask, oral or nasal airways, a laryngeal mask airway, or by any endotracheal intubation technique, and when an immediate surgical airway is not possible, should be treated by an anesthetist who institutes TTJV. Causative factors may include foreign bodies, trauma, infection, neoplasms, and laryngeal edema.

2. Lack of equipment and/or trained personnel for conventional airway management

When trained personnel are unavailable to secure an airway rapidly in an agitated, gasping patient, or if the proper armamentarium to perform endotracheal intubation, tracheostomy, or bronchoscopy is not immediately at hand, then institution of percutaneous transtracheal ventilation may be lifesaving.

B. ELECTIVE SITUATIONS

1. To facilitate operations involving the upper airway

There are several reports and recommendations for the use of the technique in planned surgical situations to avoid tracheostomy. Singh et al.[14] reported 1500 cases of transtracheal ventilation for diagnostic and surgical procedures of the upper airways. There were 1257 cases

for bronchoscopy and esophagoscopy and 135 cases for endolaryngeal surgery. Postoperative ventilatory support was carried out with this technique in 108 cases, with the patients ventilated for periods of 24 to 48 hours.

Spoerel and Greenway,[16] describing ventilation techniques during endolaryngeal surgery, similarly found adequate pulmonary ventilation with excellent conditions for microscopic surgery. Smith, Myers, and Sherman[25] reported elective transtracheal ventilation in children undergoing surgical procedures involving the head and neck. They described the use of this technique in two children, one undergoing an operation for laryngeal stenosis and one who had become obstructed and cyanosed in the recovery room. $PaCO_2$ determinations at the end of the procedures indicated that the patients were moderately hyperventilated. Similarly, since percutaneous TTJV leaves the entire airway from the vocal cords to the face accessible for surgical manipulation, it is not surprising that it has been used for virtually every conceivable type of operation on these structures in adults.[26]

Finally, Wagner, Coombs, and Doyle[27] described a case where high-frequency ventilation was used with success (thus avoiding tracheostomy) in a patient with a partial upper-airway obstruction caused by a hypopharyngeal foreign body with four sharp appendages.

2. To permit safe intubation of the trachea with a standard endotracheal tube by another route (prevent the cannot-ventilate-by-mask, cannot-intubate situation)

In situations in which an increased risk of developing a cannot-ventilate-by-mask, cannot-intubate situation can be identified, elective institution of TTJV may prevent the development of a life-threatening gas-exchange problem while a more secure permanent airway is being established. Elective placement of an intravenous catheter through the cricothyroid membrane and use of TTJV are entirely compatible with a subsequent conventional orotracheal or nasotracheal intubation, fiberoptic-aided intubation, and retrograde-intubation technique, as well as with formal tracheostomy. Indeed, one report described prophylactic TTJV that guaranteed adequate ventilation in a patient who was known to be difficult to intubate. The TTJV enabled the patient to be anesthetized, paralyzed, and intubated in a safe, nonemergent manner.[28] In another report of a 13-year-old girl with ankylosis of the temporomandibular joint secondary to a fractured mandible, TTJV was electively instituted prior to the induction of anesthesia, and the trachea was intubated with the aid of a fiberoptic bronchoscope safely and nonemergently in this well-oxygenated patient after the induction of anesthesia and paralysis.[29] In a third report, a TTJV catheter allowed enough spontaneous ventilation (in addition to the

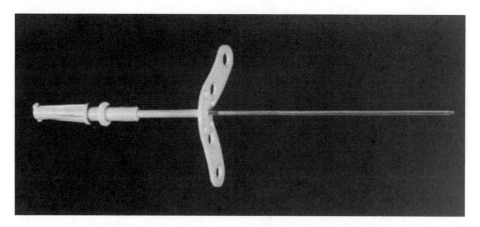

Fig. 23-1. Heimlich Micro-trach, which is a sterile, 16-gauge (1.19-mm internal diameter, 1.65-mm outer diameter), nontoxic microtracheal catheter made of clear, medical-grade polyethylene with a radiopaque stripe. A flange is inserted molded to catheter to permit secure attachment.

natural airway) in a patient with a massive upper-airway tumor that the airway could be secured in a safe and nonemergency manner.[30] Thus, it appears that TTJV can prevent the development of life-threatening gas exchange in patients who are difficult to ventilate and intubate and who require general anesthesia. The technique permits uninterrupted ventilation and oxygenation while allowing the intubationist unhurried access to the patient's upper airway.

3. To administer respiratory therapy

Use of the transtracheal approach in planned situations has recently been extended by Heimlich and Carr[31] in the form of a microcatheter (the Micro-trach) for use in patients with cystic fibrosis. In this patient population, aggressive pulmonary toilet using a bronchoscope or specially designed endotracheal tube to wash out the bronchi has been used as an effective respiratory-therapy emergency measure. Unfortunately, the procedure is dangerous and improvement is short-lived. Pulmonary lavage performed in this way requires a hospital setting, general anesthesia, and a skilled bronchoscopist and/or anesthesiologist. Even in the best of hands, the bronchial-lavage procedure may terminate in the hypoxemic death of the patient, especially if the patient is a child.

The Micro-trach is a 16-gauge catheter terminating squarely at its single outlet (Fig. 23-1). The device is designed to be inserted easily after administration of local anesthesia. The catheter is replaced at intervals varying between one and six months. Other types of indwelling transtracheal catheters require removal for cleaning several times a day. Their large length, diameter, oblique tips, and side holes predispose to mucosal injury and deposition of secretions. Indeed, mucous balls large enough to threaten airway obstruc-

tion form on such oversized catheters left in place for long periods.

Transtracheal oxygen delivery and saline instillation begin immediately after inserting the Micro-trach catheter. All patients experienced immediate relief of otherwise intractable dyspnea.[31] Oxygen administration at a rate of 0.25 to 3 L/min was therapeutically equivalent to 1 to 8 L/min delivered nasally. Over the course of the first year, a majority of the patients continued to use the Micro-trach rather than nasal cannulas or various forms of masks.

III. HOW TO DO TRANSTRACHEAL JET VENTILATION
A. INSERTION OF THE TRANSTRACHEAL CATHETER

The cricothyroid membrane is palpated with the neck of the patient extended (Fig. 23-2,*A*). Then a 12- to 16-gauge intravenous catheter with the needle pointed 30 degrees caudad off the perpendicular is used to puncture the cricothyroid membrane (Fig. 23-2,*B*). The needle stylet/catheter should have a small-angle bend (15 degrees) placed 2.5 cm from the distal end (Fig. 23-2,*B* and Fig. 23-3),[32] or be commercially precurved (Figure 23-2,*B* and Figure 23-4) and/or nonkinkable (wire coiled) (Fig. 23-2,*B* and Fig. 23-5 on p. 461). If the needle is inserted perpendicularly to the plane of the cricothyroid membrane and the long axis of the trachea, the catheter has an equal chance of turning cephalad as caudad. And since the catheter has to make a sharp 90-degree turn, the catheter has a high probability of kinking—thus, the rationale for using preangled,[32] or precurved and/or nonkinkable, catheters (Fig. 23-5). The needle should be connected to either a completely empty 20-ml syringe or a partly clear fluid-filled 20-ml syringe. An empty 20-ml syringe

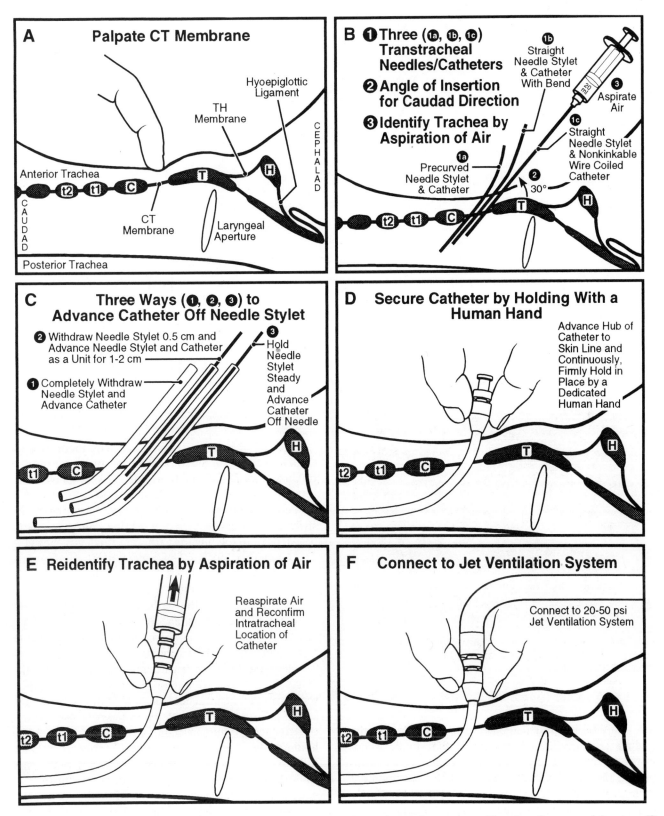

Fig. 23-2. The steps involved in transtracheal ventilation and some alternative options and considerations for some of the steps (B and C). **A,** Cricothyroid (CT) membrane is palpated first. **B,** 1. Transtracheal needle is inserted through CT membrane. Transtracheal needle/catheter can be: 1a precurved (see Fig. 23-4); 1b straight with a distal small-angle bend (see Fig. 23-3); or 1c straight with a wire coiled nonkinkable catheter (see Fig. 23-5). 2. Angle between distal end of needle/catheter and skin (i.e., angle of insertion for caudad direction) should be 30 degrees. 3. Entry into trachea should be confirmed by aspirating air. **C,** The three ways to advance catheter off needle 1, 2, and 3, are explained by labeling. **D,** Once catheter has been advanced so that hub is at skin line, it must be continuously held in place by a human hand (do not try to tape or suture hub of catheter in place). **E,** Intratracheal location should be reconfirmed by reaspirating air. **F,** Transtracheal jet-ventilation catheter is connected to jet ventilator. (*T,* thyroid cartilage; *H,* hyoid bone; *C,* cricoid cartilage; *t1,* first tracheal cartilage; *t2,* second tracheal cartilage.)

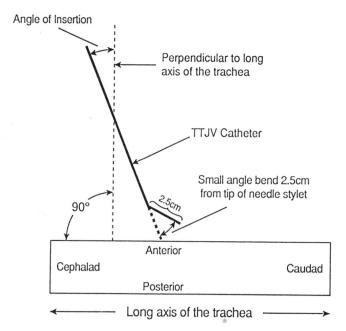

Fig. 23-3. Definition of angle of insertion and small-angle bend 2.5 cm from the distal end of needle stylet (*TTJV*, transtracheal jet ventilation).

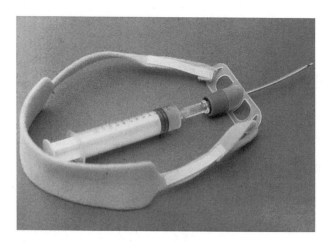

Fig. 23-4. Continuously curved transtracheal jet-ventilation needle/catheter made by International Medical and Dental Products, Park City, Utah.

will easily fill with air if the tip of the needle is in the trachea (Fig. 23-2,*B*). If the tip of the needle is not in the trachea but rather in some tissue, resistance to pulling the plunger back because of the development of negative pressure in the syringe will be felt prior to pulling the plunger of the syringe out of the syringe barrel. If an empty syringe smaller than 20 ml is used, it might be possible to pull the plunger out of the barrel of the syringe before the resistance from negative pressure is felt. If a partly clear fluid-filled syringe is used and the tip of the needle is in the trachea, then air will bubble through the liquid when the plunger is

pulled back as soon as the tip of the needle enters the trachea.

Once entry into the trachea has been identified, the catheter can be threaded over the needle stylet into the trachea (Fig. 23-2,*C*, method no. 3). A 14-gauge intravenous catheter has enough structural strength to be pushed into the trachea itself, and therefore the needle stylet of a 14-gauge catheter may be completely withdrawn prior to feeding the catheter into the trachea (Fig. 23-2,*C*, method no. 1). The needle stylet *should not* be withdrawn a short distance back into the lumen of the catheter and advanced together with the catheter, since this will only cause the catheter to hit the posterior membrane of the trachea, increasing the risk of the needle stylet perforating the catheter and/or the posterior membrane of the trachea (Fig. 23-2,*C*, method no. 2). Once the hub of the catheter reaches the skin line (Fig. 23-2,*D*), air should once again be aspirated to reconfirm the intratracheal location of the catheter (Fig. 23-2,*E*). From the moment the catheter is inserted into the trachea, a human hand should be dedicated to holding the transtracheal catheter exactly in place (allowing no movement whatsoever at any time, especially during jet ventilation) until a definitive airway (the natural airway, or a correctly positioned endotracheal tube or surgical airway) is established (Fig. 23-2,*D*).

B. MAINTAIN PATENCY OF NATURAL AIRWAY AS MUCH AS POSSIBLE

The only driving pressure for exhalation is the elastic recoil of the lung (10 to 20 cm H_2O). Thus, the inspiratory gas is driven through a relatively small

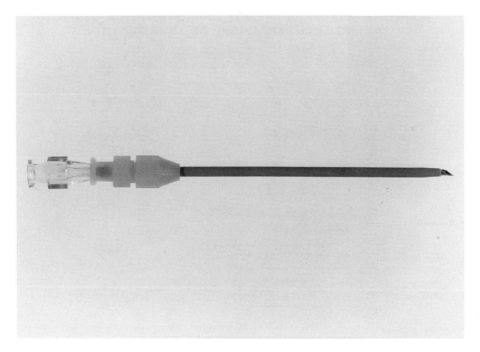

Fig. 23-5. Nonkinkable wire-coiled transtracheal jet-ventilation catheter made by Cook Critical Care.

catheter under high pressure, but the expiratory gas must escape through as large a channel as possible (i.e., the natural airway) under a relatively low driving pressure. Therefore, during TTJV the natural airway must be maintained as well as possible at all times to avoid trapping air and hyperexpansion of the lungs. This means that oropharyngeal and nasopharyngeal airways should be used and maximal jaw thrust maintained (Fig. 23-6).

C. ACCEPTABLE TRANSTRACHEAL JET-VENTILATION SYSTEMS

Many systems have been suggested for TTJV. In particular, a great deal has been written about how to connect a transtracheal catheter to a ventilatory source.[18,33-47] Distillation of this literature reveals three basic acceptable TTJV systems that work reliably and can be easily and inexpensively assembled from readily available materials and/or commercially purchased. "Acceptable" is defined as a system that has enough oxygen pressure and circuit stiffness (noncompliance) to easily achieve adequate ventilation (a normal $Paco_2$). The first acceptable TTJV system consists of a jet injector powered by central wall-oxygen pressure (50 psi) that is additionally regulated by an in-line regulator (0 to 50 psi) (Figs. 23-7 and 23-8) or remains additionally unregulated (Figs. 23-9 on p. 464 and 23-10 on p. 465). The advantage of using central pressure (50 psi) to power the jet injector (provided the system is already plugged in) is the guaranteed immediate availability of a

preassembled, reliable, tightly jointed system to connect to the transtracheal catheter. The advantage of regulated wall pressure (0 to 50 psi) is the ability to minimize barotrauma, especially in pediatric patients and when jetting through a tube exchanger (jet stylet), the distal end of which could be subcarinal. The great advantage of using a preassembled, commercially made TTJV system is the quality assurance built into a commercial product and freedom from having to assemble the ventilator system yourself (anyone who has bought an "easy to assemble" toy for a child knows how frustrating this can be). To ensure that the jet injector shown in Figs. 23-8 and 23-10, which also has industrial uses, is free of an oil coating or residue, the jet injector is always soaked in acetone (which dissolves oil) after it arrives from the manufacturer. The commercial jet injectors made for medical use (Figs. 23-7 and 23-9) do not have an oil coating or residue. All nonthreaded connections should be bound with wire or plastic ties.

The second TTJV system consists of a jet injector powered by an oxygen-tank regulator (Fig. 23-11 on p. 466). Tank regulators can be classified as high flow or low flow with respect to the steady-state pressure (pounds per square inch) and corresponding flow rates that each can generate. A high-flow tank regulator can achieve maximum steady-state pressures of 100 psi and flow rates of 320 L/min and therefore presents no problem with respect to providing adequate TTJV. A low-flow regulator (such as those that are commonly available on small [E-cylinder] oxygen transport tanks) can achieve a

MAINTAIN MAXIMAL PATENCY OF THE NATURAL AIRWAY DURING TRANSTRACHEAL JET VENTILATION

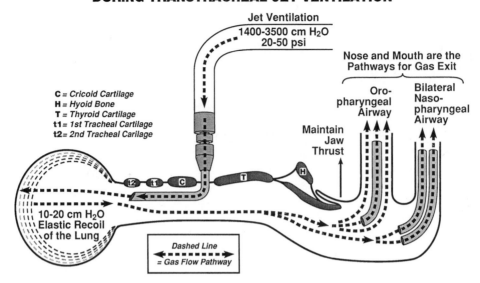

Fig. 23-6. Maximal airway patency must be maintained during transtracheal jet ventilation because pathway for exhalation of jetted oxygen is the natural airway, and the driving force for exhalation is the relatively very low elastic recoil of lungs.

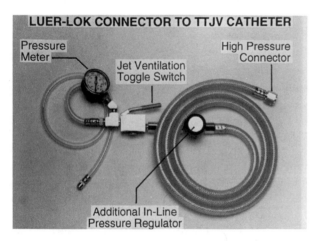

Fig. 23-7. Commercially preassembled jet-ventilation system (Mercury Medical) consisting of high-pressure connector, high-pressure hosing, additional in-line regulator, jet-ventilation toggle switch, dry gas–pressure meter, and Luer-Lok connector to transtracheal jet-ventilation (TTJV) catheter.

maximum pressure of 120 psi when the flow meter is set at the maximum of 15 L/min but no flow is allowed to occur. When flow is allowed to commence (i.e., the button on the jet injector is pressed), very high flows will occur for a moment and then exponentially decay as the pressure in the regulator exponentially decreases to steady-state values of 0 to 5 psi that permit the flow that was preset on the flow meter (0 to 15 L/min). Satisfactory tidal volumes with the 16- and 14-gauge TTJV catheters may be achieved within the first 0.5 second.[17]

The advantage of a low-flow regulator is that it is

mobile and can be used in locations that do not have a central (wall) source of high-pressure oxygen (e.g., in patients' rooms, hallways, and out-of-hospital situations). However, for this system to be effective, it must be standing by or brought to these anesthetizing locations prior to the induction of anesthesia. If a low-flow regulator must be used, the flow should be set at the maximum of 15 L/min and an I:E ratio of 1:1 used to ensure adequacy of tidal volume. But the inspiratory time should be limited to one second or less to allow the pressure in the regulator to restore itself so that the initial high-burst flow rate may once again be achieved with the next breath.[17]

The third TTJV system uses the anesthesia-machine flush valve as the jet injector. The anesthesia-machine flush valve can be powered by either a wall or tank high-pressure oxygen source and will generate a jet-ventilation pressure that approaches line pressure.[24] The fresh-gas outlet of the anesthesia machine (now an industrywide standard 15-mm male outlet) is connected to noncompliant oxygen-supply tubing by a standard 15-mm endotracheal-tube adapter that fits a 4-mm ID (internal diameter) endotracheal tube (Fig. 23-12 on p. 467). The noncompliant oxygen-supply tubing allows for bypass of the compliant reservoir bag and corrugated tubing of the anesthesia circle system. This third TTJV system is completed by connecting the oxygen-supply tubing to the TTJV catheter; although this may be accomplished in many ways, our permanent TTJV sets have a bonded Luer-Lok/hose-barb connector (Fig. 23-12, left #3). As a quick, makeshift alternative, the connection for the TTJV catheter/O_2 supply tubing can

Transtracheal Jet Ventilation (TTJV) Systems	Component-to-Component Schematic	Part	Company	Model Number
TTJV using jet injector powered by regulated central wall O_2 pressure	Wall O_2 pressure 1. 2. O_2 hose 3. 4. Regulator 5. 6. Air hose 7. Jet injector 8. 9. O_2 tubing 10. 11. TTJV Catheter	1. Chemetron wall O_2 quick disconnect + ¼" OD hose barb	Tri-Anim	11–01–0003
		2. Chemetron O_2 hose	Tri-Anim	15–11–0001
		3. ¼" ID hose barb + ⅛" NPT adapter	Western Enterpr.	MH–7
		4. Miniregulator gauge 0–50 psi	Bird Bird	2322 6765
		5. ⅛" NPT male reducing adapter + ¼" NPT female adapter	Western Enterpr.	MA–9
		6. Air hose 25'	Lawson or Sears	81070 or 9HT16224
		7. Jet injector	Lawson or Sears	11903 or 9HT16235
		8. ⅛" NPT male adapter + ¼" ID hose barb	Western Enterpr.	MH–7
		9. Tygon tubing R–3603 ⅜" OD, ¼" ID	Cole-Parmer	6408–50
		10. ¼" hose barb + male luer lok	Becton-Dickinson	9067
		11. Intravenous catheter with standard hub		

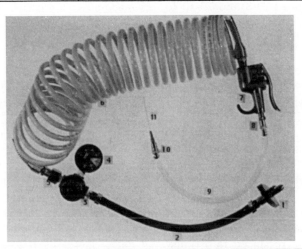

▷▷▷ = hose barb; ▨▨▨ = threaded screw connection; ▭ = male-female connection; NPT = National Pipe Thread. The parts list is the one used in our hospital.

Relevant addresses and telephone numbers of manufacturing and distributing companies for ordering parts are listed in the Appendix. Total cost = $145. Mr. Ron Rusk, personal communication.

*All nonthreaded connections should be bonded together with wire or plastic ties (see photographs). (From Benumof JL, Scheller MS. The importance of transtracheal jet ventilation in the management of the difficult airway. Anesthesiology 55:606-607, 1981; with permission.)

Fig. 23-8. Transtracheal jet-ventilation systems using regulated wall-oxygen pressure. (From Benumof JL, Scheller MS: *Anesthesiology* 55:606, 1981.)

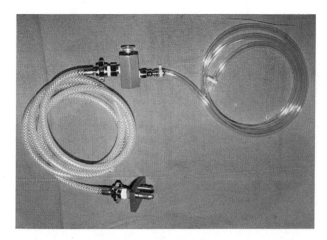

Fig. 23-9. A commercially preassembled jet-ventilation system (Instrument Industries) that has same parts as jet ventilator in Figure 23-7, except there is no additional in-line regulator and therefore no need for a pressure meter.

be accomplished by cutting the barrel of a 1-ml syringe with a scissors and inserting the cut end of the barrel into the oxygen-supply tubing and the other uncut standard male end into the standard female IV catheter hub (Fig. 23-12, right #3). The advantage of this system is that it can be quickly assembled from three readily available materials, is inexpensive, and can be used wherever there is an anesthesia machine. To be effective, it must be readily available before a cannot-ventilate/intubate situation develops (i.e., always). At the time of writing, the approximate costs for the TTJV systems in Figure 23-7 (Mercury Medical) and in Figures 23-8 and 23-10 to 23-12 were $150, $145, $83, $73, and $6, respectively.

It is important to realize that not all anesthesia machines are equal with respect to the pounds per square inch that the fresh-gas outlet delivers when the flush valve is activated. Some anesthesia machines are inadequate, by a wide margin, with respect to being able to deliver effective TTJV. Under the conditions of a widely varying lung compliance (10 to 100 ml/cm H_2O), the largest tidal volume and resultant minute ventilation are consistently obtained by activating the flush valve of the Ohmeda Modulus II and Dräger Narkomed 2 anesthesia machines (Figs. 23-13 on p. 468, 23-14 on p. 469, and Table 23-1 on p. 456).[24] Progressively smaller tidal volume and minute ventilation were produced using the Dräger Narkomed 2A (produced 18 psi) and Ohmeda Modulus II Plus (produced 7 psi) anesthesia machines (Figs. 23-13, 23-14, and Table 23-1).[24] The largest differences in flow rate, tidal volume, and minute ventilation generated by each of the anesthesia machines are due to, and explained by, the internal construction of the flush valve unique to each of them. A one-way outlet check valve is positioned between the vaporizers and flush valve in the Ohmeda Modulus II (Fig. 23-15 on p. 470) and Dräger Narkomed 2 (Fig. 23-16 on p. 471)

anesthesia machines that directs the entire flow of oxygen (45 to 75 L/min at approximately 50 psi) out the common gas outlet when the flush valve is activated.[24] There is no such valve in the Ohmeda Modulus II Plus (Fig. 23-17 on p. 472) or the Dräger Narkomed 2A (Fig. 23-18 on p. 473) anesthesia machines, so that activating the flush valves directs oxygen toward both the vaporizers and the common gas outlet.[24] Each of these anesthesia machines has a pressure-limiting mechanism so that the pressure out of the common gas outlet of both anesthesia machines is only 7 and 18 psi, respectively, resulting in dramatically lower tidal volume and subsequent minute ventilation.[24] In conclusion, the Ohmeda Modulus II Plus anesthesia machine is not an acceptable power source and the Dräger Narkomed 2A is only a marginally acceptable power source for providing total ventilatory support by activating the flush valve for jet ventilation, whereas the Dräger Narkomed 2 and Ohmeda Modulus II anesthesia machines are both acceptable power sources for jet ventilation for providing substantial partial, if not total, ventilatory support in most clinical situations.

D. SHORTCOMINGS OF ALTERNATIVE TRANSTRACHEAL VENTILATION SYSTEMS

There are two other ways to ventilate and/or oxygenate lungs by the transtracheal route that have been described, but they both fail to achieve true, and therefore, effective jet ventilation. The first of these suboptimal methods consists of using the anesthesia machine's oxygen flush valve (powered by either wall or tank oxygen) and the anesthesia circle-system corrugated tubing to deliver the oxygen to the transtracheal catheter. In this instance the compliant reservoir bag and corrugated tubing absorbs, by distention, most of the jet from the anesthesia machine's fresh-gas outlet and prevents effective ventilation of the lungs. Thus, with this system, the $Paco_2$ can be expected to increase. Unfortunately, TTJV studies using this system have not been performed, and so the exact rate of $Paco_2$ increase is not known. The second method is predictably even less effective and consists of manually ventilating the lungs by vigorously squeezing a self-inflating reservoir bag. In this instance it is impossible to achieve a significant amount of ventilation through the IV catheter and the $Paco_2$ increases at a rate of 4 mm Hg/min,[19] which is close to the rate of CO_2 increase of 6 mm Hg/min during apneic oxygen insufflation in animals anesthetized with barbiturates.[19]

Although we strongly recommend using one of the three acceptable TTJV systems discussed, and do not recommend using one of the two transtracheal systems described in the previous paragraph, it should be mentioned that both of the suboptimal methods described here can provide some, although questionably

Transtracheal Jet Ventilation Systems Using Unregulated Wall O$_2$ Pressure.*

Transtracheal Jet Ventilation (TTJV) Systems	Component-to-Component Schematic	Part	Company	Model Number
TTJV using jet injector powered by unregulated central wall O$_2$ pressure	Wall O$_2$ pressure 1. 2. 3. Air hose 4. Jet injector 5. 6. O$_2$ tubing 7. 8. TTJV Catheter	1. Chemetron wall O$_2$ quick disconnect + $\frac{1}{8}$" ID NPT male adapter	Tri-Anim	11–01–0007
		2. $\frac{1}{8}$" NPT male adapter + $\frac{1}{4}$" reducing coupling	Lawson	5308
		3. Air hose 25'	Lawson or Sears	81070 or 9HT16224
		4. Jet injector	Lawson or Sears	11903 or 9HT16235
		5. $\frac{1}{8}$" NPT male adapter + $\frac{1}{4}$" ID hose barb	Western Enterpr.	MH–7
		6. Tygon tubing R–3603 $\frac{3}{8}$" OD, $\frac{1}{4}$" ID	Cole-Parmer	6408–50
		7. $\frac{1}{4}$" hose barb male luer lok	Becton-Dickinson	9067
		8. Intravenous catheter with standard hub		

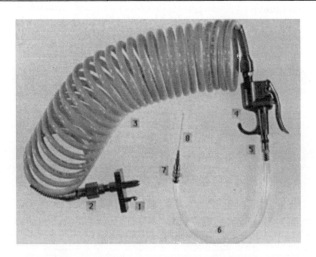

▷▷▷ = hose barb;   ▨▨▨ = threaded screw connection;   ⬜ = male-female connection; NPT = National Pipe Thread. The parts list is the one used in our hospital.

Relevant addresses and telephone numbers of manufacturing and distributing companies for ordering parts are listed in Appendix II. Total cost = $83. Mr. Ron Rusk, personal communication.

*All nonthreaded connections should be bonded together with wire or plastic ties (see photographs). (From Benumof JL, Scheller MS. The importance of transtracheal jet ventilation in the management of the difficult airway. Anesthesiology 55:606-607, 1981; with permission.)

Fig. 23-10. Transtracheal jet-ventilation systems using unregulated wall-oxygen pressure. (From Benumof JL, Scheller MS: *Anesthesiology* 55:606, 1981.)

Transtracheal Jet Ventilation Systems Using O₂ Tank Regulator.*

Transtracheal Jet Ventilation (TTJV) Systems	Component-to-Component Schematic	Part	Company	Model Number
TTJV using jet injector powered by O₂ tank regulator	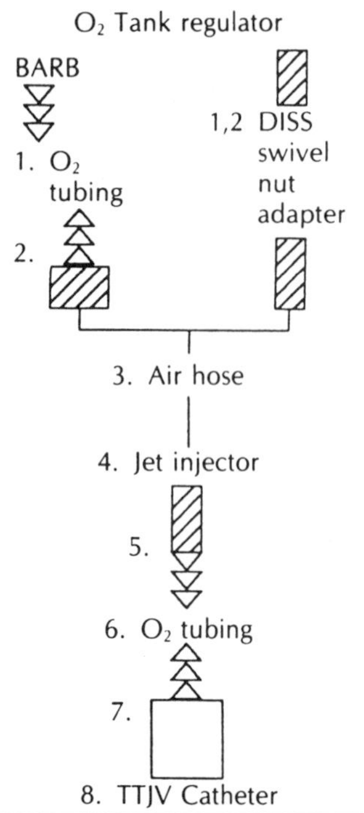 O₂ Tank regulator BARB 1. O₂ tubing 1,2 DISS swivel nut adapter 2. 3. Air hose 4. Jet injector 5. 6. O₂ tubing 7. 8. TTJV Catheter	1. Tygon tubing R–3603 + ⅜″ OD, ¼″ ID	Cole-Parmer	6408–50
		2. ¼″ ID hose barb + ¼″ NPT female adapter	Western Enterpr.	MH–7
		1,2. DISS swivel nut adapter + ¼″ NPT female adapter	Western Enterpr.	M24–35
		3. Air hose 25′	Lawson or Sears	81070 or 9HT16224
		4. Jet injector	Lawson or Sears	11903 or 9HT16235
		5. ⅛″ NPT male adapter + ¼″ ID hose barb	Western Enterpr.	MH–7
		6. Tygon tubing R–3603 ⅜″ OD, ¼″ ID	Cole-Parmer	6408–50
		7. ¼″ hose barb male luer lok	Becton-Dickinson	9067
		8. Intravenous catheter with standard hub		

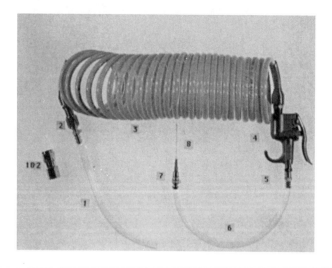

▷▷▷ = hose barb; ▨▨▨ = threaded screw connection; ▭ = male-female connection; NPT = National Pipe Thread. The parts list is the one used in our hospital.

Relevant addresses and telephone numbers of manufacturing and distributing companies for ordering parts are listed in Appendix II. Total cost = $73. Mr. Ron Rusk, personal communication.

*All nonthreaded connections should be bonded together with wire or plastic ties (see photographs). (From Benumof JL, Scheller MS. The importance of transtracheal jet ventilation in the management of the difficult airway. Anesthesiology 55:606–607, 1981; with permission.)

Fig. 23-11. Transtracheal jet-ventilation systems using oxygen-tank regulator. (From Benumof JL, Scheller MS: *Anesthesiology* 55:606, 1981.)

Transtracheal Jet Ventilation Systems Using Anesthesia Machine Fresh Gas Outlet and Flush Valve.*

Transtracheal Jet Ventilation (TTJV) Systems	Component-to-Component Schematic	Part	Company	Model Number
TTJV using anesthesia machine fresh gas outlet and flush valve	Anesthesia machine fresh gas outlet 1. 2. O₂ Supply tubing 3. 3. 4. TTJV Catheter	1. 15-mm ET tube adapter for 4-mm ID ET tube	Many companies	
		2. O₂ supply tubing	Many companies	
		3. ¼" hose barb male Luer lock or 3. cut-off 1-ml syringe	Becton-Dickinson	9067
		4. Intravenous catheter with standard hub		

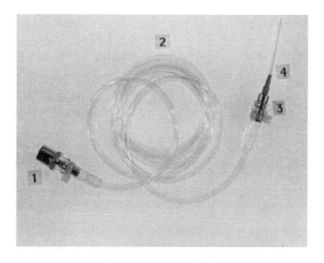

▷▷▷ = .hose barb;   ▨▨▨ = threaded screw connection;   ▭ = male-female connection; NPT = National Pipe Thread. The parts list is the one used in our hospital.

Relevant addresses and telephone numbers of manufacturing and distributing companies for ordering parts are listed in Appendix II. Total cost = $6. Mr. Ron Rusk, personal communication.

*All nonthreaded connections should be bonded together with wire or plastic ties (see photographs). (From Benumof JL, Scheller MS. The importance of transtracheal jet ventilation in the management of the difficult airway. Anesthesiology 55:606–607, 1981; with permission.)

Fig. 23-12. Transtracheal jet-ventilation systems using anesthesia machine's fresh-gas outlet. (From Benumof JL, Scheller MS: *Anesthesiology* 55:606, 1981.)

adequate, oxygenation that is certainly better than continuing with a life-threatening cannot-ventilate/intubate situation. Consequently, if either of these latter two methods must be used, it should be known that the standard 15-mm elbow connector at the end of an anesthesia circle system and at the end of a self-inflating reservoir bag can be connected to the transtracheal IV catheter in two ways: (1) by inserting the male end of a 15-mm endotracheal-tube adapter that fits a 3-mm ID endotracheal tube directly into the standard female hub of the IV catheter,[37,44] and (2) by inserting the male end of a plungerless 3- or 5-ml syringe into the standard female hub of the IV catheter, and the male end of a 15-mm endotracheal-tube adapter that fits an 8-mm and a 10-mm ID endotracheal tube, respectively, into the empty barrel of the syringe.[35,44] Still, even with these kinds of connections, if one is suddenly confronted with a cannot-ventilate/intubate situation, and is otherwise not ready for the situation, it will take significant extra time and hands to find the parts for these connections, for what is in the end analysis, not the best transtracheal ventilation system.

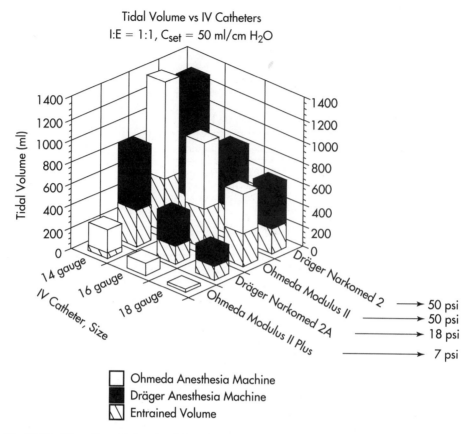

Fig. 23-13. The effect of changing IV catheter size (x-axis) on tidal volume (y-axis) for all four anesthesia machines (z-axis) at C_{set} = 50 ml/cm H_2O. As IV catheter size increases, tidal volume increases for each anesthesia machine. Ohmeda Modulus II and Dräger Narkomed 2 anesthesia machines generated the greatest tidal volumes compared to the other two anesthesia machines. Entrained volume is represented by the diagonally striped bars as a portion of total VT for each experimental condition. Contribution of entrained air to total VT ranged from 0% to 49%, with greatest contribution to total tidal volume using 14-gauge IV catheter/Ohmeda Modulus II anesthesia-machine combination. (*IV*, intravenous; *I:E*, inspiratory-to-expiratory ratio; C_{set}, set compliance of mechanical-lung model; *psi*, pounds per square inch; *VT*, tidal volume.) (From Gaughan SD, Benumof JL, Ozaki GT: *Anesth Analg* 76:800, 1993.)

One could argue that an indication to use a transtracheal catheter reservoir-bag system would be in cases in which the upper airway (i.e., cephalad to the cricothyroid membrane) was totally obstructed.[22] In cases of total upper-airway obstruction, inability to expel the TTJV gas from the lungs would greatly increase the risk of barotrauma due to gas trapping and lung hyperexpansion. With a transtracheal catheter reservoir-bag system, only small amounts of oxygen can be delivered to the alveolar space per unit of time (but, perhaps, still sufficient to maintain a life-sustaining–level of oxygenation), with a significantly reduced risk of barotrauma.[38] However, one could equally well argue that small amounts of oxygen could also be delivered to the alveolar space by true TTJV (by either jet-injector or anesthesia-machine valve with any kind of tubing) by simply using slow respiratory rates and short jet-injection times (i.e.,

low I:E ratios) and a low driving pressure (e.g., 20 psi). In any case of total upper-airway obstruction, all percutaneous transtracheal ventilation systems must be converted to a formal cricothyrotomy or tracheostomy tube, and the lungs must be well ventilated with conventional intermittent positive-pressure ventilation as soon as possible.

IV. EXAMPLES OF THE PROBLEM/THE SOLUTION

The University of California, San Diego, Medical Center installed the second acceptable TTJV system (jet-injector powered by unregulated wall pressure) in all anesthetizing locations in 1981. In the past 14 years, we have treated 11 patients whose lungs, as defined at the beginning of this chapter, could not be ventilated via mask and in whom tracheal intubation could not be

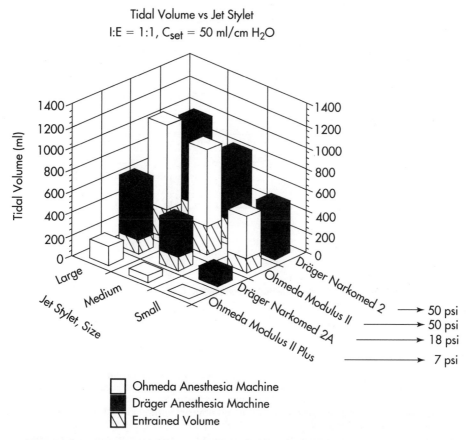

Tidal Volume vs Jet Stylet
I:E = 1:1, C_{set} = 50 ml/cm H_2O

Ohmeda Anesthesia Machine
Dräger Anesthesia Machine
Entrained Volume

Fig. 23-14. The effect of changing jet-stylet size (x-axis) on tidal volume (y-axis) for all four anesthesia machines (z-axis) at C_{set} = 50 ml/cm H_2O. As jet-stylet size increases, tidal volume increases for all four anesthesia machines. Ohmeda Modulus II and Dräger Narkomed 2 anesthesia machines generated the greatest tidal volumes of the four anesthesia machines for any given jet-stylet size. Entrained volume is represented by diagonally striped bars as a portion of total V_T for each experimental condition. Contribution of entrained air to total V_T ranged from 0% to 30% and accounted for the greatest contribution to total V_T for medium jet stylet/Ohmeda Modulus II anesthesia machine combination. (From Gaughan SD, Benumof JL, Ozaki GT: *Anesth Analg* 76:800, 1993.)

performed. All 11 patients had a brief period of severe decreased pulse-oximeter saturation (SpO_2), which was quickly reversed by the immediate administration of TTJV. The following is a brief summary of five of these cases.

Case 1. A previously healthy 34-year-old woman developed moderate edema of the face and upper airway following fluid overload during repair of a lacerated femoral vein. The patient's trachea was extubated after she was completely awake, but she immediately evidenced complete airway obstruction. Insertion of oral and nasal airways accompanied by attempts at bag and mask ventilation were of no benefit. Attempts at reintubation were unsuccessful, and TTJV was instituted as the oxygen saturation fell below 60%. There was prompt return of SpO_2 to 100% with TTJV, which was continued until a tracheostomy could be performed.

Case 2. Anesthesia and paralysis were induced with thiamylal/succinylcholine in a preeclamptic term patient

about to undergo emergency cesarean section. Following induction of anesthesia, it was not possible to ventilate the lungs with a bag and mask or to intubate the trachea due to a combination of a small mouth, receding chin, and what appeared to be generalized edema of the laryngeal aperture. Institution of TTJV promptly reversed severe hemoglobin desaturation and provided adequate ventilation until a fiberoptic-assisted intubation could be performed.

Case 3. The lungs of a 66-year-old woman with a supraglottic tumor could not be ventilated with a bag and mask, nor could the trachea be intubated following induction of anesthesia. SpO_2, which had decreased to less than 60%, was restored to 100% within four TTJV breaths. Adequate ventilation was maintained until the surgeons completed a tracheostomy.

Case 4. A previously healthy 32-year-old man, whose trachea had been easily intubated preoperatively with a blind nasotracheal technique while he was awake and

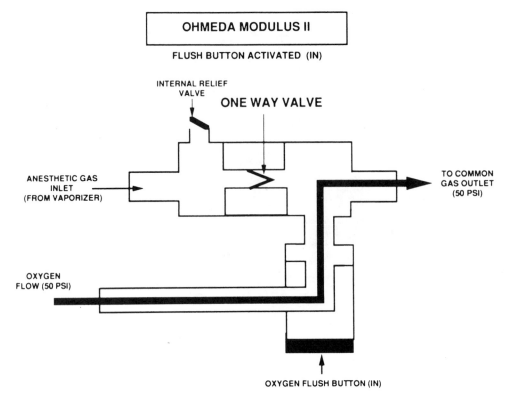

Fig. 23-15. Flush valve of Ohmeda Modulus II anesthesia machine in open (activated) position. With activation of oxygen flush button, approximately 45-75 L/min (equivalent to approximately 50 psi [pounds per square inch]) enters flush valve "chamber." Because chamber contains a one-way valve, the flow of oxygen is directed out through the common gas outlet. (From Gaughan SD, Benumof JL, Ozaki GT: *Anesth Analg* 76:800, 1993.)

who had undergone placement of nonwired arch bars for a mandibular fracture, had his trachea extubated during a period of emergence excitation (bucking on the endotracheal tube but still not responding to commands). Following extubation, it was impossible to ventilate the lungs using a bag and mask. During attempts at reintubation, no recognizable structures were visualized. SpO_2 decreased to less than 20%. Institution of TTJV resulted in prompt return of SpO_2 to 100%. TTJV was continued while racemic epinephrine and a beta-2 agonist bronchodilator were administered directly through the transtracheal catheter. After approximately 5 minutes of TTJV, the patient completely awoke and experienced no further respiratory difficulty.

Case 5. A 55-year-old woman with a history of a subglottic tumor developed dyspnea at rest. An inhalation induction was performed and despite repeated laryngoscopies, neither the vocal cords nor the glottic opening could be identified. Following an unsuccessful attempt at rigid bronchoscopy, it became impossible to ventilate the lungs with a bag and mask. SpO_2 decreased below 60%, at which time TTJV was instituted. SpO_2 promptly increased to 98%. TTJV was continued until the glottic opening could be identified by air bubbles

emanating from the trachea, which permitted insertion of an endotracheal tube.

In these five patients, different causes resulted in a common inability to ventilate the lungs via mask or to intubate the trachea (case 1, upper-airway obstruction; case 2, anatomic difficulties plus laryngeal edema; case 3, supraglottic tumor; case 4, laryngospasm; case 5, subglottic and airway edema). In all cases following decreased SpO_2, TTJV was instituted within one minute, which increased SpO_2 within another minute. In no case were arterial blood gases determined during TTJV because the purpose of the TTJV was strictly resuscitative, and in all cases the TTJV was soon converted to an effective type of permanent ventilation. In the five patients, TTJV permitted four different successful therapeutic options (tracheostomy [cases 1 and 3], intubation over fiberoptic bronchoscope [case 2], conventional orotracheal intubation [case 5], and administration of racemic epinephrine and bronchodilator and allowing the patient to further awaken [case 4]). We cannot be certain of the ultimate outcome had TTJV not been immediately available and instituted in these cases, but given the gravity of these situations, it seems reasonable to postulate that the TTJV was indeed lifesaving.

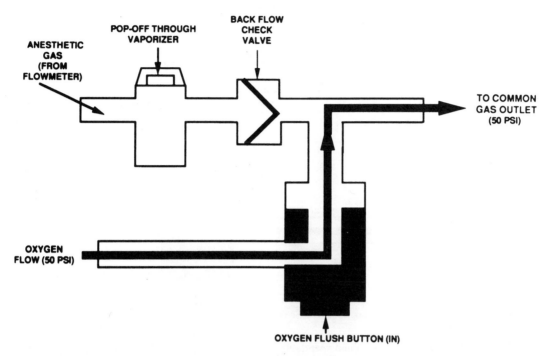

**DRÄGER NARKOMED 2
WITH BACK FLOW CHECK VALVE**

FLUSH BUTTON ACTIVATED (IN)

Fig. 23-16. Flush valve of Dräger Narkomed 2 anesthesia machine in open (activated) position. Activation of oxygen-flush button delivers approximately 50 L/min (equivalent to approximately 50 psi [pounds per square inch]) to flush valve "chamber," and one-way valve positioned between flush valve and last in-line vaporizer directs flow of oxygen out common gas outlet. Valve also prevents a pumping effect on vaporizers from back pressure generated by activation of flush button. (From Gaughan SD, Benumof JL, Ozaki GT: *Anesth Analg* 76:800, 1993.)

Finally, it is important to stress that insertion of a percutaneous TTJV catheter before a cannot-ventilate/intubate situation develops, in cases where preoperative evaluation indicates or at least increases the index of suspicion that cannot-ventilate/intubate situation might develop, is an excellent example of having a backup plan ready to go (see ASA Algorithm, Chapter 8). In addition, percutaneous insertion of a TTJV catheter may permit enough spontaneous ventilation through the catheter to be lifesaving when the natural upper airway is chronically narrowed and complete airway obstruction is imminent or has occurred.[30]

V. COMPLICATIONS OF TRANSTRACHEAL JET VENTILATION

The incidence of serious complications resulting from elective use of TTJV is relatively low and appears to be primarily limited to tissue emphysema. For example, Monnier et al.[23] provided ventilation for 65 patients undergoing laser endoscopic treatment of laryngeal and subglottic lesions with high-frequency TTJV. The can-

nulas were introduced into the trachea under endoscopic guidance. In this series only one complication occurred. This was due to dislodgment of the cannula and resulted in cervicomediastinal emphysema, which was successfully treated by needle aspiration. Smith et al.[34] also reported a 29% incidence of complications in 28 patients managed with TTJV to provide an airway in an emergency. These complications included subcutaneous emphysema (7.1%), mediastinal emphysema (3.6%), exhalation difficulty (14.3%), and arterial perforation (3.6%). None of these complications were fatal.

Barotrauma with resultant pneumothorax has been reported with both TTJV and translaryngeal jet ventilation.[20,21,48-51] Therefore, it is clearly necessary to document breath sounds as well as chest inflation and deflation following institution of TTJV and to assume that any change in cardiovascular parameters, such as hypotension, tachycardia, or bradycardia, may be secondary to pneumothorax. Clearly, the risk of pneumothorax is much increased in cases of total airway obstruction because gas cannot escape from the lungs in

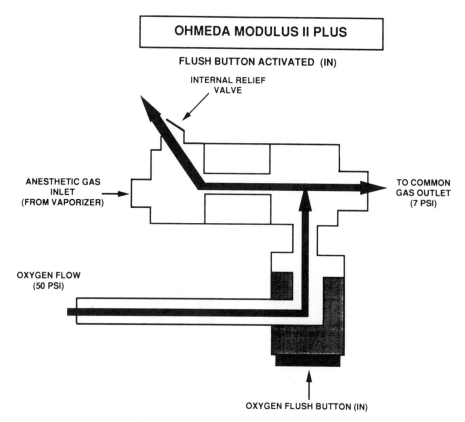

Fig. 23-17. Flush valve of Ohmeda Modulus II Plus anesthesia machine in open (activated) position. Upon activation of flush button, oxygen enters flush valve "chamber" and is directed toward both vaporizers and common gas outlet. Internal relief valve opens as pressure in chamber increases above 120-150 mm Hg (occurs at flow rates of 200 ml/min). At flow rates of 45-75 L/min, pressure directed out common gas outlet is limited to approximately 7 psi (pounds per square inch). (From Gaughan SD, Benumof JL, Ozaki GT: *Anesth Analg* 76:800, 1993.)

a normal manner (i.e., the natural airway) and in cases where the jet-ventilation catheter is a jet stylet (tube exchanger) that is subcarinal and perhaps sublobar.

Other complications, such as esophageal puncture, bleeding, hematoma, and hemoptysis, have been reported following TTJV.[47] In addition, it appears that damage to tracheal mucosa may occur following TTJV, especially if the gas is not humidified. In pigs managed with TTJV for approximately two hours with single-orifice transtracheal catheters using three different methods of nonhumidified gas delivery to the cannula, the posterior wall of the trachea clearly demonstrated macroscopic evidence of irritation and microscopic evidence of mucosal erosion.[18] However, Klain and Smith[19] did not find any tracheal damage in dogs, the lungs of which were subjected to 50 hours of nonhumidified high-frequency TTJV in which 14-gauge multiorifice catheters were used. Nonetheless, the possibility of causing tracheal mucosal ulceration should certainly be considered, particularly if TTJV is attempted through single-orifice catheters without humidification for prolonged periods of time.

VI. CONCLUSION

Presently, the baseline incidence of intraoperative deaths caused by a cannot-ventilate/intubate situation is 1% to 28%, which cannot be remedied by simply improved monitoring. The quickest, easiest, and most efficacious solution to the problem is TTJV through a percutaneously inserted intravenous catheter. The mechanism of efficacy is by mass movement of gas from the jet itself as well as by air entrainment by the Venturi effect, and the lungs of healthy and critically ill patients have been successfully ventilated by this method. The systems of choice, in descending order of preference, are a jet injector powered by regulated wall- or tank-oxygen pressure, a jet injector powered by unregulated wall- or tank-oxygen pressure, and an anesthesia-machine flush valve using noncompliant tubing from the fresh-gas outlet. Much less efficacious transtracheal ventilation systems consist of an anesthesia-machine flush valve using the compliant tubing of the anesthesia circle system (with reservoir bag) and connecting a reservoir bag directly to the transtracheal catheter. In our hospital, the use of TTJV in patients whose lungs could

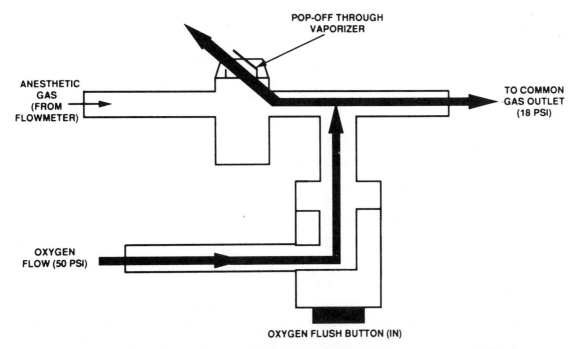

DRÄGER NARKOMED 2A WITHOUT BACK FLOW CHECK VALVE

FLUSH BUTTON ACTIVATED (IN)

POP-OFF THROUGH VAPORIZER

ANESTHETIC GAS (FROM FLOWMETER)

TO COMMON GAS OUTLET (18 PSI)

OXYGEN FLOW (50 PSI)

OXYGEN FLUSH BUTTON (IN)

Fig. 23-18. Flush valve of Dräger Narkomed 2A anesthesia machine in open (activated) position. With activation of flush button, oxygen enters flush valve "chamber" and is directed toward both vaporizers and common gas outlet. Pressure-compensation device is incorporated into vaporizers to vent all pressures greater than 18 psi, and thus pressure out common gas outlet is limited to 18 psi (pounds per square inch). (From Gaughan SD, Benumof JL, Ozaki GT: *Anesth Analg* 76:800, 1993.)

not be ventilated or intubated may have significantly reduced morbidity and mortality. Additional applications of TTJV are to facilitate upper-airway surgery, intubation via conventional laryngoscopy, antegrade fiberoptic bronchoscopy or via initial retrograde intubation technique, cricothyrotomy, and tracheostomy. Nevertheless, there are a number of serious TTJV complications, and this lifesaving procedure should only be undertaken in desperate emergencies or in carefully thought-out elective situations. However, because desperate cannot-ventilate/intubate emergencies will continue to occur in association with anesthesia, we recommend that every anesthetizing location have the immediate availability of TTJV.

REFERENCES

1. Keenan RL, Boyan CP: Cardiac arrest due to anesthesia, *JAMA* 253:2373, 1985.
2. Taylor G, Larson CP, Prestwich R: Unexpected cardiac arrest during anesthesia and surgery: an environmental study, *JAMA* 236:2758, 1976.
3. American Society of Anesthesiologists Committee on Professional Liability (K Posner, project director, and F Cheney, chairman): Personal communication, June, 1990.
4. Bolander FMF: Deaths associated with anesthesia, *Br J Anaesth* 47:36, 1975.
5. Harrison GG: Death attributable to anesthesia, *Br J Anaesth* 50:1041, 1978.
6. Davis DA: An analysis of anesthetic mishaps from medical liability claims, *Int Anesthesiol Clin* 22:31, 1984.
7. American Heart Association: *Textbook of Advanced Cardiac Life Support,* Washington, DC, 1987, American Heart Association.
8. Donegan J: Cardiopulmonary resuscitation. In Miller R, editor: *Anesthesia.* New York, 1986, Churchill Livingstone.
9. Holmgreen WC: Difficult intubation: suspected. In Brady L, Smith RB, editors: *Decision making in anesthesiology,* Philadelphia, 1987, B.C. Decker.
10. Holmgreen WC, Niskioka GR: Difficult intubations: unsuspected. In Brady L, Smith RB, editors: *Decision making in anesthesiology,* Philadelphia, 1987, B.C. Decker.
11. Gammage GW: Airway management. In Civetta JM, Taylor RW, Kirby RR, editors: *Critical Care,* Philadelphia, 1988, J.B. Lippincott.
12. Spoerel WE, Narayanan PS, Singh NP: Transtracheal ventilation, *Br J Anaesth* 43:932, 1971.
13. Jacobs HB: Needle-catheter brings oxygen to the trachea, *JAMA* 222:1231, 1972.

14. Singh NP, Agrawal AR, Dhawan, R: Resuscitation centre for management of respiratory insufficiency cases, *Indian J Chest Dis Allied Sci* 13:99, 1971.

15. Smith RB, MacMillan BB, Petruscak J et al: Transtracheal ventilation for laryngoscopy, *Ann Otol Rhinol Laryngol* 82:347, 1973.

16. Spoerel WE, Greenway RE: Technique of ventilation during endolaryngeal surgery under general anesthesia, *Can J Anaesth* 20:369, 1973.

17. Gaughan SD, Ozaki GT, Benumof JL: Comparison in a lung model of low- and high-flow regulators for transtracheal jet ventilation, *Anesthesiology* 77:189, 1992.

18. Thomas T, Zornow M, Scheller MS et al: The efficacy of three different modes of transtracheal ventilation in hypoxic hypercarbic swine, *Can J Anaesth* 35:(suppl) 61, 1988.

19. Klain M, Smith RB: High frequency percutaneous transtracheal jet ventilation, *Crit Care Med* 5:280, 1977.

20. Cote CJ, Eavey RD, Todres D et al: Cricothyroid membrane puncture: oxygenation and ventilation in a dog model using an intravenous catheter, *Crit Care Med* 16:615, 1988.

21. Weymuller EA, Paugh D, Pavlin EG et al: Management of the difficult airway problems with percutaneous transtracheal ventilation, *Ann Otol Rhinol Laryngol* 96:34, 1987.

22. Jacobs HB: Transtracheal catheter ventilation: clinical experience in 36 patients, *Chest* 65:36, 1974.

23. Monnier PH, Ravussin P, Savary M et al: Percutaneous transtracheal ventilation for laser endoscopic treatment of laryngeal and subglottic lesions, *Clin Otolaryngol* 13:209, 1988.

24. Gaughan SD, Benumof JL, Ozaki GT: Can an anesthesia machine flush valve provide for effective jet ventilation? *Anesth Analg* 76:800, 1993.

25. Smith RB, Myers EN, Sherman H: Transtracheal ventilation in pediatric patients, *Br J Anaesth* 46:313, 1974.

26. Layman PR: Transtracheal ventilation in oral surgery, *Ann R Coll Surg Engl* 65:318, 1983.

27. Wagner DJ, Coombs DW, Doyle SC: Percutaneous transtracheal ventilation for emergency dental appliance removal, *Anesthesiology* 62:664, 1985.

28. McLellan I, Gordon P, Khawaja S et al: Percutaneous transtracheal high frequency jet ventilation as an aid to difficult intubation, *Can J Anaesth* 35:404, 1988.

29. Baraka A: Transtracheal jet ventilation during fiberoptic intubation under general anesthesia, *Anesth Analg* 65:1091, 1986.

30. Dallen LT, Wine R, Benumof JL: Spontaneous ventilation via transtracheal large-bore intravenous catheters is possible, *Anesthesiology* 75:531, 1991.

31. Heimlich HJ, Carr GC: Transtracheal catheter technique for pulmonary rehabilitation, *Ann Otol Rhinol Laryngol* 94:502, 1985.

32. Sdrales L, Benumof JL: Prevention of kinking of percutaneous transtracheal intravenous catheter, *Anesthesiology* 82:288, 1995.

33. Carden E, Becker G, Hamood HL: Percutaneous jet ventilation, *Ann Otol Rhinol Laryngol* 85:652, 1976.

34. Smith BR, Babinski M, Klain M et al: Percutaneous transtracheal ventilation, *J Am Coll Emerg Physicians* 5:765, 1976.

35. Stinson TW: A simple connector for transtracheal ventilation, *Anesthesiology* 47:232, 1977 (letter).

36. Dunlap LB: A modified, simple device for the emergency administration of percutaneous transtracheal ventilation, *J Am Coll Emerg Physicians* 7:42, 1978.

37. Fisher JA: A "last ditch" airway, *Can J Anaesth* 26:225, 1979.

38. Carlton DM, Zide MF: An easily constructed cricothyroidotomy device for emergency airway management, *J Oral Surg* 38:623, 1980.

39. Delisser EA, Muravchick S: Emergency transtracheal ventilation, *Anesthesiology* 55:606, 1981.

40. Hilton PJ: A simple connector for cricothyroid cannulation, *Anaesthesia* 37:220, 1982 (letter).

41. Scuderi PE, McLeskey CH, Comer PB: Emergency percutaneous transtracheal ventilation during anaesthesia using readily available equipment, *Anesth Analg* 61:867, 1982.

42. Gildar JS: A simple system for transtracheal ventilation, *Anesthesiology* 58:106, 1983.

43. Aye LS. Percutaneous transtracheal ventilation, *Anesth Analg* 62:619, 1983 (letter).

44. Patel R. Systems for transtracheal ventilation, *Anesthesiology* 59:165, 1983 (letter).

45. Pottecher T, Bing J, Cuby C et al: Ventilation translaryngee de sauvetage par aiguille de Tuohy: utilisation en cas d'impossibilite d'intuber et de ventiler un patient curatise, *Ann Fr Anesth Reanim* 3:54, 1984.

46. Ravussin P, Freeman J: A new transtracheal catheter for ventilation and resuscitation, *Can J Anaesth* 32:60, 1985.

47. Benumof JL, Scheller MS: The importance of transtracheal jet ventilation in the management of the difficult airway, *Anesthesiology* 71:769, 1989.

48. O'Sullivan TJ, Healy GB: Complications of Venturi jet ventilation during microlaryngeal surgery, *Arch Otolaryngol Head Neck Surg* 111:127, 1985.

49. Oliverio R, Ruder CB, Fermon C et al: Report on pneumothorax secondary to ball-valve obstruction during jet ventilation, *Anesthesiology* 51:255, 1979.

50. Smith RB, Schaer WB, Pfaeffle H: Percutaneous transtracheal ventilation for anesthesia: a review and report of complications, *Can J Anesth* 22:607, 1975.

51. Egol A, Culpepper JA, Snyder JV: Barotrauma and hypotension resulting from jet ventilation in critically ill patients, *Chest* 88:98, 1985.

APPENDIX

Addresses and Telephone Numbers of Companies Listed in Figs. 23-8 and 23-10 to 23-12.

Tri-Anim Health Services, Inc.
  1630 Flower Street
  P.O. Box 3823
  Glendale, California 91201
  (818)545-7329

Cole-Parmer Instrument Co.
  7425 North Oak Park Avenue
  Chicago, Illinois 60648
  (800)323-4340

Western Enterprises
  33672 Pin Oak Parkway
  Avon Lake, Ohio 44012
  (216)933-2171

Lawson Products
  1237 West Walnut Street
  Compton, California 90220
  (213)637-1237

Division of Becton-Dickinson & Co.
  Rutherford, New Jersey 07070
  (201)460-2000

Chapter 24

PERFORMANCE OF RIGID BRONCHOSCOPY

Anthony E. Magit
Terence M. Davidson

I. CASE EXAMPLE

The patient is an 18-month-old female with a 24-hour history of wheezing, asymmetric breath sounds, and a chest x-ray showing mediastinal shift to the left. The child had a 3-day history of rhinorrhea and mild upper airway congestion without fever. Last night the child was eating a piece of raw broccoli and had an episode of choking. The child was brought to the operating room for rigid bronchoscopy with the presumptive diagnosis of retained broccoli in the airway being responsible for the wheezing and abnormal chest x-ray. After general anesthesia had been introduced via inhalation of halothane via mask, the bronchoscope was introduced into the airway without difficulty, and the findings consisted of diffuse tracheobronchial edema consistent with an acute upper respiratory infection. No foreign body was seen. Initial attempts at ventilating the patient with a mask after removing the ventilating bronchoscope were unsuccessful due to persistent desaturations. The patient was wheezing and was intubated with a 4-0 endotracheal tube to facilitate delivery of a bronchodilator into the lower airway. After 15 minutes, the wheezing resolved, and the patient was extubated in the operating room. The patient went on to have an uneventful 48-hour hospital course with resolution of her acute upper respiratory infection.

II. DISCUSSION

This case illustrates the dilemma facing the clinician when a patient with a suspected foreign body has an underlying condition complicating general anesthesia, specifically a lower respiratory infection. Adult and pediatric patients with poor pulmonary reserve, whether intrinsic or secondary to a transient condition, are prone to desaturation during bronchoscopy when positive pressure may not be possible due to an air leak around the bronchoscope. Additionally, the patient had an irritable airway, and bronchodilators could not be delivered through the bronchoscope, requiring the brief intubation for the purpose of delivering the medication.

Spontaneous ventilation is the accepted anesthetic technique for foreign body removal. Spontaneous ventilation provides a degree of airway protection, since the patient can generate positive pressure on expiration and potentially prevent objects from becoming lodged distally. Precise communication between the anesthetist and endoscopist concerning the adequacy of ventilation and endoscopic findings is the cornerstone of the team approach to airway management. Once a foreign body was not found, the goals of the procedure changed, and the management issues focused on treating a reactive airway and creating an extubatable patient.

III. OVERVIEW

Direct examination of the tracheobronchial tree can be performed with rigid or flexible bronchoscopes. The applications for diagnostic and therapeutic bronchoscopy have increased over the past quarter century, given the advances in flexible endoscopes and the capability to perform bronchoscopy using conscious sedation in adults and in children. Despite the prevalence of skilled flexible bronchoscopists, rigid bronchoscopy maintains a central position in the diagnosis and management of airway problems in adults and children because of the unique advantages of rigid bronchoscopy. There are absolute and relative indications for rigid bronchoscopy. An absolute indication for rigid bronchoscopy is the retrieval of a suspected foreign body in a child. Management of tracheal masses (i.e., hemangiomas, papillomas, cysts) can be achieved with operative bronchoscopy with laser or surgical instruments manipulated within the lumen of the rigid bronchoscope. An unstable airway in conjunction with distorted anatomy secondary to infection, tumor, or trauma may be successfully managed with rigid bronchoscopy when orotracheal or nasotracheal intubation is unsuccessful.

IV. INSTRUMENTATION

Rigid bronchoscopy has emerged from the era when illumination was provided by a prism inserted into the lumen of the bronchoscope, with the bronchoscopist relying upon his or her unaided eye. Glass rod telescopes, also called endoscopes, inserted into the lumen of the bronchoscope are the preferred method of visualizing the airway during bronchoscopy (Fig. 24-1). With telescopes and video cameras, bronchoscopy has become a highly sensitive and thorough means of examination. The bronchoscope is designed with a ventilating port for attaching ventilator tubing (Fig. 24-2). Oxygen and anesthetic agents are introduced into the airway through the bronchoscope, around the indwelling endoscope. A second side port provides a means of introducing flexible suction catheters or delicate instruments into the lumen of the bronchoscope without disrupting the connector that attaches the endoscope to the bronchoscope (Fig. 24-3). Endoscopes are available with several viewing angles. The 0-degree endoscope is the most commonly used scope, though 30- and 90-degree scopes are also used.

Pediatric bronchoscopes are available in 3 lengths and various diameters (Fig. 24-4, Table 24-1). The bronchoscopes are named according to the diameter of their internal lumen. Premature infants and neonates may

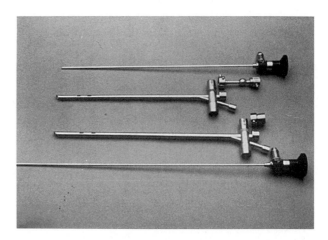

Fig. 24-1. Pictured from top to bottom are the 30-cm length telescope, the long locking bridge; a 26-cm length bronchoscope, the short locking bridge; a 30-cm length bronchoscope, and the 35-cm length telescope. The 35-cm length telescope is used with optical forceps. (Courtesy Karl Storz, Endoscopy America, Inc., Culver City, CA.)

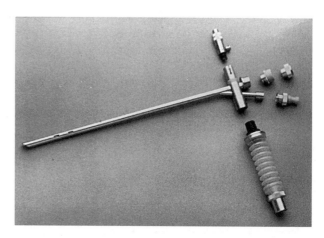

Fig. 24-2. Pictured in clockwise fashion around the rigid ventilating bronchoscope starting at 11 o'clock are prismatic light deflector, window or telescope sealing cap, instrument channel cap, and anesthesia attachment. All openings need to be plugged when ventilating the patient. (Courtesy of Karl Storz, Endoscopy America, Inc., Culver City, CA.)

require the 2.5 or 3.0 mm bronchoscope, while the average, full-term infant should have an airway that will allow atraumatic passage of the 3.5 mm bronchoscope. Adolescents and adults typically tolerate at least the 6.0 mm bronchoscope.

Various forceps are available for removing foreign objects or biopsing pathologic tissue (Fig. 24-5). As previously mentioned, larger instruments can be inserted directly into the lumen of the bronchoscope, with the bronchoscopist viewing directly into the lumen of the bronchoscope without a telescope. Alternatively, instruments can be used in conjunction with a telescope. This

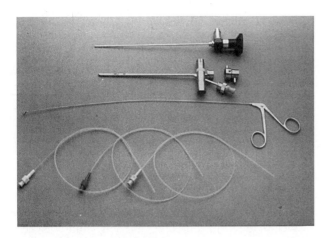

Fig. 24-3. Neonate bronchoscope (1.9 mm × 18.5 cm) with 2.5-mm bronchoscope. Flexible alligator or biopsy forceps can be inserted into lumen through side port. Variously sized suction catheters can also be introduced into lumen of bronchoscope through side port. (Courtesy of Karl Storz, Endoscopy America, Inc., Culver City, CA.)

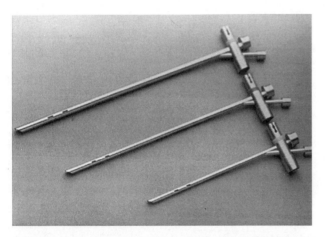

Fig. 24-4. Three lengths of pediatric bronchoscopes are depicted (30 cm, 26 cm, and 20 cm). (Courtesy of Karl Storz, Endoscopy America, Inc., Culver City, CA.)

Table 24-1. Pediatric bronchoscopes

Bronchoscope	True external diameter
2.5 mm	4.0 mm
3.0 mm	5.0 mm
3.5 mm	5.7 mm
4.0 mm	7.0 mm
6.0 mm	8.2 mm

can be done with instruments passed through the side port of the scope while using a standard telescope or by using the optical forceps. The optical forceps consist of a telescope incorporated into a forceps (Fig. 24-6). Optical forceps are available in 3 styles: alligator, peanut,

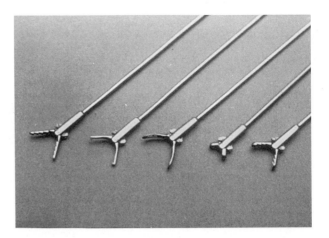

Fig. 24-5. Various types of nonoptical forceps. (Courtesy of Karl Storz, Endoscopy America, Inc., Culver City, CA.)

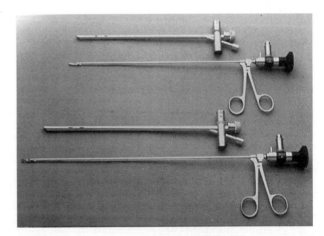

Fig. 24-6. *Top,* 26-cm bronchoscope with optical forceps and 30-cm telescope in place. This optical forceps can also be used with a 20-cm bronchoscope. *Bottom,* 30 cm bronch tube with longer optical forceps and 35-cm telescope. (Courtesy of Karl Storz, Endoscopy America, Inc., Culver City, CA.)

and biopsy (Fig. 24-7). Familiarity with the bronchoscopy instruments is essential to the proper and safe use of this equipment.

V. GENERAL TECHNIQUES

Bronchoscopy proceeds in an orderly fashion. In children, the anesthetist usually administers anesthesia through a mask as intravenous access is established (Fig. 24-8). After the patient is anesthetized and the airway is secured, the larynx is exposed with a laryngoscope. The glottis is visualized by placing the laryngoscope blade on the laryngeal surface of the epiglottis or by placing the laryngoscope blade in the vallecula. A measured dose of lidocaine can be administered topically or systemically at this time to lessen laryngeal reactivity. After the topical anesthetic is delivered, the patient is reoxygenated via a mask prior to introducing the bronchoscope. Responsibility for the airway is then given to the endoscopist who

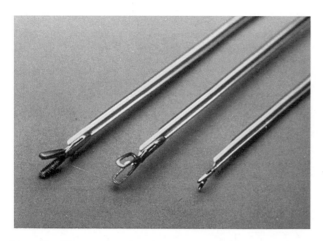

Fig. 24-7. Three styles of optical forceps: alligator, peanut, and biopsy. (Courtesy of Karl Storz, Endoscopy America, Inc., Culver City, CA.)

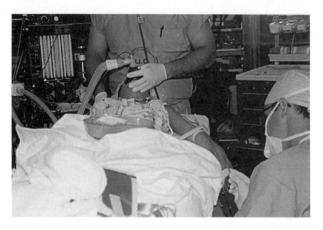

Fig. 24-8. Anesthetic is administered by mask and airway managed while intravenous access is established prior to bronchoscopy.

exposes the glottis using the anesthesia laryngoscope, a diagnostic laryngoscope, or a bronchoscope. The patient should be positioned with the head extended and the neck flexed. For adults and children, a slotted laryngoscope is an effective instrument for directly elevating the epiglottis and exposing the glottis. The removable segment of the laryngoscope is detached from the laryngoscope prior to passing the bronchoscope. Some pediatric laryngoscopes are designed with an open side to permit placement of the bronchoscope. The blade of the anesthesia laryngoscope can be placed either in the vallecula or directly on the laryngeal surface of the epiglottis. When the laryngoscope blade is placed in the vallecula, the base of tongue is elevated to rotate the epiglottis anteriorly to expose the glottis (Fig. 24-9, *A,B,C*). The laryngoscope is held in the left hand while the bronchoscope is placed in the oral cavity with the right hand (Fig. 24-10).

With the glottis visualized through the bronchoscope,

the bronchoscope is rotated 90 degrees so that the bevel of the bronchoscope is parallel to the vocal cords. In this way, the leading edge of the bronchoscope passes between the true vocal cords avoiding direct contact with the sensitive superior vocal cord surface. In the immediate subglottis, the bronchoscope is directed slightly posterior, since the trachea usually assumes a posterior direction at this level. Once through the glottis with the trachea visualized, the bronchoscope is turned so that the bevel is posterior. In this position, the ventilation connector will be posterior. The ventilator tubing is then attached to the connector on the bronchoscope, and ventilation proceeds through the bronchoscope. While advancing the bronchoscope, the left thumb is kept between the upper incisors, or the upper alveolar ridge in an edentulous patient, and the scope. The scope is advanced using the left thumb and forefinger. Advancing the scope is this way minimizes the force with which the scope is advanced. The scope must not be rocked on the teeth, which could result in damaging or loosening the teeth.

Ventilating through the bronchoscope can begin once the bronchoscope is in the subglottis. Suctioning of secretions is accomplished either with a rigid suction catheter passed directly through the lumen of the bronchoscope or with a flexible suction catheter passed through a side port. Use of the rigid suction necessitates removal of the telescope and loss of a closed ventilating system. Prior to performing rigid suctioning, the anesthetist is informed that ventilation will not be possible during suctioning, and the patient should be well oxygenated. This level of communication will lessen the chance of having the patient unexpectedly desaturate. Excessive use of the suction can result in trauma to the respiratory mucosa, from mild hyperemia to edema, resulting in a compromised airway. The bronchoscope must be centered in the lumen of the trachea and bronchi during the examination. The tendency to pass the scope along the posterior wall of the trachea, referred to as "snowplowing," must be avoided and specifically discussed during the teaching of safe bronchoscopy.

During passage of the bronchoscope through the trachea, the patient's head is maintained in a neutral position. Examination of the lower airway necessitates rotating the patient's head. The carina marks the bifurcation of the trachea into the two mainstem bronchi. This structure should be sharp in appearance and tends to have a sharper angle during expiration. Entrance into either of the mainstem bronchi is facilitated by turning the patient's head in the opposite direction to that of the bronchus to be examined. For example, prior to entering the right mainstem bronchus, the patient's head is gently rotated to the left. The left mainstem bronchus makes a larger angle with the

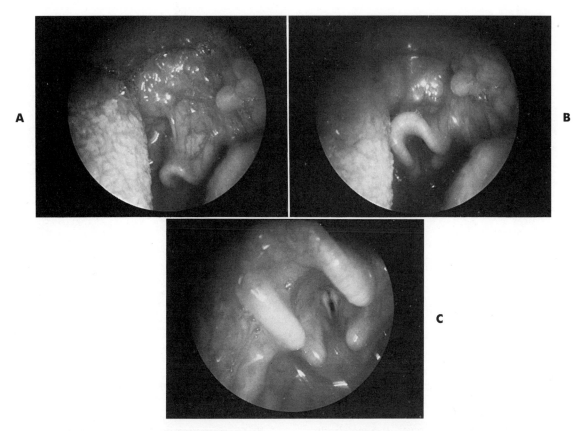

Fig. 24-9. A, Laryngoscope blade is placed in vallecula. **B,** Anterior retraction of laryngoscope elevates base of tongue and begins to rotate epiglottis. **C,** With adequate retraction, glottis is visualized without distorting the laryngeal surface of epiglottis.

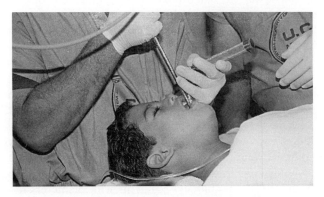

Fig. 24-10. Laryngoscope is manipulated with endoscopist's left hand while bronchoscope is introduced into right side of oral cavity.

trachea than the right mainstem bronchus, necessitating a greater degree of head rotation. The patient's chin is turned and flexed toward the right shoulder. Manipulation of the patient's head can be done by the bronchoscopist or by an assistant. During these maneuvers, the airway must be visualized through the bronchoscope to reduce the possibility of traumatizing the airway.

Angled telescopes may facilitate examination of the upper lobe segments. The 0-degree telescope is preferred for examining the basilar segments. Angled telescopes can be disorienting for the bronchoscopist, and the position of the bronchoscope must be carefully preserved during the changing of the telescopes. Passage of the bronchoscope is easier if the axis of the bronchoscope is aligned with the axis of the mainstem bronchi. Any difficulty in passing the bronchoscope needs to be investigated. The scope may be too large for the airway and excessive force can lead to mucosal edema and airway obstruction. The relationship of the scope to the tongue, lips, and teeth may be responsible for the difficulty in passing the scope. Passage of the scope should be smooth and atraumatic.

Removal of the bronchoscope should be done as carefully as its introduction into the airway. The anesthesiologist is informed that the bronchoscopic examination is near completion, and preparation is made for returning control of the patient's airway to the ventilating mask.

VI. FOREIGN BODIES

A high index of suspicion is of primary importance in the diagnosis of an airway foreign body. The development of airway distress in a previously well child with no evidence of trauma or an upper respiratory infection

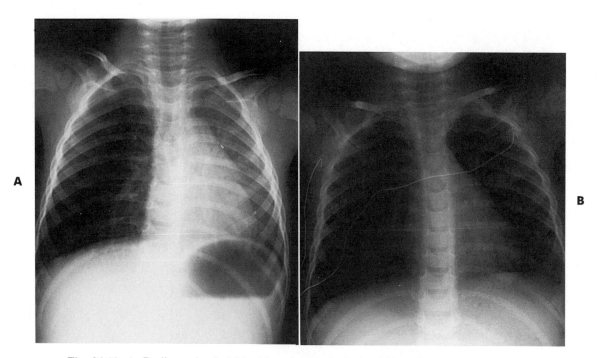

Fig. 24-11. A, Radiograph of child with a foreign body in right mainstem bronchus with hyperinflation of right lung with mediastinum shifted to the left. **B,** Immediately after removal of the foreign body, lung fields appear more symmetric with reduction of mediastinal shift.

warrants consideration of an airway foreign body. Conversely, a persistent isolated pneumonia refractory to medical management raises the possibility of an obstructing foreign body. Infants and children tend to aspirate small objects, especially toy parts. Foreign body aspiration must be strongly considered when an infant or child acutely develops signs or symptoms of airway problems. A significant percentage of adults with foreign-body aspiration have compromised upper aerodigestive tract protective mechanisms. In one series of 60 consecutive adults who aspirated a foreign object, 25 had primary neurologic disorders, trauma with loss of consciousness, or sedative or alcohol use.[1]

Physical examination may reveal asymmetric breath sounds with decreased breath sounds in the postobstructive areas. Chest radiographs may demonstrate a radiopaque object or hyperinflation of the involved lung segment secondary to a ball-valve effect of the object with subsequent air trapping (Fig. 24-11). Despite a negative radiograph, bronchoscopy is indicated if there are indications of foreign-body aspiration. Foreign-body removal in the child should be performed with a rigid bronchoscope and general anesthesia. Rigid bronchoscopy occasionally can be performed with topical anesthesia and intravenous sedation in a cooperative adult. Alternatively, flexible bronchoscopy has been successful for foreign-body removal in selected adults with rigid bronchoscopy available for flexible bronchoscopy failures.

Prior to performing bronchoscopy, the characteristics of the foreign body are reviewed.[2] If possible a duplicate foreign body is examined or a likeness is drawn if a duplicate object is not available. The duplicated object is then examined and manipulated with the forceps and bronchoscopes to determine the behavior of the object with these instruments.

Rigid bronchoscopy is superior to flexible bronchoscopy for foreign-body removal in children for several reasons. Ventilation can be maintained through the lumen of the rigid bronchoscope, while ventilation is not possible through the flexible scope. Compared to the adult airway, the smaller diameter of the pediatric airway prohibits ventilation around the flexible scope. One advantage of flexible bronchoscopy is the ability to examine distal pulmonary segments with diameters too small to allow passage of the rigid scope.

Small foreign bodies can be removed through the lumen of the bronchoscope with the bronchoscope left in position during manipulation of the foreign body. After identifying the foreign body, the bronchoscope is advanced to the object. Grasping and removing the object can be accomplished in one of three ways: use of the optical forceps, alligator or cup forceps passed through the side port of the bronchoscope, or with forceps passed directly through the lumen of the bronchoscope with or without a telescope. Instrumentation introduced through the side port can be used to remove objects in a piecemeal fashion, since the diameter of the side port severely limits the size of the forceps and therefore the objects removed with this approach. Working with optical forceps or with instruments placed directly into the lumen of the bronchoscope, sharp objects can be sheathed within the bronchoscope during removal to prevent damage to the tracheal mucosa. "Search not for the foreign body, but for the point of the foreign body," is a paraphrase of the Jackson recommendation for managing sharp foreign bodies as recounted by Holinger.[2,3] Pins and needles with the point directed toward the bronchoscopist pose a specific problem given that attempts to withdraw the object may lead to the object becoming further embedded in the tracheal mucosa. Because the sharp point becomes lodged in the mucosa, the object may need to be advanced to disengage the point and the object then sheathed by the scope.[2] Objects too large to be pulled into the lumen of the bronchoscope require that the scope be withdrawn with the object. Performing foreign-body removal in this fashion leads to an unsecured airway as the bronchoscope is withdrawn from the airway. The anesthetist must be informed as to the status of the airway and be prepared to assume control of the airway upon withdrawal of the scope. During removal of the scope, the object can become displaced during its passage through the glottis. The object may become lodged at the level of the glottis and convert a partially obstructed airway into a completely obstructed airway. If the object cannot be easily and safely grasped, it should be pushed distally to allow ventilation around the object and to allow time for a controlled reassessment of the situation.

Vegetative material (e.g., beans, peas, popcorn kernels) can become edematous when hydrated. This can make removal difficult and bloody. Holinger notes that once sufficient moisture is absorbed, the bean or pea may burst its capsule and swell to the point of occluding the trachea, resulting in asphyxiation. Granulation tissue occasionally will form around the object. Removing granulation tissue with a cup or alligator forceps prior to removal of the foreign-body removal helps define the extent of the foreign body and facilitates extraction. Periodic withdrawal of the scope into the trachea may be necessary during the removal of a foreign body to manage periods of desaturation that occur during prolonged manipulation in a mainstem bronchus or distal segment of the airway.

Staged bronchoscopy may be indicated for diffuse vegetative material. The degree of edema and local trauma may make complete removal during a single bronchoscopy impossible. Medical therapy and respiratory treatments, including chest percussion, can mobilize material not removed at the time of the initial bronchoscopy. Residual material can be removed with subsequent bronchoscopy. When significant granulation tissue and circumferential edema is found during bronchoscopy, the possibility of subsequent stenosis of the airway must be considered. Subsequent diagnostic bronchoscopy may be necessary to evaluate a potentially stenotic segment.

Early complications of tracheobronchial foreign-body aspiration include pneumonia, pneumothorax, abscess formation, and airway obstruction. Late complications of foreign-body aspiration include tracheal or bronchial stenosis, pulmonary abscess, and bronchiectasis.

VII. EMERGENCY AIRWAY

Rigid bronchoscopes are valuable tools for establishing an airway when attempts at intubation with an endotracheal tube are unsuccessful. The ability to maintain ventilation through the bronchoscope while examining the airway is unique to the rigid scope. Bypassing the upper airway with a surgical airway may be necessary when attempts at intubation with a rigid bronchoscope or endotracheal tube are unsuccessful.

In the adult patient, the bronchoscope may be passed with a laryngoscope to expose the glottis or directly into the oral cavity, with the tip of the bronchoscope placed beneath the epiglottis and used to rotate the epiglottis forward. With distortion of the airway from infection, tumor, or edema, an adequate view of the glottis may not be possible, and the bronchoscopist is faced with establishing an airway with limited anatomic landmarks. The standard positioning of an extended head with a flexed neck is preferable for initial passage of the scope through the glottis. With impending airway obstruction, patients should receive little or no anesthetic, which could suppress their respiratory drive. Evidence of air movement in the form of air bubbles should be sought and the scope passed in the direction of the bubbles. During manipulation of the bronchoscope in the pharynx, supplemental oxygen can be delivered through a catheter placed through the nose or directly into the oral cavity.

A rigid bronchoscope can facilitate management of subglottic obstruction secondary to congenital or acquired problems. Obstructing lesions of the tracheobronchial tree, like papillomas and granulomas, may be successfully managed without resorting to a tracheotomy. Removal can be accomplished with forceps or laser.

VIII. ESOPHAGEAL FOREIGN BODIES

A discussion of esophageal foreign bodies is included in this chapter because of the similarities in the clinical presentation and management of foreign bodies of the airway and esophagus. Esophageal foreign bodies can present with signs of airway obstruction due to distension of the anterior wall of the esophagus into the posterior, membranous wall of the trachea. Dysphagia and drooling with near total esophageal obstruction are hallmarks of esophageal foreign bodies.

Nonreactive foreign bodies, such as coins, can be removed nonemergently if airway obstruction or significant esophageal obstruction is not present. Reactive objects, especially batteries, require emergent removal due to the possibility of mucosal erosion.[4] Dysphagia or airway obstruction necessitates emergent removal, as would be the case for an obstructing airway foreign body. The type of esophageal foreign body typically relates to the age of the patient. Infants and children tend to swallow toy parts and coins. Adults experience difficulty with meat, often poorly masticated, and, occasionally, swallowed dentures.

Esophageal foreign bodies can be removed with rigid or flexible esophagoscopes. Adults may tolerate rigid endoscopy with intravenous sedation. Sharp objects are best managed with rigid scopes, since the scope can be used to sheath the object during extraction.

Removal of esophageal foreign bodies in infants and children should be performed with a rigid esophagoscope using general anesthesia.[5] Some authors have advocated the use of a Foley catheter without intubation to remove esophageal foreign bodies. This practice carries the risk of creating an unstable airway if control of the foreign body is lost in the pharynx. General anesthesia with laryngotracheal intubation provides the conditions to produce excellent muscular relaxation and protection of the airway during foreign-body removal.

Proper technique and positioning is crucial to the safe and efficient removal of esophageal foreign bodies. Once the patient is orotracheally intubated, the patient's head is placed in the "sniffing" position, head extended on a flexed neck, to align the scope with the cervical esophagus, which tends to be directed posteriorly.[6] The esophagoscope can be introduced into the adult esophageal inlet by passing the scope through the oral cavity and along the posterior wall of the pharynx while the endoscopist is looking through the scope. The postcricoid area is identified and the scope passed into the esophageal inlet with direct observation of the lumen through the scope. Passage of the endoscope into the esophageal inlet in the infant and child should be done using a laryngoscope to expose the postcricoid area, including the inlet of the esophagus. The laryngoscope may be placed posterior to the endotracheal tube, which is retracted anteriorly or placed into the vallecula to elevate the larynx and the endotracheal tube. A slotted laryngoscope or the anesthesia laryngoscope may be used to expose the esophageal inlet.

Passage of the endoscope within the lumen of the esophagus should be done only if the endoscopist clearly identifies a lumen. Withdrawing the telescope several millimeters from the tip of the esophagoscope provides a moisture-free zone in front of the telescope that reduces the likelihood of obscuring the endoscopist's view because of secretions accumulating on the end of the telescope. If the esophageal mucosa is edematous and the lumen not readily visualized, a soft catheter can be passed through the side port of the esphagoscope and advanced into the esophagus. The endoscopist can then follow the catheter distally into the esophagus. Once the esophagoscope has transgressed the cervical esophagus, the patient's neck is extended, either by placing a shoulder roll or by dropping the head of the operating table. Changing the position of the patient's head will keep the esophagoscope along the same axis as the esophagus, which assumes a more vertical direction distal to the thoracic inlet.

Esophageal foreign bodies are removed with optical forceps, forceps passed directly through the esophagoscope, or with instruments passed through a side port. Objects small enough to fit within the lumen of the esophagoscope can be removed while leaving the scope in the esophagus. Larger objects require that the scope be withdrawn along with the foreign body. Sharp objects, especially those with a point, can become embedded in the esophageal mucosa. Removal requires that the object be pushed distally toward the stomach to dislodge it from the mucosa and then grasped and brought within the lumen of the scope. Specific instruments are available for removing pointed objects, including straight pins, safety pins, and staples.[2]

Objects that have been present in the esophagus for a long period of time or reactive objects, such as batteries, can cause significant mucosal irritation and scarring. A barium swallow 1 to 2 weeks after the esophagoscopy may be necessary to radiographically evaluate the esophagus for the presence of strictures.

Inadvertent extubation can occur during withdrawal of the esphagoscope from the oral cavity. The endoscopist must be aware of this possibility and maintain a firm hold of the foreign body during this part of the procedure. The anesthetist should be prepared for a premature extubation and the possibility of managing a now unprotected airway.

Complications of esophageal foreign-body removal include reactive edema of the esophageal mucosa, which will resolve with time, and esophageal perforation. Esophageal perforation is treated with open surgical drainage because of the life-threatening risk of abscess formation and mediastinitis.

IX. COMPLICATIONS OF BRONCHOSCOPY

Complications of rigid bronchoscopy can be categorized as intraoperative and late. Intraoperative complications can occur as a result of poor communication between the endoscopist and anesthetist, trauma induced by the mechanical effects of the bronchoscope, and manipulation of foreign bodies.

Loss of airway control as a result of poor communication between the anesthetist and endoscopist cannot be overemphasized as a potentially devastating cause of complications. With a difficult airway and a patient with poor pulmonary reserve, the transition between ventilating with a mask and ventilating through the bronchoscope must be anticipated. Preparation includes adequately oxygenating the patient prior to transferring responsibility for managing the airway. The bronchoscopist must inform the anesthetist about the progress of the procedure. The anesthetist must be informed about the anticipated withdrawal of the bronchoscope. Insufficient warning can leave the patient poorly oxygenated and with a tenuous airway.

Iatrogenic injury to the airway can occur as a result of a rigid bronchoscope traversing the upper and lower aerodigestive tract. Teeth can be damaged or dislodged if the bronchoscopist is not vigilant in protecting dental structures. Loose and damaged teeth can become foreign bodies and a source of great frustration for the bronchoscopist. Teeth must not be used as a fulcrum for the bronchoscope and can be protected with a tooth guard and the endoscopist's left thumb and forefinger. Improper management of the bronchoscope through the glottis can result in significant laryngeal injury, including dislocated arytenoids and glottic edema. Failure to center the bronchoscope in the airway can cause avoidable mucosal injury with associated airway edema.

Foreign bodies pose unique risks with regard to airway complications. A foreign body may cause significant injury to the airway prior to any formal attempt at removal. Unnecessarily aggressive attempts at foreign-body removal may create an unextubatable airway. Reactive foreign bodies, typically vegetative matter, often lead to granulation tissue formation and mucosal injury. Conservative removal with planned secondary bronchoscopy may be required if the initial bronchoscopy is associated with bleeding and poor visualization of the airway. Not only will complete foreign-body removal not be possible in this situation, but the patient may not be able to protect his or her airway with adequate

ventilation. After a traumatic bronchoscopy, the patient may not be ready for extubation in the operating room. Attempts at foreign-body removal can lead to unintentionally forcing the object further into the lower airway, necessitating a thoracotomy for removal.

X. CONCLUSION

Rigid bronchoscopy is a versatile procedure with multiple applications. With advances in equipment and training relating to flexible bronchoscopy, rigid bronchoscopy is not frequently performed for diagnostic purposes or for managing pulmonary secretions. Rigid bronchoscopy, however, remains the primary approach for removing tracheobronchial foreign bodies in infants and children. Flexible bronchoscopy is used for retrieving aspirated foreign bodies in adults. Rigid bronchoscopy is required for flexible bronchoscopy failures.

Competence in performing rigid bronchoscopy is a valuable tool in the armamentarium of the practitioner managing difficult airways. The capacity to ventilate a patient while maneuvering through an obstructed or distorted airway is an important feature of rigid bronchoscopy. The bronchoscope can be thought of as a rigid endotracheal tube with a telescope.

REFERENCES

1. Limper AH, Prakash UBS: Tracheobronchial foreign bodies in adults, *Ann Intern Med* 112:604, 1990.
2. Holinger LD: Management of sharp and penetrating foreign bodies of the upper aerodigestive tract, *Ann Otol Rhinol Laryngol* 99:684, 1990.
3. Jackson C, Jackson CC: *Bronchoesophagology*, Philadelphia, 1950, WB Saunders.
4. Maves MD, Carithers JS, Birck HG: Esophageal burns secondary to disc ingestion, *Ann Otol Rhinol Laryngol* 93:364, 1984.
5. Benjamin B: *Diagnostic Laryngology*, Philadelphia, 1990, WB Saunders.
6. Bailey BJ, Strunk CL, Jones JK: Methods of examination. In Bluestone CD, Stool SE, editors: *Pediatric Otolaryngology*, Philadelphia, 1990, WB Saunders.

Chapter 25

PERCUTANEOUS DILATIONAL CRICOTHYROTOMY AND TRACHEOSTOMY

Richard J. Melker
Orlando G. Florete, Jr.

I. CONTROL OF THE AIRWAY

In the vast majority of instances, anesthesiologists control and maintain the airway by endotracheal intubation. However, despite extensive training and skill, every anesthesiologist occasionally encounters an airway that cannot be managed by endotracheal intubation or in which it is contraindicated. In the operating room (OR), three general scenarios have been repeatedly observed and reported during attempts to control the airway: (1) the airway can be easily controlled by mask ventilation and endotracheal intubation; (2) the airway can be mask ventilated but cannot be intubated; and (3) rarely, the airway cannot be mask ventilated or intubated. It is every anesthesiologist's nightmare to encounter a difficult airway that he/she is unable to establish and maintain.

A. ADVERSE OUTCOMES

Adverse outcomes due to respiratory-related events accounted for the largest class of injury in the American Society of Anesthesiologists (ASA) closed claims study, with brain damage or death occurring in 85% of cases.[1] Three mechanisms of injury were responsible for three fourths of the adverse respiratory events: inadequate ventilation (38%), esophageal intubation (18%), and difficult tracheal intubation (17%). Inadequate ventilation and esophageal intubation are largely preventable with better monitoring; failed tracheal intubation is not.

There are several clinical situations (i.e., orofacial or neck injury, patients who are assessed preoperatively to have difficult airways, and those who have an unexpectedly difficult airway following induction of general anesthesia) that may require alternative means of airway management. Five to 35 of 10,000 patients (0.05% to 0.35%) reportedly cannot be endotracheally intubated.[2-5] Approximately 0.01 to 2.0 out of 10,000 patients are difficult to mask ventilate and intubate.[6,7] Failure to provide adequate ventilation and oxygenation is the primary cause of cardiac arrest during general anesthesia.[8-10]

B. THE *ASA PRACTICE GUIDELINES*

Because some degree of airway difficulty is often encountered during attempted intubation and serious adverse outcomes occur, the ASA Task Force on Management of the Difficult Airway recently published *Practice Guidelines for Management of the Difficult Airway.*[11] The *ASA Guidelines* contains a difficult airway algorithm and provides strategies for evaluating, preparing for, and intubating the difficult airway. It also considers the relative merits and feasibility of alternative management choices, such as nonsurgical versus surgical techniques for the initial approach to ventilation, awake intubation versus intubation after induction of general anesthesia, and preservation versus ablation of spontaneous ventilation. Development of primary and alternative strategies for awake intubation and intubation after the induction of general anesthesia is emphasized. The algorithm describes both emergency and nonemergency pathways of managing the airway if intubation fails. The *ASA Guidelines* also suggests that equipment suitable for "emergency surgical airway access" be among the contents of a portable storage unit readily available in the OR. Among the suggested emergency airway procedures is cricothyrotomy, a technique for gaining and securing airway access through the cricothyroid space. Although the *ASA Guidelines* offers a stepwise approach to the patient with a difficult airway, it primarily focuses on difficulties encountered in the OR, with strategies to anticipate and treat in this environment. (See Chapter 8.)

C. THE HOSPITAL-WIDE ROLE OF THE ANESTHESIOLOGIST

As the recognized airway expert, the anesthesiologist is often called upon to manage the airways of critically ill patients in other hospital environments, such as the emergency department (ED), wards, diagnostic areas (i.e., radiology), or intensive care units (ICUs). The anesthesiologist may either be called right away or after other physicians have attempted unsuccessfully to secure the airway or failed to recognize the futility of standard intubation techniques. In rare instances, the availability of a physician skilled in the technique of cricothyrotomy may be lifesaving. It is altogether appropriate that this individual be the anesthesiologist. Appropriate equipment for cricothyrotomy should be available throughout the hospital or as part of an emergency airway kit.

D. RENEWED INTEREST IN CRICOTHYROTOMY

Chevalier Jackson was largely responsible for discouraging the use of cricothyrotomy for almost 5 decades.[12] Only in the 1970s, when surgeons sought a safe, effective alternative to surgical tracheostomy, did cricothyrotomy begin to gain generalized acceptance.[13,14]

Interest in cricothyrotomy as an alternative to endotracheal intubation has increased recently due largely to the development of emergency medicine as a specialty and the increasing treatment of patients in the prehospital and ED environments. Emergency physicians and prehospital providers often encounter patients with life-threatening injuries who cannot be intubated by conventional routes and who need immediate and definitive treatment.

Interest in percutaneous dilational tracheostomy and cricothyrotomy has also increased as part of a trend toward less invasive surgical procedures, often performed over guidewires. While anesthesiologists are familiar with the Seldinger technique for the insertion of vascular catheters, many may be unaware that airway devices using the same technology have been developed.

Cricothyrotomy can be performed surgically, percutaneously with or without a guidewire, or by placement of a transtracheal catheter. There remain many questions as to which of these techniques is best suited for a particular clinical situation. Cricothyrotomy is an alternative to a "surgical" airway (tracheostomy) in the emergency and nonemergency limbs of the ASA difficult airway algorithm. In the nonemergency sequence, it may be elected when intubation is unsuccessful but the patient can be adequately mask ventilated. If other alternatives of airway management such as fiberoptic bronchoscopy or blind intubation fail, either nonsurgical or surgical cricothyrotomy can be employed to secure the airway. Likewise, cricothyrotomy can be used in the emergency situation when the airway cannot be ventilated or intubated.

No guidelines similar to the *ASA Guidelines* exist for treatment of the difficult airway outside the OR. The algorithm could be modified and adapted for non-OR settings (i.e., in the ED or ICU). This chapter will review the various approaches to cricothyrotomy (used interchangeably in the medical literature with: coniotomy, cricothyroidotomy, cricothyrostomy, intercricothyrotomy, and minitracheostomy) with an emphasis on percutaneous dilational techniques and also percutaneous dilational tracheostomy. Use in truly emergent situations will be stressed. Areas of continuing controversy regarding the timing and appropriateness of cricothyrotomy by anesthesiologists will be discussed.

II. DEFINITION AND CLASSIFICATION OF CRICOTHYROTOMY

Cricothyrotomy is a technique for providing an opening in the space between the anterior inferior border of the thyroid cartilage and the anterior superior border of the cricoid cartilage for the purpose of gaining access to the airway.[15] This area is considered to be the most accessible part of the respiratory tree below the glottis.

There are many classification schemes for cricothyrotomy. The procedure has been classified, based on the urgency of the clinical situation, as either emergent or elective. Emergent cricothyrotomy may be done in the prehospital setting, in the ED, ICU, or OR. Elective cricothyrotomy is usually done prior to surgery in the OR. It may also be performed in critically ill patients in the ICU at the bedside. Depending on the technique used, the procedure may also be classified as nonsurgical or surgical. Nonsurgical approach can either be achieved by needle puncture or percutaneously over a guidewire after a small skin incision, with or without cricothyroid membrane incision.

We choose to classify cricothyrotomy into three broad technical categories, considering emergent techniques only. The first and least invasive are techniques utilizing a needle or over-the-needle catheter placed directly into the cricothyroid space without a skin incision. We prefer to call these techniques transtracheal catheter ventilation, without reference to the frequency of ventilation or the pressures required to ventilate by these techniques. While transcricoid ventilation is a more descriptive term, we bow to the convention of using the term *transtracheal ventilation*. The techniques have in common insertion without prior skin incision and use devices with a caliber insufficient to deliver tidal volumes and flow rates at peak inspiratory pressures usually provided by conventional ventilators. Therefore, special high pressure systems are often required to provide adequate ventilation with the use of this technique.

The second category includes techniques requiring an initial skin incision (and often an incision of the cricothyroid membrane), followed by introduction of a guidewire inserted through a needle or catheter placed through the incision into the cricothyroid space. An airway catheter is then introduced over a dilator threaded over the guidewire. (We use the term *airway catheter* to describe "cricothyrotomy" tubes or tracheostomy tubes inserted through the cricothyroid space.) These techniques allow the ultimate insertion of an airway considerably larger than the initial needle or catheter, often of sufficient internal diameter to allow ventilation with conventional ventilation devices, suctioning, and spontaneous ventilation. We refer to this as percutaneous dilational cricothyrotomy. Some authors substitute the term *dilatational* for dilational; we use them interchangeably.

The last category of cricothyrotomy techniques is surgical cricothyrotomy. This involves the use of a scalpel and other surgical instruments to create an opening between the skin and the cricothyroid space. A tracheostomy or endotracheal tube is then inserted. When properly performed, this technique allows insertion of a tube of an internal diameter sufficient to allow conventional ventilation, suctioning, and spontaneous ventilation.

III. HISTORICAL PERSPECTIVE

A. EARLY HISTORY OF SURGICAL AIRWAY CONTROL

Surgical manipulation of the trachea for emergent airway control is one of the oldest invasive procedures known to man.[16] It was performed in ancient Egypt and India over 3000 years ago. Tracheostomy was mentioned in the writings and illustrations of the great Greek physician, Galen (130-200 AD). He provided anatomic drawings of the airway and favored a vertical rather than horizontal incision in emergencies. He based his anatomic knowledge on dissections of animals and assumed that the structures were identical in the human body.[17]

Galen also stated that Asclepiades (124-56 BC), who practiced in Rome, recommended opening the trachea in its upper part to prevent suffocation.[18] Antyllus (approximately 150 AD) detailed both the indications and technique of tracheostomy, advocating a transverse incision between two rings.[18]

Galenic teaching persisted for over 1300 years until Andreas Wesele Vesalius (1515-1564 AD) published *de Humani Corporis Fabrica,* detailing the first correct description of human anatomy.[17] Vesalius secretly conducted extensive dissection of human cadavers and, at age 28, published his landmark work in seven volumes. Included was a detailed description of tracheostomy—control of the airway with the use of a cane or reed and assisted ventilation of the lung. Interestingly, he allegedly performed a tracheostomy and experimentally inflated the lungs of a dead Spanish nobleman. The nobleman's heart was reported to beat again. His action brought outrage in the medical and clerical community. He was condemned by the Spanish Inquisition to a pilgrimage to the Holy Land, and he died along the way in a shipwreck on an island near Greece. During the next 300 years, very few reports were published regarding the surgical control of the airway and were primarily limited to experimental control of breathing in laboratory animals. In *Respiratory Changes of Intrathoracic Pressure,* published in 1892, Samuel Meltzer described the insertion of breathing tubes through tracheostomy and successfully controlling ventilation in curarized animals.[17] In France, Armand Trousseau recognized the importance of emergency tracheostomy in airways compromised by upper airway obstruction, diphtheria, and massive infection in the oropharynx and neck.

B. CONDEMNATION OF "HIGH" TRACHEOSTOMY

In 1909, Chevalier Jackson, Sr.,[19] published his first critical assessment of the airway management techniques of that time. He advocated formal tracheostomy as the preferred method of surgical airway management and emphasized that surgical incision, rather than a tracheal stab, should be performed in cases of an obstructed larynx. Jackson followed many of his tracheotomized patients for over 30 years. In 1921, he published the results of 200 cases of chronic laryngeal and subglottic stenosis.[12] Thirty cases of laryngeal stenosis were attributed to laryngeal inflammation and cartilage necrosis associated with the primary disease process necessitating the tracheostomy. The remaining 170 patients had subglottic stenosis judged to be due to the surgical procedure, of which 158 had a previous "high" tracheostomy. In 32 cases, the opening was made through the cricothyroid membrane and thyroid cartilage. He condemned this type of procedure and advocated that emergency tracheostomy be performed lower

over the cervical trachea. Unfortunately, the high tracheostomy that Jackson referred to involved division of the cricoid (or thyroid) cartilage. Modern techniques of cricothyrotomy utilize only division and/or dilatation of the cricothyroid membrane.[20] Additionally, the underlying pathology for which cricothyrotomy was indicated in 1920 differs greatly from modern indications. Most of Jackson's patients had inflammatory lesions involving the upper airway (acute laryngeal edema from diphtheria, epiglottis, streptococcal laryngitis, syphilis, tuberculosis of the larynx, Ludwig's angina, angioneurotic edema, and other oropharyngeal infection), predisposing them to subsequent airway stenosis. Furthermore, there were no antibiotics or biocompatible tracheal tubes available at that time.

C. RENEWED INTEREST IN CRICOTHYROTOMY

For over half a century, the use of cricothyrotomy was almost universally condemned, largely because of fear of chronic subglottic stenosis. In 1969, Toye and Weinstein[21] first described a technique for percutaneous tracheostomy. It was based on the premise that a functional tracheal airway could be more rapidly and safely achieved percutaneously than with Jackson's method of surgical dissection. The technique involves inserting a needle into the trachea and dilating the resultant needle tract to allow placement of a breathing catheter.

Cricothyrotomy made a popular comeback when, in 1976, two Denver cardiothoracic surgeons, Brantigan and Grow,[13] published the results of 655 consecutive cricothyrotomies in which there were minimal complications and no reported incidence of subglottic stenosis. Subsequently, other clinical and experimental series have been reported, and cricothyrotomy has become generally accepted. The procedure was found to be faster, simpler, less invasive, and less likely to cause bleeding than tracheostomy. It also has less morbidity and mortality than emergency tracheostomy, making it desirable as an emergency technique for gaining immediate airway control. Various modifications of the original technique have been developed. The use of the Seldinger technique for insertion, as described by Corke and Cranswick in 1988,[22] enhances the safety of the procedure. The use of a guidewire and the passing of a dilator to create a channel reduces the chance of incorrect placement and damage to surrounding blood vessels. Detailed insertion instructions for a variety of cricothyrotomy and tracheostomy devices will be given later in this chapter.

IV. ANATOMY AND PHYSIOLOGY

Safe and rapid performance of cricothyrotomy requires a thorough knowledge of cricothyroid space anatomy and its relationship to other structures in the neck. The cricothyroid membrane (ligament) measures 10 mm in height and 22 mm in width and is composed mostly of yellow elastic tissue.[15] It covers the cricothyroid space and is located in the anterior neck between the thyroid cartilage superiorly and the cricoid cartilage inferiorly. The cricothyroid space can be readily identified by palpating a slight dip or indentation in the skin immediately below the laryngeal prominence.

The cricothyroid membrane consists of a central anterior triangular portion (conus elasticus) and two lateral parts. The thicker and stronger conus elasticus narrows above and broadens out below, connecting the thyroid to the cricoid cartilage. It lies subcutaneously in the midline and is often crossed horizontally in its upper third by the superior cricothyroid vessels. To minimize the possibility of bleeding, the cricothyroid membrane should be incised at its inferior third. The two lateral parts are thinner, lie close to the laryngeal mucosa, and extend from the superior border of the cricoid cartilage to the inferior margin of the true vocal cords. On either side, the cricothyroid membrane is bordered by the cricothyroid muscle. Also lateral to the membrane are venous tributaries from the inferior thyroid and anterior jugular veins. Because the vocal cords usually lie a centimeter above the cricothyroid space, they are not commonly injured, even during emergency cricothyrotomy. The anterior jugular veins run vertically in the lateral aspect of the neck and are usually spared injury; however, tributaries may occasionally course over the cricothyroid space and be damaged during the procedure. Characteristically, the cricothyroid membrane does not calcify with age and lies immediately underneath the skin.

Variations in the anatomy and dimensions of the cricothyroid membrane are common. A comprehensive study of the anatomy of the cricothyroid space was reported by Caparosa and Zavatsky,[15] describing the detailed structure of 51 human larynges. They showed that the anterior cricothyroid space is trapezoidal in shape and has a cross-sectional area of approximately 2.9 cm. The mean distance between the anterior borders of the inferior thyroid cartilage and the superior cricoid cartilage is 9 mm (range = 5 to 12 mm), whereas the width of the anterior cricothyroid space ranges from 27 to 32 mm. Kirchner[23] demonstrated that the cricothyroid space is not much larger than 7 mm in its vertical dimension and that the space may be narrowed further by contraction of the cricothyroid muscle. The vertical distance between the undersurface of the true vocal cords and the lower anterior edge of the thyroid cartilage has been reported to be 5 to 11 mm.[24]

There is also considerable variation in both the arterial and venous vessel pattern in the neck area surrounding the cricothyroid membrane. While the arteries always lie deep to the pretracheal fascia and are easily avoided during a skin incision, veins may be found in both the pretracheal fascia and between the pretracheal and superficial cervical fascia.[25] Little et al.[25] showed that the classic pattern of small bilateral cricothyroid arteries was seen only in a minority of the 27 cadavers dissected. Sixty-two percent of the cadavers had one or more vascular structures vertically crossing anterior to the cricothyroid membrane, predisposing them to damage during cricothyrotomy.

To locate the cricothyroid membrane, external visible and palpable anatomic landmarks are utilized (Fig. 25-1).[26] The laryngeal prominence (thyroid cartilage, Adam's apple) and the hyoid bone above it are readily palpable. The cricothyroid membrane usually lies one to one-and-a-half fingerbreadths below the laryngeal prominence. The cricoid cartilage is also easily felt below the cricothyroid membrane. It should take less than 5 seconds to identify these landmarks. Their importance must be emphasized because it is disastrous to place the cricothyroid tube into the thyrohyoid space instead of the cricothyroid space. Conscious effort to identify these landmarks reduces the possibility of committing this preventable error. There are instances in which the normal anatomy may be distorted and identification of the above landmarks is difficult. In such cases, the suprasternal notch may be utilized as an alternative marker. The small finger of the right hand should be placed in the patient's suprasternal notch, followed by placement of the ring, long, and index finger adjacent to each other in a stepwise fashion up the neck, with each finger touching the one below it.[27] When the head is in the neutral position, the index finger is usually on or near the cricothyroid membrane.

V. INDICATIONS AND CONTRAINDICATIONS

Cricothyrotomy is considered by many to be the standard approach to airway management when orotracheal or nasotracheal intubation and/or fiberoptic bronchoscopy have failed.[27-29] In the ED, cricothyrotomy is indicated for immediate airway control in patients with maxillofacial, cervical spine, head, neck, and multiple trauma and in other patients in whom endotracheal intubation is impossible to perform or contraindicated. It is also utilized for the immediate relief of upper airway obstruction. In the OR and in the ICU, the technique is indicated when conventional methods of intubation fail, such as in patients with traumatic facial injuries, in whom other techniques of airway access are difficult or impossible to perform. Cricothyrotomy can also be used as an alternative to tracheostomy in patients with recent sternotomy who need airway access because the incision does not communicate with the mediastinal tissue planes.

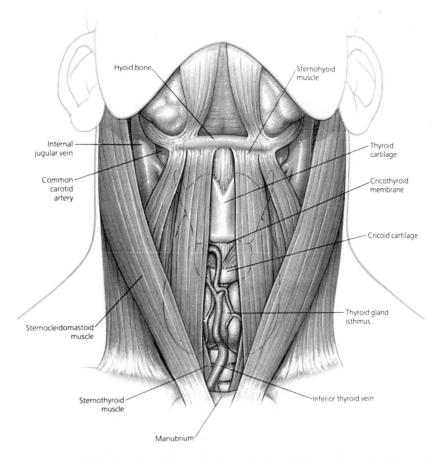

Fig. 25-1. Anatomic landmarks of the neck. (From Heffner JE, Sahn SA: *J Crit Illness* 2(5):79, 1987. Illustration by William B. Westwood, MS, AMI, copyright 1987.)

Emergency cricothyrotomy has largely replaced emergency tracheostomy in an ED setting because of its simplicity, rapidity, and minimal morbidity. Use of emergency tracheostomy is limited and indicated only in instances of direct laryngeal fractures and emergent airway management in infants and small children.[30] Laryngeal trauma may be accompanied by local edema, hemorrhage, subcutaneous emphysema, and damage to either thyroid or cricothyroid cartilage, precluding the performance of cricothyrotomy. Cricothyrotomy is difficult to perform in pediatric patients because the larynx is smaller and funnel shaped with the narrowest portion at the cricoid cartilage. Their airways contain less fibrous supporting tissue and have only loose mucous membrane attachments in the airway inlet.[31]

Absolute and relative contraindications to cricothyrotomy are rare. Patients who have been intubated translaryngeally for more than 3 days (many authors state 7 days) should not undergo cricothyrotomy because of the propensity to develop subglottic stenosis. Also, those with preexisting laryngeal diseases, such as cancer, acute or chronic inflammation, or epiglottis, have a higher morbidity when cricothyrotomy is performed. Distortion of the normal neck anatomy by disease or injury may render the technique impossible. Normal anatomic landmarks may be distorted, making identification of the cricothyroid membrane difficult. Lastly, bleeding diathesis and history of coagulopathy predispose the patient to hemorrhage, making the procedure extremely dangerous.

As previously stated, infants and children in whom anatomic landmarks are difficult to identify are largely precluded. Cricothyrotomy is technically problematic to perform in the pediatric population and should be performed with extreme caution in children below 10 years of age. It should not be performed at all in children below 6 years of age unless a wire can be placed in the cricothyroid space and placement within the trachea can be verified. Emergency tracheostomy under controlled OR conditions is the preferred choice.[32,33]

Physicians who are unfamiliar or inexperienced with the technique are discouraged from performing the procedure without adequate supervision from a more senior or knowledgeable member of the medical team.

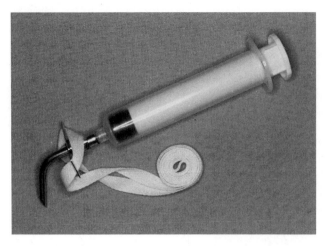

Fig. 25-2. Example of a direct puncture cricothyrotomy needle.

Inexperience has been implicated as the most important contributory factor in cricothyroid complications.[26,34]

VI. CRICOTHYROTOMY TECHNIQUES AND DEVICES

The focus of this chapter is percutaneous dilational techniques. Surgical cricothyrotomy and transtracheal catheter ventilation are discussed in detail elsewhere (Chapters 26 and 23, respectively). However, these techniques will be described briefly in the context of relative ease of use and comparative complication rates. To some extent these procedures overlap. Similarities and differences will be emphasized. Direct needle puncture cricothyrotomy, a technique that has largely fallen into disfavor, is also briefly discussed.

A. DIRECT NEEDLE PUNCTURE CRICOTHYROTOMY

Numerous large-bore, straight and curved metal needles have been developed and described for direct puncture cricothyrotomy (Fig. 25-2). With some sets, an incision is recommended before insertion; with others, it is not. The tip may have a sharp cutting edge for use without a skin incision or may be blunted, in which case an incision is needed. A sharp-tipped trocar coaxially loaded inside the cannula is another variation. The cannulae described by Safar and Penninckx[35] and Pridmore[36] and the Abelson device discussed below are typical.

Abbrecht et al.[37] evaluated the insertion forces and risk of complications caused by a number of cricothyrotomy devices, including the Abelson (Gilbert Surgical Instruments, Inc., Bellmawr, N.J.) direct puncture device. The Abelson required higher initial penetration forces, was the only device that required torquing, and had the highest complication rate of the devices tested. Ravlo et al.[38] compared another direct puncture device (essentially a large, straight hypodermic needle) to the

Nu-Trake (International Medical Devices, Inc., Northridge, Calif.) device. Both previously trained and untrained users had significantly lower success rates with the direct puncture devices. Fortunately, these have largely fallen out of favor but may still be found on "crash carts" or in other emergency equipment sets. The Abelson device is the only one commercially available today.

B. SURGICAL CRICOTHYROTOMY

Most authors state that surgical cricothyrotomy is more time consuming than percutaneous methods and requires an experienced surgeon to perform or assist the anesthesiologist. However, compared with emergency tracheostomy, it is safer, faster, and easier to perform.[33,39-41] The technique is performed as follows: after aseptically preparing the neck, the anatomic landmarks are identified, and the larynx is held in place by holding the upper pole of the thyroid cartilage firmly with the thumb and middle finger of the dominant hand. The cricothyroid space is palpated with the index finger, and, if time allows, local anesthetic is injected. A 2.0- to 3.0-cm skin incision is made in the midline of the cricothyroid space. Some authors recommend spreading the incision with Mayo scissors and making a 1.5- to 2.0-cm transverse incision at the inferior third of the cricothyroid membrane. Others recommend a single midline incision through both layers. In either case, the thyroid cartilage is identified, and the tracheal hook is inserted, applying gentle traction on the inferior margin of the thyroid cartilage. A Trousseau dilator is then inserted through the incision into the airway and spread vertically to enlarge the diameter of the cricothyroid space. If needed, the Mayo scissor can be used to enlarge the space in the transverse direction. Once the dilator is in place, the tracheal hook is removed, and an appropriately sized tracheostomy tube and stylet are inserted into the airway. After the tube is inserted, the stylet is removed, and the inner cannula (if supplied) is inserted. The cuff is inflated, and the tube is attached to a breathing circuit for positive pressure ventilation. Clinical signs and radiographic verification are observed for proper tube placement. A suction catheter may be passed through the tracheal tube. If the catheter passes easily, the tube is in the airway. (See Chapter 26.)

C. TRANSTRACHEAL CATHETER VENTILATION

Transtracheal catheter ventilation is a relatively safe and easy method to temporarily oxygenate patients who cannot be mask ventilated or intubated.[42] We consider it to be a "bridge" technique that "buys time" until the patient is either awakened or a definitive airway can be secured. The cricothyroid membrane is punctured percutaneously with a needle or, preferably, an over-the-needle catheter. In the latter case, the needle is removed, and the catheter is attached to either a high pressure oxygen source or a high-frequency jet ventilator. The mechanism by which this technique works is thought to be air entrainment and mass movement of gas. It is preferable during initial resuscitation to emergency surgical cricothyrotomy and tracheostomy because it is a much quicker procedure, the patient may not be well positioned, correct instruments for the surgical procedure may not be readily available, or the patient's anatomy may not be normal.[42-45]

As early as 1956, Jacoby et al.[46] showed that patients with complete respiratory obstruction undergoing general anesthesia could be adequately oxygenated using an oxygen flow of 4 L/min through an 18-gauge cricothyrotomy catheter. However, the technique was limited by unacceptable carbon dioxide (CO_2) retention and respiratory acidosis. Alternatively, high-frequency jet ventilation has been utilized successfully in patients without airway obstruction in the OR and in the ICU, providing more stable hemodynamic conditions than positive pressure ventilation.[47-49] Spoerel et al.[50] combined the concept of a percutaneously placed tracheal catheter and intermittent jet oxygen delivery into the respiratory tree of adults undergoing general anesthesia. His group used a 16-gauge catheter connected to a 50 pounds per square inch gauge (PSIG) oxygen source to deliver gas at an insufflation rate of 12 L/min and an inspiratory duration of 1 to 1.5 seconds. Tidal volume was estimated to be between 400 to 750 ml. Ventilation was adequate, and no significant damage to the tracheal mucosa or excessive buildup of airway pressure was noted. Other investigators, such as Ravussin and Freeman[51] and Nakatsuka and MacLeod,[52] have demonstrated that percutaneous cricothyrotomy combined with high-frequency jet ventilation provided adequate oxygenation and ventilation during general surgery on patients known to be difficult to intubate or with known distorted upper airway anatomy.

Benumof and Scheller[42] and Benumof[43] proposed that percutaneous transtracheal jet ventilation using a larger-bore intravenous catheter inserted through the cricothyroid membrane be used as the treatment of choice in situations in which the patient cannot be ventilated or intubated. Until recently, kits containing the required high-pressure circuits and equipment were not readily available. The equipment is now readily available (see Chapter 23) and consists of a 16-gauge or larger intravenous cannula and an acceptable high-pressure (50 PSIG) oxygen source either from a jet injector powered by regulated wall or oxygen tank pressure (preferred) (Mercury Medical Inc.), a jet injector powered by unregulated wall or oxygen tank pressure, or the anesthesia-machine flush valve using noncompliant oxygen tubing from the fresh gas outlet.

The technique is simple and can be performed rapidly. The patient should be continuously oxygenated with 100% oxygen by mask. After stabilizing the trachea and locating the cricothyroid cartilage by finger palpation, the cricothyroid membrane is punctured with the intravenous catheter. To confirm proper intratracheal position, air should be aspirated. The needle stylet is then withdrawn, discarded, and the catheter advanced to the hub. Intratracheal position should be rechecked again by air aspiration.

Although oxygenation may be adequate with transtracheal catheter ventilation, with near total to total upper-airway obstruction, passive exhalation may be insufficient to sustain ventilation, and air trapping and excessive hypercarbia may result. Provisions should be made to secure the airway in a more permanent fashion. Other problems associated with prolonged use of nonhumidified transtracheal jet ventilation include subcutaneous or mediastinal emphysema, pneumothorax, esophageal puncture, sore throat, infection, bleeding, hematoma formation, and mucosal ulceration. The needle or catheter may break or bend if the patient coughs or moves, resulting in respiratory obstruction. Of these complications, catheter kinking and subcutaneous air injection (sometimes massive) with loss of anatomic landmarks and pneumothorax appear to be the most serious and widely encountered. In our opinion, use of this technique with a needle or standard intravenous catheter for more than short intervals for "bridging" to another technique is inappropriate, since it is extremely difficult to secure and maintain them in the proper position, and displacement with subcutaneous air or kinking can both be lethal.

VII. PERCUTANEOUS DILATIONAL CRICOTHYROTOMY

A. GENERAL PRINCIPLES

Percutaneous dilational cricothyrotomy is fast and usually easy to perform, even on patients with short necks or with spinal injury. It does not require a surgeon's skill to gain airway access and has fewer operative and postoperative complications. A number of commercially available devices use this technology. These devices have in common the insertion of an airway catheter over a dilator, which is usually introduced over a guidewire. The guidewire is inserted through a needle or over-the-needle catheter (the Seldinger technique) after an initial skin incision. This technique, often used for the insertion of catheter introducer sheaths and central lines, is familiar to anesthesiologists. We prefer insertion of an airway over a dilator and guidewire due to the inherent safety of this technique and the ability to insert an airway of far greater diameter than the initial catheter. One device (the Nu-Trake device) introduces a "housing" similar to a dilator, but made in two parts, with the needle loaded coaxially within it. After the needle is withdrawn, metal airways with obturators are serially introduced inside the housing until the desired diameter tube is reached.

Recently, several devices have been introduced that allow insertion of the dilator directly over a needle or directly into the skin incision. While they lack the step of introducing a guidewire, they are included here since they require both a skin incision and a dilator for insertion of the airway. Percutaneous dilational cricothyrotomy is gaining popularity in the ED, ICU, and OR. It is very similar to another increasingly popular ICU technique, percutaneous dilational tracheostomy, an elective procedure.[45,53-55] Airways can be introduced rapidly by the Seldinger "over the wire" technique, which allows positive pressure ventilation without modification of standard ventilation devices.[21,56] Although the technique requires more time to perform than needle cricothyrotomy, it may be more effective in providing adequate ventilation and oxygenation.

There are a number of cricothyrotomy sets available that are inserted by the percutaneous dilational cricothyrotomy technique (Melker Emergency Cricothyrotomy Catheter Set, Patil Emergency Cricothyrotomy Catheter Set, Arndt Emergency Cricothyrotomy Set, Corke Cranswick Percutaneous Minitracheostomy Set, Cook Critical Care, Bloomington, Ind.; Portex Mini-Trach II, Concord/Portex, Kenne, N.H.; and PerTrach, Pertrach, Inc, Long Beach, Calif). Several sets (Melker, Arndt, and Corke Cranswick) are similar in design and operation. They use a skin incision, followed by insertion of a guidewire and insertion of a dilator and airway catheter (cricothyrotomy tube). The Patil set is essentially an Arndt set without the guidewire. The dilator and breathing tube are loaded on the needle and, after a skin incision, are advanced after airway positioning is verified. These sets (Arndt, Patil) come with a 3.0-mm internal diameter (ID) kink-resistant airway catheter that can be maintained in place with umbilical tape. The Melker set is available in 3.5-, 4.0-, and 6.0-mm ID airway catheter sizes and lengths of 3.8 cm, 4.2 cm, and 7.5 cm, respectively. The 4.0-mm ID airway catheter is also available in a 7.5 cm length. This allows the use of a smaller diameter tube of sufficient length for an adult neck. The Melker set also comes in a "military version" (similar to the Patil) that is modified for direct insertion through an incision without use of a guidewire. Some sets (Melker, Patil, Arndt) are available with adapters so that both jet ventilators and conventional ventilators can be attached to the airway device. The Corke Cranswick tube has a 4.0-mm ID and is 7.5 cm in length. Pertrachs are available with 5.5- and 7.1-mm ID.

A study comparing the Melker set to surgical cricothyrotomy in cadavers is underway. Preliminary reports [personal communications] indicate that the Melker set is easier to use than the Pertrach but that both techniques are more difficult to teach to paramedics than surgical cricothyrotomy.

B. INSERTION INSTRUCTIONS FOR THE MELKER, ARNDT, AND CORKE CRANSWICK PERCUTANEOUS DILATIONAL CRICOTHYROTOMY DEVICES

Many cricothyrotomy sets (Melker, Arndt, and Corke Cranswick) contain a scalpel blade, a syringe with an 18-gauge over-the-needle catheter and/or a thin wall introducer needle, a guidewire, an appropriate length and diameter dilator, and a polyvinyl airway catheter (Fig. 25-3).[34] Detailed insertion instructions for this type of device are as follows (Fig. 25-4):

1. Position the patient supine and, if no contraindication, slightly extend the neck, using a roll under the neck or shoulders. If cervical spine injury is suspected, properly immobilize the head and neck, and maintain a neutral position.
2. Open the prepackaged cricothyrotomy set and assemble the components. Whenever possible and appropriate, use aseptic technique and local anesthetic.
3. Identify the cricothyroid membrane between the cricoid and thyroid cartilages (Fig. 25-4, A).
4. Carefully palpate the cricothyroid membrane, and, while stabilizing the cartilage, make a vertical skin incision (about 1.0 to 1.5 cm) in the midline using the scalpel blade. Next make a vertical stab incision through the lower third of the cricothyroid membrane. An adequate incision eases introduction of the dilator and airway (Fig. 25-4, B). See Comments #1 and #2 following.
5. With the supplied syringe attached to the 18-gauge plastic (over-the-needle) catheter introducer needle (or alternatively, to the introducer needle), advance it through the incision into the airway at a 45-degree angle to the frontal plane in the midline in a caudad direction. When advancing the needle forward, verification of entrance into the airway can be confirmed by aspiration on the syringe resulting in free air return (Fig. 25-4, C). (Some users fill the syringe with fluid so that bubbles can be observed when the needle enters the airway. We find this unnecessary and time consuming.)
6. Remove the syringe and needle, leaving the plastic catheter or introducer needle in place. Do not attempt to advance the plastic catheter completely into the airway, this may result in kinking of the catheter and inability to pass the guidewire! Advance the soft, flexible end of the guidewire through the catheter or needle and into the airway several centimeters (Fig. 25-4, D). See Comment #3 following.
7. Remove the plastic catheter or needle, leaving the guidewire in place (Fig. 25-4, E).
8. Advance the handled (Melker, Arndt) dilator, tapered end first, into the connector end of the airway catheter until the handle stops against the connec-

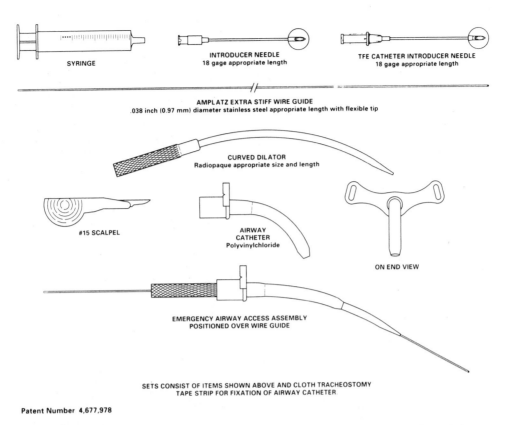

SYRINGE

INTRODUCER NEEDLE
18 gage appropriate length

TFE CATHETER INTRODUCER NEEDLE
18 gage appropriate length

AMPLATZ EXTRA STIFF WIRE GUIDE
.038 inch (0.97 mm) diameter stainless steel appropriate length with flexible tip

CURVED DILATOR
Radiopaque appropriate size and length

#15 SCALPEL

AIRWAY
CATHETER
Polyvinylchloride

ON END VIEW

EMERGENCY AIRWAY ACCESS ASSEMBLY
POSITIONED OVER WIRE GUIDE

SETS CONSIST OF ITEMS SHOWN ABOVE AND CLOTH TRACHEOSTOMY
TAPE STRIP FOR FIXATION OF AIRWAY CATHETER.

Patent Number 4,677,978

Fig. 25-3. Melker percutaneous dilational cricothyrotomy set (Cook Critical Care, Bloomington, Ind.); this is also representative of the Arndt and the Corke Cranswick sets.

tor. With other sets, insert the dilator to the recommended depth (Fig. 25-4, *F*).

NOTE: This step may be performed prior to beginning the procedure. Use of lubrication on the surface of the dilator may enhance fit and placement of the emergency airway catheter.

9. Advance the emergency airway access assembly over the guidewire until the proximal stiff end of the guidewire is completely through and visible at the handle end of the dilator. It is important to always visualize the proximal end of the guidewire during the airway insertion procedure to prevent its inadvertent loss into the trachea. Maintaining the guidewire position, advance the emergency airway access assembly over the guidewire with an in-and-out reciprocating motion. Initially, advance and retract only the dilator completely into the incision several times. Once the tract has been dilated, advance the dilator and breathing tube into the airway. Care should be taken not to advance the tip of the dilator beyond the tip of the guidewire within the trachea (Fig. 25-4, *G*).

10. As the breathing tube is fully advanced into the trachea, remove the guidewire and dilator simultaneously.

11. Fix the emergency airway catheter in place with the cloth tracheostomy tape strip in a standard fashion (Fig. 25-4, *H*).

12. Connect the emergency airway catheter, using its standard 15-22 adapter to an appropriate ventilatory device.

1. Comment #1 – Recommendation for skin incision prior to needle insertion

We recommend an incision before introducing the catheter for two reasons. First, the catheter is more likely to kink when the needle is removed if there is no skin incision, making it difficult to pass the guidewire, and, second, we have had cases reported of inability to advance the dilator because the skin incision was not next to the guidewire. Extending the incision to the guidewire solved the problem. While anesthesiologists and critical care physicians usually make a skin incision after wire introduction, we strongly recommend skin and membrane incision as the first step. We have had no cases of catheter kinking or inability to pass the dilator when the incision is made first. One set (Melker) now includes an additional introducer needle of sufficient ID to allow the guidewire to be advanced directly through a needle without the need for placing the catheter. This will eliminate any chance of kinking but increases the risk of shearing the guidewire.

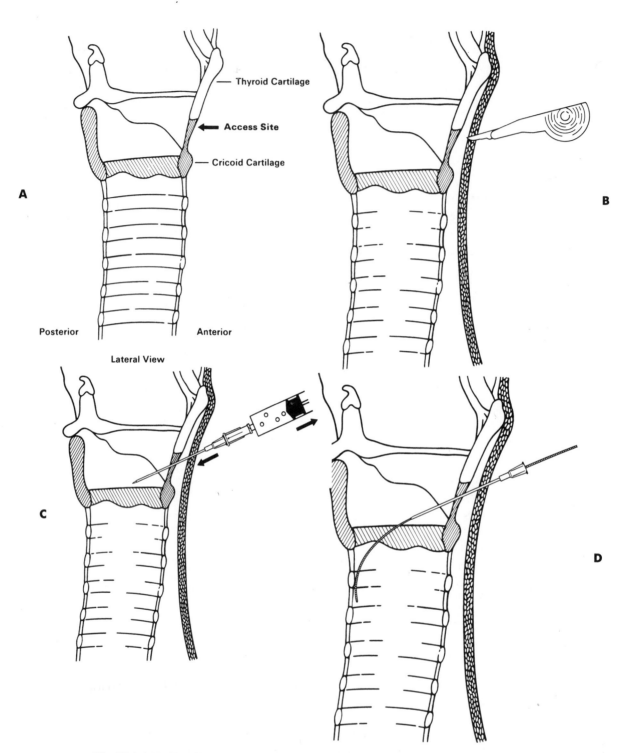

Fig. 25-4, A-H. Detailed instructions for insertion of the Melker, Arndt, and Corke Cranswick percutaneous dilational cricothyrotomy sets. (From "Melker emergency cricothyrotomy sets: suggested instructions for placement," instruction pamphlet, Cook Critical Care, 1988, Bloomington, Ind.)   *Continued.*

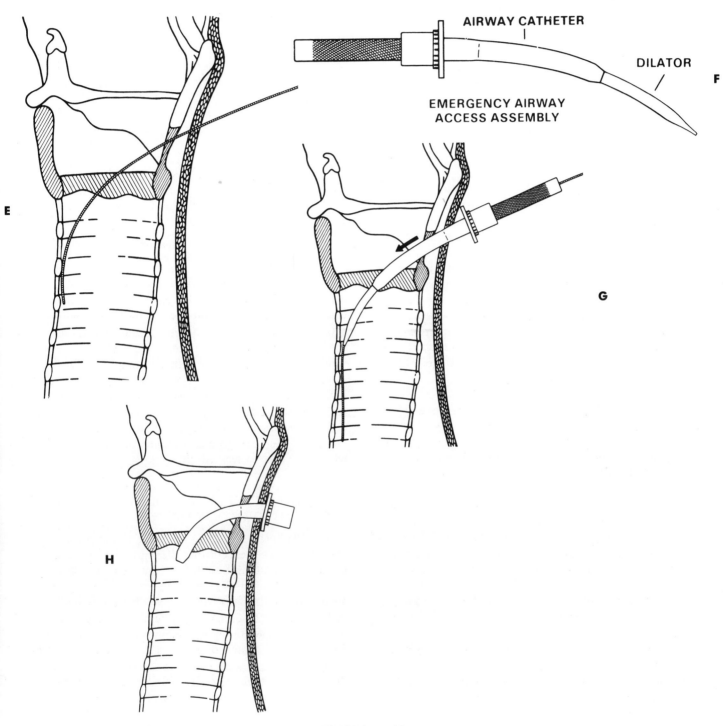

Fig. 25-4, cont'd.

Table 25-1. Success rate of guidewire introduction with or without skin incision and with an over-the-needle catheter or an introducer needle in 16 cadavers

	Easy	Difficult	Impossible
18 G* Over-the-needle catheter	8	6	2
16 G over-the-needle catheter	8	6	2
18 G needle	11	3	0
18 G over-the-needle catheter after incision	12	4	0

*G, gauge.

2. Comment #2 — Vertical versus horizontal incision

It is unclear whether a horizontal or vertical skin incision is superior. The literature is evenly divided on this matter but usually refers to surgical cricothyrotomy. However, it can be argued that a vertical incision is better during emergency cricothyrotomy because it can be extended superiorly or inferiorly if the relationship of the skin and cricothyroid membrane changes (as frequently happens). We recommend a vertical stab through the cricothyroid membrane in the inferior third to ease placement of the dilator and avoid the cricothyroid arteries, which often anastomose in the midline superiorly.

3. Comment #3 — Use of over-the-needle catheter versus introducer needle

We recently studied the success rate of 32 anesthesiology residents at guidewire introduction with or without skin incision and with an over-the-needle catheter or an introducer needle in 16 cadavers. Residents were asked to judge the ease of delineating the pretracheal anatomy and then attempted to pass a guidewire through the 18-gauge over-the-needle catheter supplied with the cricothyrotomy set (Melker), a stiff 16-gauge over-the-needle catheter, or a thin-walled introducer needle prior to skin incision. After skin incision, the 18-gauge catheter was again introduced, and guidewire insertion was again attempted. These results are shown in Table 25-1.

This study shows insertion of the guidewire through a needle to be superior when a skin incision is not used but similar in success rate to an over-the-needle catheter if an incision is used initially. Also, it appears that catheters kinked only when attempts were made to pass the total length of the catheter into the airway.

In a second study, we evaluated the rate of successfully advancing a guidewire into the airway through an over-the-needle catheter with or without a skin incision. The catheters were either advanced into the airway just to the point where air could be aspirated or totally into the airway, as with insertion of a transtracheal catheter

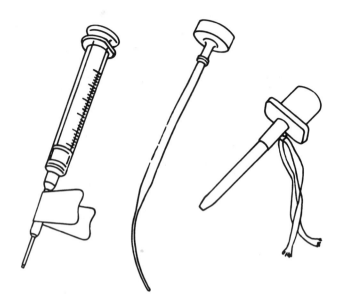

Fig. 25-5. Pertrach percutaneous dilational cricothyrotomy set (Pertrach, Inc., Long Beach, Calif.)

for "jet" ventilation. In seven cadavers, the guidewire was successfully inserted on all attempts, with or without a skin incision, when the catheter was advanced only to the point where it entered the airway. When attempts were made to advance the catheter completely into the airway, it was unsuccessful 3 of 7 times without a skin incision and 2 of 7 times with a skin incision. The catheter was successfully advanced in cases where the catheter-needle assembly could be placed at a 45-degree angle and the needle was maintained inside the airway when the catheter was advanced.

C. INSERTION INSTRUCTIONS FOR THE PERTRACH PERCUTANEOUS DILATIONAL CRICOTHYROTOMY DEVICE

The Pertrach (Fig. 25-5) is similar to the previously described devices except that the guidewire and dilator are a single unit, and, therefore, the introducer needle must be split after the distal end of the guidewire is advanced so that the dilator can be introduced (a catheter cannot be used). This is cumbersome, especially in emergency situations, and requires that the guidewire and dilator be advanced far down the airway. A recent study in cadavers showed equal success for percutaneous dilational cricothyrotomy with the Pertrach and surgical cricothyrotomy. Surgical cricothyrotomy was faster, but it was impossible to predict whether bleeding complications would have been higher with the surgical cricothyrotomies.[57] Both the manufacturer and users have reported difficulty with the needle, which is occasionally difficult or impossible to split.

Detailed insertion instructions for the Pertrach percutaneous dilational cricothyrotomy device are as follows (Fig. 25-6):

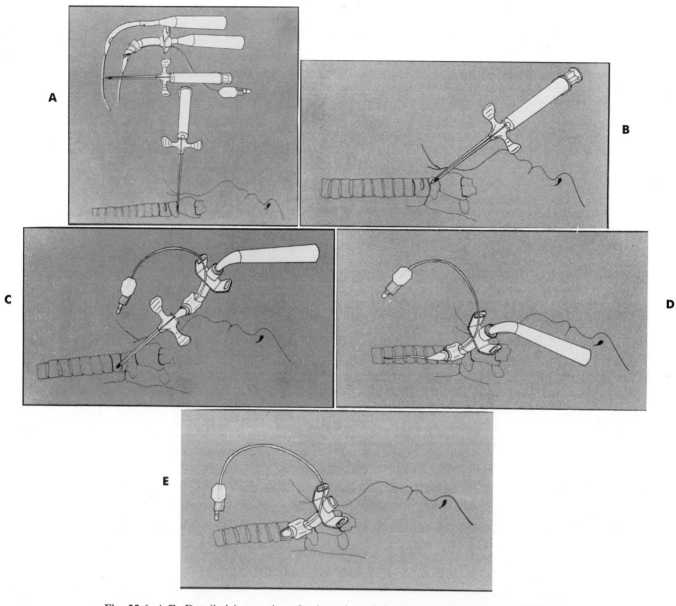

Fig. 25-6, A-E. Detailed instructions for insertion of the Pertrach percutaneous dilational cricothyrotomy set. (From "Cricothyroidotomy," instruction sheet, Pertrach, Inc., Long Beach, Calif.)

1. Test cuffed tube on dilator, lubricate cuff, deflate.
2. Make a 1 to 2 cm incision in skin over cricothyroid membrane.
3. Insert needle into incision, with syringe attached, perpendicular to the cricoid, and advance until tip is in airway (Fig. 25-6, *A*). Aspirate for air to establish position in the airway. NOTE: Before use, test the needle for air leaks by placing one finger over the end and aspirating with the attached syringe. If there is an air leak, then the above technique for insuring correct needle placement cannot be relied upon. Instead, one must adjust the needle placement by:
   a. Seeing that the needle moves freely back and forth in the tracheal lumen.
   b. Seeing that the dilator tubing can be threaded easily through the needle into the trachea.
   c. A useful sign that the needle is correctly placed is the patient coughing when the tubing is threaded in.
4. Advance needle at 45-degree angle into airway, toward the carina (Fig. 25-6, *B*).
5. Remove syringe and insert Teflon guide of dilator in needle, guiding the tubing through it (Fig. 25-6, *C*). Squeeze wings to split needle. The needle may not completely separate at this point but will enable the dilator to be advanced into the slot created by squeezing the wings. As the tubing passes down the slot, it will complete the splitting of the needle. When

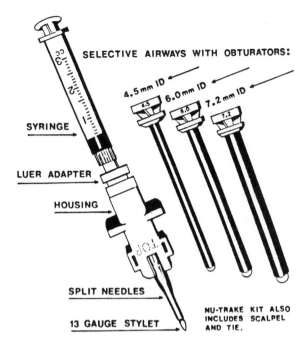

Fig. 25-7. Nu-Trake percutaneous dilational cricothyrotomy set (International Medical Devices, Inc., Northridge, Calif.)

the tip of the dilator reaches skin level, pull out the needle and discard.

6. Exert pressure and force dilator into the airway until the tube is in position, with face plate against the skin (Fig. 25-6, *D*).

7. Remove dilator and secure tube to patient. Inflate cuff, and attach respirator if needed (Fig. 25-6, *E*).

D. INSERTION INSTRUCTIONS FOR THE NU-TRAKE PERCUTANEOUS DILATIONAL CRICOTHYROTOMY DEVICE

The Nu-Trake device (Fig. 25-7) is more complicated to use, has a rigid airway, and is difficult to secure. In a recent study comparing it to the Pertrach, the Nu-Trake was found to require far greater insertion forces, often resulting in the introducer-stylet embedding in the posterior wall of the trachea.[37] Another study reports numerous complications with this device; however, these are not documented or referenced.[58] Unfortunately, the authors experienced difficulty with percutaneous dilational tracheostomy due to poor patient selection and condemn all percutaneous techniques. Bjoraker et al.[59] had anesthesiologists and residents attempt cricothyrotomy in 11 dogs with the Nu-Trake device. There was difficulty inserting the stylet and blunt needle, resulting in slippage and two subcricoid insertions. There were also frequent air leaks, and the lumen had a tendency to occlude on the posterior wall of the trachea. Subcutaneous emphysema, cricoid cartilage injury, cricotracheal ligament perforation, posterior wall perforation, and

incidental submucosal airway hemorrhage were found in 8 of 11 dogs. Hulsey[60] concludes that the Nu-Trake device "needs further development or solid clinical evidence of safety and efficacy before it can be recommended for use in emergency medicine practice." Direct comparisons of all devices presently available have not been performed. Detailed insertion instructions for the Nu-Trake percutaneous dilational cricothyrotomy device are as follows (Fig. 25-8):

1. Patient's head is hyperextended, if possible, and the cricothyroid membrane identified; palpate (Fig. 25-8, *A*).

2. Pinch 1 cm of skin, and insert sharp tip of knife blade through skin. Cut in an outward motion (Fig. 25-8, *B*).

3. The needle should puncture the membrane just beyond the entry at approximately the same angles as the lower edge of the housing. Aspirate, easy moving spring obturator denotes tracheal entrance (Fig. 25-8, *C*).

4. The stylet and syringe are removed as a unit by twisting the Luer adapter counterclockwise and lifting out (Fig. 25-8, *D*).

5. The blunt needle is gently moved further into the trachea until the housing rests on the overlying skin. A freely rocking motion confirms proper depth of insertion (Fig. 25-8, *E*).

6. In all cases, begin with the smallest airway (4.5 mm), and insert airway and obturator together PUSHING WITH THE THENAR EMINENCE resting against the cap of the obturator. Airway and obturator are PUSHED (not squeezed) downward into the needle, which is divided lengthwise and spreads apart to accommodate them (Fig. 25-8, *F*).

7. Obturator is removed, leaving a clear passage for air to reach the lungs. If airway size requires change, this can be easily performed by leaving the housing and needle guide in place, while removal and insertion of airways are made. Ties are threaded through the brackets on the sides of the housing (Fig. 25-8, *G*).

8. System in operation: Bag valve or universal (15 mm) adapter may be fitted to the top of the housing. Expansion of lungs can also be started by mouth-to-mouth respiration, with fingers closing off the vents in the housing (Fig. 25-8, *H*).

E. INSERTION INSTRUCTIONS FOR THE PATIL, THE PORTEX, AND THE MELKER MILITARY PERCUTANEOUS DILATIONAL CRICOTHYROTOMY DEVICES

The Patil set, the Portex minitrach, and the military variation of the Melker set are sold without the guidewire (Fig. 25-9 on p. 501). In this design, only a scalpel, dilator, and airway catheter are supplied. The Patil set has a metal, beveled needle loaded coaxially

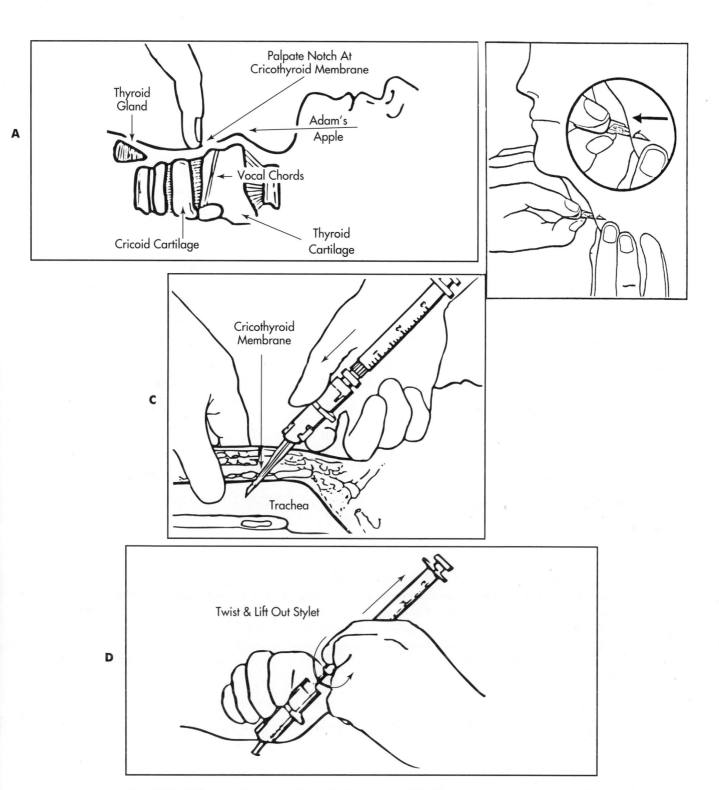

Fig. 25-8, A-H. Detailed instructions for insertion of Nu-Trake percutaneous dilational cricothyrotomy set. (From "Nu-Trake cricothyrotomy device," instruction pamphlet, International Medical Devices, Inc., Northridge, Calif.)   *Continued.*

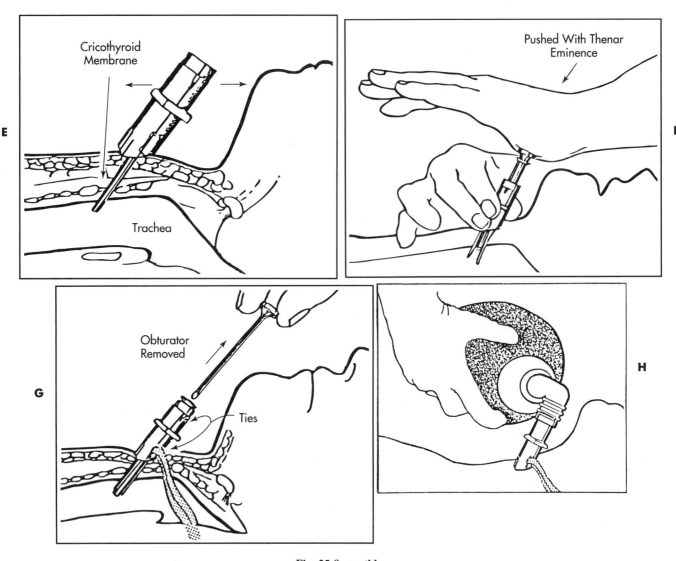

Fig. 25-8, cont'd.

inside the dilator. The devices are inserted by passing the dilator and airway catheter directly through the incision. They may lend themselves to use by prehospital providers who are unfamiliar with the Seldinger technique and often work under difficult environmental conditions. The Portex set is designed primarily for "management of sputum retention." The dilator ("introducer") is rigid and malleable, and the breathing tube is not tapered. The instructions recommend insertion of the dilator, followed by loading and passage of the breathing tube. Detailed insertion instructions for the Patil and Portex percutaneous dilational cricothyrotomy devices are as follows (Fig. 25-10):

1. Attach needle introducer assembly to the cricothyrotomy catheter. Lubricate the catheter (Fig. 25-10, *A*).
2. Prep anterior neck of patient.
3. Identify cricothyroid membrane between the cricoid and thyroid cartilages, and stabilize trachea with thumb and index finger (Fig. 25-10, *B*).

4. Make a skin incision with the #15 scalpel large enough to admit the catheter, over the cricothyroid membrane, close to the cricoid cartilage.
5. Cannulate the trachea with the catheter tip facing caudad. A loss of resistance is felt when the trachea is entered (Fig. 25-10, *C*).
6. Aspirate air into a water-filled 5-ml syringe to confirm catheter position within the tracheal lumen (Fig. 25-10, *D*).
7. Remove the needle, and advance the catheter and dilator caudad. Aspirate again to confirm position.
8. Remove the dilator, and aspirate once again to ensure correct placement within the trachea (Fig. 25-10, *E*).
9. Connect the catheter to oxygen source, and secure catheter with the tape provided.

The above instructions are designed for OR insertion under controlled circumstances. Instructions for the military design intended for emergent field use are as follows:

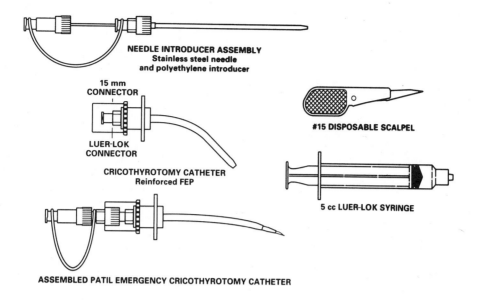

NEEDLE INTRODUCER ASSEMBLY
Stainless steel needle
and polyethylene introducer

15 mm CONNECTOR

LUER-LOK CONNECTOR

CRICOTHYROTOMY CATHETER
Reinforced FEP

#15 DISPOSABLE SCALPEL

5 cc LUER-LOK SYRINGE

ASSEMBLED PATIL EMERGENCY CRICOTHYROTOMY CATHETER

**SET CONSISTS OF ITEMS SHOWN ABOVE AND CLOTH TRACHEOSTOMY
TAPE STRIP FOR FIXATION OF AIRWAY CATHETER.**

Fig. 25-9. Patil percutaneous dilational cricothyrotomy set (Cook Critical Care, Bloomington, Ind.); this is also representative of Portex and Melker military sets.

1. Identify the cricothyroid space by palpating between the thyroid and the cricoid cartilage.
2. Under strict aseptic technique, infiltrate the cricothyroid space with anesthetic, if clinically indicated.
3. While stabilizing the cricoid cartilage, make an incision with the #15 scalpel blade through all layers of the cricothyroid space down to the airway.
4. Insert the 18-French curved dilator with the cricothyrotomy tube loaded over it into the incision in a caudad direction.
5. Advance and withdraw the dilator a few times to dilate the tract for insertion of the cricothyrotomy tube.
6. Applying steady pressure, advance the tube into the airway.
7. Maintaining the tube in the airway, withdraw the dilator.
8. Secure tube in place with tape provided.

Wain et al.[61] reported the successful use of the Portex device in 60 patients. Only one insertion was for acute airway obstruction; the others were for suctioning of secretions. Intratracheal placement was possible in every case. Two major intratracheal bleeds occurred, which necessitated endotracheal intubation. There were few minor complications.

Most presently available sets (excluding the Pertrach) have uncuffed airway catheters. In situations in which a cuffed tube is desirable, the airway catheter can be changed to a soft plastic tracheostomy tube of the same ID. For instance, a Shiley 6SCT can be used in place of the 6.0-mm ID airway catheter supplied with the Melker set.

VIII. COMPLICATIONS AND OUTCOME DATA

The reported complication rate associated with elective cricothyrotomy is between 6% and 8% and for emergent procedures, between 10% and 40%.[33,62] The morbidity and mortality of elective cricothyrotomy is similar to that with elective tracheostomy. Boyd et al.[39] found 10 complications (6.8%) out of 147 cricothyrotomies, but no differentiation was made between elective and emergency procedures. Brantigan and Grow[13] reported a 6.1% complication rate in 655 cases, most of which were correctable, self-limited, and compared favorably with the complication rate associated with tracheostomy. The same authors also implicated the presence of acute laryngeal pathology (especially prolonged intubation prior to cricothyrotomy) as the predisposing factor in the subsequent development of subglottic obstruction.[14]

Adverse effects of cricothyrotomy can be categorized into two groups: those that occur early, and those that occur late in the postoperative period (Box 25-1). Early complications include asphyxia due to failure to establish the airway, hemorrhage, improper or unsuccessful tube placement, subcutaneous and mediastinal emphysema, prolonged procedure time, pneumothorax, and airway obstruction. Esophageal or mediastinal perforation, vocal cord injury, aspiration, and laryngeal disruption may also occur. Long-term complications include tracheal and subglottic stenosis (especially in the presence of preexisting laryngeal trauma or infection), aspiration, swallowing dysfunction, tube obstruction, tracheoesophageal fistula, and voice changes. Voice change is the most common complication, occurring in up to 50% of cases.[63]

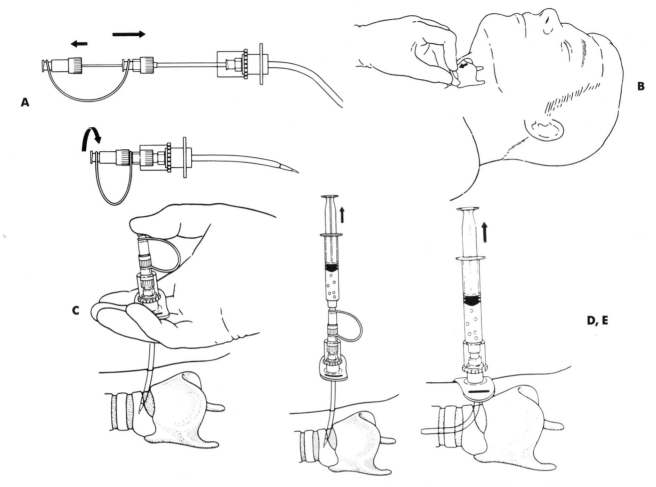

Fig. 25-10, A-E. Detailed instructions for insertion of Patil, Portex, and Melker military percutaneous dilational cricothyrotomy sets. (From Patil emergency cricothyrotomy catheter set: suggested instructions for use, Cook Critical Care, 1993, Bloomington, Ind.)

Voice problems include hoarseness, weak voice, or decreased pitch. This dysfunction in voice may be due to injury to the external branch of the superior laryngeal nerve, decreased cricothyroid muscle contractility, or mechanical obstruction due to narrowing of the anterior parts of the thyroid and cricoid cartilages.[64] Infection, late bleeding, persistent stoma, and tracheomalacia have also been reported.

Although subglottic stenosis is the most frequently reported major complication after cricothyrotomy, it is rare after tracheostomy. Pneumothorax and major blood vessel erosion are also associated with tracheostomy. Other complications associated with tracheostomy include mediastinal emphysema, accidental extubation, cardiac arrest, and death.

The complication rate for cricothyrotomy is higher in the pediatric population. Pneumothorax is the most common complication in children (5% to 7%) and is rarely seen in adults. One percent to 2% of adults will develop subglottic stenosis following tracheostomy compared with 2% to 8% in children. The mortality rate in children is up to 8.7%.

Numerous reports describing various complications associated with cricothyrotomy have appeared since the landmark paper of Brantigan and Grow.[13] Habel[65] claimed to have no major complications in his series of 30 patients who had elective cricothyrotomy. Similarly, Morain[66] found no significant complications attributable to cricothyrotomy performed in his series of 16 patients. Greisz et al.[67] had 61 elective cricothyrotomy cases, of which 30 eventually died (of unrelated causes) and 20 underwent postmortem laryngeal evaluation. They demonstrated histologic abnormalities, including overt inflammation and granular tissue formation in the majority of cases. Of the 21 extubated survivors, none had subglottic stenosis, although 14% had permanent voice change. On the other hand, Holst et al.[68] reported a 52% incidence of hoarseness, weakness, and fatigue in a series of 103 elective cricothyroidotomies. Ten percent of their patients also complained of dysphagia. Van Hasselt et al.[69] reported a similar incidence of dysphonia in their 61 elective cricothyrotomy cases.

BOX 25-1   Complications of cricothyrotomy

Early

Asphyxia
Hemorrhage
Improper or unsuccessful tube placement
Subcutaneous and mediastinal emphysema
Pneumothorax
Airway obstruction
Esophageal or mediastinal perforation
Vocal cord injury
Aspiration
Laryngeal disruption
Prolonged procedure time

Late

Tracheal and subglottic stenosis
Aspiration
Swallowing dysfunction
Tube obstruction
Tracheoesophageal fistula
Voice change
Infection
Late bleeding
Persistent stoma
Tracheomalacia

Sise et al.[33] reported a prospective analysis of morbidity and mortality in 76 critically ill and injured patients: 46 patients (61%) died, and postmortem examination was performed on 85% of them. Twenty-eight percent had airway pathologies such as ulceration, hemorrhage, and abscess at the stoma or cuff site, subglottic erosion, and mucosal separation. Seven percent had major complications, including one death, two with subglottic stenosis, and two with reversible subglottic granulation—one with partial obstruction and one with tracheomalacia. Minor complications were noted in 30% of the survivors. These included transient hoarseness, aspiration pneumonia, chronic aspiration, pain at the stoma scar, bleeding, stoma site abscess, and subglottic ulceration.

Prehospital cricothyrotomy performed by emergency medical services (EMS) personnel carries a higher risk of morbidity than the in-hospital procedure. Spaite et al.[70] reported an overall acute complication rate of 31% in 20 emergency patients. Failure to secure the airway accounted for the major complication (12%). Minor complications included right mainstem intubation, infrahyoid placement, and thyroid cartilage fracture. On the other hand, 60 surgical cricothyrotomies performed by trained aeromedical system personnel had a complication rate of 8.7%.[71] These complications included significant hemorrhage or soft tissue hematoma and incorrect placement.

Problems and complications associated with percutaneous cricothyrotomy include difficulties with insertion, esophageal or mediastinal misplacement, and bleeding.[72] The overall reported complication rate is 5%. Cricothyroid membrane calcification and blockage by secretion may make insertion difficult. Pedersen et al.[73] reported a case in which a repeat minitracheostomy could not be performed 2 months after the initial procedure. Postmortem examination of the larynx showed calcification of the cricothyroid membrane. This abnormal change was believed to be due to dystrophic ossification and heterotrophic bone formation. Displacement of the tube into the mediastinum may occur and can cause emphysema, respiratory distress, and pneumothorax.[74-76] Bleeding occurs in 2% of cases, and significant hemorrhage requiring surgical intervention has been reported.[77,78] The Seldinger technique appears to lessen the incidence of bleeding and promote a more precise technique of insertion.[79]

IX. PRACTICAL APPLICATIONS OF CRICOTHYROTOMY

A. IN THE OR AND ICU SETTINGS

Brantigan and Grow[13] reported the largest single series of elective long-term cricothyrotomy involving 655 patients. The procedure was initially utilized to decrease the incidence of sternotomy-related wound infection and subsequently was expanded for long-term mechanical ventilation. Cricothyrotomy was performed either in the OR or under local anesthesia in the patient's room. They did not observe any subglottic stenosis, and there was only a 2.6% incidence of tracheal stenosis and an overall complication rate of 6.1%. Only one patient died following a tracheostomy tube change. The authors attributed their success to the elective use of the procedure, proper usage of antibiotics, the lack of laryngeal inflammation, anatomic dissection, and better, less irritating tracheostomy tubes. They concluded that cricothyrotomy is a benign, safe, well-tolerated procedure that is not significantly associated with subglottic stenosis and offers advantages over standard tracheostomy: technical simplicity, faster performance, low complication rate, can be done at bedside, and better isolation from the median sternotomy. They recommended cricothyrotomy as the method of choice for all elective or emergency tracheal airway access. However, the authors were subsequently faulted for their lack of detailed patient follow-up.[80] Therefore, Brantigan and Grow published a follow-up paper[14] in which they reviewed 17 patients with subglottic stenosis following cricothyrotomy. They recommended that all patients have endoscopic airway assessment prior to elective placement. They also suggested tracheostomy for patients with significant laryngotracheal injury.

Other authors reported higher complication rates. Boyd et al.[39] reported a series of 147 cricothyrotomies. Fifteen cases were emergent, and the remaining 132 were done electively on postoperative median sternotomy patients. Severe glottic and subglottic stenosis was noted in 2 of the 105 survivors. Subglottic stenosis was not observed in those intubated less than 7 days prior to cricothyrotomy but was seen in 9.1% of survivors intubated for more than 7 days prior to the procedure. Esses and Jafek[40] found an overall complication rate of 28%. Kuriloff et al.[24] performed elective surgical cricothyrotomies in 48 patients undergoing cardiothoracic surgery. They showed a 52% incidence of airway complications, and six of their patients died while still cannulated. Morbidity was highest among diabetics, the elderly, and in patients in whom cricothyroid cannulation lasted longer than one month.

Percutaneous dilatational tracheostomy (and cricothyrotomy) was first described by Toye and Weinstein in 1969.[21] Subsequently, they reported their results with tracheostomy and cricothyrotomy in 100 patients.[45] Ninety-four of these were tracheotomies, and only six were cricothyrotomies. Airway access was obtained in 30 seconds to 2 minutes. When compared with standard surgical tracheostomy, there was less bleeding and a smaller resulting scar. Stoma formation was observed to develop within 24 hours and, with time, increasingly larger tracheal tubes could be inserted through the stoma. The complication rate was 14%, and there was one mortality directly attributed to the use of the device. No long-term complications were reported on subsequent follow-ups.

B. IN THE EMERGENCY DEPARTMENT SETTING

There is significantly less information available on the use of cricothyrotomy in the ED. McGill et al.[81] reviewed their experience with emergent surgical cricothyrotomies performed in the ED on 38 patients. The majority of the procedures (82%) were done after other forms of airway management failed. The remaining five patients (18%) had surgical cricothyrotomy performed as the first airway control maneuver because of severe facial or neck injury and/or airway hemorrhage. Almost a third of their patients developed immediate complications, the most common of which was incorrect placement of the tracheostomy tube. Other complications observed included prolonged insertion, unsuccessful tracheostomy tube insertion, and significant bleeding. Thirty-two percent survived and were discharged from the hospital. Only one long-term complication was reported. The patient had a longitudinal fracture of the thyroid cartilage during placement of an oversized tube through the cricoid membrane, requiring operative repair and leaving the patient with permanent dysphonia.

Table 25-2. Clinical experience with cricothyrotomy set (Melker Emergency Cricothyrotomy Catheter Set, Cook Critical Care, Bloomington, Ind.) in 15 attempted placements in adult patients

Diagnosis	Number of Patients
Multitrauma with severe facial injuries	4
Respiratory failure	3
Cardiac arrest	3
Head and neck tumor	1
Massive subcutaneous and intraoral emphysema	1
Gunshot to chest	1
Inability to intubate	2
Setting	
Prehospital	6
Emergency department	3
Intensive care unit	3
Operating room	3
Technique	
Over-the-wire	13
Direct insertion	2
Long-term complications	0
Complications during insertion	
Kinked IV catheter	3
Initial incision not at wire site	1

To date, we have reports of 15 airway control attempts using a cricothyrotomy set (Melker) in an emergency setting (Table 25-2). Thirteen were successful, and all salvageable patients did well without complications attributable to the procedure. Three attempts failed initially because of inability to pass the guidewire through the catheter. No skin incision was used in these cases. In two, kinking was recognized, and the guidewire was introduced through larger, stiffer catheters without further difficulty. In the third, the patient was intubated from above in the interim. The other failure was related to passing the dilator into the incision without placing the guidewire first. This was attempted during helicopter transport of a patient *in extremis*. The airway catheter was placed in the subcutaneous tissue. This was immediately recognized, and the airway catheter was removed. This technique had been used successfully on a previous patient and was felt to be as safe as the wire-guided technique. In another case, the physician attempted to pass the dilator over the wire without making a skin incision with the scalpel. He was unaware that a scalpel was provided or that an incision was necessary. We do not consider this to be a failure of the technique.

C. CRICOTHYROTOMY IN THE AEROMEDICAL ENVIRONMENT

We have chosen to discuss cricothyrotomy performed by hospital-based aeromedical system personnel separately from cricothyrotomy performed by EMS personnel because of the differences in training and skill levels between the groups. In general, hospital-based aeromedical providers have significantly greater training and are more familiar and comfortable with cricothyrotomy, due in no small part to active involvement of medical directors. Statistics of success and complication rates support this contention.

Boyle et al.[71] reported a 98.5% success rate in 69 patients transported by a regional helicopter program. All procedures were performed by flight nurses, and the complication rate was 8.7%. A number of other studies involving flight nurses or flight nurse-physician teams report similar results.[82-84] No studies have yet addressed the use of percutaneous dilational cricothyrotomy.

D. PREHOSPITAL (EMS) CRICOTHYROTOMY

Efficacy of cricothyrotomy is difficult to evaluate in the prehospital setting. However, it is not uncommon for paramedics to encounter clinical situations in which the airway cannot be secured by conventional means (i.e., endotracheal intubation). Training in cricothyrotomy is mandatory in most paramedic training programs, although its use is usually at the discretion of the medical director. The complication and mortality rates are higher for patients treated with surgical cricothyrotomy, owing largely to late application of the technique and the severity of injuries.[70,83] The long-term complication rates resulting from prehospital surgical cricothyrotomy have not yet been established. Johnson et al.[57] studied the proficiency of paramedic students in performing percutaneous dilational cricothyrotomy versus surgical cricothyrotomy in human cadavers. Forty-four paramedic students performed the two techniques on cadavers, but analysis of data was limited to procedures performed on subjects with intact cricoid membranes. There was no significant difference in the success rate on the first attempt between the two approaches, but the surgical procedure was significantly faster than percutaneous cricothyrotomy. Surgical cricothyrotomy was also judged to be easier to perform. However, one must be cautious in interpreting the data, since the study did not consider the presence of bleeding, which may prolong the performance of surgical cricothyrotomy. Additionally, there is a marked difference between the tone of the cricoid musculature and surrounding structures in an alive subject and in a cadaver—cadaver models may favor surgical cricothyrotomy. Also, the procedures were performed under optimal lighting conditions, all equipment was ready for use, and there was no anatomic distortion of the neck structures.

Spaite and Joseph[70] reported 20 cases of emergency prehospital surgical cricothyrotomies performed by EMS personnel. They had an 88% success rate, comparable to the success rate for cricothyrotomy performed

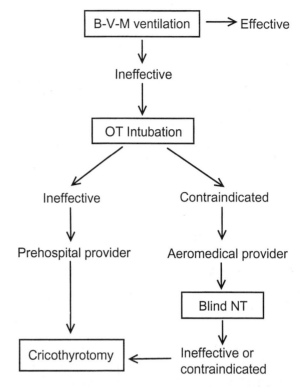

Fig. 25-11. Emergency airway protocol for prehospital care. *B-V-M,* bag-valve-mask; *OT,* orotracheal; *NT,* nasotracheal.

by physicians (92%). All patients had major injuries, and the majority had massive facial trauma or failed oral intubation with no other alternative means of airway control. They had a low incidence of serious complications (12%), primarily related to inability to secure the airway.

A committee of emergency medicine, anesthesiology, and neurologic surgery physicians at our institution developed a protocol for prehospital emergency airway control in trauma patients (Fig. 25-11). Many patients can be assisted or ventilated with a bag-valve-mask (B-V-M). The major indications for intubation include the inability to ventilate the apneic patient who has absent airway reflexes, major facial trauma precluding airway control, and severe head injury requiring hyperventilation. Orotracheal (OT) intubation is the preferred route for definitive airway control. When contraindicated, cricothyrotomy or blind nasotracheal (NT) intubation should be considered. Blind NT intubation should be performed only if the patient is breathing spontaneously. It should not be performed at all in patients with significant facial trauma above or including the maxilla, in those with nasal trauma, or in those with suspected basilar skull fractures. Placement of an intravenous (IV) catheter in the cricothyroid space is a stopgap measure. Appropriately trained rescuers should always have proper equipment available.

X. TRAINING MODELS

Because percutaneous dilational cricothyrotomy is so rarely performed, there is a need for quality teaching and training aids. While the technique closely mimics over-the-wire vascular insertion methods, it is sufficiently different that, ideally, anesthesiologists should practice on a regular basis.

Of the available animal models, dogs appear to be most similar to humans. Ruhe et al.[85] found the canine cricothyroid membrane, muscles, and cricothyroid area in toto to be similar to humans. The tracheal dimensions of the 25 kg dog are comparable to the adult human.[86]

We have performed cricothyrotomy on other animals, including pigs, sheep, and goats. Sheep and goats are acceptable; but, even in adult animals, the larynx is significantly smaller, and 3.5- or 4.0-mm ID sets must be used for teaching. Our experience with pigs has been poor. When we attempted to pass a needle or over-the-needle catheter into the cricothyroid space, we invariably hit cartilage. The space could only be entered by directing the needle cephalad, not caudad. Dissection of the larynx revealed a projection on the inferior surface of the thyroid cartilage articulating with the cricoid cartilage. This cornu had been previously described and had to be removed in order to perform cricothyrotomy studies.[64]

Our experience with cadavers has been excellent. We use both fresh and embalmed specimens. The former are superior, but much harder to find. The laryngeal structures of embalmed specimens are somewhat constricted due to muscle contraction, and it is more difficult to discern the cricothyroid space. Despite this, we have found them to be an excellent training aid.

Manikins are a less acceptable model. The Laerdal Intubation Head (Laerdal Medical Corp., Armonk, N.Y.) has palpable cricoid and thyroid cartilages and a separate larynx and tracheal model. These are good for teaching anatomy but cannot be used for practicing cricothyrotomy.

Nasco (Fort Atkinson, Wisc.) manufactures a simulator that can be used for teaching cricothyrotomy. It has a replaceable latex larynx with the cricoid and thyroid cartilages molded in. The system works well for needle cricothyrotomy, but it is difficult to insert large dilators and airway catheters; the latex tends to split and needs replacement frequently when used for percutaneous dilational cricothyrotomy. It is, however, one of the best models available.

Medical Plastics Laboratory (MPL, Gatesville, Tex.) has an intubation manikin with a large hole at the level of the cricothyroid space. It is covered with a replaceable soft latex covering. While this device is not very good for discerning anatomy, it allows easy passage of even large cricothyrotomy devices. The MPL cricothyrotomy model has rigid cricoid and thyroid cartilages and a narrow cricothyroid space. It works well for teaching anatomy but is not lifelike for cricothyrotomy, and the rigid plastic limits insertion to needles and small airway catheters.

XI. UNANSWERED QUESTIONS AND CONTROVERSY

Considerable controversy exists regarding the role of cricothyrotomy in the emergency setting. This is largely due to the lack of controlled clinical trials to evaluate differences in efficacy and morbidity among various emergency airway techniques.

Clearly, the situations in which an anesthesiologist would consider utilizing cricothyrotomy techniques are quite different than those encountered by an emergency medicine physician, trauma surgeon, or a prehospital or aeromedical provider. We believe percutaneous dilational cricothyrotomy to be the procedure of choice for anesthesiologists. It is performed in a manner very similar to the Seldinger technique for vascular access. We believe it to be safer than both transtracheal catheter ventilation and surgical cricothyrotomy. If an anesthesiologist can pass a catheter into the airway, it is relatively simple to pass a guidewire, dilator, and airway catheter. We feel it is also safer to establish an airway with a device that can be secured in place and used with conventional ventilation devices.

The cadaver studies recently performed in our laboratory suggest a relatively high failure rate due to kinking during insertion when conventional over-the-needle catheters are used. We have experienced and received reports of massive subcutaneous emphysema after attempted transtracheal ventilation with over-the-needle catheters.

A key issue is the determination of what size airway catheter to use. In situations in which the patient can awaken quickly or in whom a definitive airway is likely before the patient attempts to breathe spontaneously, a small, 3.0-mm ID, kink-resistant airway catheter is a reasonable choice. With an airway catheter of this size, ventilation can be performed with conventional equipment, and passive exhalations are likely to be complete if adequate time is permitted.

In emergency settings in which endotracheal intubation is impossible or contraindicated, particularly maxillofacial trauma, we suggest using a larger airway catheter, which will allow unimpeded air exchange and spontaneous ventilation without increased imposed work of breathing. We and others have shown that a 6.0-mm ID, 7.0-cm long cricothyrotomy tube imposes the same work as a 7.0-mm ID endotracheal tube.[56,87,88] We make a clear distinction between the truly emergent airway requiring cricothyrotomy and the difficult airway that can be treated with a number of airway adjuncts, each attempted in a controlled, orderly manner.

There are clearly other methods for emergency airway control. It is probably more important for an anesthesiologist to become familiar and facile with one, and to

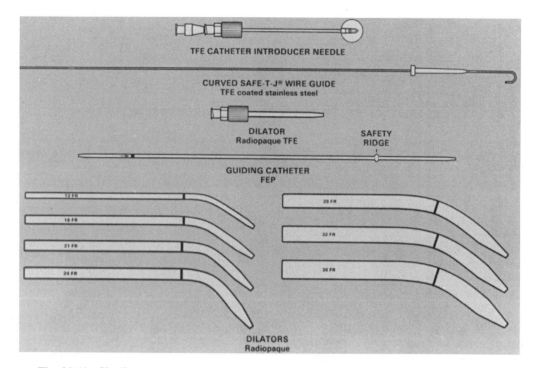

Fig. 25-12. Ciaglia percutaneous tracheostomy introducer set (Cook Critical Care, Bloomington, Ind.)

practice it periodically, than to know a myriad of techniques.

XII. PERCUTANEOUS DILATIONAL TRACHEOSTOMY

Toye and Weinstein[21] are credited with conceiving of percutaneous dilational tracheostomy. They published their initial results and a description of the Pertrach device in 1969. Their subsequent paper, published in 1988,[45] reported 94 cases of tracheostomy and 6 cases of cricothyrotomy. Only six cases were emergent, the remainder elective. Despite their results, interest in percutaneous dilational tracheostomy was sporadic, at best, until Ciaglia et al. refined the technique and published their initial findings.[53] Today, percutaneous dilational tracheostomy is an accepted alternative to formal surgical tracheostomy and is gaining in popularity, particularly for patients in the ICU who have been intubated for extended periods of time.

Percutaneous dilational tracheostomy is an elective procedure. It is included in this chapter because many anesthesiologists provide airway consultation in the ICU. Ivatury et al.[89] reported on the use of an emergency tracheostomy device (RapiTrac, Premier Medical Products, Norristown, Pa.) in 61 patients. While the device uses the Seldinger technique and a dilator, we feel cricothyrotomy to be the preferred route for emergent airway access.

The Ciaglia Percutaneous Tracheostomy Introducer (Cook Critical Care, Bloomington, Ind.) set (Fig. 25-12) is typical of devices used for this procedure. Unlike the Pertrach, which may be used for cricothyrotomy or tracheostomy, the Ciaglia and other sets are intended for subcricoid tracheostomy only. The technique is intended for use in controlled settings with the assistance of a respiratory therapist and nursing personnel.

This device is contraindicated for emergency placement, in patients with enlarged thyroids or nonpalpable cricoid cartilage, and in pediatric patients.

Detailed insertion instructions for the Ciaglia percutaneous dilational tracheostomy are as follows (Fig. 25-13):

A. PATIENT PREPARATION

1. Place the patient in the tracheostomy position. Position a pillow under the shoulders to permit full extension of head and neck. Elevate the head of the patient's bed 30 to 40 degrees.
2. Use ventilator changes and sedation to control patient respiration. Positive end-expiratory pressure (PEEP) level of 5 to 10 cm H_2O is recommended.
3. Instruct the respiratory therapist to loosen the fixation tapes of the in-place endotracheal tube and deflate the cuff, making necessary changes in tidal volume, frequency, etc., to evaluate compensation needed for air lead. Continuous oximetry monitoring should be employed.
4. Prepare and drape the anterior neck area.

B. THE PROCEDURE

1. Palpate landmark structures (thyroid notch, cricoid cartilage) to ascertain proper location for intended

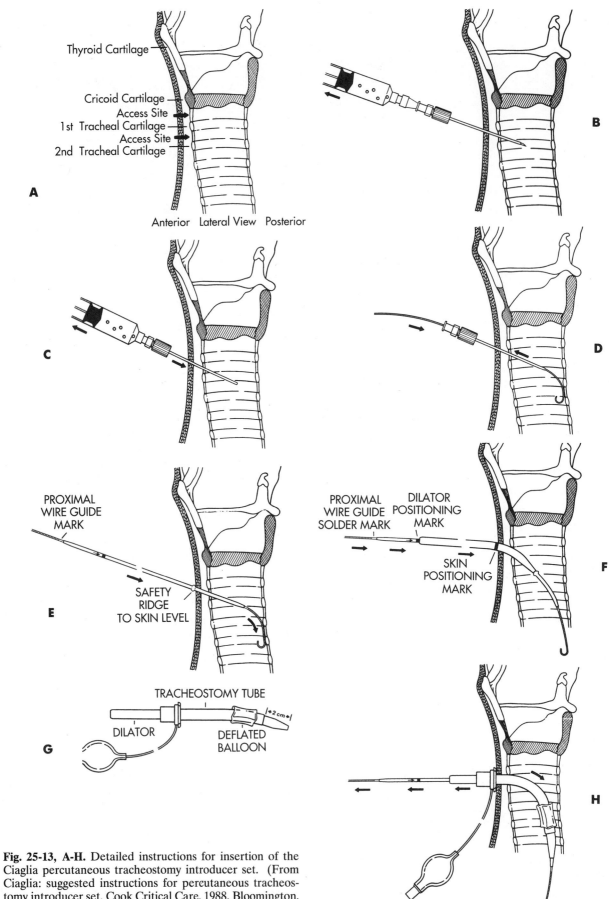

Fig. 25-13, A-H. Detailed instructions for insertion of the Ciaglia percutaneous tracheostomy introducer set. (From Ciaglia: suggested instructions for percutaneous tracheostomy introducer set, Cook Critical Care, 1988, Bloomington, Ind.)

tracheostomy tube placement. Access and ultimate tube placement is made at the level between the cricoid and the first tracheal cartilage or between the first and second tracheal cartilages whenever feasible (Fig. 25-13, *A*).

2. After introduction of local anesthesia (1% lidocaine with epinephrine), make a vertical incision from the lower edge of the cricoid cartilage downward, in the midline, for a distance of 1 to 1.5 cm.

3. If desired, use a curved mosquito clamp to gently dissect vertically and transversely down to the anterior tracheal wall. With the tip of the finger, dissect the front of the trachea, in the midline, free of any tissues, and identify the cricoid cartilage. Displace the isthmus of the thyroid downward, if present.

4. Inject additional local anesthesia to the area, and seek the tracheal air column by directing the needle, in the midline, posterior and caudad. Again, this should be done after the respiratory therapist has deflated the endotracheal tube cuff and withdrawn the endotracheal tube 1 cm. When advancing the needle forward, verification of entrance into the tracheal lumen can be confirmed by aspiration on the syringe resulting in air bubble return.

5. With the needle tip positioned in the trachea, inject 1.0 ml of lidocaine into the trachea, and remove the needle.

6. Attach a syringe half filled with lidocaine to the 17-gauge sheathed introducer needle hub, and, using the technique described in Step #4, seek the tracheal air column (Fig. 25-13, *B*). It is important not to impale the endotracheal tube with the needle. This can be checked by having the respiratory therapist gently move the endotracheal tube in and out 1 cm. If impaled, the needle is seen and felt to move also. It will be necessary to withdraw the needle and have the respiratory therapist pull back the endotracheal tube 1 cm, and then reinsert the needle.

7. When free flow of air is obtained with no impalement of the endotracheal tube, remove the inner needle of the introducer needle assembly and advance the outer Teflon sheath several millimeters. Attach a syringe and confirm position within the tracheal lumen by visualizing free flow of air into the syringe when aspirated (Fig. 25-13, *C*).

8. Remove the syringe, and introduce the 0.052 inch (1.32 mm) diameter "J" guidewire several cm into the trachea. Remove the Teflon sheath while maintaining the guidewire position within the tracheal lumen (Fig. 25-13, *D*).

9. Maintaining the guidewire position at the skin level mark on the guidewire, advance the short, 11-French introducing dilator over the guidewire to dilate the initial access site into the trachea using a slight twisting motion. Remove the dilator while maintaining the guidewire in position with the skin level mark on the guidewire at its proper level.

10. Following the direction of the arrow on the guiding catheter, advance the 8.0-French Teflon guiding catheter over the guidewire to the skin level mark on the guidewire. Insert the guiding catheter and guidewire as a unit into the trachea until the safety ridge on the guiding catheter is at the skin level. The end of the guiding catheter with the safety ridge should be introduced towards the patient. Align the proximal end of the Teflon guiding catheter at the mark on the proximal portion of the guidewire. This will assure that the distal end of the guiding catheter is properly positioned back on the guidewire, preventing possible trauma to the posterior tracheal wall during subsequent manipulations. Position the guiding catheter and guidewire as a unit so that the safety ridge on the guiding catheter is at the skin level (Fig. 25-13, *E*).

11. Begin to serially dilate the access site into the trachea. This is accomplished by first advancing the 12-French blue dilator over the guidewire-guiding catheter assembly. To properly align the dilator on the guidewire-guiding catheter assembly, position the proximal end of the dilator at the single positioning mark on the guiding catheter. This will insure that the distal tip of the dilator is properly positioned at the safety ridge on the guiding catheter to prevent possible trauma to the posterior tracheal wall during introduction. While maintaining the visual reference points and positioning relationships of the guidewire, guiding catheter, and dilator, advance them as a unit, with a twisting motion, to the skin level mark on the blue dilator. Advance and pull back the dilating assembly several times, while twisting, to perform effective dilatation of the tracheal entrance site. Remove the blue dilator, leaving the guidewire-guiding catheter assembly in position (Fig. 25-13, *F*).

12. Continue the dilatation procedure by advancing, in sizing sequence (small to large), the supplied dilators. Positioning of the dilators on the guidewire-guiding catheter assembly and dilatation of the tracheal entrance site should be done as described in Step #11.

13. Slightly overdilate the tracheal entrance site to a size appropriate for passage of the tracheostomy tube of choice to allow easy passage of the balloon portion of the tracheostomy tube into the trachea.

Tracheostomy tube Inner diameter	Appropriate dilator for initial overdilation
6 mm	24-French
7 mm	28-French
8 mm	32-French
9 mm	36-French

14. Preload the flexible tracheostomy tube to be inserted on the appropriate size blue dilator by first generously lubricating the surface of the dilator. Position the tracheostomy tube onto the dilator so that its tip is approximately 2 cm back from the distal tip of the dilator. Make sure the balloon is totally deflated. Thoroughly lubricate tracheostomy tube assembly prior to insertion (Fig. 25-13, *G*). The sizing chart below should be used as a guide to insure correct fit.

Tracheostomy tube Inner diameter	Appropriate dilator for initial overdilation
6 mm	18-French
7 mm	21-French
8 mm	24-French
9 mm	28-French

NOTE: Dual cannula tracheostomy tubes may also be placed using this technique. The inner cannula must be removed for introduction. Always check fit of dilator to tracheostomy tube prior to insertion. Follow tracheostomy tube manufacturer's instructions for testing of balloon cuff, and inflation system prior to insertion.

15. Advance the preloaded, lubricated tracheostomy tube over the guiding catheter assembly to the safety ridge, and then advance as a unit into the trachea. As soon as the deflated balloon enters the trachea, withdraw the blue dilator, guiding catheter, and guidewire (Fig. 25-13, *H*).

16. Advance the tracheostomy tube to its flange. NOTE: If using a dual cannula tracheostomy tube, insert the inner cannula at this point.

17. Connect the tracheostomy tube to the ventilator, inflate the balloon cuff, and remove the endotracheal tube. NOTE: Prior to complete removal of the endotracheal tube, test ventilation through tracheostomy tube.

18. Perform suction to determine if any significant bleeding or possible obstruction exists that has not been noted to this point.

19. If necessary, one suture may be taken at the bottom of the initial incision.

C. POSTPLACEMENT INSTRUCTIONS

Apply antibiotic ointment and dressing to the stoma site tid for 3 days. Elevate the head of the patient's bed 30 to 40 degrees for 1 hour.

D. PRECAUTIONS

1. Always confirm access into trachea by air bubble aspiration.
2. Maintain safety positioning marks of guidewire, guiding catheters, and dilators during dilating procedure to prevent trauma to posterior wall of the trachea.

3. Tracheostomy tubes should fit snugly to dilator for insertion. Generous lubrication to the surface of the dilator will enhance fit and placement of the tracheostomy tube.

To date, most studies report excellent success and low complication rates with percutaneous dilational tracheostomy. A follow-up study by Ciaglia and Graniero[90] and a study on 55 patients by Hazard et al.[55] demonstrate the utility of this procedure. A subsequent study by Hazard et al.[54] compared percutaneous tracheostomy with conventional tracheostomy in 46 patients. Complication rates were higher for conventional tracheostomy than for the percutaneous method (58% vs. 25%); predecannulation problems were higher for conventional tracheostomy (46% vs. 13%), as were late sequelae (88% vs. 27%) in survivors.

Only Wang et al.[58] report a high incidence of complications with percutaneous tracheostomy. However, they used a different device, which is no longer on the market, and a review of their patient selection demonstrates that they used patients who would probably not meet inclusion criteria in most protocols.

XIII. CONCLUSION

In the 1970s, after a 50-year hiatus, cricothyrotomy became recognized as an important procedure for emergency airway management. Despite considerable evidence that cricothyrotomy can be lifesaving and has an acceptable low complication rate, controlled trials comparing various techniques have not been, and are unlikely to be, performed. This is largely the result of the infrequency with which physicians and other health-care providers encounter patients requiring emergency cricothyrotomy.

The lack of opportunity to perform cricothyrotomy or other emergency airway procedures is a particular problem for anesthesiologists, who are the recognized airway experts. While the opportunity to perform a cricothyrotomy is rare, it must be performed expeditiously and correctly when required. We believe that percutaneous dilational cricothyrotomy should be easy for anesthesiologists to learn, since it is so similar to the Seldinger technique for insertion of catheters and sheaths, a technique used on a daily basis. The practitioner should be well trained in emergency airway techniques and have appropriate equipment available at all times.

While anesthesiologists practice primarily in the OR, there is significant likelihood that they will be called upon to perform emergency airway procedures in other settings. Additionally, they are often asked by colleagues to lecture on the subjects of the difficult airway and the emergency airway. The purpose of this chapter is to familiarize anesthesiologists with the cricothyrotomy options available.

REFERENCES

1. Caplan RA et al: Adverse respiratory events in anesthesia: a closed claims analysis, *Anesthesiology* 72:828, 1990.
2. Cormack RS, Lehane J: Difficult tracheal intubation in obstetrics, *Anaesthesia* 39:1105, 1984.
3. Glassenburg R, Vaisrub N, Albright G: The incidence of failed intubation in obstetrics: is there an irreducible minimum abstracted? *Anesthesiology* 73:A1061, 1990.
4. Lyons G: Failed intubation, *Anaesthesia* 40:759, 1985.
5. Samsoon GLT, Young JRB: Difficult tracheal intubation: a retrospective study, *Anaesthesia* 42:487, 1987.
6. Bellhouse CP, Dore C: Criteria for estimating likelihood of difficulty of endotracheal intubation with Macintosh laryngoscope, *Anaesth Intensive Care* 16:329, 1988.
7. Tunstall ME: Failed intubation in the parturient, *Can J Anaesth* 36:611, 1989 [editorial].
8. Holland R: Anesthesia related mortality in Australia, *Int Anesthesiol Clin* 22:61, 1984.
9. Keenan RL, Boyan CP: Cardiac arrest due to anesthesia, *JAMA* 253:2373, 1985.
10. Tiret L et al: Complications associated with anesthesia: a prospective survey in France, *Can Anaesth Soc J* 33:336, 1986.
11. Task Force on Guidelines for Management of the Difficult Airway: Practice guidelines for management of the difficult airway, *Anesthesiology* 78:597, 1993.
12. Jackson C: High tracheostomy and other errors: the chief causes of chronic laryngeal stenosis, *Surg Gynecol Obstet* 32:392, 1921.
13. Brantigan CO, Grow JB: Cricothyroidotomy: elective use in respiratory problems requiring tracheostomy, *J Thorac Cardiovasc Surg* 71:72, 1976.
14. Brantigan CO, Grow JB: Cricothyroidotomy revisited again, *Ear Nose Throat J* 59:289, 1980.
15. Caparosa RJ, Zavatsky AR: Practical aspects of the cricothyroid space, *Laryngoscope* 67:577, 1957.
16. Mulder DS, Marelli D: The 1991 Fraser Gurd lecture: evolution of airway control in the management of injured patients, *J Trauma* 33:856, 1992.
17. Morch ET: History of mechanical ventilation. In Kirby RR, Banner MJ, Downs JB, editors: *Clinical applications of ventilatory support,* New York, 1990, Churchill Livingstone.
18. Shapiro SL: Emergency airway for acute laryngeal obstruction, *Eye, Ear, Nose and Throat Monthly* 49:35, 1970.
19. Jackson C: Tracheostomy, *Laryngoscope* 18:285, 1909.
20. Ward Booth RP, Brown J, Jones K: Cricothyroidotomy, a useful alternative to tracheostomy in maxillofacial surgery, *Int J Oral Maxillofac Surg* 18:24, 1989.
21. Toye FJ, Weinstein JD: A percutaneous tracheostomy device, *Surgery* 65:384, 1969.
22. Corke C, Cranswick P: A Seldinger technique for mini-tracheostomy insertion, *Anaesth Intensive Care* 16:206, 1988.
23. Kirchner JA: Cricothyroidotomy and subglottic stenosis, *Plast Reconstr Surg* 68:828, 1981.
24. Kuriloff DB et al: Laryngotracheal injury following cricothyroidotomy, *Laryngoscope* 99:125, 1989.
25. Little CM, Parker MG, Tarnopolsky R: The incidence of vasculature at risk during cricothyroidostomy, *Ann Emerg Med* 15:805, 1986.
26. Heffner JE, Sahn SA: The technique of tracheostomy and cricothyroidotomy, *J Crit Illness* 2:79, 1987.
27. Walls RM: Cricothyroidotomy, *Emerg Med Clin North Am* 6:725, 1988.
28. Mace SE: Cricothyrotomy, *J Emerg Med* 6:309, 1988.
29. Roven AN, Clapham MC: Cricothyroidotomy, *Ear Nose Throat J* 62:68, 1983.
30. Piotrowski JJ, Moore EE: Emergency department tracheostomy, *Emerg Med Clin North Am* 6:737, 1988.
31. Malhotra V: Pyloric stenosis. In Yao FSF, Artusio JF Jr, editors: *Anesthesiology: problem-oriented patient management,* Philadelphia, 1993, JB Lippincott.
32. McLaughlin J, Iserson KV: Emergency pediatric tracheostomy: a usable technique and model for instruction, *Ann Emerg Med* 15:463, 1986.
33. Sise MJ et al: Cricothyroidotomy for long-term tracheal access: a prospective analysis of morbidity and mortality in 76 patients, *Ann Surg* 200:13, 1984.
34. Florete OG Jr: Airway management. In Civetta JM, Taylor RW, Kirby RR, editors: *Critical Care,* Philadelphia, 1992, JB Lippincott.
35. Safar P, Penninckx JJ: Cricothyroid membrane puncture with special cannula, *Anesthesiology* 28:943, 1967.
36. Pridmore SA: A new cricothyrotomy cannula, *Med J Aust* 1:532, 1979.
37. Abbrecht PH et al: Insertion forces and risk of complications during cricothyroid cannulation, *J Emerg Med* 10:417, 1992.
38. Ravlo O et al: A comparison between two emergency cricothyroidotomy instruments, *Acta Anaesthesiol Scand* 31:317, 1987.
39. Boyd AD et al: A clinical evaluation of cricothyroidotomy, *Surg Gynecol Obstet* 149:365, 1979.
40. Essess BA, Jafek BW: Cricothyroidotomy: a decade of experience in Denver, *Ann Otol Rhinol Laryngol* 96:519, 1987.
41. O'Connor JV et al: Cricothyroidotomy for prolonged ventilatory support after cardiac operations, *Ann Thorac Surg* 39:353, 1988.
42. Benumof JL, Scheller MS: The importance of transtracheal jet ventilation in the management of the difficult airway, *Anesthesiology* 71:769, 1989.
43. Benumof JL: Management of the difficult airway: with special emphasis on the awake tracheal intubation, *Anesthesiology* 75:1087, 1991.
44. Griggs WM et al: A simple percutaneous tracheostomy technique, *Surg Gynecol Obstet* 170:543, 1990.
45. Toye FJ, Weinstein JD: Clinical experience with percutaneous tracheostomy and cricothyroidotomy in 100 patients, *J Trauma* 26:1034, 1988.
46. Jacoby JJ, Flory FA, Jones JR: Transtracheal resuscitation, *JAMA* 162:625, 1956.
47. Fusciardi J et al: Hemodynamic effects of high frequency jet ventilation in patients with and without circulatory shock, *Anesthesiology* 65:485, 1986.
48. Turnball AD et al: High frequency jet ventilation in major airway or pulmonary disruption, *Ann Thorac Surg* 32:468, 1981.
49. Sladen A et al: High frequency jet ventilation in the postoperative period: a review of 100 patients, *Crit Care Med* 12:782, 1984.
50. Spoerel WE, Narayanan PS, Singh NP: Transtracheal ventilation, *Br J Anaesth* 43:932, 1971.
51. Ravussin P, Freeman J: A new transtracheal catheter for ventilation and resuscitation, *Can Anaesth Soc J* 32:60, 1985.
52. Nakatsuka M, MacLeod AD: Hemodynamic and respiratory effects of transtracheal high frequency jet ventilation during difficult intubation, *J Clin Anesth* 4:321, 1992.
53. Ciaglia P, Firsching R, Syniec C: Elective percutaneous dilatational tracheostomy: a new simple bedside procedure—preliminary report, *Chest* 87:715, 1985.
54. Hazard P, Jones C, Benitone J: Comparative clinical trial of standard operative tracheostomy with percutaneous tracheostomy, *Crit Care Med* 19:1018, 1991.
55. Hazard PB et al: Bedside percutaneous tracheostomy: experience with 55 elective procedures, *Ann Thorac Surg* 46:63, 1988.
56. Melker RJ, Banner MJ: Work imposed by breathing through cricothyrotomy tube. Paper presented at the Sixth World Congress on Emergency and Disaster Medicine, Hong Kong, Sept. 6-18, 1989.
57. Johnson DR et al: Cricothyrotomy performed by prehospital personnel: a comparison of two techniques in a human cadaver model, *Am J Emerg Med* 11:3:207, 1993.

58. Wang MB et al: Early experience with percutaneous tracheostomy, *Laryngoscope* 102:157, 1992.

59. Bjoraker DJ, Kumar NB, Brown ACD: Evaluation of the Nu-Trake emergency cricothyrotomy device, *Anesthesiology* 59:A517, 1983.

60. Hulsey S: Cricotomes. In Dailey RH, Simon B, Young GP, editors: *The airway: emergency management,* St Louis, 1992, Mosby.

61. Wain JC, Wilson DJ, Mathisen DJ: Clinical experience with minitracheostomy, *Ann Thorac Surg* 49:881, 1990.

62. Kress TD, Balasbramanian S: Cricothyroidotomy, *Ann Emerg Med* 11:197, 1982.

63. Cole RR, Aguilar EA: Cricothyroidotomy versus tracheostomy: an otolaryngologist's perspective, *Laryngoscope* 98:131, 1988.

64. Holst M et al: The cricothyroid muscle after cricothyroidotomy, *Acta Otolaryngol (Stockh)* 107:136, 1989.

65. Habel DW: Cricothyroidotomy as a site for elective tracheostomy, *Trans Pac Coast Otoophthal Soc* 58:181, 1977.

66. Morain WD: Cricothyroidotomy in head and neck surgery, *Plast Reconstr Surg* 65:424, 1980.

67. Greisz H et al: Cricothyroidotomy: a clinical and histopathological study, *Crit Care Med* 10:387, 1982.

68. Holst M et al: Five years' experience with elective coniotomy, *Intensive Care Med* 11:202, 1985.

69. Van Hasselt EJ, Bruining HA, Hoeve LJ: Elective cricothyroidotomy, *Intensive Care Med* 11:207, 1985.

70. Spaite D, Joseph M: Prehospital cricothyrotomy: an investigation of indications, technique, complications and patient outcome, *Ann Emerg Med* 19:279, 1990.

71. Boyle MF, Hatton D, Sheets C: Surgical cricothyrotomy performed by air ambulance flight nurses: a 5-year experience, *J Emerg Med* 11:41, 1993.

72. Ryan DW: Minitracheostomy, *Intensive Care World* 8:128, 1991.

73. Pedersen J et al: Ossification of the cricothyroid membrane following minitracheostomy, *Intensive Care Med* 15:272, 1989.

74. Tran Y, Hedley R: Misplacement of a minitracheostomy tube, *Anaesthesia* 42:783, 1987.

75. Stokes DN: Re-insertion of a minitracheostomy tube, *Anaesthesia* 42:782, 1987.

76. Silk JM, Marsh AM: Pneumothorax caused by minitracheostomy, *Anaesthesia* 44:663, 1989.

77. Wagstaff A, Sparling R, Ryan DW: Minitracheostomy, *Anaesthesia* 42:216, 1987.

78. Au J et al: Percutaneous cricothyroidostomy (minitracheostomy) for bronchial toilet: results of therapeutic and prophylactic use, *Ann Thorac Surg* 48:850, 1989.

79. Jackson IJB et al: Minitracheostomy: Seldinger — assessment of a new technique, *Anaesthesia* 46:475, 1991.

80. Mitchell SA: Cricothyroidotomy revisited, *Ear Nose Throat J* 58:54, 1979.

81. McGill J, Clinton JE, Ruiz E: Cricothyrotomy in the emergency department, *Ann Emerg Med* 11:361, 1982.

82. Miklus RM, Elliott C, Snow N: Surgical cricothyrotomy in the field: experience of a helicopter transport team, *J Trauma* 29:506, 1989.

83. Nugent WL, Rhee KJ, Wisner DH: Can nurses perform surgical cricothyrotomy with acceptable success and complication rates? *Ann Emerg Med* 20:367, 1991.

84. Xeropotamos NS, Coats TJ, Wilson AW: Prehospital surgical airway management: one year's experience from the helicopter emergency medical service, *Injury* 24:222-224, 1993.

85. Ruhe DS, Williams GV, Proud GO: Emergency airway by cricothyroid puncture or tracheostomy, *Trans Am Acad Opthalmol Otolaryngol* 64:182-203, 1960.

86. Altman PL, Dittmer DS, editors: *Respiration and circulation,* Bethesda, Md, 1972, Federation of American Societies for Experimental Biology.

87. Banner MJ et al: Excessive work imposed during spontaneous breathing through transtracheal catheters, *Anesthesiology* 77: A1231, 1992 (Abstracted).

88. Ooi R et al: Extra inspiratory work of breathing imposed by cricothyrotomy devices, *Br J Anaesth* 70:17, 1993.

89. Ivatury R et al: Percutaneous tracheostomy after trauma and critical illness, *J Trauma* 32(2):133, 1992.

90. Ciaglia P, Graniero KD: Percutaneous dilatational tracheostomy — results and long-term follow-up, *Chest* 101:464, 1992.

Chapter 26

SURGICAL AIRWAY

Terence M. Davidson
Anthony E. Magit

I. ADULT SURGICAL AIRWAY

A. INTRODUCTION

Maintaining an airway is necessary for life and in cases where orotracheal or nasotracheal intubation cannot be accomplished, emergency tracheostomy and/or cricothyroidotomy are the only means of saving an individual's life. Whether the surgery is performed emergently or electively, it demands appropriate teamwork between the surgeon and the anesthesiologist.

1. Illustrative case history

The patient is a 65-year-old obese woman who had an emergency cholecystectomy at another hospital. The patient's medical history included insulin-dependent diabetes mellitus, hypertension, and atypical chest pain. Cardiac catheterization 6 months before this admission demonstrated normal coronary arteries, ventricular hypertrophy, and diastolic dysfunction. The patient also had obstructive sleep apnea. When the patient was being anesthetized for the cholecystectomy, she was unable to be ventilated and had a respiratory arrest. Multiple attempts at mask ventilation and intubation were unsuccessful, and the patient underwent an emergency cricothyroidotomy with placement of a No. 4 Shiley tracheostomy tube. The abdominal surgery was completed and the patient recovered without incident. Attempts at decannulation in the following weeks were unsuccessful. Bronchoscopy was performed, and large amounts of stomal granulations were revealed. These were treated with laser excision, but all attempts at decannulation were unsuccessful.

The patient was then referred to the University of California, San Diego (UCSD) Medical Center. Fiberoptic bronchoscopy demonstrated large tracheal granulations and supraglottic and subglottic edema. On further inspection it was apparent that the tracheostomy tube was through the cricothyroid membrane. The patient was given systemic steroids and brought to the operating room 2 days later. The patient was anesthetized through the cricothyroid cannula. After the patient was fully anesthetized and paralyzed, the attending head and neck surgeon was unable to perform rigid laryngoscopy. A rigid bronchoscope, however, was successfully

513

passed. The cricothyroid cannula was removed, and the cervical and thoracic trachea were found to be normal. The cricothyroidotomy was converted to a tracheostomy, and the granulation tissue around the cricothyroid stoma was vaporized with a laser. Systemic steroids were administered in the perioperative and postoperative periods. One week postoperatively, the tracheostomy was changed to a smaller tube. The patient was able to breathe around the tube and a week later was successfully decannulated. The subglottic granulations did not recur and the patient has been well ever since.

2. Discussion of illustrative case

From a head and neck surgeon's perspective, this difficult airway was appropriately managed. The emergency cricothyroidotomy was performed in a timely fashion. The patient's airway and her life were preserved. Cricothyroidotomy is a temporary lifesaving procedure. In some cases the patient can be extubated within 24 hours, but in most cases longer term intubation will be required, and in these cases conversion to a proper tracheostomy is recommended. It is unusual to leave a cricothyroidotomy tube in the trachea as long as occurred in this case. Tubes placed through the cricothyroid membrane risk destroying the cricoid cartilage. When this happens, the airway collapses, subglottic stenosis ensues, and the patient is permanently disabled.

Given today's knowledge of prolonged intubation, there are proponents of prolonged nasotracheal intubation and there are proponents of tracheostomy. These are arguable. Long-term cricothyroidotomy is not a reasonable option. Although the authors do not know the original anesthesiologists and surgeons who attended this patient, it appears that the surgeons left the airway to the anesthesiologists, and the anesthesiologists left the cricothyroidotomy to the surgeons. Pretty soon, all had forgotten that a cricothyroidotomy, not a tracheostomy, had been performed. Ultimately, the prolonged failure to extubate was recognized and corrected, fortunately without long-term mishap.

B. INDICATIONS

The indications for tracheostomy are listed in Box 26-1. Any lesion or abnormality causing upper-airway obstruction may require a tracheostomy. Should such an individual require surgery, tracheostomy may be the only reasonable means to manage the airway; in the case of a neoplasm it is anticipated that this will grow and airway obstruction will occur. Upper-airway trauma requiring mandibular and maxillary surgery or in some way obstructing of the upper airway may also require elective tracheostomy.

Neurologic illness interfering with an individual's respiratory drive such as poliomyelitis or cerebrovascular illness may require prolonged intubation, and for

---

> **BOX 26-1   Indications for tracheostomy**
>
> Elective
>   Upper-airway obstruction (impending)
>   Neurologic
>   Pulmonary
> Emergency
>   Upper-airway obstruction (acute)
>   Tumor
>   Trauma
>   Failed intubation

---

these individuals tracheostomy is the most appropriate means of airway management. The most common indications for elective tracheostomy are pulmonary and are typically prolonged intubation. Another important indication is obstructive sleep apnea and obesity hypoventilation syndromes. These individuals require tracheostomy to provide continuous positive airway pressure, particularly during sleep.

Emergency tracheostomies are required for hypopharyngeal or laryngeal tumors acutely obstructing the airway, for traumatic injury to the upper respiratory tract obstructing the airway, and for failed intubation. Patients with obstructive laryngeal tumors will often have stridor and mild to moderate dyspnea. They maintain their airway by a very active inspiratory effort. Any tranquilization or narcotization can depress the respiratory drive and inspiratory effort. This acutely changes a marginal airway into an obstructed airway. Trauma to the maxilla, mandible, or larynx can also require emergency tracheostomy. In these cases an endotracheal tube is not in place and the procedure is done in a rapid fashion to sustain the individual's life. Infection such as submental or peritonsillar abscess may require emergency tracheostomy. Patients with epiglottitis and other advanced infections can be difficult to intubate and can require emergency tracheostomy.

In many cases when elective tracheostomy is performed, the patient and the surgeon will prefer that the patient be anesthetized.[4] Assuming the patient is safely intubated, careful teamwork at the time of tracheotomy and tube exchange is mandatory.

C. TRACHEOSTOMY: GENERAL CONSIDERATIONS

A surgeon and anesthesiologist accustomed to tracheostomy will perform this procedure as comfortably and smoothly as an anesthesiologist performs IV access. Surgeons and anesthesiologists not used to working together make what should have been a simple procedure an awkward, stressful, bloody, and occasionally fatal event. The operation is demonstrated in Fig. 26-1. Procedures performed with the patient under monitored

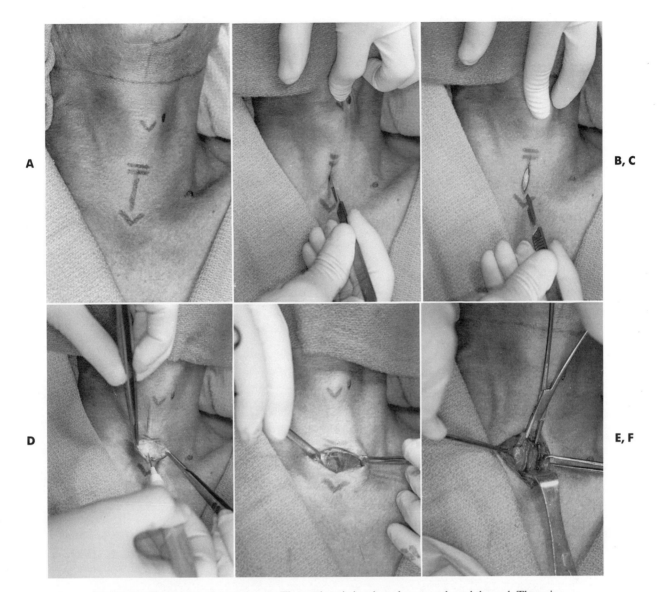

Fig. 26-1. Elective tracheostomy. **A,** The patient is intubated, prepped, and draped. There is no ether screen and the anesthesiologist is separated from the surgical field only by a towel lying over the patient's face; thus the anesthesiologist is an integral part of the surgery. The thyroid notch is marked with a V. The cricothyroid membrane is marked with the most superior horizontal line. The first tracheal ring and the sternal notch are then marked, and the incision is planned as a vertical incision from the first tracheal ring down toward the sternal notch. **B,** The vertical skin incision is made with a scalpel. **C,** The extent of the incision. **D,** The two sides of the incision are picked up by subcutaneous tissue retraction and dissection is carried posteriorly, with a cautery keeping the dissection in the midline. **E,** The anterior strap muscles have been separated. A large anterior cervical vein is evident. **F,** The second layer of strap muscles has now been divided and you are looking directly at the thyroid gland with a second and even larger anterior cervical vein overlying the thyroid isthmus. The strap muscles are pulled laterally. A hemostat has been placed deep to the thyroid isthmus separating it from the anterior tracheal wall.   *Continued.*

anesthesia care are often best performed with the patient's head and back elevated. Assuming the patient is breathing on his/her own, some tranquilization decreases the anxiety. Narcotics are not necessary for the surgery. They may supplement the patient's comfort but should never be allowed to depress the patient's airway.

The patient should be maximally oxygenated. The tracheostomy is performed. When the trachea is opened, an endotracheal tube or tracheostomy tube is inserted. The surgeon and anesthesiologist are responsible for ensuring that appropriate adapters are available, that the tracheostomy or other tube is stabilized and not

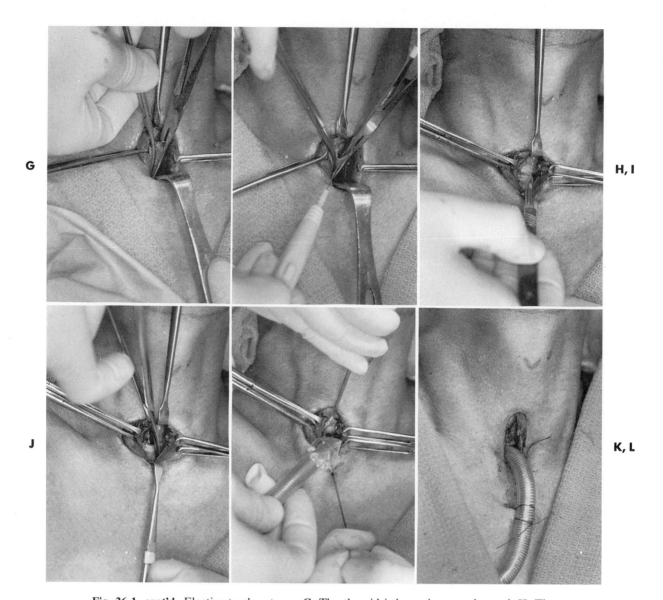

Fig. 26-1, cont'd. Elective tracheostomy. **G,** The thyroid isthmus is cross-clamped. **H,** The thyroid isthmus is transected and then suture ligated. Failure to divide the thyroid isthmus frequently results in placement of the tracheotomy too high or too low. Failure to suture ligate is the most common cause of serious postoperative hemorrhage. **I,** The fascia overlying the trachea has been swept aside. A U-shaped tracheal flap is cut. The superior horizontal limb is placed between the first and second or second and third tracheal rings. If the surgeon uses a knife, the endotracheal tube cuff must be deflated. If the surgeon uses a cautery, the patient's PO_2 must be reduced to a nonflammable level. Because of the risk of flash fire, we routinely use scalpel and scissors and do not use cautery. **J,** The vertical incisions of the inferior-based tracheal flap are cut with the scissors. **K,** The flap is sutured to the sternal skin, thereby holding the tracheotomy open. The endotracheal tube is then advanced under direct visualization, and when the tip of the tube has passed the upper margin of the tracheotomy, the endotracheal or tracheostomy tube is inserted. **L,** In this case further surgery is necessary and an armor endotracheal tube has been inserted, and held in place with a suture ligature to the anterior sternal skin.

coughed out of the airway, and that if the patient has developed hypercarbia, rapid reversal does not result in such a rapid pH change that cardiac dysrhythmia occurs. In some cases the operation is complete when the tracheostomy is finished; for others this marks the beginning of some other surgery.

In other cases the tracheostomy is performed over an endotracheal tube (ET). The operative field should be draped as shown so that the anesthesiologist can see what is happening and be an active participant in the surgery. Putting up an ether screen or other barrier obstructs the necessary teamwork.

Tracheostomies are performed equally well through horizontal and midline vertical incisions. Hemostasis is achieved throughout the surgery with cautery, ligature, or laser. Most surgeons believe that the isthmus of the thyroid should be transsected, and most surgeons perform the tracheotomy below the second tracheal ring. In all cases the first tracheal ring is left intact to protect the cricoid cartilage. Some surgeons create a small flap of tracheal ring and mucosa, whereas others resect the anterior tracheal wall, both making a small hole in the anterior tracheal wall; both are acceptable.

The authors' preference is to create an inferiorly based tracheal flap and to suture that tracheal flap to the patient's neck skin. The reason for sutures and suturing flaps to skin is primarily to provide easy access to the trachea should inadvertent decannulation occur. An additional advantage of the inferiorly based tracheal flap is that it protects the high-riding, innominate artery, minimizing the risk of innominate artery erosion and rupture.

When the trachea is opened, the ET is removed, and the tracheostomy tube is inserted, several things need to occur. First, the patient should be maximally oxygenated. If the surgeon uses a cautery to cut the tracheal mucosa, there is a risk of oxygen ignition (see Chapter 33). When the surgeon cuts into the trachea, the ET balloon should be temporarily deflated to prevent the surgeon from rupturing the balloon. Once the tracheal incisions are completed and the balloon can be visualized, it can be reinflated. The surgeon can complete the tracheal flap and suturing, or whatever else is required before the tube exchange takes place. Whenever possible, the patient should be breathing on his/her own because the patient may be able to spontaneously ventilate through the incision even if the tracheostomy tube is passed into the mediastinum (i.e., *pull* air into the lungs). When the surgeon, the patient, and the anesthesiologist are all ready, the anesthesiologist pulls back on the ET while he/she and the surgeon observe the ET through the tracheotomy. The ET is slowly pulled back so that the tip is just past the cephalad margin of the tracheal incision and is in the subglottic area proximal to the tracheostomy. The surgeon then inserts the tracheostomy tube. The endotracheal tube is kept within the larynx until all of the airway connections are made, the patient is ventilating well, and the tracheostomy tube is secured. Should anything happen to the tracheostomy tube (i.e., it gets coughed out), the ET could simply be pushed back in.

An occasional patient requiring tracheostomy has nonreversible coagulopathy. In these cases the surgery can be performed with a hand-held CO_2 laser. The thyroid isthmus still requires suture ligature. When lasers are used, the tracheal Po_2 must be 40% or lower to prevent combustion.

D. EMERGENCY TRACHEOSTOMY

Emergency tracheostomy is sometimes performed semi-emergently and sometimes performed in a full-blown emergency setting. With true full emergencies, the surgery is performed with the patient under local anesthesia or none at all. In the semiemergent situation, the neck is preinjected with lidocaine and adrenalin; when possible, this is given 10 minutes before surgery to reach its full effect. Generally, the surgeons will require that the patient's head be extended, thereby exposing the anterior neck. This can cause a worsening or complete obstruction of the airway and change a hurry-up tracheostomy into a true emergency tracheostomy.

Three different potential situations exist. The individual with an impaired but stable airway who can extend the neck without obstructing the airway can have a tracheostomy performed using local anesthesia. As in elective tracheostomy, this is performed carefully and takes 15 to 20 minutes. In other individuals the airway is diminishing with time, and a hurry-up tracheostomy is required. In these cases the cautery is often used as the exclusive surgical tool. A linear anterior cervical incision is made from the cricoid cartilage to the sternal notch, and with the Bovie on a very high setting, the tissue is cauterized directly down to the trachea. The trachea is then incised and an ET is placed. This operation requires approximately 5 minutes to perform. The ET is absolutely mandatory (see below for rationale) because once the airway and the patient are stabilized, the surgeon will reexamine the entire wound and ensure that all vessels are appropriately cauterized and that sutures are appropriately placed.

In a truly emergent tracheostomy, where the patient's airway is completely obstructed, the tracheostomy is performed in 15 to 30 seconds. Properly performed, a single incision is made through the skin. This is always a vertical incision and should extend from the cricoid cartilage to the sternal notch. The physician palpates the trachea and with the second cut of the knife incises into the trachea. Because large anterior cervical veins and arteries and the thyroid isthmus may have been cut, bleeding may be profuse. The surgeon palpates the cut trachea and, using his finger, guides the endotracheal tube into the trachea. The balloon is inflated and the neck incision is packed with gauze to tamponade bleeding.

Once the patient's airway and physiologic structures are stabilized, the surgeon can reinspect the wound, obtain appropriate hemostasis, and do whatever housekeeping is deemed necessary. For the last two situations, an ET has been used rather than a tracheostomy tube. Tracheostomy tubes typically have anterior neck flanges that prohibit the surgeon's inspection of the wound. Endotracheal tubes are therefore required. Whenever possible, an anode tube is preferred because this can be bent laterally and anteriorly without kinking and impairing airflow. Once the surgical wound has been attended to, the endotracheal tube is changed to a tracheostomy tube. A cuffed tube is always required because often the cut mucosal edges or other portions of the tracheostomy can bleed and the cuff prevents aspiration of blood. Although the standard tracheostomy tube is of an appropriate length for the average person, one needs to confirm that both lung fields are being ventilated. Occasionally, the individual's trachea is short, the tracheotomy is performed too low, or the tracheostomy tube is simply too long for the patient's anatomy. In such cases bronchial intubation has occurred and should be recognized. Tracheostomy tubes of adjustable length are available or the tracheostomy can be elevated slightly off the skin. The most important thing is to recognize the problem. The tracheostomy tube must be firmly secured because if the tube is coughed out or otherwise inadvertently removed from the trachea, recannulation by an inexperienced, or even experienced, individual can be difficult. Although there are many techniques for reinserting tracheostomy tubes, each physician should have his/her own paradigm.

First, everything possible should be done not to permit inadvertent decannulation. We always use tracheal strings, and in adults we always use an inferiorly based tracheal flap, thereby providing an obvious entrance to the trachea. It can be disastrous to blindly place a tracheostomy tube and hope that it will find its way into the airway rather than into the loose pretracheal space. The technique we prefer is to palpate the tracheal opening with the index finger of the nondominant hand. The position and attitude of the trachea and the tracheotomy are then memorized and the tracheostomy tube is then placed into the neck and by three-dimensional positional memory is advanced into the trachea. One cannot insert a tracheostomy tube directly. One must insert it from the side. Once the tracheostomy tube tip is in the trachea, the tracheostomy tube is rotated 90 degrees and advanced. Although this description may not make it obvious, a simple examination of a neck and a tracheostomy tube will clarify this small but very important point. This concept and procedure is illustrated in Fig. 26-2.

If a tracheostomy tube does not go in easily, sometimes it is easier to place an ET. If this is not easily placed, occasionally one can insert a tube changer such as an Eschmann stylet and use this to guide an ET or tracheostomy tube into the trachea.

Fig. 26-3 shows the variety of available tracheostomy tubes, and Fig. 26-4 shows the components of a fenestrated tracheostomy tube. Table 26-1 lists the sizes and dimensions of standard tracheostomy tubes.

E. EMERGENCY CRICOTHYROIDOTOMY

If a patient cannot be intubated and no intrinsic laryngeal obstruction is seen, entrance into the subglottic

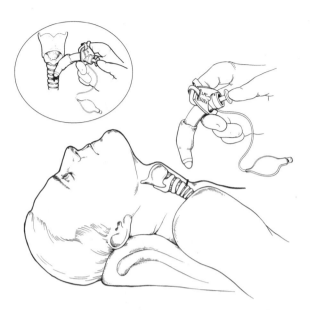

Fig. 26-2. Shiley technique for inserting the tracheostomy tube. The tracheostomy tube is inserted by holding the tracheal end of the tracheostomy tube with the trocar in place and the tip perpendicular to the anterior cervical skin. The tracheostomy tube is rotated 90 degrees in the horizontal plane. Stated differently, the tube can only be inserted through the skin and into the tracheal lumen if it is brought in from the patient's side. As soon as the tracheostomy tube is inside the tracheal lumen, it is then rotated 90 degrees and advanced to the appropriate position. (Courtesy of Shiley.)

airway through the cricothyroidotomy membrane is technically easier to accomplish and is the technique of choice for those not skilled in neck surgery. Although significant vascular structures overlie the cervical trachea and the cervical trachea is covered by the strap muscles and lies deep in the neck, the cricothyroid membrane is relatively superficial, and no important structures lie between the cricothyroid membrane and the skin. Cricothyroidotomy is performed by simply making a horizontal incision through the skin into the cricothyroid membrane. The airway is thereby entered (see Fig. 26-5 on p. 521). This opening can be widened with numerous techniques. An endotracheal tube can be inserted, resulting in an emergency airway being established. Tracheostomy tubes cannot be inserted through a cricothyroidotomy because their angles are incorrect. Cricothyroidotomy can be used for the duration of a short surgery but, as illustrated in the introductory case example, is not a means of long-term airway support.

Emergency cricothyroidotomy is a technique that most physicians can learn and successfully perform on most patients in most emergency circumstances. The two real hurdles to performing this successfully are (1) correctly identifying the cricothyroid membrane and (2) being properly prepared psychologically to perform the cricothyroidotomy. The decision process outlined in the Anesthesia Safety Foundation (ASA) difficult airway

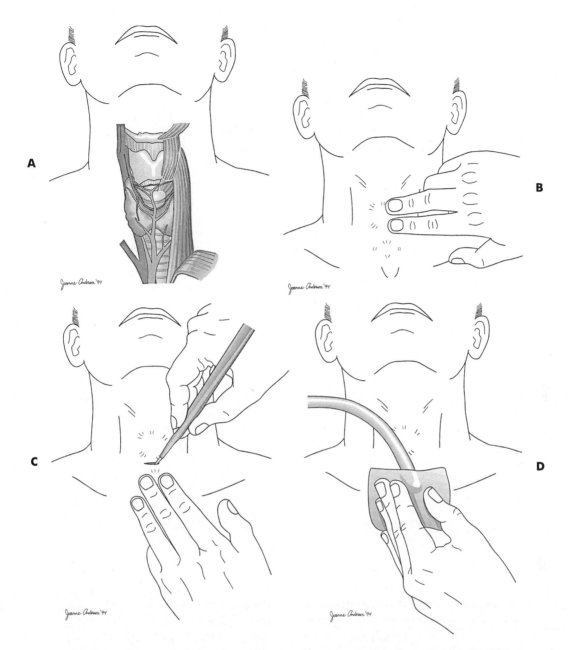

Fig. 26-3. Cricothyroidotomy. **A,** Anatomy of the cricothyroid membrane and cervical trachea. The relevant anatomy is the laryngeal cartilages including the hyoid, thyroid, and cricoid and tracheal cartilages. The muscles are the strap muscles. The overlying vasculature is rich over the cervical trachea and strikingly absent over the cricothyroid membrane. The thyroid gland with its tremendous blood supply also overlies the cervical trachea. **B,** To perform an emergency cricothyroidotomy, one palpates the thyroid cartilage, the cricoid cartilage, and then identifies the cricothyroid membrane. **C,** A scalpel or other sharp instrument is then inserted through the skin and through the cricothyroid membrane and with a single cut a 1 to 1.5 cm horizontal incision is made. **D,** The space is opened and an appropriate diameter tube inserted, thereby establishing an airway.

algorithm defines when emergency cricothyroidotomy is necessary (see Chapter 8).

Although it is certainly worthwhile to practice cricothyroidotomy in the cadaver laboratory, the availability of such resources is limited and sometimes prohibitively expensive. Nonetheless, we believe that most physicians can learn to perform a cricothyroidotomy. Reading the following section of this chapter is step 1. Step 2 is to watch a videotape presentation of an emergency cricothyroidotomy. An excellent demonstration is shown in the Anesthesia Safety Patient Foundation Videotape Series.[1]

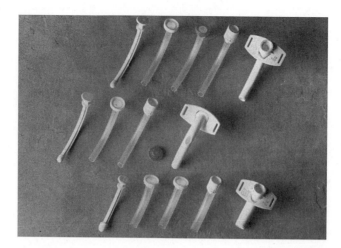

Fig. 26-4. Tracheostomy tubes. Tracheostomy tubes come in several configurations. The three tracheostomy tubes shown here are all cuffless. The same models come with low-pressure cuffs. The top series are the standard tracheostomy tubes with a normal inner cannula with 15-mm adapter, a capped inner cannula, a low-profile inner cannula, and an insertion obturator. The second row shows a fenestrated tracheostomy tube with available inner cannulas and the last row shows the shortened tracheostomy tube used in tracheotomies after laryngectomy; these are also available with an obturator. (Courtesy of Shiley.)

Table 26-1. Sizes and dimensions of standard tracheostomy tubes

Size	OD (mm)	ID (mm)	Length (mm)
4	8.5 (26 Fr.)	5.0	67
6	10.0 (30 Fr.)	7.0	78
8	12.0 (36 Fr.)	8.5	84
10	13.0 (39 Fr.)	9.0	84

OD, Outer diameter; *ID*, inner diameter.

The first step in the procedure is to find the cricothyroid membrane. This is easily accomplished in an asthenic man's neck. It is somewhat more difficult in a woman's neck. It is even more difficult in the patient with a short, thick neck. It is increasingly difficult in the patient with a fat neck and becomes extremely difficult when one is anxious and rushed. One should identify the cricothyroid membrane in 100 to 200 individuals, both when awake and after induction so that one can practice identifying the thyroid cartilage, the cricoid cartilage, and the cricothyroid membrane. Cricothyroidotomy may be required at the time when it is least expected. Under these circumstances it is hard for anyone to make the decision to perform the procedure and then to carry it out. This task is made all the more difficult if one has to struggle to identify the cricothyroid membrane. If one misidentifies the correct position, a failed outcome will ensue. It is our recommendation that when an anticipated difficult airway is encountered, a small black dot be placed on the skin immediately over the cricothyroid membrane, because this obviates the need to identify the cricothyroid membrane at some emergency later on and will greatly facilitate transtracheal jet ventilation or cricothyroidotomy.

The next key step is to have committed and then rehearsed, in one's mind, the procedure as it will occur. One must do this repeatedly so that when the time comes to perform the cricothyroidotomy the decision is made, the cricothyroid is rapidly identified, and the knife is passed through the cricothyroid membrane and into the airway. The incision is carried horizontally across the neck, the airway is opened, and an endotracheal tube is placed into the trachea. For those who watched the original *Star Wars*, the Jedi taught Luke Skywalker to practice so many times that he could visualize what he was doing even with his eyes closed, and it was only when Luke had practiced to this degree that the Jedi could say, "Let the force be with you." This same visualization and rehearsal is necessary to successfully accomplish an emergency cricothyroidotomy.

Placing a 14-gauge or even 12-gauge intravascular cannula through the cricothyroid membrane is not an acceptable alternative to a cricothyroidotomy. Unless one has the equipment and capabilities to provide jet ventilation, these small-diameter cannulas are not satisfactory ventilatory support mechanisms even for the short term.[2,3]

Percutaneous puncture cricothyroidotomy cannula trocars and equipment are available (see Chapter 25). These have no advantage over the traditional scalpel and ET. They are often not available, and their only function is misplaced psychologic comfort for the anesthesiologist. As described, one must be psychologically prepared to perform a cricothyroidotomy, and the availability of

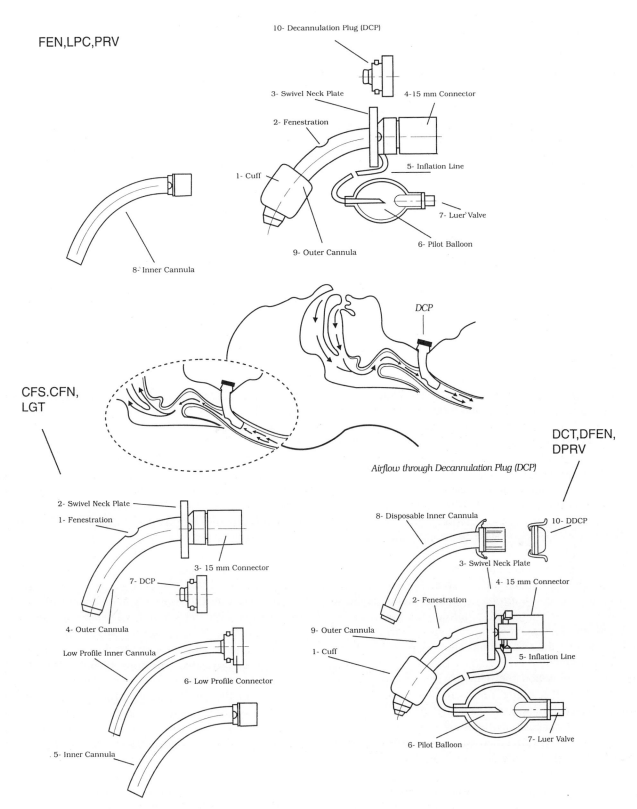

FEN,LPC,PRV

10- Decannulation Plug (DCP)

3- Swivel Neck Plate

2- Fenestration

4- 15 mm Connector

1- Cuff

5- Inflation Line

7- Luer' Valve

6- Pilot Balloon

9- Outer Cannula

8- Inner Cannula

CFS.CFN, LGT

DCP

Airflow through Decannulation Plug (DCP)

DCT,DFEN, DPRV

2- Swivel Neck Plate

1- Fenestration

3- 15 mm Connector

7- DCP

4- Outer Cannula

Low Profile Inner Cannula

6- Low Profile Connector

5- Inner Cannula

8- Disposable Inner Cannula

10- DDCP

3- Swivel Neck Plate

4- 15 mm Connector

2- Fenestration

9- Outer Cannula

1- Cuff

5- Inflation Line

6- Pilot Balloon

7- Luer Valve

Fig. 26-5. Fenestrated tracheostomy tubes. This is an engineering profile of a fenestrated tracheostomy tube. *FEN,* Fenestrated low-pressure cuffed tracheostomy tube; *LPC,* low-pressure cuffed tracheostomy tube; *PRV,* low-pressure cuffed with pressure relief valve; *CFS,* cuffless; *CFN,* cuffless fenestrated; *LGT,* laryngectomy; *DCT,* disposable cannula low-pressure cuffed tracheostomy; *DFEN,* disposable cannula cuffed tracheostomy tube, fenestrated; *DPRV,* disposable cannula cuffed tracheostomy tube with pressure relief valve. (Courtesy of Shiley.)

such instrumentation interferes with the anesthesiologists' paradigm for proceeding properly.

F. POSTOPERATIVE TRACHEOSTOMY CARE

In the past when stainless steel tracheostomy tubes were all that was available, postoperative tracheostomy care was a specialty unto itself. The inner cannula was removed and cleaned a minimum of three times a day with a bottle brush using alcohol and water. Crusting underneath the phalanges also had to be cleaned. Today, tracheostomy tubes are made of silicone elastimer (Silastic). They are well tolerated by the skin, the cervical soft tissues, and the trachea. The inner cannulas are now disposable, and in any case the Silastic cannulas are far less likely to be occluded with crusted secretions than were the old metal tubes.

In the early postoperative period, there will be intraluminal blood and mucous and the inner cannula does need to be cared for. It can be cleaned or simply discarded and a new one replaced. Because the tracheostomy tube bypasses the nose, an organ that filters, humidifies, and warms inspired air, administration of humidified, filtered air is necessary. Without this, the trachea develops a reactive mucositis. Under most circumstances the tracheostomy tube can be left open; however, a light cloth or other protective device should be considered to prevent accidental foreign body inhalation. In the past, before the availability of low-pressure cuffs, the cuffs were deflated every hour for a minimum of 5 minutes. Todays low-pressure cuffs require no attention as long as they are not overinflated to make a seal for positive pressure ventilation.

Nonetheless, it is still wise to let the cuff down for some time once or twice a day. This gives the tracheal wall mucosa some relief and it also permits the patient to speak during exhalation. As soon as bleeding and aspiration are not a problem and assuming positive pressure ventilation is not required, the cuff can be deflated and the patient can inspire air both through the tracheostomy tube and through the larynx. The patient can then exhale both through the tracheostomy tube and the larynx, and when the patient wishes to speak very often the tracheostomy tube can be occluded and excellent speech managed.

Typically, tracheostomy tubes are changed at 7 to 10 days. When a well-formed cutaneous-tracheal track has been developed, it is safe to change the tube at 1 week. When the tracheostomy tube is changed, the new tube need not have a cuff. If phonation is desirable, fenestrated tubes are routinely used. In a well-created tracheostomy, the tracheostomy tube change is simple and safe. Nonetheless, an ET, a tracheostomy changing tray, and a tracheostomy tube one or two sizes smaller than anticipated should be at hand. In a difficult tracheostomy and in a fat short neck, it is wise to defer the first tracheostomy change to 14 days and to have two

---

BOX 26-2   Complications of tracheostomy
Failure to establish an airway
Accidental extubation
Subcutaneous emphysema
Pneumothorax
Pneumomediastinum
Bleeding
Infection
Tracheal granulations
Subglottic stenosis
Tracheal stenosis

skilled individuals available at the time of changing. In any difficult tracheostomy tube change, preoxygenation for 5 to 10 minutes is advisable. It is rarely necessary to change a tracheostomy over a stylet but should such be required; their availability adds some degree of safety. The tracheostomy should be kept clean but otherwise requires very little care. Most first tracheostomies are now held in place with sutures and so the neck straps are not an issue. Once the tracheostomy tube is changed, future tracheostomies are held in place with a circumferential strap.

G. COMPLICATIONS

Complications of tracheostomy are listed in Box 26-2. Certainly, the most severe complication of an emergency tracheostomy is failure to establish an airway before brain damage or death. This would occur either because the decision to perform the procedure was not made soon enough or because the procedure was carried out too slowly. If the physician is unfamiliar with the techniques, the surgeon could go to either side of the midline and potentially incise the jugular vein or carotid artery. Probably the most common technical problem that occurs with the surgeon who has not performed tracheostomies on numerous occasions is that the initial incision is made and the superficial or anterior cervical vessels are transected, resulting in brisk hemorrhage. Instead of proceeding with a tracheal incision and insertion of the tube, the surgeon then focuses on the hemorrhage. Precious time is lost trying to clamp these bleeders and the patient becomes desaturated. The reasons for failing to perform an emergency cricothyroidotomy are usually attempts to perform the procedure somewhere other than through the cricothyroid membrane. Sometimes the thyrohyoid membrane is accidentally identified as the cricothyroid space; surgery there is difficult and often unsuccessful. The other potential complication of cricothyroidotomy is complete transection of the trachea. This would be more likely to occur in a child.

The literature on tracheostomies is typically written by head and neck surgeons or by trauma surgeons. Those who have performed enough tracheostomies to have reasonable statistics regarding complications are generally more experienced and therefore more skilled. One does not read about the individual who is called on once every 10 years to perform an emergency tracheostomy. The decision to perform a tracheostomy within this context is made late in the management of the difficult airway. The surgeon is slow in performing the procedure, and the result is that an airway is not established in a timely fashion. Although the patient may be resuscitated, he/she is too often brain injured or dies.

Accidental extubation does occur; when this happens in the early postoperative period, reestablishment of the airway, without the surgeon may be difficult. Skilled nursing care and appropriate bedside instrumentation such as a tracheostomy changing kit and a tracheostomy introducing cannula reduce the probability that accidental extubation will result in an adverse outcome. Appropriate techniques for securing the tracheostomy, such as suturing the tracheostomy, prevent this complication.

Tracheostomy tube obstruction should be prevented by appropriate suctioning and monitoring. It can occur if the patient has bleeding or tenacious secretions. Modern-day Silastic tubes with disposable inner cannulas should make this an uncommon problem. Bleeding is a complication of all surgeries, tracheostomies included. The inflated cuff prevents the aspiration of blood, but very often the bleeding is significant enough that it requires superficial tamponade and a return to the operating room. Oversewing the thyroid isthmus and meticulous attention to hemostasis during the procedure reduce the incidence of bleeding.

A rare complication of tracheostomies is an innominate artery rupture or blowout. This can occur with a high-arching innominate artery rubbing against the tracheostomy tube or if the tracheostomy tube cuff presses against the innominate artery. With today's low-pressure cuffs, this is far less likely unless the cuff is overinflated, which does occur in patients who are on high positive pressure ventilation. In these cases, the cuff is often progressively inflated a little bit more each day. The tracheal wall expands, and ultimately pressure is placed against the innominate artery. In either case pressure necrosis of the arterial wall occurs, and finally the artery ruptures with massive bleeding into the trachea. It is common in such situations to have what is called sentinel bleeding. This will be acute bleeding of 100 to 300 ml, which then stops. The sentinel bleeding should be recognized, and although it stops, cardiothoracic surgery consultation should be sought immediately and the patient brought to the operating room for exploration and repair.

If an air leak is present and the cervical skin has healed around the tracheostomy tube or if the skin has been sutured, air can escape into the paratracheal space or into the subcutaneous spaces of the neck. In the simplest of situations, subcutaneous emphysema will be noted. This must be recognized, and either the ventilatory pressures should be adjusted or the skin around the tracheostomy should be opened so that air can escape. If the air escapes into the paratracheal spaces, a pneumomediastinum can develop. The air can also extend around the lungs and a pneumothorax can develop. Prompt recognition and appropriate treatment will correct the problem and generally the air will be reabsorbed. In some situations in which the lung apex (cupula) extends into the neck, the lung itself can be cut and a pneumothorax can develop as a result. Prompt recognition and a chest tube are then indicated. A complication of long-term tracheostomy is tracheal stenosis. With today's low-pressure cuffs this is uncommon. A tracheal stenosis can be treated with a tracheal resection and repair or with placement of a Silastic stent.

The biggest controversy with tracheostomy tubes is the timing of tracheostomy for an individual who requires prolonged intubation. Consensus does not exist. The complication of long-term intubation is subglottic stenosis. The complication of tracheostomy is tracheal stenosis. Subglottic stenosis is difficult to correct and very often results in permanent damage to the larynx and to speech. Tracheal stenosis is an equally difficult problem to correct but once corrected rarely causes laryngeal or speech abnormalities.

It is the authors' strong recommendation that in those individuals in whom prolonged intubation will be required if tracheostomy is going to be performed the decision to do so should be made early and the tracheostomy should be performed as soon as the decision is made. All too often individuals who will require prolonged intubation are left intubated transorally or transnasally for 2 or more weeks and only then is the head and neck surgery service consulted and the tracheostomy requested. This places the patient at an unnecessary risk of subglottic stenosis. Therefore, if it is obvious that an individual will require prolonged intubation, the tracheostomy should be performed as soon as that decision is made. Tracheostomies are not well-received by patients not only because of aesthetic inconvenience but also because they impair their ability to speak. With today's tracheostomy tubes, including tubes with valves and fenestrations, anyone who does not require a ventilator can have a tracheostomy and phonate normally.

The last complication of tracheostomies is that once the individual is decannulated, an anterior neck scar remains. It is standard practice when decannulating a patient to simply remove the tracheostomy tube and allow the wound to heal by secondary intention. If the skin is closed primarily and the trachea remains open, any air leak that invariably ensues can cause complications with subcutaneous emphysema, pneumomediastinum, and pneumothorax. Once the wound has healed, tracheostomy scars are easily revised and the resultant scar is minimal. Many surgeons recommend a horizontal skin incision for tracheostomy with the belief that this will leave a smaller scar. We have found it easier to revise a vertical tracheostomy scar, and because it is easier to perform a tracheostomy through a vertical incision, this is the most common incision of choice.

H. CONCLUSIONS

Emergency tracheostomy and cricothyroidotomy are the last means of securing the airway. Whenever possible, tracheostomy is better performed as a planned procedure than as an emergency procedure. But when necessary, the prepared physicians should be able in most cases to enter the trachea and secure an airway fast enough to restore ventilation and save the patient's life. An anesthesiologist who has practiced identifying the cricothyroid membrane and is properly prepared psychologically to perform a cricothyroidotomy should be able to do this successfully.

The anesthesiologist who has not developed facility at identifying the cricothyroid membrane or is not properly prepared technically or psychologically to perform a cricothyroidotomy will initiate the procedure too late and will either misperform it or take so long to perform the procedure that the patient's outcome can be jeopardized.

Most tracheostomies are performed electively, and a well-coordinated anesthesia surgical team can do this safely and without stressing the anesthesiologist, the patient, or the surgeon. As with all things in life, complications do occur. Early recognition and appropriate treatment will minimize resultant disability.

II. PEDIATRIC SURGICAL AIRWAY

A. INTRODUCTION

The child or infant requiring a surgical airway poses a significantly different situation than an adult in respiratory distress. Differences exist in all aspects of clinical management, including anatomy, indications, operative techniques, postoperative management, and complications. Practices used in adult patients are not appropriate in the infant or child, and these differences have to be addressed if optimal outcomes are desired. Managing a pediatric airway may not be routine for the physician familiar with the adult airway. But the same physician may be responsible for acute airway management in the clinic, operating room, or emergency department for adults, children, and infants.

Awareness of the differences in anatomy of the infant laryngotracheal complex compared with that of the adult is essential to a logical, controlled, and safe approach to establishing an airway. The newborn larynx is situated high in the neck, with the cricoid cartilage at about the second or third cervical vertebra. The thyroid cartilage lies posterior to the hyoid bone.[5] In the newborn no space exists between the cricoid and thyroid cartilages.[6]

Establishing a surgical airway in a child may be elective or emergent. An elective surgical airway is performed after the child has been nasotracheally or orotracheally intubated. Elective situations include the need for prolonged intubation because of anatomic obstruction or the need for ventilatory support. Congenital abnormalities resulting in obstruction include supraglottic masses (i.e., hemangiomas, cystic hygromas, laryngeal cysts, craniofacial abnormalities), glottic lesions (i.e., webs, glottic stenosis), or subglottic pathologic conditions (i.e., hemangiomas, retention cysts, stenosis). Nasotracheal or orotracheal intubation is a temporary means of establishing a safe airway, and the surgical airway provides a more functional airway until definitive therapy for the obstruction is possible. Infectious causes of airway obstruction rarely require a surgical airway because nasotracheal intubation with skilled medical management and nursing care has been shown to minimize the potential for permanent airway scarring. Prolonged intubation has become an accepted means of managing infants and children requiring ventilatory support. Early experiences with prolonged intubation of infants and children during the 1960s led to numerous cases of subglottic stenosis. Because the subglottis is the only part of the lower airway with circumferential cartilaginous support, this area defined by the cricoid cartilage is prone to scarring and stenosis. With the evolution of neonatal and pediatric intensive care units capable of managing infants and children requiring prolonged intubation, iatrogenic causes have exceeded infectious causes as the most common risk factor for subglottic stenosis in infants and children. Advances in endotracheal tube management and patient care, including limiting excessive tube movement and treating gastroesophageal reflux, have led to a marked reduction in the rate of acquired subglottic stenosis. Despite these improvements, children needing prolonged ventilator support are candidates for tracheostomy as determined by the pediatrician and consulting surgeon.

Emergent cricothyroidotomy or tracheostomy is indicated when nasotracheal or orotracheal intubation is not possible. Congenital or acquired problems can result in failed attempts at intubation. As with any emergent situation, recognition of an inadequate approach to a particular situation and rapid implementation of an alternative strategy is crucial for success.

1. Illustrative case history

The patient is a 4-year-old male who has been hoarse for 2 years and has experienced the recent development of shortness of breath. He was referred by his pediatrician to an otolaryngologist for evaluation of the hoarseness and a significant exacerbation of respiratory distress. The otolaryngologist was unable to adequately examine the child with a flexible endoscope in the office and scheduled the child for general anesthesia and laryngoscopy. On entering the operating room, the anesthesiologist noted that the child had suprasternal retractions and labored breathing. The child was afebrile and was not drooling. The child had an oxygen saturation of 80% and allowed an IV line to be started with him remaining in an upright position. The child tolerated the anesthetic mask and was spontaneously breathing when laryngoscopy was attempted. On laryngoscopy, the anesthesiologist and otolaryngologist were unable to identify normal laryngeal structures, other than the tip of the epiglottis, because of diffuse papillomatous lesions. Air bubbles were seen posterior to the epiglottis; however, intubation with an endotracheal tube and stylet was unsuccessful. The oxygen saturation decreased to 40%. A rigid bronchoscope was successfully passed. Bronchoscopy confirmed that the papillomatous lesions were confined to the larynx. The child had an orderly tracheostomy performed while being ventilated through the bronchoscope.

2. Discussion of illustrative case

Establishing a surgical airway in a child is best performed after the airway is secured. Given the appearance of the papillomatous lesions and the identification of some air movement, an attempt at rigid bronchoscopy using the remaining landmarks and "following the bubbles" was the appropriate method of intubating the airway. If bronchoscopy had been unsuccessful, a temporizing measure would have been to place a 12-gauge or 14-gauge catheter through the cricothyroid membrane to establish air movement. Once adequate air movement was established, a tracheotomy could be performed. If ventilation becomes inadequate during the tracheotomy procedure, the surgeon can convert the procedure to a cricothyrotomy or emergent tracheostomy.

Maintaining spontaneous respirations was crucial to the success of securing this child's airway. Before instrumentation of the airway, or attempting intubation, the child was preoxygenated in anticipation of periods with inadequate ventilation.

B. ELECTIVE TRACHEOSTOMY

Elective tracheostomy is performed with the child intubated. General anesthesia is preferred if there are no medical contraindications. Proper positioning is critical for adequate exposure. The surgeon must identify the laryngotracheal structures through the anterior cervical skin. Accurate identification of structures may be difficult in the young child because the thyroid cartilage may lie posterior to the hyoid bone, and the cricothyroid membrane may not be palpable. The cricoid is the most prominent cartilage of the laryngotracheal complex, and this should be marked, along with the sternal notch and a line drawn vertically along the center of the tracheal rings. A subcutaneous injection with an anesthetic/vasoconstrictor solution (i.e., 1% lidocaine with 1:100,000 epinephrine) may be used.

Extension of the neck is achieved with a shoulder roll and with the anesthesiologist retracting the patient's chin superiorly. The gloved hand of the anesthesiologist may be prepped along with the anterior neck. Alternatively, extension of the neck can be maintained by taping the mandible to the head of the table.[7] Before beginning the surgical procedure, all esophageal tubes must be removed, including nasogastric tubes and esophageal stethoscopes. With the relatively small and soft noncalcified pediatric trachea, the esophageal tube may be mistaken for the endotracheal tube and an inadvertent esophagotomy could be performed.

The skin incision may be either horizontal or vertical. With a small incision, similar appearing scars result after decannulation. The advantage of a vertical orientation is the ability to extend the incision to facilitate exposure if necessary. Dissection through the subcutaneous fat is accomplished with a hemostat spreading vertically in the midline and division of the tissues with a cautery or scissors. The subcutaneous fat can be excised to expose the anterior cervical fascia. Deeper layers are serially grasped until the pretracheal fascia is encountered. The anterior jugular veins should be retracted laterally. Division and ligature of these vessels are necessary only if they are entered during the dissection. In most infants and children the thyroid isthmus can be retracted superiorly, and division and suture ligation of the isthmus is unnecessary. If retraction of the thyroid isthmus away from the intended site of the tracheotomy is not possible, the isthmus should be divided and the suture ligated. In the adult patient a tracheal hook may be used to retract the cricoid cartilage superiorly; however, this maneuver in an infant or child can result in disruption of the cricoid cartilage and should be avoided.

Once the trachea is identified, the site of the tracheotomy should be determined. Entry into the trachea should be between the second and third tracheal rings or between the third and fourth tracheal rings. A vertical incision is made into the trachea with a scalpel. Some authors have described creation of an inferiorly based flap with the tracheal flap sutured to the skin.[7] Division of the first tracheal ring should be avoided. Stay sutures should be placed on either side of the anticipated vertical incision before entering the trachea (Fig. 26-6). No cartilage should be removed in the performance of the tracheostomy. One 2-0 silk suture on a sharply curved needle is placed immediately lateral to each side of the tracheal incision. The sutures are excellent retractors during the performance of the tracheostomy.

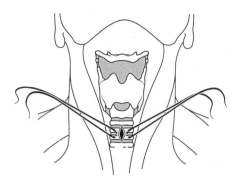

Fig. 26-6. Stay sutures are placed on either side of the vertical incision in the trachea.

If placement of the stay sutures before performing the tracheostomy is not technically possible, the trachea can be entered and the free edges of the trachea can be retracted laterally to facilitate placement of the sutures. For infants and small children, the sutures provide excellent retraction of the free edges of the trachea during introduction of the tracheostomy tube. In older children a Trousseau introducer may be used in addition to the sutures.

Once entry into the trachea has been achieved, the ET should be identified. The anesthesiologist withdraws the tube just superior to the tracheostomy, and the tracheostomy tube is introduced into the tracheal lumen with the obturator in place. The tube is introduced at a right angle to the trachea and then rotated and advanced inferiorly within the trachea. The ET is left in place until adequate ventilation is confirmed, including positive identification of carbon dioxide if a carbon dioxide monitor is being used. The tracheostomy tube is secured with tracheostomy tube ties, leaving only enough room for a single finger between the neck and tie. Suturing the tube to the skin is not recommended in infants and children. No dressing or a thin layer of gauze may be placed beneath the flanges of the tube. Bulky dressings are to be avoided. The stay sutures are labeled "right" and "left" to avoid their being crossed and are then taped to the chest. A chest radiograph is obtained postoperatively to assess the level of the tracheostomy tube tip and to evaluate the patient for pneumomediastinum or pneumothorax.

C. EMERGENCY TRACHEOSTOMY

As previously discussed, the newborn and infant airway characteristically lacks a cricothyroid membrane because there is no space between the cricoid and thyroid cartilages. Cricothyroidotomy is therefore not a surgical option for this group of patients. Emergency tracheostomy then assumes the role often reserved for emergency cricothyroidotomy in older patients. Exhaus-tive attempts should be made to secure an airway either with endotracheal intubation or rigid bronchoscopy. Administration of oxygen through a mask with adequate ventilation may allow a tracheostomy to be performed using local anesthesia. If this is not possible, a temporary airway may be achieved with placement of a 12-gauge or 14-gauge catheter into the trachea. Confirmation of catheter placement is made by withdrawing air through the catheter.

Once the decision is made to proceed with an emergency tracheostomy, the surgeon must be prepared to confront a blood-filled operative field. Neck extension facilitates identification of cervical landmarks. A vertical incision is made in the midline from the inferior border of the thyroid cartilage to the sternal notch. Palpation of the trachea may be the only means of identifying the trachea because of blood and soft tissue. Both sides of the trachea should be palpated and the dissection continued in the midline. If the patient is adequately ventilated, the dissection can follow the principles of an elective tracheostomy. If the patient's status rapidly deteriorates, the incision is carried through the soft tissues and into the trachea. Right-angled retractors may be used to retract soft tissue, strap muscles, and the anterior jugular veins laterally to isolate the trachea before entering its lumen. The free edges of the cut trachea can be retracted with forceps or hemostats during introduction of the tracheostomy tube. An alternative to a tracheostomy tube is an ET to secure the airway. A flexible anode tube provides a good alternative to a tracheostomy tube in an emergency situation.

Once the airway is secured, hemostasis can be achieved with packing.

D. EMERGENCY CRICOTHYROIDOTOMY

The principles of emergency cricothyroidotomy in an infant or child are similar to those of an adult. To ensure the success of an emergency cricothyroidotomy, the cricothyroid membrane must be clearly palpated before starting the procedure to avoid attempting to incise the cricothyroid membrane where none exists. Because the membrane may be narrow, a tracheostomy tube or small ET may not pass through this area despite vigorous retraction with hemostats. A suction catheter may be directed through a narrow cricothyroid membrane and allow ventilation while a more definitive procedure is completed.

E. POSTOPERATIVE TRACHEOSTOMY CARE

Postoperative care begins when the stay sutures are labeled and taped to the patient's chest. These stay sutures are critical to maintaining a safe airway, and the labels are the first communication between the surgeon and intensive care unit staff. Detailed information regarding the purpose of the tracheostomy and any unusual aspects of the patient's airway must be communicated to the intensive care unit staff.

Suctioning through the tracheostomy tube can result in irritation and bleeding. Routine suctioning should be limited to the lumen of the tracheostomy tube. Flexible suction catheters should be marked to prevent passage of the catheters beyond the distal opening of the tracheostomy tube. Tenacious secretions may be difficult to suction and saline solution may be used to liquify the secretions. Patency of the tracheostomy tube lumen must be maintained with vigilance because neonatal and pediatric tracheostomy tubes do not have removable inner cannulas as do adult tubes. Complete obstruction of the lumen refractory to suctioning will necessitate changing the tube in a "fresh" tracheostomy site. Therefore, extra tracheostomy tubes must be kept at the bedside. One tube should be the same size as the indwelling tube and a second, smaller tube should be readily available.

The lack of an inner cannula requires that the tracheostomy tube be changed once a week. In some situations the initial tube change may be done in the operating room if concomitant laryngoscopy or bronchoscopy is to be performed. In these situations the tube can be changed while the patient is ventilated through the bronchoscope. Most initial tube changes are performed in an intensive care unit. Safe tube changes require two experienced individuals and preparation. A surgical tracheostomy set should be at the bedside. After loosening the ties, the stay sutures are held taut at an angle of 60 degrees to retract the tracheostomy site open. A feeding tube or suction catheter can be placed into the indwelling tube and left in as a stylet while the new tube is introduced. One advantage of using a stylet with a lumen, is that the patient can exchange air during the tube change. The new tube is then secured with ties and the stay sutures are removed.

F. COMPLICATIONS

The most common early complications of tracheostomy are accidental decannulation, plugging of the tracheostomy tube, pneumothorax, and bleeding.[8-12] Obstruction is the most common complication of a tracheostomy. Obstruction is a result of obstruction within the lumen of the tube or occlusion of the distal end of the tube. If the tube appears to be lying in its proper position relative to the patient's neck, a suction catheter should be introduced to clear secretions. Thick secretions may require instillation of a saline solution. Unsuccessful suctioning attempts, including the inability to pass the catheter the entire length of the tube, should be recognized as obstruction within the tube. This requires placement of a new tube. For the first postoperative week, stay sutures are available to open the

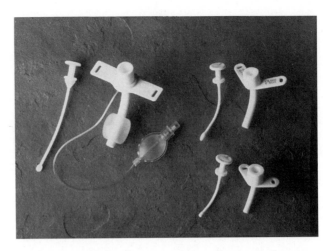

Fig. 26-7. Standard neonatal and pediatric tracheostomy tubes. Inflatable air-filled cuffed tube is pictured on left. Note the absence of an inner cannula and the single-piece construction of the uncuffed tubes. (Courtesy of Shiley.)

tracheostomy site. If the patient can be ventilated by mask, this will maintain oxygenation during the tube change. The on-call physician should be notified immediately and be present for the tube change if the patient can be ventilated. If the patient cannot be ventilated by AMBU bag, the tube is removed and replaced using the stay sutures and right-angle retractors placed in the tracheostomy. Orotracheal intubation is indicated if the tracheostomy tube cannot be replaced promptly. Unless the patient has complete obstruction above the level of the tracheostomy site or significant laryngeal trauma, intubation is the safest means of securing the airway.

Decannulation may be subtle with the outward appearance of a properly placed tube. A loosely tied tracheostomy tube may move excessively in the tracheostomy site and become dislodged from the tracheal lumen. A bulky dressing around the tracheostomy site can compromise a secure tube. A bulky dressing may prevent observation of the tip of the tracheostomy tube, which may become embedded in the soft tissues of the neck with obstruction of the lumen. Decannulation should be managed with the same approach as that of an obstructed tube.

Bleeding from the tracheostomy site may occur in the perioperative period or weeks to months after placement of the tube. Perioperative bleeding may respond to nonocclusive packing of the tracheostomy site with gauze or hemostatic material. If excessive packing is required, the patient should be placed in a setting in which the tracheostomy tube can be changed and specific bleeding sites treated with cautery or suture ligation. Excessive packing can result in subcutaneous emphysema or pneumomediastinum. Erosion of the tracheostomy tube

Table 26-2. Cross-reference for pediatric and neonatal tracheostomy tubes for Bivona, Shiley, and Portex tubes

						Uncuffed Tracheostomy Tube CROSS REFERENCE											
Bivona code no.	ID (mm)	OD (mm)	APPX Fr.	APPX Jackson	Length (mm)	Shiley code no.	ID (mm)	OD (mm)	APPX Fr.	APPX Jackson	Length (mm)	Portex code no.	ID (mm)	OD (mm)	APPX Fr.	APPX Jackson	Length (mm)
60N025	2.5	4.0	12	000	30	OONT	3.1	4.5	14	00	30	553025	2.5	4.5	13	00	30
60N030	3.0	4.7	14	00	32	ONT	3.4	5.0	15	0	32	553030	3.0	5.2	15	0	32
60N035	3.5	5.3	16	0/1	34	INT	3.7	5.5	17	1	34	553035	3.5	5.8	16	1	34
60N040	4.0	6.0	18	2	36												
60P025	2.5	4.0	12	000	38							555025	2.5	4.5	13	00	30
60P030	3.0	4.7	14	00	39	OOPT	3.1	4.5	14	00	39	555030	3.0	5.2	15	00	36
60P035	3.5	5.3	16	0/1	40	OPT	3.4	5.0	15	0	40	555035	3.5	5.8	16	01	40
60P040	4.0	6.0	18	2	41	1PT	3.7	5.5	17	1	41	555040	4.0	6.5	18	02	44
60P045	4.5	6.7	20	3−	42	2PT	4.1	6.0	18	2	42	555045	4.5	7.1	19	03	48
60P050	5.0	7.3	22	3+	44	3PT	4.8	7.0	21	3	44	555050	5.0	7.7	21	4−	50
60P055	5.5	8.0	24	4	46	4PT	5.5	8.0	24	4	46	555055	5.5	8.3	23	4+	52
60A150	5.0	7.3	22	3	60												
60A160	6.0	8.7	26	4	70	4CFS	5.0	8.5	26	4	67	550060	6.0	8.3	24	4	55
60A170	7.0	10.0	30	6	80	6CFS	7.0	10.0	30	6	78	550070	7.0	9.7	30	6	75
60A180	8.0	11.0	33	7	88							550080	8.0	11.0	33	7	82
60A190	9.0	12.3	37	8	98	8CFS	8.5	12.0	36	8	84	550090	9.0	12.4	36	8	87
60A195	9.5	13.3	40	10	98	10CFS	9.0	13.0	39	10	84	560100	10.0	13.8	40	10	98

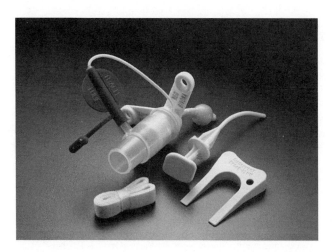

Fig. 26-8. Fome-Cuff cuff Bivona tube. Cuff inflates passively. Withdrawal of air with syringe is necessary to deflate cuff. (Courtesy of Bivona.)

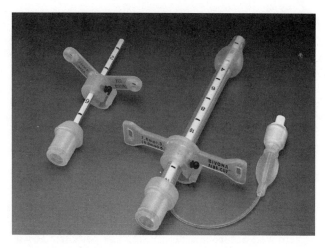

Fig. 26-9. Adjustable neck flange Hyperflex Tracheostomy Tube. Flange can be moved along the length of the tube. (Courtesy of Shiley.)

into a large vessel (i.e., the innominate) does not usually occur in the immediate postoperative period; however, a low tracheostomy would be a risk factor for this situation.

Bleeding occurring weeks to months after surgery may be due to granulation tissue. Intermittent blood-tinged sputum is best addressed with bronchoscopy and resection or laser vaporization. A large, sudden episode of hemorrhage may be sentinel bleeding indicative of erosion into a large vessel. Immediate management is to place pressure on the inferior aspect of the tracheostomy site and consult a thoracic surgeon. A cuffed tracheostomy tube may be useful to tamponade the bleeding site.

Subcutaneous air and pneumomediastinum are often the result of occlusion at the skin level. Management consists of removing occlusive dressings. If the patient does not require high ventilatory pressures, the subcutaneous emphysema and pneumomediastinum should resolve spontaneously. If not, a chest tube may be necessary to avoid a pneumothorax.

Tracheomalacia and tracheal stenosis are possible sequelae of tracheostomy tubes. Localized tracheomalacia in the form of suprastomal collapse after long-term tracheostomy tube placement may not significantly compromise the airway subsequent to decannulation. However, obstructive suprastomal collapse may develop and require an open surgical repair with a cartilage graft. Distal tracheomalacia can occur after prolonged periods of high-pressure ventilation. The risk of tracheomalacia may be reduced if an air leak is allowed. Surgical correction of distal tracheomalacia can be a challenge, requiring cartilage grafts and occasionally placement of a Silastic stent.[13] Isolated distal tracheal stenosis can be

treated with expansion grafts or primary resection and reanastomosis of the trachea.

G. TRACHEOSTOMY TUBES

Neonatal and pediatric tracheostomy tubes are available from several companies. Neonatal and pediatric tubes do not have inner cannulas because these would adversely compromise the functional inner diameter of the tube (Fig. 26-7). Cross-referenced tables facilitate size comparisons between the various tubes (Table 26-2).

Tubes are available in plastic, silicone, and silver. The silver tubes are thinner walled than their plastic and silicone counterparts. The rigidity of these tubes may be responsible for more severe tracheal damage and vessel erosion; however, a snug-fitting plastic or silicone tube can have the same adverse outcomes.[14] The standard pediatric tracheostomy tube does not have a cuff and therefore an air leak should be anticipated. Attempting to eliminate the air leak with a larger tube should be avoided. Patients requiring high airway pressures may be candidates for a foam-cuffed Bivona tube (Fig. 26-8). Animal studies have shown a reduction in the degree of tracheal dilation with foam-filled compared with air-filled cuffed tubes.[15]

Most silicone and plastic pediatric tracheostomy tubes have a 15-mm male standard connector.[16] The compatibility of the ventilating tubing and the tracheostomy tube connector must be verified before starting an elective procedure.

For emergent airway procedures, the preferred tube may be an ET. An ET's position in the tracheal lumen can be easily adjusted. An anode tube is flexible and well tolerated. Adjustable tracheostomy tubes are now available and are an excellent alternative to an ET (Bivona, Adjustable Neck Flange Hyperflex Tracheostomy Tubes) (Fig. 26-9).

H. CONCLUSIONS

Management of the pediatric airway requires familiarity with the unique anatomic features of the newborn and infant larynx and trachea. The presence of a cricothyroid membrane in a newborn or young infant should not be assumed, and this structure should be clearly palpated before any attempt at performing a cricothyroidotomy.

The reliance on palpation during airway procedures in the pediatric neck demands that all esophageal tubes be removed before any dissection. The pediatric airway is not calcified and therefore is less resistant to vigorous retraction of the cricoid and tracheal cartilages.

Care of the pediatric tracheostomy is a multispecialty endeavor. A tracheotomized child requires individuals competent in identifying a nonfunctioning tube and possessing sufficient experience to change the tube in an emergency. Education and experience are the cornerstones to ensuring that a tracheostomy is a "safe" airway.

REFERENCES

1. Davidson TM, Producer: *The difficult airway videotape, Part II. Management/the cricothyroid membrane,* Parkridge, Ill, 1992, The American Society of Anesthesiology.
2. Ooi R, Sawcett NS, Soni N et al: Extra inspiratory work of breathing imposed by cricothyrotomy devices, *Br J Anaesth* 70:17, 1993.
3. Abbrecht PH et al: Insertion forces and risk of complications during cricothyroid cannulation, *J Emerg Med* 10:417, 1992.
4. Burtner DD, Goodman M: Anesthestic and operative management of potential upper airway obstruction, *Arch Otol* 104:657, 1978.
5. Mcgill TJ, Healy GB: Congenital and acquired lesions of the infant larynx, *Clin Pediatr* 17:584, 1978.
6. Myers EN, Stool SE, Johnson JT, editors: *Tracheotomy,* New York, 1985, Churchill Livingstone, p 94.
7. Hotaling AJ, Robbins WK, Medgy DN et al: Pediatric tracheotomy: a review of technique, *Am J Otol* 13:115, 1992.
8. Crysdale WS, Feldman RI, Naito K: Tracheotomies: a 10-year experience in 319 children, *Ann Otol Rhinol Laryngol* 94:439, 1988.
9. Gilmore BB, Mickelson SA: Pediatric tracheotomy: controversies in management, *Otolaryngol Clin North Am* 19:141, 1986.
10. Kenna MA, Reilly JS, Stool SE: Tracheotomy in the preterm infant, *Ann Otol Rhinol Laryngol* 96:68, 1987.
11. Carter P, Benjamin B: Ten-year review of pediatric tracheotomy, *Ann Otol Rhinol Laryngol* 92:398, 1983.
12. Gerson CR, Tucker GF: Infant tracheotomy, *Ann Otol Rhinol Laryngol* 91:413, 1982.
13. Harrell J. Personal communication, February 1994.
14. Myers EN, Stool SE, Johnson JT, editors: *Tracheotomy,* New York, 1985, Churchill Livingstone, p 139.
15. King K, Mandava B, Kamen SM et al: Tracheal tube cuffs and tracheal dilatation, *Chest* 67:458, 1975.
16. Myers EN, Stool SE, Johnson JT, editors: *Tracheotomy,* New York, 1985, Churchill Livingstone, p 140.

Chapter 27

CONFIRMATION OF TRACHEAL INTUBATION

M. Ramez Salem
Anis Baraka

I. OVERVIEW
  A. ASA CLOSED-CLAIMS STUDIES
    1. **Pediatric versus adult anesthesia closed malpractice claims**
  B. THE MAGNITUDE OF THE PROBLEM OF ESOPHAGEAL INTUBATION
  C. IS THERE AN IDEAL TEST FOR CONFIRMATION OF TRACHEAL TUBE PLACEMENT?
II. **METHODS OF VERIFICATION OF TRACHEAL TUBE PLACEMENT**
  A. DIRECT VISUALIZATION OF THE TRACHEAL TUBE BETWEEN THE CORDS
  B. TACTILE OROTRACHEAL TUBE PLACEMENT TEST
  C. OBSERVATION AND PALPATION OF CHEST MOVEMENTS
  D. AUSCULTATION OF BREATH SOUNDS
  E. ENDOBRONCHIAL INTUBATION
  F. EPIGASTRIC AUSCULTATION AND OBSERVATION FOR ABDOMINAL DISTENTION
  G. COMBINED AUSCULTATION OF EPIGASTRIUM AND BOTH AXILLAE
  H. RESERVOIR BAG COMPLIANCE AND REFILLING
  I. RESERVOIR BAG MOVEMENTS WITH SPONTANEOUS BREATHING
  J. CUFF MANEUVERS AND NECK PALPATION
  K. SOUND OF EXPELLED GASES DURING STERNAL COMPRESSION
  L. TUBE CONDENSATION OF WATER VAPOR
  M. ELECTRONIC METAL DETECTORS
  N. VIDEO STETHOSCOPE
  O. USE OF NASOGASTRIC TUBES, GASTRIC ASPIRATES, INTRODUCERS, AND OTHER DEVICES
  P. USE OF FLEXIBLE FIBEROPTIC LARYNGOSCOPES AND BRONCHOSCOPES
  Q. TRANSTRACHEAL ILLUMINATION
  R. PULSE OXIMETRY AND DETECTION OF CYANOSIS
  S. IDENTIFICATION OF CARBON DIOXIDE IN EXHALED GAS
    1. **Capnography**
    2. **Colorimetric end-tidal carbon dioxide detection**
  T. ESOPHAGEAL DETECTOR DEVICE/SELF-INFLATING BULB
  U. CHEST RADIOGRAPHY
III. **CONCLUSIONS**

I. OVERVIEW

A. ASA CLOSED-CLAIMS STUDIES

In the past decade, the Committee on Professional Liability of the American Society of Anesthesiologists (ASA) has studied adverse anesthetic outcome based on closed claims files of nationwide insurance carriers.[1] Since the inception, it became evident that adverse outcomes involving the respiratory system constitute the single largest class of injury, representing one third of the overall claims. Generally involving healthy adults undergoing nonemergency surgery with general anesthesia, three mechanisms of injury accounted for approximately three fourths of the adverse respiratory events: inadequate ventilation (38%), esophageal intubation (18%), and difficult tracheal intubation (17%).[1] The remaining adverse respiratory events were produced by a variety of low-frequency (≤2%) mechanisms, including airway obstruction, bronchospasm, aspiration, premature and unintentional extubation, inadequate inspired oxygen delivery, and endobronchial intubation.[1]

Care was judged substandard in more than 80% of inadequate ventilation and esophageal intubation cases.[1] Almost all (>90%) claims for inadequate ventilation and esophageal intubation were considered preventable with better monitoring opposed to only 36% of claims for difficult tracheal intubation.[1] Death and permanent brain damage were more frequent in claims for inadequate ventilation and esophageal intubation (>90%) than in claims for difficult tracheal intubation (56%). Median payment was $240,000 for inadequate ventilation, $217,000 for esophageal intubation, and $76,000 for difficult tracheal intubation.[1]

In 23% of the claims for esophageal intubation, there was documentation of difficult intubation; in 73%, there was sufficient information to reconstruct the time to detection of esophageal intubation.[1] Within this subset, 3% of esophageal intubations were detected before 5 minutes, 61% in 5 to 10 minutes, and 36% after 10 minutes.[1] Auscultation of breath sounds (presumed) was documented in 63% of the claims for esophageal intubation. In 48% of cases, auscultation led to the erroneous conclusion that the tube was in the trachea.[1] This diagnostic error was eventually recognized in a variety of ways including reexamination with direct laryngoscopy, absence of the tube in the trachea at the time of an emergency tracheostomy, resolution of cyanosis after reintubation, and discovery of esophageal intubation at autopsy. Cyanosis was documented in 52% of the claims and preceded the recognition of esophageal intubation in only 34% of the cases.

1. Pediatric versus adult anesthesia closed malpractice claims

Outcome studies in pediatric patients revealed that adverse respiratory events constitute a leading cause of morbidity and mortality.[2-4] The ASA closed claims study provided a database to compare pediatric and adult cases in which an adverse outcome occurred.[4] The pediatric claims presented a different distribution of damaging events compared with adults (Tables 27-1 and 27-2). Respiratory events and mortality rate were greater in pediatric claims.[4] Anesthetic care was more often judged "less than appropriate," and the complications more frequently were considered preventable with better monitoring. The median payment to the plaintiff was greater for pediatric claims than for adult claims. Cyanosis (49%), bradycardia (64%), or both often preceded cardiac arrest in pediatric claims, resulting in death (50%) or brain damage (30%) in previously healthy children.[4]

Table 27-1. Comparison of pediatric and adult damaging events with special reference to the respiratory system

Damaging event	Pediatric (n = 238)		Adult (n = 1953)
	%	P	%
Respiratory system	43	≤0.01	30
Inadequate ventilation	20	≤0.01	9
Esophageal intubation	5	NS	6
Airway obstruction	5	NS	2
Difficult intubation	4	NS	6
Inadvertent extubation	3	NS	1
Premature extubation	3	NS	1
Aspiration	2	NS	2
Endobronchial intubation	1	NS	1
Bronchospasm	0	NS	2
Inadequate Fio₂	0	NS	<0.5

Data from Morray JP, Geiduschek JM, Caplan RA et al: *Anesthesiology* 78:461, 1993.

B. THE MAGNITUDE OF THE PROBLEM OF ESOPHAGEAL INTUBATION

Outcome studies during the past three decades have repeatedly identified adverse respiratory events, including unrecognized esophageal intubation as a leading and recurring cause of injury in anesthetic practice.[5-10] Faulty tracheal intubation was the cause of death or cerebral damage in 30.7% of anesthetic accidents reported to the Medical Defense Union of the United Kingdom from 1970 to 1977.[5] The report on Confidential Enquiries into Maternal Deaths in England and Wales in 1979 to 1981 revealed that 8 of 22 deaths attributable to anesthesia were related to difficulty in tracheal intubation. In four patients, the tube proved to be misplaced in the esophagus. A review of anesthesia-related medical liability claims in the United Kingdom from 1977 to 1982 listed esophageal intubation as a "main cause" of anesthetic accidents leading to death or brain damage, with the largest resultant claims.[6] An investigation of anesthesia mortality in Australia revealed that 69% of the deaths were related to airway management, with esophageal intubation once again identified as an important contributing factor.[10]

The predominance of esophageal intubation in these outcome studies reflects the magnitude and persistence of this problem. Virtually all anesthesiologists have experienced esophageal intubation sometime in their career, especially during their training and when they encountered difficulty in visualizing the larynx. Fortunately, most unintentional esophageal intubations are immediately and easily recognized. What has been intriguing is the rare situation when misplacement of the tube in the esophagus was not recognized, resulting in

Table 27-2. Comparison of pediatric and adult demographic, injury, and payment data

| | Pediatric (n = 238) | | Adult (n = 1953) |
	%	*P*	%
Age	28	—	—
0-14			
Sex			
Male	65	≤ .01	38
Female	32	≤ .01	62
Unknown	3	≤ .05	< .5
ASA physical status			
1	35	≤ .01	22
2	14	≤ .01	22
3	6	≤ .01	13
4	4	NS	3
5	< 0.5	NS	1
Unknown	40	NS	40
Poor medical condition and/or obesity	6	≤ .01	41
Death	50	≤ .01	35
Brain damage	30	≤ .01	11
Less than appropriate anesthetic care	54	≤ .01	44
Preventable with better monitoring	45	≤ .01	30
Median payment	$111,234	≤ .05	$90,000

Data from Morray JP, Geiduschek JM, Caplan RA et al: *Anesthesiology* 78:461, 1993.

grave consequences. Failure to recognize esophageal intubation is not limited to junior residents or inexperienced personnel. It has occurred with experienced and skilled anesthesiologists. Gannon[9] described a case in which three "consultant anaesthetists" failed to recognize that the tracheal tube was in the esophagus. There are many case reports in the literature describing anesthetic catastrophes and near disasters in patients whose esophagus had been unintentionally intubated and in whom some or many of the commonly used signs indicative of proper tube placement were misleading.[10-17]

Unintentional esophageal intubation may occur more frequently in comatose patients and in patients who suffer cardiac arrest during out-of-hospital paramedic intubation.[18,19] In one study of paramedics trained in direct laryngoscopic tracheal intubation, there were 14 esophageal intubations in 779 patients, an incidence of 1.8%.[18] Esophageal tube placement was recognized and corrected in 11 patients, but the time of recognition was not reported. Three of the 14 esophageal intubations (0.4% of the total) were not recognized and remained uncorrected. Contributing factors to this relatively high incidence of esophageal intubation include intubation under less than optimal conditions, unavailability of appropriate monitoring equipment, violation of the standard technique of auscultation of lung fields and epigastrium, and nonexpert personnel attempting intubations.

C. IS THERE AN IDEAL TEST FOR CONFIRMATION OF TRACHEAL TUBE PLACEMENT?

The ideal test for confirmation of proper tracheal tube placement should be simple and quick to perform, reliable, safe, inexpensive, and repeatable. It should not require elaborate equipment or extensive experience. It should function reliably in patients of different age groups, in the presence of various pathologic conditions, and after difficult intubations. It should yield unequivocal positive signs, should not yield false signs, and should function equally in the patient with or without cardiac arrest. An ideal test should also be readily available for use in the operating room and outside the operating room where tracheal intubation may be performed, such as hospital floors, emergency rooms, ambulances, and trauma scenes.

Unfortunately, so far, such a perfect test does not exist. Over the years many clinical signs and technical aids have been described to confirm tracheal intubation, and only recently did they receive objective scrutiny to determine their reliability.[20] Many of the studies used to assess these tests involve the placement of two tubes, one in the trachea and the other in the esophagus.[21] This scenario makes the observer's decision as to which tube was in the trachea or esophagus much easier and helps the recognition of esophageal intubation. The clinician does not have the luxury of choice between two tubes in the clinical situation.[21] In the assessment of any of these tests, the reader must understand what is meant by

---

BOX 27-1   Detection of tracheal tube placement methods and techniques

Direct visualization of the tracheal tube between the cords
Tactile orotracheal tube placement test
Observation and palpation of chest movements and auscultation of breath sounds
Endobronchial intubation
Epigastric auscultation and observation for abdominal distention
Combined auscultation of epigastrium and both axillae
Reservoir bag compliance and refilling
Reservoir bag movements with spontaneous breathing
Cuff maneuvers and neck palpation
Sound of expelled gases during sternal compression
Tube condensation of water vapor
Electronic metal detectors
Video stethoscope
Use of nasogastric tubes, gastric aspirates, introducers, and other devices
Use of flexible fiberoptic laryngoscopes and bronchoscopes
Transtracheal illumination
Pulse oximetry and detection of cyanosis
Identification of CO_2 in exhaled gas (colorimetry and capnography)
Esophageal detector devices (syringe and self-inflating bulb)
Chest radiography

BOX 27-2   Confirmation of tracheal tube placement

Traditional clinical signs

Direct visualization of the tube between the cords
Observation and palpation of chest movements and auscultation of breath sounds
Epigastric auscultation and observation for abdominal distention
Combined auscultation of epigastrium and both axillae
Reservoir bag compliance and refilling
Reservoir bag movements with spontaneous breathing
Sound of expelled gases during sternal compression
Tube condensation of water vapor

Tests based on anatomic differences

Tactile orotracheal tube placement test
Cuff maneuvers and neck palpation
Endobronchial intubation
Use of flexible fiberoptic laryngoscopes and bronchoscopes
Transtracheal illumination
Use of nasogastric tubes, gastric aspirates, introducers, and other devices
Electronic metal detectors
Video stethoscope
Chest radiography
Esophageal detector devices (syringe and self-inflating bulb)

Tests based on physiologic differences

Pulse oximetry and detection of cyanosis
Identification of CO_2 in exhaled gas (colorimetry and capnography)

---

false-negative and false-positive results. Although not all articles report agreement, most used the terms false-negative meaning tube in trachea, but the test fails, and false-positive meaning tube in the esophagus, but the result mimics that of tracheal intubation. In case of capnography, false-negative refers to the tube in the trachea, but absent waveform; false-positive implies the tube in the esophagus, but present waveform. To avoid confusion and to maintain conformity to previously used terms, these definitions will be retained throughout the discussion.

II. METHODS OF VERIFICATION OF TRACHEAL TUBE PLACEMENT

Various methods have been used to verify tracheal tube placement and to distinguish it from esophageal intubation (Box 27-1). These methods can be categorized under three main headings: traditional clinical signs, tests based on anatomic differences between the trachea and esophagus, and tests using physiologic differences (Box 27-2). Methods of verification of tracheal tube placement (or detection of esophageal intubation) can also be classified into nonfailsafe, almost

failsafe, and failsafe, depending on their reported reliability and specificity (Box 27-3).

A. DIRECT VISUALIZATION OF THE TRACHEAL TUBE BETWEEN THE CORDS

Sighting the tube passage through the larynx during intubation or confirmation of the presence of the tube between the cords after intubation is one of the most reliable methods to ensure correct tube placement. Two maneuvers can be helpful to assist direct visual confirmation of tracheal intubation, one during and the other after intubation.

If the tube is introduced directly posterior to the laryngoscope blade as shown in Fig. 27-1, *A*, the laryngoscopist's view of the cords may be obscured and the tube may inadvertently enter the esophagus. This can be avoided by directing the tube from the right corner of the mouth toward the larynx. As seen in Fig. 27-1, *B*, this maneuver can allow visualization of the tube entering the larynx, thus confirming tracheal intubation. The

BOX 27-3 **Methods of verification of tracheal tube placement**

A. Nonfailsafe methods
1. Tactile orotracheal tube placement test
2. Observation and palpation of chest movements and auscultation of breath sounds
3. Endobronchial intubation
4. Epigastric auscultation and observation for abdominal distention
5. Combined auscultation of epigastrium and both axillae
6. Reservoir bag compliance and refilling
7. Reservoir bag movements with spontaneous breathing
8. Cuff maneuvers and neck palpation
9. Sound of expelled gases during sternal compression
10. Tube condensation of water vapor
11. Electronic metal detectors
12. Video stethoscope
13. Use of nasogastric tubes, gastric aspirates, introducers, and other devices
14. Transtracheal illumination
15. Pulse oximetry and detection of cyanosis
16. Chest radiography
B. Almost failsafe methods
1. Identification of CO_2 in exhaled gas (colorimetry and capnography)
2. Esophageal detector devices (syringe and self-inflating bulb)
C. Failsafe methods
1. Direct visualization of tube between the cords
2. Use of fiberoptic laryngoscopes and bronchoscopes

This "subjective" classification scheme is based on current information and therefore may change as new data become available.

other maneuver that can be performed after intubation but before removing the laryngoscope from the mouth involves gentle posterior displacement of the tube toward the palate (Fig. 27-2).[22] This backward push on the tube against the forward traction of the laryngoscope blade exposes the cords by altering the direction of the tube as it enters the larynx. This maneuver can be helpful in cases where the cords are obscured by the tube as it enters the larynx (Fig. 27-2).

Sighting the tube entering the larynx cannot be performed in all cases of direct laryngoscopy, especially if intubation is difficult and during blind nasal intubation. Even after visualization of the tube entering the larynx, the tube may slip out of the larynx while the laryngoscope is being removed, during taping of the tube, while positioning the patient, or during transportation.[23] This tends to occur more frequently if the distal end of the tube lies just below the cords or high in the trachea. To prevent accidental extubation or endobronchial intubation, clinicians aim at placing the distal end of the tube in the middle third of the trachea. Several precautions can be undertaken to prevent tube displacement in adult patients. First, the cuffed portion of the tube should be located at least 1 to 2 cm below the cords. Second, unless head extension or flexion is needed for the surgical procedure, the head should be kept in a neutral position after intubation. Third, the laryngoscope should be removed gently after intubation while securing the tube in position. Fourth, taping of the tube should be carefully done to avoid tube movement. In adults of average height, this is usually done at the 21- to 23-cm mark after orotracheal intubation if the head is in a neutral position. In shorter individuals and in patients in whom head flexion is needed for surgery, taping of the tube may be done at or below the 20-cm mark. In contrast, in taller patients and in patients in whom head extension is needed, the tube may be taped at the 24- or even 25-cm mark. Fifth, placement of an oropharyngeal airway adjacent to the tube helps minimize its movement inside the mouth and prevents dislodgment of the tube, especially during coughing.

Excessive movement of the tube can occur during extension and flexion of the head. In a radiologic study in adults, Conrardy et al.[24] demonstrated an average of 3.8-cm movement of the tube toward the carina when the head was moved from full extension to full flexion (Fig. 27-3). In some patients this movement reached as much as 6.4 cm. With lateral head rotation, the tube moved an average of 0.7 cm away from the carina. Because the average movement of the tube when the head is moved from the neutral position to full extension is 1.9 cm, it is unlikely that extubation would occur during this movement if the distal end of the tube was correctly placed in the middle of the trachea.

Tracheal tube displacement can occur with changes in patient positioning, displacement of the diaphragm, and during surgical manipulations of the trachea or esophagus. A high incidence of mainstem intubation has been reported after the institution of a 30-degree Trendelenburg position.[25] This is due to cephalad shift of the carina causing a taped tube to relocate into a mainstem bronchus. The opposite may happen when the reverse Trendelenburg position is used. Because both trachea and esophagus are invested in the same cervical fascia, pulling on either structure can misplace a previously correctly placed tracheal tube. This can occur during repair of esophageal atresia in infants and during esophagoscopy.

The ease with which endobronchial intubation can occur with head flexion and unintentional extubation with head extension is of particular concern in the infant,

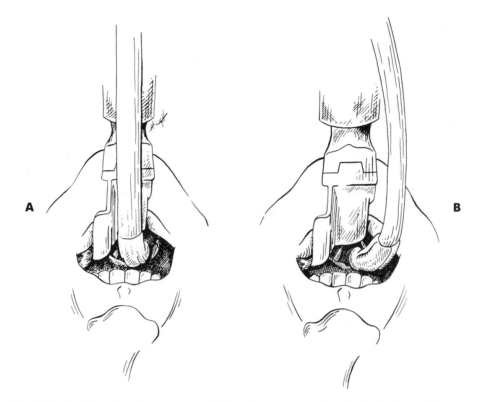

Fig. 27-1. A, When the tube is introduced directly posterior to the blade, the view of the cords may be obscured and the tube may enter the esophagus instead of the trachea. **B,** Directing the tube from the right corner of the mouth toward the larynx can allow better visualization of the tube entering the larynx.

especially in the neonate whose trachea is only 4.7 to 5.7 cm long (Fig. 27-4).[25-27] When tracheal intubation is performed in infants, precautions should be taken to ensure that the tube is placed far enough in the trachea but not in a mainstem bronchus. One precaution is to use tubes that have circumferential marks at 2.2 cm from the distal end and introduce the marker on the tube as far as the cords in term infants, to slightly above the cords in preterm infants, and to slightly below the cords in older infants. Another alternative that has been recommended is to use tubes with marks 2.2-, 2.4-, and 2.6-cm from the distal end in tubes with diameters of 2.5-, 3.0-, and 3.5-mm, respectively.

B. TACTILE OROTRACHEAL TUBE PLACEMENT TEST

Charters and Wilkinson[28] described a bimanual tactile orotracheal tube placement test to confirm laryngeal placement. The test consists of delineation of all the boundaries of the interarytenoid groove and the relationship of the tracheal tube immediately anterior to it using the gloved hand. Although intriguing, familiarity with this test is essential for its reliable implementation. Potential limitations include applicability to large males with a full set of teeth, narrow mouth, difficult intuba-

tions, nonparalyzed (potentially biting) patients with teeth, and clinicians with very small hands.[28] It is doubtful that this test will gain wide popularity.

C. OBSERVATION AND PALPATION OF CHEST MOVEMENTS

Commonly used maneuvers to confirm tracheal intubation are observation of symmetric bilateral chest movements and palpation of upper chest excursions during compression of the reservoir bag. These signs can easily distinguish tracheal from esophageal intubation in most patients. However, in obese patients, women with large breasts, and patients with a rigid chest wall, barrel chest, or less-compliant lungs, observation and palpation of chest excursions can be misinterpreted to indicate that the tube is in the esophagus.[23] More importantly, upper chest wall movements simulating ventilation of the lungs can be seen and felt with an esophageally placed tube. This phenomenon has been described in many instances of what ultimately proved to be esophageal intubation[11-16] and has been reported in patients with intrathoracic hiatal hernia and after gastric pull-up operations.[17]

Pollard and Junius[12] studied chest movements during esophageal ventilation in a male cadaver. They placed a

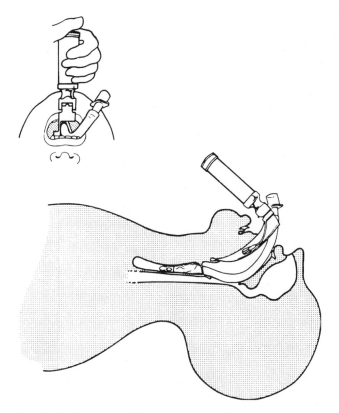

Fig. 27-2. Posterior displacement of tracheal tube restores view of larynx. (From Ford RWJ: *Can Anaesth Soc J* 30:191, 1983.)

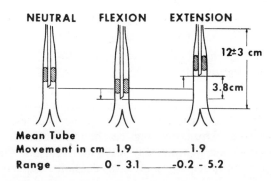

Fig. 27-3. Mean endotracheal tube movement with flexion and extension of the neck from neutral position. The mean tube movement between flexion and extension is about one-third to one-fourth the length of an adult trachea (12 ± 3 cm). (From Conrardy PA, Goodman LR, Lainge F et al: *Crit Care Med* 4:7, 1976.)

cuffed tube into the esophagus and attached it to an inflating bag. They noted that "the chest and epigastric movements observed when the bag was compressed were indistinguishable from those normally seen in ventilation of the lungs even in the upper chest area." When they dissected the body starting with the epigastrium, they noted that "the stomach was being inflated and was spontaneously deflating via the esophagus, the feel of the

inflating bag being indistinguishable from normal pulmonary ventilation." Even when the lower end of the esophagus was occluded, they noted that "chest movements still appeared identical to those seen when the lungs are inflated." After the chest was entered, they observed that "chest movements were caused by the flat esophagus distending into a firm tube that lifted the heart and upper mediastinal structures forward, thus elevating the sternum and ribs." The lifting of the chest wall by the distended esophagus is the most plausible explanation of the "chest movements" occurring during "esophageal ventilation."[12] A second possible mechanism is that gastric insufflation causes upward displacement of the diaphragm and outward movement of the lower chest. With release of bag compression, gas escapes from the stomach up the esophagus, allowing the diaphragm to move downward and the lower chest to move inward.[12,13]

D. AUSCULTATION OF BREATH SOUNDS

Auscultation of bilateral breath sounds is the most common method used to ensure proper tracheal tube placement. It can be done repeatedly anywhere tracheal intubation is performed and whenever changes in the position of the tube are suspected. In almost all cases, breath sounds heard near the midaxillary lines will leave very little doubt regarding the position of the tube. However, in numerous anecdotal reports, "deceptive" breath sounds were heard in cases that proved to be esophageal intubation.

There are several reasons why sounds heard with esophageal intubation may mimic breath sounds from the lungs. First, sounds produced by air movement through an esophageally placed tube may be interpreted as inspiratory or expiratory wheezes (rhonchi) and thus may be mistakenly identified as bronchospasm.[13] Studies of lung sounds suggest that wheezes are produced by oscillation of opposing walls of bronchi between the closed and barely open positions as gas flows into them.[29,30] The pitch of the note depends on the mass and elastic properties of the solid structure set into oscillation. This is further modified by the amount of acoustic filtering by the lungs and chest wall. In cases of esophageal intubation, the combination of esophageal wall oscillations with gas movement and acoustic filtering can produce wheezes indistinguishable from sounds arising from gas movement in the airway.[13,29,30] For this reason, it has been suggested that whenever breath sounds are heard that are abnormal in any manner, they should not be solely relied on to confirm successful tracheal intubation. Second, the high flow rate, distribution, and volume of gas delivered through the esophagus during compression of a breathing bag may lead to auscultation of predominantly bronchial breath sounds

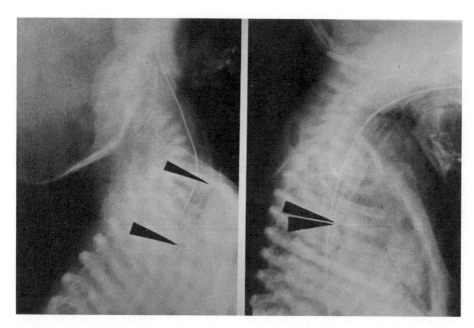

Fig. 27-4. Radiographs illustrate the effect of head position on endotracheal tube placement in newborn infants. The upper arrow indicates the tip of the endotracheal tube; the lower arrow indicates the tip of the carina. Note the marked excursion of the tip of the tube with head flexion (*right*). (From Todres ID, deBros F, Dramer SS et al: *J Pediatr* 89:126, 1976.)

and therefore may be misinterpreted as breath sounds arising from the lungs.[13] Third, the quality of breath sounds may differ depending on whether the chest is auscultated near the midline or laterally near the axilla.[12] They may also vary from patient to patient and with the presence of pulmonary disease. In infants and children, esophageal sounds can be easily transmitted to wide areas of the chest wall.[31] It should also be noted that sounds retrieved by an esophageal stethoscope are different from those heard with a precordial stethoscope and should not be used to differentiate tracheal from esophageal intubation. Fourth, in patients with a thoracic stomach or hiatal hernia, many of the clinical signs of esophageal intubation may be obscured.[17] Because of the intrathoracic location of a large size distensible viscera, bilateral breath sounds may be heard during manual ventilation.[17]

E. ENDOBRONCHIAL INTUBATION

Intentional endobronchial intubation has been used to discriminate between tracheal and esophageal intubation when doubt exists.[32] The tube is advanced until breath sounds are lost on one side, and unilateral breath sounds are heard on the other side. That should not happen if the tube is in the esophagus. The tube is then gradually withdrawn to 1 to 2 cm beyond the point at which bilateral breath sounds are heard. This technique has been used in infants and children, particularly in infants with tracheoesophageal fistulas.[33] However, it is

not recommended for routine use because it can precipitate carinal irritation and bronchospasm.[34]

F. EPIGASTRIC AUSCULTATION AND OBSERVATION FOR ABDOMINAL DISTENTION

Auscultation of the epigastric area to elicit air movement in the stomach has been recommended as a routine maneuver after tracheal intubation even before auscultating the chest.[11,15] However, normal vesicular breath sounds from the lungs can be transmitted to the epigastric area in tracheally intubated thin and small patients.[23] Consequently, on rare occasions, esophageal intubation may not be easily distinguishable from tracheal intubation if epigastric auscultation alone is used. Furthermore, there are circumstances such as obstetric emergencies, where the abdomen is prepared before induction, that preclude epigastric auscultation after intubation.

Abdominal distention caused by gastric insufflation after compression of the breathing bag in cases of esophageal intubation can be readily observed in most patients. Occasionally, this sign may not be a reliable indicator of esophageal intubation for the following reasons:[12,23,35] (1) gastric insufflation and abdominal distention might have occurred during prior mask ventilation, (2) gastric distention may not be apparent in obese patients, (3) a previously placed nasogastric tube may result in intermittent decompression of the stomach, and (4) gradual gastric filling can be difficult to distinguish from normal abdominal movements because of the esophageal reflux of gases. Conversely, gastric distention can occur in patients with congenital or acquired tracheoesophageal fistula despite the placement of a tube in the trachea.[33]

G. COMBINED AUSCULTATION OF EPIGASTRIUM AND BOTH AXILLAE

In a study of 40 adult patients who had both their trachea and esophagus intubated, blinded observers auscultating both axillae failed to diagnose esophageal intubation in 15% of cases.[36] When movement of the abdominal wall alone was used to assess tube position, false results were obtained in 90% of cases. In contrast, the combination of auscultation of the epigastrium and both axillae was found to be totally reliable in diagnosing esophageal intubation.[36] These findings emphasize the importance of combining tests to achieve a high degree of reliability in assessing tracheal tube placement.

Detection of misplaced tubes by auscultation of the chest and epigastrium is probably more difficult in infants than in adults. Uejima[31] reported two cases, a 7-month-old and a 5-year-old in whom esophageal intubation occurred. In both cases, bilateral chest movements and "breath sounds" were heard over four areas of the chest and over the epigastrium. However, these "breath sounds" were not vesicular in nature. The ease of transmission of sounds from the esophagus to the chest and epigastrium may thus mimic breath sounds, especially in infants, emphasizing again that whenever any but normal vesicular breath sounds are heard, they should not be relied on to confirm tracheal intubation.

H. RESERVOIR BAG COMPLIANCE AND REFILLING

Manual compression of the reservoir bag after tracheal intubation and cuff inflation yields a characteristic feel of the compliance of the lungs and chest wall; whereas passive exhalation on release of bag compression is accompanied by rapid bag refilling. In most esophageal intubations, compressing the reservoir bag will not inflate the chest and will not be followed by appreciable refilling. However, exceptions to this rule do occur, as has been shown in reports of accidental esophageal intubations. In these cases, repeated filling and emptying of the stomach resulted in concomitant emptying and refilling of the reservoir bag leading to the erroneous conclusion that the tube was in the trachea.[12-15,35] It is possible that high, fresh gas flow might have contributed to reservoir bag refilling in these cases. To eliminate this problem, it has been suggested that fresh gas flow is shut off temporarily during the test period. Baraka et al.[37] showed that inflation of the chest and rapid bag refilling can be repeatedly done (three to

five times in tracheally intubated patients) despite the continued interruption of the fresh gas flow. In contrast, refilling of the reservoir bag during esophageal intubation was not significant and could not be repeated if no fresh gas flow was added during the test period.

Changes in lungs or chest wall compliance may be misinterpreted by the clinician during manual compression of the reservoir bag. Similarly high airway resistance or obstruction of the tracheal tube may result in slow refilling of the breathing bag caused by slow exhalation and thus may be mistaken for esophageal intubation. For these reasons, this test alone cannot be totally relied on but can be used in conjunction with other methods.[23]

I. RESERVOIR BAG MOVEMENTS WITH SPONTANEOUS BREATHING

Movement of the reservoir bag during spontaneous breathing has been considered one of the signs indicative of tracheal intubation. Robinson[38] showed that this sign can be unreliable. In a group of anesthetized patients, the trachea and esophagus were intubated and the patients were allowed to breathe spontaneously. With the tracheal tube intentionally occluded, the high negative intrapleural pressures generated with spontaneous breathing efforts were transmitted to the esophagus, resulting in reservoir bag movements and measurable tidal volumes up to 180 ml. Therefore slight reservoir bag movements or measurements of small tidal volumes during spontaneous breathing are not reliable indicators of tracheal intubation.[38]

J. CUFF MANEUVERS AND NECK PALPATION

The higher pitched sound produced by leakage around a tube placed in the trachea with the cuff deflated during compression of the reservoir bag compared with the "flatuslike" sound of leakage around a tube placed in the esophagus has been used as a distinguishing test.[23] As has been shown in many case reports, when the cuff of an esophageally placed tube is inflated close to the cricoid cartilage, the characteristic guttural sound may be absent or may become higher pitched, resembling leakage around a tracheally placed tube.[12]

Palpation of the cuff on each side of the trachea between the cricoid cartilage and suprasternal notch while moving the tube has been proposed to confirm tracheal intubation and to ensure that the tube is not in the mainstem bronchus.[39] After intubation and cuff inflation, two or three fingers are placed above the suprasternal notch. Several rapid inflations of the cuff are performed (up to 10 ml of air). An outward force is felt by the palpating fingers if the tracheal tube is in correct position. It has been demonstrated that when the cuff is palpable, there is a high degree of confidence that the tip of the tube is greater than 2 cm from the carina;

whereas if the cuff is not palpable, the tip is precariously close to the carina.[39] Suprasternal palpation of the tube (with a stylet in it) has been also used in infants. Because it approximates the true tracheal midpoint, palpation of the distal end of the tube in the suprasternal notch between the medial ends of the clavicles, serves as a "landmark" to avoid improper positioning of the tube.[40]

Intermittent squeezing of the pilot balloon of a slightly overinflated cuff with the thumb and index finger while sensing the transmitted pulsations in the neck has been suggested as a sign for confirming tracheal tube placement.[41] A maneuver using the pilot balloon as a sensor has also been proposed.[34] After intubation, the cuff is inflated and constant pressure is applied to the pilot balloon by the index finger and thumb of one hand. A distinct increase in pressure is felt when the cuff is palpated with the other hand above the suprasternal notch. This maneuver may be more sensitive than other cuff maneuvers because pressure changes are sensed directly and not through soft tissues, and it may be safer because cuff deflation is not required.[34]

Case reports have showed that outward bulging and palpation of the cuff in the neck can also occur with inadvertent esophageal intubation.[14] In a small but controlled study, blinded observers were able to palpate the cuff above the suprasternal notch in six of seven esophageal intubations.[42] It may be concluded that a negative sign does not necessarily confirm esophageal placement of the tube because the cuff may be in the trachea but distal to the palpating fingers.[41,42] It is also possible that low-pressure, large-volume prestretched cuffs may not be palpable in the suprasternal notch despite correct tracheal tube placement.[34]

If an assistant gently palpates the trachea in the suprasternal notch or applies cricoid compression during tracheal intubation, "an old washboard-like" vibration will be appreciated as the tube rubs against the tracheal rings.[43] It has been suggested that there should be no false-positive results to this sign if the tube is misplaced in the esophagus because the esophagus is soft and lies posterior to the trachea. So far there have been no controlled studies to confirm the validity of this method.

K. SOUND OF EXPELLED GASES DURING STERNAL COMPRESSION

Pressing sharply on the sternum while listening over the proximal end of the tube to detect a characteristic feel and sound of expelled gases from the airway is occasionally used to distinguish esophageal from tracheal intubation.[12] This test is mistrusted by many because of the (1) inability to distinguish gases expelled passing through the tracheal tube from gases passing through or around a tube misplaced in the esophagus, (2) inability to distinguish gases being expelled through

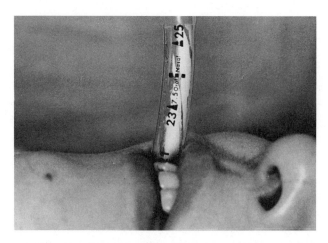

Fig. 27-5. Condensation of water vapor seen in a clear plastic tube after tracheal intubation during exhalation.

the nose, and (3) inability to distinguish esophageal and stomach gases present from prior mask ventilation.[12]

L. TUBE CONDENSATION OF WATER VAPOR

The principle of this sign is that water vapor seen in clear plastic tubes is more likely to be present in gases exhaled through a tracheally placed tube than from gases emanating from the stomach through a tube in the esophagus (Fig. 27-5). Two studies have demonstrated the observation of water condensation in all cases where tubes were placed in the trachea.[36,42] Unfortunately, water condensation can and does occur when tubes are placed in the esophagus. The fact that condensation was noticed in 85% in one study[36] and 28% in another study[42] of all cases of esophageal intubations should strongly discourage its presence from being interpreted as a reliable indicator of a successful intubation.

M. ELECTRONIC METAL DETECTORS

Cullen et al.[44] described an electromagnetic sensing technique allowing detection of a flexible circumferential foil marker band, 3-mm wide, 25 μm thick, weighing 50 mg, fused into the tracheal tube at the proximal cuff-tube junction (Fig. 27-6). This method is relatively insensitive to proximity of extraneous metallic objects and is unaffected by conducting fluids and tissue. Testing of this method demonstrated excellent correlation between the position of the foil band as detected by the electronic detector and that determined by chest radiographs. Furthermore, the detector allowed accurate location of the foil band with respect to external anatomic landmarks in the neck.[44] The cricothyroid membrane served as the most useful reference point because of its easy identification in the neck. Because the distance from the vocal cords to the cricothyroid membrane is about 1 cm in the adult, cuff location is assumed to be below the cords when the band is detected

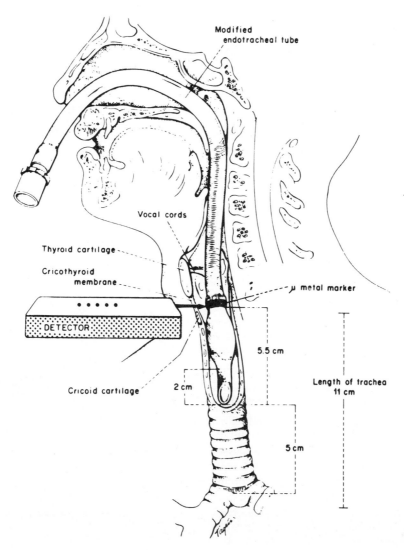

Fig. 27-6. The electronic metal detector is placed over the skin at the cricothyroid membrane to detect the micrometal marker of the endotracheal tube. Note that this places the cuff of the endotracheal tube below the vocal cords, while the tip of the tube is approximately 5 cm above the carina in the adult. (From Cullen DJ, Newbower RS, Gemer M: *Anesthesiology* 43:596, 1975.)

at the cricothyroid membrane. In this position the tube will not encroach on the carina or the right mainstem bronchus. Claimed advantages of the detector include:[44] avoidance of carinal stimulation and endobronchial intubation; the position of the tube can be checked repeatedly, especially when head position is altered; and the need for chest radiographs in the critical care setting may be decreased or eliminated. Although this method was devised primarily to ensure location of the tube in the trachea, it has been claimed that it would not yield a false reading in the event of esophageal intubation because the marker will be beyond the range of the detector.[44] However, such a study has not been done. Despite the potential usefulness of such a device, this method has not gained wide popularity.

N. VIDEO STETHOSCOPE

In search of a noninvasive method of ascertaining bilateral lung ventilation continuously, Huang et al.[45] introduced the concept of a "video stethoscope." A small plastic electrocardiographic electrode casing fitted with a microphone was affixed to the skin overlying each hemithorax in a location previously determined by auscultation of breath sounds. From each microphone the sounds were amplified and displayed on an oscilloscope screen. The distinct patterns seen allowed easy and quick identification of proper tracheal tube placement, mainstem bronchus intubation, and esophageal intubation.[45] The device permitted continuous bilateral auscultation of the chest during the operative procedure regardless of the size of the sterile field or the position of the patient. It also offered monitoring of breath sounds without the use of the earpiece, which can be uncomfortable and sometimes restricting within the operating room.

As in any electronic system, malfunction of this type of monitoring system is a possibility. Should an amplifier malfunction or the microphone become displaced, the observed pattern would simulate that of endobronchial intubation.[45] Although this technique is feasible and can provide valuable information, its testing has been limited to 25 patients, none of whom had lung disease. Furthermore, the number of patients in whom esophageal and mainstem intubation occurred was not mentioned. Obviously, before such a method can be adopted in clinical practice, it must be tested in a larger number of patients.

O. USE OF NASOGASTRIC TUBES, GASTRIC ASPIRATES, INTRODUCERS, AND OTHER DEVICES

A test devised to distinguish between placement of a tube in the trachea and a tube in the esophagus involves threading a lubricated nasogastric tube through the tube in question, applying continuous suction, and attempting to withdraw the nasogastric tube.[46] This test exploits the distinguishing features that the esophagus will collapse around the nasogastric tube when suction is applied, whereas free suction continues if applied in the trachea. In a study of 20 patients in whom both the trachea and esophagus were intubated, the ability to maintain suction and the ease of withdrawal while continuous suction is applied clearly distinguished between the two positions.[46] When the nasogastric tube was in the trachea, suction applied to it could be maintained easily because the trachea remained patent and air was entrained through the open end of the tube. This allowed the nasogastric tube to be withdrawn easily despite suctioning. In contrast, when suction was applied to the nasogastric tube in the esophagus, the esophageal wall collapsed around it, thereby obstructing suction, and interfered with easy withdrawal of the nasogastric tube.[46]

Although the length of the nasogastric tube that could be easily inserted in conjunction with feeling an impediment or resistance (5- to 15-cm distal to the tip of the tube) identified correct tracheal placement, it was found less useful in identifying esophageal intubation.[46] Similarly, the nature of the aspirate (mucus vs. bile or gastric juice) was found to be of limited value in most patients.[46] Because the total time spent to make these observations was 20 to 30 seconds, the authors concluded that the test is safe and reliable.[46] Despite their enthusiasm, this test is very rarely used because of the availability of other methods but may have a place when other tests are unavailable.

The Eschmann introducer is a 60-cm long device

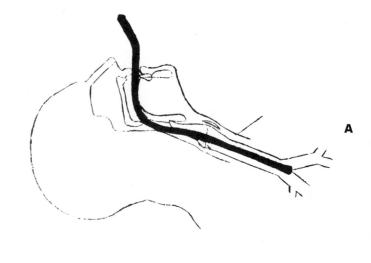

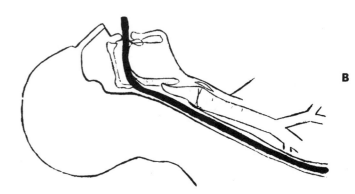

Fig. 27-7. A, Eschmann introducer in trachea. **B,** Eschmann introducer in esophagus. (From Birmingham PK, Cheney FW, Ward RJ: *Anesth Analg* 65:886, 1986.)

composed of two layers: a core of tube woven from Dacron polyester threads and an outer resin layer to provide stiffness; flexibility; and a slippery, water impervious surface.[47] Frequently, the device is referred to as a "gum elastic bougie"—despite the fact that it is not gum, elastic, or a bougie.[47] It has a 35-degree kink 2.5 cm from its distal end. Because its external diameter is 5 mm, it can be used with tracheal tubes with an inner diameter ≥ 6 mm. The device has been used for many years to facilitate intubation[47] and has recently been introduced to differentiate tracheal from esophageal intubation in emergencies when there is doubt about the location of the tube.[23]

When inserted through the lumen of the tube, the curved tip of the lubricated introducer may be felt rubbing over the tracheal rings, and resistance is encountered as the tip of the introducer meets the carina or a mainstem bronchus at approximately 28 to 32 cm in the adult.[23] If the tube is in the esophagus, the introducer passes without resistance to the distal end of the esophagus or stomach (Fig. 27-7).[23] As yet, there are no studies verifying the reliability and safety of this technique in a large number of patients. Forceful insertion of an excessive length of the introducer could conceivably result in bronchial rupture or other injuries.[47] This led the manufacturer to discourage its use as a tracheal tube changer because other devices specifically designed for this purpose are now available.

P. USE OF FLEXIBLE FIBEROPTIC LARYNGOSCOPES AND BRONCHOSCOPES

A sure method for confirmation of tracheal intubation is visualization of the tracheal rings and carina with a fiberoptic scope after intubation.[48,49] This is only convenient when a fiberoptic scope is readily available or when the instrument is used to aid intubation (see Chapter 16). It should be emphasized that visualization of the vocal cords and tracheal rings through the fiberoptic scope before threading the tube over it does not guarantee the passage of the tube into the trachea. There are three reasons why the tube may not follow the path of the scope into the trachea.[49-52] First, a stiff, large tube may carry a relatively thin scope into the esophagus even though the tip of the scope was placed in the larynx and trachea.[49,50] Second, the tip of the tube and its Murphy eye are at 90 degrees to the right when the concavity of the tube is facing anteriorly.[49,51] Consequently, the tip of the tube may be blocked from entering the larynx by the right arytenoid cartilage, vocal cord, or both. If excessive force is used, the tube may slip into the esophagus. The problem can be corrected by a 90-degree counterclockwise rotation.[49,51] Third, if the scope is inserted through a nasal tube (used as a conduit for nasal intubation), the scope may exit the tube through the Murphy eye and may actually enter the trachea, but it will be impossible to thread the tube over the scope.[49,52] To ensure that tracheal intubation has been accomplished, the scope should be withdrawn after placement of the tube and then reintroduced to visualize the tracheal rings and carina and to determine the distance from the distal end of the tube to the carina.[49] The use of fiberoptic scopes has been extended to critical care units to evaluate the position of the tip of the tracheal tube in relation to the carina and to obviate the necessity for frequent chest radiographs.[48]

Q. TRANSTRACHEAL ILLUMINATION

Clinical trials have demonstrated the usefulness of the lighted stylet (lightwand) in facilitating oral and nasal intubation[53-56] (see Chapter 18). The success of transillumination of the soft tissues of the neck anterior to the trachea in accomplishing guided intubation has culminated into the development of improved lighted stylets and introducers. It also prompted investigators to use transtracheal illumination to differentiate esophageal from tracheal tube placement and to position the tube accurately inside the trachea but above the carina.

Transmission of light through tissues depends on thickness, compactness, color, density, and light absorption characteristics of the tissue; wavelength, quality, and intensity of light; proximity of the tissue to the light source; and the ambient lighting condition in the room.[56] Typically tracheal intubation with the lighted stylet inside the tube or placement of the stylet in the lumen of the tube after intubation gives off an intense circumscribed midline glow in the region of the laryngeal prominence and sternal notch. The illumination is mostly seen opposite the thyrohyoid, cricothyroid, and cricotracheal membranes. In the event of esophageal intubation, the light is either absent or is perceived as dull and diffuse.

To enhance transillumination, darkening the room, dimming the overhead lights, or cricoid pressure (to approximate the tracheal wall to the light source and stretching the soft tissues anterior to the light source) have been recommended.[53-56] Newer lighted stylets, both battery operated or using a fiberoptic light source, have brighter lights than earlier prototypes. Consequently, dimming the overhead lights or cricoid pressure may not be necessary. Recently, a flexible intubation guide equipped with a fiberoptic bundle to illuminate its tip with a light source has been developed* (Fig. 27-8). The lubricated device is placed inside a previously cut-to-length lubricated tube so that the guide extends a minimum of 2 inches beyond the distal end of the tube when the 15-mm connector is seated in the adapter located in the guide handle. With a proximal thumb ring, the operator can maneuver the distal tip anteriorly or in any desired direction. When the introducer enters the trachea, transillumination is observed as with the lighted stylet. After the guide is advanced 2 to 3 inches in the trachea, the tube is slipped over the guide into the desired tracheal position (Fig. 27-9).

The reliability of transtracheal illumination in distinguishing esophageal from tracheal intubation in adults has been demonstrated.[56,57] In one study conducted on five cadavers only 1 of 56 intratracheal placements was misidentified as esophageal, whereas of 112 extratracheal placements (esophageal or pyriform fossa), 1 was misidentified as intratracheal.[57] In another study of 420 adult patients, tracheal transillumination was graded as excellent in 81% of patients and as good in the remaining 19%.[56] In contrast, transesophageal illumination could not be demonstrated in any patient. The authors noted occasional false-negative results (tube in trachea, but no transillumination) with the use of the newer lighted stylets and introducers in patients with neck swelling or dark skin and in obese patients. Similarly, occasional false-positive results have been noted in thin patients. Nonetheless, the use of transillumination could reduce,

---

*Lighted Flexguide. Scientific Sales International, Kalamazoo, Michigan.

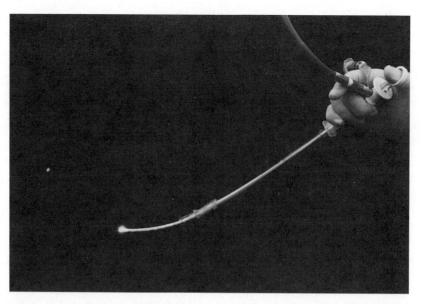

Fig. 27-8. The new Flexguide incorporates a fiberoptic bundle that can illuminate the distal tip of the device when connected to a light source through a connector in its handle. By manipulating the thumb ring, the operator can direct the lighted distal tip into the larynx.

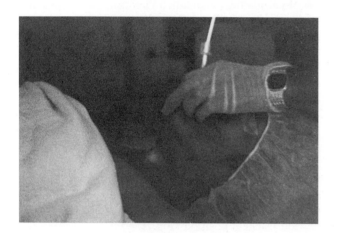

Fig. 27-9. When the lighted Flexguide enters the larynx, an intense circumscribed midline glow seen in the region of the laryngeal prominence is suggestive of tracheal intubation. After the guide is advanced in the trachea, the tube is slipped over the guide into the desired tracheal position.

if not eliminate, unrecognized esophageal intubation especially outside the operating room where other technical aids are not available.[56,57]

Transillumination can accurately help position the tracheal tube tip at a reliable distance above the carina. Two methods have been suggested. In one the flexible lighted stylet is placed inside the tube so that the stylet bulb is positioned at the tube's distal opening before intubation. By observing the maximal illumination glow at the sternal notch (a consistent anatomic landmark) during intubation, the tip of the tube could be placed consistently 5.0 ± 1.0 cm from the carina.[58] In the other, the tip of the lighted stylet is placed inside the tube just proximal to the cuff before intubation.[56] Visualization of

maximum transillumination distal to the cricoid cartilage is indicative of proper cuff positioning. In this position the distance between the tip of the tracheal tube and the carina varied between 3.7 and 4 cm in adults.[56] Use of either method could reduce the need for radiographic confirmation of the tracheal tube position in the critically injured.

Reports delineated several complications with these lighted stylets.[59-61] Loss of the bulb into the lung necessitating bronchoscopic removal has been reported.[59] A change in design involving encasing the bulb in a plastic retaining cover has virtually eliminated the possibility of this complication recurring.[53] Other reports described arytenoid subluxation.[60,61] However, no evidence exists that there is increased incidence of this complication with the use of lighted stylets because it can also occur after conventional intubation.

R. PULSE OXIMETRY AND DETECTION OF CYANOSIS

Although unrecognized esophageal intubation will ultimately lead to severe decreases in oxygen saturation (and detectable cyanosis), minutes may lapse before this happens. A disturbing finding that emerged from the ASA Closed Claims Study is that detection of esophageal intubation required 5 minutes or more in 97% of cases.[1] Furthermore, detectable cyanosis preceded the recognition of esophageal intubation in only 34% of cases. Several factors contribute to this delay (Box 27-4).

Reliance on the appearance of cyanosis as a clue to esophageal intubation can contribute to such a delay. Recognition of cyanosis usually necessitates the presence of greater than 5 g/dl of reduced hemoglobin, which

---

BOX 27-4   Factors contributing to delay of pulse oximetry in diagnosing esophageal intubation

Appearance of normal function of the ventilator

Reliance on appearance of cyanosis and lack of its recognition (anemia and infants)

Preoxygenation causing delay in decrease in SaO_2

Decrease in oxygen consumption, increased cardiac output, or both, retarding the decrease in SaO_2

Mechanical ventilation of the esophagus resulting in alveolar gas exchange

Leakage around the cuff yielding apneic oxygenation through relaxed cords

Respiratory efforts by the patient (air breathing through the unintubated trachea)

---

corresponds to an oxygen saturation between 75% and 85%.[62] Nonetheless, the detection may also depend on the concentration and type of hemoglobin and the observer's own interpretations. With severe anemia, cyanosis may not be apparent until the oxygen saturation falls to 60%. Conversely, cyanosis is usually detectable at oxygen saturation between 80% and 85%, when the hemoglobin concentration is normal or elevated. The infant with a high proportion of fetal hemoglobin may still look "pink" at a PaO_2 near 40 mm Hg because of the increased blood affinity of oxygen and leftward shifting of the fetal oxyhemoglobin dissociation curve and thus a serious reduction in PaO_2 may develop before cyanosis is apparent. Recognition of cyanosis is influenced by the limited exposure of the patient's body and the insensitivity of the human eye to changes in skin color or even the color of the blood that occurs during arterial desaturation. It could also be affected by variations in room lighting and the color of the surgical drapes.

Noninvasive monitoring of oxygen saturation (SaO_2) by pulse oximetry has proven to be a reliable indicator of arterial hemoglobin saturation.[63,64] It is undoubtedly quicker to detect accurate changes in SaO_2 by pulse oximetry than to rely on clinical detection of cyanosis. The main limitation of pulse oximetry is that it does not measure PaO_2, which may fall long before SaO_2 is affected in case of interruption of oxygen delivery. Because pulse oximetry provides continuous reliable information and is simple to use, it has gained wide popularity, and its use has proliferated to areas outside the operating rooms such as intensive care units, emergency rooms, hospital floors, and trauma scenes.

Oxygenation of the patient's lungs, which is commonly practiced before intubation, may extend the period of time before a significant decrease in SaO_2 occurs. In general, oxygen deprivation or apnea after air breathing results in a substantial fall in PaO_2 in 90 seconds; whereas PaO_2, after oxygen breathing, will remain above 100 mm Hg for at least 3 minutes of apnea and thus SaO_2 will not

change during this period.[62] Consequently, pulse oximetry after preoxygenation will not immediately indicate that the esophagus has been intubated.[65] Because of this prolonged interval with normal SaO_2 being recorded initially after the intubation attempt, misplacement of the tube may not be suspected later when SaO_2 begins to decrease.[1,65] Furthermore, the risk of misinterpretation of clinical findings suggestive of esophageal intubation may be greater when other clues such as decrease in SaO_2 or cyanosis are not yet manifest.[1] This "hazard" of preoxygenation has led some clinicians to abandon such a practice before intubation so that the recognition of esophageal intubation would be more readily appreciated.[66] One does not need to go to such extremes as to abandon a practice that has definite merits. However, it must be borne in mind that normal pulse oximetry readings after intubation should not be taken as evidence of successful tracheal intubation and that after preoxygenation desaturation as indicated by pulse oximetry is a relatively late manifestation of esophageal intubation.[1,65-68]

Both oxygen consumption and cardiac output can influence the SaO_2 through their effect on mixed venous oxygen tension ($P\bar{v}O_2$) and mixed venous oxygen content ($C\bar{v}O_2$).[62] A decrease in oxygen consumption associated with anesthetic induction, an increase in cardiac output, or both will lead to an increase in $P\bar{v}O_2$ and $C\bar{v}O_2$. The high $P\bar{v}O_2$ will retard the decrease in PaO_2 in the event of oxygen deprivation resulting from esophageal intubation and consequently may delay its recognition. Conversely in patients with low SaO_2 and in patients whose oxygen consumption is high (children, women in labor, and the morbidly obese), the onset of cyanosis and hemoglobin desaturation may occur faster.

With the vocal cords open, manual ventilation into the esophagus can result in alveolar gas exchange. In 18 of the 20 patients studied by Linko et al.[35] after intentional intubation of both the esophagus and trachea, ventilation into the esophagus caused cyclic compression of the lungs by the distending stomach and esophagus, leading to gas exchange evidenced by CO_2 recording at the proximal end of the tracheal tube. Although in this situation esophageal ventilation causes ventilation of the lungs with room air, it will considerably delay the onset of cyanosis and oxyhemoglobin desaturation.[35] Similarly respiratory efforts by the spontaneously breathing patient through the unintubated trachea may delay the recognition of esophageal intubation. Esophageal ventilation may also be effective in yielding apneic oxygenation if the cords are open and there is a leak around the cuff of the misplaced esophageal tube.

S. IDENTIFICATION OF CARBON DIOXIDE IN EXHALED GAS

The availability of capnometry (measurement of CO_2 in expired gas) and capnography (instantaneous display of the CO_2 waveform during the respiratory cycle) for intraoperative monitoring has prompted clinicians to extend their use to facilitate detection of esophageal intubation.[35,67,69-72] The principle of use stems from the fact that exhaled CO_2 can be reliably detected during controlled or spontaneous ventilation in patients with adequate pulmonary flow whose trachea is properly intubated, whereas no CO_2 would be detected from gases emanating from a tube in the esophagus. Some studies revealed that capnography and pulse oximetry could avert more than 80% of mishaps considered preventable.[73] In an amendment to its original basic intraoperative monitoring standards the ASA stated:* "When an endotracheal tube is inserted, its correct positioning in the trachea must be verified by clinical assessment and by identification of carbon dioxide in the expired gas. End-tidal CO_2 analysis, in use from the time of endotracheal tube placement, is strongly encouraged."

Identification of CO_2 in the exhaled gas has emerged as the standard for verification of proper tracheal tube placement. Furthermore, interruption of CO_2 sampling in the exhaled gas because of disconnection, obstruction, accidental tracheal extubation or total loss of ventilation will be immediately detected. Two main methods are currently used: CO_2 waveform (capnography) and colorimetric detection of CO_2.

1. Capnography

Currently available CO_2 analyzers use various principles to measure CO_2 in the inspired and exhaled gases on a breath-to-breath basis and display the CO_2 waveform: (1) mass spectrometry, (2) infrared absorption spectrometry, and (3) Raman scattering. A normal capnographic waveform in relation to the respiratory cycle is shown in Fig. 27-10.[74] A mass spectrometric tracing showing a CO_2 waveform after esophageal intubation and after correct placement of the tube in the trachea is shown in Fig. 27-11. Although capnography typically distinguishes tracheal from esophageal intubation, false-negative results (tube in trachea, absent waveform) and false-positive results (tube in esophagus or pharynx, present waveform) have been reported (Box 27-5).

Since the advent of capnography in confirming tracheal tube placement, there have been reports of markedly different problems yielding unexpected false-negative results. Disconnection of the tracheal tube from the breathing apparatus, apnea, and equipment failure may be misinterpreted as absent waveform caused by esophageal intubation.[75] A kinked or obstructed tracheal tube will interfere with sampling of exhaled gas and may lead to an absent or distorted waveform. Lack

*Standards for basic intraoperative monitoring. 1994 directory of members. American Society of Anesthesiologists, Park Ridge, Ill, p 736.

NORMAL CAPNOGRAM

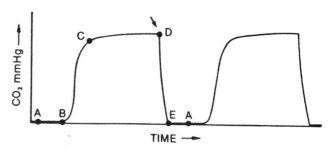

Fig. 27-10. The CO_2 waveform. *A*, Expiratory pause begins. *A→B*, Clearance of anatomic dead space. *B→C*, Dead space air mixed with alveolar air. *C→D*, Alveolar plateau. *D*, Level of end-tidal CO_2 (arrow indicates end-tidal CO_2 registered by capnogram) and beginning of inspiratory phase. *D→E*, Clearance of dead space air. *E→A*, Inspiratory gas devoid of CO_2.

of a CO_2 waveform because of severe bronchospasm has also been reported.[75] Unintentional application of PEEP to a loosely fitted or uncuffed tracheal tube may cause exhaled gases to escape around the distal lumen of the tube and result in a sampling error and absent waveform.[76] Dilution of exhaled gases by high fresh gas flow in a Mapleson D system when proximal sidestream sampling is used in infants less than 10 kg will lead to erroneous sampling.[77,78] This problem could be corrected by distal sampling from the tracheal tube, up to 12 cm mark; use of a mainstream sampling device; or use of special ventilators.[78] Dilution of exhaled gases with fresh gas flow have also been demonstrated during use of the Dryden disposable absorber in adult patients.[79] This dilution can be similarly corrected by distal sampling or by alteration of absorber design.[79] Lower sampling flow rates[80] and gas sampling line leaks[81] can result in artifactually low exhaled CO_2 values and an abnormal waveform.

Marked diminution of pulmonary blood flow will increase the alveolar component of the dead space.[62,82] Low cardiac output, hypotension, pulmonary embolism, pulmonary stenosis, tetralogy of Fallot, and kinking or clamping of the pulmonary artery during pulmonary surgery all cause a decrease in P_{ETCO_2}, reflecting an increase in alveolar dead space.[62,83] Other factors contributing to the increased alveolar dead space during anesthesia include patient age, tidal volume, use of negative phase during exhalation, short inspiratory phase, and the presence of pulmonary disease.[62,83] As a result of the widespread destruction of alveolar capillaries in patients with chronic obstructive lung disease, an increased alveolar dead space ensues. An increase in alveolar dead space is manifested as a decrease in

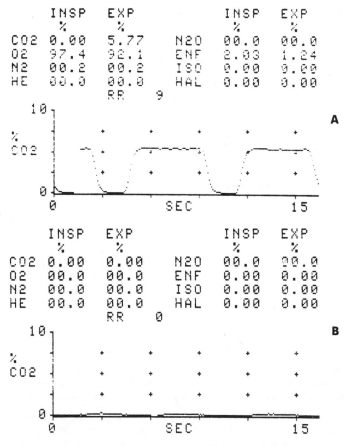

```
      INSP   EXP              INSP   EXP
       %      %                %      %
CO2   0.00   5.77      N2O    00.0   00.0
O2    97.4   92.1      ENF    2.03   1.24
N2    00.2   00.2      ISO    0.00   0.00
HE    00.0   00.0      HAL    0.00   0.00
                RR       9
```

                                              A

```
      INSP   EXP              INSP   EXP
       %      %                %      %
CO2   0.00   0.00      N2O    00.0   00.0
O2    00.0   00.0      ENF    0.00   0.00
N2    00.0   00.0      ISO    0.00   0.00
HE    00.0   00.0      HAL    0.00   0.00
                RR       0
```

                                              B

Fig. 27-11. A, Normal capnograph, tube in trachea. **B,** Absent capnograph, tube in esophagus.

$PETCO_2$ and an increase in $PaCO_2$ to $PETCO_2$ difference (normally 0 to 5 mm Hg).[62,83] If one depends on capnography alone in confirming tracheal tube placement in patients who have a very large alveolar dead space, the low $PETCO_2$ values might mislead the clinician into thinking that the tube was not placed in the trachea.

Provided that alveolar ventilation and CO_2 production are constant, changes in $PETCO_2$ should reflect changes in pulmonary blood flow (and cardiac output).[82,84] When cardiac arrest ensues, CO_2 will no longer be delivered to, or eliminated through, the lungs, even if ventilation is adequate and consequently $PETCO_2$ values may be remarkably low (<0.5%). Trevino et al.[85] demonstrated a 90% decrease in $PETCO_2$ 90 seconds after experimentally induced ventricular fibrillation. Thus a decision regarding the location of the tracheal tube on the basis of capnography findings alone during cardiac arrest may lead to a misdiagnosis.

Experimental cardiac arrest studies demonstrated a remarkably high correlation between $PETCO_2$, cardiac output, and coronary perfusion pressure during both closed-chest precordial compression, open-chest cardiac massage, and after resuscitation.[86,87] Similar observations were reported during episodes of cardiac arrest in critically ill patients.[87,88] The restoration of spontaneous circulation was heralded by a rapid increase in $PETCO_2$ within 30 seconds. This overshoot in $PETCO_2$, which is

---

BOX 27-5   Capnography

False-negative results
  Gas sampling problems
    Disconnection
    Apnea
    Equipment failure
    Kinked or obstructed tracheal tube
    Unintentional PEEP to a loosely fitted or uncuffed
      tube
    Dilution of proximal sampling by fresh gas flow in
      Mapleson D systems and Dryden absorber
    Low sampling flow rates
    Gas sampling line leaks
  Patient problems
    Severe upper- or lower-airway obstruction
    Very large alveolar dead space
      Low cardiac output, severe hypotension
      Obstruction of pulmonary circulation
        Embolism, pulmonary atresia, or stenosis; sur-
          gical interruption
      Severe lung disease
    Cardiac arrest
False-positive results
  Bag-and-mask ventilation before intubation
  After ingestion of antacids or carbonated beverages
    (Coke, 7-UP, carbonated mineral water)
  Tube in pharynx

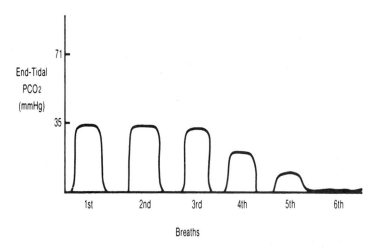

Fig. 27-12. CO_2 waveforms obtained in a 10-year-old boy with an esophageal intubation. The waveform of the first three breaths looks virtually normal before becoming flat very quickly. (From Sum Ping ST: *Anesth Analg* 66:481, 1987.)

characteristic of successful resuscitation, may exceed the prearrest value and reflects washout of CO_2 that accumulated in venous blood and in tissues during circulatory arrest.[87,88] In patients in whom resuscitative efforts failed to restore spontaneous circulation, P_{ETCO_2} remained low or even declined. These observations suggest that capnography can be used for monitoring the adequacy of blood flow generated by precordial compression during cardiopulmonary resuscitation and can serve as a prognostic indicator of successful resuscitation.[87,88]

False-positive results can occur when the tube is misplaced in the esophagus after exhaled gases are forced into the stomach during bag-and-mask ventilation preceding intubation attempts.[35,89] If enough alveolar gas reaches the stomach, CO_2 concentration higher than 2% may be initially detected, and the CO_2 waveform may be indistinguishable from that of tracheal intubation.[35,89,90] In fact, CO_2 waveforms have been observed in one third of esophageal intubations,[90] but repeated ventilation will result in rapidly diminishing CO_2 levels while the waveform becomes rather flat and irregular (Fig. 27-12).[35,89] As a result of the dilution with successive ventilation, it is very unlikely that any CO_2 would be detected after the sixth breath or after 1 minute in case of esophageal intubation, thus making it easy to distinguish esophageal from tracheal intubation.[35] Linko et al.[35] also observed that compression of the chest caused clear, peaked CO_2 elevation in 18 of 20 tracheally intubated patients but no changes in esophageal intubation. This simple, quick maneuver together with other signs can confirm proper tracheal tube placement.

False-positive results can potentially occur in the case of esophageal intubation after ingestion of carbonated beverages or antacids.[91-93] High CO_2 levels (20%) are present in all carbonated beverages.[91] Sodium bicarbon-

ate, an ingredient found in most antacids (except sodium citrate) reacts with hydrochloric acid in the stomach, releasing CO_2 levels comparable to that found in alveolar gas. With carbonated beverages, CO_2 levels as high as 5.3% can be measured initially, with esophageal ventilation rendering correct assessment of tracheal tube placement rather difficult.[91] However, rapid decline in CO_2 levels occurs with successive ventilations (Fig. 27-13). The abnormal CO_2 waveform may give an important clue in the early detection of esophageal intubation.[91] Because the observation of a normal-looking CO_2 waveform during the first few ventilations is no guarantee of correct tube placement, the waveform must be watched closely for at least 1 minute after placement of the tube.

It should be emphasized that a normal waveform is not synonymous with "the tube in the trachea."[89] A normal waveform may be observed without a tube being in the trachea during spontaneous or controlled ventilation in the following situations: face mask anesthesia, the use of laryngeal mask airway, and the use of the esophageal tracheal Combitube because ventilation will be carried out through the pharyngeal perforations.[94] A normal waveform may also be present and sustained if the distal end of the tracheal tube is in the pharynx, but not necessarily in the trachea.[95] This should be suspected by the unusual volume of cuff air required to stop the leak and an increased peak inspiratory pressure.

Although capnography has been widely used in operating rooms, its use in emergency rooms, intensive care units, and hospital floors have been rather limited for the following reasons: (1) need for warmup and careful calibration time, (2) requirement of an external power source that further decreases the ability to be used in emergency situations, and (3) it is not easily transferable to the patient's side. Portable apnea moni-

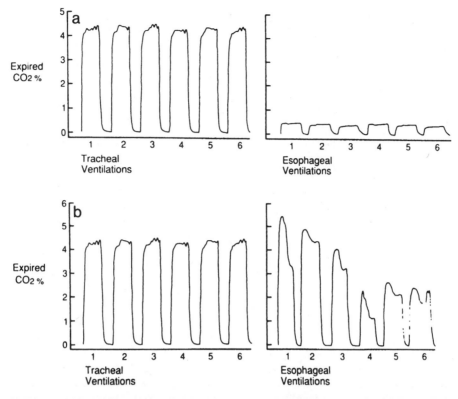

Fig. 27-13. Expired CO_2 waveform during tracheal and esophageal ventilations before (**a**) and after (**b**) addition of a carbonated beverage in the stomach. (From Sum Ping ST, Mehta MP, Symreng T: *Anesth Analg* 73:333, 1991.)

tors that use infrared spectrometry for sensing CO_2 have been used for confirmation of tracheal tube placement.[96] Although they do not accurately quantify CO_2 concentration, a moving-bar indicator with seven light-emitting diodes does provide an estimate of 1.5 percentage points per illuminated diode. Gas is aspirated through plastic tubing attached to the elbow connector proximal to the tracheal tube (Fig. 27-14), allowing it to sense CO_2 in the first exhalation after intubation. The device is cheap, portable, operates for 90 minutes by batteries, and requires neither warmup time nor calibration. This electronic instrument can also function as a breathing circuit disconnection alarm.[96]

2. Colorimetric end-tidal carbon dioxide detection

Early studies attempted to use techniques to quantitate the amount of CO_2 in exhaled gas and relied on the reaction of CO_2 with another substance such as barium hydroxide to produce a color change.[97] Berman et al.[98] introduced the Einstein CO_2 detector, which is based on the use of chemical indicators that change colors in the presence of increased hydrogen ion concentrations. The device was constructed by attaching a 15-mm adapter to one end of a De Lee mucus trap containing a mixture of 3 ml phenolphthalein and 3 ml cresol. When the exhaled gas is bubbled through the chamber, carbonic acid

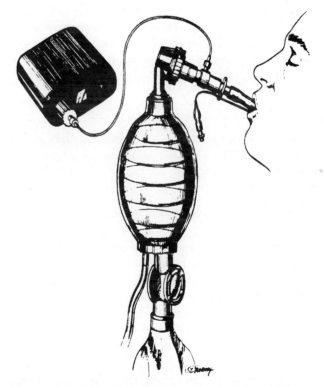

Fig. 27-14. Configuration used to sample exhaled gas from an endotracheal tube. (From Owen RL, Cheney FW: *Respir Care* 30:974, 1985.)

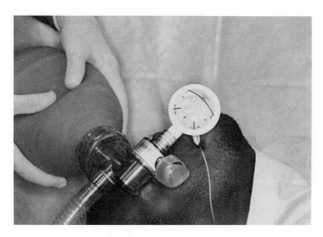

Fig. 27-15. The colorimetric carbon dioxide detector.

formation causes a dramatic color change from red to yellow within seconds. Failure of the solution to change from red to yellow should suggest esophageal intubation.[98]

A disposable CO_2 detector device (Easy Cap Endtidal CO_2 Detector)* that can be connected between a tracheal tube and a breathing circuit or a bag-and-mask assembly is now available (Fig. 27-15).[99-105] The detector contains filter paper impregnated with a colorless liquid base and pH-sensitive indicator (metacresol purple) that reversibly changes from purple to yellow as a result of pH change when exposed to CO_2 and reverts to purple when CO_2 is no longer present. The color changes are made visible through a transparent dome in the plastic housing unit of the device. In general, a purple color ("A" range) indicates CO_2 level of $\leq .5\%$. The "B" range is a dusty tan color, reflecting CO_2 levels between .5% and 2%. When the detector is exposed to CO_2 levels higher than 2%, the color brightens to a yellow-tan color, the "C" range.

Studies have shown that colorimetric P_{ETCO_2} monitoring is reliable in verifying proper tracheal tube placement in nonarrested patients.[99-105] In one study,[100] the mean minimum CO_2 concentration required for detection of the perceivable color change was .54% (4.1 mm Hg) and ranged from .25% to .60% (1.9 to 4.6 mm Hg). When a tracheal tube is correctly placed in a patient with adequate pulmonary blood flow, the detector should register "C". The color change occurs immediately with the first breath in almost all patients. In the nonarrested patient when the device registers low or absent CO_2 ("A" reading), esophageal intubation should be strongly suspected. If a "C" is obtained in an arrested patient, proper tube placement is confirmed. In contrast, an "A" reading (absence of color change) during manual ventilation in a patient with cardiac arrest is consistent with either an esophageal or a tracheal intubation in

*Nellcor, Inc., New York, NY.

patients with profound low-flow state resulting from prolonged arrest or inadequate resuscitation. In a recent study, for 28 of 106 tracheal intubations in "pulseless" patients, the detector did not show any color change, indicating a $Paco_2$ less than 4 mm Hg.[101] A multicenter trial of a colorimetric CO_2 detection device found that all cardiac arrest patients who survived to admission had a value of "C" registered on the monitor.[106] In another study, no patient in whom the detector failed to register color change survived. Thus the device may be useful as a prognostic indicator of successful resuscitation from cardiac arrest.[101]

Although the availability of such a device is considered a great leap forward, it has its own pitfalls and thus is not a substitute for the need of assessment skills. The manufacturer suggests an algorithm in case of color ranges, A, B, and C (Fig. 27-16). Following such an algorithm certainly detracts from the simplicity of the detector. Because the device has a dead space of 38 ml, the manufacturer does not recommend its use in children weighing less than 15 kg, although its efficacy in confirming tracheal intubation has been confirmed in infants older than 6 months.[107] The color change may be difficult to discern under low light conditions and may be misinterpreted by color-blind individuals. The color chart in the detector dome is color matched to fluorescent lighting. The manufacturer provides a separate color chart for use in lighting other than fluorescent, such as incandescent lighting.

Although the detector is not sensitive to temperature, it is eventually affected by humidity. Water vapor interferes with the chemical reaction and inactivates the device. It can be rendered ineffective within 15 minutes if the patient is receiving humidified gases.[108] It has been suggested that trapping the humidity with a passive moisture exchanger may extend the useful life of the device.[107] The manufacturer cautions against the use of the device in conjunction with a heated humidifier or nebulizer and emphasizes that it is not intended to be used for longer than 10 minutes after intubation. Because the indicator will permanently change colors if exposed for prolonged period to low CO_2 or other acids in the air, the device is packaged in a gas-impermeable metallic foil and is marketed as a one-time-one-use item. The packaged detector has a shelf-life of 15 months if left unopened but may not function properly if the package is accidentally opened and the device is exposed to room air for several hours. For this reason it is essential to verify that the indicator color is purple before use.

Widespread use of colorimetric CO_2 detectors has been hampered by limitations in its performance characteristics. However, a promising new colorimetric CO_2 indicator seems to have overcome some of these limitations.[109] With this improved technology,[109] it is expected that newer colorimetric CO_2 detectors will be

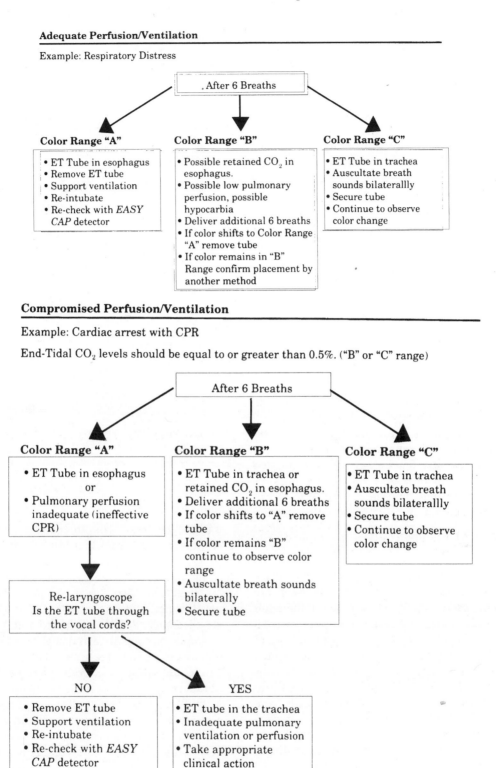

Adequate Perfusion/Ventilation

Example: Respiratory Distress

After 6 Breaths

Color Range "A"
- ET Tube in esophagus
- Remove ET tube
- Support ventilation
- Re-intubate
- Re-check with *EASY CAP* detector

Color Range "B"
- Possible retained CO_2 in esophagus.
- Possible low pulmonary perfusion, possible hypocarbia
- Deliver additional 6 breaths
- If color shifts to Color Range "A" remove tube
- If color remains in "B" Range confirm placement by another method

Color Range "C"
- ET Tube in trachea
- Auscultate breath sounds bilaterallly
- Secure tube
- Continue to observe color change

Compromised Perfusion/Ventilation

Example: Cardiac arrest with CPR

End-Tidal CO_2 levels should be equal to or greater than 0.5%. ("B" or "C" range)

After 6 Breaths

Color Range "A"
- ET Tube in esophagus
  or
- Pulmonary perfusion inadequate (ineffective CPR)

Re-laryngoscope
Is the ET tube through the vocal cords?

NO
- Remove ET tube
- Support ventilation
- Re-intubate
- Re-check with *EASY CAP* detector

YES
- ET tube in the trachea
- Inadequate pulmonary ventilation or perfusion
- Take appropriate clinical action

Color Range "B"
- ET Tube in trachea or retained CO_2 in esophagus.
- Deliver additional 6 breaths
- If color shifts to "A" remove tube
- If color remains "B" continue to observe color range
- Auscultate breath sounds bilaterally
- Secure tube

Color Range "C"
- ET Tube in trachea
- Auscultate breath sounds bilaterallly
- Secure tube
- Continue to observe color change

Fig. 27-16. Algorithms for the use of the colorimetric carbon dioxide detector. (Courtesy of Nellcor, Inc., New York, NY.)

more durable during prolonged exposure to heat, humidity, and CO_2. Furthermore, they will be cheaper and will have a longer shelf-life. Even in the nonarrested patient there are potential sources of rare errors with the use of colorimetric CO_2 monitoring. After manual

ventilation with bag and mask before intubation, CO_2 from the exhaled air may be blown into the stomach and may result in detectable CO_2 levels, yielding a false-positive yellow color if the tracheal tube is misplaced in the esophagus. Ventilating the patient with six breaths results in a washout of CO_2 to near zero if the tube is misplaced in the esophagus. Close observation of the color of the detector is essential during and after the delivery of six quick breaths so that false-positive results are avoided.

Concern over inadvertent detection of gastric CO_2 from ingested beverages after esophageal intubation and potentially vitiating colorimetric CO_2 detection have been raised.[104] In a study of carbonated beverage ingestion and esophageal intubation in the cardiac arrest porcine model, the amount of CO_2 released did not result in spurious color change of the detector in the four animals studied and did not cause difficulty in interpretation of the readings.[110] Therefore concern that false-positive results might be caused by esophageal placement in a patient who had recently ingested carbonated beverages appears to be unwarranted.[101,110]

Colorimetric CO_2 is a simple, safe, highly sensitive, reliable, and quick method for confirming tracheal tube placement in the nonarrested patient. Unlike capnography, it is portable (pocket sized) and does not require calibration or power source. It is useful in places where capnography is unavailable such as hospital floors, emergency departments, and prehospital settings. Like capnography, false-negatives results (tube in trachea, no color change) may occur. Although very rare, false-positives results (tube in esophagus, with color change) can occur with the first few breaths. In the arrested patient, interpretation of a no-color change requires caution because it may indicate circulatory arrest, inadequate resuscitation, or esophageal intubation.

T. ESOPHAGEAL DETECTOR DEVICE/SELF-INFLATING BULB

The principle of use of the esophageal detector device (EDD) is based on anatomic differences between the trachea and the esophagus.[111] The trachea in the adult is about 10 to 12 cm long and its diameter can vary from 13 to 22 mm. The trachea remains constantly patent because of C-shaped rigid cartilaginous rings joined vertically by fibroelastic tissue and closed posteriorly by unstriped trachealis muscle. The esophagus is a fibromuscular tube, 25-cm long in adults, that extends from the cricopharyngeal sphincter to the gastroesophageal junction, and there is no intrinsic structure to maintain its patency. Wee[111] introduced a new method using a simple device to distinguish esophageal from tracheal intubation. The principle underlying the use of the device is that the esophagus will collapse when a negative pressure is applied to its lumen, whereas the trachea will not. The device consists of a 60-ml syringe fitted by an adapter that can be attached to a tracheal tube connector.[111]

When the syringe is attached to a tube placed in the trachea, withdrawal of the plunger of the syringe will

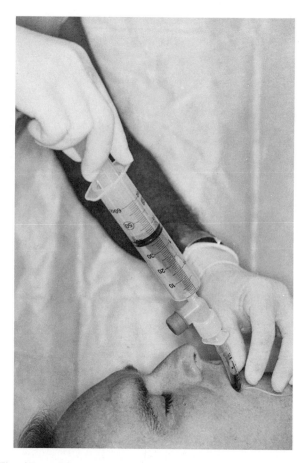

Fig. 27-17. The esophageal detector device consisting of a 60-ml syringe fitted by an adapter to a tracheal tube connector.

aspirate gas freely from the patient's lungs without any resistance apart from that inherent in the device (Fig. 27-17).[111,112] If the tube is in the esophagus, withdrawal of the plunger will cause apposition of the walls of the esophagus, occluding its lumen around the tube, and a negative pressure or resistance is felt when the plunger is pulled back. Wee[111] conducted a study in 100 patients in whom placement of tracheal and esophageal tubes was assessed using the EDD. There were 99 first-time correct identifications of tube placement, and the mean time taken by the observer to diagnose tube placement was 6.9 seconds. The application of constant but slow aspiration has been recommended to avoid the suction effect and prevent mucosal damage. Tracheal intubation is confirmed if 30 to 40 cc of gas is aspirated without resistance in adults[111,112] and 5 to 10 cc in children older than 2 years.[113]

Nunn[114] simplified the EDD by replacing the syringe with an Ellick's evacuator, which is a self-inflating bulb (SIB) with a capacity of 75 to 90 ml. After intubation, the device is connected to the tube, and the bulb is compressed. Compression is silent and refill is instantaneous if the tube is in the trachea. In contrast, if the tube is in the esophagus, compression of the SIB is accom-

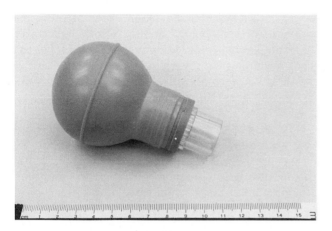

Fig. 27-18. The self-inflating bulb fitted with a standard 15-mm adapter. (From Salem MR, Wafai Y, Joseph NJ et al: *Anesthesiology* 80:42, 1994.)

panied by a characteristic flatuslike noise, and the SIB remains collapsed on release. It has been shown that the test can be accomplished easily within 3 seconds, and the outcome is unmistakable.[115] This technique has been further modified by compressing the SIB before, rather than after, connection to the tracheal tube connector.[116] Recent investigations that used the latter technique, confirmed earlier studies and demonstrated that the sensitivity, specificity, and predictive value of the SIB is 100%[117-120] (Figs. 27-18 and 27-19).

Despite the efficacy of both the EDD and the SIB in differentiating esophageal from tracheal intubation, false-negative results (tube in the trachea, but gas cannot be aspirated by the EDD or the SIB does not reinflate) have been reported. The EDD or the SIB may fail to confirm tracheal tube placement in infants in whom the tracheal wall is not held open by rigid cartilaginous rings.[121] Like capnography, the EDD or the SIB may fail to confirm tracheal tube placement if the tube is obstructed by kinking or the presence of material in the tube and in patients who have severe broncho-spasm.[122,123] Slow or no reinflation of the SIB may be encountered if the tube bevel is at the carina or in the right mainstem bronchus.[21] Slight retraction or rotation of the tube usually corrects the position of the tube and orientation of the bevel, resulting in instantaneous reinflation of the SIB.[21,124] We have noticed that the device may fail to reinflate or may reinflate slowly when connected to a properly placed tracheal tube in morbidly obese patients[124,125] and in other patients who have marked reduction in expiratory reserve volume, such as those with pulmonary edema or adult respiratory distress syndrome.

In a recent study on 2140 consecutive anesthetized adult patients,[124] the overall incidence of false-negative results (no reinflation or delayed reinflation > 4 sec) was 3.6%. It was apparent that the technique used can

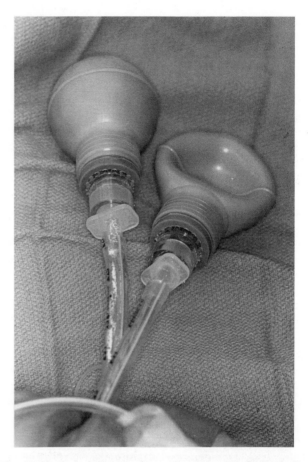

Fig. 27-19. In a demonstration, collapsed self-inflating bulbs were connected simultaneously to tracheally and esophageally placed tubes in the presence of a nasogastric tube. The bulb connected to the tube in the trachea instantaneously reinflated, whereas that connected to the tube in the esophagus remained collapsed. (From Salem MR, Wafai Y, Joseph NJ et al: *Anesthesiology* 80:42, 1994.)

contribute to false-negative results. When the SIB was fully compressed before connection to the tracheal tube, the incidence was 4.6%, whereas it was reduced to 2.4% if the SIB was compressed after connection to the tube.[124] Most of the patients (85.5%) in whom false-negative results were obtained were morbidly obese (body mass index > 35) (Table 27-3). We surmise that this phenomenon seen in morbidly obese patients and sometimes in normal individuals is due to the severely reduced functional residual capacity after anesthetic induction and muscular paralysis, leading to reduced caliber of intrathoracic airways and collapsibility of the trachea on the application of subatmospheric pressure by the SIB. It is also possible that the negative pressure generated (> −50 cm H_2O) may cause collapse and invagination of the posterior tracheal wall. Further compression can occur as a result of mediastinal compression. When the SIB is compressed after connection to the tracheal tube, a volume of gas is first introduced in the airway before subatmospheric pressure is generated by the SIB, and thus would limit the collapse of the SIB seen when it is compressed before connection to the tracheal tube.[124]

Unlike methods that rely on identification of CO_2 in exhaled gases, the EDD or SIB is not affected by ingested carbonated beverages or antacids in the event of esophageal intubation. Concern has been raised that false-positive results (tube in esophagus, but SIB reinflates) may occur as a result of gastric insufflation after bag-and-mask ventilation before intubation. In 72 patients, it has been demonstrated that even after the intentional delivery of three small breaths (300 to 350 ml each), the SIB was effective in detecting esophageal intubation in all 72 patients.[118] In another study, despite the use of mask ventilation before intubation, the authors did not observe a single instance of instantaneous reinflation of the SIB from the esophagus.[115] In a study of one pig, Foutch et al.[126] used a syringe similar to that of Wee,[111] and found that the device is effective in detecting esophageal intubation even after 1 min of bag-and-mask ventilation. These studies lead us to conclude that modest "esophageal ventilation" or prior bag-and-mask ventilation does not interfere with the reliability of the SIB in detecting esophageal intubation. Nonetheless, it is conceivable that massive inflation of

the stomach may cause reinflation of the SIB. For this reason, it is recommended that the test be undertaken before any gas is introduced through the tube. It has also been shown that the presence of a nasogastric tube or cuff deflation does not affect the performance of the device and does not contribute to false-positive results.[119]

It is essential that the SIB be of an appropriate size. Although a smaller SIB (capacity 20 ml) generates a higher negative pressure (because of its smaller radius) (Fig. 27-20), it is unreliable in detecting esophageal intubation if the SIB is compressed after connection to the tube.[127] The larger SIB (capacity 75 ml) is recommended because it does not yield false-positive results when either technique is used. SIBs may be constructed by fitting bulbs with a standard 15-mm adapter. The devices are checked before use by connecting the compressed SIB to a clamped tracheal tube; the absence of reinflation is an indication of airtightness (Fig. 27-21). Until such devices become available for single use, they should be washed and gas sterilized because they may constitute a means of spreading infectious disease. We have found that proper function of the device is not affected when a bacterial or viral filter is placed between the device and the tracheal tube connector. Therefore, if it is not sterilized, the use of the filter is recommended.

Although both the SIB and Wee's EDD are cheap and can rapidly and reliably differentiate tracheal from esophageal intubation without the use of a power source, the SIB is simpler, quicker (<4 sec), and the test can be performed with one hand. It can be used in the operating room in conjunction with capnography and outside the operating room where tracheal intubation may be performed without confirmation by capnography. Unlike capnography or colorimetric detection, the SIB functions equally well in the patient with and in the patient without cardiac arrest. Verification of tracheal placement by this method would enable physicians and emergency personnel to proceed with other resuscitative duties.

Recently, the use of the SIB has been extended to identify the location of the esophageal tracheal Com-

Table 27-3. Demography of false-negative results

Technique	T1	T2
Morbid obesity	45	20
Severe bronchospasm	2	2
Elderly w/COPD	2	2
Mainstem intubation	1	0
Pulmonary secretions	1	0
Pulmonary edema	0	1
Totals	51	25

T1, The SIB is compressed before it is connected to the tracheal tube.
T2, The SIB is first connected to the tube and is then compressed. See text for details.
From Wafai Y, Salem MR, Joseph NJ et al: *Anesthesiology* 80:A1303, 1994.

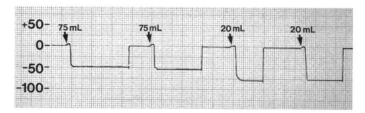

Fig. 27-20. Representative tracing of negative pressure generated by large (75 ml) and small (20 ml) SIBs when the SIB is compressed before it is connected to the tubes placed in the esophagus. The small SIB generates greater negative pressure than the large SIB. See text for details. (From Wafai Y, Salem MR, Czinn EA et al: *Anesthesiology* 79:A496, 1993.)

bitube (ETC) and facilitate its proper positioning using a simple algorithm (Figs. 27-22 and 27-23).[94] This may be of importance if the ETC is used in patients whose lungs cannot be ventilated by mask and whose trachea cannot be intubated.[94] After blind placement, the compressed SIB is connected to the distal lumen. Instantaneous reinflation implies that the ETC is in the trachea and

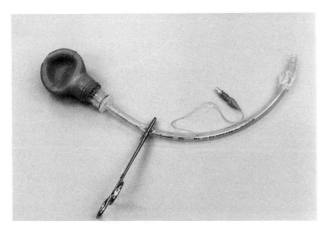

Fig. 27-21. Testing the self-inflating bulb for leakage. The compressed bulb is connected to a clamped tracheal tube. The absence of reinflation is indicative of airtightness. This test will reveal leakage from the bulb and the connector (cracked connector or loose fitting).

ventilation is carried out through the distal lumen, whereas the absence of reinflation is indicative of esophageal placement (very common). In this position, the pharyngeal balloon and the distal cuff are inflated and the compressed SIB is connected to the proximal lumen; instantaneous reinflation is expected to occur because the compressed SIB will aspirate gas from the lungs through the pharyngeal perforations. If slow or no reinflation of the SIB occurs, repositioning the ETC (1 to 2 cm pull-back) may be indicated, and rechecking with the SIB will confirm proper placement. Controlled ventilation is then carried out through the proximal lumen. Proper positioning and adequacy of ventilation can further be confirmed by the presence of breath sounds, absence of gastric insufflation, capnography or colorimetric CO_2 detection, and pulse oximetry.[94]

U. CHEST RADIOGRAPHY

Portable chest radiographs of tracheally intubated patients are commonly obtained in the critical care setting to determine the location of the distal end of the tube. A standard chest radiograph can easily detect mainstem intubation. It can also diagnose esophageal intubation if the tube is located in the lower esophagus or at the gastroesophageal junction distal to the carina (Fig. 27-24).[128] Because a tube in the esophagus is often projected over the tracheal air column on anteroposte-

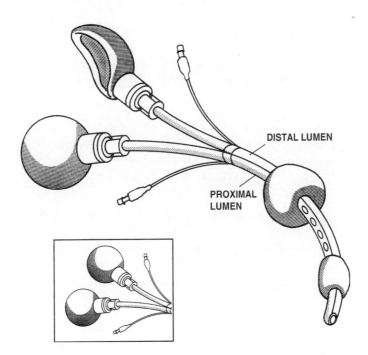

DISTAL LUMEN

PROXIMAL LUMEN

Fig. 27-22. Schematic diagram depicting outcome when the compressed self-inflating bulb is connected to the distal and proximal lumina of an esophageal tracheal Combitube in the esophageal position. Note that the bulb connected to the distal lumen remains collapsed, whereas that connected to the proximal lumen instantaneously reinflates. The insert depicts outcome when the esophageal tracheal combitube is in the trachea. Both bulbs instantaneously reinflate. (From Wafai Y, Salem MR, Baraka A et al: *Anesth Analg* 80:122, 1995.)

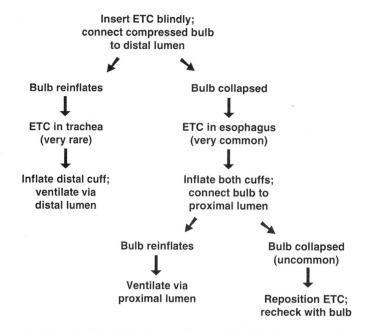

Fig. 27-23. Algorithm for identifying the position and facilitating proper placement of the esophageal tracheal Combitube *(ETC)* after blind placement. (From Wafai Y, Salem MR, Baraka A et al: *Anesth Analg* 80:122, 1995.)

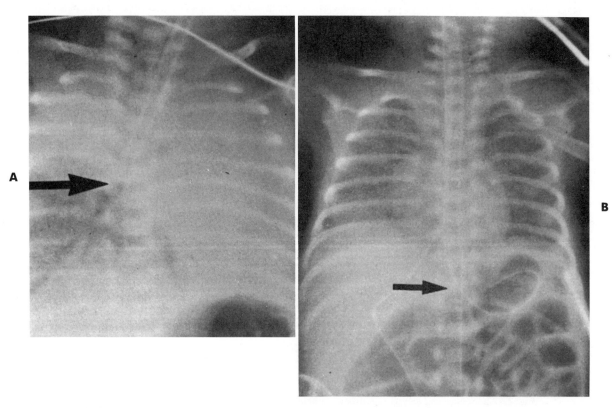

Fig. 27-24. Tracheal tube malposition. **A,** Tube in the bronchus intermedius *(arrow)*. Note the airless left lung and right upper lobe. **B,** Tube at the gastroesophageal junction *(arrow)*. Moderate intestinal dilation is seen. (From Mandel GA: Neonatal intensive care radiology. In Goodman LR, Putman CE, editors: *Intensive care radiology: imaging of the critically ill,* Philadelphia, 1983, WB Saunders.)

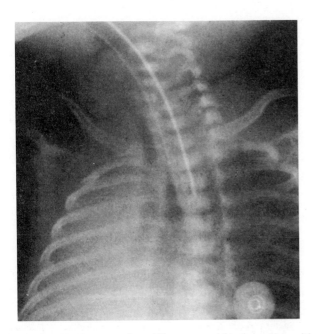

Fig. 27-25. Right posterior oblique portable chest film with patient's head turned to right shows air-filled trachea projecting to right of endotracheal tube. Tube aligns with air-filled distal esophagus. This is the best position for diagnosis of esophageal intubation. (From Smith GM, Reed JC, Choplin RH: *AJR Am J Roentgenol* 154:23, 1990.)

rior chest radiographs, the radiologic features of esophageal intubation are usually difficult to assess.[16,129] However, in the following situations it should be strongly suspected:[129] (1) if any part of the tube's borders is seen outside or lateral to the air column of the tracheobronchial tree (in the absence of a pneumomediastinum) (Fig. 27-25); (2) in the presence of esophageal air and gastric distention, particularly in the presence of a nasogastric tube; and (3) noticeable deviation of the trachea caused by an overinflated cuff. Obviously this requires a critical and thorough examination of portable chest films, which frequently are not of good quality. This can be difficult as illustrated in a case of prolonged misdiagnosis of esophageal intubation as a result of failure of several physicians, including a radiologist, to note malposition of the tube border outside the tracheobronchial tree in two consecutive radiographs.[16]

Although a lateral view of the chest could precisely reveal esophageal intubation, such views are often difficult to obtain in the critical setting. A study of chest radiographs of the tracheal tube position relative to nasogastric tube position provided evidence that the tube location could be identified correctly in 92% of the films taken with the patients in a 25-degree right posterior oblique position with the head turned to the right side.[128] Because the esophagus is located slightly to the left and behind the trachea, this projection presents the relationship *en face* with respect to the radiologic beam, resulting in avoidance of superimposition of the trachea over the esophagus. Because radiography is time consuming, cumbersome, expensive, and not yet fail-safe unless a lateral or a 25-degree right oblique view is obtained, it should not be relied on as the sole means of diagnosing esophageal intubation even in the critical care setting. However, any unusual radiologic findings suggestive of malposition of the tracheal tube should be correlated with clinical findings.

III. CONCLUSIONS

In the past unrecognized esophageal intubation has been a leading cause of injury involving the respiratory system in anesthetic practice and in the prehospital setting. Although a rare event, the outcome is so devastating that awareness of its occurrence is essential to patient safety whenever tracheal intubation is performed. A vast array of methods has been described to verify tracheal tube placement. In most patients these methods (alone or in combination) can successfully and quickly differentiate esophageal from tracheal intubation. Nevertheless, almost all these methods have been documented to fail under certain circumstances. It is crucial that the clinician performing tracheal intubation understands the basis of these tests, how to perform them correctly, and how to interpret the results. Obviously, not all these tests can be applied in every situation, but the clinician should be familiar with and use as many tests as possible. Among the most reliable tests are sighting the tube entering the larynx during direct laryngoscopy, visualization of the tracheal rings and carina with a fiberoptic scope threaded through the tube, identification of CO_2 in the exhaled gas, and the recently introduced use of the SIB. Prioritization of these tests depends on many factors, including experience, availability of devices, condition of the patient, and the place where tracheal intubation is performed. In the operating room, the use of capnography and the SIB in conjunction with clinical signs (including combined auscultation of the epigastrium and both axillae) can quickly confirm successful tracheal intubation. Outside the operating room where capnography is usually unavailable (hospital floor, emergency department, prehospital setting), the use of either the SIB or colorimetric CO_2 detection (or both) in combination with clinical signs is recommended whenever tracheal intubation is undertaken. Under no circumstances should clinical signs be ignored in the presence of information derived from monitors or technical aids.

REFERENCES

1. Caplan RA, Posner KL, Ward, RJ et al: Adverse respiratory events in anesthesia: a closed claims analysis, *Anesthesiology* 72:828, 1990.
2. Salem MR, Bennet EJ, Schweiss JF et al: Cardiac arrest related to anesthesia: contributing factors in infants and children, *JAMA* 233:238, 1975.

3. Keenan RL, Boyan CP: Cardiac arrest due to anesthesia: a study of incidence and causes, *JAMA* 253:2373, 1985.

4. Morray JP, Geiduschek JM, Caplan RA et al: A comparison of pediatric and adult anesthesia closed malpractice claims, *Anesthesiology* 78:461, 1993.

5. Utting JE, Gray TC, Shelley FC: Human misadventure in anaesthesia, *Can Anaesth Soc J* 26:472, 1979.

6. Green RA, Taylor TH: An analysis of anesthesia medical liability claims in the United Kingdom, 1977-1982, *Int Anesthesiol Clin* 22:73, 1984.

7. Morgan M: The confidential enquiry into maternal deaths in England and Wales, *Anaesthesia* 41:698, 1986 (editorial).

8. Utting JE: Pitfalls in anaesthetic practice, *Br J Anaesth* 59:877, 1987.

9. Gannon K: Mortality associated with anaesthesia: a case review study, *Anaesthesia* 46:962, 1991.

10. Holland R, Webb RK, Runciman WB: Oesophageal intubation: an analysis of 2000 incident reports, *Anaesth Intensive Care* 21:608, 1993.

11. Peterson AW, Jacker LM: Death following inadvertent esophageal intubation: a case report, *Anesth Analg* 52:398, 1973.

12. Pollard BJ, Junius F: Accidental intubation of the oesophagus, *Anaesth Intensive Care* 8:183, 1980.

13. Howells TH, Riethmuller RJ: Signs of endotracheal intubation, *Anaesthesia* 35:984, 1980.

14. Stirt JA: Endotracheal tube misplacement, *Anaesth Intensive Care* 10:274, 1982.

15. Ogden PN: Endotracheal tube misplacement, *Anaesth Intensive Care* 11:273, 1983 (letter).

16. Batra AK, Cohn MA: Uneventful prolonged misdiagnosis of esophageal intubation, *Crit Care Med* 11:763, 1983.

17. Heiselman D, Polacek DJ, Snyder JV et al: Detection of esophageal intubation in patients with intrathoracic stomach, *Crit Care Med* 13:1069, 1985.

18. Stewart RD, Paris PM, Winter PM et al: Field endotracheal intubation by paramedical personnel: success rates and complications, *Chest* 85:341, 1984.

19. Shea SR, MacDonald JR, Gruzinski G: Prehospital endotracheal tube airway or esophageal gastric tube airway: a critical comparison, *Ann Emerg Med* 14:102, 1985.

20. Charters P, Wilkinson K: Confirmation of tracheal tube placement, *Anaesthesia* 43:72, 1988, (reply).

21. Wee MY: Comments on the oesophageal detector device, *Anaesthesia* 44:930, 1989, (letter).

22. Ford RWJ: Confirming tracheal intubation: a simple manoeuvre, *Can Anaesth Soc J* 30:191, 1983.

23. Birmingham PK, Cheney FW, Ward RJ: Esophageal intubation: a review of detection techniques, *Anesth Analg* 65:886, 1986.

24. Conrardy PA, Goodman LR, Lainge F et al: Alteration of endotracheal tube position: flexion and extension of the neck, *Crit Care Med* 4:7, 1976.

25. Heinonen J, Takki S, Tammisto T: Effect of the Trendelenburg tilt and other procedures on the position of endotracheal tubes, *Lancet* 26:850, 1969.

26. Todres ID, deBros F, Dramer SS et al: Endotracheal tube displacement in the newborn infant, *J Pediatr* 89:126, 1976.

27. Bosman YK, Foster PA: Endotracheal intubation and head posture in infants, *S Afr Med J* 52:71, 1977.

28. Charters P, Wilkinson K: Tactile orotracheal tube placement: a bimanual tactile examination of the positioned orotracheal tube to confirm laryngeal placement, *Anaesthesia* 42:801, 1987.

29. Forgacs P: The functional basis of pulmonary sounds, *Chest* 73:399, 1978.

30. Banaszak EF, Kory RC, Snider GL: Phonopneumography, *Am Rev Respir Dis* 107:449, 1973.

31. Uejima T: Esophageal intubation, *Anesth Analg* 66:481, 1987 (letter).

32. Wallace CT, Cooke JE: A new method of positioning endotracheal tubes, *Anesthesiology* 44:272, 1976 (letter).

33. Salem MR, Wong AY, Lin YH et al: Prevention of gastric distension during anesthesia for newborns with tracheoesophageal fistula, *Anesthesiology* 38:82, 1973.

34. Triner L: A simple maneuver to verify proper positioning of an endotracheal tube, *Anesthesiology* 57:548, 1982 (letter).

35. Linko K, Paloheimo M, Tammisto T: Capnography for detection of accidental oesophageal intubation, *Acta Anaesthesiol Scand* 27:199, 1983.

36. Andersen KH, Hald A: Assessing the position of the tracheal tube: the reliability of different methods, *Anaesthesia* 44:984, 1989.

37. Baraka A, Tabakian H, Idriss A et al: Breathing bag refilling, *Anaesthesia* 44:81, 1989 (letter).

38. Robinson JS: Respiratory recording from the esophagus, *BMJ* 26:225, 1974.

39. Ehrenwerth J, Nagle S, Nirsch N et al: Is cuff palpation a useful tool for determining endotracheal tube position? *Anesthesiology* 65:A137, 1986 (abstract).

40. Bednarek FJ, Kuhns LR: Endotracheal tube placement in infants determined by suprasternal palpation: a new technique, *Pediatrics* 56:224, 1975.

41. Munro TN: Oesophageal misplacement of a tracheal tube, *Anaesthesia* 40:919, 1985 (letter).

42. Gillespie JH, Knight RG, Middaugh RE et al: Efficacy of endotracheal tube cuff palpation and humidity in distinguishing endotracheal from esophageal intubation, *Anesthesiology* 69:A265, 1988 (abstract).

43. Roy RC: Esophageal intubation, *Anesth Analg* 66:482, 1987 (letter).

44. Cullen DJ, Newbower RS, Gemer M: A new method for positioning endotracheal tubes, *Anesthesiology* 43:596, 1975.

45. Huang KC, Kramen SS, Wright BD: Video stethoscope: a simple method for assuring continuous bilateral lung ventilation during anesthesia, *Anesth Analg* 62:586, 1983.

46. Kalpokas M, Russell WJ: A simple technique for diagnosing oesophageal intubation, *Anaesth Intensive Care* 17:39, 1989.

47. Viswanathan S, Campbell C, Wood DG et al: The Eschmann tracheal tube introducer (gum elastic bougie), *Anesthesiol Rev* 19:29, 1992.

48. Whitehouse AC, Klock LE: Evaluation of endotracheal tube position with the fiberoptic intubation laryngoscope, *Chest* 68:848, 1975 (letter).

49. Benumof JL: Management of the difficult adult airway: with special emphasis on awake tracheal intubation, *Anesthesiology* 75:1087, 1991.

50. Moorthy SS, Dierdorf SF: An unusual difficulty in fiberoptic intubation, *Anesthesiology* 63:229, 1985 (letter).

51. Schwartz KD, Johnson C, Roberts J: A maneuver to facilitate flexible fiberoptic intubation, *Anesthesiology* 71:470, 1989.

52. Nichols KP, Zornow MH: A potential complication of fiberoptic intubation, *Anesthesiology* 70:562, 1989.

53. Ellis DG, Jakymec A, Kaplan RM et al: Guided orotracheal intubation in the operating room using a lighted stylet: a comparison with direct laryngoscopic technique, *Anesthesiology* 64:823, 1986.

54. Williams RT, Stewart RD: Transillumination of the trachea with a lighted stylette, *Anesth Analg* 65:542, 1986.

55. Fox DJ, Castro T Jr, Rastrelli AJ: Comparison of intubation techniques in the awake patient: the Flexi-lum surgical light (lightwand) versus blind nasal approach, *Anesthesiology* 66:69, 1987.

56. Mehta S: Transtracheal illumination for optimal tracheal tube placement: a clinical study, *Anaesthesia* 44:970, 1989.
57. Stewart RD, LaRosee A, Stoy WA et al: Use of a lighted stylet to confirm correct endotracheal tube placement, *Chest* 92:900, 1987.
58. Stewart RD, LaRosee A, Kaplan RM et al: Correct positioning of an endotracheal tube using a flexible lighted stylet, *Crit Care Med* 18:97, 1990.
59. Stone DJ, Stirt JA, Kaplan MJ et al: A complication of lightwand-guided nasotracheal intubation, *Anesthesiology* 61:780, 1984.
60. Debo RF, Colonna D, Dewerd G et al: Cricoarytenoid subluxation: complication of blind intubation with a lighted stylet, *Ear Nose Throat J* 68:517, 1989.
61. Szigeti CL, Baeuerle JJ, Mongan PD: Arytenoid dislocation with lighted stylet intubation: case report and retrospective review, *Anesth Analg* 78:185, 1994.
62. Nunn JF: *Applied respiratory physiology,* ed 4, Oxford, 1994, Butterworth-Heinemann.
63. Yelderman M, New W: Evaluation of pulse oximetry, *Anesthesiology* 59:349, 1983.
64. Brodsky JB, Shulman MS, Swan M et al: Pulse oximetry during one-lung ventilation, *Anesthesiology* 63:212, 1985.
65. McShane AJ, Martin JL: Preoxygenation and pulse oximetry may delay detection of esophageal intubation, *J Natl Med Assoc* 79:987, 1987.
66. Howells TH: A hazard of pre-oxygenation, *Anaesthesia* 40:86, 1985 (letter).
67. Guggenberger H, Lenz G, Federle R: Early detection of inadvertent oesophageal intubation: pulse oximetry vs. capnography, *Acta Anaesthesiol Scand* 33:112, 1989.
68. Warden JC: Accidental intubation of the oesophagus and preoxygenation, *Anaesth Intensive Care* 8:377, 1980 (letter).
69. Peters RM: Monitoring of ventilation in the anesthetized patient. In Gravenstein JS, Newbower RS, Ream AK et al editors: *Monitoring surgical patients in the operating room.* Springfield, 1989, Charles C Thomas.
70. Murray IP, Modell JH: Early detection of endotracheal tube accidents by monitoring carbon dioxide concentration in respiratory gas, *Anesthesiology* 59:344, 1983.
71. Bashein G, Cheney FW: Carbon dioxide detection to verify intratracheal placement of a breathing tube, *Anesthesiology* 61:782, 1984.
72. Duberman SM, Bendixen HH: Concepts of fail-safe in anesthesia practice. *Int Anesthesiol Clin* 22:149, 1984.
73. Tinker JH, Dull DL, Caplan RA et al: Role of monitoring devices in prevention of anesthetic mishaps: a closed claims analysis, *Anesthesiology* 71:541, 1989.
74. May WS, Heavner JE, McWhorter D et al: *Capnography in the operating room: an introductory directory,* New York, 1985, Raven Press.
75. Dunn SM, Mushlin PS, Lind LJ et al: Tracheal intubation is not invariably confirmed by capnography, *Anesthesiology* 73:1285, 1990.
76. Markovitz BP, Silverberg M, Godinez RI: Unusual cause of an absent capnogram, *Anesthesiology* 71:992, 1989.
77. Badgwell JM, Heavner JE, May WS et al: End-tidal P_{CO_2} monitoring in infants and children ventilated with either a partial rebreathing or a nonrebreathing circuit, *Anesthesiology* 66:405, 1987.
78. Badgwell JM, McLoed ME, Lerman J et al: End-tidal P_{CO_2} measurements sampled at the distal and proximal ends of the endotracheal tube in infants and children, *Anesth Analg* 66:959, 1987.
79. Benyamin RM, Salem MR, Joseph NJ: Sampling errors during use of the Dryden disposable absorber circuit. Can they be corrected? *Anesthesiology* 80:A585, 1994 (abstract).
80. Gravenstein N: Capnometry in infants should not be done at lower sampling flow rates, *J Clin Monit* 5:63, 1989 (letter).
81. Zupan J, Martin M, Benumof JL: End-tidal CO_2 excretion waveform and error with gas sampling line leak, *Anesth Analg* 67:579, 1988.
82. Kern KB, Sanders AB, Voorhees WD et al: Changes in expired end-tidal carbon dioxide during cardiopulmonary resuscitation in dogs: a prognostic guide for resuscitation, *J Am Coll Cardiol* 13:1184, 1989.
83. Salem MR: Hypercapnia, hypocapnia, and hypoxemia, *Semin Anesthesiology* 6:202, 1987.
84. Kalenda Z: The capnogram as a guide to the efficacy of cardiac massage, *Resuscitation* 6:259, 1978.
85. Trevino RP, Bisera J, Weil MH et al: End-tidal CO_2 as a guide to successful cardiopulmonary resuscitation: a preliminary report, *Crit Care Med* 13:910, 1985.
86. Sanders AB, Atlas M, Ewy GA et al: Expired P_{CO_2} as an index of coronary perfusion pressure, *Am J Emerg Med* 3:147, 1985.
87. Falk JL, Rackow EC, Weil MH: End-tidal carbon dioxide concentration during cardiopulmonary resuscitation, *N Engl J Med* 318:607, 1988.
88. Garnett AR, Ornato JP, Gonzalez ER et al: End-tidal carbon dioxide monitoring during cardiopulmonary resuscitation, *JAMA* 257:512, 1987.
89. Sum Ping ST: Esophageal intubation, *Anesth Analg* 66:481, 1987 (letter).
90. Sum Ping ST, Mehta MP, Anderton JM: A comparative study of methods of detection of esophageal intubation, *Anesth Analg* 69:627, 1989.
91. Sum Ping ST, Mehta MP, Symreng T: Reliability of capnography in identifying esophageal intubation with carbonated beverage or antacid in the stomach, *Anesth Analg* 73:333, 1991.
92. Rosenblatt WH, Kharatian A: Capnography: never forget the false positives! *Anesth Analg* 73:509, 1991 (letter).
93. Zbinden S, Schupfer G: Detection of esophageal intubation: the cola complication, *Anaesthesia* 44:81, 1989 (letter).
94. Wafai Y, Salem MR, Baraka A et al: Effectiveness of the self-inflating bulb for verification of proper placement of the esophageal tracheal Combitube, *Anesth Analg* 80:122, 1995.
95. Deluty S, Turndorf H: The failure of capnography to properly assess endotracheal tube location, *Anesthesiology* 78:783, 1993.
96. Owen RL, Cheney FW: Use of an apnea monitor to verify endotracheal intubation, *Respir Care* 30:974, 1985.
97. Smith RH, Volpitto PP: Simple method of determining CO_2 content in alveolar air, *Anesthesiology* 20:702, 1959 (letter).
98. Berman JA, Burgiuele JJ, Marx GF: The Einstein carbon dioxide detector, *Anesthesiology* 60:613, 1984 (letter).
99. Strunin L, Williams T: The FEF end-tidal carbon dioxide detector, *Anesthesiology* 71:621, 1989 (letter).
100. Jones BR, Dorsey MJ: Sensitivity of a disposable end-tidal carbon dioxide detector, *J Clin Monit* 7:268, 1991.
101. MacLeod GJ, Heller MB, Gerard J et al: Verification of endotracheal tube placement with colorimetric end-tidal CO_2 detection, *Ann Emerg Med* 20:267, 1991.
102. O'Callaghan JP, Williams RT: Confirmation of tracheal tube intubation using a chemical device, *Can J Anaesth* 33:S59, 1988 (abstract).
103. Goldberg JS, Rawle PP, Zehnder IL et al: Colorimetric end-tidal carbon dioxide monitoring for tracheal intubation, *Anesth Analg* 70:191, 1990.
104. O'Flaherty D, Adams AP: The end-tidal carbon dioxide detector: assessment of a new method to distinguish oesophageal from tracheal intubation, *Anaesthesia* 45:653, 1990.

105. Denman WT, Hayes M, Higgins D et al: The Fenem CO_2 detector device: an apparatus to prevent unnoticed oesophageal intubation, *Anaesthesia* 45:465, 1990.

106. Ornato JP, Shipley JB, Racht EM et al: Multicenter study of carbon dioxide in the prehospital setting, *Ann Emerg Med* 9:452, 1990 (abstract).

107. Kelly JS, Wilhoit RD, Brown RE et al: Efficacy of the FEF colorimetric end-tidal carbon dioxide detector in children, *Anesth Analg* 75:45, 1992.

108. Feinstein R, White PF, Westerfield SZ: Intraoperative evaluation of a disposable end-tidal CO_2 detector, *Anesthesiology* 71:A460, 1989 (abstract).

109. Gedeon A, Krill P, Mebius C: A new colorimetric breath indicator (Colobri): a comparison of the performance of two carbon dioxide indicators, *Anaesthesia* 49:798, 1994.

110. Heller MB, Yealy DM, Seaberg DC et al: End-tidal CO_2 detection, *Ann Emerg Med* 18:12, 1989.

111. Wee MYK: The oesophageal detector device: assessment of a method to distinguish oesophageal from tracheal intubation, *Anaesthesia* 43:27, 1988.

112. O'Leary JJ, Pollard BJ, Ryan MJ: A method of detecting oesophageal intubation or confirming tracheal intubation, *Anaesth Intensive Care* 16:299, 1988.

113. Wee MYK, Walker KY: The oesophageal detector device: an assessment with uncuffed tubes in children, *Anaesthesia* 46:869, 1991.

114. Nunn JF: The oesophageal detector device, *Anaesthesia* 43:804, 1988 (letter).

115. Williams KN, Nunn JF: The oesophageal detector device: a prospective trial in 100 patients, *Anaesthesia* 44:984, 1989.

116. Baraka A, Muallem M: Confirmation of correct tracheal intubation by a self-inflating bulb, *Middle East J Anesthesiol* 11:193, 1991.

117. Zaleski L, Abello D, Gold MI: The esophageal detector device. Does it work? *Anesthesiology* 79:244, 1993.

118. Salem MR, Wafai Y, Baraka A et al: Use of the self-inflating bulb for detecting esophageal intubation after "esophageal ventilation," *Anesth Analg* 77:1227, 1993.

119. Salem MR, Wafai Y, Joseph NJ et al: Efficacy of the self-inflating bulb in detecting esophageal intubation. Does the presence of a nasogastric tube or cuff deflation make a difference?, *Anesthesiology* 80:42, 1994.

120. Oberly D, Stein S, Hess D et al: An evaluation of the esophageal detector device using a cadaver model, *Am J Emerg Med* 10:317, 1992.

121. Haynes SR, Morten NS: Use of the oesophageal detector device in children under one year of age, *Anaesthesia* 45:1067, 1991.

122. Baraka A: The oesophageal detector device, *Anaesthesia* 45:697, 1991 (letter).

123. Smith I: Confirmation of correct endotracheal tube placement, *Anesth Analg* 72:263, 1991 (letter).

124. Wafai Y, Salem MR, Joseph NJ et al: The self-inflating bulb for confirmation of tracheal intubation: incidence and demography of false negatives, *Anesthesiology* 81:A1303, 1994 (abstract).

125. Baraka A, Choueiry P, Salem MR: The esophageal detector device in the morbidly obese, *Anesth Analg* 77:400, 1993 (letter).

126. Foutch RG, Magelssen MD, MacMillan JG: The esophageal detector device: a rapid and accurate method for assessing tracheal versus esophageal intubation in a porcine model, *Ann Emerg Med,* 21:43, 1992.

127. Wafai Y, Salem MR, Czinn EA et al: The self-inflating bulb in detecting esophageal intubation: effect of bulb size and technique used, *Anesthesiology* 79:A496, 1993 (abstract).

128. Mandel GA: Neonatal intensive care radiology. In Goodman LR, Putman CE, editors: *Intensive care radiology: imaging of the critically ill.* Philadelphia, 1983, WB Saunders.

129. Smith GM, Reed JC, Choplin RH: Radiographic detection of esophageal malpositioning of endotracheal tubes, *AJR Am J Roentgenol* 154:23, 1990.

Chapter 28

CASE EXAMPLES AND ANALYSIS

Charles B. Watson

I. OVERVIEW

Anesthesia, emergency life support, and critical care personnel are, by their inclination, gadget and technique oriented. Whether our fields are viewed by others as "cognitive" or "procedural," we apply our skills and knowledge to combine diagnostic data from tests and medical examination with medical techniques for care of our patients. Our patients are referred to us or brought to us in extremis (or we go to our patients, in the case of emergency medical technicians [EMTs]) in expectation of an immediate demonstration of this process.

Techniques, while they are a means to an end—in this

case, airway control—have an inherent tendency to become and end unto themselves. Technical quality assurance errors the practitioner should avoid include (1) inappropriate choice of technique, (2) failure to perform the technique properly, (3) perseverance with a technique when all objective evidence suggests that it is failing, and (4) inability to apply another technique or modify the one chosen to meet the changing needs of the situation. In anesthetic practice and during advanced airway life support (ALS), these errors commonly translate into failed recognition of an inadequate mask airway, traumatic or failed intubation, and persistent attempts to translaryngeally intubate someone as time runs out and hypoxia and/or hypercapnea evolve.

Skilled technicians gain and maintain their skills by repetitive performance of the same technique under a number of circumstances. The knowledgeable airway skills expert, on the other hand, should be able to select his approach to a problem from a number of techniques. It is not sufficient to merely know the equipment and how to use it. One must know its relative advantages and how to manage complications of its use. The preceding chapters have been written with these ideas in mind.

Variation in individual experience leads to a difficult question. Most of us learn skills such as cycling as youngsters and have not forgotten the basics. How many of us (who are not cycling enthusiasts) are technically adept when we as adults use the technique once or twice a year? Of all those who can ride a bicycle, how many do it as well as they did when they were 14 years old? In medical terms, the issue is certification and maintenance of procedural credentials. Once one learns to place a laryngeal mask airway, we would agree that routine use makes it less problematic to apply their use to the difficult situation. Is there a critical threshold of experience? Since the ability to gain expertise with a technique over time is operator dependent, and since repetition increases the probability of expertise, most external bodies have adopted a seemingly arbitrary number of clinical cases as a guideline for achievement or maintenance of a clinical skill (for example, 50 bronchoscopies is a recommended experience baseline for training with a fiberoptic bronchoscope according to the American College of Chest Physicians).

We can gain expertise through repetitive practice under most circumstances. Unfortunately, our patients are both our raison d'être and our medical experiments. No patient would like to think that his/her physician is inexperienced. Therefore, we seek to gain experience in a controlled setting after some educational effort. Happily, we can also combine case analyses and morbidity and mortality discussion experiences to formulate a knowledge base that will accelerate our learning curve and help us develop clinical wisdom. This case discussion format is offered as a means toward merging some key aspects of the technique and/or case involved with the readers' and our experience. All of the cases presented in this chapter were submitted by the authors of the chapters regarding various individual techniques. While the discussions may not be exhaustive, I anticipate that they will serve to focus the reader's thoughts on the cognitive decision-making and reflective analysis that distinguishes a technician from an experienced clinician.

II. A PROBLEM AFTER ANESTHESIA WITH MASK VENTILATION (CHAPTER 12)

A. INTRODUCTION

Mask anesthesia is widely used for short cases in healthful patients who have fasted and have no history of gastric reflux, gastroparesis, or esophageal dysfunction. The mask airway is our first line of airway support. It is readily adapted to fit a variety of facial shapes and sizes. It allows accurate administration of a known gas mixture. It permits institution of staged ventilatory support from airway-distending pressure through assisted to controlled ventilation provided with a wide range of gas flow-pressure curves, inspiratory to expiratory time ratios, and ventilatory rates. The mask may be used with a number of airway maintenance adjuvants, such as pharyngeal and nasopharyngeal airways, and permits use of nasogastric tubes or blockers. Finally, the mask can be used for both surgical anesthesia and airway life support.

B. CASE PRESENTATION

A 42-year-old white male outpatient was scheduled for a right knee arthroscopy because he has popping and locking of the knee. He was an active man (played tennis 2-3 times per week) in good health with a history of childhood asthma that never required hospitalization. He was taking no medicines. His family history was negative for anesthesia-related problems, and he had never had an anesthetic. His physical examination, complete blood count (CBC), and urinalysis were normal. He requested a general anesthetic. The surgeon indicated that the procedure would last approximately 30 to 45 minutes.

The patient was given intravenous propofol followed by inhalation of a 50% nitrous oxide-oxygen mixture with 0.5% to 2% isoflurane for anesthetic maintenance. The mask airway appeared to be easy, with a no. 3 Guedel oral airway. No reaction was noted to placement of the oropharyngeal airway. Spontaneous ventilation returned after inflation of the tourniquet. The tourniquet time was 35 minutes, after which anesthetic gasses were discontinued. During emergence, mild coughing followed by laryngospasm was treated with the triple airway maneuver (jaw thrust, neck extension, and mouth opening) with the head and shoulders rotated 45 degrees to the side.

After this period, the patient was taken to the Post-Anesthetic Care Unit (PACU). Although the initial pulse oximeter measurement was 93%, it rose to 96% with nasal oxygen. He was discharged from the first-to second-stage PACU an hour later with a documented saturation of 95% on room air. At that time he noted burning in his chest. Two hours later he was diaphoretic with chills. Tachypnea and wheezing were noted on physical exam. Oxygen and antibiotics were administered, and the patient was admitted to hospital. After 2 days he was discharged in good condition. He declined an esophageal and gastrointestinal (GI) work up for reflux.

C. DISCUSSION

Although the incidence of subclinical peri-anesthetic aspiration is relatively high (15% to 30%[1,2,3]) during general anesthesia, clinical illness associated with aspiration is less common. In fact, recent data challenge our traditional notions regarding the ideal fasting period that will minimize the risk of clinically significant perioperative aspiration.[4] Mendelson's triad—wheezing, tachypnea, and pulmonary infiltrates on the chest x-ray—was the first clinical complex described for the pulmonary aspiration syndrome (Mendelson's syndrome) noted in one of more than 660 patients during the peripartum period.[5] Aspiration of gastric or pharyngeal secretions is a less common pulmonary complication of anesthesia in current studies (recent retrospective reports cite aspiration in 1:2000-3000 to fewer than 1:5000 anesthetics[6,7,8]), but remains a significant cause of perioperative morbidity.[9]

Even though the incidence of gastric aspiration during anesthesia is low, especially in elective, nonobese, fasting patients with a normal upper airway, this complication can range in severity from mild, transient laryngospasm in the perioperative period to profound hypoxemia with a progressive adult respiratory distress syndrome (ARDS), multiple organ system failure, and cardiac arrest. It follows that those who use this technique (or any technique associated with depressed upper airway reflexes) must be prepared to identify and treat the pulmonary aspiration syndrome if they wish to prevent further morbidity or mortality.

Aspiration during anesthesia is most commonly reported during induction, prior to intubation, or during mask anesthesia. Some have argued that it can be avoided through the use of regional anesthesia, but this has not been unequivocally proven,[10] probably because of predisposing factors (age, pain, pregnancy, abdominal

pathology, obesity, and esophageal reflux) and the widespread use of reflex suppressant narcotic and sedative drugs. Other anesthesiologists recommend that all patients with predisposing factors should be translaryngeally intubated, no matter how short the planned procedure, in order to avoid aspiration. The apparently healthy patient in this case presentation is typical of those who receive a general inhalational anesthetic administered by face mask for a brief outpatient procedure. From the clinical course, it appears that aspiration occurred during the emergence from anesthesia, when coughing and laryngospasm were noted. The progressive observations of coughing, suggesting tracheal stimulation under partial anesthesia, followed by laryngospasm, as the patient's anesthetic level was decreased, ultimately culminated in progressive hypoxemia with pulmonary symptoms and findings delayed until 1 to 2 hours postoperatively.

Which patients who have coughing or laryngospasm without obvious regurgitation and aspiration should be monitored or admitted to hospital? Warner et al.,[7] from their series of more than 215,000 patients, concluded that those patients who aspirate but have no symptoms or signs within 2 hours of the episode are unlikely to have respiratory complications. The surprisingly low oxygen saturation in room air observed in this normal patient 1 hour after such a brief anesthetic should have tipped the PACU and anesthesia staff to a clinically significant problem. Additionally, cardiopulmonary pathology should have been anticipated when the patient expressed vague complaints of chest pain upon transfer to the outpatient lounge. Hospitalization was prudent when significant symptoms associated with hypoxemia and pulmonary infiltrates evolved. Although more severe acid or particulate aspiration tends to present a more acute, rapidly evolving picture both in animals and patients, no one can predict the ultimate severity of the process.

Supportive therapy with oxygen, positive airway pressure, and ventilation, if necessary, is the main treatment for aspiration pneumonitis. Since the condition is primarily associated with nonbacterial lung inflammation, most pulmonary, anesthesia, and critical care physicians withhold antibiotic therapy until they see evidence of a treatable infection. Systemic steroids, long recommended for their antiinflammatory properties, are no longer recommended in the acute period. Progressive loss of lung function and volume is associated with an acute, frank, inflammatory, noncardiogenic pulmonary edema during which lung weight increases many fold with severe aspiration pneumonitis. Typically, hemoconcentration is noted as the damaged pulmonary endothelium leaks protein and fluid into the pulmonary (and other tissue) interstitium. Consequently, diuretics play no role in the acute management of aspiration pneumonitis, and close attention must be paid to effective circulation, especially as ventilatory support is instituted.

III. DIGITAL TRACHEAL INTUBATION (CHAPTER 15)

A. INTRODUCTION

Airway control in a crisis such as large-volume vomitus, presence of massive upper airway bleeding, or technical failure of equipment makes standard techniques near impossible and may require an unorthodox approach. Although a number of new devices have recently been introduced that make this process somewhat easier, the airway expert who is outside of the well-defined environment of an operating room or a trauma emergency room may have to rely on more basic techniques.

B. CASE PRESENTATION

A call was received by the 911 center of a large, urban emergency medical system (EMS) that reported a "man not breathing" at a downtown hotel. A mobile intensive care unit from the nearest ambulance station was dispatched within 40 seconds of the call.

On arrival 3 minutes later, the EMS team was directed to the top floor of the hotel where a wedding reception was in progress. The 120 kg patient was found in complete cardiorespiratory arrest on the floor of a small restroom. According to the history given by relatives, the patient had noted chest pain while dancing after a large meal. He went into the bathroom and collapsed.

Although cardiopulmonary resuscitation (CPR) was commenced immediately, the paramedic on the scene could not intubate the patient because of the large quantity of vomitus that obscured the airway. Although suction was provided by a portable unit, the large quantity of vomitus filled the collection system rapidly, and the airway could not be cleared. "Quick-look" defibrillator paddles revealed asystole.

Attempts to obtain intravenous (IV) access were successful, as CPR with mask ventilation continued. Second and third attempts to perform laryngoscopy for translaryngeal intubation resulted in esophageal intubation. This was readily recognized and mask ventilation continued.

When the EMS physician-on-duty arrived, it became clear that direct laryngoscopy was impossible because of the continued flow of vomitus into the upper airway. Because of this, a 7.5-mm inner diameter (ID) endotracheal tube was passed digitally by insertion of the operator's hand into the mouth, tactile identification of the larynx, and direct digital guidance of the tube through the larynx. Tracheal placement was confirmed after the first attempt. After ventilation and tracheal suction, the patient's color improved. CPR continued during transport to a local hospital.

C. DISCUSSION

Direct digital intubation is an old technique,[11] introduced in the early part of this century by Kuhn,[12] that is rarely described and little taught these days. As a blind, tactile technique, it requires that the operator be able to reach and identify the larynx with his or her fingers and to digitally guide an endotracheal tube (ET) between the fingers and the larynx. The technique is bimanual. Usually the operator's dominant hand directs the tube into the larynx, while the other advances or rotates the tube to meet the pharyngeally placed fingers. A stylet helps, unless the tube is very stiff, as in Kuhn's day.

Digital intubation can be practiced in the operating room with anesthetized patients but is most applicable in the urgent setting when no equipment is available, the equipment malfunctions, or—as in this case—when vomitus or blood totally obscures any view of the airway. I have used it in the intensive care unit when the laryngoscope light fails, in the operating room under similar conditions, and in the resuscitation setting when great quantities of blood or vomit completely obscure the field. It can also be used after massive facial trauma when there is little underlying structural integrity and the pharynx is torn and filled with blood, provided that there is a palpable larynx. Also, it may be possible to use the digital approach instead of repeat laryngoscopy to confirm that the tube is passed translaryngeally even when the operators hands are too small or the teeth too prominent for routine digital endotracheal intubation.[13] Since the technique is applicable in the emergent setting, it is not surprising that it has been advocated as a field technique by emergency physicians.[14]

Digital intubation sounds easier than it is. Normally, one has to be able to reach the larynx with at least two fingers—one to lift the epiglottis, and one to guide the tube anteriorly toward the laryngeal inlet—while the other hand advances the tube into the pharynx and larynx. Small individuals find that it is difficult to reach the larynx, while large individuals often find that they can not get their hands into the mouths of smaller patients. Edentulous patients are easier to work with, since the operator does not risk cutting fingers on sharp or jagged teeth and support structures for the jaw are atrophic and easily passed by the fingers. Particulate vomitus and blood clots may block the digital approach and need to be removed manually, sometimes with the use of a gauze wrap around the gloved fingers. Tumors and abscesses may distort normal structures so much that the larynx is not easily palpated from the pharynx. Liquid blood and vomit lubricate pharyngeal and laryngeal structures so that it is often difficult to direct the tube properly. A number of trainees have objected to digital intubation on the grounds that it is easy to cut fingers and incurs a risk of acquiring blood borne or other infections.

A traditional approach to this problem has been to use conventional laryngoscopy and make blind passes at the larynx with the endotracheal tube and to leave the esophageally placed tube or tubes in as esophageal blockers or drains while mask ventilation is performed around the tubes. Diversion of the stream of vomitus or blood (out the mouth and/or through a suction catheter) sometimes enables the airway team to clear the field enough to visualize the larynx—that is, if the tube or tubes themselves do not obstruct the view. This was the concept behind and forerunner of the esophageal obturator airway[15,16] and its successors (esophageal gastric tube airway, pharyngeotracheal lumen airway, and esophageal-tracheal Combitube), although the esophageal obturator airway has fallen into disrepute.[17,18] Although the latter devices may be more effective, all perform well when applied by skilled individuals under appropriate circumstances[19] and may have been helpful had digital intubation failed in this case.

Another problem in the obtunded, spontaneously breathing patient is that the digital intubator's hand nearly occludes the airway during intubation. If intubation is not completed in a brief period, oxygenation and ventilation may be worse. Even if one cannot find the larynx with a laryngoscope, one can at least maintain an open airway and insufflate oxygen in a head down or lateral position that drains blood and vomitus away from the larynx for a spontaneously breathing patient. Ventilation of apneic patients in such a position can buy time while a cricothyrotomy or tracheotomy is being performed.

Various modifications of digital or tactile intubation include digitally assisted intubation,[20] manual palpation of a rigid stylet as it is directed blindly toward the larynx, blind intubation facilitated by a manually steered hooked guide,[21] blind intubation over a directed gum-rubber bougie,[22] cuff inflation to blindly direct a pharyngeal tube into the larynx,[23] and light wand[24] or magnet-guided digitally assisted intubation. Most require spontaneous breathing or periodic hyperventilation with oxygen during anesthesia if dramatic hypoxemia is to be avoided. Like other options for dealing with the difficult airway, blind digital intubation is more likely to work in an urgent setting if it is a familiar technique that has been practiced in the elective setting. Also, one must be prepared to proceed with a different option, such as percutaneous jet catheter ventilation, tracheostomy, or percutaneous cricothyrotomy, when digital attempts take too long or fail.

In summary, blind, digital intubation is a basic, often overlooked technique that can serve the airway consultant in difficult situations such as an airway obscured by

continuous drainage of blood or vomit. It requires experience, an obtunded patient with diminished airway reflexes, and a reasonable anatomic match between the operator's hand and the patient's airway.

IV. FIBEROPTIC ENDOSCOPY AIDED TECHNIQUES (CHAPTER 16)
A. INTRODUCTION

Fiberoptic intubation has gained considerable interest and support as a technique for avoiding and/or solving a difficult airway problem, managing lung isolation, or managing the difficult intubation. Numerous articles, reviews, and at least two monographs have been written on the subject in recent years. Two case histories illustrate advantages and potential pitfalls of this approach.

B. CASE 1 PRESENTATION

A 60-year-old man with severe fixed-neck flexion deformity due to longstanding rheumatoid arthritis is scheduled for total hip replacement. Access to the neck is extremely limited.

1. Clinical approach

Regional anesthesia with postoperative pain control is recommended by the consultant anesthesiologist after a comprehensive physical evaluation and review of this patient's history. Concern for the airway and a need for a backup plan in case of respiratory compromise or technical failure was expressed. Alternatives for airway control included "awake," sedated transnasal fiberoptic intubation or fiberoptic intubation under mask anesthesia with adjuvants like the laryngeal mask airway, the Patil mask, and various oropharyngeal airway guides. Also, general anesthesia via laryngeal mask in the lateral position was discussed as an technical alternative to intubation.

2. Discussion

This is not an unusual presentation in any center where a significant number of joint replacement procedures are performed. Patients with rheumatoid disease and deformities present for joint replacement at a younger age than the patients with traumatic and degenerative osteoarthritis, but both groups may have significant cervical disease that limits neck motion and could make airway management difficult. Of course, patients with rheumatoid disease may have involvement of rib articulation, the temporomandibular joints, and cartilagenous articulation in the larynx. A key part of their assessment should focus upon extraarticular rheumatoid involvement. In addition to the airway, this may include renal, respiratory, gastrointestinal, and cardiovascular disease. The patient's pulmonary reserve is of primary interest to the anesthesiologist. A marked deficit, together with limited mechanical function, is associated with respiratory insufficiency under low thoracic and high lumbar levels of regional anesthesia. Limited vital capacity or flows would suggest that this patient might have difficulty managing secretions in the postoperative period when he will be forced to maintain a supine position with an abduction pillow.

With both degenerative joint disease and rheumatoid disease, cervical rigidity or advanced cervical spine deformity poses an airway challenge. Ironically, the patients often have an easy mask airway but are very difficult to intubate. Similarly patients who have neck contractures due to facial or neck burns may be impossible to directly laryngoscope using standard equipment. Direct blind nasal intubation or nasal intubation assisted by use of an oral hook, a nasotracheal suction catheter, or an indirectly guided ET are the oldest solutions to the fixed neck problem.[25] The prism,[26] angulated[27] and mirror[28] laryngoscope blades have been used in the distant past. Retrograde intubation, surgical tracheostomy, or cricothyrotomy may be impossible because the acutely flexed neck will not permit access to the cricothyroid membrane and trachea. These are the reasons that such patients typically polarize anesthesia departments into two factions—those who favor general anesthesia with airway control as a primary objective, and those who believe that the subject should be avoided by use of regional anesthesia.

More recently, use of the flexible fiberoptic broncho-scope has improved our ability to manage this type of patient.[29,30] Ovassapian[31] and others, including myself, have argued that it is even relatively safe in the setting of GI bleeding, trauma, and the "full stomach." It has been helpful with patients who have fractured necks[32] and major flexion deformities of the cervical spine.[33] Fiberoptic endoscopy and intubation is known to be associated with a lower endocrine and hemodynamic stress response[34,35] when performed properly. From time to time, one encounters a patient whose extreme cervical flexion and laryngeal abnormalities make laryn-goscopy with the fiberscope difficult.[36] The transnasal approach is usually easier in this setting.[37] When even our most skillful fiberoptic endoscopist fails, we have used the bright light from the bronchoscope as a light wand or used a retrograde wire to guide the fiberscope anteriorly into the larynx. Now that the laryngeal mask airway is available, it offers the option of primary airway control in lateral position and can also serve as a guide to the larynx for the fiberoptic endoscopist.

C. CASE 2 PRESENTATION

A 50-year-old man with Ludwig's angina is presented to the anesthesia department for emergent incision and drainage of the abscess. He is 6 feet tall and weighs 200 pounds. He has moderate stridor and is unable to lie down. The otolaryngologist is reluctant to consider a tracheostomy.

1. Clinical approach

The anesthesiologist recommended conscious seda-tion and humidified, high-flow oxygen in the sitting position while transnasal fiberoptic endoscopy could be performed. He informed the patient and otolaryngolo-gist of the following options, in order of preference: transnasal fiberoptic intubation in the sitting position under conscious sedation, direct laryngoscopy with sedation and topical anesthesia in the semi-sitting position to assess the upper airway, blind nasotracheal intubation, a modified rapid sequence intubation with tracheostomy or cricothyrotomy "standby," or surgical tracheotomy.

2. Discussion

No one argues with a 6-foot, 200-pound man who is in respiratory distress. The goal is to secure and protect the airway without aspiration of pus or tracheostomy. Noninvasive oximetry can gauge the efficacy of oxygen therapy and safety of conscious sedation in the sitting position. A blood gas would be helpful if the clinical setting permits. An IV is certainly essential, especially since the patient is unlikely to have eaten or drunk adequately for a number of hours before presentation.

If the patient is profoundly hypoxemic or rapidly deteriorating, one must proceed with a rapid sequence induction, attempted intubation, and a transtracheal or transcricoid airway if intubation fails. A risk that must be recognized, in addition to that of airway loss with need for rapid transtracheal backup, is abscess rupture and aspiration of purulent secretions. This is additional incentive for an atraumatic technique like transnasal or peroral fiberoptic intubation. The procedure can be performed in an upright, sitting position with the endoscopist facing the patient. Oxygen therapy is essen-tial during this procedure because the stressed, febrile patient with a partly obstructed airway will have a markedly increased oxygen consumption with high risk of diminished lung capacity. Children and adults who are able to understand the airway problem are often quite cooperative during awake fiberoptic bronchoscopy, par-ticularly when the alternatives and risks are made clear to them.

Following intubation, there is a small, but significant, risk of postobstructive or "low pressure" pulmonary edema. This is presumably due to recurrent respiratory effort against an obstructed airway, with a transcapillary pressure gradient that favors fluid sequestration in the pulmonary interstitium due to very low intrapleural and pulmonary interstitial pressures with normal pulmonary capillary pressures. The reason for rapid onset immedi-ately following relief of the obstruction is obscure.

Whatever the etiology, the problem responds to continuous distending airway pressure in the form of continuous positive airway pressure breathing (CPAP), intermittent mandatory ventilation (IMV), pressure support (PS) ventilation, or controlled mechanical ventilation (CMV) with positive end-expiratory pressure (PEEP), and time.

Both of these cases represent very difficult airway-intubation challenges. The former patient would not need intubation unless pulmonary reserve is markedly limited. The latter patient is in urgent need of airway control. Although the clinical presentation must affect exact choice of technique, both of these patients are candidates for fiberoptic intubation.

V. RETROGRADE TRACHEAL INTUBATION (CHAPTER 17)

A. INTRODUCTION

The retrograde approach is misnamed, as has been pointed out by others,[38] because the endotracheal tube is passed anterograde over a stylet or catheter. Retrograde cannulation is a basic skill that can be mastered by any clinician who has used stylets and guidewires and who can perform a transtracheal injection or aspiration. This is another useful technique for the semielective setting when the anterior trachea can be palpated and other approaches have failed.

B. CASE PRESENTATION

A 34-year-old white female with advanced juvenile rheumatoid arthritis was scheduled for thoracotomy and wedge resection of a central nodular mass. Her pulmonary history was benign. Fiberoptic-guided transbronchial biopsy of a "silent" lesion that was noted on her chest x-ray failed. The bronchoscopist, an experienced radiologist, and a consultant pulmonary physician were unable to visualize the larynx or gain access to the trachea on account of severe flexion deformity of the cervical spine. On this occasion, 2 days prior to scheduled surgery, the epiglottis was visualized but the larynx was "high" and "anterior" so that the endoscopist could not pass anteriorly around the epiglottis.

Over the past 15 years, this patient had had eight peripheral orthopedic procedures. She had regional anesthesia for her last two procedures because it was noted that she was "impossible" to intubate by experienced staff on two previous occasions, 6 and 5 years prior to this admission, when she had prolonged mask anesthetics. On one occasion, an elective procedure had been aborted because she could not be intubated after many attempts by experienced personnel.

On examination, the patient had a rigid, flexed cervical spine, limited mouth opening, and multiple peripheral stigmata of rheumatoid disease. Her larynx appeared to be very prominent, and a number of tracheal rings could be palpated despite her neck flexion. The mouth could only open to admit two fingers, and the examiner could only insert one finger between the hyoid bone and the inside of the mandible.

The patient was taken to the operating room where IV sedation with fentanyl and droperidol was administered. Oxygen was administered by nasal cannulae as both superior laryngeal nerve and transtracheal injections were performed with 3 ml of 2% lidocaine using a 22-gauge needle. Nasal analgesia was obtained by using 1.5 ml 4% cocaine solution on cotton-tipped applicators. Viscous lidocaine was gargled and swallowed to supplement oropharyngeal anesthesia. A 14-gauge needle was advanced through the cricoid membrane in a cephalad direction until air could be aspirated. Afterwards, a 16-gauge, styletted, 24-inch central venous catheter (CVC) (Intracath, Deseret Medical, Inc., Sandy, Utah) was passed via the needle in retrograde fashion into the pharynx. A #12, red rubber suction catheter was passed from the left naris, and both catheters were digitally retrieved from the pharynx via the mouth. The CVC was knotted through the end-side hole of the suction catheter and passed retrograde through the nasopharynx as the red, rubber suction catheter was withdrawn. Then, as one individual maintained tension on the CVC, a lubricated, 6.0-mm ID, cuffed red rubber tube (Rusch) was passed nasally over the catheter until it would no longer advance. The CVC was withdrawn from the cricothyroid membrane, and the tube was advanced with a gentle rotating motion until it reached a tracheal position as demonstrated by audible respiration through the tube, the patient's inability to phonate after cuff inflation, and the breath sounds that were audible bilaterally with controlled positive pressure ventilation. General anesthesia was induced with sodium thiopental and halothane in nitrous oxide and oxygen, and the patient was positioned for thoracotomy. At the end of the procedure, the patient was taken to the recovery room and extubated when wide awake in the sitting position. The biopsy was benign. There was no hoarseness or sore throat noted in the postoperative period or at discharge from hospital.

C. DISCUSSION

This patient presented a number of years ago with a physical examination that suggested that tracheostomy would be difficult and a history confirming the fact that both direct and indirect intubation would be difficult. Both the patient and her medical team were highly motivated to participate in airway control. Retrograde endotracheal intubation was a satisfactory option because the alternative, elective tracheostomy, was less palatable to all concerned. In more recent times, it is likely that either an otolaryngologist or an anesthesiologist with fiberoptic intubation skills would have assessed this patient's laryngeal apparatus to ensure that arytenoid subluxation was not a problem before and after intubation. Indeed, a smaller fiberoptic instrument with a greater angle of flexion would be more likely to succeed where the older, 6-mm OD instruments might not. Nevertheless, patients with such distorted supraglottic anatomy in whom fiberoptic visualization is not possible do exist, and the retrograde technique offers a satisfactory elective option short of cricothyrotomy.

A problem that has been reported with retrograde cannulation is failure to pass an ET once the tip is in the laryngeal inlet, either due to angulation of the larynx and trachea, to the tube's catching on fixed structures like arytenoid cartilages during passage, or to abnormality of the larynx. In this case, a small, relatively stiff tube was passed over the retrograde cannula. In other cases, a "gliding" knot attached to the Murphy eye of the tube,[39] a guidewire, tapered multilumen catheter of large external diameter,[40] a fiberoptic bronchoscope passed inside the ET into the laryngeal inlet and below the cricoid level as a stylet, an endotracheal tube changer passed over a guidewire as a stylet for tube passage,[41] and a specially designed tapered stylet that advances into the trachea over the retrograde guide (Cook, Inc., Bloomington, Ind.) have been used to overcome this problem. The basic idea has been to insert a stylet for intubation that fits more closely over a retrograde guide but is smaller and less likely to "hang up." Alternatively, a thinner jet ventilation catheter has been easier to pass.[40] The fiberoptic approach allows the operator to be certain that the stylet (a fiberoptic bronchoscope) is passed below the cricoid and is within the trachea.

The retrograde technique has been advocated or reported for the difficult pediatric patient,[42,43] for victims of facial, head, or neck trauma,[44,45] for double-lumen tube insertion,[46] for difficult burn patients,[41] and for patients with supraglottic or pharyngeal masses. Enthusiasm for the systems now available should be tempered by the realization that the retrograde technique is blind. Laceration of the posterior membranous portion of the trachea, laryngeal injury, aspiration, and injection of masses or foreign bodies[47] into the trachea have all been reported.[48] Anesthesia staff and their patients tend to avoid using this technique because it seems to be invasive; however, it is certainly less invasive than surgical cricothyrotomy or tracheostomy.

Retrograde intubation is an older airway management technique that has been revitalized by new variations. Newer, off-the-shelf equipment makes the technique both more aesthetically acceptable and more successful. It is, however, a blind technique and may be associated with trauma. Consequently, retrograde intubation should not be the first choice in approaching the stable patient with a known difficult airway.

VI. THE ILLUMINATING STYLET (LIGHTWAND) (CHAPTER 18)

A. INTRODUCTION

Transillumination is a useful technique for identifying the location of an illuminated body in the airway and elsewhere. It is used to assist the inexperienced in locating the tip of a fiberoptic bronchoscope when lost in secretions or disoriented by unfamiliar anatomy. A number of rigid, malleable, and steerable systems allow placement of a stylet in the larynx over which an ET can be passed. Blind, light guided passage of an atraumatic stylet over which an ET can be passed could replace direct laryngoscopy for routine intubations.

B. CASE PRESENTATION

A 23-year-old healthy male was scheduled for cervical laminectomy for cervical spine radiculopathy. The preoperative examination demonstrated a restricted mouth opening and guarded neck extension. Under general anesthesia, only the tip of the epiglottis could be seen at laryngoscopy. The patient was effectively ventilated using a no. 4 laryngeal mask airway (LMA). Through the LMA, placement of the ET using the fiberscope was quite difficult. Staff experienced with the light wand (Trachlight) was called to assist with ET intubation. Intubation was successfully performed using this technique in less than 8 seconds.

C. DISCUSSION

Over the years, a number of fiberoptic light systems have been used to transilluminate the pharynx, larynx, and trachea for intubation and tube positioning.[49-54] These techniques have been around for over 30 years as an alternative option for difficult laryngoscopy and intubation.[55,56] Trials of newer devices in the operating room and field settings have demonstrated that these systems can be used "blindly" with a high success rate, provided that the mouth can be opened.[57,58] Newer light-wand systems have been adapted for nasal intubation.[59] There is even discussion of light-wand transillumination for intubation of patients who have acute cervical spine injuries, despite the fact that an indirect technique may carry foreign material into the trachea or lacerate previously injured tissues.[60,61]

Intubation over a lighted stylet that is positioned by transillumination represents a significant breakthrough for the airway expert. Refined versions of the system, such as the Flexi-Lum, Trach-Light (Laerdal, Inc.), and Tube-stat (Concept Corp., Clearwater, Fla.), are convenient and simple. The equipment involved is no more expensive than the direct laryngoscope. It is reusable and technically straightforward. The procedure takes no more time than direct laryngoscopy and is probably less traumatic, since the tissues of the pharynx are not deformed by application of the rigid laryngoscope blade with distracting pressures required to open the mouth, extend the neck, and lift the head. Because the passage of stylet and ET is blind, there remains a potential for laryngeal or tracheal injury, and the technique should be practiced in uncomplicated patients as a routine before using it with the difficult airway.[62]

An interesting question about this case is why fiberoptic intubation failed while transillumination was successful. One of the problems with use of the laryngeal mask airway (LMA) as an intubation guide is the fact that the orifice of the LMA is not immediately opposite the larynx.[63] A central position is only observed in 59% of adults[64] and 49% of children,[65] while the epiglottis is observed to protrude in the mask grille 49% to 66% of the time. Fiberoptic intubation through an LMA has been more successful than blind intubation through the LMA.[66] I have found that, when the larynx is angled away from the grille of the LMA, it may be necessary to deflate the cuff of the LMA and withdraw it a bit so that the flexible fiberoptic bronchoscope (FFB) can negotiate the angle around the epiglottis into the larynx more effectively.[67] This would suggest that, when the flexible fiberscope cannot visualize or enter the larynx, a blind stylet will be unlikely to do so unless it simply forces the epiglottis downward into the larynx so that the stylet can gain access. We have no information about the difficulty the endoscopist encountered. We are possibly comparing an inexperienced endoscopist with an experienced lightwand user. Clearly, experience is required with either technique, although lightwand intubation is easier to learn.

The modern versions of the lightwand are highly effective for endotracheal intubation and technically easy to use. Frequent use brings greater facility with the technique and greater assurance that it will be helpful in the difficult airway situation.

VII. THE LARYNGEAL MASK AIRWAY (CHAPTER 19)

A. INTRODUCTION

Dr. A.I. Brain's innovative creation was quite slow to achieve recognition in the United States, despite a large clinical data base and the personal testimonials of a number of competent airway experts. The LMA's acceptance has now reached an accelerated stage. These cases demonstrate that the LMA, in addition to providing an adequate anesthetic airway under many circumstances, provides a bridge between the mask and endotracheal tube—a safe airway guide for difficult intubation.

B. CASE 1 PRESENTATION

A 55-year-old female presented for total knee replacement under general anesthesia. Preoperative evaluation revealed a Mallampati Class 1 airway, and no difficulties were anticipated. Following induction of general anesthesia (IV thiopental and atracurium) and control of the airway with mask ventilation, laryngoscopy was difficult. Only the epiglottis could be seen. An attempt to pass a gum-elastic bougie resulted in esophageal intubation. Following this, a #4 LMA was inserted. Effective ventilation was easy to manage. A lubricated 6.0-mm ID, cuffed ET was passed blindly through the LMA into the trachea. Controlled ventilation was provided via this tube for the duration of the operation. After surgery, anesthesia was discontinued, and the LMA and ET were removed together when the patient was fully awake. No complications followed an uneventful recovery.

C. CASE 2 PRESENTATION

A 54-year-old man was scheduled for coronary artery bypass grafting (CABG). The preoperative evaluation revealed significant coronary disease, but the airway was unremarkable. Pancuronium was given for paralysis following a thiopental and phenoperidine induction. Ventilation by face mask was judged difficult, although adequate. Laryngoscopy revealed no useful landmarks, and blind passage of a gum-elastic bougie resulted in esophageal intubation. A size #4 LMA was passed. This provided an effective airway. A gum-elastic bougie was passed via the LMA and used for attempted intubation after removal of the LMA. Unfortunately, esophageal placement was again demonstrated.

The LMA was replaced and used for ventilation with an isoflurane-oxygen gas mixture, while cricothyrotomy was performed with an epidural needle. A catheter was passed retrograde into the pharynx and used as a guide for intubation after removal of the LMA. Esophageal intubation was thought to be due to a release of tension on the catheter as the endotracheal tube was passed. The LMA was replaced and, using adequate tension on the catheter from both ends, endotracheal intubation was successful. Approximately 45 minutes elapsed from initial laryngoscopy to endotracheal intubation, during which there was no evidence of arterial desaturation, electrocardiographic ST segment change, or inadequate anesthesia. Operation and recovery were uneventful, excepting a prolonged, paralytic ileus that was thought to be unrelated to the airway management difficulty. The patient had no recall of anesthesia or the intubation procedures.

D. DISCUSSION

Brain described an extensive experience with his new concept for airway control in 1983.[68] Case reports and interprofessional communication about this spread into North America thereafter,[69,70] but it took over 10 years for the LMA to reach wide acceptance in the United States. This was partly due to the delayed presentation of an approved LMA for the American market and partly due to the aesthetics of the airway. Most anesthesia personnel and nursing support staff are initially sceptical when they actually see the airway because they cannot believe that it effectively isolates the larynx and that it is atraumatic.[71] Clinical acceptance has been greatly facilitated by careful documentation in both the American and international literature. Additionally, actual experience has shown that one LMA, if properly cared for, can provide 200 to 400 clinical uses.

In the first case, the LMA provided the route through which an ET could be blindly passed into the trachea. In the second, the LMA contributed a measure of security while retrograde cannulation for intubation could be performed. A stable airway that allows administration of anesthesia and effective ventilation and oxygenation while other measures to achieve endotracheal intubation can be devised offers increased safety for our patients and a stress-free environment for the anesthesia and surgical teams. Numerous attempts have been made to achieve this with modified face masks in the past.[72,73] Recent prospective trials,[74,75,76] reviews,[77] and case reports* have clearly demonstrated the utility of the LMA in these settings. The LMA now has a clear role for airway management of patients with either a difficult airway or difficult intubation and has been referenced in the American Society of Anesthesiologists' recently published difficult airway algorithm.[84]

The remarkable finding that the LMA provides an adequate airway despite an eccentric, suboptimal position or epiglottis herniation into the grille-covered aperture of the airway, as confirmed by a number of authors (see preceding discussion of light-wand mediated intubation), suggests that blind intubation may not be effective. In the second case, it is doubtful that any blindly inserted device would have passed through the LMA into the trachea, since the gum-elastic bougie[85] failed. A number of groups (cited previously) have demonstrated that the LMA can serve as a convenient guide to the larynx for a flexible fiberoptic bronchoscope (FFB). It has even been proposed to pulmonologists as an airway of choice to facilitate FFB when patients have obstructing tumors and stridor.[86]

To my knowledge, no one has previously described use of the LMA for retrograde intubation. Earlier descriptions of retrograde intubation have emphasized the fact that it is a three-handed technique: two hands are required to maintain tension on the retrograde wire or catheter, while another advances the tube and rotates it, if necessary, if it hangs up at the larynx.[87] The Cook Retrograde Intubation Set (Cook Critical Care, Bloomington, Ind.) provides a tapered stylet that is passed down into the larynx over a guidewire. The stylet passed over a guidewire may have a higher success rate than

*References 78, 79, 80, 81, 82, 83.

passage over an epidural or styletted CVC. If the retrograde catheter had been passed through the LMA, it might have avoided the intubation failure that the author noted with the first attempt at anterograde passage of the endotracheal tube over the retrograde catheter. From this stage, it would be relatively simple to place a larger tube than a 6.0-mm ID (LMA #3 and 4) or a 2.5- to 5.0-mm ID (LMA #1, 2, and 2.5) by exchanging it over appropriately sized Cook or other "tube changer."

Each anesthesiologist, nurse anesthetist, emergency medical physician, emergency medical technician, and advanced life support provider should be taught use of the LMA. No airway expert should be ignorant of its potential uses in cases where the airway is difficult, laryngoscopy is problematic, or repeated attempts to perform translaryngeal intubation have failed.

VIII. NEW LARYNGOSCOPE BLADES (CHAPTER 20)

A. INTRODUCTION

Anesthesiologists and other physicians who practice acute medicine are tinkerers, ever trying to improve on the techniques that precede them. While most of the medical community groups rigid laryngoscopes into those that employ straight versus curved blades, there is a constant evolution of blade variants. Most are eponymous. Dr. S.D. Cooper offers several case reports that illustrate the advantages of several of the new variants.

B. CASE 1 PRESENTATION

A 54-year-old man is scheduled for an elective Bankhart procedure of his right shoulder. His past medical history is unremarkable. Your preoperative airway examination is notable for Class 2 visualization of the oropharynx with mouth opening during neck extension and a heavy, full beard. On closer examination, the beard hides a receding chin with a hyomental distance of only 2 cm.

1. Assessment

This patient has a very short hyomental distance. A short distance between hyoid and jaw normally correlates with a very short hyothyroid distance and an anteriorly angled larynx. Typically, in this circumstance the endoscopist passes any laryngoscope blade too far into the hypopharynx, consequently missing the laryngeal inlet. Also, as Roberts has shown, an anteriorly tilted larynx requires special effort for full visualization and passage of an endotracheal tube. Mask anesthesia is also likely to be difficult because of the beard and receding jaw.

C. CASE 2 PRESENTATION

You have just induced general anesthesia IV in a 35-year-old female who is scheduled for total abdominal hysterectomy. Her past medical history is significant for smoking and uterine fibroids. She reports no drug allergies. General anesthesia is induced with midazolam (2 mg), fentanyl (5 ml), propofol (120 mg) and vecuronium (7 mg). The mask airway was good prior to administration of the neuromuscular blocking agent, but now you are experiencing progressive difficulty.

Little red welts begin to appear on the patients chest and arms. All you see is a mass of swollen, glistening oropharyngeal tissues. You suspect a delayed hypersensitivity or anaphylactoid reaction.

1. Assessment

The LMA comes immediately to mind as a way to bypass a difficult upper airway, but, with evidence of tissue swelling and hives, endotracheal intubation would offer the advantages of a tight cuff seal that will allow higher pressures during ventilation and prevent laryngeal edema from closing the airway. The Bainton blade (or pharyngolaryngoscope) would be useful in this setting. This tubular blade prevents pharyngeal tissues from obscuring the endoscopist's vision, provided he or she can recognize structures that are in view. Blades like the Flagg, Wisconsin-Foregger, Guedel, Magill, and Foregger versions can be rotated 90 degrees and inserted directly into the larynx to allow passage of an ET when the larynx is edematous. Some are designed so that a tube can be passed directly along the inner channel into the larynx when tissue edema or loss of visualization after placement of the laryngoscope blade presents a problem.

D. CASE 3 PRESENTATION

The anesthesiologist on call is paged to the trauma unit for airway control of a young adult male who went through the windshield of a motor vehicle during a head-on collision. On arrival the patient is immobilized on a spine board, in a cervical collar, and his head is secured in the midline with sandbags on either side. He has a low-flow mask providing oxygen at 4 L/min and is spitting blood with exhalation. As a history and evaluation are attempted, he appears inebriated and uncooperative.

1. Assessment

The Bullard laryngoscope would be an excellent option in this situation[88] because its use does not require much mouth opening, jaw lift, or neck movement,[89] and it has a 2.2 mm suction port that would facilitate clearance of bloody secretions from the field of view. Despite obvious evidence of alcohol use, altered mentation could be due to traumatic central nervous system (CNS) injury or other drug ingestion. If a neuroanesthetic (IV induction, hyperventilation and paralysis with a nondepolarizing relaxant, and direct intubation with stabilization of head and neck) is needed because of the patient's agitation or changing CNS level, a cricothyrotomy or surgical tracheostomy "standby" should be planned.

E. DISCUSSION

All three of these patients present unique airway management challenges that are likely to occur in clinical practice. Case #2 is a bit more unusual, but the challenge is quite similar to those posed by the morbidly obese patient, the patient with angioneurotic edema, and patients with airway burns. To some extent, these cases present an outline of several types of intubation difficulty: the short, high laryngeal placement with anterior angulation, redundant soft tissues that fall into the field and obstruct the endoscopist's view, the abnormal laryngeal inlet that frustrates the endoscopist because it can be seen but not entered, the mouth that will not open, obstructing blood and secretions, and/or the immobile neck. Approaches to each of these problems vary, and it should be clear that, given interindividual variability in airway anatomy, no single technical approach to placement or type of laryngoscope will be ideal for all patients.

No matter how many times the process is rediscovered, there are really four ways to deal with the high, anterior larynx. First, one may change laryngeal angulation so that it lines up with the endoscopist's line of sight by using the appropriate choice of curved or straight laryngoscope blade with effective mouth opening, correct neck flexion, and atlantoaxial joint extension, and posterior pressure on the larynx.[90,91,92,93] Because there is significant variability from patient to patient, the correct blade characteristics may be unique to each difficult patient. This justifies the orderly progression some anesthetists make from blade to blade when encountering difficult laryngoscopy. Second, one can learn to use angled stylets or other apparatus (see light wand, etc., preceding) for laryngoscope directed, blind intubation.[94] This is what most anesthesia staff actually do when they document poor visualization. Third, one can use an angled, mirror, or prism blade that "sees around corners" so that the larynx is viewed indirectly during intubation.[95,96,97,98] Another variant on this approach is use of the indirect, mirror laryngoscope, a technique favored by older otolaryngologists who have expertise with the mirror and head lamp. A more recent report of this technique described the use of a dental mirror, probably because the otolaryngologist's tool was unfamiliar to the anesthesia staff involved.[99] Finally, one can use a FFB, angled telescope (Bullard laryngoscope[100,101,102]), or malleable fiberoptic telescope. The latter devices tend to provide a better view of the larynx, provided blood and secretions can be kept off the larynx.

Redundant soft tissue in the airway is best dealt with by use of either a flanged (Macintosh), a partly enclosed (Flagg), or a fully enclosed (Bainton[103]) laryngoscope blade that tends to retract tissue and to protect the light from blockage by infolding tissue. The enclosed designs really derive from the original Jackson laryngoscope and later versions of suspension laryngoscopes used for endoscopic surgery. The utility of enclosed blades explains the occasional observation that a rigid bronchoscope can succeed in passing the laryngeal inlet when a standard laryngoscope fails. Aside from the fact that another airway expert is entered fresh into the fray, the bronchoscopist wields a rigid, circular scope that can both retract tissues and serve as an airway. It has been forced through closed or swollen vocal cords to create an airway on numerous occasions when no one could pass a styletted ET.

As with the tube bronchoscope, tube or half-round style blades, like the Flagg, can be inserted between the cords and rotated to open them, while the endotracheal tube is passed along the channel within the curved flange. One technical problem with enclosed blades is that, the more fully enclosed the blade, the more difficult it is to remove the instrument after intubation. For this reason, some of the fully enclosed ear, nose, and throat (ENT) endoscopes (for example, suspension laser laryngoscopes) have one or more articulated sides that may be removed by the operator during use.

Until recently, fiberoptic endoscopes were somewhat specialized. The malleable stylet or telescope provides excellent optics but has a large outer diameter, in keeping with its optics, and lack of suction capability. It was good for transoral and transnasal laryngoscopy, especially for patients and their doctors who remembered mirror laryngoscopy. A tube can either be passed over it into the trachea or passed off it into the laryngeal inlet under direct visualization. The Bullard instrument was well suited to the difficult pediatric airway because the external diameter of flexible and malleable fiberoptic instruments was too great. It was only a second generation of this instrument with a specially shaped stylet that functioned as well in adults as earlier flexible scopes. Now there is a generation of ultra-thin flexible instruments in the 1.5- to 2.5-mm range and at least one commercially marketed pediatric intubating FFB below an outer diameter of 3.5 mm.

Blood, vomitus, and secretions obscure all types of fiberoptic systems at some point. A large suction channel is a desirable feature, as is simplicity of use, steering capability, handling ease, price, and low maintenance cost. Both the malleable stylet and Bullard laryngoscope require skills that most anesthesia personnel already possess or find easy to acquire. The malleable fiberoptic telescope is cheapest. The Bullard laryngoscope has good optics and suction but only provides a remote picture of the airway so that an intubating stylet can be passed into it. The Bullard laryngoscope can also be used to guide nasotracheal intubation, just as the malleable

stylet and FFB can.[104] Also, all three fiberoptic devices are good choices for patients, such as #3, who have fixed necks,[105] when direct laryngoscopy appears to fail because of limited jaw and neck mobility.

My own choice for intubation is the more versatile, full-length FFB when airway difficulty is anticipated. It turns corners and can be passed transnasally, periorally, and via a tracheotomy stoma. The FFB can be used for atraumatic nasopharyngeal, pharyngeal, and laryngeal diagnosis, for observation as another maneuver is performed, as a stylet for endotracheal intubation, and for guided suction or blockade of lower airways. The instrument is ubiquitous in our offices and hospitals. It is understood by a broad spectrum of acute care physicians, and it comes in a variety of sizes. Available options include a diverse number of light sources, teaching attachments, video systems, biopsy-brush sampling systems, and suction-injector adapters. Although cleaning, maintenance, and repair expenses are significant, a large hospital experience shared among similar flexible fiberoptic endoscopes (e.g., gastroscopes, sigmoidoscopes, choledochoscopes, colonoscopes, and nasopharygoscopes) insures that many support staff are trained to care for the FFB. Fiberoptic intubation would be my preference in Case #3 if the level of consciousness permits time for the procedure.[106] Other authors[107] and I have argued that a flexible fiberoptic device that passes an ET over a stylet without deforming anatomy (e.g., FFB) is crucial for endotracheal intubation of the trauma patient with an unstable neck, but clinical data suggest that direct laryngoscopy may not be so deforming as we think.[108] Also, there are no data that clearly show fiberoptic intubation to be superior to careful intubation by direct laryngoscopy.[109]

It is difficult to master all of the types of laryngoscope blades that have been designed by innovative airway experts. I believe that it is more important to understand airway problems and bring a technical arsenal and a well-thought out plan (i.e., the ASA difficult airway algorithm)[84] to bear on them. Flanged and semienclosed straight blades have a place in our armamentarium, as do a variety of curved blades. Flexible, malleable, and rigid fiberoptic endoscopes have unique characteristics that enable their use under different circumstances. The FFB remains the most versatile of these, especially now that ultrathin varieties have been designed.

Rather than identify the ideal laryngoscope blade, the clinician should incorporate a staged sequence of thoughtful steps during intubation attempts. These range from the search for the ideal head-pharyngeal-neck axis during laryngoscopy with different types of blades to the use of LMA, FFB, retrograde intubation, and/or cricothyrotomy when unexpected difficulty occurs. All of the fiberoptic systems work well when used in an appropriate setting by experienced personnel.

Clearly, the crisis situation is not the first time or place to attempt use of an unfamiliar piece of equipment.

IX. RIGID BRONCHOSCOPY, SHARED AIRWAY (CHAPTER 24)

A. INTRODUCTION

Obstructing airway lesions present a major challenge for the anesthesia team. One must combine one's best understanding of the problem with technical expertise and a wide cornucopia of techniques from which to choose. When the problem is compounded by a need to share the airway with another caregiver for diagnostic or therapeutic purposes, special problems often arise.

B. CASE PRESENTATION

The patient is an 18-month-old female with a 24-hour history of wheezing, asymmetric breath sounds, and a chest x-ray consistent with a left-shifted mediastinum. Prior to presentation at the pediatrician's office, the child was afebrile during a 3-day course of runny nose and mild upper airway congestion. The night before coming to see her pediatrician, the child had an episode of choking while eating a piece of raw broccoli. Respiratory distress was not noted at that time. The child was presented to the operating room for rigid bronchoscopy that was to be both diagnostic and therapeutic, since it was presumed that broccoli in the airway was responsible for the wheezing and the x-ray findings.

Anesthesia was induced uneventfully by mask with halothane in nitrous oxide-oxygen. After controlling ventilation with halothane in 100% oxygen, a rigid bronchoscope was introduced without difficulty. The findings were consistent with diffuse tracheabronchial edema due to laryngotracheobronchitis in the absence of any foreign body. After bronchoscopy, the mask airway was compromised. Initial attempts to ventilate the patient were associated with wheezing and persistent arterial desaturation. For this reason, the child was reintubated with a 4.0-mm ET, and bronchodilator therapy was instilled into the lower airway via the ET. Wheezing abated after 15 minutes so that the patient could be extubated in the operating room. She was treated symptomatically and observed in hospital for 48 hours, during which she progressed to an uneventful recovery from her respiratory infection.

C. DISCUSSION

This child presents a number of challenges. It is presumed that she has active airway inflammation with a superimposed stimulus to airway reactivity. While the diagnosis was not clear in advance,[110] the anesthesiologist must assume that she might have a crumbling foreign body that is obstructing an airway. X-ray changes could be due either to unilateral hyperinflation and air trapping or to lung volume loss associated with near total

obstruction and resorption of distal gasses.[111] Both conditions are likely to cause hypoxemia. Hypoxemia is most commonly associated with an increased number of low ventilation/perfusion ratio lung units. There may be more rapid desaturation of this patient than others with apnea or atelectasis because of the increased oxygen consumption caused by her 3-day systemic infectious process. Additionally, although wheezing and hypoxemia might be due to airway reaction to the foreign body alone, one must remember that reactive airway disease is noted with croup (laryngotracheobronchitis), epiglottitis, and tracheitis.[112,113]

The otolaryngologist and anesthesiologist have a shared concern in cases like this. There is a general issue concerning use of positive pressure, endotracheal intubation, and other maneuvers that might dislodge a laryngeal or tracheal foreign body. Noninvasive oxygen therapy is well advised prior to anesthesia—excitement increases gas flows, resistance, and turbulence through narrowed airways. As a critical resistance is reached, flow will cease, and distal atelectasis with hypoxemia is likely. In addition, excitement increases oxygen requirement at a time when supply is limited. During or after anesthetic induction, vigorous positive pressure ventilation will force gas past a partially obstructing lesion or foreign body. The foreign body may then act like a ball valve in exhalation, trapping gas and hyperinflating distal lung segments. Regional hyperinflation can cause pneumothorax, pneumopericardium or pneumomediastinum and cardiovascular collapse. These problems, in addition to secretion plugging with infection, most likely account for the greater complication rate associated with delayed diagnosis and removal of laryngeal and tracheal foreign bodies.[114,115]

The anesthetic induction should be gradual, whether IV or inhalational. It is helpful to maintain spontaneous ventilation until the patient is deeply anesthetized. Even though newer paralytic agents may have a safer therapeutic index for cardiovascular and pulmonary complications and a better metabolic profile, succinylcholine offers positive advantages. The drug can be given for a rapidly reversible test of controlled ventilation or to permit rigid bronchoscopy with the fastest paralytic "offset" now available in case of difficulty. It can also be titrated for a variable length of time as a continuous infusion. I recommend that the anesthetist attempt to visualize the hypopharynx and larynx with a laryngoscope prior to bronchoscopy, unless there is a pharyngeal foreign body. This will allow the anesthesia team to know how difficult intubation and bronchoscopy will be. Forewarned is forearmed.

Since the anesthetist must literally surrender his patient to the otolaryngist for endoscopy, it is well to plan ahead. This should not take a great deal of time, but it is essential that the airway management role and options of all team members be worked out in advance. Also, the case should be performed in an operating room environment where there is access to emergency equipment and personnel. Ketamine or one of the potent, volatile anesthetic vapors that has bronchodilating properties offers significant advantages for the bronchoscopy patient. It is of paramount importance that the patient be adequately anesthetized (probably deeply) whenever the rigid bronchoscope is within, or being moved about, the tracheobronchial tree, and the stimulus for bronchospasm or sustained forceful exhalation is great.

In this case the patient had inflammatory airway disease of probable infectious etiology. The 3-day course and bronchoscopic findings fit this diagnosis, as do the events following bronchoscopy. For poorly understood reasons, airway inflammation increases bronchoreactivity, as does airway instrumentation. (One hypothesis is that narrowed, edematous airways restrict flow more when they constrict than normal airways do. Another is that the smooth muscle is more reactive.) The rigid bronchoscope is a rather traumatic instrument that deforms and rubs against soft tissues. Unlike the suspension laryngoscope, the rigid bronchoscope is often levered against the teeth (protected by a dental guard) or the operator's gloved finger set against the upper teeth. Endobronchial insertion and periods of segmental or unilateral lung inflation are common—as is manipulation of all levels of the airway with swabs, biopsy forceps, and rigid suction cannulas. The anesthetist can help the bronchoscopist during this process by monitoring oxygenation with a pulse oximeter and intermittently ventilating the patient so that end-tidal carbon dioxide levels can be used to assess adequacy of ventilation. Also, if there is a loose laryngeal fit around the bronchoscope with a large leak, the anesthesia team can increase effective ventilation by maintaining full paralysis and/or applying gentle pressure on the anterior neck that seals soft tissues around the bronchoscope. Increased bronchospasm postbronchoscopy can most likely be attributed to decreasing anesthetic levels in hopes of awakening the patient promptly and to bronchoscopic trauma superimposed upon the underlying disease. The bronchospasm could have been treated with deeper inhalational anesthesia (assuming the patient's cardiovascular system will tolerate this) or, as in this case, with an inhaled or injectable bronchodilator.

Croup or laryngotracheobronchitis that presents in toddlers and children under doubtful circumstances may be due to foreign body. Management of inflamed or infected airways is difficult and frought with peril. Foreign body extraction is one of those difficult situations where the anesthetist and endoscopist must share the already compromised airway. Nowadays, some enlightened otolaryngologists will perform FFB in pediatric cases before rigid endoscopy, but the clinical problems are similar. Bronchospasm, barotrauma, and other consequences of airway instrumentation can manifest themselves both during and after bronchoscopy. Deep anesthesia can minimize these complications. Every anesthesia practitioner, whether a bronchoscopist or not, should be aware of the technical problems that occur during airway endoscopy.

X. THE COMBITUBE (CHAPTER 22)

A. INTRODUCTION

The Combitube or esophageal tracheal airway (ETA) was studied and introduced to the anesthesia, emergency medicine, and critical care community as an airway management alternative when mask ventilation is ineffective and endotracheal intubation is difficult or impossible.[116-119] Many have thought the device to be merely an improved esophageal obturator airway after its introduction in the mid-1980s. It was introduced at approximately the same time as the pharyngeal tracheal lumen airway and as emergency medical technicians and their hospital control services experienced widespread disenchantment with the esophageal obturator airways in current use.[120] These are most likely the reasons that the device has failed to achieve widespread use in the United States over the last 10 years. The following case demonstrates that the ETA does, indeed, have something to offer those responsible for anesthesia care and emergency airway control.

B. CASE PRESENTATION

A 63-year-old man with severe chronic obstructive lung disease was admitted to the ICU. A diagnosis of acute pulmonary embolus was suspected, and thrombolytic therapy was administered. Baseline coagulation parameters were within the normal range. Thrombolytic therapy was initiated with 230 mg of anisoylated plasminogen streptokinase activator complex (APSAC). Due to confusion over the thrombolytic protocol, an additional infusion of 230 mg APSAC was administered.

Four hours later, the patient began to bleed from the pharynx. This was so dramatic that endotracheal intubation was indicated to prevent aspiration. Multiple attempts at direct translaryngeal intubation failed because of the copious active bleeding. Both blind and fiberoptic attempts were also unsuccessful. Cricothyroidotomy was considered but felt to be inadvisable because of the ongoing hemorrhagic diathesis.

At this point, the Combitube was inserted. Mechanical ventilation could be performed successfully. After the coagulation abnormality was stable, the Combitube was replaced with a conventional endotracheal airway. Direct laryngoscopy during translaryngeal intubation revealed sublingual, right pharyngeal, and palatal hematomata. Two days later, the patient was weaned from the respirator. He was discharged from the hospital a week later with no signs of neurologic deficit.

C. DISCUSSION

This case nicely illustrates the unique applications of the Combitube. The device is clearly not just another emergency esophageal obturator. Its use for pharyngeal tamponade is a logical extension of the concept illustrated by earlier uses for balloon catheters like the Foley catheter in control of nasopharyngeal bleeding or the Blakemore-Sengstaken and other esophageal or gastric obturators for bleeding below the pharynx. Earlier work has suggested that the ETA could be used as a definitive airway in place of translaryngeal or transtracheal intubation for an extended period.[121] Here, the ETA both tamponaded bleeding and provided a secure tube for mechanical ventilation until an ET could be placed.

Heretofore, our best alternatives for intubation in the presence of active bleeding into the upper airway have employed an extreme head down or lateral Trendelenburg position for drainage with or without endotracheal intubation.[122] Direct, indirect, or fiberoptic awake intubation can be managed in cooperative adults. "Crash" intubation in Trendelenburg position under anesthesia is also used in children[123] and adults when the situation is more stable. Often, the only clue to the laryngeal location during laryngoscopy is bubbling exhaled gas through the blood. I recommend cricoid pressure with the idea that swallowed blood will not be regurgitated into the field during intubation under anesthesia. An experienced assistant can often provide cricoid pressure that enables the operator to intubate while assuring that the ET cuff is properly inflated by palpating it below the cricoid cartilage following intubation.

Fiberoptic intubation has most often worked for us in the emergency setting, provided oxygenation can be maintained during spontaneous breathing,[124] but it is notoriously difficult[125] when blood interferes. I think that retrograde cricothyroid guidewire or catheter-guided intubation would have been inappropriate in this situation because of the ongoing, life-threatening risk of blood aspiration. Additionally, as with tracheostomy and cricothyrotomy, it can induce more bleeding from within the trachea. While one might propose insertion of a laryngeal mask on the grounds that, as an alternative airway, it will partly protect the larynx from blood and also provide an intubation pathway, the LMA is not so likely to control pharyngeal bleeding by direct tamponade as the ETA.

Since there was significant sublingual and lateral pharyngeal hematoma accumulation that might have extended to make later endotracheal intubation or tracheostomy nearly impossible, the decision to follow this patient clinically without inserting a tracheal airway would be viewed as controversial by some.[126] For this reason, the options of cricothyroid jet ventilation, percutaneous cricothyrotomy with a cuffed endotracheal tube, or a formal, surgical tracheostomy must be considered as alternatives early in the course of such a patient's care. The choice of the ETA as a bridge to translaryngeal intubation must have been (and should be) purely clinical. A deteriorating situation despite effective ventilation through the Combitube or rapidly expanding neck hematoma that showed signs of distorting the larynx and upper trachea would mitigate in favor of a surgical airway in spite of the coagulopathy. A cuffed tracheostomy tube will, at least, diminish the risk that upper airway bleeding will drain below the stoma site into the trachea.

This case illustrates use of the esophageal tracheal Combitube as an interim airway that tamponaded upper airway bleeding while preventing aspiration, surgical airway bleeding, or further trauma due to direct laryngoscopy in an anticoagulated patient. While the issues of the Combitube as the ideal field EMT airway[127] and as a long-term airway for controlled ventilation are not relevant to this case, it is clear that the device has a unique niche in our airway management armamentarium. Most acute airway practitioners should be aware of this airway, and every anesthesia department and emergency room should consider having appropriately sized ETAs on the emergency airway cart.

XI. PERCUTANEOUS DILATIONAL CRICOTHYROTOMY AND TRACHEOTOMY

A. INTRODUCTION

Percutaneous dilatational cricothyrotomy and tracheotomy is an elaborate name for percutaneous airway insertion using a modified Seldinger technique. The airway can be an oxygen delivery or suction catheter, a jet ventilation cannula, or a normal-sized, cuffed endotracheal tube.

B. CASE PRESENTATION

DG was a 17-year-old male driver involved in a head-on collision. He had not been drinking, and it was not known whether he was using a seat belt. When EMS arrived on the scene, he was out of the car walking and had not lost consciousness. The steering wheel was bent. He was given a Glasgow Coma Scale (GCS) of 13, which means that he could move everything, withdraw from pain, and follow commands but was confused and somewhat disoriented. He was hemodynamically stable when taken to the nearest medical center. Clinical examination raised the question of closed head trauma and cervical spine injury because of severe midface injuries and tenderness to palpation over cervical vertebrae. He had an equivocal Babinski reflex bilaterally. Cervical spine films demonstrated a pedicle fracture of C6, a probable C5 facet fracture, laminar fractures at C6 and C7, a possible C3 facet fracture, and widening of the spinal canal in the midcervical level.

Despite significant facial injury, the patient was transported to the radiology department for computerized tomography (CT) scanning without airway control. The head CT revealed diffuse cerebral edema with effacement and a right basal ganglia hemorrhage. The CT was aborted, and the patient transported to the surgical intensive care unit (SICU) when his mental status declined, and he became combative. In the SICU, multiple attempts at direct translaryngeal intubation with neck stabilization by the neurosurgeon failed. Attempted fiberoptic intubation failed. Effective bag-mask hyperventilation with oxygen was provided before and during intubation attempts. This was documented by physical examination and with pulse oximetry. He was given sodium thiopental and succinylcholine to control intracranial pressure and permit laryngoscopy.

Because fiberoptic intubation failed and airway pressures and soft tissue edema in the airway seemed to increase, a cricothyrotomy was rapidly performed, and a 6.0-mm ID ET was placed using the Seldinger technique. Despite normoxia and effective ventilation via the cricothyroid tube, further attempts at oral and fiberoptic intubation also failed. The cricothyrotomy was surgically converted to a formal stoma after approximately 2 hours so that hyperventilation and tracheal toilet could be optimized. Follow-up CT of the head and spine demonstrated extensive cervical and facial injuries that required operative stabilization. Airway endoscopy was performed on postinjury day #12. This showed no injury or complications attributable to cricothyrotomy, and the patient was transferred to a rehabilitation facility 2 days later.

C. DISCUSSION

This case report illustrates the role of urgent cricothyroid airway placement when conventional techniques fail. Lifesaving airway intervention can be performed with ubiquitous equipment from the emergency room and operating room setting.[128-130] A single needle placement can be used to oxygenate,[131] partially ventilate,[132] jet ventilate,[133] or dilate a transtracheal track so that a rigid or flexible tube can be placed for conventional ventilation. Once placed, a cricothyroid airway can stabilize the situation as definitive translaryngeal, transtracheal, or cricothyroid airways are placed.

The case also shows how issues involved in the setting—edema, physician anxiety, bloody secretions, crisis demands, equipment failures, etc.—can make an airway procedure impossible that may not be quite so difficult at another time, in another setting. Endoscopic evaluation of this patient was not impossible. The patient was uneventfully bronchoscoped 2 weeks later for evaluation of possible injury associated with airway intubation attempts. The case presents a powerful argument for elective control of the traumatized airway before evolving insults or secondary injury intensifies the difficulty.[134] It cannot have been easy to gain control of this combative patient with a bloody upper airway, unstable neck, increased intracranial pressure, and midface fractures once he became combative and hypoxic in the CT scanner. That is why many trauma experts recommend intubation of any trauma patient with a GCS of 13 or less prior to CT. Although intubation with the least head and neck displacement is an ideal, one should evaluate patients individually and even employ the less theoretically attractive approach when the patient's condition warrants it.[135] Our protocol involves direct laryngoscopy and intubation with a thiobarbiturate, paralytic dose of a nondepolarizing agent and manual-in-line neck stabilization after a priming dose of nondepolarizing relaxant and hyperventilation. If this approach does not succeed immediately, tracheotomy or cricothyrotomy are performed. When midface or other trauma is associated with basilar skull fracture or CSF leakage into the airway, a direct transtracheal airway is preferred.[136]

In recent years, a number of convenient, off-the-shelf systems have been investigated for placement of large gauge catheters, jet injector catheters and cuffed or uncuffed tracheotomy tubes with standard 15-mm ventilator adaptors (e.g., Melker, Patil, Arndt,[137] marketed by Cook Critical Care and other manufacturers[138-140]). Additionally, there are now several percutaneous dilatational kits for both emergency and elective, permanent cricothyroidotomy and tracheostomy (e.g., Pertrach, Rapidtrach,[141] and others). Early reports[142,143] suggest their safety and efficiency may be as good as the more labor intensive, expensive surgical tracheostomy. Reports regarding field placement of this equipment and opinions about the equipment are more mixed.[144-147]

Cricothyroid ventilation for resuscitation is an old concept.[148] In modern times, emergency cricothyrotomy has been publicized in the cinema, on television, and even through the sales of an executive accessory for the successful surgeon, the pocket cricothyrotomy knife. More recently, it has gained both recognition and support from organizations like the American Society of Anesthesiologists and the American College of Surgeons. The former group has included generic transtracheal catheter techniques as part of its airway management algorithm. The latter includes it in the Advanced Trauma Life Support course, as do other emergency groups. What is new in this area is a major educational effort designed to bring these techniques into every operating room and emergency room. Complementing this is a generation of percutaneous dilatational crico-thyrotomy kits that utilize a modified Seldinger technique. These systems are technically feasible and can be used by a mix of anesthesia and emergency personnel whose surgical training is minimal.

XII. CONFIRMING TRACHEAL INTUBATION (CHAPTER 27)

A. INTRODUCTION

As the following case demonstrates, it is not always easy to be certain that the ET has been placed properly. Newer monitors have made this easier, but the issue is still not always clear at first. Direct visualization of the larynx as an endotracheal tube is passed is not always possible, and both clinical monitors and clinical examination can provide equivocal data for some time after tube placement.

B. CASE PRESENTATION

A 42-year-old female was scheduled for laparoscopic cholecystectomy. Past medical history was unremarkable. After application of routine monitors, including pulse oximetry and mass spectrometry, the patient's lungs were denitrogenated for 3 minutes with an FiO_2 of 1.0. Anesthesia was induced with etomidate and, after paralysis with vecuronium, orotracheal intubation was performed with a 7.5-mm ID ET, and the cuff was deflated. Auscultation revealed bilateral breath sounds during manual ventilation. The SaO_2 was 97%.

When mechanical ventilation was initiated, the ventilator bellows collapsed, and the oxygen saturation decreased to 94%. Repeated auscultation of the chest again demonstrated equal breath sounds with manual ventilation. The mass spectrometer alarm sounded because no CO_2 was detected and no wave could be observed on the monitor. Following this, the O_2 saturation decreased to 87%. Esophageal intubation was suspected and confirmed by direct laryngoscopy. The tube was withdrawn and placed translaryngeally under direct vision. Tracheal placement was further confirmed by auscultation of the chest and epigastrium and by the presence of a normal CO_2 waveform on the mass spectroscopy monitor. Oxygen saturation increased to 99%. The stomach was decompressed with a nasogastric tube. Further anesthesia and surgical care was uneventful.

C. DISCUSSION

Several technical steps might have reduced the delay in recognition that the tube was esophageal. First, if the laryngoscopist had visualized the tube as it was passed above the arytenoids, through the cords, and seen it in place, there could be little doubt of the location. Unfortunately, anesthesia caregivers often have a less ideal view of the larynx and find that the tube obscures the larynx as it is passed somewhere below the epiglottis. In my experience, this is more common when the Macintosh blade is used for intubation. Also, in most teaching institutions, the intubation is often performed by an anesthesia resident, a nurse anesthetist, a student nurse anesthetist, a medical student, a paramedic, or some other resident trainee whose skills may be in doubt.

The second step is to feel the lungs as they are inflated. Humidified expiratory gasses mist the transparent endotracheal tube as the anesthetist's hand feels the tidal return of gasses refill the ventilation reservoir bag. If the reservoir bag is easily emptied but gas does not return, something is clearly amiss. Auscultation, the next step, should routinely begin with the right chest, where an endobronchial intubation is most likely to generate the loudest breath sounds for comparison with those elsewhere. Breath sounds should be sought from the lateral chest, below the axillae, on the right and left sides in turn. Large breasts or chest flab may need to be manually retracted. Precordial breath sounds can be confusing or transmit from right to left. Finally, one should listen over the epigastrium, as was done after the second instance of intubation, to ensure that sounds are not louder there, as might be the case with esophageal intubation, and only transmitted to the chest through tissues.

It should not be surprising to see either gradual arterial desaturation after esophageal intubation or acute desaturation briefly following endotracheal intubation. The relationship between lung oxygen stores (FiO_2 and FRC dependent), minute oxygen consumption, and patency of the airway from either the esophagus or trachea defines the temporal saturation profile. Esophageal intubation with large lung oxygen stores and a low oxygen consumption rate under anesthesia or retrograde ventilation via the pharynx may maintain saturation for a time. Tracheal intubation of someone with high oxygen consumption and low oxygen stores (i.e., an infant, a morbidly obese patient, a patient with chest trauma and multitrauma, an asthmatic in bronchospasm, etc.) or intubation of someone who is "light" and responds with sustained cough and breath holding, thereby reducing lung volume, is likely to result in desaturation that appears slow to respond to ventilation.

Many of us who teach have developed the habit of looking for a capnographic display following a trainee's intubation. Some of the delay in recognizing esophageal intubation in this case may have been due to a slow monitoring response time or to residual CO_2 from the stomach. One may see CO_2 from the stomach and esophagus, but not for long and not in concentrations that resemble end-tidal concentrations for more than a breath or two.[149] The side-stream capnometer that continuously aspirates gasses from an endotracheal tube or tube adapter on the breathing system provides delayed data that, not infrequently, lags a breath or two behind the events. The mass spectrometer is normally a shared system that samples aspirated gas from several operating rooms. Therefore, the display of data, whether numeric or graphic, lags even further behind the side-stream capnometer. Some institutions where there was a shared mass spectrometry system actually installed individual capnometers on the anesthesia systems because of inadequate response times in the salad days of anesthesia reimbursement. A mainstream capnometer that measures gas composition from a sensor directly connected between the endotracheal tube and the anesthesia circuit provides the most immediate response.

Bellows collapse when a recently intubated patient is placed on the ventilator can be caused by several things. Ventilation of a less elastic space, such as the pharynx or stomach, is not ordinarily followed by exhalation. Any other leak will empty the anesthesia system and preclude gas return into the bellows. An inadequate cuff seal or tube fit at the larynx will also leak most of a tidal breath into the pharynx and atmosphere, thus preventing return of gas into the anesthetic system and ventilator bellows. Misplacement of a nasogastric tube or esophageal stethoscope into the trachea is not uncommon. If the ET cuff is damaged or a nasogastric tube is placed upon low suction, gas does not refill the ventilator bellows, and either low peak ventilatory pressures or the negative pressure alarm may alert the anesthetist to the problem. In some operating rooms, a thermocouple or capnometry sampling tube interface with the anesthesia circuit can cause this problem. Ventilators that are set up for manually adjusted pressure-limited modalities can simulate the older system that required the pressure relief valve to be secured prior to ventilation by "popping off" a significant portion of each tidal breath so that the circle will not refill. The least common problem is an intrinsic leak in the ventilator. Periodic leak tests of the anesthesia machine and ventilator should detect this problem before the system grossly fails to ventilate a patient.

Experienced clinicians encounter doubts or apparently conflicting evidence regarding ET placement from time to time, as in this case. The capnometer is one of the most effective tools for resolving apparent clinical conflict that we have, but, since recognition may be delayed by anomalous clinical settings and the monitoring time lag, there is no substitute for seeing the tube pass through the larynx into the trachea and auscultating the chest and epigastrium. Sometimes one needs to assimilate a constellation of clinical data before diagnosis is clear. One classic quality assurance error that has led to airway misadventures is a failure to reassess tube position by assimilation of more data as the clinical picture evolves. Recognition of a misplaced endotracheal tube is different from documentation that the tube is appropriately placed. Critical care and anesthesia personnel should be able to use several confirming criteria for tube placement.

XIII. CONCLUSION

There has been a significant reduction in anesthesia-related morbidity and mortality noted in the last 2 decades.[150] Recent events, such as the introduction of a new type of airway, the LMA, the evolution of simple, safe cricothyrotomy technique, ventilatory monitors, airway management strategies[84] and the elucidation of problems associated with determination of endotracheal tube positioning have contributed to this progress. The vital role that airway management plays in life support makes this an important area for the acute care physician. Newer airway management equipment and continued evolution of airway placement techniques have lead to recent changes in practice, whether in the operating room, the ambulance, or emergency room. Although not all innovations lead to an evolution of practice, the discriminating clinician will evaluate each in context and continue to build on this ever-growing airway knowledge base.

REFERENCES

1. Blitt CD, Gutman HL, Cohen DD et al: "Silent" regurgitation during general anesthesia, *Anesth Analg* 49:707, 1970.
2. Turndorf H, Rodis ID, Clark TS: "Silent" regurgitation during general anesthesia. *Anesth Analg* 53:700, 1974.
3. Illing L, Duncan PG, Yip R: Gastroesophageal reflux during anesthesia, *Can J Anaesth* 39:466, 1992.
4. Coté CJ: NPO after midnight for children—a reappraisal, *Anesthesiology* 72:589, 1990.
5. Mendelson CL: The aspiration of stomach contents into the lungs during obstetric anesthesia, *Am J Obstet Gynecol* 52:191, 1946.
6. Olsson GL, Hallen B, Hambraeus-Jonzon K: Aspiration during anaesthesia: a computer-aided study of 185,358 anaesthetics, *Acta Anaesthesiol Scand* 30:84, 1986.
7. Warner MA, Warner ME, Weber JG: Clinical significance of pulmonary aspiration during the perioperative period, *Anesthesiology* 78:56, 1993.
8. Lichtiger M, Wetchler B, Philip BK: The adult and geriatric patient. In Wetchler B, editor: *Anesthesia for ambulatory surgery*, Philadelphia, 1985, JB Lippincott.
9. Cheney FW, Posner DL, Caplan RA: Adverse respiratory events infrequently leading to malpractice suits: a closed claims analysis, *Anesthesiology* 75:932, 1991.
10. Brown DL: Anesthetic choice. In Brown DL, editor: *Risk and Outcome in Anesthesia*, ed 2, Philadelphia, 1992, JB Lippincott.
11. Roberts J: Oral intubation techniques. In *Fundamentals of Tracheal Intubation*, New York, 1983, Grune and Stratton.
12. Goerig M, Franz Kuhn (1866-1929) zum 125. Geburtstag, *Anasthesiol Intensivmed Notfallmed Schmerzther* 26:416, 1991.
13. Horton WA, Perera S, Charters P: An additional tactile test: further developments in tactile tests to confirm laryngeal placement of tracheal tubes, *Anaesthesia* 43:240, 1988.
14. Hardwick WC, Bluhm D: Digital intubation. *J Emerg Med* 1:317, 1984.
15. Michael TA: Comparison of the esophageal obturator airway and endotracheal intubation in prehospital ventilation during CPR, *Chest* 87:814, 1985.

16. Pons PT: Esophageal obturator airway, *Emerg Med Clin North Am* 6:693, 1988.
17. Gertler JP, Cameron ED, Shea K et al: The esophageal obturator airway: obturator or obtundator? *J Trauma* 25:424, 1985.
18. White RD: Controversies in out-of-hospital emergency airway control: esophageal obstruction or endotracheal intubation? *Ann Emerg Med* 13:778, 1984.
19. Pepe PE, Zachariah BS, Chandra NC: Invasive airway techniques in resuscitation, *Ann Emerg Med* 22:393, 1993.
20. Sutera PT, Gordon GJ: Digitally assisted tracheal intubation in a neonate with Pierre-Robin syndrome, *Anesthesiology* 78:983, 1993.
21. Singh A: Blind nasal intubation: a report of the use of a hook in three cases of ankylosis of the jaw, *Anaesthesia* 21:827, 1966.
22. Latto IP: Management of difficult tracheal intubation. In Latto IP, Rosen M, editors: *Difficulties in tracheal intubation,* Eastbourne, East Sussex, UK, 1985, Ballière-Tindall, p 99.
23. Van Elstraete AC, Pennant JH, Gajraj NM et al: Tracheal tube cuff inflation as an aid to blind nasotracheal intubation, *Br J Anaesth* 70:691, 1993.
24. Ducrow M: Throwing light on blind intubation, *Anaesthesia* 33:827, 1973.
25. Latto IP: Management of difficult tracheal intubation. In Latto IP, Rosen M, editors: *Difficulties in tracheal intubation,* Eastbourne, East Sussex, UK, 1985, Ballière-Tindall, p. 116-120.
26. Huffman HP, Elam JO: Prisms and fiberoptics for laryngoscopy, *Anesth Analg* 50:64, 1971.
27. Bellhause CP: An angulated laryngoscope for routine and difficult trauma intubation, *Anesthesiology* 69:126, 1988.
28. Siker ES: A mirror laryngoscope, *Anesthesiology* 17:48, 1956.
29. Watson CB: Fiberoptic bronchoscopy for anesthesia, *Anesthesiology Review* 9:17, 1984.
30. Beamer WC, Prough DS: Technical and pharmacologic considerations in emergency translaryngeal intubation, *Ear Nose Throat J* 62:463, 1983.
31. Ovassapian A, Krejcie TC, Yelich SJ: Awake fibreoptic intubation in the patient at high risk of aspiration, *Br J Anaesth* 62:13, 1989.
32. Watson CB: Fiberoptic endoscopy and anesthesia in a general hospital, *Anes Clin N A* 9:129, 1991.
33. Ovassapian A, Land P, Schafer MF et al: Anesthetic management for surgical correction of severe flexion deformity of the cervical spine, *Anesthesiology* 58:370, 1983.
34. Latorre F, Hofmann M, Kleemann PP et al: Fiberoptische Intubation und Stress, *Anaesthetist (Berlin)* 42:423, 1993.
35. Smith JE: Heart rate and arterial pressure changes during fiberoptic tracheal intubation under general anesthesia, *Anaesthesia* 43:629, 1988.
36. Ovassapian A, Yelich SJ, Dykes MHM: Fiberoptic nasotracheal intubation—incidence and causes of failure, *Anesth Analg* 62:692, 1983.
37. Ovassapian A: *Fiberoptic airway endoscopy in anesthesia and critical care,* New York, 1990, Raven Press.
38. Benumof Procedural Text. Ward CF and Salvatierra CA: Special intubation techniques for the adult patient, Ch. 7. In Benumof J: *Clinical procedures in anesthesia and intensive care,* Philadelphia, 1992, JB Lippincott.
39. Abou-Madi MN, Trop D: Pulling versus guiding: a modification of retrograde guided intubation, *Can J Anaesth* 36:336, 1989.
40. Dhara SS: Retrograde intubation—a facilitated approach, *Br J Anaesth* 69:631, 1992.
41. Hines MH, Meredith JW: Modified retrograde intubation technique for rapid airway access, *Am J Surg* 159:597, 1990.
42. Audenaert SM, Montgomery CL, Stone B et al: Retrograde-assisted fiberoptic tracheal intubation in children with difficult airways, *Anesth Analg* 73:660, 1991.
43. Williamson R: Paediatric intubation—retrograde or blind? *Anaesthesia* 43:801, 1988 (letter).
44. Barriot P, Riou B: Retrograde technique for tracheal intubation in trauma patients, *Crit Care Med* 16:712, 1988.
45. Mahiou P, Bouvet F, Korach JM et al: Combined retrograde intubation and laryngeal nerve block in conscious trauma patients, *Ann Fr Anesth Reanim* 8(suppl):R26, 1989.
46. Alfery DD: Double-lumen endobronchial tube intubation using a retrograde wire technique, *Anesth Analg* 76:1374, 1993 (letter).
47. Contrucci RB, Gottlieb JS: A complication of retrograde endotracheal intubation, *Ear Nose Throat J* 69:776, 1990.
48. Guggenberger H, Lenz G, Heumann H: Erfolgsrate und Komplikationen einer modifizierten retrograden Intubationstechnik bei 36 Patienten (Success rate and complications of a modified retrograde intubation tecnic in 36 patients), *Anaesthesist (Berlin)* 36:703, 1987.
49. Ducrow M: Throwing light on blind intubation, *Anaesthesia* 33:827, 1978.
50. Katz RL, Berci G: The optical stylet—a new intubation technique for adults and children with specific reference to teaching, *Anesthesiology* 51:251, 1979.
51. Ainsworth QP, Howells TH: Transilluminated tracheal intubation, *Br J Anaesth* 62:494, 1989.
52. Stewart RD, La Rosee A, Stoy WA et al: Use of a lighted stylet to confirm correct endotracheal tube placement, *Chest* 92:900, 1987.
53. Watson CB, Clapham M: Transillumination for correct tube positioning: use of a new fiberoptic endotracheal tube, *Anesthesiology* 60:253, 1984 (letter).
54. Stewart RD, La Rosee A, Kaplan RM: Correct positioning of an endotracheal tube using a flexible lighted stylet, *Crit Care Med* 18:97, 1990.
55. Zbinden S, Schupfer G: Tube-Stat: ein nutzliches Hilfsmittel bei schwieriger Intubation, *Anaesthesist (Berlin)* 38:140, 1989.
56. Rayburn RL: Light wand intubation, *Anaesthesia* 34:667, 1979.
57. Ellis DB, Stewart RD, Kaplan RM et al: Success rates of blind orotracheal intubation using a transillumination technique with a lighted stylet, *Ann Emerg Med* 15:138, 1986.
58. Weiss FR, Hatton MN: Intubation by use of the light wand: experience in 253 patients, *J Oral Maxillofac Surg* 47:577, 1989.
59. Verdile VP, Chiang JL, Bedger R et al: Nasotracheal intubation using a flexible lighted stylet, *Ann Emerg Med* 19:506, 1990.
60. Weiss FR: Light-wand intubation for cervical spine injuries. *Anesth Analg* 74:622, 1992 (letter).
61. Hastings RH, Marks JD: response to letter from Weiss, *Anesth Analg* 74:622, 1992.
62. Debo RF, Colonna D, Dewerd G et al: Cricoarytenoid subluxation: complication of blind intubation with a lighted stylet, *Ear Nose Throat J* 68:517, 1989.
63. Nandi PR, Nunn JF, Charlesworth CH et al: Radiological study of the laryngeal mask, *Eur J Anaesthesiol Suppl* 4:33, 1991.
64. Pothmann W, Fulledrug B, Schulte am Esch J: Fiberoptische Befunde zum Sitz der Kehlkopfmaske, *Anaesthesist (Berlin)* 41:779-84, 1992.
65. Rowbottom SJ, Simpson DL, Grubb D: The laryngeal mask airway in children: a fiberoptic assessment of positioning, *Anaesthesia* 46:489, 1991.
66. Silk JM, Hill HM, Calder I: Difficult intubation and the laryngeal mask, *Eur J Anaesthesiol Suppl* 4:47, 1991.
67. Watson CB: Laryngeal mask airway assisted tracheal intubation, *Anesthesiology News* 21:2, March 1995.
68. Brain AI: The laryngeal mask—a new concept in airway management, *Br J Anaesth* 55:801, 1983.
69. Broderick PM, Webster NR, Nunn JF: The laryngeal mask airway, *Anaesthesia* 44:238, 1989.
70. Sarna MC, Clapham MC: Failed tracheal intubation managed

with laryngeal mask airway. In Watson CB, editor: Problems in airway management, *Anesthesiology News* 10:36, 1989.

71. Alexander CA, Leach AB, Thompson AR et al: Use your Brain, *Anaesthesia* 43:893, 1988 (letter).

72. Mallios C: A modification of the Laerdal anaesthesia mask for nasotracheal intubation with the fiberoptic laryngoscope, *Anaesthesia* 35:599, 1980.

73. Patil V, Stehling L, Zauder H: *Fiberoptic endoscopy in anesthesia*, Chicago, 1983, Year Book Medical.

74. Loken RG, Moir CL: The laryngeal mask airway as an aid to blind orotracheal intubation, *Can J Anaesth* 39:518, 1992.

75. Pennant JH, Pace NA, Gajraj NM: Role of the laryngeal mask airway in the immobile cervical spine, *J Clin Anesth* 5:226, 1993.

76. Silk JM, Hill HM, Calder I: Difficult intubation and the laryngeal mask, *Eur J Anaesthesiol Suppl* 4:47, 1991.

77. Pennant JH, White PF: The laryngeal mask airway: its uses in anesthesiology, *Anesthesiology* 79:144, 1993.

78. Watson CB: Assisted tracheal intubation, *Anesthesiology News*: 21-2, March 1995.

79. Brimacombe J, Berry A: Placement of a Cook airway exchange catheter via the laryngeal mask airway, *Anaesthesia* 48:4, 1993 (letter).

80. Smith JE, Sherwood NA: Combined use of laryngeal mask airway and fiberoptic laryngoscope in difficult intubation, *Anaesth Intensive Care* 19:471, 1991 (letter).

81. Hasham F, Kumar CM, Lawler PG: The use of the laryngeal mask airway to assist fiberoptic orotracheal intubation, *Anaesthesia* 46:891, 1991.

82. Calder, Ordman AJ, Jackowski A et al: The Brain laryngeal mask airway: an alternative to emergency tracheal intubation, *Anaesthesia*, 45:137, 1990.

83. Chadd GD, Crane DL, Phillips RM: Extubation and reintubation guided by the laryngeal mask airway in a child with Pierre-Robin syndrome, *Anesthesiology* 77:401, 1992.

84. Practice guidelines for management of the difficult airway. A report by the American Society of Anesthesiologists Task Force on the Management of the Difficult Airway, *Anesthesiology* 78:597, 1993.

85. McCarroll SM, Lamont BJK, Buckland MR et al: The gum-elastic bougie: old but still useful, *Anesthesiology* 68:643, 1987.

86. McNamee CJ, Meyns B, Pagliero KM: Flexible bronchoscopy via the laryngeal mask: a new technique, *Thorax* 46:141, 1991.

87. Waters DJ: Guided blind endotracheal intubation, *Anaesthesia* 18:158, 1963.

88. Abrams KJ, Desai N, Katsnelson T: Bullard laryngoscopy for trauma airway management in suspected cervical spine injuries, *Analg Anesth* 74:623, 1992 (letter).

89. Saunders PR, Giesecke AH: Clinical assessment of the adult Bullard laryngoscope, *Can J Anaesth* 36:S118, 1989.

90. Marks RR, Hancock R, Charters P: An analysis of laryngoscope blade shape and design: new criteria for laryngoscope evaluation, *Can J Anaesth* 40:1903, 1993.

91. Eldor J, Gozal Y: The length of the blade is more important than its design in difficult tracheal intubation, *Can J Anaesth* 36:94, 1989.

92. Horton WA, Fahy L, Charters P: Defining a standard intubating position using "angle finder," *Br J Anaesth* 62:6, 1989.

93. Gentry WB, Shanks CA: Reevaluation of a maneuver to visualize the anterior larynx after visualization, *Anesth Analg* 77:161, 1993.

94. Cormack RS, Lehane J: Difficult tracheal intubation in obstetrics, *Anaesthesia* 39:1105, 1984.

95. Biro P: Ein modifizierter Macintosh-Spatel fur schwierige Intubationed: der Spiegel-Spatel (A modified Macintosh blade for difficult intubation: the mirror blade), *Anaesthesist (Berlin)* 42:105, 1993.

96. McCoy EP, Mirakhur RL: The levering laryngoscope, *Anaesthesia* 48:516, 1993.

97. Miskovska M, Pachl J, Rhina B: A modified laryngoscope blade for difficult intubation—preliminary experience, *Middle East J Anesthesiol*, 11:563, 1992.

98. Scherer R, Habel G: Ein modifizierter Macintosh-Spatel mit abwinkelbarer Spitze fur schwierige Intubationen (A modified Macintosh blade with an angulated tip for difficult intubations), *Anasth Intensivther Notfallmed* 25:432, 1990.

99. Patil VU, Sopchak AM, Thomas PS: Use of a dental mirror as an aid to tracheal intubation in an infant, *Anesthesiology* 78:619, 1993 (letter).

100. Borland LM, Casselbrant M: The Bullard laryngoscope: a new indirect oral laryngoscope, *Anesth Analg* 70:105, 1990.

101. Gorback MS: Management of the challenging airway with the Bullard laryngoscope, *J Clin Anesth* 3:473, 1991.

102. Mendel P, Bristow A: Anaesthesia for procedures on the larynx and pharynx: the use of the Bullard laryngoscope in conjunction with high frequency jet ventilation, *Anaesthesia* 48:263, 1993.

103. Bainton CR: A new laryngoscope blade to overcome pharyngeal obstruction, *Anesthesiology* 67:767, 1987.

104. Shigematsu T, Miyazawa N, Yorozu T: Nasotracheal intubation using Bullard laryngoscope, *Can J Anaesth* 38:798, 1991.

105. Baraka A, Muallem M, Sibai AN et al: Bullard laryngoscopy for tracheal intubation of patients with cervical spine pathology, *Can J Anaesth* 39:513, 1992.

106. Watson CB, Gorback MS: Fiberoptic intubation. ch. 6, In Emergency Airway Management, ch 6, Philadelphia, 1990, BC Decker.

107. Watson CB, Norfleet EA: Anesthesia for trauma. In Meyer A, editor: *Critical care management of the trauma patient, Crit Care Clin* 2:717, 1986.

108. Majernick TG, Bieniek R, Houston JB et al: Cervical spine movement during orotracheal intubation, *Ann Emerg Med* 15: 417, 1986.

109. Hastings RH, Marks JD: Airway management for trauma patients with potential cervical spine injuries, *Anesth Analg* 73:471, 1991.

110. Gay BB, Atkinson GO, Vanderzalm T et al: Subglottic foreign bodies in pediatric patients, *Am J Dis Child* 140:165, 1986.

111. Wiseman NE: The diagnosis of foreign body aspiration in childhood, *J Pediatr Surg* 19:531, 1984.

112. Walker P, Crysdale WS: Croup, epiglottitis, retropharyngeal abscess, and bacterial tracheitis: evolving patterns of occurrence and care, *Int Anesthesiol Clin* 30:57, 1992.

113. Weiss ST, Tager IB, Munoz A et al: The relationship of respiratory infections in early childhood to the occurrence of increased levels of bronchial responsiveness and atopy. *Am Rev Respir Dis* 1312:573, 1985.

114. Esclamado RM, Richardson MA: Laryngotracheal foreign bodies in children: a comparison with bronchial foreign bodies. *Am J Dis Child* 141:259, 1987.

115. Lima JA: Laryngeal foreign bodies in children: a persistent, life-threatening problem, *Laryngoscope* 99:415, 1989.

116. Hammargren Y, Clinton JE, Ruiz E: A standard comparison of esophageal obturator airway and endotracheal tube ventilation in cardiac arrest, *Ann Emerg Med* 14:943, 1985.

117. Frass M, Frenzer, Rauscha F et al: Ventilation with the esophageal tracheal Combitube in cardiopulmonary resuscitation: promptness and effectiveness, *Chest* 93:781, 1988.

118. Frass M, Frenzer R, Mayer G et al: Mechanical ventilation with the esophageal tracheal Combitube (ETC) in the intensive care unit, *Arch Emerg Med* 4:219, 1987.

119. Frass M, Frenzer R, Ilias W et al: Esophageal tracheal Combitube (ETC): Tieresperimentelle Ergebnisse mit einem neuen

Notfalltubus, *Anasth Intensivther Notfallmed (West Germany)* 22:142, 1987.

120. Hunt RC, Sheets CA, Whitley TW: Pharyngeal tracheal lumen airway training: failure to discriminate between esophageal and endotracheal modes and failure to confirm ventilation, *Ann Emerg Med* 18:947, 1989.

121. Frass M, Rodler S, Frenzer R et al: Esophageal tracheal Combitube, endotracheal airway, and mask: comparison of ventilatory pressure curves, *J Trauma* 29:1476, 1989.

122. Montgomery T, Watson CB, Mackie A: Anesthesia for tonsillectomy and andenoidectomy, *Otolaryngol Clin North Am* 20:(2)331-334, 1987.

123. Capper JW, Randall C: Post-operative haemorrhage in tonsillectomy and adenoidectomy in children, *J Laryngol Otol* 98:363, 1984.

124. Cicala RS, Kudsk KA, Butts A et al: Initial evaluation and management of upper airway injuries in trauma patients, *J Clin Anesth* 3:91, 1991.

125. Mlinek EJ, Clinton JE, Plummer D et al: Fiberoptic intubation in the emergency department, *Ann Emerg Med,* 19:359, 1990.

126. Bohrer H, Kick O: Management of difficult intubation in the case of upper airway obstruction due to carotid endarterectomy rebleeding, *J Cardiothorac Vasc Anesth* 6:776, 1992 (letter).

127. Pepe PE, Zachariah BS, Chandra NC: Invasive airway techniques in resuscitation, *Ann Emerg Med* 22:393, 1993.

128. Jacobs HB: Emergency percutaneous transtracheal catheter and ventilation, *J Trauma* 12:50, 1972.

129. Patel R: Systems for transtracheal ventilation, *Anesthesiology* 59:165, 1983.

130. Roven AN, Clapham MCC: Cricothyroidotomy, *Ear Nose Throat J* 3:68, 1983.

131. Jacobs HB: Needle catheter brings oxygen to trachea. *JAMA* 222:1231, 1972 (letter).

132. Safer P, Pennick J: Cricothyroid membrane puncture with special cannula, *Anesthesiology* 28:943, 1967.

133. Klain M, Smith RB: High frequency percutaneous transtracheal ventilation, *Crit Care Med* 5:280, 1977.

134. Campbell WH: Controversies in trauma management, *J Emerg Med* 7:391, 1989 (editorial).

135. Rosen P, Wolf RE: Therapeutic legends of emergency medicine, *J Emerg Med* 7:387, 1989.

136. Knuth TE, Watson CB: Priorities in initial resuscitation and perioperative management: multitrauma patients with head, chest and other major injuries (submitted for publication 1994).

137. Arndt G, Fender M, Hecht M et al: An evaluation of the air contrast cricothyrotomy system (ACCS) in a large swine model, *Anesth Analg* 80:S14, 1995.

138. Boyce JR, Peters G: Vessel dilator cricothyrotomy for transtracheal jet ventilation, *Can J Anaesth* 36:350, 1989.

139. Matthews HR, Fischer BJ, Smith BE et al: Minitracheostomy: a new delivery system for jet ventilation, *J Thorac Cardiovasc Surg* 92:673, 1986.

140. Helms U, Heilmann K: Ein neues Krikothyreoidotomie-Besteck fur den Notfall (A new cricothyrotomy set for emergencies), *Anaesthesist (Berlin)* 34:47, 1985.

141. Ciaglia P, Firsching R, Syniec C: Elective percutaneous dilatational tracheostomy: a new simple bedside procedure—preliminary report, *Chest* 87:715, 1985.

142. Toye FJ, Weinstein JD: Clinical experience with percutaneous tracheostomy and cricothyroidotomy in 100 patients, *J Trauma* 26:1034, 1986.

143. Bodenham A, Cohen A, Webster N: A clinical evaluation of the "Rapitrach": a bedside percutaneous tracheostomy technique, *Anaesthesia* 47:332, 1992.

144. Nugent WL, Rhee KJ, Wisner DH: Can nurses perform surgical cricothyrotomy with acceptable success and complication rates? *Ann Emerg Med* 20:367, 1991.

145. Johnson DR, Dunlap A, McFeeley P et al: Cricothyrotomy performed by prehospital personnel: a comparison of two techniques in a human cadaver model, *Am J Emerg Med* 11:207, 1993.

146. Spaite DW, Joseph M: Prehospital cricothyrotomy: an investigation of indications, technique, complications, and patient outcome, *Ann Emerg Med* 19:279, 1990.

147. Heffner JE: Percutaneous tracheotomy—novel technique or technical novelty? *Intensive Care Med* 17:252, 1991 (editorial).

148. Shroff PK, Skerman JH, Benumof JL: Transtracheal ventilation. In Benumof JL, editor: *Clinical Procedures in Anesthesia and Intensive Care,* ch 9, Philadelphia, 1992, JB Lippincott.

149. Linko K, Paloheimo M, Tammisto T: Capnography for detection of accidental oesophageal intubation, *Acta Anaesthesiol Scand* 27:199-202, 1983.

150. Eichorn JH: Risk reduction in anesthesia, *Problems in Anesthesia* 6:278-294, 1992.

Part V

THE DIFFICULT AIRWAY SITUATIONS

Chapter 29

THE DIFFICULT PEDIATRIC AIRWAY

Jalil Riazi

I. INTRODUCTION

Pediatric patients display a wide spectrum of diseases, which can present challenging airway problems for the anesthesiologist. Such diseases can have an impact on the facility of endotracheal intubation, mask ventilation, or both. To optimize the successful management of the difficult airway (DA), it is important to understand the anatomic features of the pediatric airway and to be familiar with disease processes and the common syndromes that adversely affect the airway. Knowledge of the embryologic development of the airway facilitates comprehension of airway diseases and syndromes. Many of the DA situations in pediatrics are easily recognizable, whereas others are less evident and reveal themselves unexpectedly during administration of anesthesia.

When managing the pediatric airway, it must be realized that infants and small children are at a physiologic disadvantage compared with adults.[1] They have increased oxygen consumption and less oxygen reserve and are more apt to develop gastric distention with mask ventilation. Gastric distention can elevate the diaphragm, reduce functional residual capacity (FRC)

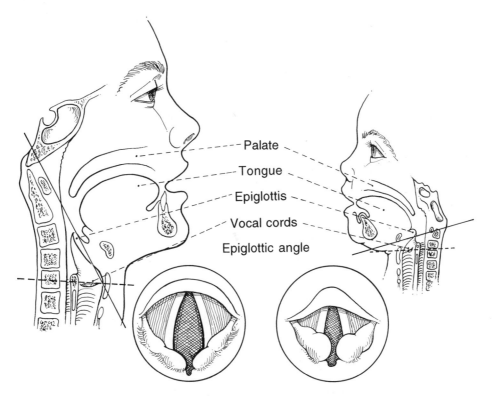

Fig. 29-1. Comparison of the adult and the infant airway. The dashed line demonstrates the relative position of the glottis to the cervical spine. The solid lines show that in the infant, the angle created between the body of the epiglottis and the glottis is more acute than in the adult.

Labels: Palate, Tongue, Epiglottis, Vocal cords, Epiglottic angle

and oxygen reserve, decrease lung compliance, interfere with positive pressure ventilation, and increase the risk of regurgitation and aspiration. Even in the absence of gastric distention, general anesthesia results in a significantly greater decrease in FRC in infants compared with older children.[2] Infants and young children may be more susceptible to upper airway obstruction during general anesthesia because of increased sensitivity of certain inspiratory muscles to anesthetic agents.[3] In infants the parasympathetic system predominates, bradycardia is the main response to hypoxemia, and heart rate is a major determinant of cardiac output. Thus failure to maintain a patent airway in these patients can more readily result in morbidity and mortality.

Morbidity and mortality rates during anesthesia are higher in pediatric patients than in adults.[4-6] Within the pediatric population the incidence of anesthesia-related cardiac arrest and death is greater in newborns and infants than in older children.[4,6] Respiratory events are the major reason for morbidity and mortality and also represent the primary cause of poor outcome in closed claims studies involving pediatric patients.[7] Inadequate ventilation, difficulty with endotracheal intubation, and airway obstruction were the major causes of adverse outcome. Characteristic features of airway anatomy and physiology in infants and small children, together with lack of complete familiarity with these, increase the likelihood of such adverse events.[8,9]

II. ANATOMY OF THE PEDIATRIC AIRWAY

In children, airway anatomy progressively approaches its adult counterpart over the first years of life. Newborns and infants demonstrate the greatest difference from the adult in airway anatomy. In the infant the nares are small and constitute the primary route of breathing in the first 6 months of life. The tongue is relatively large; the larynx is comparably small for the size of the mouth. The larynx is positioned more cephalad; the glottic opening is at the level of C3-4 interspace in the full-term infant and descends to the adult level of C5 at age 6 years (Fig. 29-1).[10] The epiglottis is short, often omega- or U-shaped, and much softer than in the adult. Its attachment at the base of the tongue creates a shallow vallecular notch and angles it in the direction of the glottis.[10] The shape of the epiglottis reaches adult configuration by around 3 years of age. In the infant the arytenoids (Figs. 29-2 and 29-3) are large compared with the glottic opening. The vocal cords are inclined such that the anterior attachments to the laryngeal cartilage are more caudad than the posterior connections. There is progressive reduction in size from the hyoid to the cricoid, so the larynx and its support form a conic shape. The cricoid is in continuity with the trachea and represents the narrowest part of the larynx. Infants 3 months of age and younger have a short trachea with an average tracheal length of 5.7 cm.[11] Its descent into the thorax is in a posterior direction, as opposed to the more

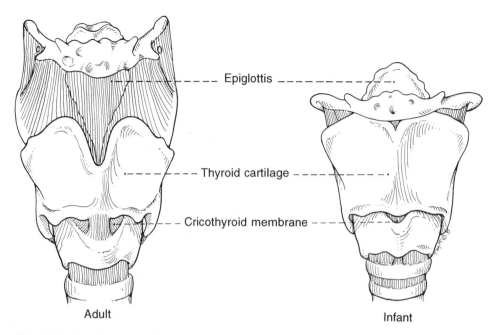

Fig. 29-2. Anterior view of the adult and the infant larynx, showing reduced size of the thyrohyoid and cricothyroid ligaments in the infant.

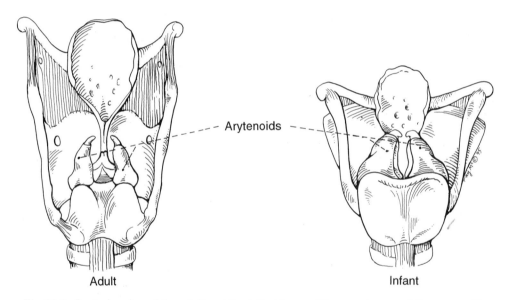

Fig. 29-3. Posterior view of the adult and the infant larynx. The prominence of the arytenoids and the conic shape of the larynx in the infant are evident.

vertical direction in the adult. In children the tonsils and adenoids enlarge to reach a maximum size at age 4 to 6 years. Furthermore, in the infant the head and occiput are relatively large, while the neck is relatively short. The head-to-body ratio diminishes with advancing age.

The distinctive features of the pediatric airway can contribute to a technically more difficult tracheal intubation. The large head and occiput influence how the patient should be positioned to optimize visualization of the glottis during direct laryngoscopy. The infant's large occiput promotes cervical flexion, so simple head extension may be sufficient to produce a "sniffing" position. Placing support beneath the occiput results in excessive flexion of the neck. The relatively large tongue and enlarged tonsils make the oropharynx prone to obstruction. The cephalad position of the larynx translates into a more "anterior-appearing" glottis during laryngoscopy. The shallow vallecula is less accommodating to the tip of a laryngoscope blade, and the shorter size and more posterior-directed axis of the epiglottis make it harder to lift during laryngoscopy. The prominence of the arytenoids, the more caudad insertion of the anterior commissure, and the narrow cricoid ring may present obstacles to smooth passage of the endotracheal tube (ET).

III. PEDIATRIC AIRWAY EQUIPMENT

When managing the pediatric airway, the anesthesiologist has access to nearly all classes of airway equipment available for use in adults, although by necessity, the equipment is reduced in size. Many of the pieces of specialized equipment designed to deal with DA situations in pediatric patients have temporally followed their availability for use in adults; some still are not made for the infant or small child (e.g., the Combitube). This section summarizes basic airway equipment and adjuncts used in managing the difficult pediatric airway.

A. FACE MASKS

To avoid adverse outcome in a child with a DA, the ability to mask ventilate is generally more important than accomplishing endotracheal intubation. To successfully provide adequate oxygenation and ventilation by mask, it is necessary to have a face mask of appropriate size for the child's face, with a fit that allows minimal to no leakage and a patent airway passage to the lungs. The face masks most commonly used in pediatric patients are clear plastic, constructed with a rim of air that cushions and provides a leak-free contact with the face. There are a number of brands that differ in contour. The transparent nature is less intimidating to the child and permits visualization of the nose and mouth beneath. Used less commonly are the Rendell-Baker face mask, Ohio rubber masks, and a number of others with minor variations in shape. The Rendell-Baker mask is shaped to conform to the contours of the face without the benefit of a cushioned rim. It has the advantage of comporting a smaller dead space, as is the case with most Ohio rubber masks. The Patil-Syracuse mask is designed to allow fiberoptic laryngoscopy through a second (endoscopic) orifice on the mask while the patient breathes oxygen or inhaled anesthetics. This orifice is covered with a rubber diaphragm and approximates the mouth when the mask is in position on the patient's face. This mask is not available in a size for use in infants.

B. OROPHARYNGEAL AIRWAYS

Oropharyngeal airways are used to treat or prevent upper airway obstruction caused by the tongue abutting against the palate or posterior pharyngeal wall. When used solely for the purpose of a bite block, oral airways can unnecessarily result in pharyngeal or oral injury, especially in long procedures or when the face is prone or not visible during the procedure. Under such circum-

stances a bite block between the molars serves the same purpose with less trauma. The oropharyngeal airways most commonly used are the Guedel and the Berman. It is important to select the oral airway of appropriate size and to insert it while depressing the tongue in order to avoid laryngeal injury or exacerbation of airway obstruction by the tongue.

C. NASOPHARYNGEAL AIRWAYS

Nasopharyngeal airways are used to bypass obstruction from the nose to the hypopharynx. They are preferred in awake patients and in those with oral or dental disease that may make the use of oropharyngeal airways undesirable. Nasopharyngeal airways are made of rubber or plastic; for pediatric patients they are available in sizes as small as 12 French (12F). In children the adenoids are prone to trauma during insertion of nasal airways, which should be well lubricated and advanced gently, preferably in a previously vasoconstricted nasal passage. Nasopharyngeal airways are themselves prone to lumen obstruction, and their use is contraindicated in several pathologic conditions, including coagulopathy and basal skull fractures.

D. ENDOTRACHEAL TUBES

The ETs available for use in pediatric patients are classified according to internal diameter. The most common ETs are made of polyvinyl chloride and comply with tissue implantation tests. There are a variety of ETs with special indications, which differ in material and shape. Laser-resistant ETs are useful for laser surgery of the mouth or airway disease. Nasal and oral Ring-Adair-Elwyn (RAE) tubes are preshaped to angle them away from the surgical field, reducing the chance of kinking. Endotrol (Mallinckrodt Critical Care, Glens Falls, N.Y.) endotracheal tubes incorporate a finger-activated cable that can be pulled to direct the tip of the tube anteriorly. Reinforced ETs are equipped with a spiral wire within the tube wall, which gives them resistance to kinking or compression from outside pressure. They are useful when tracheomalacia or extrinsic pressure on the trachea may cause standard ETs to dent and become obstructed.

The double-lumen ET and its indications and method of positioning are detailed in Chapter 21. The size limitation, as for other tubes (e.g., Endotrol), makes it unavailable for use in infants and young children.

E. STYLETS

Stylets are pliable yet firm structures that are inserted into an ET to give it rigidity and the desired shape to facilitate endotracheal intubation. Stylets should be available for every endotracheal intubation, in particular, for patients with anticipated DAs. Stylets are also useful for routine use with small endotracheal tubes that tend to warm up and lose their rigidity faster. Tight-fitting stylets with high friction should be lubricated for easy removal following intubation. Care should be taken to ensure that the tip of the stylet is within the ET so that it does not injure airway structures.

The elastic-gum bougie and stylets with controllable, flexible tips are available for use in children. The former are available in sizes as small as a 5F, which easily fits within a 2.5-mm ET. The cannula of a Laryngotracheal Anesthesia Kit (Abbott Laboratories, North Chicago, Illinois) has also been used to guide an ET into the trachea.[12]

F. ENDOTRACHEAL TUBE EXCHANGERS

Endotracheal tube exchangers are valuable adjuncts to the management of the DA in the child. They are long, semirigid catheters that can fit inside ETs. Endotracheal tube exchangers typically have an inner channel of their own that allows analysis for concentration of carbon dioxide, administration of oxygen, or passage of a vascular guidewire. Thus they can be used to change an ET, give a trial of extubation while maintaining the ability to reintubate the trachea, facilitate intubation with the wire technique (see Techniques of Endotracheal Intubation), and remove a laryngeal mask airway (LMA) following an LMA-assisted endotracheal intubation. Endotracheal tube exchangers are made in sizes small enough to pass through a 3-mm ET.

G. LARYNGEAL MASK AIRWAY

A detailed description of the LMA is provided in Chapter 19. The LMA is available in sizes 1, 2, 2½, and 3 for use in pediatric patients weighing less than 6.5 kg, 6.5 to 20 kg, 20 to 30 kg, and 30 to 70 kg, respectively. The LMA has several applications for the child with a DA. It can be used to ventilate the lungs (when endotracheal intubation and ventilation by face mask are difficult or undesirable), guide a flexible fiberoptic bronchoscope (FFB) to the glottis, and facilitate endotracheal intubation (see LMA-Assisted Endotracheal Intubation).

H. LARYNGOSCOPE BLADES

The numerous laryngoscope blades developed for use in pediatric patients fall into two categories, straight and curved, the most common being the Miller and the Macintosh, respectively. There are numerous additional blades, such as the Seward and Wis-Hipple, but these represent modifications of the straight or curved blades. Selection of a particular blade depends on the age of the child and on individual preference and level of experience of the physician. Because of the anatomic peculiarities of the infant airway, however, that is, the reduced space in the vallecula and the posterior angulation of the epiglottis, the straight blade is preferred for its ability to better expose the glottis in newborns and infants.

Straight and curved blades both work well for small children; the latter is more useful for older children. Laryngoscope blades are available with a built-in side channel that allows insufflation of oxygen to the patient during laryngoscopy, thus reducing the risk of hypoxemia.[13]

The anterior commissure laryngoscope used by otolaryngologists can be used to accomplish direct laryngoscopy and endotracheal intubation in children whose larynx is difficult to expose. This laryngoscope is essentially a tubular straight blade with a slightly bent tip (Hollinger modification). Laryngoscopy is performed by lifting the epiglottis. An ET loaded onto a stylet or small telescope can be passed through the laryngoscope and into the trachea. The tubular laryngoscope is also useful for visualization of the glottis in presence of pharyngeal swelling,[14] and small versions for use in pediatric patients have been described.[15]

I. BULLARD LARYNGOSCOPE

The pediatric Bullard laryngoscope is a special blade with about a 90-degree curve and is equipped with fiberoptic and mirror technology to allow indirect visualization of the vocal cords with minimal mouth opening and without the need to align the oral, pharyngeal, and laryngeal axes. The trachea is intubated by advancing an ET that was previously loaded onto the device's intubating stylet, which fastens to the right side of the laryngoscope. As an alternative, a styletted ET separate from the device can be advanced in the direction of the vocal cords using the Bullard laryngoscope to visualize the glottis and the ET. The pediatric Bullard laryngoscope has been used with high success rate in securing DAs in children.[16] A smaller size for use in neonates and infants is also available.

J. FLEXIBLE FIBEROPTIC BRONCHOSCOPE

The FFB has been available for more than 20 years, and the indications for its use in pediatric patients have increased to include diagnosis and therapy of multiple upper and lower airway disease entities.[17,18] The primary application of the FFB by the anesthesiologist, however, is for endotracheal intubation. The fiberscopes most commonly used in children vary in outer diameter from 2.2 to 4.0 mm. There are 4.0-, 3.5- and 2.8-mm scopes containing suction channels and a flexible tip. The 2.2- and 2.7-mm ultrathin fiberscopes have a distal bending tip but lack a suction port.[19,20] The 2.2-mm ultrathin fiberscope is small enough to pass through a 2.5-mm ET and thus can be used to intubate the trachea of the smallest infants. Fiberoptic bronchoscopes smaller than 2.2 mm (e.g., 1.8 mm) are available but lack a flexible end. The working length of most FBs is 60 cm, with a distance of about 75 cm from the suction port to the distal tip.

K. ORAL AIRWAY GUIDES FOR THE FLEXIBLE FIBEROPTIC BRONCHOSCOPE

Oral airway guides for the FFB, such as the Ovassapian airway and the Williams airway intubator, are not available in small sizes for use in the infant or small child. To accomplish the goal provided by these instruments, it is possible to cut the posterior part of an appropriately sized Guedel airway to create a midline passageway for the FFB. As an alternative, an LMA appropriate for the child's age can be placed (after topical or general anesthesia) to guide the FFB to the glottis. Not only is the LMA excellent for this purpose, but also it permits the pediatric patient to breathe oxygen or potent inhalation agents during the fiberoptic laryngoscopy.

L. FIBEROPTIC BRONCHOSCOPE SWIVEL ADAPTERS

These instruments are in the form of an elbow and connect between the breathing circle and an anesthesia mask or an LMA. At the angle of the elbow they contain a port through which fiberoptic laryngoscopy and endotracheal intubation can be carried out. They are especially useful in infants, in whom they can serve the function of the Patil-Syracuse mask.

M. FLEXIBLE GUIDEWIRES

In securing the DA, guidewires are valuable accessories for use with either the FFB or the retrograde techniques (see Techniques of Endotracheal Intubation). The "wire technique" of endotracheal intubation using the FFB requires a long wire that is thin enough to pass through the suction channel of the scope, yet firm enough to guide an ET or an ET exchanger. Guidewires of 100 cm or longer have sufficient length to work well in FFBs with a distance of approximately 75 cm from suction port to tip. A 0.035-inch wire is an ideal fit for FFBs of 3.5 and 4.0 mm, which have suction channel diameters of 1.2 mm and 1.5 mm, respectively.

Guidewire selection for use with the retrograde technique will be determined in part by the size of the needle or catheter placed through the cricothyroid membrane. Guidewires of 0.030, 0.025, and 0.021 inch are suitable for use in 18-, 20-, and 22-gauge catheters, respectively (see Tables 17-5 and 17-6).

N. LIGHTWAND

The lightwand has been demonstrated to be useful for securing the DA in pediatric patients.[21] The principles and technique of its use are similar to those for adults. Recent developments have made the newer lightwands thin enough to use with ETs as small as 2.5 mm.

O. RIGID VENTILATING BRONCHOSCOPE

Rigid bronchoscopes are long cylindric metal tubes that are made for insertion into the trachea. They are made in various sizes, have adapters proximal for lighting, ventilation, and administration of anesthetic agents, and allow passage of a suction catheter or extraction forceps for removal of foreign bodies. The rigid ventilating bronchoscope should be available for use when anesthetizing children with mediastinal masses, since it can be used to stent the airway in case of collapse during anesthesia.

IV. ASSESSMENT OF THE PEDIATRIC AIRWAY

The ability to distinguish the difficult from the normal airway is key to optimal preparation and proper selection of techniques in airway management. When the airway is evaluated to be normal, it also helps avoid the use of time-consuming and potentially more traumatic methods of endotracheal intubation.

A detailed history and physical examination form the foundation for recognizing the DA. The history should include review of previous anesthetic records and emphasize prior airway management during anesthesia, since this may be the only clue to a DA. The history should elicit information regarding congenital, traumatic, inflammatory, or other acquired problems that may adversely affect the airway. There are numerous congenital anomalies and syndromes that become evident with a DA. A basic understanding of these congenital diseases helps direct attention to associated airway abnormalities. Questions should be directed at problems with snoring, apnea, daytime somnolence, hoarse voice, and prior surgery or radiation treatment to the face or neck.

The physical examination must focus on anomalies of the head, neck, and spine. Specifically, one should evaluate the size and shape of the head; gross features of the face; size and symmetry of the mandible, as well as presence of submandibular disease; size of the tongue and shape of the palate; prominence of the upper incisors; and range of motion in the jaw, head, and neck.

As in the adult, the goal of airway evaluation in pediatric patients is aimed at determining the likelihood of visualizing the glottic opening during direct laryngoscopy. Recognition of a DA requires clinical assays with good predictive value, as well as patient cooperation to allow precise evaluation to take place. There are several simple and complex clinical evaluations directed at predicting patients with a DA. These techniques have been detailed in Chapter 7. Their predictive value in small pediatric patients has not been demonstrated. Furthermore, in the infant and young or uncooperative child, appropriate evaluation is hampered. Therefore in pediatric patients the anesthesiologist is often faced with administering anesthesia with less objective airway information than is necessary to accurately predict a DA. This places the pediatric anesthesiologist at a disadvantage in confronting an unexpected DA and underscores the added significance of airway history, when available. It also emphasizes that the pediatric anesthesiologist must always be prepared to deal with a difficult laryngoscopy.

Occasionally, history and physical examination may dictate that additional studies be performed to better elucidate specific features of the airway. These include awake direct laryngoscopy; indirect examination of the glottis by a dental mirror, pharyngoscope, or broncho-scope; flow-volume loops; radiologic imaging (x-ray, computed tomographic [CT] scan, and magnetic reso-nance imaging [MRI]); and blood gas studies.

V. CLASSIFICATION OF THE DIFFICULT PEDIATRIC AIRWAY

In the pediatric population there is a diverse group of pathologic entities that can adversely influence the process of endotracheal intubation, mask ventilation, or both. Such a list can be categorized in various ways. In this chapter these anomalies are classified by anatomic location, that is, the region of the airway primarily affected by that disease. In many circumstances, how-ever, the disease process involves more than one component of the airway, and airway difficulty is caused by more than one mechanism. The conditions that can affect airway management in the pediatric patient are outlined in Box 29-1.

VI. MANAGEMENT TECHNIQUES
A. GENERAL PRINCIPLES

The general principles of managing the DA in the adult and the American Society of Anesthesiologists (ASA) guidelines for DA also apply to the pediatric patient. When managing a pediatric airway, it is crucial to concentrate on *recognition* of DA, appropriate *prepa-ration* (of equipment, personnel, and the patient), and development of primary and alternate *management strategies* for dealing with the recognized and the unrecognized DA. It is also vital to understand the principles and be technically familiar with the various *methods* of endotracheal intubation and emergency lung ventilation. The strategies presented in the DA algo-rithm, such as summoning help early, awake endotra-cheal intubation, limiting the number of attempts at direct laryngoscopy, and restoring the patient to spon-taneous ventilation or awake state, are equally important in management of the pediatric patient.

Anesthetic management of the child with a DA may not necessarily require endotracheal intubation. Local, conductive, and regional nerve blocks or mask anesthe-sia may provide suitable alternatives. However, one should always have primary and alternative plans for securing the DA should the need arise.

BOX 29-1   Anomalies according to anatomic location

I. Head Anomalies
  A. Mass lesions
    1. Encephalocele
    2. Soft tissue sarcoma
  B. Gross enlargement (macrocephaly)
    1. Severe hydrocephaly
    2. Mucopolysaccharidosis [Hurler's syndrome]
  C. Disease affecting access to the airway
    1. Certain conjoined twins [thoracopagus]
    2. Presence of a head stereotactic frame
II. Facial anomalies
  A. Maxillary and mandibular disease
    1. Maxillary hypoplasia
      a. Apert's syndrome
      b. Crouzon's disease
    2. Mandibular hypoplasia and hyperplasia
      a. Pierre Robin syndrome
      b. Treacher Collins syndrome
      c. Goldenhar's syndrome
  B. Temporomandibular joint disease
    1. Reduced mobility
    2. Ankylosis (traumatic, congenital, inflamma-tory, infectious)
III. Mouth and tongue anomalies
  A. Microstomia
    1. Congenital (whistling face syndrome)
    2. Acquired (burns, chemical injection)
  B. Tongue disease
    1. Enlargement
      a. Beckwith-Wiedemann syndrome
      b. Down syndrome
      c. Congenital hypothyroidism
      d. Pompe's disease
    2. Swelling
      a. After surgery
      b. Burn injury
      c. Trauma
      d. Ludwig's angina
    3. Tumors
      a. Hemangioma
      b. Lymphangioma
IV. Nasal, palatal, and pharyngeal anomalies
  A. Nasal anomalies
    1. Choanal atresia
    2. Masses
      a. Encephaloceles
      b. Gliomas
      c. Foreign body
  B. Palatal anomalies
    1. Arch anomaly
    2. Cleft palate
    3. Swelling
    4. Hematoma

Continued.

BOX 29-1   Anomalies according to anatomic location—cont'd

 C. Pharynx
  1. Enlarged adenoids
  2. Enlarged tonsils
  3. Others (tumors, peritonsillar abscess)
 D. Pharyngeal wall
  1. Retropharyngeal and parapharyngeal abscess
  2. Pharyngeal bullae or scarring
   a. Epidermolysis bullosa
   b. Erythema multiforme bullosum
 V. Laryngeal anomalies
  A. Supraglottic disease
   1. Laryngomalacia
   2. Epiglottitis
  B. Glottic disease
   1. Congenital lesions
    a. Vocal cord paralysis
    b. Laryngeal web, cyst, and laryngocele
   2. Papillomatosis
   3. Granuloma formation
   4. Foreign body (see Tracheal and bronchial anomalies)
  C. Subglottic disease
   1. Congenital stenosis
   2. Infectious (croup)
   3. Inflammatory disease
    a. Edema
    b. Traumatic stenosis
 VI. Tracheal and bronchial anomalies
  A. Tracheobronchial tree
   1. Tracheomalacia
   2. Croup
   3. Bacterial tracheitis
   4. Mediastinal masses
   5. Vascular malformations
   6. Foreign body aspiration
   7. Others
    a. Tracheal stenosis
    b. Webbing
    c. Fistula
    d. Diverticulum
 VII. Neck and spine anomalies
  A. Neck
   1. Masses
    a. Lymphatic malformation
    b. Hemangioma
    c. Teratoma
   2. Skin contracture
    a. After burn
    b. Inflammatory
     i. Scleroderma
     ii. Epidermolysis bullosa
     iii. Erythema multiforme bullosum

Continued.

BOX 29-1   Anomalies according to anatomic location—cont'd

 B. Spine
  1. Limited cervical spine mobility
   a. Congenital disease (Klippel-Fiel syndrome)
   b. Acquired disease
    i. Surgery (fusion)
    ii. Trauma (vertebral fracture)
    iii. Inflammatory disease (juvenile rheumatoid arthritis)
  2. Cervical spine instability
   a. Congenital disease (Down syndrome)
   b. Acquired disease
    i. Trauma (subluxation, fracture)
    ii. Inflammatory disease (juvenile rheumatoid arthritis)

1. Monitoring

Appropriate monitoring of oxygenation and ventilation is critical during airway management in the pediatric patient. Electrocardiography, pulse oximetry, capnography, noninvasive blood pressure measurement, and auscultation of breath sounds should be carried out. Temperature should also be monitored because some airway lesions (e.g., encephalocele) can be associated with defective temperature regulation.[22] During the early phases of induction of anesthesia in the uncooperative child or when minimal disturbance is preferred, pulse oximetry and a precordial stethoscope may suffice. Results of pediatric closed claim studies[7] suggested that pulse oximetry or capnography, or both, had the potential to prevent 89% of ventilation-related adverse outcomes.

2. Positioning

Patient positioning is important in optimizing conditions necessary for endotracheal intubation in the pediatric patient. To align the axes of the mouth, pharynx, and larynx during direct laryngoscopy, the head should be extended at the atlantoaxial joint while the cervical spine is flexed with respect to the thoracic vertebrae, achieving head extension with concurrent neck flexion. The smaller the child, the larger the occiput and the head-to-body size ratio. The prominent occiput causes both the head and neck to flex, making laryngoscopy difficult. Extension of the head, often aided by padding below the shoulders, produces a "sniffing" position.

The position of the child's body can also be critical in successful airway management. Although most endotracheal intubation is accomplished with the patient in the supine position, at times this may not be desirable. The child with epiglottitis or a symptomatic mediastinal mass may not tolerate a supine position. Induction and endotracheal intubation may have to be carried out with the patient in a semiseated or lateral position. The lateral head-down (right tonsil) position is an option for children with bleeding after tonsillectomy or a ruptured retropharyngeal abscess. Patients with large occipital encephalocele have been intubated in the left lateral position.[22]

3. Sedation

The use of sedatives and opioids in a pediatric patient with anticipated DA should be based on evaluation of the individual patient's need for sedation, availability of alternate techniques, condition of the airway, and overall patient clinical status. If, despite presence of airway difficulty, sedation is necessary, it is best to have the sedative agent slowly titrated to the desired effect. Use of agents that can be pharmacologically antagonized provides the option of reversing drug effect should it become necessary. It is important to recognize that premedication can produce apnea or exacerbate airway obstruction in infants and children.[23,24]

In pediatric patients who will not tolerate separation from parents or who do not cooperate with awake techniques of endotracheal intubation, some degree of pharmacologic aid may be necessary. Oral, nasal, rectal, or sublingual midazolam may be used to premedicate pediatric patients. Premedication may also be accomplished with ketamine that is administered orally or intramuscularly. Intravenous access allows incremental administration of these medications. The use of opioids carries a higher risk of apnea and is not recommended in the child with a DA. Rectal methohexital behaves as an induction agent and frequently causes the child to fall asleep. If the patient displays airway obstruction during sleep or mask ventilation is likely to be difficult, the use of methohexital is not appropriate. When premedication is given to a child with a DA, the anesthesiologist should remain with the patient and have available appropriate equipment and medications to manage airway compromise. Under special circumstances parental presence during induction of anesthesia may be useful and obviate the need for premedication.

4. Topical anesthesia

Preparation of the airway for awake endotracheal intubation is detailed in Chapter 9. In pediatric patients, topical anesthesia of the airway structures may be carried out by applying local anesthetic via spray, nebulizer, or swabs; by viscous, lidocaine-soaked, gloved fingers; or infrequently by nerve block. An FBB with a suction port can be used to inject local anesthetic agents

---

> **BOX 29-2   Techniques of endotracheal intubation in the pediatric patient**
>
> I. Direct (visual) laryngoscopy
> II. Nonvisual ("blind") endotracheal intubation
>   A. Blind nasotracheal and blind orotracheal intubation
>   B. Tactile or digital endotracheal intubation
>   C. Lightwand
> III. Indirect (visual) endotracheal intubation
>   A. Flexible fiberoptic bronchoscope
>   1. Standard-size pediatric fiberscope
>   2. Ultrathin fiberscope
>   3. Wire technique
>   4. Retrograde-assisted intubation
>   5. Laryngeal mask airway–assisted intubation
>   B. Bullard laryngoscope
>   C. Prism devices for the laryngoscope blade
>   D. Dental mirror
> IV. Retrograde endotracheal intubation
> V. Laryngeal mask airway–assisted endotracheal intubation
> VI. Surgical access
>   A. Cricothyrotomy
>   B. Tracheostomy

---

to the glottis and trachea under visualization.[25] Lidocaine is the agent of choice, although cocaine and tetracaine can also be used. In infants and young children gentle titration of sedative agents may be required, although these should not be given to those at risk of airway obstruction. In uncooperative patients administration of local anesthesia is best tolerated when administered by nebulizer.[26] Care should be taken to administer a nontoxic dose of local anesthetic.

B. TECHNIQUES OF ENDOTRACHEAL INTUBATION

The techniques available for intubating the trachea of a child with a DA are similar to those for the adult, except for refinements that are necessary because of size limitations. Restrictions in equipment size and anatomic features distinctive to the pediatric airway have prompted development of innovative methods of securing the DA in infants and small children. The various methods of endotracheal intubation in pediatric patients are outlined in Box 29-2. Many times endotracheal intubation can be carried out with the patient awake. Awake endotracheal intubation has the advantage of allowing spontaneous respiration and conservation of muscle tone in the oropharynx, which help keep the airway patent and, in most circumstances, the protective reflexes intact. However, awake endotracheal intubation requires a certain degree of patient cooperation which, in the pediatric population, may have to be accomplished with the judicious titration of pharmacologic agents aimed at producing a working environment without excessive respiratory depression.

The choice of a particular technique of endotracheal intubation is influenced by the familiarity and expertise of the anesthesiologist and by whether the DA is anticipated. The selection should also be based on an understanding of the potential complications associated with each method. Recognition of a DA allows advanced formulation of a therapeutic approach to endotracheal intubation. An unrecognized DA is generally confronted during or after induction of anesthesia or possibly following administration of muscle relaxants. At this stage awake intubation techniques are not immediate options, and the anesthesiologist is faced with more critical options that appear later in the DA algorithm management scheme.

1. Direct (visual) laryngoscopy

The aim of laryngoscopy is to achieve direct visualization of the glottis by alignment of the axes of the mouth, pharynx, and larynx. The sniff position produced by appropriate support below the head and shoulders improves the likelihood of successful direct laryngoscopy. Newborns and infants or children with enlarged heads may not require padding below the occiput. If the glottis is not visible, external pressure on the larynx in the posterosuperior direction may place part or all of the glottis in direct view. This may be accomplished by a two-person team, one performing laryngoscopy while the other applies appropriate laryngeal pressure (directed by the laryngoscopist). In some circumstances, even without direct view of the glottic structures, modifying the shape of the ET to produce a hockey stick shaped–tip may allow its passage behind the epiglottis in an anterior direction into the trachea. In older children the Endotrol tube, angled or flexible guides such as Eschmann's bent stylet (Eschmann Health Care, Kent, England) and the Flexiguide (Scientific Sales International, Kalamazoo, Michigan), may be used to intubate the trachea when little or no part of the laryngeal inlet is visible. The choice of laryngoscope blade that is suitable for the patient's size and disease and the availability of different blade types and sizes are important factors in successful direct laryngoscopy.

2. Nonvisual ("blind") endotracheal intubation

a. BLIND NASOTRACHEAL AND BLIND OROTRACHEAL INTUBATION

When direct laryngoscopy fails to accomplish intubation of the trachea and before multiple attempts result in trauma and swelling of the pharynx and larynx, one must resort to other intubation techniques. Nonvisual or "blind" methods are efforts to secure the airway without viewing the glottis. Blind nasotracheal and, to much lesser extent, blind orotracheal intubation are used in this way.

Blind nasotracheal intubation is a useful method to learn, although it is not as practical in pediatric patients as it is in adults. Intubation is accomplished by advancing the ET through a nostril into the pharynx and then directing it through the glottic opening into the trachea. Listening for breath sounds in a spontaneously breathing patient is used to assist in guiding the ET. Multiple modifications to blind nasotracheal intubation have been described. These include using end-tidal CO_2 or a whistle device to identify proximity to the glottis; using a prebent stylet;[27-29] combining the prebent stylet with a malleable lighted stylet or an FFB; inflating the cuff of an ET to push the tip in an anterior direction; and using an Endotrol tube.

The indications for blind nasotracheal intubation include endotracheal intubation of a patient with a DA and emergency airway management in critically ill patients who are breathing spontaneously and are at high risk for administration of anesthetic agents or muscle relaxants. Nasotracheal intubation has several contraindications in children, including facial fractures, coagulopathy, and nasal polyps. In trauma patients apnea is an additional contraindication to blind nasotracheal intubation. Complications involving nasal trauma, bleeding, central nervous system (CNS) penetration, and bacteremia have been described.[30,31] The pediatric patient with enlarged lymphoid tissue may be at risk for trauma to the adenoids, bleeding, and impaction of ET with adenoid tissue. If time allows, the nostril to be used should be vasoconstricted to minimize bleeding. Obstruction to passage of the ET into the trachea may be due to impingement at the pyriform fossae or the vocal cords or, rarely, anterior impingement at the vallecula.

b. TACTILE OR DIGITAL ENDOTRACHEAL INTUBATION

Digital endotracheal intubation is not widely practiced but can be a valuable adjunct in airway management. Digital intubation has been described as the preferred method of intubation by some authors, even in the normal airway.[32] However, its application for the anesthesiologist is to secure the DA following unsuccessful attempts of other techniques or when necessary DA equipment is not available.[33] The technique is simple, and for the right-handed physician it is accomplished by standing to the right of the patient (Fig. 29-4). With the oropharynx anesthetized with local anesthetic the gloved left index finger is passed in the midline along the surface of the tongue until it reaches the posterior aspect of the epiglottis. The right hand then advances the ET (which may be styletted into a C shape), using the left index finger as a guide, until the tip reaches the epiglottis. The left index finger manipulates the ET behind the epiglottis in the direction of the glottic

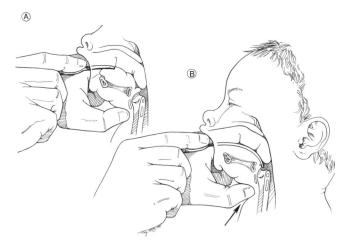

Fig. 29-4. Tactile endotracheal intubation. **A,** The left index finger is in midline position, feeling the posterior surface of the epiglottis and serving as a guide for the endotracheal tube (ET) (in grey) that is being inserted by the right hand. **B,** Once the tip of the ET reaches the epiglottis, it is maneuvered into the glottic opening by the left index finger. The arrow shows use of the left thumb to push the larynx in posterior direction to facilitate intubation.

aperture as the right hand pushes it into the trachea. The left thumb may be used to push the larynx in a posterior direction to facilitate intubation.

c. LIGHTWAND OR LIGHTED STYLET

The lightwand technique is a "blind" method with the addition of a high-intensity light source that, when directed into the trachea, transmits a bright red glow through the skin at the level of the subglottic region (Fig. 29-5). This information helps indicate the correct direction of the lightwand and ET toward the laryngeal inlet. The utility of the technique for rapid endotracheal intubation in pediatric patients with DAs has been demonstrated.[21,34] Earlier uses of the lightwand were limited by the size of the ET. Current lightwands—with fiberoptic light source (Fiberoptic Medical Products, Inc., Allentown, Pa.) and small diameters that allow their use with ETs as small as 2.5 mm—have expanded their application to newborns with DAs.

3. Indirect visual methods of endotracheal intubation

a. FLEXIBLE FIBEROPTIC LARYNGOSCOPY

Although the FFB has limitations, it remains one of the most useful methods of managing the DA, and every anesthesiologist caring for pediatric patients should be familiar with it. Excellent optics, a flexible distal end, and a suction channel, allow endotracheal intubation under indirect visual guidance. With technical advances that have allowed the introduction of 2.2-mm ultrathin fiberscopes, small infants who tolerate only a 2.5-mm ETT can now have endotracheal intubation with this device. Because the technique of using this apparatus is described in Chapter 16, only some specific applications of the fiberscope for the pediatric patient are described here.

i. Standard-size fiberscope. The 3.5- to 4.0-mm FFBs are easy to work with and have a bending tip and suction port, which can be used to administer oxygen, inject local anesthetic, or suction secretions. The drawback to these FFBs is that they only pass through ETs of 4.5 mm and larger. Thus their use is typically directed at children, not infants.

ii. Ultrathin fiberscope. The ultrathin fiberoptic bronchoscopes equipped with a flexible tip are 2.2 and 2.7 mm in outer diameter. They do not have a suction channel. The 2.2-mm scope can pass through a 2.5-mm ET.[19]

iii. Wire technique with standard-size flexible fiberoptic bronchoscope. The larger FFBs can be used to intubate the trachea of newborns and infants with the aid of a flexible vascular guidewire.[35,36] This technique is of particular use for the infant with a DA when the ultrathin fiberscope is not available or when the glottis can be visualized with the FFB but not entered. The method (Fig. 29-6) involves using an FFB with a suction channel to visualize the vocal cords, then passing a vascular wire (e.g., 0.035 inch diameter, 145 cm long), soft tip first, via the suction port through the vocal cords and into the trachea. The fiberscope is removed, leaving the wire in the trachea. The wire may then be used to "railroad" a small ET into the trachea. If a 4-mm or larger ET is to be used, a tube exchanger should first be passed over the wire to provide a better guide for the ET. This technique has also been described using the nasal route.[37]

iv. Retrograde-assisted flexible fiberoptic laryngoscopy. Another application of the FFB in children is to couple its use with the retrograde technique.[38] The cricothyroid membrane is identified, and an angiocath attached to a syringe is advanced slightly cephalad or perpendicular to

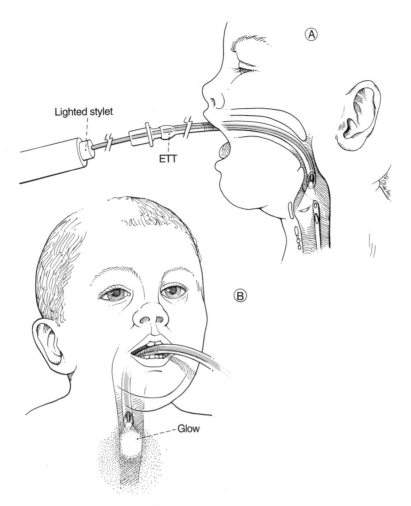

Lighted stylet

ETT

Glow

Fig. 29-5. Lightwand technique. **A,** Lateral midsagittal view showing the desired position of the lightwand. **B,** Anterior view demonstrating the (red) glow seen through the skin in the suprasternal region.

the skin until air is aspirated. The catheter is gently pushed in a cephalad direction as the needle is withdrawn. A guidewire with a flexible tip of adequate length (at least 100 cm) is pushed through the catheter in a cephalad direction and retrieved at the mouth or nose. The wire should be secured with a hemostat at the laryngeal end. This guidewire may be used to intubate the trachea in two ways. If the child is large enough to accommodate the smallest ET that will pass over a FFB with a suction channel (e.g., a 4.5-mm ET and a 3.5-mm FFB), the fiberscope is preloaded with the ET and the suction port passed over the cephalad tip of the wire and advanced under view past the vocal cords to the cricothyroid membrane. The wire may be removed in a caudad direction, and the fiberscope and ET passed into the trachea. As an alternative, if the ET to be used will accommodate the simultaneous presence of a fiberscope and the wire, the ET may be advanced over the wire and into the hypopharynx (Fig. 29-7). The fiberoptic bronchoscope is then passed through the ET, but *alongside*

the wire; the wire can be used as a visual guide for advancing the FFB through the vocal cords, but this time *past* the cricothyroid membrane into the distal trachea. The wire is removed in the same manner as before, and the ET advanced over the bronchoscope. When puncturing the cricothyroid membrane in infants and young children, one must appreciate the reduced size of this membrane and the close proximity of the vocal cords and posterior wall of the trachea to the insertion site of the angiocatheter.

v. Laryngeal mask airway–guided flexible fiberoptic laryngoscopy. The standard adult oral airway guides for FFBs are not available in sizes for use in infants and young children. Alternatives are Guedel airways of appropriate size, with the posterior part cut out, and the LMA. The LMA, when positioned properly, provides an excellent route for directing the fiberscope to the laryngeal inlet.[39,40] By connecting the LMA to a swivel adapter with a port that allows passage of the FFB, the child can breathe 100% oxygen with or

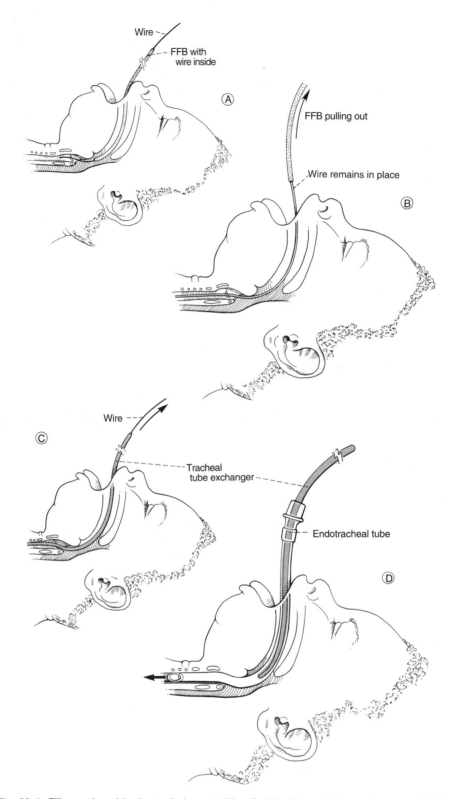

Fig. 29-6. Fiberoptic guidewire technique. **A,** The flexible fiberoptic bronchoscope (FFB) is used to visualize the vocal cords while a guidewire (soft tip first) is advanced through its suction channel into the proximal trachea. **B,** The guidewire is advanced to the carina and the FFB *(arrow)* is removed. **C,** An ET exchanger is passed over the guidewire to the carina. The arrow shows the wire being removed (optional). **D,** The ET *(arrow)* is advanced into the trachea over the tube exchanger, which is then withdrawn.

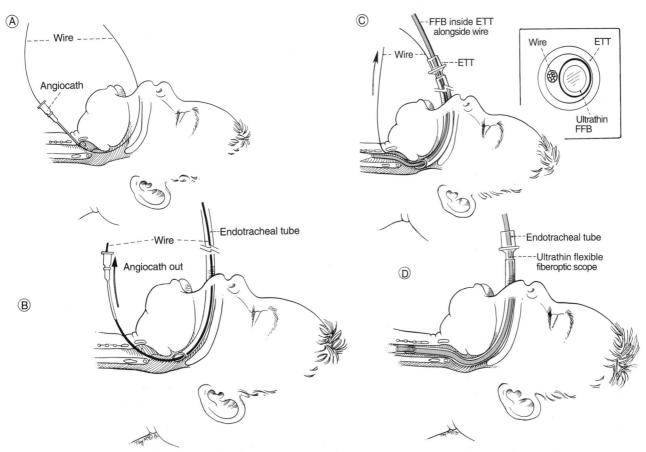

Fig. 29-7. Retrograde-assisted flexible fiberoptic laryngoscopy. **A,** Angiocath is placed through the cricothyroid membrane in a cephalad direction. A guidewire is advanced an appropriate length and retrieved in the oral cavity. **B,** Endotracheal tube is advanced over the guidewire into the hypopharynx. Arrow shows the angiocath being removed, although it may be better to leave it in place. Not shown is a hemostat securing the wire at the laryngeal end. **C,** Flexible fiberoptic bronchoscope is placed inside the ET alongside the guidewire *(inset)* and advanced through the glottis under indirect view. Once the FFB is at the carina, the guidewire is removed. **D,** The ET is advanced as in standard fiberoptic intubation.

without halothane during endoscopy, and endotracheal intubation.

b. BULLARD LARYNGOSCOPE

The Bullard laryngoscope is a beneficial instrument that can be used for endotracheal intubation in children and infants with DAs.[16] The advantages of this device are that it is easy to use, allows indirect visualization of the glottis, can be inserted through a small mouth opening, and requires minimal movement of the jaw and neck. The pediatric Bullard laryngoscope is employed in the same manner as in the adult. It is held in the left hand with the handle parallel to the patient as the blade is inserted into the mouth. The blade is advanced into the mouth while moving the laryngoscope handle up, perpendicular to the patient (Fig. 29-8). The glottis will be visible once the tip of the blade is maneuvered posterior to the epiglottis. The ET can be passed through the vocal cords while viewing both. This technique can be used in awake children after topical anesthesia to the airway or following general anesthesia with or without muscle relaxation.

c. PRISM DEVICES FOR THE LARYNGOSCOPE BLADE

In circumstances when direct laryngoscopy does not expose the glottis, a prism may be attached to a curved or Bellhouse blade[41] to produce refraction of light and indirect visualization of the vocal cords. This view of the glottis can be used to direct a hockey stick–shaped ET, an Endotrol tube, or a flexible stylet into the trachea.

d. DENTAL MIRROR–ASSISTED LARYNGOSCOPY

The laryngeal or dental mirror, employed for the indirect examination of the larynx, can be used during direct laryngoscopy to view an anterior larynx otherwise not visible during direct laryngoscopy.[42] The technique involves performing direct laryngoscopy followed by insertion of the laryngeal mirror, which is angled to

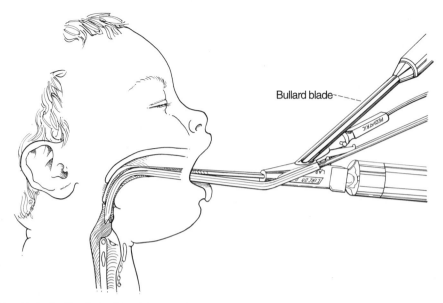

Fig. 29-8. Pediatric Bullard blade in final intubating position with ET armed onto stylet.

reflect the image of the glottis. An appropriately curved, styletted ET is then passed through the vocal cords. The technique does require practice to allow coordination between the hand advancing the ET tube and the mirror image of the glottic aperture.

4. Retrograde endotracheal intubation

Retrograde endotracheal intubation has been widely used in adults (see Chapter 17) with DAs. This technique has also been used successfully in pediatric patients[43,44] and should be considered when conventional and less time-consuming methods of endotracheal intubation are not likely to be successful. In children, retrograde intubation may be carried out with the patient awake (following topical anesthesia of the airway) or anesthetized, preferably with the patient breathing spontaneously. The technique involves placing a needle or Teflon catheter through the cricothyroid membrane until air is retrieved. The use of a catheter has several advantages. It can shield the puncture site from contact with a nonsterile wire, it can allow reinsertion of the wire if this becomes necessary, and it may induce less trauma than a needle if contact is made with the vocal cords or laryngeal wall. In pediatric patients special care must be taken with regard to the size of the catheter and the direction and distance of insertion through the cricothyroid membrane. Clinicians have described the use of 18- or 20-gauge needles and 22-gauge catheters in infants. To expose the cricothyroid membrane and underlying laryngeal structures to the least degree of trauma, the smallest catheter that can accomplish the objective of retrograde intubation should be used. A 22-gauge

catheter will accommodate a 0.018-inch guide-wire. If the wire is too thin to guide the ET through the glottis, an ET exchanger may first be passed over the wire to allow easier railroading of the ET.[45]

The use of the retrograde technique for infants has been considered dangerous,[46] although without supporting data. This technique has been used in infants safely.[43,44,47] The size and direction of catheter or needle advancement through the cricothyroid membrane are important, since the vocal cords lie so close to the insertion site. In newborns and infants the cricothyroid membrane is minimally developed, and the distance that separates it from the vocal cords may be in the order of 5 mm.[38] When the cricothyroid membrane is punctured in the infant and air retrieved, the needle should not be advanced more than 2 to 3 mm in the cephalad direction. As described earlier, the retrograde technique can be combined with the FFB to facilitate endotracheal intubation.

5. Laryngeal mask airway–assisted endotracheal intubation

The LMA has been used to intubate the trachea by both the indirect visual and the blind technique. The proper technique of LMA insertion has been discussed in Chapter 19. As previously stated, the LMA can be used to direct the FFB to the glottis.[39]

Many other methods of using the LMA for securing the DA have been described, including blind passage of a gum elastic bougie and blind orotracheal intubation.[48] However, "blind" insertions through the LMA may not be prudent in pediatric patients, since use of the FFB is simple and there may be a high incidence of the epiglottis obstructing the path to the laryngeal inlet, despite a patent airway on clinical examination.[49] Other authors[50] have used the LMA in children with a DA to establish an airway for administering inhalation anesthesia, followed by tracheal intubation, in this case with the aid of a lighted stylet.

The LMA has also been used in patients with tracheal stenosis when endotracheal intubation may have aggravated airway obstruction postoperatively.[51] In children, tonsillar hypertrophy can create difficulty in advancing the LMA.[52]

6. Surgical access

When emergency airway access is needed or when other techniques of endotracheal intubation have failed, surgical access to the trachea may be necessary. This can be accomplished by cricothyrotomy or tracheostomy. Emergency cricothyrotomy requires satisfactory exposure of the neck and identification and puncture of the cricothyroid membrane, through which a tube of appropriate size is inserted. This may be accomplished with readily available material[53] or specially made equipment (NU-TRAKE and PEDIA-TRAKE, [Bivona Inc., Gary, Indiana]). Limitations in patient age, importance of prior training, and potential complications of these devices must be appreciated.[54] Tracheostomy is best carried out by an experienced surgeon. In rare circumstances, when severe glottic or supraglottic airway obstruction is present, elective tracheostomy may be the best initial approach to airway control.

C. TECHNIQUES OF LUNG VENTILATION

To prevent hypoxic insult to the pediatric patient, it is more important to know the available options of how to emergently ventilate the lungs than how to intubate the trachea. In the hypoxic pediatric patient, ventilation and oxygenation are required, not necessarily endotracheal intubation. The different methods of ventilation are shown in Box 29-3.

If use of a proper-size mask and positive pressure ventilation does not achieve air exchange, the head and jaw position should be assessed for proper positioning. An oral or a nasopharyngeal airway, or both, should be placed. In large patients a better seal may be obtained by holding the mask with both hands while a second person attempts ventilation by squeezing the bag. In pediatric patients, especially during inhalation induction of anesthesia, laryngospasm must be considered and treated by continuous positive pressure or by administration of succinylcholine, or both, if the previously described measures are unsuccessful or if hypoxemia ensues. The LMA may permit ventilation and oxygenation when endotracheal intubation and ventilation by face mask are unsuccessful. The Com-

---

BOX 29-3 **Techniques of lung ventilation (other than by endotracheal intubation)**

Face mask ventilation

Optimal head and jaw position

Oral and nasopharyngeal airways

Two-person mask ventilation

In children undergoing mask ventilation, may be necessary to rule out laryngospasm with administration of succinylcholine

Laryngeal mask airway

Combitube in adolescents

Rigid bronchoscope

Transtracheal jet ventilation

Surgical airway

Cricothyroidotomy

Tracheostomy

---

bitube (see Chapter 22) is useful for similar situations but because of size restrictions cannot be used in infants or children. A rigid bronchoscope is indicated for the patient with mediastinal mass who cannot be ventilated despite intubation with an ET.

Transtracheal jet ventilation (TTJV) refers to ventilation and oxygenation via catheter access through the cricothyroid membrane (translaryngeal) or the membrane separating the first and second tracheal rings.[55] Gas flow is provided by a high-pressure source, with either normal or high-frequency rates. In children, its use has allowed oxygenation and variable amounts of ventilation. Transtracheal jet ventilation is useful for emergency airway access when it is not possible to intubate the trachea or ventilate the lungs by other readily available means and as a substitute for endotracheal intubation or tracheostomy. It has also been used electively when supraglottic approach to the airway has been difficult.[56]

Transtracheal jet ventilation can lead to serious complications.[57] Complications relate to the needle puncture or the high-pressure jets of gas and include vocal cord, tracheal wall, and esophageal injury; pneumomediastinum; pneumothorax; and severe subcutaneous emphysema. To avoid barotrauma, it is critical to ensure that the catheter tip is not outside the tracheal lumen in the soft tissues of the neck and that a route of escape is available for the gas. Transtracheal jet ventilation should not be carried out unless necessary. Cricothyroidotomy and tracheostomy are generally performed as a last resort and are discussed earlier in this chapter.

VII. AIRWAY DISEASES AND THEIR MANAGEMENT

A. HEAD ANOMALIES

1. Pathologic conditions

Certain pathologic conditions of the head can adversely affect airway management. Mass lesions and gross enlargement of the head can interfere with mask ventilation or direct laryngoscopy, or both. Certain conjoined twins may be attached in a manner that interferes with access to the airway by direct laryngoscopy.

Mass lesions of the head include soft tissue tumors and neural tube defects. The most frequent soft tissue tumor of the head and neck region is rhabdomyosarcoma.[58] Encephaloceles, or neural tube defects of the head, usually occur in the occipital area, although they may involve the frontal and nasal regions. Patients with encephaloceles may have other diseases that complicate airway management. These include a high incidence of Klippel-Feil syndrome (cervical vertebral synostosis), hydrocephalus, and cleft palate. Micrognathia and subglottic stenosis have also been described in conjunction with encephaloceles.

Gross enlargement of the head in pediatric patients can result from numerous conditions. Macrocephaly can be due to hydrocephaly, various storage diseases, phakomatoses, cranioskeletal dysplasias, and megalencephaly, among other conditions. Some of these diseases involve disease that affects the airway by more than one mechanism. For example, children with hydrocephalus who also have Arnold-Chiari malformation may demonstrate vocal cord paralysis that manifests as airway obstruction.

Hurler's syndrome (Fig. 29-9) is the most severe form of a rare group of storage diseases in which excess amounts of intracellular mucopolysaccharides accumulate in various tissues of the body, affecting their structure and function. These patients can have multiple abnormalities that may complicate airway management. The head becomes excessively enlarged and has prominent frontal areas. The facies is generally flat. The soft tissues of the pharynx, larynx, and trachea enlarge and become less compliant. Tonsils and adenoids are often hypertrophied. These patients may display macroglossia, reduced mandibular size, and less distensible submandibular soft tissue. The neck is short and gradually becomes less mobile, as does the jaw. There may be thoracic kyphoscoliosis, atlantoaxial instability, and odontoid hypoplasia, although the latter is primarily a finding in Morquio's syndrome, another of the mucopolysaccharidoses.

Conjoined twins occur with very rarely and are believed to result from incomplete fission during twinning. Conjoined twins are classified according to the major site of union. Some forms of conjoined twins may

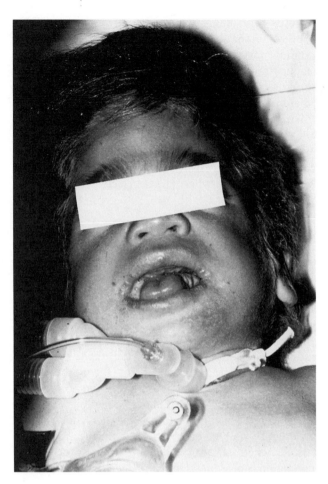

Fig. 29-9. Hurler's syndrome. Macrocephaly, a prominent forehead, and short neck are evident. In addition, there may be reduced neck and jaw mobility, macroglossia, and hypertrophy of lymphoid tissue. This child needed tracheostomy because of upper airway obstruction.

be attached in a manner that can present major obstacles to airway management. Face-to-face encroachment of the heads or close proximity of the chests (thoracopagus) can prevent direct laryngoscopy and easy access to the airway. Presence of stereotactic frames on the head may result in similar difficulty by limiting approach to the airway for endotracheal intubation and, possibly, mask ventilation.

2. Airway implications

Macrocephaly can cause positioning problems because of the large head size. However, the underlying cause of macrocephaly must be sought, since associated anomalies may have considerable airway implications. In mucopolysaccaridoses an enlarged tongue, small mandible, and hypertrophied tonsils and adenoids predispose these patients to airway obstruction following premedication or during mask ventilation. Mucopolysaccharide storage in the trachea and bronchial walls may reduce their lumen size and render these structures more prone to collapse. Direct laryngoscopy may prove difficult or impossible in permitting visualization of the glottis, because of a large tongue, micrognathia, reduced submandibular soft tissue compliance, a short neck, and limited neck and jaw mobility. Caution must be exercised to avoid hyperextension of the head in those with odontoid hypoplasia. In addition, reduced total lung and FRC lower available oxygen reserve during airway management. These patients may come to medical attention with pulmonary hypertension.

Encephaloceles, when large, affect airway management by interfering with mask fit or laryngoscopy.[59] Some forms of conjoined twins may make patient positioning difficult and also necessitate that one twin be held in a compromising position while the airway of the other is being secured. In addition, it is important to understand the cardiovascular communication in conjoined twins. In those with shared circulation, administration of anesthetic agents or muscle relaxants to one twin can have dramatic and unpredictable affects on the second.

3. Airway management

Airway management in children with macrocephaly requires proper head and neck positioning and care relating to associated airway anomalies, which are a frequent finding in patients with mucopolysaccharidosis. If careful evaluation suggests presence of a DA, awake methods of endotracheal intubation should be initially attempted.

In children, awake tracheal intubation may require careful use of sedatives, in addition to topical anesthesia to the oropharynx, larynx, and nasopharynx (for nasotracheal intubation). A limited number of attempts at direct laryngoscopy may be made. If these are not successful, one of the various techniques of nonvisual or indirect laryngoscopy as detailed earlier may be used to secure the airway. If the patient does not comply with awake endotracheal intubation without the use of an amount of sedative that risks respiratory compromise, general anesthesia may be induced, as long as mask ventilation is possible. The patient may be allowed to breathe a potent vapor anesthetic until a level of anesthesia is achieved that allows endotracheal intubation. Options include fiberoptic laryngoscopy in a patient breathing spontaneously through a mask or an LMA, use of the lighted stylet, use of a Bullard laryngoscope, or the retrograde technique. In children in whom mask ventilation is known to be easy, muscle relaxants may be used if their use notably improves the chance of endotracheal intubation.

Airway management in conjoined twins requires much preparation and presence of two anesthesia teams with separate anesthesia machines and equipment. For conjoined twins with difficult access to the airway it is

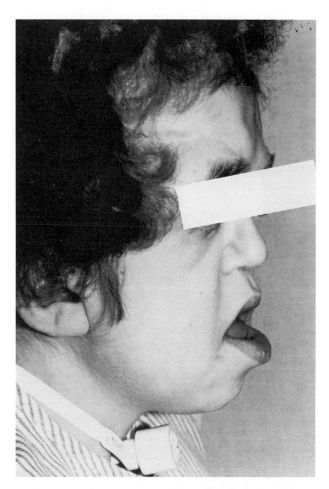

Fig. 29-10. Pfeiffer's syndrome. Maxillary retrusion gives the facies a concave appearance and impression of prognathia, whereas the mandible is typically smaller than normal.

prudent to secure the airways of both twins before administering medications that may cause respiratory suppression or apnea. If sedation or analgesia is given to a twin following endotracheal intubation, it should be titrated in small increments to minimize adverse effects on the remaining twin.

B. FACIAL ANOMALIES

1. Maxillary and mandibular disease

a. PATHOLOGIC CONDITIONS

Maxillary or midfacial diseases affecting airway management include hypoplasia, trauma, and mass lesions. Maxillary hypoplasia results from premature synostosis of facial and cranial sutures and usually manifests as one of multiple abnormal features in a group of rare, but complex syndromes called acrocephalosyndactylies. Included among these are craniosynostoses such as Apert's, Pfeiffer's, and Hallermann-Streiff syndromes and Crouzon's disease (Fig. 29-10). These patients have characteristic head and facial features that typically include a flat occiput and a tall, flat forehead with bitemporal bulging; cloverleaf-shaped head; maxillary hypoplasia resulting in a concave face; flat, depressed nasal bridge; hypertelorism; and proptosis. The midface retrusion gives the appearance of prognathia, although in reality the mandible is smaller than normal. In addition, there may be associated anomalies of the CNS (increased intracranial pressure and absent corpus callosum), the extremities, and in a small percentage of patients, the heart.[60]

Both the upper and lower airways may be adversely affected in these patients.[61] Maxillary retrusion may be associated with choanal stenosis or atresia, reduction in nasopharyngeal space,[62] and palate deformity (narrow, high-arched, or cleft). The soft palate may also be cleft and exist as a bifid uvula. These features may cause respiratory compromise or obstructive apnea early in life, although as the child grows obstruction can become worse because of continued restriction in growth of the maxillary region. Children may be forced to become mouth breathers. Some develop cor pulmonale as a result of chronic hypoxemia. Lower airway disease in the acrocephalosyndactylies occurs in the form of tracheomalacia, bronchomalacia, solid cartilaginous trachea lacking tracheal rings, and tracheal stenosis. Patients with tubular cartilaginous tracheas have displayed propensity to easy tracheal injury, edema, stenosis, and potential for lower airway infection (tracheitis and bronchitis) and mucous plugging, since tracheal ciliary activity may be deficient. In certain forms of craniosynostosis the cervical spine and the lower airway may also be abnormal.[63] Patients with Apert's, Pfeiffer's syndrome and Crouzon's disease may have cervical spine fusion at one or more levels.[64,65] Up to 68% of patients with Apert's syndrome display cervical fusion; 31% have multiple or block fusions.[63] The most common vertebrae affected in patients with Apert's syndrome are C5 and C6, whereas C2-3 is the primary level involved in patients with Crouzon's disease, 25% of whom exhibit cervical fusion. Radiologic findings of cervical fusion vary with age.

Mandibular hypoplasia is one of the main anomalies of the mandible with profound ramification on the airway. Micrognathia results in posterior regression of the tongue and a small hyomental space. It is a feature in many rare syndromes,[66] including Pierre Robin, Treacher Collins, Goldenhar's, Nager's and Escobar syndromes (Figs. 29-11 and 29-12). Although micrognathia is a finding that these syndromes share in common, they often present additional clinical features with adverse effect on the airway.

Pierre Robin syndrome includes a triad of findings: micrognathia, glossoptosis, and cleft palate. It results from failure of mandibular growth during the first several (9) weeks of embryogenesis. This causes posterior displacement of the tongue, which prevents normal

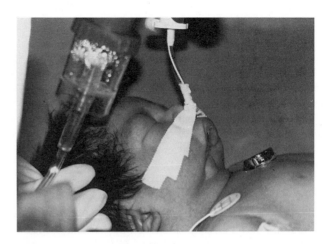

Fig. 29-11. Pierre Robin syndrome. The marked micrognathia in this newborn caused upper airway obstruction from birth. The infant had nasotracheal intubation using the ultrathin FFB after topical anesthesia of the airway. He received an elective tracheostomy.

growth and closure of the palate. Treacher Collins syndrome results from deficient vascular supply to the first visceral arch during the initial 3 to 4 weeks of gestation. In addition to micrognathia, patients with Treacher Collins syndrome have characteristic facial anomalies (ocular, ear defects, and so forth), including a small mouth, large tongue, and palate deformities. Goldenhar's syndrome or oculoauriculovertebral dysplasia is a rare abnomality of first and second branchial arches that involves defective development of multiple organ systems. Pertinent to the airway are mandibular, vertebral, and palatal involvement. Patients with Goldenhar's syndrome can manifest mandibular hypoplasia, cleft or high-arched palate, cervical vertebral anomalies, and scoliosis. Facial hypoplasia is commonly unilateral.

The other extreme, mandibular enlargement, can also complicate direct laryngoscopy. Cherubism is a familial disease of childhood in which patients acquire mandibular and sometimes maxillary enlargement. The mandibular rami hypertrophy, limiting the submandibular space for displacement of the tongue and making visualization of the glottis during direct laryngoscopy difficult.[67]

b. AIRWAY IMPLICATIONS

The airway implications of midfacial hypoplasia relate primarily to choanal stenosis and nasopharyngeal and oropharyngeal obstruction. Furthermore, palate deformity may make laryngoscopy difficult, and optimal mask fit could be a problem.[68] Abnormalities of the trachea may predispose it to collapse, injury, swelling, and infection. Cervical spine fusion at one or more levels may compound the airway problem by limiting cervical movement.

Patients with micrognathia display multiple airway problems from early infancy. They encounter airway obstruction from the regressed tongue abutting against

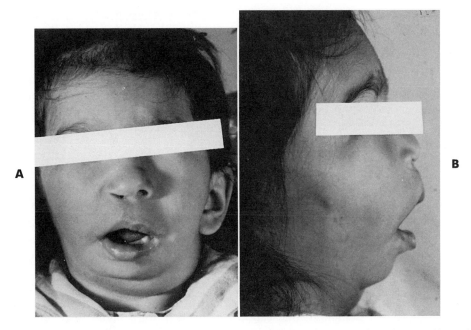

Fig. 29-12. Goldenhar's syndrome. **A,** Anterior and, **B,** lateral views showing micrognathia and asymmetric involvement (right hemifacial microsomia). External ear structures are absent on right. This child's glottis was not visible with direct laryngoscopy but was readily intubated with use of the pediatric Bullard laryngoscope.

the hypopharynx. This frequently has to be treated by insertion of a nasopharyngeal tube, by anterior suturing of the tongue, or by tracheostomy. If these patients require endotracheal intubation, direct laryngoscopy is difficult because of reduced mandibular size and problem in forward displacement of the tongue. Presence of a small mouth and a cleft or high-arched palate can exacerbate the difficult direct laryngoscopy. Micrognathia may also hamper placement of a tight-fitting mask. Patients with Goldenhar's syndrome may have cervical spine diseases that limit neck mobility.

c. AIRWAY MANAGEMENT

Airway management in these patients requires a complete history and physical examination, seeking out events such as snoring, airway obstruction, any previous anesthetic difficulties in managing the airway, and associated presence of choanal stenosis, upper airway obstruction, tracheomalacia, and cervical spine fusion. There should be a detailed examination of the airway, looking at the extent of mouth opening, tongue size, hyomandibular distance, and head and neck mobility. In small or uncooperative pediatric patients complete examination is often hampered. In children who will not easily separate from the parent, the use of premedication should be determined on an individual basis. If the child has history of significant airway obstruction or obstructive apnea, premedication is best avoided; if used, the child must be closely observed by a qualified physician equipped to manage airway obstruction. Un-

der such circumstances parental presence is an acceptable alternative to premedication.

If the child's airway is determined to be difficult to manage, awake endotracheal intubation preceded by adequate topical anesthesia of the airway structures is preferable as consistent with the DA algorithm.[69-71] Awake direct laryngoscopy may help determine the likelihood of visualizing the glottis following general anesthesia. In small children, awake endotracheal intubation may be difficult, and it may be necessary to use sedation or general anesthesia. Sedation in children with a DA should be used with extreme caution. The minimal dose providing the desired effect should be used, titrated in small increments through an intravenous line. If general anesthesia is chosen, inhalation induction with halothane and oxygen is ideal. An anticholinergic agent helps prevent bradycardia during deep inhalation anesthesia and diminish oral secretions. Allowing spontaneous ventilation provides an added safety element should mask ventilation prove difficult. Following deep inhalation anesthesia, direct laryngoscopy may be performed, but the number of attempts should be limited to avoid pharyngeal swelling and airway obstruction.[72] As an alternative, one of several methods of indirect laryngeal visualization, or "blind" techniques such as lightwand, may be used to secure the airway. In selected patients in whom mask ventilation is easy, muscle relaxants can be used if this will facilitate endotracheal intubation. An LMA may be placed to allow induction of inhalation anesthesia followed by endotracheal intubation.[50] With the LMA properly positioned an FFB may be guided into the trachea, or the LMA may be removed while endotracheal intubation is accomplished by indirect or blind techniques.[73] It must be realized that face mask fit may not be ideal in patients with facial diseases, and there must be alternate plans of intervention should airway obstruction occur during inhalation anesthesia.

2. Temporomandibular joint disease
a. PATHOLOGIC CONDITIONS

Temporomandibular joint disease is underrecognized in pediatric patients. When severe, it can lead to reduced jaw mobility or ankylosis. The most common cause of ankylosis is trauma, but it may be congenital or may result from infection and inflammatory diseases.[74,75] Temporomandibular joint disease is common in children with Still's disease, the systemic form of juvenile rheumatoid arthritis, which can also result in cervical spine and cricoarytenoid arthritis. Conditions that can mimic temporomandibular joint involvement and result in acute limitation of jaw mobility include masseter spasm, status epilepticus, and trismus. Clinical manifestations depend on the severity of joint disease. There may be jaw or head pain, reduced mandibular movement, malocclusion, speech difficulty, and asymmetric facies. Severe forms may affect normal development of the mandible, resulting in micrognathia. The disease may be bilateral or may involve just one side. Diagnosis is made by history, clinical examination, and radiologic studies. Treatment may be conservative, or surgery with aggressive physical therapy may be required.[74]

b. AIRWAY IMPLICATIONS

Disease processes afflicting the temporomandibular joint may affect airway management by limiting jaw movement and mouth opening. This can make direct view of the glottis during laryngoscopy unlikely.[76] Airway management is further compounded if there is associated micrognathia.

c. AIRWAY MANAGEMENT

Children with joint disease affecting the jaw should be considered as having a DA. A thorough history and physical examination should disclose potential problems with the temporomandibular joint. For children who do not cooperate in opening the mouth one must seek information from recent surgical procedures and parents' description of extent of mouth opening.

The anesthetic plan in accordance with the DA algorithm should initially consider awake endotracheal intubation. Older children may be prepared for this procedure by adequate titration of sedatives and appropriate topical anesthesia to the areas of the airway to be traversed by the ET. Young children and infants are often best managed following general anesthesia, provided mask ventilation is expected to be without

problems. Alternative methods of endotracheal intubation include use of the FFB via the nasal or oral route; Bullard laryngoscope, as long as the mouth opens far enough to allow the blade to pass into the mouth; and the lighted stylet, which has been successfully used in such circumstances by placement through the side of the mouth.[77] Other options are blind nasotracheal intubation or one of its variations and the retrograde technique.

C. MOUTH AND TONGUE ANOMALIES

1. Microstomia
a. PATHOLOGIC CONDITIONS

Microstomia refers to presence of a small mouth opening. Microstomia is uncommon and may be congenital or acquired. It may be a component of certain syndromes (e.g., Freeman-Sheldon [whistling face], Hallermann-Streiff, and otopalatodigital syndromes). Acquired forms of microstomia in children are primarily a result of burn injury or mouth contact with caustic agents.

b. AIRWAY IMPLICATIONS

Microstomia can limit the space needed for simultaneous insertion of a laryngoscope blade, visualization of the glottis, and passage of an ET during direct laryngoscopy. When microstomia is caused by ingestion of caustic chemicals, there may, in addition, be scarring of the oral cavity that disrupts normal landmarks.

c. AIRWAY MANAGEMENT

Direct laryngoscopy may be difficult or impossible in patients with microstomia. A trial of direct laryngoscopy may be made in the awake or anesthetized patient. If endotracheal intubation is not feasible, indirect visual or nonvisual methods of endotracheal intubation such as nasal or oral flexible fiberoptic laryngoscopy, use of the Bullard laryngoscope or lighted stylet, blind nasal intubation, and retrograde technique (nasal or oral route) can be used. Successful intubation with laryngoscopy using a rigid tubular blade in a child who is breathing potent vapor anesthetic spontaneously through a nasopharyngeal airway has been described.[78] In this case bilateral commissurotomies were necessary to allow insertion of the laryngoscope into the mouth.

2. Tongue disease
a. PATHOLOGIC CONDITIONS

Multiple diseases and disorders are associated with tongue enlargement. Among these are congenital diseases such as Beckwith-Weidemann, Down, and Hurler's syndromes, Pompe's disease, and hypothyroidism. The tongue may also enlarge as a result of swelling caused by various insults such as burns, trauma, prolonged surgical traction, and infection. A serious infectious cause of tongue swelling is Ludwig's angina. This disorder is rare in children but can result in a rapidly

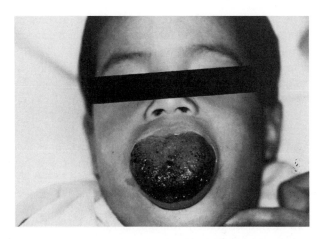

Fig. 29-13. Tongue lymphangioma. The dramatic macroglossia extends the tongue outside the mouth in this 2-year-old child. Tracheostomy was required because of airway obstruction.

progressive infection of the sublingual and submandibular space, which can lead to swelling of the tongue and hypopharyngeal space and cause upper airway obstruction.[79,80] Treatment is directed at ensuring airway patency, antibiotic therapy, and surgical drainage.

The tongue can be a site of tumors. Hamangioma and lymphangiomatous growth (Fig. 29-13) involving the tongue are rare occurrences that may cause severe airway compromise. Although lymphatic malformation preferentially afflicts the submandibular space and the neck, it may extend cephalad and invade the tongue and surrounding structures such as the vallecula, epiglottis, and soft palate. Lymphangiomatous involvement of the tongue is generally diffuse and may result in dramatic macroglossia, extending the tongue outside the mouth beyond the lip margins. Dramatic enlargements of this kind frequently involve airway obstruction, as well as dysphagia and speech, orthodontic, and aesthetic problems. Lymphangioma of the tongue can display acute enlargement following trauma or upper respiratory tract infections. Of the multiple therapeutic methods advocated, surgical laser resection is the mainstay. Laser resection may have to be repeated, since there is tendency for recurrence. Spontaneous resolution is uncommon. In many patients tracheostomy for extended periods is required. If the condition is left untreated for extended periods, pulmonary hypertension and cor pulmonale may develop.

The base of the tongue can be a site of extrinsic masses such as ectopic tonsillar or thyroid tissue and of thyroglossal duct cyst. Because of the location, when such lesions enlarge, they can displace the epiglottis posteriorly onto the glottic aperture and impede air exchange. Lingual tonsils can hypertrophy after tonsillectomy or in patients with atopic disease.[81] This can lead to chronic upper airway obstruction and pose problems with direct laryngoscopy or mask ventilation during anesthesia.[82] Treatment is surgical excision.

b. AIRWAY IMPLICATIONS

Any enlargement of the tongue or reduction in size of the oral cavity or submandibular space may contribute to airway obstruction and difficulty with direct laryngoscopy. Airway obstruction may be mild, manifesting itself as sleep apnea, or severe, resulting in airway obstruction in the awake state. It is also a determinant of the successful visualization of the glottis during direct laryngoscopy. Thus the tongue can be a source of airway obstruction and an impediment to laryngoscopy.

c. AIRWAY MANAGEMENT

Airway management in patients with macroglossia must take into consideration the relative size of the tongue and degree of airway obstruction. In children with extensive enlargement of the tongue or severe airway obstruction, endotracheal intubation should be attempted by means of an awake technique. The nasotracheal route of intubation is preferred and generally easier to perform. Among the various options are nasal flexible fiberoptic laryngoscopy and blind nasal, retrograde, and lightwand techniques. Occasionally in severe disease tracheostomy may be necessary as the initial airway access. In children with mild enlargement of the tongue and minimal signs of airway obstruction, endotracheal intubation may be attempted following administration of general anesthesia.

D. NASAL, PALATAL, AND PHARYNGEAL ANOMALIES

Nasal obstruction in pediatrics may result from a number of causes, including choanal atresia, developmental defects, tumors, polyps, foreign body, and a combination of choanal stenosis with nasal mucosal edema.[83-85] These lesions may become evident at time of birth or later in childhood. They can result in airway obstruction and feeding difficulty and complicate airway management.

1. Choanal atresia
a. PATHOLOGIC CONDITIONS
Choanal atresia (Fig. 29-14) is a congenital anomaly of the nasal choana that results in lack of continuity between the nasal cavity and the pharynx. This entity is rare and develops as a result of failure of resorption of the nasobuccal membrane at the sixth to seventh week of gestation. Congenital choanal atresia is most commonly bony and unilateral, as opposed to membranous and bilateral. It is often associated with other congenital anomalies such as cleft palate, Treacher Collins syndrome, or CHARGE association (coloboma; heart disease; atresia choanae; retarded growth, development, or CNS anomalies; genital hypoplasia; and ear anomalies or deafness). Other airway abnormalities, when part

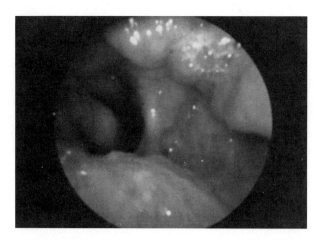

Fig. 29-14. Unilateral choanal atresia. Posterior view of nasal choana. The FFB shows turbinates on the left and choanal atresia on the right.

of the CHARGE association, may be present.[86] If bilateral, choanal atresia is a medical emergency that becomes evident after birth with severe respiratory distress and cyanosis. These signs resolve with cry and recur when crying stops or the infant attempts to feed. In unilateral disease the signs and symptoms are less evident and thus may result in delayed diagnosis. These patients come to medical attention with unilateral nasal discharge and mouth breathing. Respiratory distress occurs when the second nostril becomes obstructed, as during an upper respiratory tract infection. Older children display nasal discharge, inability to blow the nose on the affected side, nasal speech, and mouth breathing.

Diagnosis is based on history and physical examination, inability to pass a nasal catheter into the nasopharynx, flexible fiberoptic examination, and radiologic studies. CT scan is useful in demonstrating the atretic area. Treatment is directed at providing the patient with a patent airway. Infants may receive treatment with placement of an oral airway. Feeding may take place in form of gavage. Surgical correction is not an emergency and is carried out by an endonasal or a transpalatal approach. It is aimed at removing the bony or membranous obstruction and part of the vomer and stenting the newly created path. In infants the transpalatal approach is less common because of risk of injury to the palatal growth center. Endotracheal intubation is usually not needed unless there are associated congenital anomalies. Tracheostomy is not necessary.

b. AIRWAY IMPLICATIONS

The newborn with bilateral choanal atresia can come to medical attention with respiratory distress immediately after birth. Unilateral disease may involve variable degrees of airway obstruction in the infant, depending on the patency of the other nasopharyngeal pathway.

Associated airway anomalies, when present, could complicate airway management. There should be careful evaluation for other airway abnormalities such as micrognathia, laryngomalacia, and subglottic stenosis,[86] which may occur in patients with CHARGE association.

c. AIRWAY MANAGEMENT

Infants with bilateral choanal atresia may come to medical attention with respiratory distress that requires immediate therapy. Placement of an oropharyngeal airway provides a patent airway, although endotracheal intubation may be necessary. If micrognathia or subglottic stenosis is present, a difficult endotracheal intubation should be anticipated. Awake endotracheal intubation or induction of general anesthesia followed by limited attempts at direct laryngoscopy, indirect visual techniques, or nonvisual intubation techniques may be used. Should tracheal stenosis exist, then smaller-than-usual ETTs must be available.

2. Nasal masses

a. PATHOLOGIC CONDITIONS

Nasal mass lesions are rare disorders in the pediatric population with an incidence from 1 in 20,000 to 1 in 40,000 live births.[87,88] Nasal mass lesions include a diverse group of lesions that include anomalies of embryogenesis, such as encephaloceles, gliomas, dermal and nasolacrimal duct cysts, tumors, and inflammatory processes.[83] Encephaloceles represent herniation of CNS tissue at the level of the cranium. Although most encephaloceles are located in the occipital area, some occur anteriorly and may contain various quantities of brain tissue. Encephaloceles may have other associated midline defects. Gliomas also contain brain tissue but lack intracranial communication. Dermal cysts become evident as hard intranasal masses that result from herniation of dura and subsequent contact with the skin. These midline defects may manifest as a nasal obstruction without a facial mass. There is risk of local abscess formation and intracranial infection. Diagnosis is made by history and physical examination.

Tumors located in the nasal area in children are rare occurrences. They include hemangiomas, neurofibromas, angiofibromas, hamartomas, lipomas, and rhabdomyosarcomas. Radiologic studies such as CT scan, MRI, and angiography can elucidate the size and position of the mass and display coexistence of any cranial bone defect. The mainstay of treatment is surgery.

Foreign body in the nostril is a finding in small children. The objects may be various toy objects or food particles. The condition can result in obstruction on the affected side. It typically manifests as nasal discharge, which may be purulent, foul smelling, or bloody. Diagnosis is made by history, examination of the nares, and, occasionally, radiologic evaluation.

b. AIRWAY IMPLICATIONS

Nasal masses can affect the airway in various ways. They can cause nasal airway obstruction, affect mask fit, and interfere with direct laryngoscopy and endotracheal intubation. Nasotracheal intubation and passage of catheters through the nose should be avoided. If there is a palate defect, the mass may extend into the mouth and interfere with endotracheal intubation.[89] Airway implications of nasal foreign bodies are related to nasal obstruction on the affected side and potential for aspiration of the object.

c. AIRWAY MANAGEMENT

When a mass lesion is noted in the nasal area, it should be considered a sign of possible problems with mask ventilation and endotracheal intubation. If mask fit or direct laryngoscopy is assessed to be difficult, then an awake method of endotracheal intubation is warranted. As an alternative, an LMA may be placed in an awake patient with the patient anesthetized with inhalation anesthetics and endotracheal intubation accomplished by direct laryngoscopy or indirect or nonvisual techniques. Allowing the patient to breathe spontaneously in such situations provides an added margin of safety.

3. Palatal anomalies

Anomalies of the palate include cleft and high-arched deformities and hypertrophy of the alveolar ridge area. In children undergoing palate repair, difficulty with endotracheal intubation was encountered in 6.5% of those in one study.[90] Deformities of the palate are frequently associated with congenital malformations, most commonly craniofacial anomalies with airway ramifications of their own,[91,92] for example, Pierre Robin, Treacher Collins, Goldenhar's and Klippel-Feil syndromes. Although cleft palate deformity can contribute to difficulty with airway management, its presence should prompt careful patient evaluation for existence of craniofacial anomalies. The palate can also have edema or hematoma formation. Swelling limited to the soft palate or uvula can cause posture-dependent airway obstruction in children.[93] Edema may result from a variety of insults, such as instrumentation of the airway, burn injury, allergy, and infectious agents.

4. Enlarged adenoids

a. PATHOLOGIC CONDITIONS

Adenoids and tonsils are lymphoid tissue located in the nasal and oral pharynx. In response to recurrent stimulation by infectious agents such tissue can hypertrophy. Adenoidal hypertrophy peaks at 4 to 6 years of age and disappears by adolescence. Although it is a disease of the older child, it can occur in the infant. One of the major complications of adenoidal hyperplasia is airway obstruction. Signs and symptoms of airway obstruction include snoring and restless sleep, somnolence during the day, noisy breathing, mouth breathing, hyponasal speech, persistent nasal secretions, apnea, choking during feeds, respiratory distress, and behavioral disturbances.[94] If the condition is left untreated, failure to thrive; a characteristic long adenoid facies with open mouth, palate, and dental malformations; and cardiovascular changes (cor pulmonale) reflective of chronic hypoxemia and hypercarbia may develop.[95,96]

The diagnosis is made by history and physical examination. History may reveal one or more symptoms of nasal obstruction noted earlier. Physical examination should search for adenoid facies, mouth breathing, and low weight for age. Examination of the oropharynx may show associated enlarged tonsils. Radiologic studies such as lateral neck film can display shadows consistent with adenoidal enlargement. In selected patients, mirror examination or nasopharyngoscopy may allow visualization of adenoidal hyperplasia. In patients suspected of having airway obstruction, polysomnography is helpful in documenting the frequency of obstructive apnea and any accompanying hypoxemia. Cine-CT scans have been used to show the mechanics of airway obstruction.

Airway obstruction resulting from adenoid tissue is determined not by the absolute size of the adenoids, but rather by their size relative to volume of the pharynx.[94] Patients with preexisting diseases that reduce nasopharyngeal size or alter its integrity may have airway obstruction with only mild degrees of adenoidal hyperplasia, for example, children with craniofacial anomalies (in whom the nasopharynx may be reduced in size) and those with nasal polyps, septal or tubinate malformations, mucopolysaccharidoses, or deficient pharyngeal support (Down syndrome).

The treatment of adenoidal hyperplasia as the primary cause of a major contributing factor in airway obstruction is adenoidectomy. The tonsils are often resected simultaneously. Tonsillectomy and adenoidectomy are among the most common surgical procedures in children. There are multiple indications for excision of tonsils and adenoids.[97] Of these surgical indications, upper airway obstruction is of the most concern for the anesthesiologist because these patients may have airway obstruction both during induction of anesthesia and in the postoperative period.

b. AIRWAY IMPLICATIONS

Adenoidal hyperplasia can result in airway obstruction during anesthesia. Upper airway obstruction may occur after premedication, during induction of anesthesia, or following endotracheal extubation. Visualization of the glottis during direct laryngoscopy may be difficult if there is associated tonsillar hypertrophy. Resection of tonsils and adenoids may not result in imme-

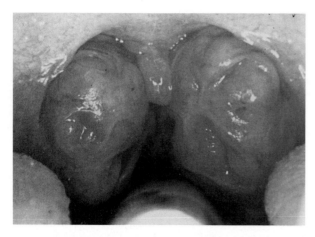

Fig. 29-15. Tonsillar hyperplasia. Enlarged "kissing" tonsils meeting in midline in a patient with history of airway obstruction. The uvula, *above,* is being compressed by the tonsils, and the ET, *below,* is shown pressing on the tongue.

diate improvement of airway obstruction. Bleeding and edema can make the child susceptible to postoperative airway obstruction. Although best recognized for causing chronic upper airway obstruction, adenotonsillar hypertrophy can result in acute airway obstruction.[98-100]

c. AIRWAY MANAGEMENT

Airway management of adenoidal hypertrophy is discussed with management of tonsillar disease in the next section.

5. Tonsillar disease

a. PATHOLOGIC CONDITIONS

The tonsils constitute part of the ringlike lymphoid tissue located at the level of the pharynx. Because of its location, tonsillar disease can influence airway patency. The tonsils can be involved in hypertrophy, inflammation, recurrent infection, and abscess formation.

Tonsillar hyperplasia (Fig. 29-15) is a physiologic phenomenon of childhood that peaks at about 7 years of age. It can cause obstructive sleep apnea in which children typically have restless sleep with an irregular breathing pattern, snoring, intermittent periods of apnea, as well as daytime somnolence, irritability, and poor school performance. Long-standing subobstruction of the airway can be associated with repeated hypoxic episodes and may result in pulmonary hypertension, cor pulmonale, and right-sided heart failure. Adenotonsillar hypertrophy can demonstrate acute exacerbation that necessitates emergency securing of the airway.[99,101] Lingual tonsils are a rare occurrence, but their hypertrophy can result in airway obstruction and interfere with endotracheal intubation.[81,102]

Physical examination may show mouth breathing and enlarged tonsils meeting in the midline. Occasionally the tonsils may appear normal while causing airway obstruction by extending into the hypopharynx or nasopharynx[97]

or when there are associated diseases with adverse influence on the upper airway, such as obesity, Down syndrome, and craniofacial anomalies. Polysomnography can be used to confirm obstructive sleep apnea when the diagnosis is questionable. Airway obstruction has become an increasingly important cause for adenotonsillectomy in children and in some reports exceeds recurrent tonsillitis as the indication for surgery.[103,104,106] Children with obstructive sleep apnea benefit from tonsillectomy, which is often associated with adenoidectomy, especially if there is evidence of nasopharyngeal obstruction.

b. AIRWAY IMPLICATIONS

Airway manifestations of tonsillar hypertrophy involve potential for airway obstruction during anesthesia. Patients with obstructive sleep apnea are susceptible to similar airway obstruction as the oropharyngeal muscle tone relaxes with deepening levels of anesthesia. One should also be cautious of children with history of tonsillitis, since they are prone to having enlarged, inflamed tonsils with potential for airway subobstruction.

c. AIRWAY MANAGEMENT

Management of the airway in pediatric patients with adenotonsillar disease requires detailed history of airway obstruction and associated diseases that could make the airway more problematic. There should be careful examination of the oropharynx for size of the tonsils. Airway management in patients with adenotonsillar hyperplasia depends on the degree of airway obstruction and presence of other diseases that affect the pharyngeal space. Patients with obstructive sleep apnea are at risk for airway obstruction when anesthetized.

In children with history of severe airway obstruction, premedication should be avoided. Awake endotracheal intubation (FFB, Bullard, lighted stylet, digital, and so forth) can be considered but only for those with marked airway obstruction who may have difficulty maintaining a patent airway once anesthetized. The majority of children will not cooperate with this method of endotracheal intubation without an amount of sedation that could potentiate airway obstruction. In these patients general anesthesia, preferably induced by inhaling oxygen and halothane, is required. Children may show airway obstruction during induction, which necessitates positive end-expiratory pressure (PEEP) or gentle assisted ventilation to maintain airway patency. Oral or nasopharyngeal airways may be helpful once adequate depth of anesthesia has been achieved; care must be taken not to traumatize the adenoids. As an alternative, induction may be carried out by the intravenous route but ability to ventilate by mask should be demonstrated before inducing muscle relaxation, since tonsillar hypertrophy may interfere with visualization of the glottis during direct laryngoscopy and necessitate mask ventilation for a prolonged period.

If the patient has airway obstruction during anesthesia, a sequence of maneuvers should be carried out to reestablish air exchange. Continuous positive airway pressure (CPAP) should be applied, the head and jaw should be repositioned, and oral or nasopharyngeal airways should be used. If these are unsuccessful and laryngospasm is considered possible, succinylcholine may be given, if not contraindicated. Should airway obstruction persist, attempts should be made to awaken the patient. If hypoxemia develops before the patient resumes spontaneous ventilation, an LMA may be inserted and a quick attempt at direct laryngoscopy can be made and followed by surgical techniques of ventilation. Tracheostomy may rarely be necessary in the treatment of patients with acute airway obstruction caused by tonsillar hypertrophy or peritonsillar abscess.

Patients who are markedly symptomatic for upper airway obstruction, have positive history of obstructive apnea, or have diseases with upper or lower airway manifestations such as obesity, Down syndrome, neuromuscular disease, and bronchopulmonary dysplasia are at risk for postoperative airway complications.[105,106] Children with severe cor pulmonale are prone to postoperative respiratory arrest if central respiratory drive is altered by administration of oxygen.[96] These patients should be monitored in the hospital following surgery for signs of airway obstruction and hypoxemia. Young age (less than 3 years old) has also been used as an indication for postoperative monitoring after tonsillectomy.[106]

6. Other pharyngeal diseases

The nasopharynx can be the site of tumors and cysts. Teratomas (Fig. 29-16) can rarely occur in the oral and nasopharynx and cause airway obstruction. With prenatal diagnosis and planning and multidisciplinary approach the outcome can be favorable.[107] Upper airway obstruction has also been described in patients who have undergone pharyngeal flap surgery to correct hypernasal speech.[108,109] The procedure is aimed at reducing air escape through the nose during speech. However, it also may reduce the oropharyngeal and hypopharyngeal space, potentiating airway obstruction, especially if there is associated tonsillar hypertrophy or craniofacial syndromes affecting the oropharynx.[109] Up to 10% of patients with pharyngeal flap surgery can have airway obstruction of variable duration.

Peritonsillar abscess in children becomes evident as a purulent mass circumscribed by the tonsillar capsule. It occurs more frequently in older children.[110] Signs and symptoms include fever, sore throat, tonsillar mass, dysphagia, pooling of saliva, muffled voice, trismus, and variable degrees of toxic appearance. Peritonsillar abscess requires intravenous antibiotic therapy. If symptoms of airway obstruction develop or patients fail to

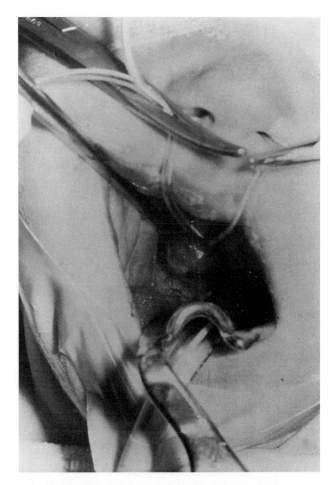

Fig. 29-16. Nasopharyngeal teratoma. The tongue and soft palate are retracted to reveal a teratoma, which became evident with airway obstruction in this infant.

respond to medical therapy, incision and drainage with tonsillectomy are recommended.[111] Peritonsillar abscess affects the airway in a manner similar to tonsillar hypertrophy, except that patients may display trismus. There may be associated edema of the supraglottic area, uvula, and soft palate that exacerbates airway obstruction. Patients are prone to airway obstruction during either spontaneous or manual mask ventilation. During direct laryngoscopy care should be taken not to rupture the abscess. When the abscess is large, it can interfere with visualization of the vocal cords. Tonsillar tumor is a rare occurrence in pediatric patients and is often misdiagnosed as peritonsillar cellulitis or abscess until mass growth is evident.[112]

7. Retropharyngeal and parapharyngeal abscesses

a. PATHOLOGIC CONDITIONS

The various spaces and potential spaces in the pharynx and neck are in anatomic continuity with one another. The retropharyngeal, parapharyngeal, peritonsillar, and submandibular spaces intercommunicate, and infection in one can extend to the others. Retropharyngeal abscess is a rare but potentially fatal infection of the pharyngeal wall. It occurs primarily in pediatric patients; more than half of the patients were less than 12 months old in one study.[113] In children it commonly results from suppurative involvement of lymph nodes located in the retropharyngeal space. These nodes drain lymph from the pharynx, nasopharynx, paranasal sinuses, and middle ear. Other causes of retropharyngeal abscess include spread of infection from pharyngitis or peritonsillar abscess, penetrating trauma, and foreign body ingestion.

Clinical presentation varies with patient age. Most children show fever, some degree of toxic appearance, a hyperextended or stiff neck, dysphagia, drooling, trismus, muffled voice, and respiratory distress. Infants and young children may have stridor. Older children with mediastinal involvement may, in addition, complain of chest pain. Physical examination may display cervical lymphadenopathy and pharyngeal swelling. A lateral radiograph of the neck typically shows widening of the retropharyngeal prevertebral soft tissue. Computed tomography not only can demonstrate the abscess and its extension, but also can help differentiate it from cellulitis. Ultrasound imaging can also demonstrate the disease and distinguish its suppurative from presuppurative stage.[114] Chest radiographs may show mediastinal involvement and tracheal deviation.[115] Complications of retropharyngeal abscess involve airway obstruction, abscess rupture, pneumonia, sepsis, and extension of disease into the mediastinum and the carotid sheath, which causes mediastinitis, jugular vein thrombosis, or erosion into the carotid artery. Treatment consists of airway support, antibiotic therapy, and early incision and drainage.

b. AIRWAY IMPLICATIONS

The danger of retropharyngeal abscess relates to the potential for rapid progression to airway obstruction. In one report 5 of 65 patients required tracheostomy.[116] There is also an ever present risk of abscess rupture and aspiration of pus into the airway. The clinical presentation of children with retropharyngeal abscess can mimic epiglottitis and croup.

c. AIRWAY MANAGEMENT

All patients with the diagnosis of retropharyngeal abscess must be considered to have a DA. The management techniques depend on the severity of airway distress and degree of patient cooperation. In older, cooperative children with marked respiratory distress one may proceed according to the DA algorithm with an awake method of endotracheal intubation or secure an airway by surgical access. In small or uncooperative children anesthesia is required. General anesthesia may be induced by inhalation of halothane and oxygen with emergency plans of securing the airway in case obstruction is encountered. If not in place, an intravenous line

should be secured and atropine administered. It is advantageous to maintain spontaneous ventilation, since neuromuscular blockade may relax the pharyngeal musculature and potentiate airway obstruction in an already reduced pharyngeal space. After adequate anesthetic depth has been achieved, gentle direct laryngoscopy should be attempted, taking care not to rupture the abscess. If endotracheal intubation is not possible following limited attempts at direct laryngoscopy, surgical airway should be considered for those with large lesions. In children with minimal respiratory distress and adequate mask air exchange, other intubation techniques (indirect visual or nonvisual) may be tried first. It is important to take special precautions not to traumatize the abscess during endotracheal intubation. "Blind" attempts at intubation, insertion of an LMA or oral airway, or overzealous direct laryngoscopy all may result in rupture of abscess.

8. Pharyngeal bullae or scarring

a. PATHOLOGIC CONDITIONS

Inflammatory lesions of the pharynx can be a source of problem airways. Diseases such as epidermolysis bullosa, erythema multiforme bullosum, burn injury, or trauma can result in pharyngeal mucosa that is friable and prone to injury, making laryngoscopy and endotracheal intubation difficult.

Epidermolysis bullosa is a collective term used to describe a group of genetically transmitted skin disorders characterized by blistering and skin denudation following friction injury or minor trauma to the skin. There are three subtypes (epidermolysis bullosa simplex, junctional, and dystrophic), which vary in severity and area of skin disruption. The dystrophic form, which is scar forming, is further divided into a dominant and recessive type. As a result of repeated skin infection, injury, and healing, patients with the dystrophic form develop contractures. Contractures may involve skin of the neck and mouth. In addition, esophageal constrictures may develop, which necessitate repeated dilations. In contrast, junctional epidermolysis bullosa is non–scar forming, but there is generalized mucosal involvement that includes the larynx, the lower airway, and the pharynx.[117] The long-term outcome in patients with epidermolysis bullosa depends on the subtype. Therapy in these patients is primarily preventive, although systemic treatments aimed at palliation have been used with varying success.

Stevens-Johnson syndrome, a severe form of erythema multiforme, is an inflammatory bullous process with a high mortality rate that results in skin and mucosal desquamation. It generally follows the administration of certain drugs, which act as a trigger for an immunologic reaction. Although multiple organ systems are affected, edema of the neck and mouth, as well as desquamation and swelling of oropharyngeal mucosa, can create problems with laryngoscopy, endotracheal intubation, and mask ventilation. Acute burn injury and trauma to the oropharynx can result in rapid swelling of the mucous membranes and make visualization of the glottis difficult during direct laryngoscopy, since the redundant tissue has a tendency to collapse around the laryngoscope blade, obstructing the view.

b. AIRWAY IMPLICATIONS

Epidermolysis bullosa can cause airway compromise as a result of swelling, bullous lesions, and ulcerations. In addition, there is increased susceptibility to injury of oral, pharyngeal, laryngeal, and subglottic mucosa. Laryngeal involvement is more common with the junctional subtype, but all groups should be considered prone to such involvement.[116] Patients may have laryngeal stenosis, which influences air exchange and the ET size that can be used. Some patients may have microstomia and reduced neck and jaw mobility from skin contractures of the neck and mouth corners as a result of recurrent skin injury, particularly in the dystrophic forms. Scar formation in the tongue can result in ankylostomia. In patients with epidermolysis bullosa who have instrumentation of the trachea, laryngeal or tracheal bullae and airway obstruction may develop following extubation. In patients who undergo tracheostomy decannulation is rarely accomplished.[118]

c. AIRWAY MANAGEMENT

Airway management in patients with epidermolysis bullosa can be fraught with difficulty.[119,120] Airway manipulation should be minimized, and if general anesthesia is necessary, endotracheal intubation should be avoided if possible. Repeated general anesthetics have been successfully administered by spontaneous respiration of inhalation agents using a well-lubricated face mask.[121] The appropriateness of regional anesthesia must be considered. Some cases may be amenable to the use of ketamine or intravenous sedatives and analgesic. If endotracheal intubation is necessary and direct laryngoscopy is thought to be difficult because of limited mouth opening, an awake method of endotracheal intubation should be considered. Mask ventilation in the patient is easy, general anesthesia may first be induced in preparation for use of an indirect visual method of endotracheal intubation (FFB or Bullard laryngoscope). For patients with Stevens-Johnson syndrome, trauma, or burn injury, tubular laryngoscope blades are helpful in preventing soft tissue invasion onto the viewing field of the glottis. Blind techniques (e.g., blind oral intubation or lighted stylet) have been used successfully[119] but may result in trauma to the laryngeal structures if multiple unsuccessful attempts are required. All airway instruments and an undersized ET should be lubricated before use. Patients with esophageal disease may be prone to regurgitation.[119] In caring

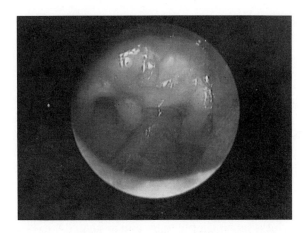

Fig. 29-17. Vallecular cyst. This lesion was found in a 2-month-old infant with significant respiratory distress and intermittent apneic spells. Anesthesia was induced with inhalation agents. Patient displayed difficult mask ventilation, and the trachea was intubated by direct laryngoscopy with great difficulty. The disrupted contour of the anterior aspect of the epiglottis and presence of the ET can be seen.

for patients with epidermolysis bullosa, it is important to take general precautions to protect the entirety of the skin from trauma, friction injury, and adhesive products. Areas susceptible to pressure (e.g., below the face mask) should be generously lubricated. Patients receiving systemic corticosteroid therapy may need perioperative supplementation.

E. LARYNGEAL ANOMALIES

Congenital laryngeal anomalies include a variety of abnormalities that can cause airway problems for the newborn and infant[122] (Fig. 29-17). By far the most frequent disorder is laryngomalacia, followed by vocal cord paralysis and subglottic stenosis.

1. Laryngomalacia

a. PATHOLOGIC CONDITIONS

Laryngomalacia is the most common congenital laryngeal anomaly and the most frequent reason for stridor in the infant.[123] It results from collapse of the supraglottic larynx during inspiration. Its cause is not known but may be due to increased laxity of the supraglottic laryngeal cartilages or their deficient neuromuscular control. Symptoms appear at birth or in the first weeks of life and include inspiratory stridor with positional dependency (being more marked in the supine position and less so when the infant is placed prone or when the head is extended). During inspiration the flaccid supraglottic area tends to be drawn inward, narrowing the superior laryngeal inlet and resulting in a coarse, striderous noise with difficulty on inspiration. This may be associated with retractions. Expiration is generally normal. Patients may also display feeding problems. Approximately 10% of infants have significant respiratory symptoms, including apnea and cyanosis, or display failure to thrive.[124] Although radiologic studies may be useful, endoscopy is the method for confirming the diagnosis. During inspiration one typically observes a flexible epiglottis, together with excessive aryepiglottic folds and corniculate mounds, being pulled inward. This disorder is most often self-limited and tends to resolve within the first 2 years of life. For this group of patients treatment may be conservative. Those with severe disease require surgical intervention. This subpopulation of patients with laryngomalacia in the past received treatment with tracheostomy, although recently epiglottoplasty or laser excision of redundant supraglottic tissue (epiglottis, aryepiglottic folds, and arytenoids) has been successful in preventing tracheostomy.[125,126] Laryngomalacia has been reported to be associated with subglottic stenosis, tracheomalacia, vascular compression (innominate artery), and gastroesophageal reflux.[127]

b. AIRWAY IMPLICATIONS

Laryngomalacia may result in airway obstruction during mask ventilation, especially in patients with severe disease, or during crying and agitation. Associated airway anomalies, when present, must be taken into consideration. Patients with long-standing disease may have cor pulmonale. A portion of the patients have gastroesophageal reflux and may be prone to aspiration. If a laser procedure is anticipated, appropriate measures for laser surgery need to be taken.

c. AIRWAY MANAGEMENT

Management of patients with laryngomalacia depends on the severity of airway obstruction, presence of other airway disease, and the surgical plan. Diagnostic procedures may be accomplished without endotracheal intubation. All patients with laryngeal anomalies must be considered at risk for airway obstruction. In patients with marked respiratory distress the trachea should be secured with the patient awake. Appropriate application of topical anesthesia to the tongue and glottic area allows patient compliance and helps reduce cardiovascular response to airway instrumentation. Sedation should be avoided in patients with marked respiratory compromise, since there may be risk of complete airway obstruction.

As an alternative, general anesthesia may be induced with inhalation of halothane and oxygen. Spontaneous respiration is necessary to allow the surgeon to evaluate supraglottic dynamics. Direct laryngoscopy may be attempted after deep levels of anesthesia have been achieved. If surgery is necessary, it can be performed with an ET in place, with jet Venturi ventilation, or with spontaneous ventilation. Anesthesia may be maintained by intravenous agents, inhalation anesthesia, or both. Administration of inhalation anesthesia has been described in several ways.[128] Halothane has been insufflated directly into the mouth, via a nasopharyngeal tube,

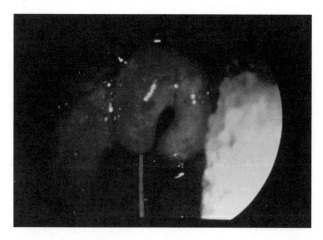

Fig. 29-18. Epiglottitis. The swollen, erythematous epiglottis with a friable texture can be seen after endotracheal intubation *(white line)* following deep inhalation anesthesia with halothane.

or via the side arm of the laryngoscope, among other ways. The potential disadvantages of these techniques are the contamination of the operating room with potent inhalation agents, the possibility of laryngospasm, and laryngeal mobility during surgery.

2. Epiglottitis

a. PATHOLOGIC CONDITIONS

Epiglottitis, more accurately referred to as supraglottitis, is an acute inflammatory disease of the epiglottis, arytenoids, and aryepiglottic folds (Fig. 29-18). It constitutes a potentially fatal airway emergency that can quickly progress to complete obstruction of the airway.[129] Epiglottitis nearly always results from bacterial infection. In children the bacterial cause is most commonly Haemophilus influenzae B (Hib). Since the introduction of Hib vaccine, epiglottitis that is due to Hib, as well as the overall incidence of epiglottitis, appears to be decreasing.[130] The age-group with the highest predilection is children between the ages of 2 and 6 years, although the condition can occur in infants, older children, and adults.[131-133] Recent studies have suggested the age range to be increasing.[131]

The clinical presentation of epiglottitis varies according to age. The signs and symptoms of epiglottitis in children differs from those in adults both in nature and in speed of onset.[131] Within the pediatric population the clinical picture typically seen in the child is more suggestive of epiglottitis than that in the infant. The child may complain of sore throat and display dysphagia, drooling, open mouth, muffled voice, respiratory distress, preference for sitting and leaning the body and chin forward, high fever, and toxic, anxious appearance.[134] However, pediatric patients less than 2 years of age can lack fever and toxic appearance while having a history of upper respiratory infection and croupy cough and thus are at risk for misdiagnosis.[135] Epiglottitis is generally diagnosed based on clinical findings. If the diagnosis is questionable and the patient's condition permits, a lateral neck film can aid in the diagnosis by demonstrating a swollen, enlarged epiglottis shadow and a distended hypopharynx.[136-138] Radiologic studies must be carried out in the presence of a physician equipped and skilled in managing the pediatric airway. Definitive diagnosis is made following direct visualization of the epiglottis.

b. AIRWAY IMPLICATIONS

The inflamed epiglottis and arytenoids place the pediatric patient at risk of rapid progression to complete airway obstruction, hypoxemia, and death.[129] In children the disease is quickly progressive,[129,139] often taking just a few hours from onset of symptoms to complete airway obstruction. During examination children should not have their oropharynx manipulated, nor should children be placed in a supine position, because of the risk of glottic obstruction.[129,140]

c. AIRWAY MANAGEMENT

When epiglottitis is suspected, it should be treated as an airway emergency with a systematic, multidisciplinary management approach.[141,142] It is important not to disturb the child with irritating procedures such as attempts at intravenous line placement and oral examination. These patients are at risk for acute laryngospasm.[143] Although conservative methods of management for children with epiglottitis have been described,[144,145] because of the increased risk for airway obstruction, patients should have prophylactic securing of the airway.[146,147] This procedure should be performed in the operating room.[141] If the child is having a stressful response to parental separation, parental presence during induction of anesthesia should be strongly considered. Sedating a child with epiglottitis may result in disastrous consequences. A surgeon skilled in performing emergency tracheostomy must be present in the operating room at the time of induction of anesthesia.

In the DA management algorithm awake endotracheal intubation is not an acceptable option in treatment of children with epiglottitis. The primary method of airway management is typically inhalation induction of anesthesia followed by endotracheal intubation. The past preference for tracheostomy is reserved for the scenario of complete airway obstruction or the inability to secure the airway by means of an ET.[148]

The preferred agents for induction of anesthesia are halothane and oxygen. Following gentle placement of minimal monitors (pulse oximeter and precordial stethoscope) an inhalation induction is performed with the child in his or her preferred position, usually sitting. Nitrous oxide is not recommended, but if used to facilitate induction, it should be weaned as soon as the patient is asleep and breathing high concentrations of halothane. After the child is adequately anesthetized, he or she may be reclined with a slightly head-up position, the remaining monitors attached, and an intravenous line placed. The patient should be rehydrated, and atropine may be used to decrease the likelihood of bradycardia under deep levels of halothane anesthesia and to help reduce oral secretions. The neck may be prepared for tracheostomy, in the event that airway obstruction occurs. Spontaneous ventilation should be preserved, although CPAP may be necessary to support airway patency. After an adequate level of anesthesia has been established to allow airway manipulation (this may require 10 to 15 minutes or more of breathing halothane), direct laryngoscopy is performed. Glottic opening will be reduced in size and sometimes is difficult to appreciate. Expiratory gas bubbles during spontaneous ventilation or induced by gentle pressure on the child's chest may reveal the glottic opening. A styletted, uncuffed ET one or two sizes smaller than that normal for the child's age should be inserted into the trachea, and correct placement confirmed by auscultation and capnography. Some practitioners prefer to initially place an orotracheal tube and then change it to a nasotracheal route for increased stability.[142,149] If there is airway obstruction during induction of anesthesia or if tracheal intubation is unsuccessful, one should progress, according to the DA algorithm, to surgical airway tracheostomy.

After the airway has been secured, throat and blood cultures are obtained and suitable antibiotic therapy is started. Corticosteroid use has been advocated by some authors to reduce the supraglottic edema of the acute phase and to prevent postextubation croup.[144,149] Pulmonary edema may complicate the postintubation period.[150] Patient management is in the intensive care unit with adequate sedation and analgesia and appropriate measures to ensure that the ET is not accidentally removed. Following clinical improvement, usually after 24 to 48 hours of antibiotic therapy, the epiglottis is reevaluated for possible controlled tracheal extubation, preferably in the operating room with the patient under anesthesia.[147,151]

3. Congenital glottic lesions

a. PATHOLOGIC CONDITIONS

Congenital forms of airway obstruction may result from various pathologic conditions. In addition to laryngomalacia, congenital laryngeal anomalies include vocal cord paralysis, laryngeal webs (or atresia), laryngocele, subglottic stenosis, and hemangioma.

Vocal cord paralysis is the second most common cause of congenital airway obstruction in infants.[152] It may be bilateral or limited to one side. Causes include birth trauma to the vagus nerve; CNS disease such as a bleed, hydrocephalus, Arnold-Chiari malformation, and encephalocele; surgery or disease within the chest or neck, inducing trauma or compression of the recurrent laryngeal nerve(s); and idiopathic. In unilateral vocal cord paralysis, the left side is more frequently involved. Clinical manifestations of vocal cord paralysis depend on whether it is unilateral or bilateral. In unilateral disease the affected vocal cord stays in the abducted position and may display few symptoms (such as mild stridor and discrete changes in tone of cry) or no symptoms. Bilateral vocal cord paralysis is often associated with inspiratory stridor, marked airway obstruction, cyanosis, and apnea resulting from midline or a slightly abducted position of both vocal cords. Diagnosis is made by endoscopy or direct laryngoscopy. There is risk of aspiration in both unilateral and bilateral vocal cord paralysis.

Most acquired forms of vocal cord paralysis resolve spontaneously, whereas the majority of the congenital forms do not.[153] Therefore treatment is conservative when there is minimal respiratory distress. Unilateral disease rarely requires treatment, whereas a large portion of those with bilateral vocal cord palsy require tracheostomy.[154] Identifying and treating the underlying cause may correct the problem over time and obviate the need for tracheostomy. If vocal cord paralysis is permanent, Teflon injection of the paralyzed vocal cord and arytenoidectomy have been used as treatment modalities.

Laryngeal web, cyst, and laryngocele are rare diseases that become evident with various degrees of airway obstruction depending on the size and extent of the lesion. Laryngeal webs result from incomplete resorption of the laryngeal inlet epithelial covering, which causes airway obstruction. The obstruction is typically at the glottic level but may exist at the supraglottic or infraglottic regions. Signs and symptoms become evident shortly after birth; therefore the diagnosis is suspected early. Diagnosis is confirmed by direct laryngoscopy or endoscopy. Infants may display respiratory distress, retractions, stridor, and weak cry. Treatment is lysis of the web. Some patients require tracheostomy. When the web is complete, there is complete laryngeal atresia, a condition incompatible with survival unless it is recognized immediately and the obstruction bypassed.[122]

Laryngoceles are saclike lesions originating from the laryngeal ventricles and may be filled with air or fluid. Congenital laryngeal cysts are more often localized to the supraglottic region. Both may cause airway compression and become evident with stridor or altered tone of cry or as severe respiratory distress requiring urgent treatment. Radiologic studies of the neck (x-ray, ultrasound or CT scan) may aid in diagnosis and localization of the lesion. Treatment may be needle aspiration of the cystic structure, but complete resection of the cyst is often necessary to minimize chance of recurrence.

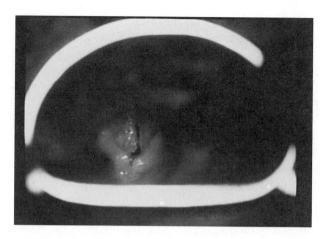

Fig. 29-19. Laryngeal papillomatosis. The glottis is visualized through a suspension laryngoscope, revealing papillomatosis involvement of primarily the left vocal cord. Jet Venturi system of ventilation was used during laser treatment of this lesion.

b. AIRWAY IMPLICATIONS

Congenital laryngeal lesions can cause airway obstruction and may alter the anatomy of the glottic region and make endotracheal intubation difficult. Bilateral vocal cord paralysis may cause airway obstruction during induction or emergence from anesthesia. Unilateral vocal cord palsy rarely causes problems with air exchange or aspiration. Patients with ventriculoperitoneal shunt malfunction and increase in intracranial pressure may have vocal cord palsy and come to medical attention with airway obstruction.

c. AIRWAY MANAGEMENT

Anesthetic management of patients with congenital glottic lesions depends on the severity of obstruction. In lesions with minimal obstruction routine airway management may be satisfactory. In case of moderate symptoms or respiratory distress one should proceed with minimal sedation, awake endotracheal intubation, or spontaneous ventilation of inhalation anesthetic agents to allow laryngoscopy and evaluation of the glottis before securing the airway and providing muscle relaxation. Preparations should be made to access the airway from the cricothyroid membrane in case of airway obstruction. Primary access by tracheostomy is an option for some patients with severe glottic airway obstruction.

4. Laryngeal papillomatosis
a. PATHOLOGIC CONDITIONS

Juvenile laryngeal papillomatosis of the airway can lead to recurrent, often severe airway compromise in pediatric patients[155] (Fig. 29-19). It has an incidence of 0.6 per 100,000 children. Papillomatosis typically afflicts children 2 years of age and older but may occur in infancy,[156] when the prognosis appears to be poor. Airway papillomatosis affects primarily the larynx but can involve any part of the respiratory tract. It may extend to the epiglottis, palate, tracheobronchial tree, and rarely, the lung parenchyma, which, when involved, carries a high mortality rate. The disease is caused by the human papilloma virus (HPV), which is also responsible for genital condyloma and cutaneous warts. Both intra-uterine and hematogenous routes appear to play a role in transmitting the virus to the infant.[157,158]

Signs and symptoms of respiratory papillomatosis are a result of abnormal tissue growth on the larynx and trachea, which causes variable degrees of obstruction to air flow. Afflicted children may display hoarseness, altered voice, and stridor, which can progress to aphonia, respiratory distress, airway obstruction, and death. There is no definitive treatment for papillomatosis of the airway, although some cases may spontaneously resolve. The major mode of therapy remains surgical ablation, even though it may leave long-term scarring of the underlying structures.[159] Surgery can be carried out by forceps or more commonly by laser. There are various medical treatment modalities such as interferon and photodynamic therapy,[160-162] but these are generally directed at severe forms of the disease. Children with aggressive papillomatosis may need laser therapy as frequently as every 2 weeks.

b. AIRWAY IMPLICATIONS

Children with respiratory papillomatosis come to the anesthesiologist with moderate to severe degrees of airway obstruction and thus are at risk for complete airway occlusion, hypoventilation, and hypoxemia. Additional challenges of management in these patients lie in the necessity to share the airway with the surgeon and allow the surgeon clear access to a preferably immobile surgical target, while ensuring adequate patient anesthetic depth, oxygenation, and ventilation. The risks associated with laser surgery of the airway must be recognized, and appropriate precautions taken.[163]

c. AIRWAY MANAGEMENT

Airway papillomatosis typically becomes evident as a recognized DA. The management goals are to provide adequate level of anesthesia, maintain airway patency, and allow the surgeon appropriate access to the lesion. Pediatric patients require general anesthesia, but this does not imply the need for endotracheal intubation. Sedation should be avoided in patients with severe obstruction and respiratory distress. If sedation is used, it must be carried out with proper patient monitoring and availability of trained personnel and necessary equipment to manage airway compromise. In selected patients parental presence during induction of anesthesia is a good alternative to premedication.

Induction of anesthesia or muscle relaxation in children with airway papillomatosis can reduce airway patency or lead to complete airway obstruction. During induction of anesthesia the patient should be allowed to breathe spontaneously until the airway is evaluated for extent of disease involvement and ease of securement. Halothane in oxygen is an ideal agent for inhalation induction. Continuous positive airway pressure of 5 to 10 cm H_2O may help maintain the airway patency. An intravenous line should be secured if not already in place. The child may undergo direct laryngoscopy while spontaneous ventilation under deep inhalation anesthesia is maintained, to evaluate the airway and its securability prior to muscle relaxation. An anticholinergic agent may be administered to reduce the chance of bradycardia in response to high levels of inspired halothane.

Alternative methods of ventilation and oxygenation during laser surgery include the jet Venturi system, the use of an endotracheal tube, intermittent mask ventilation, or spontaneous ventilation.[163] Anesthesia may be maintained with intravenous medications such as propofol, opioids and benzodiazepines or inhalation agents when an ET or spontaneous ventilation is used. During jet ventilation and when an ET is in place, patients may be relaxed with short- or intermediate-acting nondepolarizing muscle relaxants to improve chest wall compliance and to immobilize the vocal cords during laser therapy.

Jet Venturi ventilation is established after induction of anesthesia and placement of a suspension laryngoscope with a Luer-Lok system for attachment to a wall oxygen source.[164,165] An appropriate rate of jet ventilation for the child's age is provided. Nitrous oxide may be mixed with oxygen to provide supplemental anesthesia. For children the jet Venturi system should be equipped with a pressure regulator to allow reduction of wall oxygen pressure (50 psi) to a level that produces adequate chest movement. This pressure level varies with patient size, lung and chest wall compliance, and accurate directioning of the tip of the jet ventilator system. The patient should be relaxed during this mode of ventilation for more effective chest movement. With correct use of the jet Venturi system the patient can receive adequate oxygenation and ventilation.[166] The major advantage of this method of anesthesia is the surgeon's unhindered view of, and access to, the surgical site. The disadvantages include potential complications of the high-pressure ventilation (air leak), hypoventilation, gastric distention, and distal displacement of resected tissue, viral particles, and blood.[167,168] Subglottic jet Venturi ventilation has been described in adults[169] and therefore may be applicable to adolescents.

A second method of anesthetizing these children for laser surgery of airway papillomatosis is by intubating the trachea following deep inhalation anesthesia. Maintenance anesthesia may be accomplished with any combination of intravenous or inhalation agents. Muscle relaxation facilitates laser therapy. The surgeon may then alternate between removing the ET during short periods of laser therapy and replacing it for oxygenation and ventilation. Another option is to leave in place a laser-resistant ET or one wrapped with a protectant metallic tape that reflects the laser beam while laser exision is performed. The use of an ET may impede access to the lesion. As an alternative, after ensuring that the patient's airway is easy to intubate and mask ventilate, it is possible to relax the child and allow the surgeon to carry out brief periods of laser therapy between periods of mask ventilation (apneic technique).[170,171] The patient can also be allowed to breathe spontaneously during laryngoscopy and laser therapy.[163] A nasopharyngeal tube attached to the circle system provides oxygen; anesthesia may be maintained with potent vapor anesthesia or infusion of intravenous agents. Insufflation through a suction catheter inserted into the Andrews anterior commissure retractor allows more directed administration of oxygen and potent vapor anesthetics.[172] The potential advantage of this technique is reduced chance of advancing resected tumor and viral particle into the distal airway. The disadvantages are the risk for laryngospasm and vocal cord movement during laser therapy and operating room contamination that is due to lack of a good scavenging system for the vapor anesthetic. Spontaneous ventilation of vapor anesthetics using a subglottoscope has also been described.[173] If endotracheal intubation or jet Venturi ventilation is unsuccessful, surgical airway access will be necessary. Elective tracheostomy is not recommended because of the potential for extension of papillomatosis to the tracheobronchial tree.[155]

5. Laryngeal granulomas
a. PATHOLOGIC CONDITIONS
Laryngeal granulomas occur primarily in adults and are rarely seen in pediatric patients. They result from prolonged or traumatic endotracheal intubation, although cases following shorter-term intubation have also been described. Lesions are usually in the arytenoid end of the vocal cord and develop from a series of reactions following vocal cord abrasion. Granulomas may occasionally be pedunculated, which increases the chance of airway obstruction. Symptoms are often progressive and include hoarseness, inspiratory stridor, altered voice, and dyspnea. Pedunculated lesions may produce symptoms that change with phase of respiration and position.

b. AIRWAY IMPLICATIONS
The effect of laryngeal granulomas on the airway relate to the degree of laryngeal inlet narrowing and respiratory distress. When interarytenoid adhesions form, the size of the glottic opening may be significantly reduced, limiting the size of ET that may be placed. Pedunculated lesions may produce a ball-valve effect.

c. AIRWAY MANAGEMENT
Management strategy for patients with laryngeal granulomas varies depending on the degree of airway symptoms. Patients with minimal symptoms may require no special precautions, whereas those with symptoms should raise concern about potential for upper airway obstruction and reduction in size of the laryngeal inlet. The latter should be managed by inhalation induction of anesthesia with spontaneous ventilation or by awake laryngoscopy following application of topical anesthesia to the upper airway. Endotracheal tubes one or two sizes smaller than for the patient's age should be at hand.

6. Congenital and acquired subglottic disease
a. PATHOLOGIC CONDITIONS
The cricoid cartilage is the narrowest part of the larynx in infants and small children. The region of the cricoid can be involved in various types of disease, both congenital and acquired. Congenital subglottic stenosis is the abnormal narrowing of the cricoid lumen as a result of a narrow cricoid cartilage or cephalad position of the first tracheal ring. The cricoid cartilage may develop in atypical shapes (flattened, elliptic, or distorted) and thickness, which affects its internal diameter. In severe forms the newborn manifests inspiratory stridor and respiratory distress. In milder forms signs may not appear until later in infancy or following infection or laryngeal trauma that causes edema in an already narrow airway. The subglottic area is susceptible to trauma, and in acquired forms of stenosis trauma is usually related to endotracheal intubation. Diagnosis is by endoscopy. Treatment depends on the severity of stenosis. Occasionally, there can be spontaneous resolution, although this tends to be so in congenital forms of subglottic stenosis, not in acquired forms. Treatment options include observation, tracheostomy, stenting, excision of excess tissue, and cricoid and laryngotracheal reconstruction.

Congenital laryngeal hemangioma generally involves the subglottic region and may cause severe airway problems (Fig. 29-20). Many patients display cutaneous hemangiomas of the face. The most common symptom is stridor. However, patients may show change in tone of cry, dyspnea, cyanosis, and difficulty in feeding. Diagnosis is made by endoscopy, which generally reveals a unilateral subglottic mass. Treatment depends on the severity of symptoms. In subglottic hemangiomas with minimal symptoms, treatment is conservative observation, since there is tendency for spontaneous regression over the first 2 years of life. In moderate to severe forms, corticosteroid therapy or surgical intervention such as tracheostomy or laser excision may be necessary.

Croup is a term used to describe the clinical triad of barking cough, stridor, and hoarseness.[174] *Croup* encompasses a group of diseases[175] but most commonly refers to laryngotracheobronchitis, a disease that is primarily viral in origin and afflicts children between the ages of 1 and 3 years. The most frequently implicated viral agent is the parainfluenza virus.[176] The viral infection results in

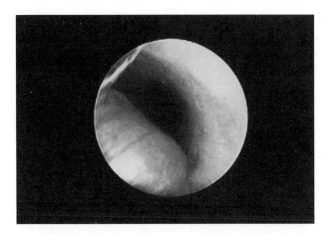

Fig. 29-20. Subglottic hemangioma. The picture demonstrates a posteriorly located hemangioma that is markedly reducing the size of the tracheal lumen. This child was symptomatic, and treatment was with laser excision and tracheostomy.

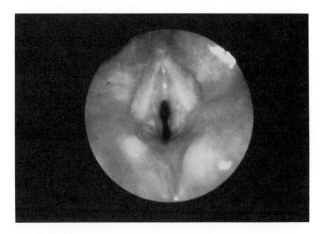

Fig. 29-21. Croup. The glottis is visualized through a fiberoptic scope. The prominent subglottic edema with interposition of the anterior commissures is evident.

narrowing of the subglottic region at the level of cricoid from mucosal swelling[177] (Fig. 29-21). The illness is often compounded by extension of inflammation to the lower airways, which results in increased secretions and ventilation perfusion mismatch.[178] Croup is a self-limited disease that generally resolves in 3 to 5 days. It typically begins with an upper respiratory tract infection that progresses to a brassy, barking cough, inspiratory stridor, and hoarseness with exacerbation of symptoms at night. As the disease advances, children may have respiratory distress, retractions, and hypoxemia. There is generally an associated low-grade fever. Diagnosis is based on history and physical examination. An antero-posterior neck film may reveal a "pencil" or "steeple" sign, a nonspecific finding corresponding to a narrowing of the subglottic area.[136] Treatment consists of adequate hydration, and cool mist with possible need for supplemental oxygen, corticosteroid therapy, and in case of dyspnea, nebulized racemic epinephrine. Racemic epinephrine is used in a dose of 0.5 ml 2.25% solution in 2 to 3 ml saline. The dose can be repeated as required as frequently as every 20 to 30 minutes with the patient under close cardiovascular monitoring. The benefits of racemic epinephrine are temporary, and there can be rebound respiratory distress following its use. If children require supplemental oxygen or treatment with racemic epinephrine, they should be hospitalized for observation. Effectiveness of corticosteroid therapy has long been the center of controversy, but it may have beneficial effects on early symptoms of croup, need for racemic epinephrine use, and endotracheal intubation.[179,180] Dexamethasone 0.3 to 0.5 mg/kg is the recommended dose. Rarely, severe respiratory distress or fatigue develops, despite maximal medical treatment, and endotracheal intubation and respiratory support are needed.[181] Spasmodic croup is similar to viral laryngotracheitis in age distribution, viral origin, and clinical presentation. It differs in

its acute onset at night and lack of fever. Symptoms respond to mist and cool night air but may recur a few nights in a row. Spasmodic croup responds to racemic epinephrine and corticosteroid treatment.

b. AIRWAY IMPLICATIONS

The airway concern in congenital subglottic anomalies, as in the other congenital laryngeal lesions, is obstruction to air exchange. Subglottic hemangiomas further present the risk of uncontrolled bleeding and airway obstruction resulting from acute enlargement of the hemangioma.

The airway implications of croup relate to subglottic edema, tracheal and bronchial inflammation, and increased mucosal secretions. Subglottic edema narrows the airway and restricts air flow. Associated tracheal and bronchial inflammation can add to the child's respiratory distress, ventilation-perfusion mismatch, and depletion of oxygen reserve. The combined effect of such airway pathology can lead to increased work of breathing and fatigue, causing hypercarbia, hypoxemia, and respiratory failure. Most children respond to medical therapy. Up to 3% of children require endotracheal intubation and airway support.[178] Because of the narrowed subglottic region, ETs that are small for the age of the child should be available.

c. AIRWAY MANAGEMENT

Children with severe croup who fail to respond to medical therapy require endotracheal intubation. The issues of concern are the reduced diameter of the subglottic region and the inflammation/reaction of the lower airway that results in less oxygen reserve and potential for hypoxemia. Further trauma to the airway should be minimized by performing a gentle, controlled intubation. Children may be anesthetized with any induction agent, and use of muscle relaxant, when possible, allows a less traumatic intubation. Awake intubation of the trachea should be reserved for patients in extreme respiratory distress and minimal air exchange. Trachea should be secured with special care to minimize trauma and bleeding of the vascular lesion.

F. TRACHEOBRONCHIAL TREE ANOMALIES

1. Tracheomalacia

a. PATHOLOGIC CONDITIONS

Tracheomalacia is the excessive compliance of the cartilaginous support of the trachea that predisposes it to collapse. Tracheomalacia may be limited to a small part of the trachea or extend over its entire length. Tracheomalacia may be classified as congenital or acquired.[182,183] Congenital causes include intrinsic pliancy of the tracheal cartilage rings, and in utero factors such as vascular rings and tracheoesophageal fistula. The latter affects the normal development of tracheal wall shape and integrity. Acquired lesions may be due to extrinsic compression by the innominate artery, aorta, or mass lesions of the mediastinum and neck. Tracheomalacia has a high rate of association with tracheoesophageal fistula and its repair[184] and with the period after closure of long-term tracheostomies.[185] Tracheomalacia must be part of the differential diagnosis in infants with respiratory problems that follow repair of congenital esophageal anomalies. Symptoms include cough, expiratory stridor, dysphagia, recurrent respiratory infections, and in severe cases cyanosis and recurrent, life-threatening episodes of obstructive apnea. Stridor is not always a finding in tracheomalacia.[186] Symptoms may worsen during eating as the swallowed food compresses into the posterior part of the trachea. The anomaly may be diagnosed by use of radiologic imaging, barium swallow, and bronchoscopy, which may reveal an elliptic narrowing of the trachea with a possible pulsatile component in case of vascular compression. Treatment may not be necessary in mild congenital forms that tend to resolve with time. Symptomatic forms and those associated with structural anomalies require treatment. Surgical techniques include vascular resection and suspension procedures (e.g., aortopexy), internal or external stenting, cricoid-tracheal suspension in posttracheostomy tracheomalacia, and tracheoplasty for localized defects.

b. AIRWAY IMPLICATIONS

Airway manifestations of tracheomalacia involve the potential for airway compression at the site of disease. Patients with tracheomalacia are prone to tracheal collapse, especially during exhalation, when there is a rise in intrathoracic pressure.[187] The circumstances for airway collapse vary depending on the origin. Children with tracheomalacia can have "dying spells" during these episodes. Acquired forms of tracheomalacia may have additional anesthetic implications relating to the causative factor (e.g., mediastinal mass).

c. AIRWAY MANAGEMENT

Patients with moderate to severe disease require surgical repair. The major concern is with airway obstruction during induction of anesthesia. The trachea may be secured by means of any one of several methods: awake endotracheal intubation, inhalation induction preserving spontaneous ventilation, or intravenous induction. One should be prepared to deal with airway obstruction by having a rigid bronchoscope or reinforced ET available to push past the site of tracheal obstruction.

2. Croup

See Congenital and Acquired Subglottic Disease.

3. Bacterial tracheitis

a. PATHOLOGIC CONDITIONS

Bacterial tracheitis is a rare disease of childhood with a high degree of morbidity and mortality.[188] It generally follows a viral respiratory tract illness. The most common bacterial pathogens are *Staphylococcus aureus* and *Haemophilus influenzae*. Patients come to medical attention with crouplike cough, fever, and stridor, which progress to toxic appearance, cyanosis, and respiratory distress. The signs and symptoms are nonpathognomonic and may be mistaken for croup or epiglottitis.[189] However, these patients do not manifest drooling, do not tolerate the supine position, and do not show response to treatment with racemic epinephrine or corticosteroids. Endoscopy, which is diagnostic, reveals a normal-appearing epiglottis with subglottic edema, friable trachea and bronchi with ulcerations, and copious mucopurulent secretions. Secretions are often so thick that tracheostomy and stripping of inspissated secretions are necessary. Patients are prone to pneumonitis, pneumothorax (or pneumomediastinum), and respiratory insufficiency leading to death. In a review of 118 cases one report found an 11% incidence of cardiopulmonary arrest resulting from airway obstruction.[190] Associated toxic shock syndrome has been described.[191] Diagnosis is made by history and endoscopy. Chest x-ray may show subglottic narrowing, radiopaque streaks within the trachea, and pulmonary infiltrates. Treatment often necessitates endotracheal intubation for ventilatory support and pulmonary toilet.[190] Humidification of airway gases helps prevent drying of secretions. Tracheostomy has been recommended.[192] Appropriate antimicrobial therapy is essential.

b. AIRWAY IMPLICATIONS

The major problem faced by children with bacterial tracheitis is acute large airway obstruction caused by presence of mucosal edema, thick tracheal secretions, and pseudomembranes.[190] Patients are susceptible to bronchospasm, pneumonia, pneumothorax, and pneumomediastinum. These patients have reduced tracheal lumen size and diminished oxygenation, ventilation, and oxygen reserve.

c. AIRWAY MANAGEMENT

In patients suspected of having bacterial tracheitis rigid bronchoscopy is often required for diagnosis and

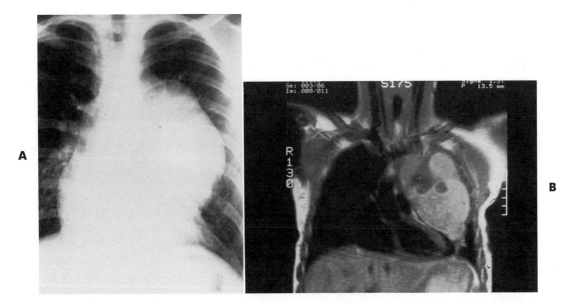

Fig. 29-22. Mediastinal mass. **A,** Chest radiograph, anteroposterior view, showing large mediastinal mass compressing the left lung and masking the left cardiac silhouette. **B,** Magnetic resonance imaging shows the relationship of the mass to the heart, lung, and great vessels. This 11-year-old, who came to medical attention with chest pain, was given anesthesia in the left lateral position and was spontaneously breathing halothane, and the trachea was intubated with an FFB using a reinforced ET. The mass was a teratoma.

therapeutic removal of secretions.[188,193] Bronchoscopy should be carried out with the patient under general anesthesia, much in the way patients with epiglottitis are treated. Inhalation induction with halothane and oxygen is preferred. One should be prepared to deal with complete airway obstruction. Most patients continue to have endotracheal intubation for positive pressure ventilation and pulmonary toilet, which should be carried out with utmost vigilance. Rigid bronchoscopy may have to be repeated on a frequent basis for monitoring of progress and removal of secretions.[188] Affected children who require endotracheal intubation generally remain intubated for several days.[188] Adequate sedation should be provided, and care taken to prevent premature tracheal extubation.

4. Mediastinal masses

a. PATHOLOGIC CONDITIONS

Mediastinal mass lesions (Fig. 29-22) and administration of anesthesia can be a potentially fatal combination. Masses within the mediastinum can cause sudden cardiopulmonary collapse that is often refractory to the most aggressive treatment.[194-196] Airway obstruction can occur during induction, after endotracheal intubation, following change in patient position, and subsequent to emergence and endotracheal extubation.[196,197] Thus any mediastinal mass, even if asymptomatic, should be properly evaluated, and special precautions taken during all phases of anesthesia.

The mediastinum is a compartment within the thoracic cavity bound by the medial aspect of the lungs and plurae, the sternum, the vertebral column, the thoracic inlet, and the diaphragm.[198] The mediastinum is divided into superior and inferior sections; the latter are further divided into the anterior, middle, and posterior mediastina. The prevalence of mediastinal masses within pediatric patients varies with age and anatomic location. In newborns and infants neurogenic tumors are the most frequent. Other diseases and disorders in infants include bronchogenic cysts, cystic hygroma, hemangiomas, and diaphragmatic hernias. Neurogenic tumors are also the most frequent mediastinal mass disease in small children. In older children and adolescents lymphomas constitute the major cause of mediastinal disease and are primarily located in the anterior mediastinum. In this older age-group teratomas, thymomas, neurogenic tumors, and mesenchymal tumors are also found.

The clinical presentation of mediastinal tumors depends on the lesion's mass effect, location, infiltrative nature, and patient posture. The effect on the respiratory pathway may cause cough, dyspnea, orthopnea, stridor, diminished breath sounds, wheezing or prolonged expiratory time, and cyanosis.[199] Although some children may be asymptomatic, children younger than 2 years of age frequently have symptoms of airway compression.[200] Cardiovascular manifestations can include fatigue, shortness of breath, orthopnea, pulsus paradoxus, syncope (especially with Valsalva-type maneuvers), or no symptoms at all. These signs and symptoms may be more pronounced in the supine position. In symptomatic patients the possibility of respiratory and cardiovascular compression should be considered and investigated. If there is associated superior vena cava syndrome, patients may complain of feeling light-headed and of having visual disturbances, syncope, or respiratory distress. Symptoms generally worsen with a head-down position. Examination may reveal distended veins in the upper extremity, head, face, and neck, as well as papilledema or edema of the conjunctiva.[201] The involved area may appear cyanotic or purple.

Laboratory evaluations are used to confirm the diagnosis of mediastinal mass and to elucidate the size, location, and mass effect on vital mediastinal structures. Anteroposterior and lateral chest films are highly accurate in demonstrating the mass and its position within the mediastinum.[202] Computed tomographic scan and MRI of the thorax more precisely delineate the mass and its relation to surrounding structures. Flow-volume loops, obtained with the patient in the sitting and supine positions, can help assess dynamic airway compression by revealing flattening of the inspiratory and expiratory phases.[197] Flexible fiberoptic bronchoscopy after topical anesthesia has been recommended as a method of evaluating the dynamic effects of the mass on the airway. If there is suggestion of cardiovascular involvement, echocardiography may determine whether there is compression or infiltration of vital structures (pericardium, heart, pulmonary arteries, and aorta) and the degree to which it is influenced by position.[203] It is important to note that in small children many of these tests require sedation, which may not be without risks of its own. Thus each patient must be evaluated on an individual basis to determine whether these evaluations should be carried out outside the operating room area. Treatment of mediastinal masses depends on the disease and involves a combination of surgery, radiation therapy, chemotherapy and corticosteroid therapy.

b. AIRWAY IMPLICATIONS

Mediastinal masses, especially those within the anterior mediastinum, can adversely affect vital structures such as the tracheobronchial tree, pericardium, heart, great vessels, and vena cava by mass effect or through infiltration.[199] The respiratory manifestations result from extrinsic compression or softening of the airway structures. This can be at the level of the trachea, carina, or bronchus, resulting in various levels of dynamic airway obstruction. Experience has shown that in patients with mediastinal mass, dynamic physiologic changes can develop on induction of anesthesia, on muscle relaxation, or following patient positioning, which may have detrimental effects on cardiac output and airway patency. These changes take place through a combination of factors that result in mechanical compression of cardiorespiratory structures in the mediastinum. Relaxation of muscles of respiration, loss of negative transpulmonary pressure, reduced lung and mediastinal volume, decreased airway size and support, as well as positive pressure ventilation and cardiovascular effects of potent inhalation agents, combine to cause airway and cardiovascular collapse following induction of anesthesia and muscle paralysis.[185,197] The likelihood of airway collapse during general anesthesia correlates with the degree of airway narrowing on CT scan.[185]

Equally important in the management of these patients is the influence of mediastinal mass on the cardiovascular system. Cardiovascular structures such as the pericardium, pulmonary artery, cardiac chambers, or aorta can be compressed by the mass causing obstruction to blood flow. It is important to realize that during general anesthesia a patient with mediastinal mass may have complete airway obstruction or cardiovascular collapse even if previously asymptomatic.[195] The reason for the adverse effect of general anesthesia and muscle relaxation on air exchange and cardiac output may be the loss of muscle tone and diminished structural support of the tumor within the thoracic cavity.[195] The superior vena cava is particularly prone to compression because of its weak supporting walls. Clinical implications of superior vena cava syndrome relate to decreased blood return from the upper part of the body to the heart. This can cause a reduction in cardiac output, increased blood loss during surgery, and a delay for medications administered via upper extremity veins to reach the central circulation. Fluids administered in the same manner may not readily reach the heart, but rather may cause further distention of the head, neck, and intrathoracic venous system and exacerbate symptoms.

c. AIRWAY MANAGEMENT

Anesthetic management of children with mediastinal masses requires a thorough preoperative evaluation and specialized preparation. The history and physical examination should focus on signs and symptoms of airway or cardiovascular involvement in different postures. These can determine optimal positioning of the patient during induction of anesthesia. Patients with history of syncope may be especially prone to cardiovascular decompensation on induction.[194] However, severity of symptoms is not always a good indicator of cardiopulmonary involvement, so all children with mediastinal mass should receive adequate preparation and utmost care.[195,204] The rigid bronchoscope should be present in the operating room.[195] Children with cardiovascular symptoms should be considered for a femoral-femoral bypass.

Pediatric patients with mediastinal mass who require premedication should receive the least amount necessary while being continuously observed in an environment where emergency airway support can be provided. Excessive sedation may mimic effects of anesthesia on the mediastinal disease. All patients should have a secure intravenous line in place (in the lower extremity in case of superior vena cava syndrome) before receiving an anesthetic.

With respect to the DA algorithm, children with a mediastinal mass should be considered potentially difficult to ventilate. In addition, they are at risk of cardiovascular compromise. Unless general anesthesia is necessary for therapeutic surgical resection of the lesion, it should be avoided in children with mediastinal mass, if at all possible. If the surgery is for a node biopsy, it should be performed with the patient under local anesthesia.[205] Diagnostic thoracoscopy has been performed in spontaneously breathing children over 3 years of age with use of intercostal nerve blocks and intravenous ketamine.[206] If the diagnosis is known and the lesion is sensitive to radiation therapy, prior irradiation may shrink tumor size, reduce mass effect, and diminish the risk associated with administration of anesthesia.[207] In high-risk children, empirical treatment with chemotherapy and irradiation has been recommended.[208]

If general anesthesia is necessary and the child will tolerate awake endotracheal intubation, the airway may be secured by any one of several techniques (such as direct laryngoscopy, FFB, or Bullard) following appropriate topical anesthesia of the airway. Since small or anxious children may not cooperate with awake endotracheal intubation, they may first have to be anesthetized. It is important to maintain the child as much as possible in a posture best tolerated in the awake state (e.g., semiseated). Induction of anesthesia in the lateral position has been suggested.[195] Anesthesia may be induced with halothane and oxygen. It is recommended that patients maintain spontaneous respiration and not receive muscle relaxation.[197] When adequate depth of anesthesia has been achieved to allow laryngoscopy, the trachea is intubated with a reinforced ET.

If respiratory or cardiovascular collapse is encountered during anesthesia induction and endotracheal intubation, appropriate steps include the following:

1. Stenting the airway by advancing a reinforced ET or a rigid bronchoscope past the level of obstruction[205]
2. Changing the patient to the lateral decubitus or prone position, thus causing the mass to shift its weight distribution[195,205]
3. Femoral-femoral bypass[209]

Other methods that have been successful include traction on the airway as performed during direct laryngoscopy,[204] endotracheal extubation and spontaneous mask ventilation with PEEP,[205] and placement of two ETs, one in each bronchus.[208]

5. Vascular malformations (vascular rings)

a. PATHOLOGIC CONDITIONS

In children vascular anomalies are rare entities that can be a source of significant airway problems.[210,211] Because of the close relationship between the great vessels of the chest and airway structures, anatomic malformations in the former can have adverse affects on the airway. Such vascular anomalies result from abnormal persistence of structures of the aortic arch complex, and although the term vascular ring is used to describe them, they do not always form a complete circle. Vascular rings can compress the trachea, bronchi, and often the esophagus, causing a variety of respiratory complications.

The most common form of vascular ring requiring surgical correction is the double aortic arch. It results from presence of both fourth aortic arches that encircle the trachea and esophagus.[211] Patients with this anomaly are frequently symptomatic. Another vascular anomaly forming a complete ring around the trachea is a right aortic arch with aberrant left subclavian artery. In this anomaly the left subclavian artery originates from the descending aorta, travels behind the esophagus, and with the ligamentum arteriosum completes a circle. This malformation has an association with tetralogy of Fallot. Other vascular anomalies include aberrant innominant artery, pulmonary artery sling, retroesophageal subclavian artery, and left aortic arch with an aberrant right subclavian artery. Vascular rings have an association with other congenital anomalies.[212]

The most frequent symptoms include stridor, recurrent respiratory tract infection, cyanosis, dysphagia, and cough.[212] Symptoms generally manifest in the first year of life and worsen during cry or an upper respiratory infection. Some patients may have marked manifestations in form of respiratory distress, apnea, and cardiorespiratory arrest, while others may have minimal to no symptoms and the condition may go unrecognized. Esophageal compression can cause dysphagia, increased oral secretions, recurrent aspiration, and failure to thrive.

Diagnosis is suggested by history and physical examination and confirmed by radiologic studies and endoscopy. A plain chest radiograph may show the direction of the aortic arch and shift or indentation of the trachea. A chest film in presence of esophageal barium contrast is one of the most informative examinations and helps make the diagnosis in case the esophagus is involved. It will not aid in the diagnosis of aberrant innominate artery. Angiography is sometimes indicated to better elucidate the vascular abnormality and define associated congenital heart disease. Pulmonary function tests, MRI, echocardiography, and bronchoscopy also have a role in the diagnosis of vascular ring anomalies. In most circumstances bronchoscopy is not necessary, but it can assist in the search for additional tracheoesophageal anomalies and in the diagnosis of aberrant innominate artery by showing a pulsatile constriction of the trachea.[213]

Treatment of vascular anomalies depends on the severity of patient symptoms. Asymptomatic children

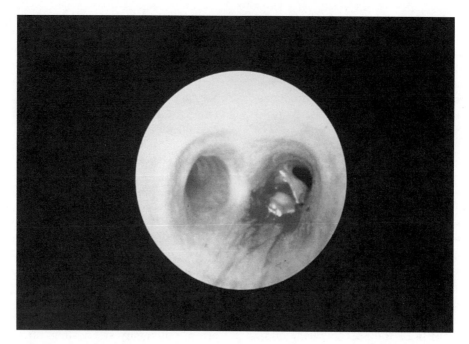

Fig. 29-23. Foreign body aspiration. Foreign body (pecan) in the right mainstem bronchus. Partial obstruction, mucosal irritation, and bleeding are evident.

may not require any treatment. Those with respiratory difficulty need surgical correction. Most surgeons approach the repair through a left thoracotomy, with occasional need for right thoracotomy or median sternotomy. Double aortic arch defects typically must undergo surgical correction early in life. Although an aberrant innominate artery may be suspended to the chest wall, most surgical repairs involve excision of the constrictive vessel. This does not always correct the structural changes incurred by the airway, which may persist as tracheal stenosis, tracheomalacia, and bronchomalacia and cause symptoms for variable periods.[212] Persistent tracheal wall defect may necessitate corrective surgery or tracheostomy. Surgical resection of tracheal stenosis has been performed using cardiopulmonary bypass.[214]

b. AIRWAY IMPLICATIONS

Mediastinal vascular malformations can be a source of airway compression. The severity depends on the type of anomaly and the degree of airway constriction. Severe constriction of the tracheobronchial tree leads to lower airway obstruction and respiratory distress. Longstanding airway compression can result in tracheomalacia or bronchomalacia. Patients with left pulmonary artery sling may have tracheal stenosis or complete tracheal rings that can persist despite vascular repair.[214] These patients are prone to recurrent respiratory infections, which may further limit adequate ventilation and oxygenation. Tendency toward airway collapse may persist even after surgical repair of the constricting vessel.[212]

c. AIRWAY MANAGEMENT

Patients having surgery for correction of symptomatic vascular ring anomalies are at risk for complete airway obstruction during anesthesia.[212] Tracheal compression and tracheomalacia, combined with traction on the lung during surgery, may cause airway collapse and difficulty with ventilation.[212] Appropriate preparation should include availability of a rigid bronchoscope to serve as a stent in case of complete airway collapse. Spontaneous respiration and avoidance of muscle relaxation may help maintain the airway patent until the trachea is intubated. Placing a reinforced ET past the compressed region of the trachea helps keep the airway patent.

Patients may not improve in the immediate postoperative period and could be prone to airway collapse from persistent tracheomalacia. Associated congenital anomalies and their anesthetic implications, as well as ramifications of compressing one of the lungs during surgical access to the vessels, should be considered.

6. Foreign body aspiration

a. PATHOLOGIC CONDITIONS

In children, foreign body (FB) aspiration is responsible for several hundred deaths each year and represents one of the major causes of accidental death in the home.[215-217] Children between ages 1 and 2 years are the most common victims.[218-220] Food particles are by far the most frequent objects aspirated[220-222] (Fig. 29-23). The majority of FBs become lodged in the main bronchi; the remainder are localized in the trachea or larynx or occur in multiple sites.[220] Signs and symptoms of aspiration and radiologic findings vary with the location of the FB. Those lodged in the laryngotracheal region manifest primarily as stridor, dyspnea, and cough, whereas bronchial FBs mainly cause cough, decreased air exchange on the affected side, wheezing, and dyspnea.[220,223] Other clinical findings may include fever, rales, tachypnea, retractions, cyanosis, apnea, and recurrent pneumonia and bronchospasm in chronic forms. Chest x-rays may show a radiopaque object, atelectasis, mediastinal shift, or air trapping on the affected side when inspiratory and expiratory or right and left decubitus radiographs are compared. However, most chest films are negative in the first 24 hours following FB aspiration, in particular, if the object is in the upper airway.[223] Lateral neck radiographs may be helpful in presence of laryngotracheal FBs by revealing subglottic abnormalities.[223] Thus the location of the FB within the airway can often be determined by a combination of physical examination[224] and radiographic studies.[225] Magnetic resonance imaging has also been useful in the diagnosis of FB aspiration.[226]

Many incidents of aspiration go unwitnessed, potentially delaying diagnosis. The time interval from aspiration to diagnosis also varies widely.[220] Although the majority are detected within 24 hours, over a third may take as long as a month to diagnose and a few may go undiagnosed for a year or longer. Misdiagnosis of FB aspiration is associated with a worsened outcome.[227]

b. AIRWAY IMPLICATIONS

Airway manifestations of FB aspiration depend on the object's size relative to that of the airway, the location, and the nature of the FB. The acute risk of FB aspiration is obstruction to air flow affecting ventilation and oxygenation. Many who require immediate care die at the scene. Obstruction may occur at the level of a segmental bronchus, main bronchus, carina, trachea, or larynx. Peripheral airway obstruction can result in atelectasis, bronchospasm, and air trapping because of a ball-valve effect with possible mediastinal shift. Airway obstruction can be severe when the FB is lodged in the larynx or trachea or at the level of the carina, where air entry can be restricted to both lungs. Laryngeal FBs are associated with high morbidity and mortality rates.[228] Chronic sequelae of FB aspiration include atelectasis, pneumonia, bronchospasm, hemoptysis, lung abscess, and bronchiectasis. Esophageal FBs can become evident with symptoms and complications of airway obstruction.[229,230]

c. AIRWAY MANAGEMENT

Emergency management of FB aspiration at the scene of accident (Heimlich maneuver, back and chest blows, and the like) are not discussed here but are detailed in other writings.[231] Children who make it to the hospital should undergo prompt evaluation and be scheduled for removal of the FB in the operating room. This can usually be performed after the required period of receiving nothing by mouth has passed. However, emergency removal of the FB is indicated if the child is in respiratory distress, if the FB is in a compromising location (e.g., larynx), or if its nature merits removal as soon as possible (e.g., sharp objects or agents such as peanuts, which are caustic to the respiratory mucosa and risk fragmentation if allowed to remain in the airway). Foreign bodies in place for a long time generally do not require emergency removal. Use of antibiotics and corticosteroids before removal of FB may reduce complication rates.[232]

Appropriate preparation includes readiness to manage total airway obstruction during the procedure. In children the method of providing optimal conditions for FB removal is through general anesthesia. Anesthetic management of these patients should be aimed at providing adequate ventilation and oxygenation, a smooth induction, and sufficient anesthetic depth to allow rigid bronchoscopy without cough, laryngospasm, bronchospasm, or displacement of the FB. In the child with respiratory distress or an FB in a compromising location it is important to avoid excessive agitation that could displace the object and cause complete obstruction. Patients with marked respiratory distress should not receive premedication. Agitation may be a sign of hypoxemia and this possibility should be ruled out by oximetry rather than treated by administration of sedatives. Parental presence to make anesthesia induction less distressing should be considered. In long-standing aspiration or for frightened children with minimal respiratory distress, premedication with midazolam (rectal, nasal, or oral), rectal methohexital, or ketamine (oral or intramuscular) may be helpful. The premedicated child should be closely observed, and appropriate suction and airway equipment kept at hand. The otorhinolaryngologist should be present in the operating room at the start of induction.

There is more than one method of anesthetizing children who have aspirated an FB. This relates to several controversial issues regarding treatment of FB aspiration in the pediatric patient. These include the use of inhalation versus intravenous induction, spontaneous versus controlled ventilation; use of muscle relaxants, rapid sequence induction, and cricoid pressure. Inhalation induction has the advantage of allowing titration of anesthetic depth, maintenance of spontaneous respiration, and minimal effect on moving the FB. However, it does not protect the patient against aspiration and requires the experience of knowing when the patient has reached the necessary anesthetic depth to allow laryngoscopy without cough and laryngospasm. Inhalation induction may be carried out with oxygen and halothane. Nitrous oxide is not recommended in patients with respiratory distress or hypoxemia or in those at risk for complete airway obstruction. Using 100 percent oxygen will provide a larger safety margin should complete airway obstruction occur. Once an appropriate depth of anesthesia is achieved, an intravenous line may be started if not already in place. Administration of an anticholinergic agent helps reduce oral secretions and maintain heart rate under deep levels of halothane anesthesia that are necessary to allow direct laryngoscopy. Continuous positive airway pressure of 5 to 10 cm H_2O or gentle assisted ventilation may sometimes be necessary to keep the airway patent. Once the depth of anesthesia permits, direct laryngoscopy is performed. Lidocaine 3 to 5 mg/kg can be injected at the vocal cords and into the trachea and allowed to take effect for 2 to 3 minutes for added anesthesia and reduction of airway reflexes in response to bronchoscopy. One hundred percent oxygen should be used during such procedures. A rigid bronchoscope equipped with a sidearm is then advanced into the airway by the surgeon under direct view to retrieve the foreign object. If the FB is not quickly retrieved, the patient may need to be actively ventilated and oxygenated through the sidearm of the rigid bronchoscope. If the leak around the bronchoscope is large, it may be difficult to ventilate the patient and high oxygen flows or change to a larger-size bronchoscope may be necessary. The anesthetic may be continued with inhalation or intravenous agents. Muscle relaxation may be necessary to prevent coughing and to immobilize the vocal cords in order to facilitate removal of the FB and minimize trauma to the airway. Patients with an FB in place for a long period may be treated with muscle relaxation and positive pressure ventilation from the onset of anesthesia. Once the FB is removed, the trachea may be intubated with an ET and the patient allowed to emerge from anesthesia.

If airway obstruction is encountered during inhalation induction, one must quickly differentiate between upper airway obstruction from soft tissue and tongue, laryngospasm, and foreign body by changing head and jaw position, providing CPAP by mask, using succinylcholine, and performing immediate bronchoscopy. If airway obstruction occurs during rigid bronchoscopy, the foreign body is most likely in the larynx or at the level of the carina, where it must be immediately removed or displaced into a mainstem bronchus.

Rapid sequence induction with cricoid pressure is an alternative method of induction preferred by some authors.[233,234] It has the advantages of protecting the airway from aspiration of stomach contents and allowing the use of muscle relaxants, which immobilize the vocal cords, prevent cough, and generally permit better lung ventilation and oxygenation. The potential disadvantages are inability to ventilate following muscle relaxation and concern for displacing the FB into a more compromising position as a result of positive pressure ventilation or endotracheal intubation, or both. Rapid sequence induction should not be performed if one has assessed that ventilation and oxygenation may be difficult after muscle relaxation. Cricoid pressure may cause harm if the FB is in the larynx or is potentially penetrating (e.g., open safety pin). Other alternatives of retrieving FB from the airway include tracheal incision[235] for large or pointed objects with little chance of passing the glottis, elective use of transtracheal jet ventilation[236] in cases with high risk for complete upper airway obstruction, and occasionally, thoracotomy and bronchotomy.[237]

After removal of FB, most children should be in a position to have the trachea extubated. This procedure depends on the amount of injury to the airway, the child's size, and anticipated degree of airway swelling. Some children may display stridor and croupy cough that benefit from use of humidified air, racemic epinephrine, and corticosteroids. Complications associated with FB removal from the airway include bronchospasm, laryngospasm, airway obstruction, pneumothorax, bronchial rupture, fragmentation of the foreign body, and hemorrhage.[238] In patients who may have residual gastric content the stomach should be aspirated by passing an orogastric tube before tracheal extubation. The success rate for FB removal by bronchoscopy is 95% to 98%; in the remainder of cases surgical removal (tracheostomy or thoracotomy) is required. In a small percentage of children a second bronchoscopy is needed for removal of residual FB or granulation tissue.

7. Other tracheal diseases

The trachea may be the site of other rare congenital or acquired diseases. These include tracheal stenosis[239] (Fig. 29-24) that involves either a limited portion or an extensive length of the trachea, tracheal granulation tissue or webbing, tracheal fistula, and tracheal diverticulum associated with tracheoesophageal fistula repair.[240] Origins or causes may be vascular rings, prolonged intubation, tracheal papillomatosis, and presence of annular cartilage rings. There may be associated tracheomalacia. Symptoms include stridor, cough, respiratory infections, and severe respiratory distress. Treatment includes laser excision (may have to be repeated), segmental tracheal resection, and rib cartilage grafting for stenoses involving prolonged segments of the trachea. These anomalies can cause difficulty with distal advancement of the ET or the ability to ventilate after intubation. When managing patients with such disease, small ETs should be available. If possible, endotracheal intubation should be avoided so as not to cause trauma and further narrowing of the airway.[51]

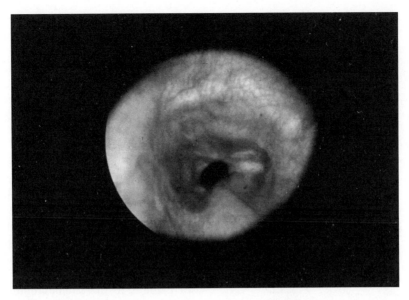

Fig. 29-24. Tracheal stenosis. Significant narrowing of the tracheal lumen below the third tracheal ring limits air exchange.

G. NECK AND SPINE ANOMALIES

1. Neck

a. PATHOLOGIC CONDITIONS

Mass lesions of the neck make up a diverse group of anomalies with potential for profound airway ramifications. The lesions include lymphatic and vascular malformations, bronchial and thyroglossal duct abnormalities, thyroid lesions, teratomas, dermoid cysts, neurogenic tumors, and abscesses, in addition to other rare anomalies.[102,241]

The most frequent congenital mass of the neck is the thyroglossal duct cyst.[102] This duct, involved in the embryogenesis of the thyroid gland, may persist and lead to cyst formation in early childhood. The lesion is almost always midline and in the proximity of the hyoid bone. Thyroglossal duct cysts are a potential source for infection and malignant transformation. Branchial apparatus defects result from abnormal embryologic remnants and can lead to formation of cysts, fistulas, and sinuses in various areas of the neck.[102] Bronchial cysts become evident as lateral cervical masses as they enlarge with time. Their size and location determine the degree of encroachment on the airway.

Lymphatic malformations or lymphangiomas represent sequestered lymphatic tissue devoid of the normal drainage into the lymphatic channels, giving it potential for abnormal growth and enlargement.[242] Lymphatic malformation can occur anywhere in the body, although most instances are found in the neck. The malformations have been classified into three types by Landing and Farber.[243] Those composed of large multiloculated cysts are called cystic hygroma. Cystic hygromas (Fig. 29-25) are typically found in infants and small children. Lymphatic lesions, like hemangiomas, can enlarge over a short time. Cystic hygromas of the neck respond to respiratory tract infections by acute enlargement, which may lead to exacerbation of airway obstruction. They can be associated with various syndromes, and when diagnosed in utero, they carry a poor prognosis.[244,245] A small percentage of children with large cystic hygromas of the neck have extension into the mediastinum, oropharynx, or laryngeal structures.[242]

In children the neck can also be a site for soft tissue tumors. Rhabdomyosarcoma is the most common of these,[58] although it can become evident at sites other than the neck. Rhabdomyosarcomas are generally found in children under 6 years of age and are susceptible to metastasis and local recurrence. Teratomas are rare in the neck region, although they can cause airway obstruction, and carry a high mortality rate.[107,246]

Neck abscesses in children occur primarily in children under 5 years of age; nearly half of these are infants between 6 and 12 months of age.[247] The great majority of neck abscesses are in the lateral neck; the remainder are in the midline. The origin is usually not evident, although most are preceded by a recent upper respiratory tract infection. Rarely, they are caused by cystic lesions of the neck such as thyroglossal and bronchial cleft cysts or dental infection. *Staphylococcus aureus* and group A β-hemolytic streptococci are the two most common isolated bacterial agents.

Clinical presentation of neck masses varies with the type of lesion, its size, and degree of encroachment on the airway. Inherent in their location, most of these pathologic entities can cause variable degrees of airway obstruction and feeding difficulty.[248] When there is

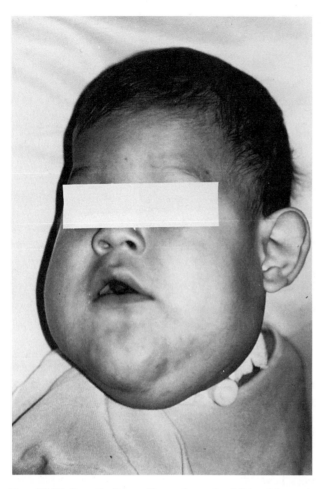

Fig. 29-25. Lymphatic malformation. A child with cystic hygroma of the neck and submandibular space, which caused airway obstruction that necessitated placement of a tracheostomy. This lesion is prone to recurrence and acute exacerbation during respiratory tract infections.

airway compression, children may display stridor, cough, and respiratory distress. In addition to having swelling, patients with neck abscesses may be febrile. Diagnosis of neck mass is based on history and physical examination. Radiologic studies (plain radiographs, CT scan, MRI, and ultrasound) and endoscopy can help elucidate the nature and size of the lesion and its relationship to airway structures. For example, ultrasound can differentiate between a solid and a cystic mass,[249] and CT scan findings of a cystic hygroma reveal a reproducible multilocular cystic image.

Treatment of neck masses depends on the nature of the lesion and its effect on the airway. To avoid airway compromise, large, benign lesions are best treated with surgical resection. Thyroglossal duct cysts and bronchial apparatus defects pose a risk for infection and should be removed. Whereas cystic hygromas rarely regress spontaneously, most are difficult to fully resect and tend to recur.[248] Abscesses should receive early antibiotic therapy and surgical drainage. Malignant disease is treated with a combination of surgery, irradiation, and chemotherapy.

Skin contractures reduce extensibility of the tegument and when localized to the neck, can influence airway management. Causes include recovery from burn, surgery, inflammatory states (e.g., epidermolysis bullosa), and radiation therapy.

b. AIRWAY IMPLICATIONS

All mass lesions of the neck can affect the airway and complicate its management. Even thyroglossal duct cysts and bronchial cysts can enlarge to a size that can cause airway obstruction. Neck masses can encroach on the airway and cause variable degrees of obstruction to air flow, or they can distort airway structures and interfere with direct laryngoscopy and visualization of the glottis. Mask placement can be suboptimal if the lesion is large or extends to the submandibular region or face. Skin contractures in the neck region restrict head extension on the cervical spine, thus interfering with alignment of the axes necessary for visualization of the glottis during direct laryngoscopy.

c. AIRWAY MANAGEMENT

Airway management of pediatric patients with neck lesions must take into consideration the extent of airway involvement and whether mask ventilation or direct laryngoscopy will be adversely affected. If airway difficulty is assessed to be likely, then according to the DA algorithm, an awake technique of endotracheal intubation should be selected. After appropriate topical anesthesia, one of several available methods using the FFB, Bullard laryngoscope, lighted stylet, or digital technique may be used to intubate the trachea. Children who will not cooperate with this technique without an inappropriately high level of sedation should be considered for general anesthesia. This should be performed while maintaining spontaneous ventilation. If mask fit is adequate, general anesthesia can be induced by inhalation induction. Should the neck mass influence feasible mask fit, then it may be possible to place an LMA into the oropharynx and induce general anesthesia by use of halothane and oxygen. The trachea may subsequently be secured with a fiberscope through the LMA or with use of a lighted stylet or Bullard laryngoscope after removal of the LMA. After induction of general anesthesia it is possible to attempt direct laryngoscopy, although attempts should be limited. One should be prepared to use transtracheal jet ventilation or emergency tracheostomy should complete airway obstruction occur.

When there is prenatal diagnosis of a neck mass, several authors have described a multidisciplinary approach to securing the newborn airway immediately upon delivery.[107,250-252] The fetal head and neck are delivered by cesarean section, and while preserving uteroplacental perfusion, the trachea is intubated. Some authors recommend use of halothane anesthesia in the mother to prevent uterine contraction and premature detachment of the placenta.[251]

2. Limited cervical spine mobility

a. PATHOLOGIC CONDITIONS

Diseases of the cervical spine complicate airway management by restricting neck movement and impeding proper head positioning for direct laryngoscopy. They include lesions that render the cervical spine instable and those that restrict its flexion. The latter group of anomalies comprises congenital and acquired diseases such as juvenile rheumatoid arthritis, traumatic injury, and surgical fusion. Klippel-Feil syndrome exemplifies congenital cervical spine anomaly of this type. Patients with classic Klippel-Feil syndrome have a triad of clinical findings: cervical vertebral fusion, short neck, and low-set occipital hairline. Cervical fusion may be limited to a single level (two vertebrae) or involve all cervical vertebrae.[253] The syndrome is associated with other organ system dysfunction that can increase the likelihood of airway obstruction.[254] Anomalies of the CNS, such as that of the cervicomedullary junction, and Arnold-Chiari malformation are among the most common.

Juvenile rheumatoid arthritis is a devastating inflammatory disease that affects multiple organ systems (including cardiac, pulmonary, renal, and hematologic and the CNS) and can handicap children from early age. It has a bimodal age distribution corresponding to age 2 years and late in the first decade of life.[255] Juvenile rheumatoid arthritis is divided into systemic (Still's disease), polyarticular, and pauciarticular forms, which differ with respect to initial presentation, pattern of joint involvement, eye disease, and laboratory findings. In addition to peripheral joint disease, the cervical spine and temporomandibular and cricoarytenoid joints can be affected. The diagnosis is made by clinical evaluation with the aid of hematologic and radiologic studies. The prognosis for joint disease in the systemic form is poor. Treatment comprises a combination of corticosteroid and nonsteroidal antiinflammatory agents, gold, penicillamine, and hydroxychloroquine.

b. AIRWAY IMPLICATIONS

Direct laryngoscopy is less likely to expose the glottis in patients with Klippel-Feil syndrome, and there is increased risk of airway obstruction and cervical spine injury. The cervical spine fusion and short neck in these patients limit cervical flexion and neck extension. If there is associated Arnold-Chiari malformation, vocal cord dysfunction may potentiate airway obstruction. These patients are also more likely to sustain cervical spine injury, especially to vertebrae adjacent to the fused segments.[256]

Airway manifestations of juvenile rheumatoid arthritis are related to several factors. Cervical spine disease is common in the systemic and polyarticular forms of juvenile rheumatoid arthritis. The disease includes joint erosion and spine fusion, which usually start at the high cervical level and extend as low as the thoracic spine. Some patients may have complete cervical spine ankylosis.[257] These patients are at low risk for atlantoaxial subluxation. Spine disease can stunt the normal growth of the cervical region, resulting in a short neck. The combination of reduced cervical mobility, short neck, and potential for atlantoaxial subluxation can limit head and neck mobility and make endotracheal intubation difficult.[258] Furthermore, in a significant portion of children with juvenile rheumatoid arthritis torticollis can develop during the acute attack, further limiting neck mobility.

In childhood arthritis other anomalies that affect the airway must be evaluated. Temporomandibular joint disease is a common occurrence, and when severe, it can limit mouth opening. In addition, it can be associated with abnormal mandibular growth and result in micrognathia,[255] which can further hamper successful direct laryngoscopy.

Cricoarytenoid arthritis is rare in pediatric patients[259,260] but when present, can manifest as stridor and life-threatening airway obstruction. Children with cricoarytenoid arthritis have increasing hoarseness over a period of several weeks that progresses to respiratory distress and airway obstruction. Symptoms tend to be worse during sleep and sedation. Several of the cases described have required tracheostomy. Definitive diagnosis is made during laryngoscopy, which may reveal edematous arytenoids found fixed in adduction and reduced vocal cord mobility.[260] Cricoarytenoid arthritis is responsive to corticosteroid therapy.

c. AIRWAY MANAGEMENT

In patients with an unyielding cervical spine the ability to align the airway axes, which is necessary for visualization of the glottis during direct laryngoscopy, is limited. Other airway anomalies that may coexist (temporomandibular joint disease, cricoarytenoid arthritis, and so forth) must be sought and considered in the management plan.

For many patients with cervical spine disease, clinical evaluation is often strongly suggestive that direct laryngoscopy will be unsuccessful. Additional information may be acquired by direct laryngoscopy in the awake state, with the oropharynx topically anesthetized. These data can help determine how the process of endotracheal intubation should proceed. If such evaluation is highly in favor of a complicated airway, the "awake endotracheal intubation" limb of the DA algorithm should be followed. Awake techniques can include tactile intubation and the FFB or one of its variations. Bullard laryngoscope and the lightwand are particularly suited, since, like the fiberscope, they require limited neck and jaw movement. Blind and retrograde intubation should also be considered.

If awake endotracheal intubation is not appropriate, general anesthesia may be necessary. The way this is accomplished will be influenced by the ease of mask ventilation. If mask ventilation in the patient is easily accomplished, general anesthesia may be induced by inhalation or intravenous agents and ventilation can be spontaneous or controlled. Patients in whom mask ventilation is difficult should be allowed to breathe vapor anesthesia spontaneously through a face mask or an LMA. The trachea may then be secured with the FFB, blind nasotracheal intubation, Bullard laryngoscope, lightwand, or retrograde techniques. Use of an LMA facilitates directing the fiberscope to the laryngeal inlet.

3. Congenital cervical spine instability

a. PATHOLOGIC CONDITIONS

Cervical spine instability can lead to catastrophic neurologic injury and death during airway management. A variety of congenital diseases are associated with cervical spine instability, including Down syndrome, familial cervical dysplasia, and mucopolysaccharidoses such as Hurler's and Morquio's syndromes.[261] Acquired cervical spine instability may be due to traumatic injury and to juvenile rheumatoid arthritis.

Down syndrome or trisomy 21 is a chromosomal defect that results in characteristic phenotypic features and potential for organ system anomalies. The latter can include variable degrees of mental retardation, congenital heart disease (endocardial cushion defect), gastrointestinal anomalies (duodenal atresia), and skeletal abnormalities. In addition, nearly a third of Down syndrome patients demonstrate upper airway obstruction during sleep.[262] This is likely to be due to a relatively large tongue for the size of the oral cavity. Other airway-related diseases include a short neck and reduced tracheal length and lumen size.

Children with Down syndrome have a much higher incidence of cervical spine disease than do age- and sex-matched normal children.[263] Cervical spine instability occurs in 9% to 31% of patients with Down syndrome.[264] Atlantoaxial instability is thought to result from extension of the generalized ligamental laxity (in Down syndrome) to the transverse atlantal ligament that maintains the odontoid process close to the anterior arch of the atlas.[265] Ligamental laxity in the cervical spine may also contribute to instability at the atlantooccipital region.[266] However, others have found that general laxity is not related to laxity at the transverse (atlantal) ligament.[267] Atlantoaxial instability is generally considered as an atlantodens interval of 5 mm or greater. Intervals in excess of 5 mm are associated with a greater incidence of symptoms and higher potential for spinal cord compression.[268] Atlantoaxial instability may be associated with abnormal neurologic findings such as neck pain, hyperreflexia, ankle clonus, positive Babinski's sign, gait disturbances, muscle weakness, and torticollis. Only 1% to 2% of Down syndrome patients have symptomatic atlantoaxial instability,[269] but these patients are at increased risk for further neurologic injury and should be evaluated for cervical stabilization. Those with asymptomatic atlantoaxial instability may not require cervical fusion before surgery but management should be in a manner that avoids excessive movement of the cervical spine. Studies have shown that atlantodens interval changes minimally over time.[269] Children with Down syndrome can display other abnormalities of the cervical spine, including os odontoideum, reduced width of spinal canal, atlantooccipital laxity or fusion, and hypoplasia of the atlas.

Diagnosis is suspected by history and physical examination and confirmed by radiologic studies. Evaluation should concentrate on neurologic function in an effort to detect children with symptomatic instability. Radiologic evaluation of atlantoaxial instability is made by plain lateral neck radiographs in the neutral, flexion, and extension positions. Flexion position allows the greatest translation between the atlas and the odontoid, providing the best test for integrity of the transverse atlantal ligament. However, it does not distinguish all atlantoaxial instability; thus the other two images are necessary.[269]

b. AIRWAY IMPLICATIONS

Patients with symptomatic atlantoaxial instability are at risk for further neurologic injury during neck flexion or extension. These patients should be evaluated for cervical fusion. There are no data to support that Down syndrome patients with asymptomatic atlantoaxial instability are at higher risk for subluxation than their counterparts with normal atlantodens interval. Experts, however, recommend that the neck be prevented from maximal flexion (and probably extension).[269,270] In addition, patients with Down syndrome are at increased risk for upper airway obstruction.

c. AIRWAY MANAGEMENT

Airway management of children with Down syndrome should take into consideration the potential for upper airway obstruction and cervical spine instability. Patients with symptomatic atlantoaxial instability should not undergo elective anesthesia until evaluated by a neurosurgeon. If they must undergo *emergency* surgery, precautions similar to those for any patient with an unstable cervical spine should be taken. Although the use of limited attempts at blind nasotracheal intubation has been recommended, endotracheal intubation should be accomplished after induction of anesthesia with in-line stabilization of the cervical spine with direct laryngoscopy, ensuring minimal movement of the neck. As an alternative, techniques that require minimal neck mobility, such as the Bullard blade or lighted stylet, may be used. If these are unsuccessful in the emergency setting, one should proceed with a surgical airway.

Down syndrome patients with asymptomatic atlanto-axial instability should have endotracheal intubation in ways that avoid excessive movement of the neck. This can be accomplished with the patient awake or after induction of general anesthesia, using direct laryngoscopy or one of various indirect visual or blind techniques. Awake techniques have the benefit of allowing evaluation and documentation of the effect of endotracheal intubation on the patient's neurologic status.

4. Acquired cervical spine instability

a. PATHOLOGIC CONDITIONS

Acquired cervical spine instability in children can result from diverse mechanisms, including inflammatory diseases and trauma. This section is primarily devoted to traumatic causes of cervical spine instability.

Cervical spine injury in the pediatric patient is uncommon,[271] especially in young children, whose injuries tend to be at the high cervical level. Most of such injuries in children are due to trauma; motor vehicle accidents represent the major source.[272] Trauma to the cervical spine can result in crush fractures from hyperflexion and dislocation of the vertebral body with or without fracture, rendering the spine unstable. Trauma patients such as those with Down syndrome should be considered at high risk for cervical spine injury.

The diagnosis of cervical spine injury is more difficult in children than in adults. In pediatric patients standard lateral radiographs of the neck may fail to detect those at risk of spinal cord injury.[273] Therefore any child with a possibility of neck injury should have cervical spine precautions (spine board, cervical collar, and lateral head support), and receive detailed radiologic and neurologic evaluation before the C-spine is labeled as "cleared." In addition, any child with head, face, or neck injury who complains of neck pain or displays unexplained refractory shock should be considered as having spinal cord involvement until proven otherwise. It is important to recognize that children with cervical spine trauma may have increased intracranial pressure or multiorgan injury and that airway management must be altered accordingly.

b. AIRWAY IMPLICATIONS

Airway management in patients with trauma to the cervical spine risks causing or extending injury to the spinal cord[274] as a result of excessive movement of the neck during endotracheal intubation. Thus head extension and cervical flexion to optimize positioning for direct laryngoscopy are limited. Furthermore, evaluation of the airway is generally incomplete, since patients are unable to sit for examination of the oropharynx. If there is

trauma to the face, there may be facial fractures, swelling of oropharyngeal structures, and presence of blood that mask view of the glottis. All trauma patients should be considered to have a full stomach and to be at risk for pulmonary aspiration.

c. AIRWAY MANAGEMENT

Management of the airway in traumatic cervical spine instability presents either an immediate or a nonimmediate need for securing the airway. The method selected should consider the aforementioned issues and their influence on the process of endotracheal intubation. A major difference between cervical spine injury resulting from trauma and cervical spine instability of congenital source is that the former is more frequently associated with need for emergent endotracheal intubation and full-stomach precautions.

If the need for endotracheal intubation is *immediate,* the patient should receive 100% oxygen by mask. Patients who are apneic should have positive pressure mask ventilation while cricoid pressure is applied. In case the airway is obstructed there should be a quick attempt to establish a patent airway by anterior displacement of the mandible or insertion of an oropharyngeal airway. If the airway appears normal, direct laryngoscopy with cricoid pressure and in-line cervical stabilization can be attempted after administration of appropriate induction agents. Should airway evaluation suggest a DA, or if there is severe facial trauma, one should proceed with tracheostomy or cricothyrotomy. This could be preceded by a limited attempt at endotracheal intubation with one of several techniques (e.g., direct laryngoscopy or Bullard laryngoscopy).

In patients who are breathing spontaneously, blind nasotracheal intubation has been recommended, as long as there is no facial trauma. Nasal intubation in small children may injure the adenoids, cause bleeding, and obstruct the ET. If endotracheal intubation fails, the DA algorithm should be followed (help, mask ventilation, further attempts depending on the ease of mask ventilation and oxygenation, and surgical airway). In trauma patients one should proceed to surgical airway management more promptly in light of potential for increased intracranial pressure and risk of aspiration.

As an alternative, if ventilation and oxygenation in the patient with potential C-spine injury is adequate, the need for endotracheal intubation is *not immediate.* Time should be taken to fully evaluate the cervical spine for potential injury. If the cervical spine is uninjured and the patient airway appears normal on evaluation, the trachea may be intubated by induction of anesthesia, direct laryngoscopy, and application of cricoid pressure. In-line cervical stabilization should be used even when radiologic studies are normal unless the neurosurgeon or trauma surgeon has evaluated the patient and removed the neck collar. Airway management according to the

DA algorithm may be followed. If the cervical spine is unstable or the studies are inconclusive and the airway appears normal, general anesthesia may be induced, using in-line cervical stabilization and cricoid pressure to secure the airway by direct laryngoscopy. If intubation fails, one may proceed according to the "unrecognized" limb of the DA algorithm while maintaining cricoid pressure. If cervical spine is unstable and a DA is anticipated, one may proceed with an awake method (FFB, Bullard laryngoscope, retrograde, or lightwand). If this method is unsuccessful, surgical techniques of securing the airway should be employed.

ACKNOWLEDGMENT

I wish to extend my appreciation to Dr. Carol J. MacArthur of the Department of Otolaryngology Head and Neck Surgery at University of California, Irvine Medical Center for her assistance in the preparation of this chapter.

REFERENCES

1. Eigen H, Grosfeld JL: Pulmonary physiology in the surgical infant. In Otherson HB, editor: *The pediatric airway,* Philadelphia, 1991, WB Saunders.
2. Motoyama EK, Brinkmeyer SD, Mutich RL et al: Reduced FRC in anesthetized infants: effect of low PEEP, *Anesthesiology* 57:A418, 1982.
3. Motoyama EK: Anesthesia and the upper airway in infants and children, *Int Anesthesiol Clin* 30:17, 1992.
4. Olsson GL, Hallen B: Cardiac arrest during anaesthesia: a computer-aided study in 250543 anaesthetics, *Acta Anaesthesiol Scand* 32:653, 1988.
5. Keenan RL, Boyan CP: Cardiac arrest due to anesthesia, *JAMA* 253:2373, 1985.
6. Tiret L, Nivoche Y, Hatton F et al: Complications related to anesthesia in infants and children, *Br J Anaesth* 61:263, 1988.
7. Morray JP, Geiduschek JM, Caplan RA et al: A comparison of pediatric and adult anesthesia closed malpractice claims, *Anesthesiology* 78:461, 1993.
8. Keenan RL, Shapiro JH, Kane FR et al: Bradycardia during anesthesia in infants, *Anesthesiology* 80:976-82, 1994.
9. Keenan RL, Shapiro JH, Dawson K: Frequency of anesthetic cardiac arrest in infants: effect of pediatric anesthesiologists, *J Clin Anesth* 3:433, 1991.
10. Tucker HM: Embryology and developmental anatomy. In Tucker HM, editor: *The Larynx,* ed 2, New York, 1993, Thieme.
11. Fearon B, Whalen JS: Tracheal dimensions in the living infant, *Ann Otol Rhinol Laryngol* 76:965, 1967.
12. Rosenberg MB, Levesque PR, Bourke DL: Use of the LTAR Kit as a guide for endotracheal intubation, *Anesth Analg* 56:287, 1977.
13. Todres ID, Crone RK: Experience with a modified laryngoscope in sick infants, *Crit Care Med* 9:544, 1981.
14. Bainton CR: A new laryngoscope blade to overcome pharyngeal obstruction, *Anesthesiology* 67:767, 1987.
15. Diaz JH, Guarisco JL, LeJeune FE: A modified tubular pharyngolaryngoscope for difficult pediatric laryngoscopy, *Anesthesiology* 73:357, 1990.
16. Borland LM, Casselbrant M: The Bullard laryngoscope: a new indirect oral laryngoscope (pediatric version), *Anesth Analg* 70:105, 1990.
17. Noviski N, Todres D: Fiberoptic bronchoscopy in the pediatric patient, *Anesthesiology Clin North Am* 9:163, 1991.
18. Wood RE, Postma D: Endoscopy of the airway in infants and children, *J Pediatr* 112:1, 1988.
19. deBlic J, Delacourt C, Scheinmann P: Ultrathin flexible bronchoscopy in neonatal intensive care units, *Arch Dis Child* 66:1383, 1991.
20. Fan LL, Sparks LM, Dulinski JP: Application of an ultrathin flexible bronchoscope for neonatal and pediatric airway problems, *Chest* 89:673, 1986.
21. Holzman RS, Nargozian CD, Florence FB: Lightwand intubation in children with abnormal upper airways, *Anesthesiology* 69:784, 1988.
22. Creighton RE, Relton JES, Meridy HW: Anaesthesia for occipital encephalocele, *Can Anaesth Soc J* 21:403, 1974.
23. Yemen TA, Pullerits J, Stillman R et al: Rectal methohexital causing apnea in two patients with meningomyeloceles, *Anesthesiology* 74:1139, 1991.
24. Smith JA, Santer LJ: Respiratory arrest following intramuscular ketamine injection in a 4-year-old child, *Ann Emerg Med* 22:613, 1993.
25. Kleeman PP, Jantzen J, Bonfils P: The ultrathin bronchoscope in management of the difficult paediatric airway, *Can J Anaesth* 34:606, 1987.
26. Vuckovic DD, Rooney SM, Goldiner PL et al: Aerosol anesthesia of the airway using a small disposable nebulizer, *Anesth Analg* 59:803, 1980.
27. Berry F: The use of a stylet in blind nasotracheal intubation, *Anesthesiology* 61:469, 1984.
28. Brown RE, Vollers JM, Rader GR et al: Nasotracheal intubation in a child with Treacher Collins syndrome using Bullard intubating laryngoscope, *J Clin Anesth* 5:492, 1993.
29. Dohi S, Inomata S, Tanaka M et al: End-tidal carbon dioxide monitoring during awake blind nasotracheal intubation, *J Clin Anesth* 2:415, 1990.
30. Cameron D, Lupton BA: Inadvertent brain penetration during neonatal nasotracheal intubation, *Arch Dis Child* 69:79, 1993.
31. Knuth TE, Richards JR: Mainstem bronchial obstruction secondary to nasotracheal intubation: a case report and review of the literature, *Anesth Analg* 73:487, 1991.
32. Hancock PJ, Peterson G: Finger intubation of the trachea in newborns, *Pediatrics* 89:325, 1992.
33. Suetra PT, Gordon GJ: Digitally assisted tracheal intubation in a neonate with Pierre Robin syndrome, *Anesthesiology* 78:983, 1993.
34. Krucylak CP, Schreiner MS: Orotracheal intubation of an infant with hemifacial microsomia using a modified lighted stylet, *Anesthesiology* 77:826, 1992.
35. Stiles CM: A flexible fiberoptic bronchoscope for endotracheal intubation in infants, *Anesth Analg* 53:1017, 1974.
36. Scheller JG, Schulman SR: Fiber-optic bronchoscopic guidance for intubating a neonate with Pierre-Robin syndrome, *J Clin Anesth* 3:45, 1991.
37. Howardy-Hansen P, Berthelsen P: Fiberoptic bronchoscopic nasotracheal intubation of a neonate with Pierre Robin syndrome, *Anaesthesia* 43:121, 1988.
38. Audenaert SM, Montgomery CL, Stone B et al: Retrograde-assisted fiberoptic tracheal intubation in children with difficult airways, *Anesth Analg* 73:660, 1991.
39. Maekawa N, Mikawa K, Obara H: The laryngeal mask may be a useful device for fiberoptic airway endoscopy in pediatric anesthesia, *Anesthesiology* 75:169, 1991.
40. Reynolds PI, O'Kelly SW: Fiberoptic intubation and the laryngeal mask airway, *Anesthesiology* 79:1144, 1993.
41. Bellhouse CP: An angulated laryngoscope for routine and difficult tracheal intubation, *Anesthesiology* 69:126, 1988.
42. Patil VU, Sopchak AM, Thomas PS: Use of a dental mirror as an aid to tracheal intubation in an infant, *Anesthesiology* 78:619, 1993.
43. Borland LM, Swan DM, Leff S: Difficult pediatric endotracheal

intubation: a new approach to the retrograde technique, *Anesthesiology* 55:577, 1981.

44. Cooper CMS, Murray-Wilson A: Retrograde intubation: management of a 4.8-kg, 5-month infant, *Anaesthesia* 42:1197, 1987.

45. Freund PR, Rooke A, Schwid H: Retrograde intubation with a modified Eschmann stylet, *Anesth Analg* 67:605, 1988.

46. Levin RM: Anesthesia for cleft lip and cleft palate, *Anesth Rev* 6:25, 1979.

47. Scwartz D, Singh J: Retrograde wire-guided direct laryngoscopy in a 1-month-old infant, *Anesthesiology* 77:607, 1992.

48. Thomson KD: A blind nasal intubation using a laryngeal mask airway, *Anaesthesia* 48:785, 1993.

49. Rowbottom SJ, Simpson DL, Grubb D: The laryngeal mask airway in children: a fiberoptic assessment of positioning, *Anaesthesia* 46:489, 1991.

50. Markakis DA, Sayson SC, Schreiner MS: Insertion of the laryngeal mask airway in awake infants with the Robin sequence, *Anesth Analg* 75:822, 1992.

51. Asai T, Fujise K, Uchida M: Use of the laryngeal mask in a child with tracheal stenosis, *Anesthesiology* 75:903, 1991.

52. Mason DG, Bingham RM: The laryngeal mask airway in children, *Anaesthesia* 45:760, 1990.

53. Scuderi PE, McLeskey CH, Comer PB: Emergency percutaneous transtracheal ventilation during anesthesia using readily available equipment, *Anesth Analg* 61:867, 1982.

54. Bjoraker DG, Kumar NB, Brown ACD: Evaluation of an emergency cricothyroidotomy instrument, *Crit Care Med* 15:157, 1987.

55. Smith RB: Transtracheal ventilation during anesthesia, *Anesth Analg* 53:225, 1974.

56. Ravussin P, Bayer-Berger M, Monnier P et al: Percutaneous transtracheal ventilation for laser endoscopic procedures in infants and small children with laryngeal obstruction: report of two cases, *Can J Anaesth* 34:83, 1987.

57. Poon YK: Case history number 89: a life-threatening complication of cricothyroid membrane puncture, *Anesth Analg* 55:298, 1986.

58. Healy GB, Upton J, Black PML et al: The role of surgery in rhabdomyosarcoma of the head and neck in children, *Arch Otolaryngol Head Neck Surg* 117:1185, 1991.

59. Marquez X, Roxas R: Induction of anesthesia in infants with frontonasal dysplasia and meningoencephalocele: a case report, *Anesth Analg* 56:736, 1977.

60. Marsh JL, Galic M, Vannier MW: The craniofacial anatomy of Apert syndrome, *Clin Plast Surg* 18:237, 1991.

61. Cohen MM Jr, Kreiborg S: Upper and lower airway compromise in the Apert syndrome, *Am J Med Genet* 44:90, 1992.

62. McGill T: Otolaryngologic aspects of Apert syndrome, *Clin Plast Surg* 18:309, 1991.

63. Kreiborg S, Barr M, Cohen MM Jr: Cervical spine in Apert syndrome, *Am J Med Genet* 43:704, 1992.

64. Sagehashi N: An infant with Crouzon's syndrome with a cartilaginous trachea and a human tail, *J Craniomaxillofac Surg* 20:21, 1992.

65. Stone P, Trevenen CL, Mitchell I et al: Congenital tracheal stenosis in Pfeiffer syndrome, *Clin Genet* 38:145, 1990.

66. Jones KL, editor: Smith's recognizable pattern of human malformation, ed 4, Philadelphia, 1988, WB Saunders.

67. Maydew RP, Berry FA: Cherubism with difficult laryngoscopy and tracheal intubation, *Anesthesiology* 62:810, 1985.

68. Mixter RC, David DJ, Perloff WH et al: Obstructive sleep apnea in Apert's and Pfeiffer's syndromes: more than a craniofacial abnormality, *Plast Reconstr Surg* 86:457, 1990.

69. Nargozian C: Apert syndrome: anesthetic management, *Clin Plast Surg* 18:227, 1991.

70. Scheller JG, Schulman SR: Fiber-optic bronchoscopic guidance for intubating a neonate with Pierre-Robin syndrome, *J Clin Anesth* 3:45, 1991.

71. Finer NN, Muzyka D: Flexible endoscopic intubation of the neonate, *Pediatr Pulmonal* 12:48, 1992.

72. Benumof JL: Management of the difficult adult airway: with special emphasis on awake tracheal intubation, *Anesthesiology* 75:1087, 1990.

73. Benumof JL: Use of the laryngeal mask to facilitate fiberoptic endoscopy intubation, *Anesth Analg* 74:313, 1992.

74. Posnick JC, Goldstein JA: Surgical management of temporomandibular joint ankylosis in the pediatric population, *Plast Reconstr Surg* 91:791, 1993.

75. Alfrey DD, Ward CF, Harwood IR et al: Airway management for a neonate with congenital fusion of the jaw, *Anesthesiology* 51:340, 1979.

76. Adekeye EO: Ankylosis of the mandible: analysis of 76 cases, *J Oral Maxillofac Surg* 41:442, 1983.

77. Hartman RA, Castro T, Matson M et al: Rapid orotracheal intubation in the clenched-jaw patient: a modification of the lightwand technique, *J Clin Anesth* 4:245, 1992.

78. Diaz JH, Guarisco JL, LeJeune FE: Perioperative management of pediatric microstomia, *Can J Anesth* 38:217, 1991.

79. Sethi DS, Stanley RE: Deep neck abscesses: changing trends, *J Laryngol Otol* 108:138, 1994.

80. Barkin RM, Bonis SL, Elghammer RM et al: Ludwig angina in children, *J Pediatr* 87:563, 1975.

81. Cohle SD, Jones DH, Puri S: Lingual tonsillar hypertrophy causing failed intubation and cerebral anoxia, *Am J Forensic Med Pathol* 14:158, 1993.

82. Guarisco JL, Littlewood SC, Butcher RB: Severe upper airway obstruction in children secondary to lingual tonsil hypertrophy, *Ann Otol Rhino Laryngol* 99:621, 1990.

83. Sweet RM: Lesions of the nasal radix in pediatric patients: diagnosis and management, *South Med J* 85:164, 1992.

84. Morgan DW, Evans JNG: Developmental nasal anomalies, *J Laryngol Otol* 104:394, 1990.

85. Derkay CS, Grundfast KM: Airway compromise from nasal obstruction in neonates and infants, *Int J Pediatr Otorhinolaryngol* 19:241, 1990.

86. Stack CG, Wyse RKH: Incidence and management of airway problems in the CHARGE Association, *Anaesthesia* 46:582, 1990.

87. Hughes GB, Shapiro G, Hunt W et al: Management of the congenital midline mass, *Head Neck Surg* 2:222, 1980.

88. Harley EH: Pediatric congenital nasal masses, *Ear Nose Throat J* 70:28, 1991.

89. Carlan SJ, Angel JL, Leo J et al: Cephalocele involving the oral cavity, *Obstet Gynecol* 75:494, 1990.

90. Rinaldi PA, Dogra S, Sellman GL: Difficult intubation in paediatric palatoplasty, *Anaesthesia* 48:358, 1993.

91. Rollinick BR, Pruzansky S: Genetic services at a center for craniofacial anomalies, *Cleft Palate Craniofac J* 18:304, 1981.

92. Shprintzen RJ, Siegel-Sadewitz VL, Amato J et al: Anomalies associated with cleft lip, cleft palate, or both, *Am J Med Genet* 20:585, 1985.

93. Haselby KA, McNiece WL: Respiratory obstruction from uvular edema in a pediatric patient, *Anesth Analg* 62:1127, 1983.

94. Potsic WP: Assessment and treatment of adenotonsillar hypertrophy in children, *Am J Otolaryngol* 13:259, 1992.

95. Levy AM, Tabakian BS, Hanson JS et al: Hypertrophied adenoids causing pulmonary hypertension and severe congestive heart failure, *N Engl J Med* 277:506, 1967.

96. Brown OE, Manning SC, Ridenour B: Cor pulmonale secondary to tonsillar and adenoidal hypertrophy: management considerations, *Int J Pediatr Otorhinolaryngol* 16:131, 1988.

97. Kearns DB, Pransky SM, Seid AB: Current concepts in pediatric adenotonsillar disease, *Ear Nose Throat J* 70:15, 1991.

98. Livesey JR, Solomons NB, Gillies EAD: Emergency adenotonsillectomy for acute postoperative upper airway obstruction, *Anaesthesia* 46:36, 1991.

99. Shechtman FG, Lin PT, Pincus RL: Urgent adenotonsillectomy for upper airway obstruction, *Int J Pediatr Otorhinolaryngol* 24:83, 1992.

100. Wolfe JA, Rowe LD: Upper airway obstruction in infectious mononucleosis, *Ann Otol Rhinol Laryngol* 89:430, 1980.

101. Spector S, Bautista AG: Respiratory obstruction caused by acute tonsillitis and acute adenoiditis, *NY State J Med* 56:2118, 1956.

102. Guarisco JL: Congenital head and neck masses in infants and children, *Ear Nose Throat J* 70:40, 1990.

103. Rosenfeld RM, Green RP: Tonsillectomy and adenoidectomy: changing trends, *Ann Otol Rhinol Laryngol* 99:187, 1990.

104. Potsic WP: Tonsillectomy and adenoidectomy, *Int Anesthesiol Clinics* 26:58, 1988.

105. Price SD, Hawkins DB, Kahlstrom EJ: Tonsil and adenoid surgery for airway obstruction: Perioperative respiratory morbidity, *Ear Nose Throat J* 72:526, 1993.

106. Tom LWC, DeDio RM, Cohen DE et al: Is outpatient tonsillectomy appropriate for young children? *Laryngoscope,* 102:277, 1992.

107. Zerella JT, Finberg FJ: Obstruction of the neonatal airway from teratomas, *Surg Gynecol Obstet* 170:126, 1990.

108. Kravath RE, Pollak CP, Borowiecki B et al: Obstructive sleep apnea and death associated with surgical correction of velopharyngeal incompetence, *J Pediatr* 96:645, 1980.

109. Shprintzen RJ: Pharyngeal flap surgery and the pediatric upper airway, *Int Anesthiol Clin* 26:79, 1988.

110. Oski FA: *Principles and practice of pediatrics,* Philadelphia, 1994, JB Lippincott.

111. Parker GS, Tami TA: The management of peritonsillar abscess in the 90s: an update, *Am J Otolaryngol* 13:284, 1992.

112. Yano-Villalvazo S, Hernandez-Suarez L, Valenzuela-Espinoza A et al: Carcinoma of the tonsils in pediatrics, *Bol Med Hosp Infant Mex* 49:313, 1992.

113. Coulthard M, Isaacs D: Retropharyngeal abscess, *Arch Dis Child* 66:1227, 1991.

114. Ben-Ami T, Yousefzadeh DK, Aramburo MJ: Pre-suppurative phase of retropharyngeal infection: contribution of ultrasonography in the diagnosis and treatment, *Pediatr Radiol* 21:23, 1990.

115. Hartmann RW: Recognition of retropharyngeal abscess in children, *Am Fam Physician* 46:193, 1992.

116. Thompson JW, Ahmed AR, Dudley JP: Epidermolysis bullosa dystrophica of the larynx and trachea, *Ann Otol Rhinol Laryngol* 89:428, 1980.

117. Holzman RS, Worthen HM, Johnson KL: Anaesthesia for children with junctional epidermolysis bullosa (lethalis), *Can J Anaesth* 34(4):395, 1987.

118. Lyos AT, Malpica A, Levy ML et al: Laryngeal involvement in epidermolysis bullosa, *Ann Otol Rhinol Laryngol* 103:542, 1994.

119. Griffin RP, Mayou BG: The anaesthetic management of patients with dystrophic epidermolysis bullosa: a review of forty-four patients over a 10-year period, *Anaesthesia* 48:810, 1993.

120. James I, Wark H: Airway management during anesthesia in patients with epidermolysis bullosa dystrophica, *Anesthesiology* 56:323, 1982.

121. Heyman MB, Zwass M, Applebaum M et al: Chronic recurrent esophageal strictures treated with balloon dilatation in children with autosomal recessive epidermolysis bullosa dystrophica, *Am J Gastroenterol* 88:953, 1993.

122. Cotton RT, Richardson MA: Congenital laryngeal anomalies, *Otolaryngol Clin North Am* 14:203, 1981.

123. Hollinger LD: Etiology of stridor in the neonate, infant and child, *Ann Otol Rhinol Laryngol* 89:397, 1980.

124. Polonovski JM, Contencini P, Viala P et al: Aryepiglottic fold excision for the treatment of severe laryngomalacia, *Ann Otol Rhinol Laryngol* 99:625, 1990.

125. McClurg FLD, Evans DA: Laser laryngoplasty for laryngomalacia, *Laryngoscope* 104:247, 1994.

126. Jani P, Koltai P, Ochi JW et al: Surgical treatment of laryngomalacia, *J Laryngol Otol* 105:1040, 1991.

127. Nussbaum E, Maggi: Laryngomalacia in children, *Chest* 98:942, 1990.

128. Baxter MR: Congenital laryngomalacia, *Can J Anaesth* 41:332, 1994.

129. Bass JW, Fahardo JE, Brian JH et al: Sudden death due to epiglottitis, *Pediatr Infect Dis J* 4:447, 1985.

130. Gorelick MH, Baker MD: Epiglottitis in children, 1979 through 1992: effects of *Haemophilus influenzae* type b immunization, *Arch Pediatr Adolesc Med* 148(1):47, 1992.

131. Ryan M, Hunt M, Snowberger T: A changing pattern of epiglottitis, *Clin Pediatr* (Phila) 31:532, 1992.

132. Baxter JD: Acute epiglottitis in children, *Laryngoscope* 77:1358, 1967.

133. Rowe LD: Advances and controversies in the management of supraglottitis and laryngotracheobronchitis, *Am J Otolaryngol* 1:235, 1980.

134. Lazoritz S, Saunders BS, Bason WM: Management of acute epiglottitis, *Crit Care Med* 7:285, 1979.

135. Brilli RJ, Benzing G, Cotcamp DH: Epiglottitis in infants less than two years of age. *Pediatr Emerg Med* 5:16, 1989.

136. Rapkin RH: The diagnosis of epiglottitis: simplicity and reliability of radiographs of the neck in the differential diagnosis of the croup syndrome, *J Pediatr* 80:96, 1972.

137. Podgore JK, Bass JW: The "thumb sign" and "little finger sign" in acute epiglottitis, *J Pediatr* 88:154, 1976.

138. Gevin JL, Lee FA: Radiologic case of the month: acute epiglottitis, *Am J Dis Child* 130:195, 1976.

139. Bass JW, Steele RW, Wiebe RA: Acute epiglottitis: an acute surgical emergency, *JAMA* 229:671, 1974.

140. Bates JR: Epiglottitis: diagnosis and treatment, *Pediatr Rev* 1:173, 1979.

141. Oh TH, Motoyama EK: Comparison of nasotracheal intubation and tracheostomy in management of acute epiglottitis, *Anesthesiology* 46:214, 1977.

142. Hannallah R, Rosales JK: Acute epiglottitis: current management and review, *Can Anaesth Soc J* 25:84, 1978.

143. Contrell RW, Bell RA, Morioka WF: Acute epiglottitis: intubation versus tracheostomy, *Laryngoscope* 88:994, 1978.

144. Glicklich M, Cohen RD, Jona JZ: Steroids and bag and mask ventilation in the treatment of acute epiglottitis, *J Pediatr Surg* 14:247, 1979.

145. Schuller DE, Birck HG: The safety of intubation in croup and epiglottitis: an eight-year follow-up, *Laryngoscope* 85:33, 1975.

146. Johnson GK, Sullivan JL, Bishop LA: Acute epiglottitis, *Arch Otolaryngol* 100:333, 1974.

147. Battaglia JD, Lockhart CH: Management of acute epiglottitis by nasotracheal intubation, *Am J Dis Child* 129:334, 1975.

148. Crysdale WS, Sendi K: Evolution in the management of acute epiglottitis: a 10-year experience with 242 children, *Int Anesthesiol Clin* 26:32, 1988.

149. Schloss MD, Gold JA, Rosales JK et al: Acute epiglottitis: current management, *Laryngoscope* 93:489, 1982.

150. Soliman MG, Richer P: Epiglottitis and pulmonary edema in children, *Can Anaesth Soc J* 25:270, 1978.

151. Henry RL, Bingham AL, Halliday JA: The management of epiglottitis in a small pediatric intensive care unit, *J Quality Clin Pract* 14:17, 1994.

152. Holinger PH, Brown WT: Congenital webs, cysts, laryngoceles and other anomalies of the larynx, *Ann Otol Rhinol Laryngol* 76:744, 1967.

153. Emery PJ, Fearon B: Vocal cord palsy in pediatric practice: a review of 71 cases, *Int J Pediatr Otorhinolaryngol* 8:147, 1984.

154. Gentile RD, Miller RH, Woodson GE: Vocal cord paralysis in children 1 year of age and younger, *Ann Otol Rhinol Laryngol* 95:622, 1986.

155. Strong M, Vaughan C, Healy G et al: Recurrent respiratory papillomatosis, *Ann Otol Rhinol Laryngol* 85:508, 1976.

156. Chipps BE, McClurg FL Jr, Freidman EM et al: Respiratory papillomas: presentation before six months, *Pediatric Pulmonol* 9(2):125, 1990.

157. Sedlacek T, Lindheim S, Eder C et al: Mechanism for human papillomavirus transmission at birth, *Ann J Obstet Gynecol* 161:55, 1989.

158. Tseng CJ, Lin CY, Wang RL et al: Possible transplacental transmission of human papillomavirus, *Am J Obstet Gynecol* 166(1):35, 1992.

159. Ossoff R, Werkhaven J, Dere H: Soft-tissue complications of laser surgery for recurrent respiratory papillomatosis, *Laryngoscope* 101:1162, 1991.

160. Lusk R, McCabe B, Mixon J: Three-year experience of treating recurrent respiratory papilloma with interferon, *Ann Otol Rhinol Laryngol* 96:158, 1987.

161. Abramson A, Waner M, Brandsma J: The clinical treatment of laryngeal papillomas with hematoporphyrin therapy, *Arch Otolaryngol Head Neck Surg* 114:795, 1988.

162. Shikowitz M: Comparison of pulsed and continuous wave light in photodynamic therapy of papillomas: an experimental study, *Laryngoscope* 102:300, 1992.

163. Hermans JM, Bennett MJ, Hirshman CA: Anesthesia for laser surgery, *Anesth Analg* 62:218, 1983.

164. Scamman FL, McCabe BF: Supraglottic jet ventilation for laser surgery of the larynx in children, *Ann Otol Rhinol Laryngol* 95:142, 1986.

165. Borland LM, Reilly JS: Jet ventilation for laser laryngeal surgery in children: modification of the Saunders jet ventilation technique, *Int J Pediatr Otorhinolaryngol* 14:65, 1987.

166. Scamman FL, McCabe BF: Evaluation of supraglottic jet ventilation for laser surgery of the larynx, *Anesthesiology* 61:A447, 1984.

167. O'Sullivan TJ, Healy GB: Complications of Venturi jet ventilation during microlaryngeal surgery, *Arch Otolaryngol* 111:127, 1985.

168. Wegrzynowicz ES, Jensen NF, Pearson KS et al: Airway fire during jet ventilation for laser excision of vocal cord papillomata, *Anesthesiology* 76:468, 1992.

169. Rontal E, Rontal M, Wenokur ME: Jet insufflation anesthesia for endolaryngeal laser surgery: a review of 318 consecutive cases, *Laryngoscope* 95:990, 1985.

170. Weisberger EC, Miner JD: Apneic anesthesia for improved endoscopic removal of laryngeal papillomata, *Laryngoscope* 98:693, 1988.

171. Keon TP: Anesthetic considerations for laser surgery, *Int Anesthesiol Clin* 26:50, 1988.

172. Johans TG, Reichert TJ: An insufflation device for anesthesia during subglottic carbon dioxide laser microsurgery in children, *Anesth Analg* 63:368, 1984.

173. Matt BH, McCall JE, Cotton RT: Modified subglottoscope in the treatment of recurrent respiratory papillomatosis, *Laryngoscope* 100:1022, 1990.

174. Baugh R, Gilmore BB Jr: Infectious croup: a critical review, *Otolaryngol Head Neck Surg* 95:40, 1986.

175. Wald ER: Croup. In Oski F, editor: *Pediatrics,* ed 2, Philadelphia, 1994, JB Lippincott.

176. Denny FW, Murphy TF, Clyde WA et al: Croup: an 11-year study in a pediatric practice, *Pediatrics* 71:871, 1983.

177. Walker P, Crysdale WS: Croup, epiglottitis, retropharyngeal abscess, and bacterial tracheitis: evolving patterns of occurrence and care, *Int Anesthesiol Clin* 30:57, 1992.

178. Levinson H, Tabachnik E, Newth CJL: Wheezing in infancy, croup, and epiglottitis, *Curr Probl Pediatr* 12:38, 1982.

179. Super DM, Cartelli NA, Brooks LJ et al: A prospective randomized double-blind study to evaluate the effect of dexamethasone in acute laryngotracheitis, *J Pediatr* 115:3239, 1989.

180. Kairys SW, Olmstead EM, O'Connor GT: Steroid treatment of laryngotracheitis: a meta-analysis of the evidence from randomized trials, *Pediatrics* 83:683, 1989.

181. Lenney W, Milner AD: Treatment of acute viral croup, *Arch Dis Child* 53:704, 1978.

182. Otherson HB, Filler RM: Tracheomalacia. In Otherson HB, editor: *The pediatric airway,* Philadelphia, 1991, WB Saunders.

183. Benjamin B: Tracheomalacia in infants and children, *Ann Otol Rhinol Laryngol* 93:438, 1984.

184. Filler RM, Messineo A, Vinograd I: Severe tracheomalacia associated with esophageal atresia: results of surgical treatment, *J Pediatr Surg* 27:1136, 1992.

185. Azizkhan RG, Lacey SR, Wood RE: Anterior cricoid suspension and peristomal tracheomalacia following tracheostomy, *J Pediatr Surg* 28:169, 1993.

186. Duncan S, Eid N: Tracheomalacia and bronchopulmonary dysplasia, *Ann Otol Rhinol Laryngol* 100:856, 1991.

187. Wittenborg MH, Geypes MT, Crocker D: Tracheal dynamics in infants with respiratory distress, stridor, and collapsing trachea, *Radiology* 88:653, 1967.

188. Kasian GF, Bingham WT, Steinberg J et al: Bacterial tracheitis in children, *Can Med Assoc J* 140:46, 1989.

189. Eckel HE, Widemann B, Damm M et al: Airway endoscopy in the diagnosis and treatment of bacterial tracheitis in children, *Int J Pediatr Otorhinolaryngol* 27:147, 1993.

190. Donnelly BW, McMillan JA, Weiner LB: Bacterial tracheitis: report of eight new cases and review, *Rev Infect Dis* 12:729, 1990.

191. Surh L, Read S: Staphylococcal tracheitis and toxic shock syndrome in a young child, *J Pediatr* 105:585, 1984.

192. Liston SL, Gehrz RC, Siegel LG et al: Bacterial tracheitis, *Am J Dis Child* 137:764, 1983.

193. Rabie McShane D, Warde D: Bacterial tracheitis, *J Laryngol Otol* 103:1059, 1989.

194. Keon TP: Death on induction of anesthesia for cervical node biopsy, *Anesthesiology* 55:471, 1981.

195. Bray RJ, Fernandez FJ: Mediastinal tumor causing airway obstruction in anesthetised children, *Anaesthesia* 37:571, 1982.

196. Montange F, Truffa-Bachi J, Pichard E: Airway obstruction during anesthesia in a child with a mediastinal mass, *Can J Anaesth* 37:271, 1990.

197. Sibert KS, Biondi JW, Hirsch NP: Spontaneous respiration during thoracotomy in a patient with a mediastinal mass, *Anesth Analg* 66:904, 1987.

198. Snell RS, Katz J: *Clinical anatomy for anesthesiologists,* Norwalk, Conn, 1988, Appleton & Lange.

199. Pullerits J, Holzman R: Anaesthesia for patients with mediastinal masses, *Can J Anaesth* 36:681, 1989.

200. King RM, Telander RL, Smithson WA et al: Primary mediastinal tumors in children, *J Pediatr Surg* 17:512, 1982.

201. Janin Y, Becker J, Wise L et al: Superior vena cava syndrome in childhood and adolescence: a review of the literature and report of three cases, *J Pediatr Surg* 17:290, 1982.

202. Harris GJ, Harman PK, Trinkle JK et al: Standard biplane roentgenography is highly sensitive in documenting mediastinal masses, *Ann Thorac Surg* 44:238, 1987.

203. Canedo MI, Otken L, Stefadouros MA: Echocardiographic features of cardiac compression by a thymoma simulating cardiac tamponade and obstruction of the superior vena cava, *Br Heart J* 39:1038, 1977.

204. deSoto H: Direct laryngoscopy as an aid to relieve airway obstruction in a patient with a mediastinal mass, *Anesthesiology* 67:116, 1987.

205. Azizkhan RG, Dudgeon DL, Buck JR et al: Life-threatening airway obstruction as a complication to the management of mediastinal masses in children, *J Pediatr Surg* 20:816, 1985.

206. Ryckman FC, Rogers BM: Thoracoscopy for intrathoracic neoplasia in children, *J Pediatr Surg* 17:521, 1982.

207. Piro AH, Weiss DR, Hellman S: Mediastinal Hodgkin's disease: a possible danger for intubation of anesthesia, *Int J Radiat Oncol Biol Phys* 1:415, 1976.

208. John RE, Narang VPS: A boy with an anterior mediastinal mass, *Anaesthesia* 43:864, 1988.

209. Hall KD, Friedman M: Extracorporeal oxygenation for induction of anesthesia in a patient with an intrathoracic tumor, *Anesthesiology* 42:493, 1975.

210. Park S: Vascular abnormalities, *Pediatr Clinic North Am* 28:949, 1981.

211. Braunstein PW, Sade R: Vascular malformations with airway obstruction. In Otherson HB, editor: *The pediatric airway,* Philadelphia, 1991, WB Saunders.

212. Roesler M, de Leval M, Chrispin A et al: Surgical management of vascular ring, *Ann Surg* 197:139, 1983.

213. Benjamin B: Endoscopy in congenital tracheal anomalies, *J Pediatr Surg* 15:164, 1980.

214. Jonas RA, Spevak PJ, McGill T et al: Pulmonary artery sling: primary repair by tracheal resection in infancy, *J Thorac Cardiovasc Surg* 97:548, 1989.

215. Eller WC, Haugen RK: Food asphyxiation, *N Engl J Med* 289:81, 1973.

216. Cohen SR, Lewis GB Jr, Herbert WI et al: Foreign body in the airway: five-year retrospective study with special reference to management, *Ann Otol Rhinol Laryngol* 89:437, 1980.

217. Kosloke AM: Bronchoscopic extraction of aspirated foreign bodies in children, *Am J Dis Child* 136:924, 1982.

218. Menendez AA, Gotay CF, Seda FJ et al: Foreign body aspiration: experience at the University Pediatric Hospital, *Puerto Rico Health Sciences J* 10(3):127, 1991.

219. Mu L, He P, Sun D: Inhalation of foreign bodies in Chinese children: a review of 400 cases, *Laryngoscope* 101:657, 1991.

220. Blazer S, Naveh Y, Friedman A: Foreign body in the airway, *Am J Dis Child* 134:68, 1990.

221. Pasaoglu I, Dogan R, Demircin M et al: Bronchoscopic removal of foreign bodies in children: retrospective analysis of 822 cases, *Thorac Cardiovasc Surg* 39(2):95, 1991.

222. Baraka A: Bronchoscopic removal of inhaled foreign bodies in children, *Br J Anaesth* 46:124, 1974.

223. Esclamado RM, Richardson MA: Laryngotracheal foreign bodies in children, *Am J Dis Child* 141:259, 1978.

224. Parsons DS, Kearns D: The two-headed stethoscope: its use for ruling out airway foreign bodies, *Int J Pediat Otorhinolaryngol* 22(2):181, 1991.

225. Mu LC, Sun DQ, He P: Radiologic diagnosis of aspirated foreign bodies in children: review of 343 cases, *J Laryngol Otol* 104(10):778, 1990.

226. Kitinaka S, Mikami I, Tokumaru A et al: Diagnosis of peanut inhalation by MRI, *Pediatr Radiol* 22(4):300, 1992.

227. Moskowitz D, Gardiner LJ, Sasaki CT: Foreign body aspiration: potential misdiagnosis, *Arch Otolaryngol Head Neck Surg* 108:806, 1982.

228. Lima J: Laryngeal foreign bodies in children: a persistent, life-threatening problem, *Laryngoscope* 99:415, 1989.

229. Brady PG: Esophageal foreign bodies, *Gastroentrol Clin North Am* 20(4):691, 1991.

230. Byard RW, Moore L, Bourne AJ: Sudden and unexpected death: a late effect of occult intraesophageal foreign body, *Pediatr Pathol* 10:837, 1990.

231. Emergency Cardiac Care Committee and Subcommittee, American Heart Association: Guidelines for cardiopulmonary resuscitation and emergency cardiac care. V: Pediatric basic life support, *JAMA* 268:2258, 1992.

232. Steen KH, Zimmermann T: Tracheobronchial aspiration of foreign bodies in children: a study of 94 cases, *Laryngoscope* 100:525, 1990.

233. Kain ZN, O'Connor TZ, Berde CB: Management of tracheobronchial and esophageal foreign bodies in children: a survey study, *J Clin Anesth* 6:28, 1994.

234. Keon TP: Bronchoscopy for a foreign body. In Stehling L, editor: *Common problems in pediatric anesthesia,* ed 2, St Louis, 1992, Mosby.

235. Ohkouchi Y, Inomoto Y, Suzuki C et al: Bronchoscopy for airway foreign bodies: consideration based on an extraordinarily large one, *Fukushima J Med Sci* 38:99, 1992.

236. Eyrich JE, Riopelle JM, Naraghi M: Elective transtracheal jet ventilation for bronchoscopic removal of tracheal foreign body, *South Med J* 85:1017, 1992.

237. Chua RN, Engle WA, Brown JW et al: The use of bronchotomy and retrograde dilatation to repair acquired obliterative bronchial obstruction, *J Pediatr Surg* 27:98, 1992.

238. Wilkinson KA, Beckett W, Brown TC: Pneumothorax secondary to foreign body inhalation in a 20-month-old child, *J Paediatr Child Health* 28:67, 1992.

239. Narcy P, Contencin P, Fligny I, Francois M: Surgical treatment for laryngotracheal stenosis in the pediatric patient, *Arch Otolaryngol Head Neck Surg* 116:1047, 1990.

240. Dinner M, Ward R, Yun E: Ventilation difficulty secondary to a tracheal diverticulum, *Anesthesiology* 77:586, 1992.

241. Torsiglieri AJ, Tom LWC, Ross AJ et al: Pediatric neck masses: guidelines for evaluation, *Int J Pediatr Otorhinolaryngol* 16:199, 1988.

242. MacDonald DJF: Cystic hygroma: an anaesthetic and surgical problem, *Anaesthesia* 21:66, 1966.

243. Landing BH, Farber S: Tumors of the cardiovascular system. In Committee on Pathology of the National Research Council: *Atlas of tumor pathology,* Washington, DC, 1956, Armed Forces Institute of Pathology.

244. Edwards MJ, Graham JM: Posterior nuchal cystic hygroma, *Clin Perinatol* 17:611, 1990.

245. Langer JC, Fitzgerald PG, Desa D et al: Cervical cystic hygroma in the fetus: clinical spectrum and outcome, *J Pediatr Surg* 25:58, 1990.

246. Byard RW, Jimenez CL, Carpenter BF et al: Congenital teratomas of the neck and nasopharynx: a clinical and pathological study of 18 cases, *J Paediatr Child Health* 26:12, 1990.

247. Hawkins DB, Austin JR: Abscesses of the neck in infants and young children, *Ann Otol Rhinol Laryngol* 100:361, 1991.

248. Ricciardelli EJ, Richardson MA: Cervicofacial cystic hygroma, *Arch Otolaryngol Head Neck Surg* 117:546, 1991.

249. Mahboubi S, Potsic WB: Computed tomography of cervical cystic hygroma in the neck, *Int J Pediatr Otorhinolaryngol* 18:47, 1989.

250. Schwartz MZ, Silver H, Schulman S: Maintenance of the placental circulation to evaluate and treat an infant with massive head and neck hemangioma, *J Pediatr Surg* 28:520, 1993.

251. Schulman SR, Jones BR, Slotnick N et al: Fetal tracheal intubation with intact uteroplacental circulation, *Anesth Analg* 76:197, 1993.

252. Tanaka M, Sato S, Naito H et al: Anaesthetic management of a neonate with prenatally diagnosed cervical tumour and upper airway obstruction, *Can J Anaesth* 41:236, 1994.

253. Nguyen VD, Tyrrel R: Klippel-Feil syndrome: patterns of bony fusion and wasp-waist sign, *Skeletal Radiol* 22:519, 1993.

254. Rosen CL, Novotny EJ, D'Andrea LA et al: Klippel-Feil sequence and sleep-disordered breathing in two children, *Am Rev Respir Dis* 147:202, 1993.

255. Jacobs JC: *Pediatric rheumatology for the practitioner.* New York, 1981, Springer-Verlag.

256. MacMillan M, Stauffer ES: Traumatic instability in the previously fused cervical spine, *J Spine Disord* 4:449, 1991.

257. Cabane J, Michon A, Ziza JM et al: Comparison of long-term evolution of adult onset and juvenile onset Still's disease, both followed up for more than 10 years, *Ann Rheum Dis* 49:283, 1990.

258. D'Arch EJ, Fell RH: Anesthesia in juvenile chronic polyarthritis. In Arden GP, Ansell BM, editors: *Surgical management of juvenile chronic polyarthritis,* London, 1978, Academic.

259. Malleson P, Riding K, Petty R: Stridor due to cricoarytenoid arthritis in pauciarticular onset juvenile rheumatoid arthritis, *J Rheumatol* 13:952-3, 1986.

260. Futran ND, Sherris D, Norante JD: Cricoarytenoid arthritis in children, *Otolaryngol Head Neck Surg* 104:366, 1990.

261. Birkinshaw KJ: Anaesthesia in a patient with an unstable neck, *Anaesthesia* 30:46, 1975.

262. Stebbens VA, Dennis J, Samuels MP et al: Sleep-related upper airway obstruction in a cohort with Down's syndrome, *Arch Dis Child* 66:1333, 1991.

263. Pueschel SM, Scola FH, Tupper TB et al: Skeletal anomalies of the upper cervical spine in children with Down syndrome, *J Pediatr Orthop* 10:607, 1990.

264. Pueschel SM, Moon AC, Scola FH: Computerized tomography in persons with Down syndrome and atlantoaxial instability, *Spine* 17:735, 1992.

265. Semine AA, Ertel AN, Goldberg MJ et al: Cervical spine instability in children with Down syndrome (trisomy 21), *J Bone Joint Surg (Am)* 60:649, 1978.

266. Tredwell SJ, Newman DE, Lockitch G: Instability of the upper cervical spine in Down syndrome, *J Pediatr Orthop* 10:602, 1990.

267. Cremers MJG, Beijer HM: No relation between general laxity and atlantoaxial instability in children with Down syndrome, *J Pediatr Orthop* 13:318, 1993.

268. Pueschel SM, Herndon JH, Gelch MM et al: Symptomatic atlantoaxial subluxation in persons with Down syndrome, *J Pediatr Orthop* 4:682, 1984.

269. Pueschel SM, Scola FH: Atlantoaxial instability in individuals with Down syndrome: epidemiologic, radiologic, and clinical studies, *Pediatrics* 80:555, 1987.

270. Harley EH, Collins MD: Neurologic sequelae secondary to atlantoaxial instability in Down syndrome: implications in otolaryngologic surgery, *Arch Otolaryngol Head Neck Surg* 120:159, 1994.

271. Kewalramani LS, Orth MS, Kraus JF et al: Acute spinal-cord lesions in a pediatric population: epidemiological and clinical features, *Paraplegia* 18:206, 1980.

272. Jaffe D, Wesson D: Emergency management of blunt trauma in children, *New Engl J Med* 324:1477, 1991.

273. Pang D, Pollack IF: Spinal cord injury without radiographic abnormality in children: The SCIWORA syndrome, *J Trauma* 29:654, 1989.

274. Hastings RH, Kelley SD: Neurologic deterioration associated with airway management in a cervical spine-injured patient, *Anesthesiology* 78:580, 1993.

Chapter 30

THE DIFFICULT AIRWAY IN OBSTETRIC ANESTHESIA

Edward T. Crosby

I. INTRODUCTION

Airway management and difficulties related to it now represent the single largest risk factor for anesthetic-related maternal mortality. A difficult or failed intubation increases the risk of both pulmonary aspiration and hypoxemic cardiorespiratory arrest with subsequent maternal morbidity or mortality. General anesthesia for cesarean section and, in particular, emergency cesarean section represents the highest risk anesthetic intervention in obstetric anesthesia and accounts for the bulk of the poor maternal outcomes reported. Physician recognition of the factors associated with or predisposing to maternal airway disasters and appropriate preparation for dealing with both anticipated and unanticipated difficulties is essential to reduce anesthesia-attributable maternal morbidity and mortality. The following discussion will offer insights into the occurrence of anesthesia-

Maternal Mortality (deaths per 100,000 births)

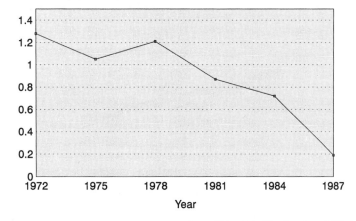

Fig. 30-1. Anesthesia attributable maternal mortality 1970-1987, England and Wales. (Data from Report on confidential enquiries into maternal deaths in the United Kingdom 1985-87, London, 1991, Her Majesty's Stationery Office.)

related maternal mortality in addition to offering assessment and management guidelines related to airway care in obstetric anesthesia.

II. THE OBSTETRIC AIRWAY IN PERSPECTIVE
A. MATERNAL MORBIDITY AND MORTALITY

The last decades have witnessed an enormous reduction in maternal mortality from all causes including that attributable to anesthesia. The Confidential Enquiries into Maternal Deaths (in England and Wales and the United Kingdom) represent the most accurate and in-depth analyses of maternal mortality (see Addendum to this chapter). They have charted the causes and incidence of maternal mortality every 3 years since 1952. The reports are characterized by a virtually 100% retrieval rate so that the causes of all maternal deaths over the last 4 decades in England and Wales are known. The maternal mortality in the United Kingdom decreased from 118.7 to 45.6 deaths per million pregnancies between 1970 and 1987.[1] Maternal mortality attributable to anesthetic care decreased from 12.8 deaths per million estimated pregnancies to 1.9 per million over this same period (Fig. 30-1). The actual reduction in mortality rate directly due to anesthesia care is probably greater than that suggested by this statistic, since the number of anesthetics provided for operative obstetric procedures continues to rise[1] (Fig. 30-2). The majority of anesthetic deaths in the later reports prior to 1987 have been associated with induction of general anesthesia and result from two main causes: inhalation of gastric contents, and failure to intubate the trachea with resultant hypoxia and cardiac arrest.[1,2] Deaths from aspiration pneumonitis had become less common in the later reports, but, when they occurred, they were often precipitated by difficult or failed intubation. Hypoxemic cardiac arrest following failed endotracheal intubation is now the most common cause of direct anesthetic maternal mortality, having superceded deaths attributable to aspiration in latter reports. Two factors appear to predominate in these deaths: failure to acknowledge that the patient cannot be intubated and must be oxygenated, and a reluctance to accept that the endotracheal tube is, in fact, in the esophagus. The operative procedure most commonly involved with episodes of mortality across the last decade has been emergency cesarean section, accounting for up to three quarters of all deaths.[1] Anesthesia was the single leading cause for direct obstetric deaths associated with cesarean section until the 1982-84 report, when it fell to third after embolism and hypertensive disease. In the latest report (1985-87), it has been pushed to fifth by hemorrhage and other direct causes of maternal mortality. However, the majority of anesthesia-attributable maternal mortalities are still deemed to be avoidable.[1,3]

With the decline in the deaths directly related to anesthesia, there has been an increase in the number of deaths in which anesthetic care has been felt to be contributing. A number of these deaths involved airway obstruction, aspiration of gastric contents into an unprotected airway concurrent with sedation given for the management of hypertensive disorders of pregnancy and postoperative airway complications.[1] These deaths are considered to be anesthesia-related as anesthesiologists are now accepting increasing responsibility for sick parturients in both the antepartum and postpartum periods. These new responsibilities include assisted antepartum management of the disorders of pregnancy and assessment and management of preexistent respiratory and circulatory system disorders. A consistent finding in reports on the Confidential Enquiries has been that mortality was linked to care being provided by junior and inexperienced anesthesia and obstetric personnel.

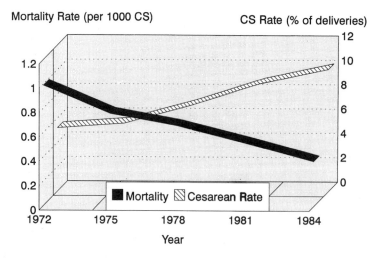

Fig. 30-2. Mortality associated with cesarean section 1970-84, England and Wales. (Data from Report on confidential enquiries into maternal deaths in the United Kingdom 1985-87, London, 1991, Her Majesty's Stationery Office.)

Anesthesia care provided in the cases of anesthesia-attributable maternal mortality has been consistently, though not uniformly, rated as substandard by the assessors reviewing the maternal deaths. Finally, it has also been concluded in the last report that many of the problems associated with avoidable maternal mortality involved a failure of communication between the obstetrician and the anesthesiologist.[1]

An accurate assessment of maternal mortality, both overall and that attributable to anesthesia, is more difficult to derive from North American sources, since there are no data comparable in scope or detail to the Confidential Enquiries. Reports tend to reflect experience on a state or regional basis, although recent initiatives have attempted to broaden the reporting base. The Maternal Mortality Collaborative, a special interest group of the American College of Obstetricians and Gynecologists (ACOG), established voluntary surveillance of maternal mortality in 1985.[4] The goals of the Collaborative were to improve the detection of maternal deaths in the United States, to collect and analyze data relating to maternal mortality, and to make the results available for educating physicians. The first detailed report was published in 1988. Nineteen areas reported, including sixteen states, New York City, San Jose County in California, and Puerto Rico. The investigators noted that the Collaborative reported 37% more maternal deaths from those areas in the years 1980-85 than did the National Center for Health Statistics. This higher compliance rate for reporting may represent an increased comfort level for physicians reporting to groups such as the Maternal Mortality Collaborative compared with public agencies. Underreporting and misclassification of maternal deaths have been deficiencies identified by others in the estimation of maternal mortality in the

United States.[5-7] There is some evidence for overreporting of unpreventable causes of maternal mortality, such as amniotic fluid embolism in the United States, with some of these reports not being validated by independent state maternal mortality committees.[6] Medicolegal concerns may encourage some incorrect diagnosis being reported and would favor the reporting of unpreventable causes of maternal mortality. The impact, if any, of incorrect diagnoses on estimates of anesthesia-attributable maternal mortality in the United States is not known.

Maternal mortality was estimated by the Collaborative at 14.1 deaths per 100,000 live births, and anesthesia complications were recorded as the sixth leading cause of maternal mortality. The specific details of the anesthetic-attributable mortality are not available from the published reports of the Collaborative. However, the Collaborative's ranking of anesthesia as the sixth leading cause of maternal mortality was consistent with that reported a decade earlier by Kaunitz, reviewing countrywide (U.S.A.) data.[6] Anesthesia contributed to 4% of maternal mortalities, and the rates were highest in the smallest and largest centers. These findings were attributed to the presumed decreased capabilities (both physician and institutional) in the smaller centers, and a higher incidence of referred cases and high risk parturients seen in the larger centers. Sachs similarly reported that anesthesia was responsible for, or contributed to, 4.2% of all maternal deaths in the state of Massachusetts over the 4 decades from 1954-85.[8] The maternal mortality rate was 0.6 deaths per 100,000 live births in the years 1982-85. The primary causes of anesthesia-attributable deaths were aspiration and cardiorespiratory arrest. Aspiration deaths during mask anesthesia occurred exclusively in the early part of the experience and were largely supplanted by deaths due to failed intubation or aspiration associated with difficult endotracheal intubation.

Malpractice claims filed against anesthesiologists for care involving obstetric anesthesia taken from the ASA Closed-Claim Database provide an alternate, although biased, assessment of maternal anesthetic risk in the United States.[9] Among the claims, difficult endotracheal intubation, inadequate ventilation, aspiration, and esophageal intubation were the most common events cited. Half of the cases of pulmonary aspiration were associated with difficult endotracheal intubation, esophageal intubation, or inadequate ventilation. The expected standard of care was not felt to have been met in 39% of all claims, and 56% of those claims resulted in payments. That is, in over half the cases where the anesthesiologist was considered to be responsible for the outcome and liable for damages, the delivered care was deemed by the assessors to be substandard.

Maternal deaths related to anesthesia have been significantly reduced over the last decades. There is considerable evidence that further reductions are possible, as avoidable deaths continue to account for many of the maternal deaths attributed to anesthetic care in North America and the United Kingdom.[1,10] Reductions in maternal mortality in the years ahead will be dependent upon well-trained anesthesiologists, cognizant of the risks inherent to obstetric care, involving themselves early in the care of parturients, especially those at risk, carrying out adequate patient and airway assessments, anticipating difficulties in airway management, and developing the expertise to manage such difficulties. Management schemes to effectively deal with failed intubations early enough to avoid maternal morbidity and mortality must be evolved and implemented.

B. DIFFICULT INTUBATION IN OBSTETRIC ANESTHESIA

There is a lack of conformity in the literature with respect to the terminology related to the assessment and management of the difficult airway. The definitions proposed by American Society of Anesthesiologists Task Force on Management of the Difficult Airway will be utilized for the purposes of the following discussion[11] (Box 30-1).

The incidence of the difficult airway, difficult laryngoscopy, and difficult intubation is not well defined. Rocke reported that some difficulty was experienced during intubation in 7.9% (119 to 1500) of parturients undergoing general anesthesia for cesarean section.[12] Two percent of the patients (30 to 1500) were deemed to be very difficult to intubate. In a nonobstetric surgical population, Rose noted that 2.5% of patients required two laryngoscopies to achieve endotracheal

---

BOX 30-1   Definitions regarding the difficult airway

Difficult airway
- A conventionally trained anesthetist experiences difficulty with mask ventilation, endotracheal intubation, or both.

Difficult mask ventilation
- It is not possible for the unassisted anesthesiologist to maintain SaO_2 >90% using 100% O_2 and positive pressure mask ventilation in a patient whose SaO_2 was >90% before anesthetic intervention.
- It is not possible for the unassisted anesthesiologist to prevent or reverse causes of inadequate ventilation during positive mask ventilation.

Difficult laryngoscopy
- It is not possible to visualize any portion of the vocal cords with conventional laryngoscopy.

Difficult endotracheal intubation
- Proper insertion of the endotracheal tube with conventional laryngoscopy requires more than three attempts or more than 10 minutes.

From Caplan RA, Benumof, JL, Berry FA et al: *Anesthesiology* 78:597, 1993.

---

intubation and that 1.8% required more than three.[13] These data, if an accurate reflection, suggest that some degree of difficulty with intubation is experienced more frequently during obstetric anesthesia than general surgical anesthesia (7.9% versus 2.5%) but that very difficult intubations are seen with a similar frequency in obstetric and nonobstetric surgical populations (2% versus 1.8%). The incidence of difficult mask ventilation is again not well defined but appears to be much less than that of difficult intubation. In a nonobstetric population, Rose reported an incidence of 0.01%, whereas Benumof cited an incidence of 0.0001% to 0.02%, although neither the source nor the patient populations were reported.[13,14]

Difficulty with intubation is the factor most commonly associated with obstetric anesthesia disasters in the United States and Europe.[1,3,10,15,16] The incidence of failed intubation in obstetric anesthesia has been reported to be between 0.05% and 0.35%, with a composite figure of 0.2% quoted by Davies.[12,17-20] Although the incidence of failed intubation in obstetric anesthesia is generally said to be several-fold higher than that seen in the nonobstetric surgical population, Rose has reported an incidence of failed intubation of 0.3% in 18,500 general surgical patients.[13] Clearly different institutional patterns of practice and patient populations occur and make these cross-institutional comparisons inconclusive.

Parturients who were difficult to intubate were often reported not to present with the features of a difficult airway, and intubation difficulties were then quite unexpected.[10,20] The question of whether or not an adequate assessment had been made in these patients is a pertinent one, since follow-up evaluation of parturients who had presented as difficult intubations demonstrated patient features suggesting that difficulties should have been anticipated on the basis of patient examination.[20,21] There are a number of factors that may conspire to yield the higher incidence of intubation difficulties and failure in the obstetric population. The adoption of a failed intubation drill should and probably does occur earlier in this group than in others. Determined efforts to intubate the trachea despite the requirement for persistent or prolonged attempts with the potential for hypoxemia, gastric insufflation, and aspiration is discouraged, and this notion has been well propagated. Pregnant patients are more likely to have full and intact dentition, reducing the area (interdental distance) in which the laryngoscopist may maneuver. Obesity is common in parturients, and morbid obesity is not rare. Obesity results in relative neck extension when the patient is supine, leading to more anterior placement of the larynx.[22,23] The neck is somewhat foreshortened, and redundant pharyngeal and palatal folds are evident in the airways of obese patients. The breasts of the parturient are enlarged and engorged and may interfere with placement of the laryngoscope in the mouth.[24] Further, the hand of the assistant providing cricoid pressure is, by necessity, situated higher in the field (placed above the breasts) and may also interfere with laryngoscopy. Proper application of cricoid pressure, as described by Sellick, requires some degree of neck extension, resulting in anterior displacement of the larynx.[25] Although this extension can and should be minimized so as not to complicate intubation, in very obese patients it may be difficult to achieve cricoid pressure without some degree of neck extension. The supine wedged position may result in a change in orientation of the trachea relative to the underlying cervical spine, and cricoid pressure may be more likely to result in tracheal displacement and intubation difficulties. Pregnancy is an edematous state, and the tongue and supraglottic soft tissues may be engorged.[22] Although not usually a problem, severe airway edema has been associated with excessive weight gain in pregnancy, preeclampsia, iatrogenic fluid overload, excess airway manipulations, and maternal expulsive efforts.[26-38] Severe airway edema may develop over a short period of time, especially when associated with maternal efforts.[30] As tissues of the supraglottic airway expand due to edema, the airway lumen is compromised, and mask ventilation, laryngoscopy, and endotracheal intubation will be more difficult. Edema of the face and neck may alert the physician to the potential for significant but asymptomatic airway edema, but these features are not consistently present.[26] Because of mucosal congestion and the increased friability of the airway tissues, repeated attempts at intubation may result in airway bleeding and edema and a rapidly worsening situation. A fatal airway hemorrhage was reported in a parturient when blind nasotracheal intubation was attempted after failed direct laryngoscopic intubation.[39] Blind nasal intubation should be used sparingly in obstetric patients because of the enhanced risk of hemorrhage from the friable membranes and the impact of such bleeding on subsequent airway management.[40]

There are a number of changes during pregnancy that impact on the ability of the parturient to tolerate periods of apnea without hypoxemia. Up to one third of parturients experience early airway closure in the supine position, and this is more likely to occur in the obese parturient.[41,42] Airway closure increases ventilation-perfusion mismatching and predisposes the parturient to lower partial pressures of oxygen in the blood. Oxygen consumption is increased by 20% or more in the term pregnant patient, and there is a more rapid decrease in arterial oxygen content during induction of general anesthesia in pregnant patients.[22] Parturients are less tolerant of any apneic period with respect to arterial oxygenation and prone to rapidly develop hypoxemia in the event that there is a delay in accomplishing intubation and commencing assisted ventilation.[43,44]

Physician anxiety has been cited as a factor in failed obstetric intubations. In commentary on the Confidential Enquiries, it has been suggested that, in the haste to achieve rapid intubation, laryngoscopy is attempted too early, by inexperienced physicians, assisted by untrained aides.[45] This opinion is supported by the finding that less experienced physicians are more likely to attempt laryngoscopy well before adequate muscle relaxation has been achieved in obstetrical patients than in general surgical patients.[46] The administration of small doses of induction agents, coupled with inadequate delay to permit the administered muscle relaxants to take effect, leads to poor conditions for laryngoscopy. With these early and inappropriate intubation attempts, the mouth is more difficult to open, interdental distance is reduced, laryngoscopy is compromised, and there is increased potential for patient retching, gastric regurgitation, and aspiration. The Confidential Enquiries also reveal that aspiration has occurred because cricoid pressure was not provided at all, was poorly provided, or was released when the patient vomited, ostensibly to prevent esophageal rupture. This has been linked to a lack of trained assistants to provide support to the anesthesiologist providing care to the patient.[1]

C. ACID ASPIRATION SYNDROME

1. The effects of pregnancy on gastroesophageal physiology

The physiologic changes of pregnancy include a number of hormonal alterations that influence gastroesophageal physiology. Maternal gastrin levels are elevated in pregnancy.[47] Gastrin induces copious secretions of water, electrolytes, and enzymes from the stomach, pancreas, and small intestine. Decreased plasma motilin levels have also been reported in pregnant patients.[48] Motilin is a hormonal peptide that has gastrointestinal smooth muscle stimulating effects. It accelerates gastric emptying, stimulates the lower esophageal sphincter (LES), and reduces intestinal transit time. Finally, the increased serum progesterone levels seen in pregnancy are associated with a reduction of the LES pressure and an increase in gastrointestinal transit time.[49-51] Published works have demonstrated no consistent delays in gastric emptying across populations of term parturients.[52-54] However, Sandhar recorded a doubling of gastric emptying time at term in two of the patients studied, when compared with control values measured 6 weeks postpartum.[52] Hirschheimer also reported that gastric emptying slowed in some mothers during early labor.[54] Established labor may cause unpredictable delays in gastric emptying that are further potentiated by the use of narcotic analgesics. Once labor is initiated, solid foodstuffs may remain in the stomach for prolonged periods.[53] There is ultrasound documentation of solid food in the stomachs of 66% of laboring parturients, irrespective of the time of last oral intake.[55] Gastric emptying has returned to normal by 24 hours postpartum.[56] However, the pattern of emptying during the first postpartum day has not been elucidated, and the same precautions against aspiration should be taken with newly delivered mothers as with laboring patients. Mothers undergoing tubal ligation within 9 hours of delivery had gastric aspirates of pH < 2.5, and 60% had gastric volumes greater than 25 ml.[57] The high incidence of reflux as measured by lower esophageal pH studies returns to normal by the second postpartum day.[58]

Symptoms suggestive of gastroesophageal reflux occur in almost 80% of pregnant women at term.[59] The symptom of heartburn correlates with reflux, and moderate to severe reflux occurs in 80% of parturients with heartburn and in 30% of those without symptoms.[60] Pregnant women suffering from heartburn have the longest delay in gastric emptying.[48] The LES pressure is lower in parturients with heartburn than in those without the symptom.[61] The presence of heartburn indicates an increased risk of regurgitation, particularly when the supine position is assumed.[62] Gastroesophageal reflux occurs when the LES pressure is inadequate to prevent retrograde flow of gastric contents across the sphincter

into the esophagus. During pregnancy the growth of the uterus from the pelvis into the abdomen may increase average intragastric pressures from 7 to 17 cm H_2O.[63] The supine position and especially the lithotomy and Trendelenburg positions may further increase intragastric pressures. The presence of multiple gestations, polyhydramnios, or gross obesity may be associated with intragastric pressures in excess of 40 cm H_2O.[64] The mean LES barrier pressures are lower in parturients when compared to nonpregnant controls.[59] However, the LES tone increases to average values of 44 cm H_2O during pregnancy, providing some protection from the increased intragastric pressure. Patients with heartburn may experience a paradoxical decrease in LES tone during gestation.[63] Medications commonly used in anesthesia that reduce the LES tone and barrier pressures include narcotics, benzodiazepines, and anticholinergic agents.[65-68] Intravenous anticholinergic administration may cause sufficiently large decrements in LES pressure as to allow free reflux into the esophagus.[69]

The upper esophageal sphincter (UES) is formed by the lamina of the cricoid cartilage anteriorly and striated muscle, primarily cricopharyngeus, posteriorly. The UES forms a barrier to prevent material regurgitated from the stomach into the esophagus from entering the pharynx and, from there, the lungs. The UES pressure is about 40 mm Hg and varies with different levels of arousal, decreasing to about 8 mm Hg with sleep.[70] The UES can prevent regurgitation of esophageal contents during light levels of anesthesia, in the absence of neuromuscular relaxants.[71] Intravenous induction of general anesthesia with pentothal and muscle relaxation with succinylcholine causes an abrupt fall in the UES pressure to less than 10 mm Hg, which may be low enough to allow regurgitation, especially in the setting of high intragastric pressures and LES incompetence.[72] Inhalational induction with halothane maintains UES tone, and coughing and straining during light levels of inhalational anesthesia may actually increase UES pressure and prevent regurgitation. Cricoid pressure is used to replace the UES during rapid sequence induction in patients at risk for pulmonary aspiration. (See also Chapter 10.)

2. Airway pressure and gastric distention

Intermittent positive pressure ventilation by mask may result in gastric insufflation, increasing intragastric pressure and causing regurgitation. The average intragastric pressure in spontaneously breathing, nonpregnant subjects is 11 cm H_2O (range 9 to 16 cm H_2O).[73] In paralyzed anesthetized patients, the average intragastric pressure required to cause reflux is 23 to 35 cm H_2O, consistent with pressures known to exist in normal pregnant patients.[63,64,74,75] There is a relationship between the airway pressures required to ventilate the lungs and those which force air into the stomach.[76] In subjects ventilated by bag and mask without cricoid pressure, airway pressures below 15 cm H_2O rarely cause stomach inflation, pressures between 15 to 25 cm H_2O will result in gastric insufflation in some patients, and pressures greater than 25 cm H_2O do so in most patients.[77,78] Application of cricoid pressure during mask-bag ventilation will increase the maximum pressure reached during mask ventilation, without air entering the stomach, to about 45 cm H_2O.[77] Gastric distention, as may occur with forceful mask ventilation, may increase intragastric pressures by 10 mm Hg.[79] The requirement for high pressure mask and bag ventilation in the difficult to ventilate pregnant patient will result in increased intragastric pressure and an augmented risk of regurgitation.

3. Aspiration pneumonitis in obstetrics

In 1946 Mendelson published his classic treatise on acid aspiration pneumonitis in paturients.[80] He calculated an incidence of 0.15%, the syndrome occurring in 66 of the 44,016 parturients Mendelson reviewed. The incidence of aspiration associated with cesarean section reported by Olsson, after reviewing 2643 operations, was 0.15%, no different than that reported 4 decades earlier by Mendelson.[81] All aspirations documented by Mendelson occurred in patients receiving face-mask anesthesia for labor and delivery. More than half of the patients required longer administration and greater depth of anesthesia for the operative intervention than was the norm for his institution. Sixty-eight percent of the aspirations were recognized at the time that they occurred; the remainder were not known to have occurred until the patients subsequently became symptomatic (silent aspiration). Patients who had liquid aspiration (both witnessed and silent) developed a syndrome characterized by bronchospasm, hypoxemia, and atelectasis. They were acutely ill; their condition gradually stabilized over 24 to 36 hours; then they recovered. Two patients who died aspirated solid material, obstructing their airways and resulting in suffocation. Three others who aspirated solid material had either partial obstructions or their obstructions were relieved and they survived. The incidence of fatal pulmonary aspiration syndrome reported by Mendelson in obstetrics was 0.005% (2 of 44,016 parturients). Mendelson concluded his report by encouraging the oral administration of warm alkaline solutions during labor to balance gastric acidity, discouraging the involvement of new and inexperienced anesthesia personnel as the primary care providers in obstetric anesthesia, and advocating the wider use of local anesthesia in obstetric anesthesia practice. In the years following Mendelson's report, routine endotracheal intubation for general anesthesia became a common, albeit not exclusively employed, technique to provide airway maintenance during obstetrical interventions. However, antacid therapy was inconsistently applied, and the continued involvement in some jurisdictions of inexperienced personnel as the primary care providers in obstetric anesthesia remained evident, and was criticized, for decades.[3,82] Two techniques subsequently evolved in anesthesia to manage patients at risk for regurgitation and aspiration.[25] Inhalational induction in the supine or lateral positions with a head-down tilt was utilized. Vomiting was said to occur in lighter planes of anesthesia when protective reflexes were still present. Difficulties during induction predisposed to regurgitation and episodes of hypoxemia resulted. Muscle relaxants were considered to be contraindicated because of the increased risk of gastric reflux following esophageal relaxation and the requirement to maintain spontaneous ventilation. Alternatively, the use of a barbiturate muscle-relaxant induction with rapid intubation in the head-up position was recommended and, for a limited time, was used.[25,83,84] This technique did predispose to hemodynamic instability and even cardiovascular collapse in compromised patients. Additionally, if regurgitation occurred in the interval between loss of consciousness and muscle relaxation, entry of stomach contents into the lungs was promoted by the sitting position.

4. Cricoid pressure

Sellick proposed the application of cricoid pressure as a simple maneuver, employed during induction of anesthesia to control regurgitation of gastric or esophageal contents and also to prevent inflation of the stomach, a potent cause of regurgitation.[25] To perform the maneuver in the manner described by Sellick, the neck was extended, increasing the anterior convexity of the cervical spine and stretching the esophagus. This prevented lateral displacement of the esophagus when cricoid pressure was applied. Before induction of anesthesia, the cricoid was palpated and lightly held between the thumb and second finger. As induction commenced, pressure was exerted on the cricoid cartilage, mainly by the index finger. As the patient lost consciousness, Sellick recommended firm pressure, sufficient to seal the esophagus without obstructing the airway. He noted that during cricoid pressure, the lungs may be ventilated without the risk of gastric distention. Cricoid pressure was initially felt to be contraindicated by Sellick in the setting of active vomiting, in the belief that the esophagus may be damaged by vomit under high pressure. He later modified this stand, stating that he felt the risk of rupture to be almost nonexistent.[85] This particular item has continued to represent a focus of controversy in anesthesia. There are instances reported in which fatal aspiration has occurred because cricoid pressure was released when the patient began vomiting during induction of anesthesia.[86] There is a single case report in the literature associating rupture of the esophagus with cricoid pressure.[87] It involved an elderly female, subjected to laparotomy after repeated episodes of hematemesis. The patient vomited on induction; she was positioned laterally, cricoid pressure was released, and the trachea was intubated after pharyngeal aspiration. At surgery, a longitudinal split was found in the lower esophagus. It was concluded, by the reporting authors, that the esophageal rupture represented an esophageal injury attributable to the cricoid pressure. However, the diagnosis of spontaneous rupture of the esophagus as a result of the repeated episodes of hematemesis represents a more likely diagnosis; the stomach (gastric cardia) adjacent to the area of esophageal injury was noted to be bruised and swollen during the surgery, suggesting a temporally more remote injury. Other authors are in agreement with Sellick's revised views on not releasing cricoid pressure during induction should the patient vomit.[61,88,89] That is, while there is ample evidence that fatal aspiration may result if cricoid pressure is released should vomiting occur at induction, there is no evidence that esophageal rupture is a significant risk should the pressure be maintained. They concluded that the pressure should not be released.[61,85,88]

Although cricoid pressures required to consistently prevent reflux have been determined and devices that measure applied pressure are available, application of this knowledge in routine clinical practice is difficult. Based on studies utilizing water-filled esophageal catheters in anesthetized patients, values of applied pressure of 40 to 44 Newtons (about 4 kg of applied pressure) have been recommended to prevent passive regurgitation of esophageal contents.[90,91] Vanner reported that difficulty in breathing occurred in about half of awake patients with such forces applied, and Lawes reported that airway obstruction occurred in about 10%.[92,93] Lesser applied forces (20 to 30 N) are probably sufficient in the majority of patients. Training using a modified intubation mannequin equipped with a force-measuring device, demonstrates that cricoid (force) application techniques do improve with training.[94] Upper esophageal sphincter pressure rapidly decreases with anesthetic induction, usually before loss of consciousness.[91] Therefore, cricoid pressure should be applied concurrent with the start of anesthetic induction. The pressure should be uncomfortable to the awake patient, but the airway should not be compromised. As induction is completed, the force may be increased, but, again, caution should be employed so as not to obstruct the airway. Usually extreme pressure is required to compromise the airway, although there are reports of more modest levels of cricoid pressure resulting in airway

obstruction, usually due to benign airway pathology.[95] The pressure is maintained until the trachea has been intubated, the cuff of the endotracheal tube inflated, and the intratracheal placement of the tube confirmed. Only then should the request to release the pressure be made. In the event of difficult laryngoscopy, cricoid pressure may be transiently decreased or removed in order to determine if laryngoscopy is improved and intubation can be effected. Maintenance of adequate cricoid pressure for prolonged periods may be difficult.[96]

The effectiveness of cricoid pressure in preventing aspiration has been challenged by Whittington, who reported two cases of aspiration in parturients despite cricoid pressure having been employed at induction.[86] In both instances, muscle relaxation was maintained during anesthesia maintenance for cesarean section by large doses of pancuronium. The first patient vomited and aspirated after extubation, and the second demonstrated signs of inadequate relaxant reversal, then respiratory failure, and subsequently manifested signs of pulmonary aspiration. In neither case was there any intraoperative evidence of the massive, fatal aspirations that were clearly evident after extubations complicated by aspiration. Cricoid pressure cannot provide absolute protection against aspiration, and there are a number of factors that would explain occasional failures. The landmarks on the patient's neck may not be identified properly, and, as a result, pressure may not be exerted on the cricoid cartilage itself. Cricoid pressure may not be arranged before induction, allowing for an interval between loss of consciousness and application of cricoid pressures, during which the patient is at risk for aspiration.[97] Nonmedical personnel are often relied upon to assist the anesthesiologist during induction of general anesthesia and may be inadequately trained to do so.[1,98] Cricoid pressure may be released inadvertently before the trachea is intubated and the cuff filled.[97] Howells has demonstrated that only about half of a population of trained assistants applied sufficient pressure to result in esophageal occlusion.[97] Finally, there is a steady decline in the applied force when cricoid pressure is sustained for more than 30 seconds, suggesting that the maneuver may become less effective in preventing aspiration during instances of difficult intubation as time passes.[96] Cricoid pressure may also complicate the process of intubation, delaying or preventing intubation and thereby increasing the risk of aspiration. The airway may be obstructed by cricoid pressure, although this is unusual and extreme forces must be applied to do so.[93] Inappropriately applied cricoid pressure may distort the airway, either angulating the larynx or deviating it from midline. Flexion of the head on the neck may occur as a result of cricoid pressure, and this may impede laryngoscopy. An attempt to maintain extension of the head on the neck during the application of cricoid pressure

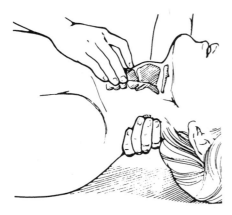

Fig. 30-3. Bimanual cricoid pressure. Assistant's left hand is placed behind the neck lifting up, and the right hand is used to apply cricoid pressure. The lifting action (countercricoid pressure) places the head in an improved sniffing position for laryngoscopy. (From Crowley DS, Giesecke AH: *Anaesthesia* 45:588, 1990.)

will improve the conditions for laryngoscopy.[99] Bimanual cricoid pressure with the free hand of the assistant placed behind and supporting the neck of the parturient or, alternatively, the use of a small support placed behind the patient's neck have been recommended to overcome the tendency to head flexion[100,101] (Fig. 30-3).

Following publication of Sellick's report, the use of cricoid pressure increasingly evolved as the most important mechanism to prevent pulmonary aspiration in parturients undergoing general anesthesia. Rapid sequence induction with cricoid pressure has become the accepted standard of care for the parturient undergoing general anesthesia. The impact that this has had on maternal deaths from anesthesia has been twofold. First, deaths from aspiration have clearly been reduced and eliminated altogether in some reports. This is, in part, due to the abandonment of face-mask anesthesia in obstetrics and cannot be entirely attributed to the implementation of cricoid pressure. Second, deaths due to hypoxemic cardiac arrest following failed intubation with either inability or failure to ventilate the patient and aspirations resulting from failed or esophageal intubations have become the single most common and, by far, the predominant causes of anesthesia-related maternal mortality.

III. ISSUES IN PATIENT MANAGEMENT

A. PREOPERATIVE ASSESSMENT OF THE AIRWAY—PREDICTION OF DIFFICULT INTUBATION

Mallampati reported a correlation between the visibility of oropharyngeal structures and the degree of difficulty of laryngeal exposure during laryngoscopy and concluded that difficult laryngeal visualization could be predicted in most cases by assessing the visibility of the faucial pillars and uvula.[102] Preoperative oropharyngeal examination and classification using a three-tier (Class I = soft palate, pillars, and uvula visualized; Class II = soft palate and pillars visualized; Class III = soft palate visualized) grading system was proposed. Prospective application of the system by Mallampati revealed that, in the majority of patients with poor visualization of pharyngeal structures, laryngoscopy was difficult. Samsoon and Young reviewed a series of obstetric and general surgical patients who were known difficult intubations and assigned Mallampati classifications.[20] They added a further tier (Class IV = no pharyngeal structures visualized) to the Mallampati grading scheme. Samsoon observed that, among patients in whom laryngoscopy was known to be difficult, Class III and Class IV assignments predominated. Samsoon also noted that, among obstetric patients, none of the difficult to intubate patients had presented with features that had in the past been associated with difficult intubation, such as poor cervical spinal movement, dental problems, and limited mouth opening. The Mallampati classification system was further evaluated by Tham who studied the effects of posture, phonation, and observer on Mallampati classification.[103] Phonation produced a marked improvement of view and a more favorable classification, whereas the supine position resulted in a somewhat worse view and a higher grade assignment.

Wilson developed a five-factor evaluation mechanism after reviewing the features of patients who had proven to be difficult to intubate.[104] Patient weight, head and neck movement, jaw movement, mandibular size, and prominence of the upper incisors were each graded (0 to 2), and a rank sum score was determined. Of the five factors identified by multivariate analysis as contributing to difficult intubation, obesity was the weakest predictor. Although Wilson measured body weight, high body mass index (BMI) has been advocated as a more accurate index of both obesity and the likelihood of difficult intubation.[104,105] It is also a marker for both an increased incidence of cesarean delivery and increased maternal risk for maternal morbidity and mortality.[23,105-107] This has particular relevance in obstetric anesthesia practice, since a significant proportion of the patients have increased BMI. However, Bond reported that there was no correlation between high BMI and grade of laryngoscopy.[105] No attempt was made to control for other factors contributory to difficult intubation. Additionally, there was a 21% incidence of laryngoscopies of Class III or greater in the control group to which the high BMI group was being compared, an unusually high incidence and one that could mask difficulties in the high BMI group.

Eighty-five of the first 2000 anesthesia-related incidents reported to the Australian Incident Monitoring Study involved difficult or failed intubations.[108] Only three of the 85 incidents reported involved obstetric patients. Obesity, limited neck mobility, limited mouth opening, and inadequate assistance were major factors contributing to intubation difficulties. Reflux of gastric contents with aspiration occurred in seven of the 85 incidents. Thirteen of the 85 patients were also difficult to ventilate. There were no deaths in the series. There were also 35 cases of esophageal intubation in the first 2000 incidents. Eighteen of the 35 esophageal intubations occurred in the setting of difficult intubation, although in 15 there was no perceived difficulty in intubation. One death and three aspirations resulted. Five of the eighteen difficult intubations occurred in the setting of emergency situations. Abandonment of the procedure was not always feasible, emphasizing the need for a failed intubation drill. The gum-elastic bougie was the most useful aid to intubation in the patients successfully intubated.[109]

Rocke reported the factors, assessed preoperatively, that were associated with difficult intubation in 1500 parturients undergoing emergency and elective cesarean section under general anesthesia.[12] He utilized prospective application of the Samsoon-Young modified Mallampati classification for airway assessment as well, noting the presence of the following maternal characteristics: short neck, obesity, missing maxillary incisors, protruding maxillary incisors, single maxillary tooth, receding mandible, facial edema, and swollen tongue. In the series, 32% of patients had a Class I airway, 42% of patients had a Class II airway, 21% a Class III airway, and 5% a Class IV airway. Grade 1 laryngoscopy occurred in 98% of Class I airways, 87% of Class II, 75% of Class III, and 71% of Class IV. An easy, first attempt intubation occurred in 96% of Class I airways, 91% of Class II, 82% of Class III, and 76% of Class IV airways. Although difficulty with intubation increased with increasing airway class, most patients with Class IV airways were not difficult to intubate. Only 4% and 6% of Class III and IV airways, respectively, were considered to be very difficult intubations. There were two failed intubations (1:750), one each in Class II (0.2%) and Class III (0.3%). Rocke speculated on the possibility that a Class IV assignment in the obstetric patients has a different significance than a similar determination in a nonobstetric patient, given that so few of the Class IV patients proved to be difficult intubations. After using univariate and stepwise multiple logistic regression analysis to eliminate associated factors, the following emerged as etiologic factors (relative risk in brackets) predicting difficult or failed intubation: airway Class II (3.23); airway Class III (7.58); airway Class IV (11.30); short neck (5.01); receding mandible (9.71); and protruding maxillary incisors (8.0). Obesity and a short neck were linked factors, with obesity being eliminated as a risk factor if short neck was excluded.

Capillary engorgement and edema of the airway as a consequence of the pregnancy, complications related to the pregnancy, and maternal expulsive efforts may predispose the parturient to difficult intubation.[26-38] The lack of compressibility of the edematous tissues may make it difficult to achieve the forward and downward movement of the hyoid necessary to elevate the epiglottis during intubation. However, postpartum reevaluation of patients who presented difficulties at laryngoscopy usually demonstrate that features suggestive of difficult intubation persist.[21] That is, in the majority of parturients who present difficulties at laryngoscopy and intubation, these difficulties do not result from the pregnancy but rather from the patients prepregnant anatomic characteristics.

All parturients being considered for an anesthetic, whether regional or general or presenting with a condition that predisposes them to higher risk for cesarean section, should undergo airway evaluation and have a Mallampati-Samsoon classification assigned. Davies encourages evaluation of the airway in the supine position, although Tham has reported that there is little difference in designated class with supine versus upright position.[17,103] In fact, based on Tham's data, routine assessment in the supine position would result in decreased specificity of the Mallampati assessment. Further airway evaluation should include determination of the patient's body habitus, mouth opening (interdental distance), prominence of upper incisors, ability to protrude the lower jaw beyond the upper incisors, mandibular length, thyromental distance, and neck extension. The latter assessment may be carried out with a simple bedside maneuver.[110] The distance from the sternal notch to the tip of the chin is measured with the patient both in the neutral and maximally extended position. With extension, the distance should increase. An increase of less than 5 cm is associated with a high sensitivity, specificity, and positive predictive value for difficult laryngoscopy. An increase of greater than 5 cm should reassure the examiner that neck mobility is normal. After airway assessment, a summary conclusion should be generated as to the anticipated difficulty in performing laryngoscopy, and the patient can be advised of both the conclusion and its implications.

Although the majority of reports implicate airway class as a predictor of difficult intubation, it is clear that the use of Mallampati classification used alone is an imprecise mechanism for the preoperative detection of the difficult-to-intubate patient. The combination of the Mallampati classification with other risk criteria, especially short neck, small jaw, short interdental distance, prominent upper incisors, and neck mobility, improves the specificity and sensitivity of the preoperative assessment. Rocke has constructed a figure predicting the probability of difficult intubation based on the findings of

Risk Factors

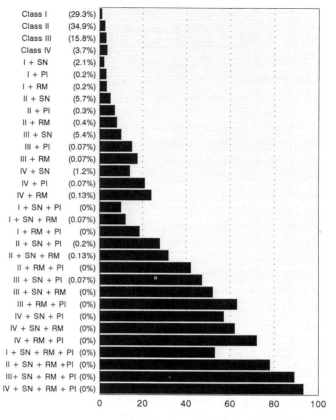

Fig. 30-4. The probability of experiencing a difficult intubation (grades 3 and 4 combined) for the varying combinations of risk factors and the observed incidence of these combinations. *SN,* short neck; *PI,* protruding maxillary incisors; *RM,* receding mandible. (From Rocke DA, Murray WB, Rout CC et al: *Anesthesiology* 77:63, 1992.)

preoperative evaluation and, although not yet prospectively verified, its application is encouraged[12] (Fig. 30-4).

B. ACID ASPIRATION – STRATEGIES FOR RISK REDUCTION IN THE PARTURIENT

Strategies to reduce the risk of acid aspiration focus on: (1) reducing the potential for significant gastric volume and acidity in parturients; (2) reducing the use of general anesthesia in obstetrics and relying on other forms of analgesia that maintain maternal consciousness; (3) appropriate assessment of the maternal airway (even when urgent interventions are otherwise required); and (4) evolving management schemes to deal with failures to intubate and/or ventilate in elective and emergent situations. The concept of critical or threshold volumes and pH of gastric contents is debated.[62] However, that the incidence and intensity or severity of aspiration pneumonitis increases as pH decreases and gastric volume increases is widely accepted. There are four major risk factors for acid aspiration: (1) a full stomach with acid gastric contents; (2) an increased

intraabdominal or intragastric pressure; (3) a decreased lower esophageal sphincter barrier pressure; and (4) a delay or inability to protect the airway should protective mechanisms (UES) be lost.

Reduction of the acidity of the gastric contents may reduce morbidity should aspiration occur. There are two mechanisms to reduce gastric acidity. Antacids effectively neutralize acid contents of the stomach. Nonparticulate antacids are favored, since there is evidence that particulate antacids are themselves capable of causing lung injury should aspiration occur.[111] Sodium citrate is the most widely used and recommended antacid in obstetric anesthesia practice.[62] Thirty ml of 0.3 M sodium citrate given 15 to 20 minutes before induction of general anesthesia is effective in raising the pH of stomach contents, beginning about 5 minutes after administration and lasting for 40 to 60 minutes.[112,113] The effect may be relatively prolonged in anesthetized patients, with beneficial effects persisting several hours after administration.[114] The histamine (H$_2$) blocking agents, cimetidine and ranitidine, have also been consistently shown to reduce gastric volume and acidity in parturients.[62] The use of ranitidine is favored because of its longer duration of action, fewer side effects, and lesser inhibition of the mixed function oxidase system when compared with cimetidine. An orally administered dose of ranitidine 150 mg, given 90 minutes before surgery will reliably increase pH in the majority of parturients. A small number of patients will continue to have gastric pH below 2.5 despite ranitidine administration. The incidence of at-risk patients will increase in the setting of urgent cesarean section compared with elective surgeries, despite ranitidine administration.[115] The coadministration of sodium citrate with intravenous ranitidine provides more effective prophylaxis than antacid alone, although 30 minutes is required from the time of injection to see this enhanced effect.[116] Combination therapy is thus likely to provide little real benefit, compared to antacid administration alone, in the setting of emergency cesarean section. The use of effervescent cimetidine-sodium citrate is also more effective than sodium citrate alone in increasing and maintaining maternal gastric pH above 2.5.[117] Omeprazole, which selectively blocks the proton pump in the gastric parietal cell (the terminal step in the production of gastric acid), is more effective than ranitidine in decreasing pH in parturients presenting for elective cesarean section when given orally both the evening before and the morning of surgery.[118] Intravenous omeprazole reduces both the gastric pH and volume in parturients presenting for emergency cesarean section, but, once again, about 30 minutes are required for this effect.[119] Maternal and fetal side effects have not been a significant issue with respect to the use of the acid suppressing agents. The use of anticholinergic agents to reduce gastric acid secretion has been widely and wisely abandoned.[111] Their effect on gastric secretion is variable, and there is little evidence that they reduce gastric acid secretion. Further, anticholinergic agents adversely affect the esophageal sphincter pressure, thus reducing the barrier to esophageal reflux.

Metoclopramide is a prokinetic agent that, when administered to parturients undergoing cesarean section, results in an increased barrier pressure at the LES and may promote gastric emptying.[120] Metoclopramide (10 mg administered intramuscularly) decreased gastric emptying time in primigravid women, including some who had received meperidine during labor.[121] Whether or not metoclopramide consistently promotes gastric emptying in all parturients has not been fully resolved. Cohen was unable to demonstrate this effect in individual parturients, although overall there was a decrease in the number of patients with gastric volumes greater than 25 ml and pH less than 2.5.[120] Anticholinergic agents may counteract the effects of metoclopramide on both gastric peristalsis and the LES. Metoclopramide

may not reliably reverse narcotic-induced inhibition of gastric motility, but there is evidence that intravenous administration is more effective than intramuscular injection in antagonizing the delay in gastric emptying caused by morphine.[122] Despite the narcotic antagonism to the gastric emptying effects of metoclopramide, there is still evidence for enhanced gastric emptying after administration of metoclopramide in laboring patients who have received narcotics.[123] The usual dose of metoclopramide is 10 mg, given either orally or intramuscularly, 60 to 90 minutes before surgery. In an emergency, 10 mg injected slowly intravenously will begin to have an effect in 1 to 3 minutes. Acute use of dopamine antagonists before cesarean section does not appear to produce adverse effects in either the mother or newborn. (See also Chapter 10.)

C. MANAGEMENT OF INDUCTION OF GENERAL ANESTHESIA

The following recommendations pertain to the parturient presenting for elective or nonelective cesarean section who, after appropriate preoperative assessment, is deemed to have *an airway that will not likely be difficult to intubate.* Patients in whom difficulty with intubation is anticipated should undergo operative delivery under regional anesthesia or, if general anesthesia is deemed to be indicated, should have general anesthesia induced after awake intubation. A detailed discussion on the preparation of the patient for awake intubation can be found in Chapter 9.

1. Aspiration prophylaxis (Box 30-2)

Patients presenting for elective cesarean section under general anesthesia should receive oral ranitidine (150 mg) the evening before surgery and 90 minutes before surgery and 30 ml of oral sodium citrate or its equivalent 10 to 20 minutes before surgery. The use of effervescent cimetidine, 400 mg of cimetidine with sodium citrate (half of a tablet of Tagamet 800 effervescent), is an effective alternative. Metoclopramide 10 mg is administered in the same manner as ranitidine to parturients who experience symptomatic reflux. Patients undergoing urgent cesarean section under general anesthesia should receive therapy with oral antacids and parenteral ranitidine before induction of anesthesia, with induction delayed as long as feasible to allow for a pharmacologic effect. Patients who present for emergency cesarean section under general anesthesia should receive oral sodium citrate or effervescent cimetidine before anesthetic induction. Intravenous administration of ranitidine and metoclopramide can be considered after induction of anesthesia to reduce gastric volume and acidity at the time of extubation, although there is no data available to attest to the effectiveness of this.

BOX 30-2   Pharmacologic prophylaxis — aspiration pneumonitis

Labor

- All women in active labor are under restricted oral intake — primarily clear fluids and ice chips.
- Patients in normal or augmented labor do not receive routine prophylaxis.
- Metoclopramide and ranitidine are used primarily in parturients who have significant reflux symptoms or excess nausea and vomiting while in labor.

Elective cesarean section

- Sodium citrate (30 ml of 0.3 M solution) is given 10-20 min preoperatively, irrespective of the type of anesthesia planned.
- For patients who have significant symptoms of reflux, ranitidine 150 mg or metoclopramide 10 mg is given orally at hs the night before surgery and 90 min before surgery.

Nonelective cesarean section

- Sodium citrate is given, per os, before moving the patient to the operating room, irrespective of the type of anesthesia planned.
- Parenteral administration of ranitidine and metoclopramide are given to those patients with symptomatic reflux or who have recently eaten, respectively, and for whom a general anesthesia is planned provided a delay of anesthetic induction is feasible (to allow for pharmacologic effect).

Emergency cesarean section

- Sodium citrate 30 ml is given per os in the labor suite before transporting the patient to the operating room.
- Ranitidine and metoclopramide are not routinely given preinduction but may be administered intraoperatively or on specific indication.

BOX 30-3   The difficult intubation kit for obstetric anesthesia

Essential

Airways oral and pharyngeal
Laryngoscopes   short, polio handles
                       Macintosh, Miller blades
Bougie
Lighted stylet
Laryngeal mask airways size no. 3 and no. 4
Combitube
Retrograde catheter kit
Cricothyrotomy kit (preassembled oxygen insufflation kit)
Endotracheal tubes sizes 5-7, including half sizes

Optional

Fiberoptic laryngoscope or bronchoscope
Bullard laryngoscope

---

2. Equipment

A number of items of equipment should be immediately available for all cases and brought into the room for anticipated difficulties or once difficulties are experienced. Equipment specifically modified for use in obstetric anesthesia has been described.[124] A list of essential and optional items to be included in a difficult intubation kit is provided in Box 30-3. It is recommended that clinicians familiarize themselves with these items before they are required in emergent situations.

3. Positioning

The table should be at a height that is most convenient for the anesthesiologist performing laryngoscopy. The height of the table can be adjusted to suit the obstetrician once the airway has been secured. The patient is placed in the wedged supine position with the right hip elevated 10 to 12 cm. The head should be positioned in the sniffing position with a small pillow under the occiput. Folded sheets or flannels may be used to accomplish this positioning and are particularly useful in the very obese patient (Fig. 30-5). The obstetric patient is typically prepped and draped for surgery before the induction of general anesthesia to minimize the induction-delivery interval. The drapes on the ether screen (or its equivalent) should be arranged so that they do not overlie the neck and head region, so as not to interfere with laryngoscopy.

4. Preoxygenation

Denitrogenation occurs more quickly in the pregnant patient than in the nonpregnant patient because of the decreased functional residual capacity and higher minute ventilation that occur in pregnancy.[125-127] However, oxygen consumption in the term parturient is higher than in nonpregnant patients, and the lung stores of oxygen are reduced.[128,129] The parturient sustains a threefold more rapid reduction in arterial oxygen content during apneic periods, as would occur following induction of anesthesia, before endotracheal intubation is achieved.[130] In the event of delayed intubation, frank hypoxemia may become manifest. The usual method for preoxygenating patients before anesthetic induction involves having the patient breathe 100% oxygen through a snug-fitting face mask for 3 to 5 minutes. Norris reported that four maximal capacity breaths are as effective in preoxygenating parturients, although an additional study by Norris showed that the four-breath method does not as completely denitrogenate parturients when compared to tidal breathing.[126,131] Further, nonpregnant patients preoxygenated with four vital

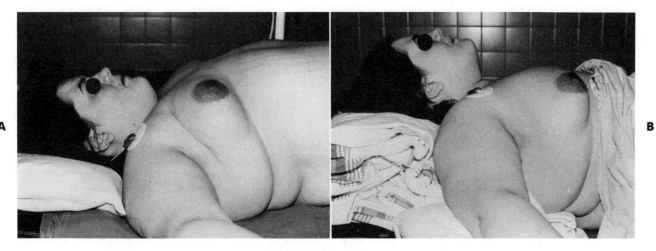

Fig. 30-5. Enhanced positioning of the obese parturient for laryngoscopy. **A,** Standard positioning on the operating table. **B,** Improved positioning achieved with elevation of the torso and head. (From Davies JM, Weeks SA, Crone LA et al: *Can J Anaesth* 36:668, 1989.)

capacity breaths desaturated more quickly than patients preoxygenated for 3 minutes.[132] For these reasons, and whenever possible, it is recommended that the tidal breathing technique be employed and that the four-breath technique should be reserved for situations that require haste. Two to 3 minutes of tidal breathing provide adequate denitrogenation in parturients.[126]

5. Cricoid pressure

Women undergoing cesarean section under general anesthesia lose their protective airway reflexes during induction of anesthesia, and the airway is unprotected during the interval to tracheal intubation. Cricoid pressure remains an effective technique for preventing gastroesophageal reflux and gastric insufflation during this time. The cricoid cartilage should be identified by the assistant during preoxygenation, before induction of anesthesia, and the accuracy of the landmark should be confirmed by the anesthesiologist. It must be acknowledged that the assistant's exclusive responsibility is to the anesthesiologist until he/she is released from this obligation by the anesthesiologist. As induction of anesthesia begins, the cricoid pressure should be applied. In some patients, application of cricoid pressure may cause forward flexion of the head on the neck, thus impairing laryngoscopy. In the event that this occurs, posterior neck support applied with the assistant's other hand (bimanual cricoid pressure) often overcomes this tendency to flexion (see Fig. 30-3). Alternatively, a contracricoid device placed behind the patient's neck before induction of anesthesia may achieve the same purpose. These maneuvers reduce both the neck flexion induced by cricoid pressure and the frequency with which a difficult intubation attributable to the application of cricoid pressure will be encountered.

Should the patient make retching motions after administration of anesthetic induction agents, I ask that the assistant maintain cricoid pressure. The risk of esophageal rupture, albeit real, appears extremely small.[61,85,87] The risk of aspiration should cricoid pressure be released, although also undefined, seems of greater magnitude. The retching motions quickly subside as the succinylcholine takes effect. If it is elected to release cricoid in this scenario, the patient should be immediately turned onto the left lateral position, placed head down, the oropharynx suctioned, and the patient intubated in the left lateral position.

6. Induction of anesthesia

Rapid sequence induction implies rapid administration of both the induction agent and muscle relaxant. Succinylcholine is the muscle relaxant of choice in rapid sequence induction, barring a contraindication to its use. It is the muscle relaxant capable of achieving the most rapid and effective muscle relaxation. Adequate time should be allowed for muscle relaxation before attempting laryngoscopy. If sufficient time is not allowed, masseter muscle tone may be increased, making mouth opening more difficult and compromising laryngoscopy.[133] The use of vecuronium for rapid-sequence induction in patients undergoing cesarean section has been reported.[134] Patients were given 10 $\mu g/kg^{-1}$ as a priming dose followed 4 to 6 min later by 100 $\mu g/kg^{-1}$ or 200 $\mu g/kg^{-1}$ as a single bolus. Onset time to 100% twitch suppression was 177 and 175 seconds, respectively. Duration of effect, measured to 25% twitch height recovery was 73 and 115 minutes, respectively. There would appear to be little advantage to using the higher dose of vecuronium. Because of the delayed onset time and prolonged recovery compared to that expected from succinylcholine, use of intermediate agents should only be considered when succinylcholine is contraindicated.

7. Laryngoscopy, intubation, and postoperative extubation

Once adequate muscle relaxation is achieved, laryngoscopy should be performed and the trachea intubated. Confirmation of intratracheal placement is by the observation of end-tidal carbon dioxide in the volume of gas exhaled through the endotracheal tube. Once confirmation of correct placement is made, cricoid pressure is released, the surgeon is given the go-ahead, and the tube is secured.

The patient is ideally extubated on her side, head slightly down, awake and following commands, and without residual paralysis from muscle relaxants. The oropharynx is gently suctioned, and the patient is asked to take a big breath. At the end of the spontaneous inspiration, the cuff is deflated and the trachea extubated. A vigorous cough results, expelling secretions from the upper airway.

IV. THE FAILED INTUBATION—MANAGEMENT OPTIONS AND SPECIAL SITUATIONS

A. THE FAILED INTUBATION DRILL—A HISTORICAL PERSPECTIVE

Tunstall proposed a failed intubation drill for obstetric anesthesia in 1976 and offered revised versions in 1986 and 1987.[135-137] Tunstall's recommendations, following failed intubation, were to maintain cricoid pressure, turn the patient onto her left side in the head-down position, and continue positive pressure ventilation by hand with a mask and bag. If ventilation was easy using nitrous oxide, oxygen, and a volatile agent, it was recommended to gradually establish a plane of surgical anesthesia with spontaneous ventilation and a face mask. Performance of an elective cesarean section with spontaneous ventilation and face mask anesthesia was considered acceptable provided that a clear airway could be achieved. If the airway remained partially obstructed, Tunstall considered it prudent to allow the patient to awaken and then to proceed with an alternate course of management. If an adequate (unobstructed) airway could not be established, Tunstall recommended insertion of an esophageal gastric tube airway.[137] A cricothyroid membrane puncture and transtracheal oxygenation was recommended if oxygenation remained impossible despite the aforementioned interventions. Once a patient who had been both a failed intubation and a difficult airway was awoken, Tunstall considered an inhalational induction with spontaneous respiration and face mask anesthesia an appropriate subsequent course of management.

A number of authors have since advanced protocols for the management of failed intubation in obstetric anesthesia.[17,138-141] Two conclusions have been consistent through most recent protocols and also with the recommendations proposed by Tunstall. An early acceptance of failure to intubate must occur and a maximum of two to three intubation attempts have been recommended. Further, it is desirable to evolve and implement a standard protocol for managing failed intubation that recognizes the paramount importance of ensuring oxygenation. However, most other authors have not shared Tunstall's willingness to proceed with a nonurgent cesarean section with an unsecured, albeit open airway.[17,138-141] There is general agreement that, if the fetus is in good condition, the mother should be allowed to awaken after failed intubation, and an alternative method of anesthesia should be employed. A preoperative determination of the need to continue with general anesthesia, should unanticipated difficulties arise, may be useful in order to identify situations for which continuation of general anesthesia would be warranted. In the absence of a threat to maternal health, some would argue that there are no compelling reasons to carry on with a general anesthetic despite fetal concerns.[40,142] However, the overriding argument advanced in defense of this reasoning relates to the experience of the anesthetic care providers who are likely to have to deal with this situation. In the event that no experienced anesthesiologist is available to provide care, a decision to continue with general anesthesia despite failed intubation cannot be supported. This is rarely the case in North American practice.

B. MANAGEMENT GUIDELINES—FAILED INTUBATION—ELECTIVE CESAREAN SECTION

No approach to the failed intubation in obstetric anesthesia may be formulated that does not have some limitations. The following comments represent guidelines for the management of the parturient, presenting for elective or nonemergent cesarean section, who is difficult or impossible to intubate (Fig. 30-6, *A,B*). Preoperative airway evaluation should already have determined a low probability of difficulty during laryngoscopy. The presence of two or more risk factors for difficult intubation should prompt consideration of either avoidance of general anesthesia or awake intubation prior to induction of general anesthesia. A decision should have been made preoperatively as to the course of action if difficulties are experienced during laryngoscopy and intubation (e.g., see Fig. 30-6, *B,C*). Following induction of anesthesia and laryngoscopy, visual assessment will reveal whether or not the parturient will be difficult, if not impossible, to intubate. Cricoid pressure may be transiently released at this time, and it can be determined whether or not the release of cricoid pressure or pressure in a slightly different location (i.e.,

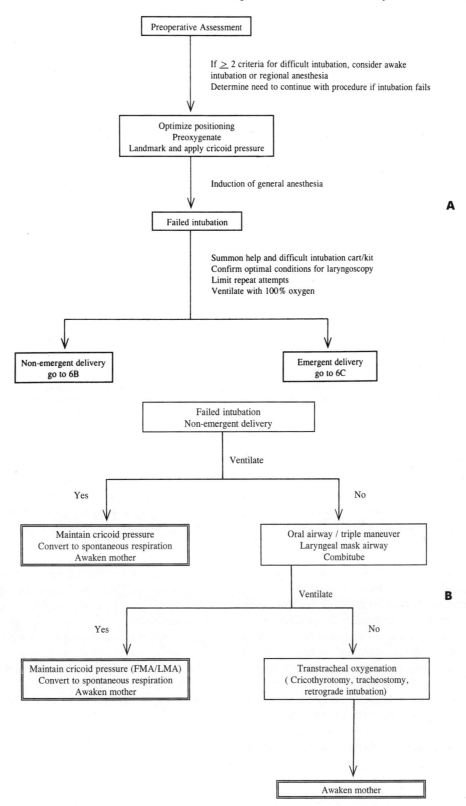

Fig. 30-6. Management algorithms for failed intubation in the parturient. **A,** Outlines initial assessment and management of the obstetric airway. Decision points in the management of failed intubation include the determination of the urgency of the delivery and the ability to oxygenate the mother. For elective or nonemergent delivery, **B,** Outlines management schemes following failed intubation with goals being to oxygenate and awaken the mother. **C,** Provides guidelines in the emergent situation where goals are to oxygenate and anesthetize the mother and deliver the infant. Boxes with double borders represent end points for the algorithm.

Continued.

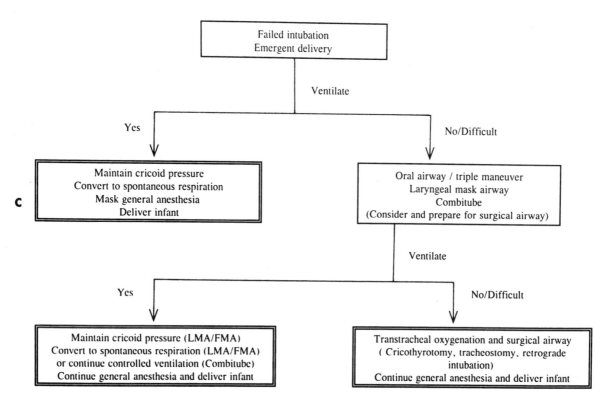

Fig. 30-6, cont'd.

determine optimal laryngeal manipulation, see Chapter 14) will facilitate intubation. If there is no improvement, cricoid pressure should be immediately reapplied and maintained. The operating room (OR) team is alerted to the situation, and experienced help is summoned immediately. The position of the patient is not changed initially, and the face mask is reapplied and positive pressure ventilation with 100% oxygen commenced. Maternal oxygenation and airway protection are the paramount goals from this point forward. Many intubation difficulties may be overcome if positioning is optimized, and a counter cricoid maneuver is employed to offset the flexion of the head caused by application of cricoid pressure. The efficacy of these maneuvers can be ascertained. In the event that ventilation is difficult, an oral airway should be inserted. Simple methods to improve the airway include the chin lift, two-handed jaw thrust, or triple maneuver (head tilt, jaw thrust, mouth opened). A second person should assist with ventilation.

Patient positioning, cricoid pressure (bimanual), the intubating instrument, and the personnel (second laryngoscopist) may all be modified during subsequent attempts at intubation. Oxygenation must be assured during this period. Useful aids to blind intubation when direct laryngoscopy reveals a grade 3 or 4 view include the gum-rubber bougie and the lighted stylet. If three properly controlled attempts at intubation have failed, a decision must be taken on further management. In the

absence of fetal compromise and in the setting of an elective cesarean section, the procedure is abandoned, and the mother is allowed to awaken. If ventilation is easy with mask and bag, it can be artificially maintained until spontaneous ventilation returns. Cricoid pressure is ideally maintained during this period. Positioning the mother in the left lateral, head-down position can be considered, once spontaneous ventilation has resumed and is encouraged. If ventilation remains impossible, insertion either of a laryngeal mask airway (LMA) or a Combitube should be considered. It may be necessary to transiently release cricoid pressure to insert the laryngeal mask, and it will be necessary to do so to insert the Combitube. Transtracheal oxygenation through a cricothyroid puncture should be reserved for the unlikely event that neither an LMA or Combitube is available or effective.

C. MANAGEMENT GUIDELINES—FAILED INTUBATION—NONELECTIVE CESAREAN SECTION

The decision to abandon the anesthesia-surgery and awaken the mother is influenced both by the ability to oxygenate the mother and the degree of urgency of the cesarean section. It is difficult to justify putting the mother at continued risk by continuing an anesthetic after failed intubation has occurred when the procedure is elective. However, in situations where the mother, the fetus, or both are at risk due to obstetric circumstances, continuation of the anesthetic and delivery may be lifesaving to one or both. If a decision is made to continue with the procedure, then the best possible airway is sought. A tenuous airway is not generally acceptable, and it is prudent to proceed to the next step to ensure a secure airway. (During the wake-up drill for the abandoned elective situation, I will accept a tenuous airway in an oxygenating mother.)

Once a decision has been taken to carry on following failed intubation, mask-and-bag ventilation is attempted, facilitated by an airway, if necessary, with cricoid pressure maintained (Fig. 30-6, *A,C*). If ventilation is successful, spontaneous ventilation is allowed to return, and the cesarean section is carried out with the patient under face mask general anesthesia (FMA). Minimal fundal pressure to effect delivery of the fetus is encouraged to reduce intragastric pressures. If ventilation is difficult (tenuous airway) or impossible, either an LMA or a Combitube should be employed. A transtracheal or translaryngeal (retrograde intubation) is generally reserved for situations where an acceptable airway cannot otherwise be obtained nonsurgically. However, rather than tolerate an undue delay in achieving a nonsurgical airway, earlier invasive airway intervention is readily defensible.

Emergency induction of general anesthesia for urgent cesarean section, the "crash section," is a particularly high-risk intervention in obstetric anesthesia, with much of the measured maternal mortality resulting from this intervention.[1,16,143] There is little time for more than rapid gathering of a pertinent history, a perfunctory patient examination, a hurried equipment check, followed by induction of general anesthesia and operative delivery. Because of the inherent risk involved, it should be reserved for situations where such haste and risk are warranted. A strategy for identifying patients likely to deliver by cesarean section early in labor and initiating epidural anesthesia will reduce the requirement for urgent induction of general anesthesia.[144] (Box 30-4). The need for nonelective or emergency cesarean section could be anticipated in 87% of parturients reviewed by Morgan, and epidural anesthesia was provided in 70% of patients.[144] However, not all epidural blocks established for labor analgesia could be rapidly or successfully converted to provide surgical anesthesia for cesarean delivery. In 194 patients, an epidural catheter was placed and activated after they were deemed likely to deliver by cesarean section, and a catheter was placed in a further 57 patients when the decision to deliver them by cesarean section was actually made. Twenty-seven (12%) of these patients were given general anesthesia for delivery, fifteen because the epidural block was inadequate for surgery, the rest for reasons not explicitly stated. Ostheimer reported that epidural blockade

---

> **BOX 30-4 Factors increasing the likelihood of nonelective cesarean section**
>
> Obstructed labor—failed augmentation
> Abnormal fetal heart rate (FHR) trace
> Abnormal fetal blood sampling
> Breech presentation
> Persistent malpresentation other than breech
> Nonengaged fetal head
> Multiple gestation pregnancy
> Suspected intrauterine growth retardation
> Fetal macrosomia
> Vaginal birth after cesarean section
> Suspected cephalopelvic disproportion
> Obesity

---

provided inadequate anesthesia for cesarean delivery in 18.2% of patients.[145] Preston reported that 5% of functioning labor epidural blocks could not be extended to provide adequate anesthesia for cesarean delivery.[146] Many of the blocks performed in the latter two series were performed by residents and fellows, and these failure rates will be influenced by the experience of the anesthesiologist. Subarachnoid block is associated with significantly lower failure rates when compared with epidural anesthesia.

There should be an attempt to distinguish those nonelective cesarean deliveries that are not urgent from those that are urgent and those that are truly emergent. For the latter two categories (urgent and emergent) the distinction will be influenced not only by maternal and fetal factors but also the experience and interaction of the obstetrician and anesthesiologist. Nonurgent, nonelective cesarean sections would include presentations such as: the primiparous patient with a fetus in breech presentation, scheduled for elective cesarean section, who presents in early labor before the scheduled date for delivery; or a mother in failed (obstructed) labor, without evidence of significant maternal or fetal compromise. In these scenarios, a full assessment of the maternal-infant pair is in order, and, in most instances, regional anesthesia can be offered and provided for operative delivery. Elective induction of general anesthesia may be considered for those patients desiring it, provided that the airway assessment reveals a low probability of difficult intubation and no other contraindication against general anesthesia. More urgent scenarios could include: fetal heart rate (FHR) traces with persistent deceleration patterns but with intact FHR variability, or limited antepartum hemorrhage with no evident maternal or fetal compromise. Again, there is time for a complete maternal-fetal assessment, determination of risk, and establishment of a management plan. Regional anesthesia or general anesthesia may be offered. The crash section, with the implication of the emergency induction of general anesthesia in a parturient who may not have been optimally assessed, should be reserved for fetal-maternal conditions that are so grievous that any delay to achieve delivery may result in mortality or very significant morbidity. These scenarios are discussed subsequently.

D. EMERGENCY CESAREAN SECTION FOR FETAL DISTRESS

The normal FHR pattern has a baseline heart rate of 120 to 160 beats/min. Heart rates below 120 beats/min are arbitrarily deemed to be bradycardia, and those above 160, tachycardia. The duration of bradycardia and its depth is proportional to the duration and severity of the asphyxial insult to the fetus. Bradycardia between 100 and 120 beats/min with normal variability is generally well tolerated. Rates of 80 to 100 beats/min, again with preserved variability, can be managed conservatively. Rates below 80 and especially below 60 beats/min represent obstetric emergencies that necessitate immediate delivery. Tachycardia is caused by a large number of maternal and fetal conditions, the most common of which is maternal fever in the former and is nonspecific with respect to the latter.[147,148] If variability is preserved and tachycardia is the isolated finding, it is felt by many authors to be well tolerated by the fetus.[149,150] FHR variability is represented by the variation in the FHR and is classified as either short term or long term. The presence of normal FHR variability is almost invariably associated with fetal vigor at birth.[151] If the FHR demonstrates normal variability, the fetus is at low risk for immediate morbidity from asphyxia, even in the presence of decelerations and bradycardia. A decrease or loss of variability in the presence of these patterns is a sign that the physiologic compensations available to the fetus are being overwhelmed as a result of the severity of asphyxia. Fetal distress as applied to interpretation of FHR traces is a widely used but poorly defined term. This confusion of definition compounds the difficulty of making an accurate diagnosis and initiating appropriate treatment. A normal FHR recording correctly predicts a healthy newborn in 95% of cases, yet the predictive value of tracings defined as pathologic lacks diagnostic specificity: in 50% of cases, fetal distress is diagnosed in a completely healthy fetus.[148] This fact should be balanced against the maternal risks inherent in the emergency cesarean section done for fetal distress.

The most common asphyxial stresses imposed on the fetus during labor are inadequate uterine blood flow, insufficient umbilical blood flow, and, more rarely, a decrease in uterine arterial oxygenation. Each of these stresses produce characteristic fetal heart rate patterns: late decelerations, variable decelerations, or prolonged bradycardia. Late decelerations mirror the contraction, with the onset, nadir, and recovery delayed 10 to 30 seconds after the similar features of the contraction. They are seen when an acute insult such as maternal hypotension is imposed on a previously normoxic fetus. Contractions superimposed on this new insult result in transient decreases in uterine blood flow sufficient to result in relative fetal hypoxemia. Between contractions, the FHR is normal and variability is maintained. Late decelerations may also be evident in the absence of variability. This characteristic of absent variability concurrent with late decelerations suggests fetal decompensation. Efforts made to abolish late decelerations when variability is maintained by optimizing placental blood flow (correcting hypotension) or inducing maternal hyperoxia are generally successful in abolishing the decelerations. Late decelerations occurring in the absence of variability are generally more persistent and often do not respond to efforts made to abolish them, and early delivery is recommended. Variable decelerations are characterized by a duration and magnitude of dip in the FHR that varies from deceleration to deceleration and with an abrupt onset and cessation. They are described as severe when the dip is more than 60 beats below baseline, when the dip is to 60 beats/min or less, and when the deceleration lasts more than 60 seconds (Rule of 60s). If variability is evident on the FHR trace, it is likely that the fetus is compensated. Vigorous efforts should be made to eliminate severe variable decelerations, since placental function and fetal condition will eventually deteriorate. Mild (decrease of 20 to 30 beats/min persisting for 30 sec or less) to moderate (30 to 60 beats/min drop lasting 60 sec or less) decelerations are better tolerated for prolonged periods, whereas severe decelerations are rarely tolerated for more than 30 minutes.[150] Should operative delivery be deemed necessary, the presence of persistent FHR variability implies that sufficient time exists for both careful maternal assessment and regional anesthesia. Absent variability and severe decelerations (either late or variable type) imply poor fetal condition, and rapid delivery is mandated. However, there is time for assessment of the maternal airway, and, if difficulty is anticipated, regional anesthesia or awake intubation is recommended. Subarachnoid anesthesia is an appropriate option if maternal assessment suggests that maternal airway difficulties are probable in the setting of fetal distress.[152,153] Rapid induction of general anesthesia is an alternative option if maternal assessment is consistent with no anticipated airway difficulties.

The severity of the FHR abnormality should be considered when the urgency of the delivery and the type of anesthesia to be administered are determined. Cesarean deliveries that are performed for a nonreassuring fetal heart pattern do not necessarily preclude the use of regional anesthesia, a conclusion recently endorsed by the American College of Obstetricians and Gynecologists[153] (Appendix). Emergency induction of general anesthesia for nonreassuring fetal heart pattern ("fetal distress") should be reserved for those situations where it is likely that the fetus is at risk of imminent asphyxial morbidity or mortality. These situations could include acute, severe bradycardia, persistent below 80 beats/min, or severe, deep, and prolonged decelerations, either late or variable, with absent FHR variability. In these instances, it is likely that general anesthesia will often result in a more rapid delivery of the fetus. However, if it is recognized that the airway is likely to be difficult, regional anesthesia is not contraindicated, and subarachnoid anesthesia, in particular, is to be recommended. If the trachea cannot be intubated once general anesthesia has been induced, alternative methods of airway management should be employed to effect prompt delivery of the infant in this setting. If the airway cannot be controlled despite multiple attempts, consideration should be given to waking the mother up and proceeding with regional anesthesia, despite the apparent fetal compromise.

E. MATERNAL HEMORRHAGIC EMERGENCIES

Obstetric hemorrhage as a cause of maternal death remains prominent in the majority of mortality reports.[1,4] The most common causes of maternal hemorrhage include placenta previa, abruptio placentae, placenta accreta, and uterine rupture.[154] Placenta previa is defined as a placenta implanted in the lower uterine segment with varying degrees of encroachment on the internal cervical os. The primary presenting complaint is painless vaginal bleeding with the initial bleed usually being self-limited and rarely fatal. However, 10% to 25% of parturients with placenta previa develop hypovolemic shock, and shock is more common in patients with total previa.[155,156] Abruptio placentae is defined as the separation of all or part of the normally implanted placentae after the twentieth week of gestation and before the birth of the fetus. The presentation and clinical manifestations of abruptio placentae depend primarily on the degree of placental separation and the amount of hemorrhage. Uterine rupture may occur spontaneously in a uterus with no scars but is more commonly manifest as scar separation through a previous cesarean scar. The rupture may be initially silent, but severe abdominal pain, maternal shock, and fetal distress or demise often result. Emergent cesarean section may be required to obtain fetal or maternal salvage in these hemorrhagic syndromes. General anesthesia is often mandated for management as maternal hemodynamic instability, hypovolemic shock, clotting abnormalities, or severe fetal compromise may all contraindicate regional anesthesia. Provided that an airway may be

obtained after failed intubation, general anesthesia should be continued, the fetus delivered, and the hemorrhagic condition surgically ablated. A second, experienced anesthesiologist should be summoned to assist with patient care as the primary physician is likely to be well occupied with the airway. Regional anesthesia may be employed for delivery in parturients with abruptio placentae or placenta previa when there is limited hemorrhage without evidence of significant ongoing loss and no maternal hemodynamic instability. In these instances, the fetus is usually not compromised.

Retained or adherent placenta is a common early postpartum complication. The intravenous administration of nitroglycerin may allow for spontaneous or assisted removal of a placenta trapped by a closed cervix but will often be ineffective for adherent placenta.[157] If bleeding is limited and the mother is stable hemodynamically, spinal saddle block provides good conditions for assisted removal. Conscious sedation and analgesia using nitrous oxide supplemented with intravenous narcotics (fentanyl 1-2 μ/kg^{-1}) and low-dose ketamine (0.25 mg/kg^{-1}) incrementally provide good conditions for manual removal and uterine curettage. A patient and gentle obstetrician and an encouraging anesthesiologist do much to complement this technique. In the event that hemorrhage has been considerable and is persistent, ketamine induction of general anesthesia may be lifesaving. Again, provided that an airway can be maintained after failed intubation, general anesthesia should be continued and the uterus evacuated. A second anesthesiologist is again invaluable in this setting and should be summoned immediately once failed intubation is recognized.

F. AIRWAY MANAGEMENT DURING EMERGENT VAGINAL DELIVERY

There are a number of obstetric scenarios for which there will be an immediate requirement for vaginal delivery. The most commonly encountered situation is that of severe fetal decompensation as manifest by FHR abnormalities, usually severe decelerations. These are often a result of head compression as the fetus negotiates the terminal portion of the passageway. In many instances, a saddle block or a pudendal block with perineal infiltration will allow for forceps extraction. If there are any concerns about the maternal airway, this management scheme is encouraged. Incremental low-dose ketamine or fentanyl supplementation may be used. Less commonly, immediate induction of general anesthesia will be required to effect vaginal delivery. An assessment of the maternal airway must precede induction. If there is concern about difficult intubation, general anesthesia should be avoided. In the event that intubation is difficult or impossible once general anesthesia has been established, the patient should be managed as would be the patient presenting for emergent cesarean section. That is, the airway should be controlled and protected, and the delivery effected.

Shoulder dystocia and a trapped after-coming head during breech delivery are two less commonly encountered situations requiring immediate vaginal delivery. Because of the nature of the occurrence and the urgency of the situation, general anesthesia is almost always required to effect delivery. An intravenous bolus of nitroglycerin will sometimes provide sufficient uterine relaxation to release the trapped breech head and may be administered as the patient is prepared for general anesthesia. If airway assessment suggests the likelihood of difficult intubation, turning the patient into the lateral position and performing a subarachnoid block represents the best alternative. The situation otherwise should be managed as would the emergency cesarean section. Failure of a second twin to deliver after the uneventful delivery of the first or the acute deterioration in the condition of the second twin may also prompt a request for immediate induction of anesthesia to allow for delivery, either vaginal or abdominal. Ideally, this scenario is anticipated, and an epidural catheter is both placed and activated. However, it may happen that the mother presents to hospital already having delivered the first infant or delivers precipitously soon after admission, with no time available to establish epidural anesthesia. Electronic FHR monitoring should be initiated and may provide reassurance as to the condition of the fetus. Concurrent with the initiation of the FHR monitoring, an evaluation of the maternal airway must be made. If the maternal airway is suspect, subarachnoid anesthesia remains the technique of choice to allow for prompt delivery. If there are no concerns about the maternal airway, general anesthesia remains a prudent choice. Should general anesthesia be induced and the intubation cannot be achieved, the ability to manage the airway and the condition of the fetus will determine the next step.[40]

G. AIRWAY MANAGEMENT FOR THE MORBIDLY OBESE PARTURIENT

Morbidly obese parturients experience more antenatal medical complications and are more likely to be delivered by cesarean section than are nonobese parturients.[23,107] Intrapartum complications occur more frequently in obese patients; thus, the likelihood of an urgent or emergent cesarean section is also greater.[23] Morbid obesity is implicated as a risk factor for maternal mortality, and it is likely that both antepartum and intrapartum factors figure in the deaths.[1,143,158] Expiratory reserve volume, functional residual capacity, and residual volume are all decreased in obesity and further decreased in pregnancy.[23] The resultant decreased alveolar size reduces lung compliance and shunts ventilation to the nondependent, more compliant portions of the lung. Obese patients tend to breathe at smaller tidal volumes and faster respiratory rates. The smaller tidal volumes tend to exaggerate this shift in ventilation away from the more dependent, well-perfused portions of the lungs.[23] Ventilation-perfusion mismatch results, and maternal Pao_2 is reduced in the obese parturient compared with nonobese mothers.[159,160] There is a greater tendency to hypoxemia in the obese parturient, and the supine position exaggerates the hypoxemia. Morbidly obese parturients are more likely to become hypoxemic during induction of general anesthesia, and, if intubation is delayed, severe hypoxemia will result. Although there is a correlation between increasing weight or body mass index and difficult intubation, obesity alone is not a strong predictor of difficult intubation.[12,104,106] It is likely that the same anatomic changes that make intubation more difficult in pregnancy are responsible for the same outcome in obesity and that the combination of the two compound the effect. In addition, the morbidly obese have redundant palatal and pharyngeal tissues that compromise mask ventilation, laryngoscopy, and intubation. It is more difficult to determine accurate landmarks on the thick, obesity-foreshortened neck, and misapplied cricoid pressure may permit gastric insufflation; regurgitation and compromising laryngoscopy and intubation. Further, it may be more difficult to achieve mask ventilation with higher airway pressures being required. Gastric insufflation results, and there is an increased risk for pulmonary aspiration.

Airway assessment of all laboring morbidly obese parturients is recommended early in the labor. The use of regional anesthesia is encouraged for both the provision of labor analgesia and anesthesia for operative delivery. If general anesthesia is to be employed in the morbidly obese parturient, consideration can be given to awake intubation, especially if other characteristics of the maternal airway enhance the possibility of difficult intubation. (I do not consider morbid obesity alone to be an indication for routine awake intubation.) Positioning is all important to optimize the conditions for laryngoscopy and intubation in the morbidly obese patient.[17] Three to 5 minutes of preoxygenation is recommended. It is often difficult to achieve adequate response to peripheral nerve stimulation in the morbidly obese parturient, and I perform laryngoscopy at 45-seconds elapsed time after administration of the succinylcholine. A failed first attempt at intubation should prompt immediate consideration of awakening the patient.

H. THE ROLE OF THE LARYNGEAL MASK AIRWAY IN THE FAILED INTUBATION DRILL

The laryngeal mask airway (LMA) is a novel device recently introduced into anesthetic practice.[161] A full discussion of LMA can be found in Chapter 19. The LMA is inserted blindly into the pharynx and forms a low-pressure seal around the laryngeal inlet. It is easily placed, and a clear, unobstructed airway may be obtained in virtually all patients, even when used by physicians with little or no prior experience.[162] Insertion of the LMA is not more difficult in patients with class III or IV airways or in those patients in whom laryngoscopy reveals grades 3 or 4 views.[163] The airway is occasionally completely or partially obstructed after placement of the LMA, and this is usually related to downfolding of the epiglottis or infolding of the aryepiglottic folds.[164] The most outstanding feature of the LMA is its ability to rapidly provide a clear airway, and there are now numerous reports of the LMA relieving hypoxia after failed intubation and ventilation in obstetric anesthesia.[165-170] It has also been utilized in parturients who could not be intubated but whose airways could be managed with face-mask anesthesia.[171,172] This latter application has generated much controversy for two reasons, in particular. First, there is evidence that the LMA is more likely to promote gastric regurgitation when compared to face-mask anesthesia.[173,174] The LMA results in a decrease in the LES barrier pressure in anesthetized, spontaneously breathing patients compared with a face mask that promotes an increase in barrier pressure. The postulated mechanism is that the LMA causes reflex relaxation of the LES by distention of the hypopharyngeal muscles, similar to the effect of a food bolus. Although El Mikatti did not find an increased incidence of regurgitation in patients managed with an LMA compared with face-mask anesthesia, it was commented that two LMA patients not included in the study analysis had signs of regurgitation after vigorous coughing during light anesthesia.[175] There were no similar events in the patients managed with a face mask. Second, it has been suggested that the inflated cuff of the LMA may prevent escape of regurgitated material into the pharynx and deflect it instead into the airway.[176] This effect would diminish or negate the protective effect of the left lateral position during a failed intubation drill.

When the patients' lungs can be ventilated adequately with a face mask after failed intubation, the LMA confers no advantage and may, in fact, promote gastric regurgitation. The liberal use of an LMA in this scenario has been discouraged.[177] The airway should be maintained with a face mask, and cricoid pressure and spontaneous ventilation should be allowed to resume. Once spontaneous ventilation has returned through an open airway, there again would be little advantage to be gained by passing an LMA.[178] When adequate ventilation cannot be maintained after failed intubation, the LMA could be tried. An attempt to pass it should be made early in the course of management, after it has

been determined that intubation is impossible and ventilation is difficult or impossible with the face mask. The laryngeal reflexes are likely still to be blunted by the residual effects of the anesthetic induction, and the patient is less likely to respond unfavorably to airway placement if it is attempted early.[162] The stimulation related to passage of a laryngeal mask is approximately the same as that for an oropharyngeal airway.[179] Because there should be less gastric distention if there have not been persistent and forceful attempts to ventilate a patient with an obstructed airway, the risk of regurgitation may be reduced.[76]

Whether or not cricoid pressure should be released during insertion of the LMA is controversial, but it is reasonable and prudent to do so for brief periods to assess the result on laryngoscopy, intubation, and ventilation. The presence of the LMA does not appear to compromise effective application of cricoid pressure, although cricoid pressure may make the insertion of the LMA more difficult.[180-183] The likelihood of successful placement of the LMA so that effective ventilation can be established is reduced by the application of cricoid pressure. It is also more difficult to pass an endotracheal tube through the LMA and into the trachea, both blindly and assisted by a fiberoptic scope, with cricoid pressure applied.[181,184] Cricoid pressure causes an anterior tilt to the larynx, and this is likely the cause of difficulty in intubating the trachea.[184] The anterior angulation of the larynx may also result in closure of the vocal cords and airway obstruction, and, although this has been reported, it is presumably rare.[185] The LMA is not an alternative to the endotracheal tube in obstetric anesthesia. Rather, it should be considered an alternative to the face mask when it is not possible to ventilate and oxygenate a parturient through a face mask after failed intubation.[186] After this determination has been made, an attempt to pass the LMA should be made early, with cricoid pressure maintained. If it is not possible to pass the LMA with cricoid pressure maintained, the pressure should be briefly released, a second pass made, and the cricoid pressure reapplied. Again, if it is not possible to establish an open airway, the LMA should be removed and the face mask reapplied with cricoid pressure now released. An attempt to ventilate the patient without cricoid pressure can now be made, and consideration should be given to the use of either a Combitube or surgical airway depending upon the success achieved with the face mask and the obstetric circumstances.

If ventilation is reestablished with the LMA, the mother should be allowed to awaken. The option to wake the patient should only be excluded by the urgency to proceed for fetal or maternal welfare. In this circumstance, general anesthesia may be provided via the LMA, with cricoid pressure maintained and the mother breathing spontaneously. Other factors, such as the mother's preoperative reluctance to undergo elective cesarean delivery with regional anesthesia, should in no way compel the anesthesiologist to carry on with general anesthesia with a controlled but unprotected airway. Once the airway has been opened with the LMA and the decision made to proceed with general anesthesia for cesarean delivery because of compelling maternal or fetal factors, it is controversial whether further steps should be taken to protect the airway. Intubation through the LMA with a small gauge (6.0 mm) endotracheal tube, both blind or assisted with a bougie, tube changer, or fiberoptic scope have all been described.[167,181,187,188] Such interventions are compromised by the maintenance of cricoid pressure, and it is difficult to justify release of the pressure if an adequate airway has already been achieved with the LMA and the airway is protected by cricoid pressure. Clearly, if not readily successful, attempts to pass an endotracheal tube should not be persistent, given that an adequate airway has already been established with the LMA.

If it is not possible to open the airway with the LMA, consideration should be given to the use of the Combitube, transtracheal oxygenation, or the creation of a surgical airway. Recent published commentary supports the use of the LMA prior to creation of a surgical airway in the cannot-intubate-cannot-ventilate situation.[189,190]

I. THE ROLE OF THE COMBITUBE IN THE FAILED INTUBATION DRILL

The Combitube (Sheridan Catheter Corporation, Argyle, N.Y.) is a new emergency airway, which can be used in the esophageal as well as tracheal positions.[191-193] A full discussion on the Combitube can be found in Chapter 22. It is a double-lumen tube, combining the function of an esophageal obturator airway and a conventional endotracheal airway. The esophageal lumen has an open upper end, perforations at the pharyngeal level, and a closed distal end. The tracheal lumen has open proximal and distal ends. The lumens are separated by a partitioning wall, and each lumen is linked via a short tube with a connector. An oropharyngeal balloon is situated proximal to the pharyngeal perforations, and it serves to seal the oral and nasal cavities after insertion. At the lower end, a second cuff serves to seal either the trachea or esophagus. To place the tube, the lower jaw and tongue are lifted, and the tube is inserted until the printed ring marks lie between the teeth or alveolar ridges. The oropharyngeal balloon is inflated with 100 ml of air and the distal balloon with 10 to 15 ml of air. There is an expectation of esophageal placement with blind insertion, and ventilation begins through the esophageal lumen. Auscultation of breath sounds over the chest and confirmation of expired carbon dioxide confirms ventilation. In the event of negative auscultation over the lungs, the Combitube has been placed in the trachea, and ventilation is carried out through the tracheal lumen.

Although experience with the Combitube is limited and its use in obstetric anesthesia has yet to be reported, it is clearly an alternative to the LMA in the parturient in whom intubation has failed and ventilation is difficult. It can be placed quickly and allows for protection of the airway, thus preventing aspiration. It probably offers a greater degree of airway protection than does the LMA, although the two have not been formally compared.[194,195] The stomach can be evacuated, usually through the tracheal lumen. Cricoid pressure would have to be released transiently to allow for placement of the Combitube, and the airway would be at risk from aspiration during the brief period before cuff inflation.

The Combitube has evolved from the esophageal obturator and esophageal gastric airways. Both had been criticized because of difficulty in obtaining effective ventilation, the potential for esophageal trauma on insertion, aspiration on removal, and inadvertent tracheal placement resulting in total airway obstruction. Despite these limitations, failed intubation in obstetric anesthesia was considered by Tunstall an indication for their use.[136] The Combitube is indicated in a similar fashion in the failed intubation drill.

V. CONCLUSION

Muir recently posed the question: "Is general anesthesia for obstetric patients obsolete?"[196] In response to her own query, she notes that, although uncommonly used in academic centers, general anesthesia remains a widely employed technique for operative delivery, including elective cesarean section. General anesthesia may be induced rapidly, provides reliably good operative conditions, maintains hemodynamic stability, and usually renders the patient unaware. Further, there remain situations in obstetric anesthesia for which general anesthesia represents the anesthetic technique of choice and many more for which it is an ideal choice, though not exclusively so. General anesthesia continues to be a useful, occasionally lifesaving (fetal and maternal) technique that will occupy the anesthetic landscape for the foreseeable future. The major limitation to the use of general anesthesia is the requirement to control the airway and protect it from the threat of acid aspiration. Rapid sequence induction, cricoid pressure, and endotracheal intubation are the mechanisms usually employed to achieve these goals. However, it must be recognized that the appropriate end points are controlling and protecting the airway and ensuring maternal oxygenation and not necessarily achieving endotracheal intubation. These goals can be achieved through a variety of techniques and modalities, some recently introduced to anesthesia. The safety of general anesthesia will be enhanced with assessment of at-risk patients by obstetricians and appropriate referral for anesthetic consultation, routine preoperative (elective and emergent situations) maternal airway assessments, strict avoidance of general anesthesia when the airway is deemed to be difficult, automatic implementation of a practiced-failed intubation drill when intubation difficulties become manifest, and ensuring physician familiarity with new and novel equipment designed to aid in the management of the difficult airway. Such cooperative management schemes are effective in identifying at-risk patients and will be instrumental in reducing maternal morbidity and mortality in the future.

VI. ADDENDUM

After this chapter had been submitted for publication, the Report on Confidential Enquiries into Maternal Mortalities in the United Kingdom 1988-90 was released. The relevant findings of this report are briefly summarized as follows.*

There has been a leveling since 1985 of the previous downward trend in the maternal mortality rate. Maternal deaths due to hemorrhage and sepsis have increased, and the number resulting from hypertensive disorders, thrombosis, and thromboembolism has not changed. However, it is rewarding to note that deaths directly attributable to anesthesia continue to decline, in absolute numbers, as a percentage of all direct maternal deaths (2.7%) and when expressed as a rate per million pregnancies (1.7 deaths per million pregnancies). In the last triennium, there were no direct maternal deaths resulting from either failed intubation or esophageal intubation, although gastric aspiration continues to figure prominently in maternal deaths. Inadequate postoperative care and a lack of direct supervision of inexperienced junior staff by consultants were cited as important factors contributing to both substandard care and maternal mortality.

VII. APPENDIX: ANESTHESIA FOR EMERGENCY DELIVERIES

Failed intubation and pulmonary aspiration of gastric contents continue to be leading causes of maternal morbidity and mortality from anesthesia. The risk of these complications can be reduced by careful antepartum assessment to identify patients at risk, greater use of regional anesthesia when possible, and appropriate selection and preparation of patients who require general anesthesia for delivery.

A. ANTEPARTUM RISK MANAGEMENT

The obstetric care team should be alert to the presence of risk factors that place the parturient at increased risk for complications from emergency general or regional anesthesia. These factors include, but are not limited to, marked obesity,

severe facial and neck edema, extremely short stature, a short neck, difficulty opening the mouth, a small mandible, protuberant teeth, arthritis of the neck, anatomic abnormalities of the face or mouth, a large thyroid, asthma, serious medical or obstetric complications, and a history of problems with anesthetics.

When such risk factors are identified, a physician who is credentialed to provide general and regional anesthesia should be consulted in the antepartum period to allow for joint development of a plan of management including optimal location for delivery. Strategies thereby can be developed to minimize the need for emergency induction of general anesthesia in women for whom this would be especially hazardous. For those patients at risk, consideration should be given to the planned placement in early labor of an intravenous line and an epidural or spinal catheter, with confirmation that the catheter is functional. If a patient at unusual risk of complications from anesthesia is identified (e.g., prior failed intubation), strong consideration should be given to antepartum referral of the patient to allow for delivery at a hospital that can manage such anesthesia on a 24-hour basis.

B. EMERGENCY ANESTHESIA

The need for expeditious abdominal delivery cannot always be anticipated. When preparing for the rapid initiation of anesthesia, the maternal and the fetal status must be considered. Oral nonparticulate antacids should be administered immediately prior to the induction of general or major regional anesthesia to decrease the mother's risk of developing aspiration pneumonitis.

Although there are some situations in which general anesthesia is preferable to regional anesthesia, the risk of general anesthesia must be weighed against the benefit for those patients who have a greater potential for complications. Examples of circumstances in which a rapid induction of general anesthesia may be indicated include prolapsed umbilical cord with severe fetal bradycardia and active hemorrhage in a hemodynamically unstable mother.

In some cases, a nonreassuring FHR pattern is diagnosed as "fetal distress," and delivery is performed immediately. The term *fetal distress* is imprecise, nonspecific, and has little positive predictive value. The severity of the fetal heart rate abnormality should be considered when the urgency of the delivery and the type of anesthesia to be administered are determined. Cesarean deliveries that are performed for a nonreassuring FHR pattern do not necessarily preclude the use of regional anesthesia.

From American College of Obstetricians and Gynecologists: Committee Opinion No. 104, Washington, D.C., 1992, ACOG. Reprinted with permission.

REFERENCES

1. Report on confidential enquiries into maternal deaths in the United Kingdom 1985-87, London 1991, Her Majesty's Stationery Office.
2. Report on confidential enquiries into maternal deaths in England and Wales 1982-84, London 1989, Her Majesty's Stationery Office.
3. Morgan M: Anaesthetic contribution to maternal mortality, *Br J Anaesth* 59:842, 1987.
4. Rochat RW, Koonin LM, Atrash HK et al: Maternal mortality in

*Report on confidential enquiries into maternal mortalities in the United Kingdom 1988-90, London, 1994, Her Majesty's Stationery Office.

the United States: report from the maternal mortality collaborative, *Obstet Gynecol* 72:91, 1989.

5. Rubin G, McCarthy B, Shelton J et al: The risk of childbearing re-evaluated, *Am J Public Health* 71:712, 1981.

6. Kaunitz AM, Hughes JM, Grimes DA et al: Causes of maternal mortality in the United States, *Am J Obstet Gynecol* 65:605, 1985.

7. Friede AM, Rochat RW: Maternal mortality and perinatal mortality: an epidemiologic perspective. In Sachs B, editor: Clinical obstetrics: a public health perspective, Littleton, Mass., 1986, PSG.

8. Sachs BP, Yey J, Acker D et al: Cesarean section-related maternal mortality in Massachusetts, 1954-85, *Obstet Gynecol* 71:385, 1988.

9. Chadwick HS, Posner K, Ward RJ et al: A review of obstetric anesthesia malpractice claims, *Anesthesiology* 71:A942, 1989.

10. Cormack RS, Lehane J: Difficult tracheal intubation in obstetrics, *Anaesthesia* 34:1105, 1984.

11. Caplan RA, Benumof JL, Berry FA et al: Practice guidelines for management of the difficult airway. A report by the American Society of Anesthesiologists Task Force on Management of the Difficult Airway, *Anesthesiology* 78:597, 1993.

12. Rocke DA, Murray WB, Rout CC et al: Relative risk analysis of factors associated with difficult intubation in obstetric anesthesia, *Anesthesiology* 77:63, 1992.

13. Rose DK, Cohen MM: The airway: problems and predictions in 18,500 patients, *Can J Anaesth* 41:372, 1994.

14. Benumof JL: Difficult laryngoscopy: obtaining the best view, *Can J Anaesth* 41:361, 1994.

15. Hood DD, Dewan DM: Obstetric anesthesia. In Brown DL, editor: *Risk and outcome in anesthesia,* ed 2, Philadelphia, 1992, JB Lippincott.

16. Hogberg U: Maternal deaths in Sweden, 1971-80, *Acta Obstet Gynecol Scand* 65:161, 1986.

17. Davies JM, Weeks S, Crone LA et al: Difficult intubation in the parturient, *Can J Anaesth* 36:668, 1989.

18. Lyons G: Failed intubation: six years' experience in a teaching maternity unit, *Anaesthesia* 40:759, 1985.

19. Lyons G, MacDonald R: Difficult intubation in obstetrics, *Anaesthesia* 40:1016, 1985.

20. Samsoon GLT, Young JRB: Difficult tracheal intubation: a retrospective study, *Anaesthesia* 42:487, 1987.

21. Fahy L, Horton WA, Sprigge JS et al: X-ray laryngoscopy in patients with a history of difficult laryngoscopy during pregnancy, *Br J Anaesth* 62:234P, 1989.

22. Cheek TG, Gutsche BB: Maternal physiologic alterations during pregnancy. In Shnider SM, Levinson G, (editors): *Anesthesia for obstetrics,* ed 3, Baltimore, 1993, Williams and Wilkins.

23. Dewan DM: Anesthesia for the morbidly obese parturient, *Prob Anesth* 3:56, 1989.

24. Kay NH: Mammomegaly and intubation, *Anaesthesia* 37:221, 1982.

25. Sellick BA: Cricoid pressure to control regurgitation of stomach contents during induction of anaesthesia, *Lancet* 2:404, 1961.

26. Brimacombe J: Acute pharyngolaryngeal oedema and pre-eclamptic toxaemia, *Anaesth Intensive Care* 20:97, 1992.

27. Brock-Utne JG, Downing JW, Seedat F: Laryngeal oedema associated with pre-eclamptic toxaemia, *Anaesthesia* 32:556, 1977.

28. Dobb G: Laryngeal oedema complicating obstetric anaesthesia, *Anaesthesia* 33:839, 1978.

29. Ebert RJ: Post partum airway obstruction after vaginal delivery, *Anaesth Intensive Care* 20:365, 1992.

30. Farcon EL, Kim MH, Marx GF: Changing Mallampati score during labour, *Can J Anaesth* 41:50, 1994.

31. Jouppila R, Jouppila P, Hollmén A: Laryngeal oedema as an obstetric anaesthesia complication, *Acta Anaesthesiol Scand* 24:97, 1980.

32. MacKenzie AI: Laryngeal oedema complicating obstetric anaesthesia, *Anaesthesia* 33:271, 1978.

33. Procter AJM, White JB: Laryngeal oedema in pregnancy, *Anaesthesia* 38:167, 1983.

34. Rocke DA, Scoones GP: Rapidly progressive laryngeal oedema associated with pregnancy aggravated hypertension, *Anaesthesia* 47:141, 1992.

35. Salt PJ, Nutbourne PA, Park GR et al: Laryngeal oedema after caesarean section, *Anaesthesia* 38:693, 1983.

36. Seager SJ, MacDonald R: Laryngeal oedema and pre-eclampsia, *Anaesthesia* 35:360, 1980.

37. Spotoft H, Christensen P: Laryngeal oedema accompanying weight gain in pregnancy, *Anaesthesia* 36:71, 1981.

38. Tillmann Hein HA: Cardiorespiratory arrest with laryngeal oedema in pregnancy-induced hypertension, *Can Anaesth Soc J* 31:210, 1984.

39. Crowhurst JA: Failed intubation management at caesarean section, *Anaesth Intensive Care* 19:305, 1991.

40. Malan TP Jr, Johnson MD: The difficult airway in obstetric anesthesia: techniques for airway management and the role of regional anesthesia, *J Clin Anesth* 1:104, 1988.

41. Bevan DR, Holdcroft A, Loh L et al: Closing volume and pregnancy, *BMJ* 1:13, 1974.

42. Awe RJ, Nicotra MB, Newsome TD et al: Arterial oxygenation and alveolar-arterial gradients in term pregnancy, *Obstet Gynecol* 53:182, 1979.

43. Archer GW, Marx GF: Arterial oxygen tension during apnoea in parturient women, *Br J Anaesth* 46:358, 1974.

44. Baraka AS, Hanna MT, Samar SI et al: Proxygenation of pregnant and nonpregnant women in the head-up versus supine position, *Anesth Analg* 75:757, 1992.

45. Morgan M: The confidential enquiry into maternal deaths, *Anaesthesia* 41:689, 1986.

46. Carnie JC, Street MK, Kumar B: Emergency intubation of the trachea facilitated by suxamethonium: observations in obstetric and general surgical patients, *Br J Anaesth* 58:498, 1986.

47. Attia RR, Ebeid AM, Fischer JE et al: Maternal, fetal and placental gastrin concentrations, *Anaesthesia* 37:18, 1982.

48. Christofides ND, Ghatei MA, Bloom SR et al: Decreased plasma motilin concentrations in pregnancy, *BMJ* 285:1453, 1982.

49. Fisher RS, Roberts GS, Grabowski CJ et al: Inhibition of lower esophageal sphincter circular muscle by female sex hormones, *Am J Physiol* 23:E243, 1978.

50. Bruce LA, Behsudi FM: Progesterone effects on three regional gastrointestinal tissues, *Life Sci* 25:729, 1979.

51. Wald A, Van Thiel DH, Hoechspetter L et al: Gastrointestinal transit: the effect of the menstrual cycle, *Gastroenterology* 80:1497, 1981.

52. Sandhar BK, Elliott RH, Windram I et al: Peripartum changes in gastric emptying, *Anaesthesia* 47:196, 1992.

53. O'Sullivan G: Gastric emptying during pregnancy and the puerperium, *Int J Obstet Anesth* 2:216, 1993.

54. Hirschheimer A, January D, Daversa JJ: An x-ray study of gastric function in labor, *Am J Obstet Gynecol* 36:671, 1938.

55. Carp H, Jayaram A, Stoll M: Ultrasound examinations of the stomach contents of parturients, *Anesth Analg* 74:683, 1992.

56. Whitehead EM, Smith M, Dean Y et al: An evaluation of gastric emptying times in pregnancy and the puerperium, *Anaesthesia* 48:53, 1993.

57. James CF, Gibbs CP, Banner T: Postpartum perioperative risk of aspiration pneumonia, *Anesthesiology* 61:756, 1984.

58. Vanner RG, Goodman NW: Gastro-oesophageal reflux in pregnancy at term and after delivery, *Anaesthesia* 44:808, 1989.

59. Hey VMF, Cowley DJ, Ganguli PC et al: Gastro-esophageal reflux in late pregnancy, *Anaesthesia* 32:372, 1977.

60. Bainbridge ET, Temple JG, Nicholas SP et al: Symptomatic

gastro-oesphageal reflux in pregnancy: a comparative study of white Europeans and Asians in Birmingham, *Br J Clin Pract* 37:53, 1983.

61. Vanner RG: Mini-symposium on the gastrointestinal tract and pulmonary aspiration: mechanisms of regurgitation and its prevention with cricoid pressure, *Int J Obstet Anesth* 2:207, 1993.
62. Cheek TG, Gutsche BB: Pulmonary aspiration of gastric contents. In Shnider SM, Levinson G, editors: *Anesthesia for obstetrics,* ed 3, Baltimore, 1993, Williams and Wilkins.
63. Lind JF, Smith A, McIver DR et al: Heartburn in pregnancy: a manometric study, *Can Med Assoc J* 98:571, 1968.
64. Spence AA, Moir DD, Finlay WEI: Observations on intragastric pressure, *Anaesthesia* 22:249, 1967.
65. Brock-Utne JG, Rubin J, Welman S et al: The action of commonly used antiemetics on the lower oesophageal sphincter, *Br J Anaesth* 50:295, 1978.
66. Brock-Utne JG, Rubin J, Welman S et al: The effect of glycopyrrolate (Robinul) on the lower oesophageal sphincter, *Can Anaesth Soc J* 25:144, 1978.
67. Hall AW, Moossa AR, Clark J et al: The effects of premedication drugs on the lower oesophageal high pressure zone and reflux status of rhesus monkeys and man, *Gut* 16:347, 1975.
68. Hey UMF, Ostick DG, Mazumder JK et al: Pethidine, metoclopramide and the gastro-oesophageal sphincter: a study in healthy volunteers, *Anaesthesia* 36:173, 1981.
69. Dow TGB, Brock-Utne JG, Rubin J et al: The effect of atropine on the lower oesophageal sphincter in late pregnancy, *Obstet Gynecol* 51:426, 1978.
70. Kahrilas PJ, Dodds WJ, Dent J et al: Effect of sleep, spontaneous gastroesophageal reflux, and a meal on upper esophageal sphincter pressure in normal human volunteers, *Gastroenterology* 92:466, 1987.
71. Vanner RG: Gastro-oesophageal reflux and regurgitation during general anaesthesia for termination of pregnancy, *Int J Obstet Anesth* 1:123, 1992.
72. Vanner RG, Pryle BJ, O'Dwyer JP et al: Upper oesophageal sphincter pressure and the intravenous induction of anaesthesia, *Anaesthesia* 47:371, 1992.
73. Roe RB: The effect of suxamethonium on intragastric pressure, *Anaesthesia* 17:179, 1962.
74. Clark CG, Riddoch ME: Observations on the human cardia at operation, *Br J Anaesth* 34:75, 1962.
75. Greenan J: The cardio-oesophageal junction, *Br J Anaesth* 33:432, 1961.
76. Ovassapian A: The difficult airway. In Ovassapian A, editor: *Fiberoptic airway endoscopy in anesthesia and critical care,* New York, 1990, Raven Press.
77. Lawes EG, Campbell I, Mercer D: Inflation pressure, gastric insufflation and rapid sequence induction, *Br J Anaesth* 59:315, 1987.
78. Ruben H, Krudsen EJ, Carngati G: Gastric inflation in relation to airway pressure, *Acta Anaesthesiol Scand* 5:107, 1961.
79. Smith G, Dalling R, Williams TIR: Gastroesophageal pressure gradients produced by induction of anaesthesia and suxamethonium, *Br J Anaesth* 50:1137, 1978.
80. Mendelson CL: The aspiration of stomach contents into the lungs during obstetric anesthesia, *Am J Obstet Gynecol* 52:191, 1946.
81. Olsson GL, Hallen B, Hambraeus-Jonzon K: Aspiration during anaesthesia: a computer-aided study of 185,358 anaesthetists, *Acta Anaesthesiol Scand* 30:84, 1986.
82. Sweeney B, Wright I: The use of antacids as a prophylaxis against Mendelson's syndrome in the United Kingdom: a survey, *Anaesthesia* 41:419, 1986.
83. Snow RG, Nunn JF: Induction of anaesthesia in the foot down position for patients with a full stomach, *Br J Anaesth* 31:493, 1959.
84. Hodges RJH, Tunstall ME, Bennett JR: Vomiting and the head-up position, *Br J Anaesth* 32:619, 1960.
85. Sellick BA: Rupture of the oesophagus following cricoid pressure? *Anaesthesia* 37:213, 1982.
86. Whittington RM, Robinson JS, Thompson JM: Fatal aspiration (Mendelson's) syndrome despite antacids and cricoid pressure, *Lancet* 2:228, 1979.
87. Ralph SJ, Wareham CA: Rupture of the oesophagus during cricoid pressure, *Anaesthesia* 46:40, 1991.
88. Forrester PC: Active vomiting during cricoid pressure, *Anaesthesia* 40:388, 1985.
89. Notcutt WG: Rupture of the oesophagus following cricoid pressure? *Anaesthesia* 36:911, 1981.
90. Wraight WJ, Chamney AR, Howells TH: The determination of an effective cricoid pressure, *Anaesthesia* 38:461, 1983.
91. Vanner RG, O'Dwyer JP, Pryle BJ: Upper oesophageal sphincter pressure and the effect of cricoid pressure, *Anaesthesia* 47:95, 1992.
92. Vanner RG: Tolerance of cricoid pressure by conscious volunteers, *Int J Obstet Anesth* 1;195, 1992.
93. Lawes EG, Duncan PW, Bland B et al: The cricoid yoke – a device for providing consistent and reproducible cricoid pressure, *Br J Anaesth* 58:925, 1986.
94. O'Leary SD, Maryniak JK, Tucker JH: Teaching effective cricoid pressure application using a force measuring device, *Can J Anaesth* 41:A5, 1994.
95. Georgescu A, Miller JN, Lecklitner ML: The Sellick maneuver causing complete airway obstruction, *Anesth Analg* 74:457, 1992.
96. Lawes EG: Cricoid pressure with or without the "Cricoid Yoke," *Br J Anaesth* 58:1376, 1986.
97. Howells TH, Chamney AR, Wraight WJ et al: The application of cricoid pressure: an assessment and survey of its practice, *Anaesthesia* 38:457, 1983.
98. Mehta S: Deaths associated with anaesthesia in obstetrics, *Anaesthesia* 36:910, 1981.
99. Baxter AD: Cricoid pressure in the sniffing position, *Anaesthesia* 46:327, 1991.
100. Crowley DS, Giesecke AH: Bimanual cricoid pressure, *Anaesthesia* 45:588, 1990.
101. Crawford JS: The contracricoid cuboid aid to tracheal intubation, *Anaesthesia* 37:345, 1982.
102. Mallampati SR, Gatt SP, Gugino LD et al: A clinical sign to predict difficult tracheal intubation: a prospective study, *Can Anaesth Soc J* 32:429, 1985.
103. Tham EJ, Gildersleve CD, Sanders LD et al: Effects of posture, phonation and observer on Mallampati classification, *Br J Anaesth* 62:32, 1992.
104. Wilson ME, Spiegelhalter D, Robertson JA et al: Predicting difficult intubation, *Br J Anaesth* 61:211, 1988.
105. Bond A: Obesity and difficult intubation, *Anaesth Intensive Care* 21:828, 1993.
106. Dupont X, Hamza J, Jullien P et al: Risk factors associated with difficult airway in normotensive parturients, *Anesthesiology* 73:A998, 1990.
107. Garbaciak J, Richter M, Miller S et al: Maternal weight and pregnancy complications, *Am J Obstet Gynecol* 152:238, 1985.
108. Williamson JA, Webb, RK, Szekely S et al: Difficult intubation: an analysis of 2000 incident reports, *Anaesth Intensive Care* 21:602, 1993.
109. Williamson JA, Runciman WB: Difficult intubation, *Br J Anaesth* 72:366, 1994.
110. Chow FL, Duncan PG, Code WE: Can bedside neck extension predict difficult intubation? *Can J Anaesth* 40:A4, 1993.
111. Tordoff SG, Sweeney BP: Acid aspiration prophylaxis in 288 obstetric anaesthetic departments in the United Kingdom, *Anaesthesia* 45:776, 1990.

112. Viegas OJ, Ravindran RS, Schumacker CA: Gastric fluid pH in patients receiving sodium citrate, *Anesth Analg* 60:521, 1981.

113. Gibbs CP, Banner TC: Effectiveness of Bicitra as a preoperative antacid, *Anesthesiology* 61:97, 1984.

114. Viegas OJ, Ravindram RS, Stoops CA: Duration of action of sodium citrate as an antacid, *Anesth Analg* 61:624, 1982.

115. Colman RD, Frank M, Loughnan BA et al: Use of IM ranitidine for the prophylaxis of aspiration pneumonitis in obstetrics, *Br J Anaesth* 61:720, 1988.

116. Rout CC, Rocke DA, Gouws E: Intravenous ranitidine reduces the risk of acid aspiration of gastric contents at emergency cesarean section, *Anesth Analg* 73:156, 1993.

117. Ormezzano X, Francois TP, Viaud JY et al: Aspiration pneumonitis prophylaxis in obstetric anesthesia: comparison of effervescent-sodium citrate mixture and sodium citrate, *Br J Anaesth* 64:503, 1990.

118. Ewart MC, Yau G, Gin T et al: A comparison of the effects of omeprazole and ranitidine on gastric secretion in women undergoing elective caesarean section, *Anaesthesia* 45:527, 1990.

119. Rocke DA, Rout CC, Gouws E: Intravenous administration of the proton pump inhibitor omeprazole reduces the risk of acid aspiration at emergency cesarean section, *Anesth Analg* 78:1093, 1994.

120. Cohen SE, Jasson J, Talafre ML et al: Does metoclopramide decrease the volume of gastric contents in patients undergoing cesarean section? *Anesthesiology* 61:604, 1984.

121. Howard FA, Sharp DS: Effect of metoclopramide on gastric emptying during labour, *BMJ* i:446, 1973.

122. McCammon RL: The role of antacids, histamine H2 receptor blockers, and metoclopramide in the prophylaxis of aspiration, *Sem Anesth* 7:192, 1988.

123. Murphy DF, Nally B, Gardiner J et al: Effect of metoclopramide on gastric emptying before elective and emergency caesarean section, *Br J Anaesth* 56:1113, 1984.

124. Datta S, Briwa J: Modified laryngoscope for endotracheal intubation of obese patients, *Anesth Analg* 60:120, 1981.

125. Byrne F, Odeno-Dominah A, Kipling R: The effect of pregnancy on pulmonary nitrogen washout: a study of preoxygenation, *Anaesthesia* 42:148, 1987.

126. Norris MC, Kirkland MR, Torjman MC et al: Denitrogenation in pregnancy, *Can J Anaesth* 36:523, 1989.

127. Russell GN, Smith CL, Snowden SL et al: Preoxygenation and the parturient patient, *Anaesthesia* 42:346, 1987.

128. Clapp JF III: Oxygen consumption during treadmill exercise before, during and after pregnancy, *Am J Obstet Gynecol* 161:1458, 1989.

129. McMurray RG, Katz VL, Berry MJ et al: The effect of pregnancy on metabolic responses during rest, immersion and aerobic exercise in the water, *Am J Obstet Gynecol* 158:481, 1988.

130. Archer GW Jr, Marx GF: Arterial oxygen tension during apnoea in parturient women, *Br J Anaesth* 46:358, 1974.

131. Norris MC, Dewan DM: Preoxygenation for cesarean section: a comparison of two techniques, *Anesthesiology* 62:827, 1985.

132. Gamber AM, Hertzka RE, Fisher DM: Preoxygenation techniques: comparison of three minutes and four breaths, *Anesth Analg* 66:468, 1987.

133. Saddler JM, Bevan JC, Plumley MH et al: Jaw tension after succinylcholine in children undergoing strabismus surgery, *Can J Anaesth* 37:21, 1990.

134. Hawkins JL, Johnson TD, Kubicek MA et al: Vecuronium for rapid-sequence intubation for cesarean section, *Anesth Analg* 71:185, 1990.

135. Tunstall ME: Failed intubation drill, *Anaesthesia* 31:850, 1976.

136. Tunstall ME, Sheikh A: Failed intubation protocol: oxygenation without aspiration, *Clin Anesth* 4:171, 1986.

137. Tunstall ME, Geddes C: Failed intubation in obstetric anaesthesia: an indication for use of the "esophageal gastric tube airway," *Br J Anaesth* 56:659, 1984.

138. Hewett E, Livingstone P: Management of failed endotracheal intubation at caesarean section, *Anaesth Intensive Care* 18:330, 1990.

139. Lawlor M, Johnson C, Weiner M: Airway management in obstetric anesthesia, *Int J Obstet Anesth* 3:225, 1993.

140. Rosen M: Difficult and failed intubation in obstetrics. In Latto IP, Rosen M, editors: *Difficulties in tracheal intubation,* London, 1985, Ballière Tindall.

141. Shnider SM, Levinson G: Anesthesia for cesarean section. In Shnider SM, Levinson G, editors: *Anesthesia for obstetrics,* ed 3, Baltimore, 1993, Williams and Wilkins.

142. Harmer M, Rubin AP: Only maternal, not fetal, survival should persuade the anaesthetist to proceed with general anaesthesia for caesarean section after failed intubation, *Int J Obstet Anesth* 2:100, 1993.

143. Endler GC, Mariona FG, Sokol RJ et al: Anesthesia-related maternal mortality in Michigan, 1972 to 1984, *Am J Obstet Gynecol* 159:187, 1988.

144. Morgan BM, Magni V, Goroszenuik T: Anaesthesia for emergency caesarean section, *Br J Obstet Gynecol* 97:420, 1990.

145. Ostheimer GW: The labor and delivery suite. In Ostheimer GW, editor: *Manual of obstetric anesthesia,* New York, 1984, Churchill Livingstone.

146. Preston R, Halpern SH, Petras A: Quality assurance in obstetrical anaesthesia, *Can J Anaesth* 41:A28, 1994.

147. Huddleston JF: Electronic fetal monitoring. In Eden RD, Boehm FH, Haire M, editors: *Assessment and care of the fetus: Physiological, clinical and medicolegal principles,* Norwalk, 1990, Appleton & Lange.

148. Katz M, Meizner I, Insler V: *Fetal well-being: Physiological basis and methods of clinical assessment,* Boca Raton, 1990, CRC Press.

149. Intrapartum fetal heart rate monitoring, Technical Bulletin 132, 1989, American College of Obstetricians and Gynecologists, Washington.

150. Parer JT: Diagnosis and management of fetal aphyxia. In Shnider SM, Levinson G, editors: *Anesthesia for obstetrics,* ed 3, Baltimore, 1993, Williams and Wilkins.

151. Parer JT, Livingstone EG: What is fetal distress? *Am J Obstet Gynecol* 162:1421, 1990.

152. Marx GF, Luykx WM, Cohen S: Fetal-neonatal status following caesarean section for fetal distress, *Br J Anaesth* 56:1009, 1984.

153. Committee on Obstetrics: Maternal and fetal medicine. *Anesthesia for emergency deliveries,* Committee Opinion 104, 1992, American College of Obstetricians and Gynecologists.

154. Skerman JH, Huckaby T, Walker EB et al: Perinatal management of maternal and fetal emergencies. In Diaz JH, editor: *Perinatal anesthesia and critical care,* Philadelphia, 1991, WB Saunders.

155. Hibbard LT: Placenta previa, *Am J Obstet Gynecol* 104:172, 1969.

156. Morgan J: Placenta previa: report on a series of 538 cases, *J Obstet Gynecol Br Commonw* 72:700, 1965.

157. Peng ATC, Gorman RS, Shulman SM et al: Intravenous nitroglycerin for uterine relaxation in the postpartum patient with retained placenta, *Anesthesiology* 71:172, 1989.

158. Maeder E, Barno A, Mecklenburg F: Obesity: a maternal high risk factor, *Obstet Gynecol* 45:669, 1975.

159. Blass NH: Regional anesthesia in the morbidly obese, *Reg Anesth* 4:20, 1979.

160. Eng M, Butler J, Bonica J: Respiratory function in pregnant obese women, *Am J Obstet Gynecol* 123:241, 1975.

161. Brain AIJ: The laryngeal mask—a new concept in airway management, *Br J Anaesth* 55:801, 1983.

162. Brodrick PM, Webster NR, Nunn JF: The laryngeal mask airway: a study of 100 patients during spontaneous breathing, *Anaesthesia* 44:238, 1989.

163. Mahiou P, Narchi P, Veyrac P et al: Is laryngeal mask easy to use in case of difficult intubation? *Anesthesiology* 77:A1228, 1992.

164. Payne J: The use of the fibreoptic laryngoscope to confirm the position of the laryngeal mask, *Anaesthesia* 44:865, 1989.

165. Brimacombe J, Berry A: The laryngeal mask airway—the first ten years, *Anaesth Intensive Care* 21:225, 1993.

166. Christian AS: Failed obstetric intubation, *Anaesthesia* 45:995, 1990.

167. Hashman FM, Andrews PJD, Juneja MM et al: The laryngeal mask airway facilitates intubation at cesarean section: a case report of difficult intubation, *Int J Obstet Anesth* 2:181, 1993.

168. McClune S, Regan M, Moore J: Laryngeal mask airway for caesarean section, *Anaesthesia* 45:227, 1990.

169. McFarlane C: Failed intubation in the obese obstetric patient and the laryngeal mask, *Int J Obstet Anesth* 2:183, 1993.

170. Storey J: The laryngeal mask for failed intubation at caesarean section, *Anaesth Intensive Care* 20:118, 1992.

171. Chadwick IS, Vohra A: Anaesthesia for emergency caesarean section using the Brain laryngeal airway, *Anaesthesia* 44:261, 1989.

172. Priscu V, Priscu L, Soroker D: Laryngeal mask for failed intubation in emergency cesarean section, *Can J Anaesth* 39:893, 1992.

173. Barker P, Langton JA, Murphy PJ et al. Regurgitation of gastric contents during general anaesthesia using the laryngeal mask airway, *Br J Anaesth* 69:314, 1992.

174. Rabey PG, Murphy PJ, Langton JA et al: Effect of the laryngeal mask airway on lower oesophageal sphincter pressure in patients during general anaesthesia, *Br J Anaesth* 69:346, 1992.

175. El Mikatti N, Luthra D, Healy TEJ et al: Gastric regurgitation during general anaesthesia in the supine position with the laryngeal and face mask airways, *Br J Anaesth* 69:529P, 1992.

176. Nanji GM, Maltby JR: Vomiting and aspiration pneumonitis with the laryngeal mask airway, *Can J Anaesth* 39:69, 1992.

177. Freeman R, Baxendale B: Laryngeal mask airway for caesarean section, *Anaesthesia* 45:1094, 1990.

178. King TA, Adams AP: Failed tracheal intubation, *Br J Anaesth* 67:225, 1991.

179. Smith I, White PF: Use of the laryngeal mask airway as an alternative to a face mask during outpatient arthroscopy, *Anesthesiology* 77:850, 1992.

180. Ansermino JM, Blogg CE: Cricoid pressure may prevent insertion of the laryngeal mask airway, *Br J Anaesth* 69:465, 1992.

181. Asai T, Barclay K, Power I et al: Cricoid pressure impedes placement of the laryngeal mask airway and subsequent tracheal intubation through the mask, *Br J Anaesth* 72:47, 1994.

182. Heath ML, Allagain J: Intubation through the laryngeal mask: a technique for unexpected difficult intubation, *Anaesthesia* 46:545, 1991.

183. Strang TI: Does the laryngeal mask airway compromise cricoid pressure? *Anaesthesia* 47:829, 1992.

184. Brimacombe J: Cricoid pressure and the laryngeal mask airway, *Anaesthesia* 46:986, 1991.

185. Brimacombe J, Berry A: Mechanical airway obstruction after cricoid pressure with the laryngeal mask airway, *Anesth Analg* 78:604, 1994.

186. Brimacombe J, Berry A, White A: An algorithm for use of the laryngeal mask airway during failed intubation in the patient with a full stomach, *Anesth Analg* 77:398, 1993.

187. Allison A, McCrory J: Tracheal placement of a gum elastic bougie using the laryngeal mask airway, *Anaesthesia* 45:419, 1990.

188. Heath ML: Endotracheal intubation through the laryngeal mask airway: helpful when laryngoscopy is difficult or dangerous. *Eur J Anaesthesiol Suppl* 4:41, 1991.

189. McCrirrick A: The laryngeal mask for failed intubation at caesarean section, *Anaesth Intensive Care* 19:135, 1991.

190. Reynolds F: Tracheostomy in obstetric practice—how about the laryngeal mask airway? *Anaesthesia* 44:870, 1989.

191. Frass M, Frenzer R, Rauscha F et al: Evaluation of esophageal tracheal Combitube in cardiopulmonary resuscitation, *Crit Care Med* 15:609, 1986.

192. Frass M, Frenzer R, Zahler J: Ventilation via the esophageal tracheal Combitube in a case of difficult intubation, *J Cardiothor Anesth* 1:565, 1987.

193. Frass M, Frenzer R, Mayer G et al: Mechanical ventilation with the esophageal tracheal Combitube (ETC) in the intensive care unit, *Arch Emerg Med* 4:219, 1987.

194. Brimacombe J, Berry A: The oesophageal tracheal Combitube for difficult intubation, *Can J Anaesth* 41:656, 1994.

195. Baraka A, Salem R: The Combitube oesphageal-tracheal double lumen airway for difficult intubation, *Can J Anaesth* 40:1222, 1993.

196. Muir HA: General anaesthesia for obstetrics, is it obsolete? *Can J Anaesth* 41:R20, 1994.

Chapter 31

ANESTHETIC AND AIRWAY MANAGEMENT OF LARYNGOSCOPY AND BRONCHOSCOPY

John V. Donlon, Jr.

I. INTRODUCTION

Perhaps nowhere else in anesthesia is the need for cooperation, communication, attention to detail, and knowledge of equipment more important than in the planning and execution of the anesthetic management for endoscopy procedures of the larynx, trachea, and bronchi.

The surgeon and the anesthesiologist are both working in the same anatomic field. On the one hand, the anesthesiologist is concerned about maintaining a patent airway, oxygenation, and carbon dioxide removed and preventing aspiration while minimizing laryngeal motion and cardiac dysrhythmias. On the other hand, the surgeon needs a clear view of a motionless field for a reasonable time. At times these goals conflict. It is essential that anesthesiologist and surgeon work as a team, communicate in advance of the procedure, and understand each other's options. There is a wide variety of equipment available for endoscopy procedures, therefore there is a wide variety of anesthesia techniques. No one technique or piece of equipment is to be preferred for all cases. Each case must be individualized for the patient's age, physical condition, and specific airway disease and the intended surgical procedure. Of the variety of available anesthetic techniques for endoscopy the anesthesiologist must choose the safest for each particular patient.

In this chapter we will review the goals for all endoscopy anesthetics and outline preoperative airway evaluation and patient preparation.

II. GOALS FOR ENDOSCOPY ANESTHESIA

The following areas should be considered goals in anesthesia for endoscopy:

- Control of the airway
- Decreased airway reflexes
- Topical anesthesia
- Amnesia
- Unobstructed view of immobile surgical field
- No time restriction on surgeon
- Prevention of aspiration
- Smooth emergence
- Safe extubation
- Minimization of secretions
- Prevention of adrenergic reflexes

The ideal anesthetic technique should always be *safe.* Most patients presenting themselves for endoscopy procedures have actual or potential airway disease and may have varying degrees of compromised airway. Safety usually means ensuring that the anesthetic techniques chosen will always provide *control of the airway.* While sharing the airway with the surgeon, the anesthesiologist must be able to control it and provide adequate oxygenation and ventilation as needed. An alternate plan to establish an airway (such as needle cricothyrotomy or surgical airway) should be arranged before proceeding.

Given the choice, the safest anesthesia techniques for endoscopy are those that allow a known concentration of oxygen and agent to be delivered with controlled ventilation directly to the airway, for example, small endotracheal tube and rigid ventilating bronchoscope.

Uncertain inspired oxygen concentrations, hypoxia, and carbon dioxide retention can occur with some techniques such as jet Venturi, high-frequency jet ventilation, apneic methods, spontaneous respirations under deep general anesthesia, and fiberoptic bronchoscopy.[1,2]

Ideally the techniques should be kept as simple as possible. A wide variety of equipment, adapters, connectors, and alternative techniques are available. Care must be taken not to jerry-rig a setup. The anesthetic technique must be consistent with the endoscopy equipment used.

Decreased airway reflexes are essential to the smooth administration of anesthesia during endoscopy procedures. Instrumentation of the larynx, trachea, or bronchi is a powerful stimulus and can easily elicit coughing, bucking, larygospasm, gagging, dysrhythmias, or hypertensive responses that can lead to serious complications.

The anesthetic technique *must* ablate these reflex responses via the judicious use of narcotics, muscle relaxants, volatile agents, and local anesthetics. These reflexes are potent and difficult to suppress. The minimum alveolar concentration of halothane necessary to prevent 95% of patient motion and adrenergic response to tracheal intubation is 1.90% or 1.7 times minimum alveolar concentration (MAC) for surgical stimulation.[3]

A good baseline of *topical local anesthesia* to the pharynx, larynx, and trachea should be the basis of all anesthetic techniques for endoscopy, even when a general anesthesia technique is planned.

Amnesia for the procedure is especially important during local anesthetic techniques and when a total intravenous anesthesia (TIVA) technique is planned.

The surgeon usually requires an *unobstructed view* of an *immobile* surgical field. A safe anesthetic choice may require temporary compromise of this goal. For example, a small endotracheal tube (5 mm internal diameter [ID]) technique allows the use of muscle relaxants to ensure immobility, but will obscure the surgeon's view of the posterior commissure area. On the other hand, a jet ventilation technique for laryngoscopy presents an unobstructed view but the jet may cause vocal cord motion.

At times, during part of the procedure the surgeon may require an active-dynamic larynx (evaluation of tracheomalacia, phonation, or vocal cord paresis). The ideal anesthetic for these procedures must be able to move easily and quickly from airway immobility to spontaneous respirations and back if necessary.

There should be *no time restrictions* for the surgeon inherent in the anesthesia technique. Certain techniques such as apneic oxygenation and deep spontaneous mask general anesthesia require that the surgeon interrupt his or her work every 2 minutes to permit reoxygenation and deepening of anesthesia. Anesthesia techniques that control the airway and permit continuous oxygenation and ventilation allow the surgeon endoscopist to work uninterrupted and unhurried.

Prevention of aspiration is a concern to be addressed by any general anesthetic technique. For endoscopy procedures the use of a small endotracheal tube or ventilating bronchoscope is most likely to secure an airway. Other techniques are less ideal in this regard, leaving the airway relatively unprotected from regurgitation of stomach contents.

When an unprotected airway technique (e.g., jet ventilation) is used, the stomach should be decompressed and pretreatment with a potent antiemetic such as metoclopramide to aide forward emptying and increase gastric sphincter tone, and even pretreatment with bicitrate, should be considered.

A *smooth emergence* with rapid return of protective airway reflexes is important after endoscopy procedures. The need to maintain deep general anesthesia, suppression of airway reflexes, and muscle paralysis until the very end of the procedure often makes this ideal goal a challenging prospect.

· When *extubation* is deemed safe, patients must be extubated awake, breathing spontaneously. Short-acting, rapid-offset agents (succinylcholine, mivacurium chloride, alfentanil, and propofol) are available and can be used judiciously with appropriate topical local anesthesia to meet these conditions of rapid, safe emergence.

Every effort must be made to *minimize secretions.* Instrumentation of the upper airways, especially when succinylcholine is being used, elicits a profound outpouring of secretions. These secretions can stimulate airway reflexes, obscure the surgeon's view, and require the surgeon to frequently interrupt his or her work, prolonging the procedure. Frequent suctioning of the trachea removes oxygen from the lungs and may cause atelectasis. Therefore the ideal anesthetic technique for endoscopy must include the use of an antisialogogue such as intravenous (IV) atropine 0.006 mg per kg or IV glycopyrrolate 0.003 mg per kg. Concern that IV atropine will cause thickened, tenacious secretions appears to be unwarranted.[4]

Patients scheduled for endoscopy of the upper airway often are smokers and have a history of coronary artery disease and chronic lung problems. The incidence of myocardial ischemia after endoscopic surgery of the larynx is between 1.5% and 4%.[5] Therefore it is important to *prevent adrenergic reflexes* that can cause dysrhythmias and hypertension and to avoid hypercarbia and hypoxia. Narcotics or beta-adrenergic blockers such as labetalol or esmolol can be used to obtund these cardiovascular reflexes in patients at risk.

III. PREOPERATIVE AIRWAY EVALUATION

Patients presenting themselves for diagnostic or therapeutic endoscopy of the upper airways, trachea, or bronchi can be expected to have airway disease.

This disease may be minimal and incidental or sufficiently significant to cause airway compromise and difficult intubations. Thus a thorough preoperative airway evaluation is especially important in avoiding potential airway problems in patients scheduled for airway endoscopy.

Endoscopy patients are frequently heavy smokers with a history of chronic bronchitis. They are more likely to cough and to have airway secretions, bronchospasm,

hemoptysis, and dysphagia. These patients may have distorted airway anatomy that is due to previous neck or laryngeal surgery and scarring (fibrosis), or trismus or edema of the upper airways that is due to radiation treatments.

A wide range of potentially airway-limiting disease is possible, including tracheomalacia; friable, exophytic supraglottic masses such as cricoid chondroma or hemangiomas; and large, sessile vocal cord polyps, vocal cord paralysis, and peritonsillar or retropharyngeal infections.

(The general principles for evaluating the relative difficulty of viewing and intubating a patient's airway have been discussed in Chapter 7).

Before proceeding with endoscopy surgery the anesthesiologist should feel comfortable that he or she understands what to expect in the way of airway disease. This knowledge will help in choosing the safest anesthetic method. In evaluating airway disease the following key factors must be addressed:

1. Is the problem located above or below the glottis? Large supraglottic lesions (epiglottic cancer, pappilomatosis, and cancer of pyriform fossa) can obstruct the view of the vocal cords, making intubation very difficult. A subglottic lesion (e.g., cricoid, chondroma, or hemangioma) may narrow the trachea, but the view of the glottic opening is unobstructed.

2. Is the lesion mobile (floppy or soft) or fixed (rigid)? That is, will the degree of airway obstruction change during sedation or induction as a result of change in position or relaxation of tissues? Patients with large, fixed lesions such as a tracheal web, tracheal stenosis, or cricoid chondroma have a limited airway, but it is not likely to become worse during induction. Patients with large, supraglottic soft tissue tumors such as papillomatosis or epiglottic cancer and large, sessile vocal cord polyps are likely to have increasing airway obstruction in response to heavy sedation or the induction of general anesthesia.

3. To what extent if any does the airway disease limit airflow? Vocal cord carcinoma in situ, small vocal cord polyps, or mild tracheal stenosis may not alter airway dynamics, but larger lesions, especially lesions that limit functional airway diameter to 4.5 mm or less (in an adult) can cause turbulent flow and increased resistance to air flow and affect ventilation mechanics. Knowing the size of the airway helps in making decisions regarding bronchoscope or endotracheal tube size or the efficacy of a jet ventilation technique.

The preoperative evaluation of the endoscopy patient's airway should determine as closely as possible the location, size, and mobility of the airway disease, the degree of airway obstruction, and the difficulty of intubation.

In addition to the usual, detailed *physical examination* of the airway, special attention must be paid to the presence and quality of stridor, dysphagia, breathing patterns during sleep, and voice changes. *Stridor* indicates the presence of airway obstruction. Stridor at rest implies an airway diameter limited to 4.5 mm or less. Patients with chronic airway limitations have learned to adjust their activity level to avoid stridor but will admit to stridor on minimal exertion. The patient may have a preferred position for best breathing, and stridor may be dependent on position, if the airway lesion is very mobile. Inspiratory stridor is usually associated with lesions *above* the glottis, whereas expiratory stridor is more common when the disease that is limiting air flow is *below* the glottis.

The patient's breathing pattern while sleeping (snoring or sleep apnea) may indicate his or her likely response to sedation or induction of general anesthesia.

A weak, wispy voice indicates decreased air flow. Hoarseness indicates a problem at the vocal cord level.

Clinical history and old records may provide useful information. Has the patient had previous endoscopy examinations? Were they difficult? What were the anatomic findings? Has the patient needed a tracheostomy? Has the patient completed a recent course of head or neck radiation treatments?

Special radiographic studies such as computed tomographic (CT) scans or magnetic resonance imaging (MRI) studies of the neck or larynx may help define the location, size, and anatomic distortions of airway disease such as cricoid chondroma, radiation edema, and extent of retropharyngeal abscess or exophytic laryngeal tumors.

A final source of information is a laryngoscopic examination of the airway (direct or indirect method) in an awake patient following a topical laryngeal local anesthetic block and, if necessary, careful sedation. The *indirect* examination is often performed as an office evaluation by the ear, nose, and throat surgeon with a fiberscope. If this information is not available, and if there is any question regarding ability to maintain and secure the airway, a *direct* laryngoscopic examination should be performed just before anticipated general anesthesia. Such an examination shows a dynamic larynx with motion, sounds, and air bubbles.

IV. PATIENT PREPARATION

Patients presenting themselves for endoscopic procedures frequently have medical conditions such as coronary artery disease, coronary ischemia, dysrhythmias, hypertension, chronic lung disease, hypoxia, and hypoventilation. The adrenergic stress of the endoscopic examination can exacerbate these conditions, with serious consequences. Therefore cardiac and pulmonary medical conditions must be evaluated, optimally treated, and monitored in these patients.

Monitoring during the procedure should always include electrocardiogram, blood pressure readings, pulse oximetry, end-tidal CO_2 values (if possible), precordial stethoscopy, and muscle relaxation. Transcutaneous CO_2 monitors may be useful when the usual end-tidal expired CO_2 is not available (Venturi jet ventilation and apneic oxygenation). Carbon dioxide monitoring must include waveforms, in addition to peak values. Waveform information can help determine, for example, that a low CO_2 value is actually due to dilution by dead space gas and air trapping and does not reflect hyperventilation. The patient could, in fact, be hypercarbic.[6]

During jet ventilation techniques the motion of the chest wall should be visible and should be observed throughout the procedure.

Documentation of the extent of muscle relaxation is essential to avoid sudden movements, coughing, bucking, or vocal cord motion during endoscopic procedures. A train-of-four (TOF) or double-burst stimulus pattern may be used.[7] All muscles are not the same in their response to muscle relaxants.[8,9] The laryngeal muscles, the orbicularis oculi, and the adductor pollicis muscles have different time courses of muscle relaxant effects. Since laryngeal muscles recover from the effects of nondepolarizing muscle blockade more rapidly than pollicis muscles, it is possible to have laryngeal motion when the adductor pollicis muscle TOF indicates complete blockade.[10] The response of the orbicularis oculi more accurately reflects the response of laryngeal muscles to muscle relaxants and would be the preferable muscle to monitor during endoscopy.[10,11]

The use of *antisialagogues* is essential in the preparation of patients for endoscopy procedures of the upper airways. Antisialagogues attenuate the volume of airway secretions without increasing their viscosity.[4] The vagolytic effect of antisialagogues helps prevent vagally mediated dysrhythmias associated with mechanical stimulation of the airway. A dry airway ensures more effective topical local anesthesia and minimizes the need for frequent suctioning, thereby facilitating the surgeon's work and expediting the procedure.

Preoperative *sedation* must be carefully considered and titrated intravenously in a monitored, observed patient. Patients with stridor and compromised airways may be more fatigued than their anxiety indicates. It is tempting to give them an anxiolytic; however, this maneuver may result in increased airway obstruction, somnolence, and hypoxia as the soft tissue relaxation and sedation effects of the anxiolytic unmask an underlying fatigue and hypercarbia.

Preoperative narcotic medication may be considered. Narcotics ease anxiety, slow the respiratory rate, and suppress airway reflexes without significant loss of muscle tone. Narcotics affect the CO_2 response curve and depress the respiratory drive, and they must be administered via IV titration in a continually monitored, observed patient. Either IV morphine 0.04 to 0.07 mg/kg or IV fentanyl 0.5 μ/kg in increments may be given. Relative overdoses may easily be reversed with increments of IV naloxone 0.03 mg/kg.

All patients having endoscopy procedures should have *local anesthesia* applied to the pharynx, larynx, glottis, and if necessary, trachea. This practice should be considered an important part of any general anesthetic technique for endoscopy.

Local anesthesia helps decrease the airway reflexes and adrenergic responses to mechanical instrumentation of the airway. This allows a more conservative use of the more potent agents, a smoother operative-emergence course, less myocardial depression, and a more likely rapid emergence.

Before selecting an anesthesia technique the surgeon and the anesthesiologist must concur on a management *plan,* understanding each other's needs, options, and the sequence of events during the proposed procedure. Any possible change in the procedure, depending on the result of endoscopy findings, must be considered and planned for.

V. ANESTHETIC MANAGEMENT TECHNIQUES
A. LOCAL ANESTHESIA OF THE LARYNX AND TRACHEA[2,6,12-15]

Suppression of laryngeal and tracheal sensation and reflexes by local anesthetics (topical or specific injections) should be the basis of, and an important component of, *all* anesthetic techniques for endoscopy.

Local anesthesia of the larynx and trachea combined with careful IV sedation can provide sufficient, safe conditions for selected endoscopic procedures in selected patients without the need for general anesthesia.

1. Indications
The indications include brief diagnostic examinations of the airway, requirement of patient phonation or a dynamic airway, minimal instrumentation, and no expected bleeding. The technique is often used for office fiberoptic examinations of the upper airway and when evaluation of voice quality during vocal cord injections is necessary.

Local anesthesia of the larynx with careful IV sedation is a useful preanesthesia technique in the evaluation of difficult or compromised airways before further compromising the airway by general anesthesia or muscle relaxation.

The *advantage* of this technique is that the patient maintains his or her own airway, spontaneous respira-

tions, and cooperation. The surgeon has an unobstructed view of a dynamic larynx.

The *disadvantage* is the need for patient cooperation. (Some patients may not be good candidates for this technique.) The procedures cannot be prolonged or involve significant instrumentation or bleeding. There is the possibility of toxic reaction to the dose of local anesthetic.

The *technique* may be primarily topical, or by specific local anesthetic injections or a combination of both. It must be based on an understanding of the anatomy and sensory innervation of the larynx and trachea. The technique of anesthetizing the larynx with local anesthetics is carried out slowly and precisely in three separate steps (see Techniques).

2. Anatomy
The sensory innervation of the larynx is principally derived from the glossopharyngeal and the vagus cranial nerves, (IX and X, respectively). The lingual, pharyngeal, and tonsillar branches of the glossopharyngeal nerve innervate the posterior one third of the tongue, the oropharynx, tonsillar surfaces, and the anterior surface of the epiglottis.[2]

The two major sensory components of the vagus nerve in the larynx are the superior laryngeal nerve (SLN) and the recurrent laryngeal nerve. The SLN divides into internal and external branches at the hyoid bone. The *external* branch is a motor nerve for the cricothyroid muscle but has no sensory function. The *internal* branch of the SLN enters the thyroid membrane, then divides into a superior and an inferior twig. The superior portion provides sensory innervation to the lower pharynx, vallecula, pyriform fossae, and posterior surface of the epiglottis. The inferior twig of the internal branch of the SLN is the sensory nerve for the aryepiglottic folds and laryngeal mucous membranes, including the false vocal cords.[2]

The internal branch of the SLN lies just beneath the surface mucosa in the depths of the pyriform fossae. It may be blocked here by the precise mucosal application of a topical local anesthetic. An SLN block does not interfere with sensory innervation of the true vocal cords or upper trachea.

The recurrent laryngeal nerve provides sensory innervation from the true vocal cords or upper trachea. The recurrent laryngeal nerve also supplies motor innervation to all intrinsic muscles of the larynx except the cricothyroid (vocal cord tensor).

3. Techniques
Many methods have been described using both intraoral and external approaches.[16-18] Good surface mucosal anesthesia may be obtained by direct topical

application of local anesthetics using water-soluble ointments, lozenges, atomized spray, gargling, ultrasonic nebulizers, curved forceps and gauze, or syringe or transtracheal injection.

An intraoral SLN block can be performed by holding gauze pledgets soaked with lidocaine (2% to 4%) into each pyriform fossa.

An external SLN block can easily be accomplished by infiltrating 2 ml local anesthetic into the thyroid membrane above the superior cornu of the thyroid cartilage and below the greater cornu of the hyoid bone.[16-19] The presence of tumor or infection in the neck-larynx area may preclude the option of a transcutaneous, external SLN block.

Local anesthesia for the mucous membranes of the true vocal cords and below into the upper trachea is best achieved either by atomized spray of these areas under direct vision or by a transtracheal injection of local anesthetic. A percutaneous midline puncture of the cricothyroid membrane is made with a 22-gauge needle-catheter, and after aspirating air, 4 ml 2% lidocaine is injected.[2] The patient will cough and disperse the anesthetic to the subglottic area.

Topical application of local anesthetic to mucous membranes is most effective when these membranes are dry. Therefore pretreatment with antisialogogues enhances the effectiveness of the topical anesthetic.

Although topical application of local anesthetics ablates superficial sensation to the mucous membranes, it may be inadequate to block the deeper pressure responses such as the gag reflex.

The gag reflex is mediated through the glossopharyngeal nerve (IX). The glossopharyngeal nerve can be blocked by a specific injection of 2 ml lidocaine 1% to 2%, about 8-mm deep at the palatoglossal arch, 1 cm from the lateral margin of the root of the tongue.[6,20]

A short (⅝-inch) needle must be used and the injection made just lateral to the tongue, always on the medial aspect of the pharyngeal wall to avoid the internal carotid artery, which descends lateral to the pharyngeal wall.[12]

A blunted gag reflex and topical anesthesia of the upper trachea remove the reflexes that protect the airway from aspiration. This consequence must be appreciated, especially when dealing with patients at high risk for regurgitation (hiatus hernia, obesity, full stomach, and so forth).

The author performs a topical laryngeal block in the following precise, deliberate stages over a 15-minute period:

First stage: Open the patient's mouth and extend the tongue. With the aide of a tongue depressor, place 5% oral lidocaine ointment at base of tongue. As an alternative, an atomizer may be used to spray the base of the tongue and the posterior oropharyngeal surface, with special attention to the anterior tonsillar pillar area.

Second stage: After several minutes, reapproach the patient and use a tongue depressor and curved atomizer-nebulizer to spray local anesthetic beyond the curve of the base of the tongue, down into the depths of the pharynx, especially along the left and right sides toward the tonsils and pyriform areas.

Third stage: After several minutes, gently and slowly insert a laryngoscope past the base of the tongue to view the tip of the epiglottis. The vallecula, epiglottis, and aryepiglottic areas are sprayed with local anesthetic under direct vision. A forceps with anesthetic-soaked gauze is placed and held into each pyriform fossa for 30 seconds. For bronchoscopic procedures, local anesthetic is also sprayed through the vocal cords into the upper trachea.

Patient cooperation is important. It is obtained by constant reassurance and explanation, by proceeding slowly and gently, with the judicious use of added sedation before each stage, and with the patience to allow each application of local anesthetic to be effective before proceeding.

4. Toxic limits of local anesthetics

Although the absorption of local anesthetic through the pharyngeal and laryngeal mucosa is slow—peak levels are achieved 20 minutes after application[21]—local anesthetics can be rapidly absorbed from the trachea, small airways, and alveoli,[6] attaining blood levels similar to those following IV administration.[18] Toxic effects of lidocaine occur when plasma levels reach 5 to 6 μg/ml.[22] Early signs of toxic response to local anesthetics include tremor, bradycardia, nystagmus, and seizures.

Lidocaine 3 to 5 mg/kg total dose can be safely used when application is limited to the pharynx and larynx *above* the vocal cords.[6] The amount of lidocaine delivered into the tracheal areas should be limited to 1 to 1.5 mg/kg.

B. GENERAL ANESTHESIA WITHOUT ENDOTRACHEAL INTUBATION

General anesthesia without endotracheal intubation relies on potent inhalation or IV agents to provide patient cooperation, comfort, amnesia, and relaxation during endoscopic procedures.

The standard method is to administer a potent volatile agent via a mask to achieve a deep level of general anesthesia and suppress airway reflexes while maintaining spontaneous respirations. The endoscopist can then have an unobstructed view of a dynamic larynx.

Variations of this method include using a small catheter to insufflate agent and oxygen into the hypopharynx during the procedure and even the use of muscle relaxation and intermittent mask ventilation in an apneic oxygenation technique.

1. Indications and advantages

General anesthesia without endotracheal intubation for endoscopic procedures is best adapted to brief diagnostic examinations, especially in pediatric patients and when there will be minimal bleeding or instrumentation. This technique is also useful when the airway is relatively unobstructed, with a fixed lesion (e.g., tracheal web), when there is a need to evaluate the dynamics of the airway during spontaneous respirations (e.g., tracheomalacia), or when a full view of the glottic area and posterior commissure is necessary.

The *advantage* of this technique is the safety of spontaneous respirations, especially if the airway air flow is limited by disease. The surgeon has a cooperative patient, no fear of sudden movement, and the leisure to evaluate an active, dynamic larynx with an unobstructed view.

2. Disadvantages

There are several *disadvantages* inherent in the use of general anesthesia without endotracheal intubation. Insufflation techniques contaminate the operating room air with nitrous oxide and potent volatile agents. Operating room air pollution may be minimized by scavenging exhaled gases near the mouth or at the proximal end of the laryngoscope or bronchoscope.

It is difficult to maintain a stable depth of anesthesia with this technique. There are periods when air entrainment dilutes the inspired concentration of the potent anesthetic gas, and also periods of apnea, and periods of interrupted anesthesia while the endoscopist has control of the airway. Thus there are frequent changes and uncertain levels of general anesthesia.

There is no control of ventilation with this technique. Hypoventilation that is due to deep anesthesia, a narrow or limited airway, or the effect of IV agents can lead to hypercarbia, atelectasis, and dysrhythmias during prolonged procedures.[23,67]

With this technique the endoscopist view is time limited by the need to reventilate, oxygenate, and reestablish a sufficient depth of general anesthesia.

The constant vocal cord motion, a consequence of this technique, may be an impediment to the endoscopist.

This technique removes protective airway reflexes while leaving the airway unprotected. This technique is not suited for endoscopic manipulations that will cause bleeding. This technique requires a relatively patent airway. It is not useful in the presence of large, supraglottic soft tissue masses or floppy lesions that can obstruct the airway in response to the relaxing effects of general anesthesia.

This technique—mask, volatile agent, breathe-down general anesthetic—requires patience. At least 10 to 15 minutes may be required to achieve a sufficient depth of general anesthesia to suppress airway reflexes, especially in patients with limited air flow.

3. Method

Patients should receive an antisialogogue to dry airway secretions. Nitrous oxide may be included in the initial breathe-down procedure to expedite the uptake of general anesthetic but should be discontinued in favor of a 98% oxygen-volatile anesthetic mixture 3 minutes before endoscopic manipulation. This serves to denitrogenate the functional residual volume of the lung and provide an oxygen reservoir during any apneic periods.

A thorough topical local anesthesia of the pharynx and larynx should be considered a part of this technique and should be applied at least 5 minutes before handing the airway over to the endoscopist.

This local anesthesia decreases the reliance on *deep levels* of general anesthesia to suppress airway reflexes, minimizes the myocardial depression associated with high concentrations of volatile agents, and helps provide a more predictable level of adequate anesthesia for the procedure.

The manipulation of the endoscopist must be interrupted if the pulse oximeter indicates oxygen saturation levels falling below 96% in a patient with a previously normal saturation level (98% to 100%). In patients with initial saturation levels of less than 98%, a decrease of 3% to 4% should be considered significant and should result in reinstitution of ventilation.[24] In pediatric patients the endoscopists should be limited to 2-minute periods of viewing and working to ensure normocarbia and maintenance of adequate depth of general anesthesia.

These view-work periods may be lengthened by using one side channel of a ventilating laryngoscope to insufflate oxygen and anesthetic agent.

At the conclusion of endoscopies using a no-endotracheal-tube technique, intubation may be desirable to secure and protect the airway during emergence until adequate airway reflexes are present.

C. GENERAL ANESTHESIA USING A SMALL ENDOTRACHEAL TUBE

In 95% of patients scheduled for microlaryngoscopy the airway disease does *not* involve the posterior commissure area. Endoscopy procedures for these patients can safely and adequately be performed without compromising the surgeon's view by using a small (5-mm, internal diameter), long (31 cm) microlaryngoscopy tube (MLT) endotracheal tube.[25]

General anesthesia using a small endotracheal tube permits a wide variety of anesthesia management options. A potent volatile anesthetic, nitrous oxide–narcotic, or TIVA technique is possible. Respirations may be spontaneous, assisted, or controlled. Muscle relaxants may be used.

1. Indications

The use of a small endotracheal tube during endoscopy of the upper airway is indicated when the posterior commissure does not need to be examined; if airway bleeding, edema, or secretions are likely; if the airway is already limited and loss of patency is a possibility; if the endoscopic procedure or its duration is uncertain, or duration; for longer (30- to 60-minute) procedures; when there is a risk of gastric regurgitation (full stomach, hiatus hernia, or vocal cord paralysis) and aspiration and a need to protect the airway; or if positive pressure or assisted ventilation may be required (obesity or severe COPD with CO_2 retention).

2. Disadvantages

It has been documented that an adult can be adequately ventilated via a 5-mm ID, 31-cm long endotracheal tube using controlled ventilation.[25] The increased resistance to air flow inherent in these endotracheal tubes, however, is apparent during spontaneous respirations. A disadvantage of using a small endotracheal tube is that it obscures the view of the posterior commissure area and prevents full range of motion of the vocal cords. The tube also causes irritation of the trachea, which can lead to coughing or bucking on emergence.

3. Method

Pretreatment with an antisialogogue is important to control airway secretions. Airway secretions are especially likely in response to the combination of instrumentation of the airway and succinylcholine drip for muscle relaxation.

Thorough topical local anesthesia of the larynx should be considered an essential part of this technique. Good topical airway analgesia helps suppress airway reflexes and the adrenergic responses to airway instrumentation and allows a reduction of potent anesthetic drugs, thereby enhancing rapid emergence at the conclusion of the procedure.

An anesthetic regimen of nitrous oxide–narcotic and muscle relaxant is usually adequate. A low concentration of potent volatile agent may be added to control hypertension or to ensure lack of recall when the nitrous oxide concentration is decreased in favor of oxygen. The likelihood of awareness under anesthesia may also be decreased by adding an IV benzodiazepine and using at least 66% nitrous oxide. Controlled hyperventilation is used to maintain end-tidal carbon dioxide values in the range of 32 to 35 mm Hg.

Potent short-acting narcotics such as fentanyl, sufentanil, or alfentanil must be used to depress airway reflexes and blunt the discomfort of airway instrumentaton.

Muscle relaxants are used to provide jaw relaxation and to prevent laryngospasm and sudden patient movement. Muscle relaxants are chosen as appropriate to the expected length of the procedure. The effect of muscle relaxants is monitored with TOF or double-burst pattern stimuli.

D. GENERAL ANESTHESIA WITHOUT AN ENDOTRACHEAL TUBE BY MEANS OF JET VENTILATION TECHNIQUES

1. History

Since 1967 jet ventilation techniques and equipment have been developed for laryngoscopy and bronchoscopy procedures during general anesthesia.[2,6,12-14,26-28]

The ventilating bronchoscope was first described in 1953 by Muendrich and Hoflehner.[29] The anesthesia breathing circuit was connected to a large sidearm near the proximal end of a rigid bronchoscope and an eyepiece was used to seal the proximal end. Thus anesthetic gases could be delivered to the trachea while the endoscopist had time to examine the airway. A leak around the bronchoscope allowed egress for the gases, and ventilation could be assisted or controlled. A disadvantage of this system was the inability to ventilate the patient whenever the endoscopist removed the eyepiece to place instrumentation or suction within the bronchoscope.

In 1967 Sanders[26] developed the jet ventilation technique, relying on air entrainment (Venturi effect) to continue ventilation despite an open bronchoscope. Sanders used a 14- to 16-gauge jet placed down a sidearm of a rigid bronchoscope. Sanders used intermittent (eight per minute) jets of oxygen at 50 psi driving pressure to entrain air (Fig. 31-1). He demonstrated that this technique could maintain oxygen pressure (Po_2) between 200 and 300 mm Hg, while Pco_2 level did not rise.

In 1973 Carden and Schwesinger[30] developed a sidearm injector that allowed the jetted gas to be a mixture of oxygen and nitrous oxide. The Carden sidearm adapter permitted the use of a lower driving pressure (30 psi) to generate adequate (55 cm H_2O) airway pressures,[31] providing superior ventilation and lower arterial CO_2 levels.

The jet is most effective when delivered directly into the trachea. Peak airway pressures are reduced, and vocal cord motion is avoided. However, there is an increased risk of barotrauma with midtracheal jet techniques and therefore a definite need for gas egress through an adequate glottic opening to ensure that a clear expiratory phase is possible and no air trapping occurs.

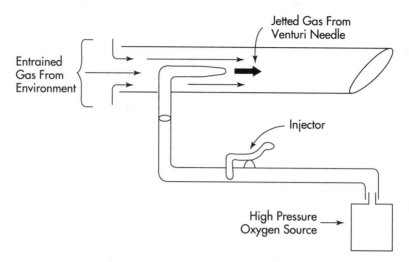

Fig. 31-1. This schematic diagram of a rigid Venturi bronchoscope shows that the jet of gas exiting from a Venturi needle placed within the lumen and parallel to the long axis of the bronchoscope entrains gas from the environment. The jetted gas comes from a high pressure source and an intermittent (12/min) injector. The flow of gas from the tube into the patient is equal to the volume of gas through the jet plus the air entrained. (From Benumof JL: Anesthesia for special elective diagnostic procedures. In Benumof JL, editor: *Anesthesia for thoracic surgery,* Philadelphia, 1987, WB Saunders.)

Benjamin,[13] Johnson and Myers,[32] and Smith,[33] among others, have developed midtracheal jet techniques using, respectively, a special Benjet small (2.8 to 4.0 mm) rigid catheter, a 3.5-mm (diameter) pediatric chest tube, and a small catheter placed through the glottis into the trachea. These techniques are contraindicated in the presence of significant laryngeal obstruction, an obstructing carcinoma, bilateral vocal cord paralysis, or large papillomas of the upper airway.

In 1975 Babinski et al.[14] applied the concept of high-frequency jet ventilation to a ventilation laryngoscope and showed that ventilation at a rapid rate (60 to 150 breaths per minute) with small tidal volumes could provide adequate ventilation at low airway pressures. Babinski et al.[14] used a 3.5-mm rigid catheter placed at midtrachea level.

In 1971 Oulton and Donald[34] reported the effective use of a Jako laryngoscope adapted with an 11-gauge jet to provide adequate jet ventilation (Po_2, 214 mm Hg; Pco_2, 35 mm Hg) during endoscopic laryngoscopy. Albert et al.[35] used a similar technique with a smaller jet nozzle (19-gauge) and demonstrated a greater Venturi effect (air entrainment) with increased tidal volumes and lower Pco_2 levels. The increased air entrainment, however, diluted the inspired oxygen concentration, resulting in a lowering of Po_2 levels compared with the 11-gauge jet size.

Disadvantages of supraglottic jet ventilation techniques include forcing tumor, tissue, or blood down into the respiratory tract; need for precise alignment of the laryngoscope along the axis of the trachea for good

ventilation; possibility of vocal cord motion in response to the jet; and possibility of jet gases causing gastric dilation.

Weeks[15] and Koufman et al.[36] adapted an operating Jako laryngoscope by placing a 3-mm ID (no. 12) Rosen ear suction device into one of the scope's two light source channels to serve as the port for jet ventilation. Jet alignment was optimal, and this proximal larger-base injector allowed large tidal volumes to be generated at low ventilating pressures, thereby minimizing barotrauma and gastric dilation. An 800-ml tidal volume could be delivered in a patient with an 8-mm airway using a ventilating pressure of only 25 psi. Weeks[15] used this technique in patients of all ages and degrees of airway obstruction for endoscopy procedures lasting 10 to 60 minutes. Blood gas levels always remained within safe limits: Po_2, 211 to 222 mm Hg; Pco_2, 37 to 42 mm Hg; and pH, 7.37 to 7.40. Complications were rare; laryngospasm (2.5% incidence) was the most common.

Cozine et al.[37] by a retrospective nationwide survey compared the complications rates for ventilation through an endotracheal tube versus Venturi jet ventilation for endoscopic CO_2 laser surgery of the larynx. The results indicated a threefold increase in the complication rate when Venturi jet ventilation was used (1.2% versus 0.36%).[37] These complications were usually related to barotrauma (pneumothorax or mediastinal air), gastric dilation, and inadequate ventilation during inhalation or exhalation. Complication rates with Venturi jets have been reported to be as high as 7%.[38] The incidence of complications with jet Venturi systems seems to be related to the level of experience. The fewer the Venturi jet ventilation procedures routinely performed, the higher the complication rate.[37]

2. Indications, advantages, and disadvantages

The indications for jet ventilation techniques include patients with relatively patent airways when the surgeon needs a completely unobstructed view, especially of the posterior commissure area.

Patient selection is important when considering the use of jet ventilation. Patients with significantly compromised airways are susceptible to barotrauma, pneumothorax, and hypoventilation and are not good candidates for jet ventilation. Obese patients and patients with poor lung compliance are difficult to adequately ventilate using jet techniques, and hypercarbia or hypoxia may develop.[3] Small pediatric patients are at increased risk for barotrauma and pneumothorax, and management should be careful.

Disadvantages of jet ventilation techniques include potential contamination of operating room air; vocal cord motion; blowing tumors, blood, or debris into the depths of the lungs; gastric dilation; uncertainty of oxygen concentrations delivered; inability to monitor end-tidal CO_2; and the fact that the fractional inspired oxygen concentration (Fio_2) and air entrainment depend on jet location, nozzle size, driving pressure, and airway resistance.

A jet ventilation laryngoscope must be aligned with a patent glottic opening to be effective. The jet will not be effective while the surgeon is viewing the depths of the pyriform fossa. Laryngoscope jet ventilation is not effective in the presence of a limited airway (e.g., severe papillomatosis). Jet ventilation techniques rely on passive recoil of the lung for exhalation. This exhalation phase needs adequate egress and time to prevent air trapping and pressure build-up in small airways.

3. Method

The jet ventilation method should be used only by anesthesiologists who understand the mechanics of the system and the limitations and complications inherent in the technique.

The oxygen source is usually set at 30 to 50 psi and jetted at a frequency of about 8 to 10 jets per minute to allow time for exhalation.[39] High-frequency techniques of jet ventilation and positive pressure ventilation have been developed and used for laryngoscopies and bronchoscopy.[2,14,40-42] They require special equipment and familiarity with the mechanics of the technique. Advantages of high-frequency jet ventilation at ventilation rates of 100 to 150 jets per minute are smaller tidal volumes, less vocal cord motion, and reduced airway barotrauma.

Usually TIVA technique is used in association with jet

ventilation equipment. Oxygen (100%) is used as the jet gas. The effective Fio_2 is about 0.8 to 0.9 because of dilution from entrainment of ambient air. A Carden sidearm blender allows nitrous oxide to be added to the jet gas.[30] It is recommended to provide a minimum of 50% oxygen in the jet gas to ensure adequate patient oxygenation and a margin of safety.

Anesthesia is provided by a mixture of either thiopental sodium (pentothal) or propofol with a potent narcotic such as fentanyl or alfentanil and muscle relaxation.

After induction, a propofol drip at a rate of 100 to 200 μg/kg per minute can provide the deep sedation component of TIVA.[43] Narcotics are necessary to suppress airway reflexes and blunt adrenergic responses to pain. Sudden patient motion, coughing, or bucking during endoscopic instrumentation of the upper or lower airway can have disastrous consequences such as mucosal bleeding or perforation. Therefore adequate, documented muscle relaxation is an essential part of this procedure.

The possibility of patient recall during TIVA is real and can be decreased by adding a benzodiazepine such as midazolam to the anesthetic management.

As with all anesthesia regimens for endoscopic procedures, a thorough topical local anesthesia of the larynx and, if necessary, glottis and trachea is accomplished as the basis for the general anesthesia technique.

Before beginning to use the jet, the upper airway must be examined by direct laryngoscopy to ensure that adequate egress exists for the jetted gas. All jetting equipment, connectors, and adapters must be on hand and functional before initiating general anesthesia.

Airway pressures and end-tidal CO_2 values cannot be monitored during jet ventilation. The adequacy of the mechanics of ventilation is determined by observing the chest wall or sternum rise and fall with each jetted ventilation. Therefore the patient's chest must be clearly visible throughout the procedure. Jet ventilation techniques require adequate muscle relaxation to minimize the active resistance of chest wall muscle to inhalation.

Techniques using high-pressure jet ventilation should be used only by an anesthesiologist experienced with the equipment and technique.

E. COMBINED TECHNIQUES WITH GENERAL ANESTHESIA

Combined techniques with general anesthesia include initial use of a small, MLT endotracheal tube, followed by a nonendotracheal tube technique (e.g., intermittent apneic anesthesia or jet ventilation) when the surgical field moves to the posterior larynx and subglottic area and have been described by Weisberger and Mines.[24]

Combined techniques with general anesthesia are

useful when dealing with significant supraglottic obstructing diseases such as papillomatosis that also require visualization of the posterior commissure area. In cases with severe upper airway obstruction, intubation is necessary initially to secure the airway, establish an adequate depth of general anesthesia, and permit a thorough evaluation of the airway by the endoscopist before proceeding.

After a brief, direct examination of the upper airway, general anesthesia is carefully induced either by mask or intravenously and the airway secured with a small-diameter MLT endotracheal tube. Most of the surgical manipulation and tissue resection is accomplished with the endotracheal tube in place. Once the patency of the upper airway has been reestablished, the operating laryngoscope is set up to view the glottic area, the patient receives hyperventilation for 2 minutes with 100% oxygen to create a reserve of oxygen in the functional residual capacity of the lung, and the endotracheal tube is removed. Thus the surgeon has an unobstructed posterior view of the posterior commissure, subglottic area, and posterior aspect of the vocal cords and may proceed to work in these areas.

The anesthesia technique is now changed to either a jet ventilation or an intermittent apneic anesthesia method.

The jet ventilation methods and precautions have been described previously. With the intermittent apneic technique the trachea is reintubated, a small endotracheal tube is placed into the trachea through the operating laryngoscope and mechanical ventilation resumed, if the pulse oximeter reading falls below 96%, a transcutaneous oxygen reading is less than 150 mm Hg, or 3 to 3½ minutes of apnea has elapsed. This apneic period should be limited to 1½ minutes in patients younger than 5 years of age. Reintubation is easy because the glottis is already in the field of view of the operating laryngoscope. After 2 to 3 minutes of hyperventilation and reoxygenation to a saturation level of 99% and deepening general anesthesia, the small endotracheal tube may be removed and surgical manipulation recommended. At the end of the surgical procedure the patient is reintubated to secure the airway during emergence and the return of protective airway reflexes.

Before the removal of the operating laryngoscope the vocal cords and glottic area may be sprayed with lidocaine 2% to 4% to minimize the likelihood of laryngospasm. The reversal (spontaneous or pharmacologic) of muscle relaxation must be documented. After extubation patients receive humidified oxygen in the postanesthesia care unit, and treatments with nebulized racemic epinephrine may be necessary to control airway edema.

F. PEDIATRIC ENDOSCOPY

Most pediatric endoscopy procedures are performed with the patient under general anesthesia. General anesthesia ensures a cooperative patient, avoids the psychologic stress of awake endoscopy, reduces trauma to the airway, and allows the endoscopist time to examine the disease in detail.

Many approaches are available for pediatric endoscopy, including awake, general anesthesia and apneic oxygenation; spontaneous or controlled ventilation; jet ventilation; and small endotracheal tube methods. The safest choice depends on factors such as the age and health of the patient, the location and extent of the airway disease, and the planned procedure.[6,12]

Advances in anesthesia monitoring, anesthetic drugs, and pediatric endoscopic equipment have significantly decreased the morbidity and mortality rates of pediatric endoscopy.[12]

Parsons et al.[12] and Woods[6] have reviewed in detail the equipment and anesthetic techniques for a wide variety of endoscopy procedures in children.

Endoscopic examinations can be performed with a flexible endoscope in an awake child via the nasal or (in patients under 6 months of age) the oral route following topical local anesthesia (lidocaine 1% to 2%) of the nasal passages or oropharynx. A nasal vasoconstrictor such as oxymetazoline should be used to avoid nasal bleeding. These examinations are usually only diagnostic and do not include surgical intervention. Therefore the surgeon can evaluate the disease in a dynamic, cooperative airway, especially when it is important to evaluate vocalization dynamics.

Rigid bronchoscopy can safely be performed in stridorous newborns without general anesthesia using oxygen insufflation alone. The choices for sedation to allay anxiety and gain cooperation of children for a flexible endoscopic examination include narcotics and benzodiazepines.

Narcotics have a calming effect, depress airway reflexes, and slow respirations but may cause nausea. Appropriate choices would include IV fentanyl 0.5 μg/kg or IV morphine 0.07 mg/kg. If necessary, narcotic effects can be reversed with titrated doses of naloxone.

Benzodiazepines such as IV midazolam 0.03 mg/kg decrease anxiety and produce some amnesia and sedation. Reversal of oversedation with benzodiazepines is possible with flumazenil.[44]

Benjamin[45] and Parsons et al.[12] have described a technique for small children (less than 35 kg) using spontaneous ventilation of halothane and oxygen via a large, wide-bore cannula placed in the left-side channel of a Parsons pediatric laryngoscope. The technique also relies on topical lidocaine (4 mg/kg maximum dose, without epinephrine) applied to the vocal cords and supraglottic area to inhibit laryngospasm. A bronchoscopic examination can be performed through the Pediatric laryngoscope using a Hopkins telescopic endoscope.[46]

In children weighing more than 35 kg, Benjamin[13] used a jet ventilation technique via a special 2.8-mm (outside diameter) Benjet tube placed through the vocal cords to the midtrachea. Johnson and Myers[32] used a 3.5-mm pediatric chest tube in a similar fashion.

Children are at increased risk for barotrauma during jet ventilation for endoscopy. Before jetting begins, a direct laryngoscopic examination should be performed to ensure that adequate egress exists for the jetted gases. The inspiratory/expiratory ratio of ventilation should be at least 1:4 to allow adequate time for complete passive exhalation. The respiratory frequency for small children should be about 20 breaths per minute. Driving pressures of only 5 to 10 psi are used initially and increased gradually until sufficient expansion of the thorax occurs with each jetted ventilation.[6] Chest wall muscle relaxation is essential to ensure low resistance to inspiration and adequate tidal volumes at reasonable airway pressures. Intermediate-acting nondepolarizing muscle relaxants, such as atracurium besylate, vecuronium bromide, or mivacurium chloride, are used and their effect documented by monitoring muscle relaxation with TOF or double-burst stimuli.

Children, because of their high metabolic rates, small functional residual capacity, and high cardiac output, are likely to have a significant decrease in oxygen tension during laryngoscopy and intubation. Hypoxemia and the vagal stimulation of airway instrumentation can lead to serious cardiovascular problems. Insufflation of 100% oxygen via a large side-bore catheter in a Parsons pediatric laryngoscope or anesthesia laryngoscope blades fitted with oxygen insufflation ports (Oxyscope, Mercury Medical Products, St. Petersburg, Florida) effectively reduces the fall in oxygen tension during laryngoscopy in small children.[12,47] Atropine can effectively maintain heart rate despite vagal stimulation.

G. FOREIGN BODIES IN THE AIRWAYS

Endoscopy for the extraction of foreign bodies from the airway is a delicate, dangerous procedure. Woods[6] has discussed the details and precautions of anesthetic management when retrieving foreign bodies from the larynx, trachea, or bronchi.

Laryngeal foreign bodies are always symptomatic and frequently present with a classic brassy cough.

Foreign bodies lodged in the larynx are more likely to cause total airway obstruction than are foreign bodies below the glottis. If radiopaque, the nature and location of the foreign body can be demonstrated by x-ray if the patient's condition (i.e., no cyanosis, no decreased

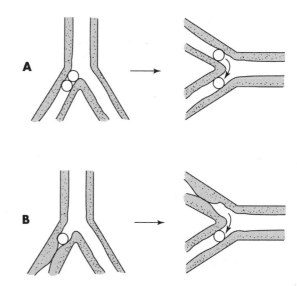

Fig. 31-2. Mechanisms of bilateral bronchial obstruction following foreign body aspiration. **A,** Two objects are in the right main bronchus, and when the patient assumes the left lateral decubitus position, one of them enters the opposite bronchus. **B,** There is swelling distal to a foreign body. When the object is dislodged and enters the opposite bronchus, total obstruction results. (From Woods AM: Pediatric endoscopy. In Berry FA, editor: *Anesthetic management of difficult and routine pediatric patients,* ed 2, New York, 1990, Churchill Livingstone.)

consciousness, or no significant stridor) permits time for radiographic evaluation. The patient should be accompanied to the radiology department by personnel trained in emergency airway management.

Foreign bodies located in the bronchi may dislodge from cough or change in position and cause total airway obstruction (Fig. 31-2).[6] Therefore prompt removal is important. A cough (either before or during surgery) may move a foreign body from a bronchus into the trachea to cause complete obstruction. An emergency intraoperative maneuver may be to push the foreign body back down into one bronchus to reestablish some ventilation. A change in body position can also dislodge one of multiple foreign bodies with movement into an unobstructed bronchus.[6,48]

The challenge to the anesthesiologist during foreign body extraction is to provide good ventilation without worsening the airway. Usually these patients have full stomachs, but cricoid pressure may cause further airway damage. A foreign body with sharp edges can tear the mucosa. If time and the patient's condition permit, an awake flexible endoscopic examination can be performed. If cyanosis or altered levels of consciousness are present, an immediate awake direct laryngoscopy must be performed.

If the child is breathing adequately, a slow, gentle, spontaneous-respiration mask induction using 100% oxygen and halothane is performed. No muscle paralysis or positive pressure ventilation is used, lest the laryngeal foreign body be forced into the glottis or upper trachea and cause sudden total airway obstruction. This induction in a patient with marginal air flow is slow and 15 to 20 minutes may be required, to reach a sufficient depth of general anesthesia to suppress airway reflexes (end-tidal halothane value, 1.5%).[6] Before endoscope insertion, topical local anesthesia of the oropharynx helps prevent airway reflexes. The endoscopist has about 3 minutes to find and extract the laryngeal foreign body before the anesthesiologist must reoxygenate and reanesthetize by mask with spontaneous respiration.

Woods[6] preferred a spontaneous respiration technique during bronchial foreign body removal. A recent survey by Kain et al.[49] indicated that in children most anesthesiologists prefer a mask induction without cricoid pressure for management of a foreign body in the airway. Choice of induction technique was not affected by pressure of symptoms or type of object. Anesthesiologists with more experience, especially with pediatric cases, were more likely to choose the inhalation induction method. Kosloske[50] routinely used muscle paralysis and controlled ventilation. The risk of controlled, positive pressure ventilation is to force the foreign body deeper into the small airways. The risk of a nonparalyzed, spontaneous breathing technique is sudden motion by the patient. Therefore adequate depth of general anesthesia and good topical local anesthesia of the larynx and glottis are essential with a spontaneous respiration–potent agent technique.

Instrumentation such as forceps, suctioning, or telescopes placed into the ventilating bronchoscope impair air flow, cause turbulent air flow, increase resistance, and decrease ventilation.[6] The placement of the bronchoscope is important. If the bronchoscope remains deep in a bronchus for more than 60 seconds, the nonventilated lung may become atelectatic; hypercarbia and light anesthesia may ensue. Therefore the bronchoscope must be pulled back to the midtracheal level from time to time to permit adequate ventilation.

After extraction of the foreign body the airway is intubated, the patient receives ventilation with 100% oxygen and positive pressure to expand the lungs, and a nasogastric tube is placed and removed to decompress the stomach.

In the presence of significant airway edema the airway is left intubated and the patient is observed for 12 to 24 hours in an intensive care setting. Otherwise, extubation is performed with the patient awake and with protective airway reflexes present, and treatment is with humidified oxygen and nebulized racemic epinephrine to control edema. A chest x-ray should be obtained before the patient is discharged from the postanesthesia care unit.

> **BOX 31-1   Local anesthetic techniques for nasotracheal fiberoptic bronchoscopy**
>
> 1. Cocaine (10%) to nasal mucosa
> 2. Soft nasopharyngeal airways liberally coated with lidocaine ointment
> 3. Local anesthetic spray to nasopharyngeal, oropharyngeal, laryngeal and tracheal mucosal surfaces
>   a. Tetracaine 0.5% with epinephrine
>   b. Lidocaine 4%
> 4. Superior laryngeal nerve block
>   a. Externally by needle
>   b. Internally by swab soaked in local anesthesia
> 5. Transtracheal block
> 6. Local anesthesia spray down suction channel of fiberoptic bronchoscope

From Benumof JL: Anesthesia for special elective diagnostic procedures. In Benumof JL, editor: *Anesthesia for thoracic surgery,* Philadelphia, 1987, WB Saunders.

H. USE OF MUSCLE RELAXANTS DURING ENDOSCOPIC PROCEDURES

Good muscle relaxation is an important component of many of the anesthetic techniques used for endoscopic procedures. Jaw muscle relaxation is needed to facilitate placement of ventilating laryngoscopes and rigid bronchoscopes. Muscle relaxation minimizes the likelihood of laryngospasm, coughing, bucking, gagging, or unwanted vocal cord motion and relaxes the glottis to facilitate the passage of the bronchoscope. Relaxation of the chest wall muscles is necessary during jet ventilation techniques to ensure adequate tidal volumes at minimal peak airway pressures.

All muscles are not the same in their response to nondepolarizing muscle relaxants.[9] The time course of the onset of relaxation and the recovery phase differs between adductor pollicis, orbicularis oculi, diaphragm, masseter, and laryngeal muscles. In general the onset of relaxation and recovery of laryngeal muscles is more rapid than that of the adductor pollicis.[10] Therefore monitoring the relaxation of the adductor pollicis may not accurately predict the extent of relaxation of the laryngeal muscles. It is possible to document a TOF ratio of zero at the adductor pollicis while the laryngeal muscles have already significantly recovered. Studies have shown that the orbicularis oculi has a more rapid onset and short recovery time to a nondepolarizing muscle relaxant, compared with the adductor pollicis response.[10,11] Monitoring the orbicularis oculi response may more accurately reflect the degree of relaxation of the laryngeal muscles during endoscopic procedures.[11] Recovery of the orbicularis oculi precedes recovery of the adductor pollicis and may underestimate the degree of residual blockade and ventilatory ability at the time of reversal.[11]

Table 31-1. Ventilation characteristics and anesthetic implications of the three different types of bronchoscopes

Type of bronchoscope	F_{IO_2}	Concentration of inhalation anesthesia	Constancy of minute ventilation	Suitable duration of procedure	Preferred type of anesthesia
Flexible fiberoptic	Known	Known	Constant	Long	Local or general anesthesia
Rigid ventilating	Known	Known	Inconstant	Short (15 to 20 min)	Inhalational or intravenous general anesthesia
Rigid Venturi	Unknown	Unknown	Constant	Long	Intravenous general anesthesia

From Benumof JL: Anesthesia for special elective diagnostic procedures. In Benumof JL, editor: *Anesthesia for thoracic surgery,* Philadelphia, 1987, WB Saunders.

The different muscle groups demonstrate varied sensitivities to nondepolarizing muscle relaxants. In addition, there may be differences in the way nondepolarizing muscle relaxants such as vecuronium, mivacurium, atracurium, and rocuronium interact with each muscle group. The usual correlation of relaxation of the orbicularis oculi and diaphragm may not be true for mivacurium.[11]

The anesthesiologist should appreciate the sometimes subtle differences in the use and monitoring of muscle relaxants when planning anesthetic management for endoscopy procedures.

VI. SPECIAL BRONCHOSCOPY CONSIDERATIONS

There are different indications for the use of rigid or flexible bronchoscopes. Anesthesia techniques vary depending on which type of bronchoscope is used for endoscopy (Table 31-1).

Rigid bronchoscopes are useful for foreign body removal, for evaluation of hemoptysis, vascular tumors, and endobronchial lesions, and for obtaining large biopsy specimens. The rigid bronchoscope allows better visualization, suctioning, and control of bleeding. Ventilation is more reliably ensured with a rigid, ventilating bronchoscope, especially when it is necessary to displace a large, obstructing soft tissue tumor to create an airway. Rigid bronchoscopy is stimulating to the airway and requires extremes of neck extension for proper placement. Sudden, unexpected patient motion or cough during rigid bronchoscopy can cause significant tracheal or laryngeal damage. Therefore, although successful rigid bronchoscopy with the patient under local topical anesthesia and sedation has been reported,[51] general anesthesia techniques are usually preferred.[2]

Flexible fiberoptic bronchoscopes (FOBs) are useful for evaluating lesions of the smaller airways located peripherally or in the upper lobes. The small diameter and flexibility of these scopes facilitate their use in awake or lightly sedated patients in the intensive care unit or as an office procedure. The FOB is also useful as an aid to management of a difficult airway that is due to trismus, base of tongue lesions, poor neck mechanics, facial trauma, and the like.[2] (See Box 31-1.)

Good topical anesthesia of the larynx and trachea is usually sufficient for most FOB examinations (See Box 31-1). The sedative agent may be titrated as necessary to allay anxiety and gain cooperation in selected patients. Narcotics such as IV fentanyl 1 to 2 µg/kg or a benzodiazepine such as IV midazolam 0.02 to 0.04 mg/kg may be used while level of consciousness, respirations, oxygenation, electrocardiogram, and blood pressure are monitored during the procedure.

The topical laryngeal block (described previously) must be thorough and include nasal passages, base of tongue, glossopharyngeal nerve (IX), SLN at the pyriform fossa, glottic area, vocal cords, epiglottis, and upper trachea (Fig. 31-3). Local anesthesia may be injected directly into the trachea by the transtracheal approach or by injecting down the suction channel of the flexible bronchoscope as necessary. Recall that lidocaine is absorbed very rapidly from the trachea and small airways, resulting in blood levels similar to those with IV injections. Intratracheal lidocaine injection should be limited to 1 mg/kg total dose.[52]

A. GENERAL ANESTHESIA VIA AN ENDOTRACHEAL TUBE FOR FLEXIBLE FIBEROPTIC BRONCHOSCOPY

General anesthesia may be indicated for flexible fiberoptic bronchoscopy if the procedure will be prolonged or the patient is uncooperative because of anxiety, if there is a communication or language barrier, or if there is an abnormal mental condition. Adult FOB sizes range from 5.0 to 6.0 mm (outside diameter). To ensure adequate air flow around the FOB and minimal turbulence, endotracheal tubes no smaller than 8.0 or 8.5 mm should be used.[53] A 5.7-mm (outside diameter) FOB reduces the cross-sectional area of a 8.0-mm endotracheal tube by 52% (Fig. 31-4);[42] that is, the result is the functional equivalent of a 5.5-mm endotracheal tube. Hypoventilation, CO_2 retention, gas trapping, positive end-expiratory pressure, and barotrauma can occur when smaller (less than 8.0 mm) endotracheal tubes are used during flexible fiberoptic bronchoscopy.[2] Consequently, ventilation must be assisted or controlled during flexible fiberoptic bronchoscopy through an endotra-

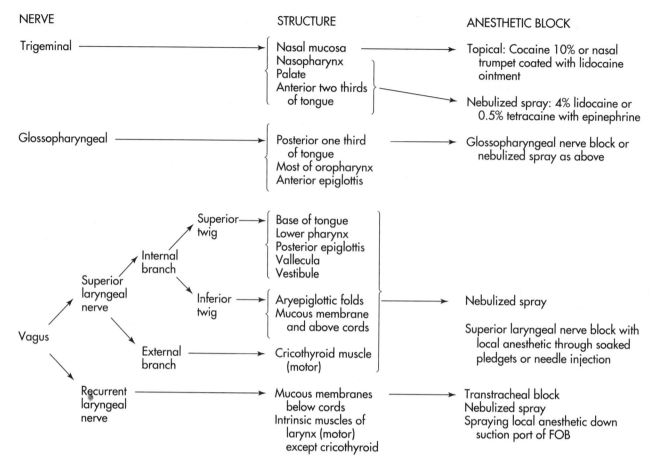

NERVE · STRUCTURE · ANESTHETIC BLOCK

Trigeminal → Nasal mucosa / Nasopharynx / Palate / Anterior two thirds of tongue → Topical: Cocaine 10% or nasal trumpet coated with lidocaine ointment / Nebulized spray: 4% lidocaine or 0.5% tetracaine with epinephrine

Glossopharyngeal → Posterior one third of tongue / Most of oropharynx / Anterior epiglottis → Glossopharyngeal nerve block or nebulized spray as above

Vagus → Superior laryngeal nerve → Internal branch → Superior twig → Base of tongue / Lower pharynx / Posterior epiglottis / Vallecula / Vestibule

Inferior twig → Aryepiglottic folds / Mucous membrane and above cords → Nebulized spray / Superior laryngeal nerve block with local anesthetic through soaked pledgets or needle injection

External branch → Cricothyroid muscle (motor)

Recurrent laryngeal nerve → Mucous membranes below cords / Intrinsic muscles of larynx (motor) except cricothyroid → Transtracheal block / Nebulized spray / Spraying local anesthetic down suction port of FOB

Fig. 31-3. Nerves to be blocked during local anesthesia for fiberoptic bronchoscopy. (From McGoldrick KE, Ho MD: Endoscopy procedures and laser surgery of the airway. In McGoldrick KE, editor: *Anesthesia for ophthalmic and otolaryngologic surgery,* Philadelphia, 1992, WB Saunders.)

cheal tube to ensure adequate ventilation. Sufficient time for expiration must be allowed to prevent air trapping. Jet ventilation of oxygen may be added through the suction port of the FOB if necessary.[54] A laryngeal mask airway (LMA) is an appropriate conduit for an FOB. An FOB can be advanced through an LMA to provide a dynamic view of the vocal cords, glottis, and trachea. Since the internal diameter of the LMA is 2 to 4 mm greater than the equivalent endotracheal tube, the larger free cross-sectional area ensures adequate ventilation during bronchoscopy.[55]

General anesthesia techniques for fiberoptic bronchoscopy are based on solid topical local anesthesia of the upper airways. The goals include providing sufficient depth of general anesthesia for amnesia, immobility, and suppression of airway and adrenergic reflexes, yet allow the patient to awaken rapidly with return of protective airway reflexes. When used alone, significant concentrations (1.7 MAC) of potent volatile agents are required to suppress airway reflexes and prevent laryngospasm.[3] Nitrous oxide concentrations should be limited to a

maximum of 50% to ensure adequate oxygenation. Propofol and alfentanil are short-duration agents and can be used in drip form to provide amnesia, sedation, pain relief, and suppression of reflexes without prolonging recovery. Desflurane is the latest development in volatile halogenated anesthetic agents, which promise to have a rapid emergence. Desflurane is pungent and has been shown to be irritating to the airway when used for mask inductions.[56] Many patients scheduled for bronchoscopy are smokers with chronic bronchitis and hyperactive airways and are therefore susceptible to bronchospasm.

B. GENERAL ANESTHESIA FOR RIGID VENTILATING BRONCHOSCOPE

General anesthesia for jet ventilation bronchoscopy relies on thorough topical local anesthesia of the larynx, glottis, and trachea and excellent muscle relaxation. The basic anesthetic is a TIV approach, using propofol or thiopental sodium, midazolam, and narcotic such as fentanyl or alfentanil.[43]

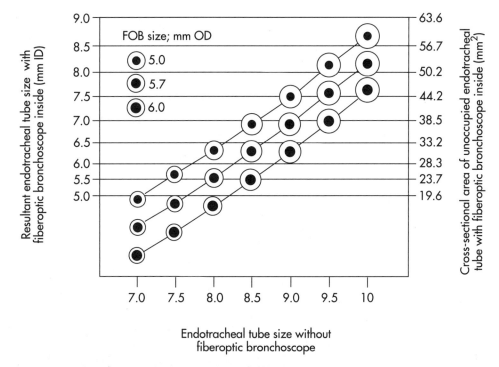

Fig. 31-4. Resultant cross-sectional area and equivalent endotracheal tube size following placement of 5.0-, 5.7-, or 6.0-mm fiberoptic bronchoscopes within variously sized endotracheal tubes. (From Lindholm CE, Ollman B, Synder JV et al: Cardiorespiratory effect of flexible fiberoptic bronchoscopy in critically ill patients, *Chest* 74:362, 1978.)

Ventilation can be either spontaneous or controlled. Intermittent ventilation with apneic oxygenation allows only brief (2-minute) periods of bronchoscopic manipulation and can result in hypercarbia, hypoxemia, and inadequate levels of anesthesia. Spontaneous ventilation techniques can also result in either hypoventilation (deep level of anesthesia) or the risk of patient movement or bronchospasm (light level of anesthesia). These methods of ventilation are contraindicated in obese patients and in patients with obstructed airways and decreased pulmonary function.

Controlled ventilation is the preferred method of ventilation for anesthesia during rigid bronchoscopy. Muendrich and Hoflehner[29] developed the sidearm ventilating bronchoscope in 1953, which allows reliable ventilation with a known amount of oxygen and volatile agent in a semiclosed system (Fig. 31-5). Removal of the viewing eyepiece to permit surgical instrumentation or suctioning produces an open bronchoscope system and interrupts ventilation. The development of the Hopkins lens telescope,[6,46] eyepiece diaphragm, and side ports for suction and biopsy instruments (see Bronchoscopy, Chapter 24) helps maintain the semiclosed system and permits continuous ventilation while the endoscopist works.

Care must taken in using Hopkins telescopes within pediatric bronchoscopes. The space between the bronchoscope sheath and the telescope determines the resistance to air flow and may create turbulent flow patterns (Fig. 31-6). Under conditions of turbulent flow, resistance increases further as flow rates increase. Air trapping and barotrauma may occur. Adequate expiration times (greater than 5 seconds) should be maintained to allow complete egress of exhaled gases. The use of a 2.8-mm (diameter) telescope in a 3.5-mm pediatric bronchoscope sheath should allow sufficient gas egress to avoid air trapping, even during controlled ventilation in a paralyzed patient.[6,57] When a 2.5-mm bronchoscope is used in small infants, lung emptying is facilitated by using low-flow oxygen (1 L/min), removing the telescope frequently, and leaving the pop-off valve open and by an occasional positive pressure breath.

In 1967 Sanders[26] used a 16-gauge needle at the proximal end of an open bronchoscope to inject oxygen under high pressure toward the trachea. This jet of oxygen entrained ambient air (Venturi effect) to provide mechanical ventilation. By using this technique it is possible to allow simultaneous instrumentation and uninterrupted ventilation through an open bronchoscope. In 1973 Carden[58] modified this system to use a sidearm adapter to inject oxygen at lower driving pressures, resulting in improved oxygenation and lower CO_2 values compared with conventional ventilating bronchoscopes. The proximal eyepiece of the Carden bronchoscope does not need to be removed, permitting constant uninterrupted minute ventilation. Jet ventilation tech-

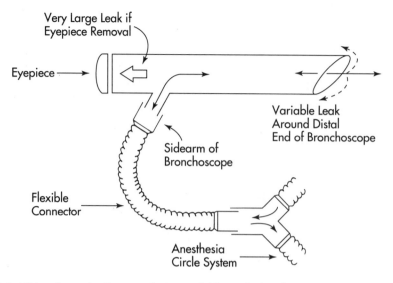

Fig. 31-5. This schematic diagram shows a rigid ventilating bronchoscope system, which consists of the anesthesia circle system attached to a flexible connector that is attached to the sidearm of the bronchoscope. With the proximal eyepiece in place, most of the inspired gas goes into the patient. However, since the bronchoscope cannot fully fill the area of the trachea, there is a variable leak around the distal end of the bronchoscope. Exhaled gases are through the anesthesia circle system. When the eyepiece is removed there is a very large leak out the proximal end of the bronchoscope. (From Benumof JL: Anesthesia for special elective diagnostic procedures. In Benumof JL, editor: *Anesthesia for thoracic surgery,* Philadelphia, 1987, WB Saunders.)

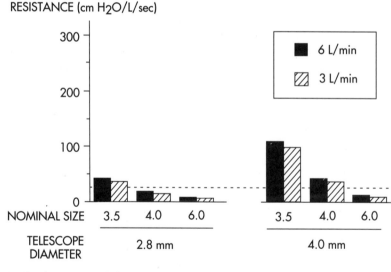

Fig. 31-6. Resistance to airflow through pediatric ventilating bronchoscopes. Replacing 4.0-mm telescope with a smaller-diameter 2.8-mm telescope in child bronchoscopes significantly decreases airflow resistance in the nominal-size 3.5 bronchoscope. The dotted line represents the upper limit of normal respiratory resistance for an infant. (From Woods AM: Pediatric endoscopy. In Berry FA, editor: *Anesthetic management of difficult and routine pediatric patients,* ed 2, New York, 1990, Churchill Livingstone.)

niques require adequate time and sufficient lumen patency for complete egress of injected gases through the bronchoscope.

The effective inspired oxygen concentration varies depending on the amount of entrained ambient air.

Hypoxemia is more likely with this jet ventilation system[1] than with the known inspired oxygen concentration using the ventilating bronchoscope. Tidal volumes achieved with jet ventilation are variable and depend on thoracic compliance. Adequate muscle relaxation is an essential component of any anesthetic technique for jet ventilation bronchoscopy. The chest wall excursion must be observed closely to determine the adequacy of ventilatory mechanics.

High-frequency jet ventilation[14] and high-frequency positive pressure ventilation[41] techniques have been used with rigid Venturi bronchoscopes to establish effective ventilation with small tidal volumes at low airway pressures.

Carden and Schwesinger[30] added a nitrous oxide–oxygen blender to the sidearm injector of a Sanders Venturi bronchoscope to permit a balanced anesthetic to be used. To ensure adequate oxygenation, nitrous oxide concentrations should not exceed 50%. Disadvantages of using nitrous oxide are limited oxygen concentrations, pollution of operating room air, and optical distortion caused by the refractive index of the nitrous oxide–oxygen gas mix.

C. COMPLICATIONS

Complications associated with anesthesia for bronchoscopy include hypoxia, bronchospasm pneumothorax, dysrhythmias, toxic effects of local anesthetics, and unpleasant recall.[59-67]

Hypoxia can be caused by oversedation and hypoventilation during spontaneous respiration techniques, change in respiratory mechanics during flexible fiberoptic bronchoscopy, atelectasis as a result of repeated suctioning, excess secretions in patients with chronic bronchitis, and bronchospasm. Therefore oxygen monitoring and a safety margin of oxygen saturation is an essential part of any anesthetic technique for endoscopy. The incidence of bronchospasm associated with bronchoscopy is 16.4 per 1000 procedures, or 10 times the incidence of bronchospasm during general anesthesia for nonbronchoscopy procedures.[61] Bronchospasm is equally likely during rigid or flexible bronchoscopy. Patients with a history of reactive airways (asthma, bronchitis, or smokers) are more likely to have bronchospastic episodes during anesthesia. Inadequate depth of anesthesia, permitting responsive airway reflexes, is a common cause of bronchospasm.

Difficult or prolonged bronchoscopies with either flexible or rigid bronchoscopes can result in pneumothorax.[60] The risk of tracheal tear and pneumothorax is increased if the patient coughs[6] or moves during rigid bronchoscopy. Therefore complete, documented muscle relaxation is important during rigid bronchoscopy. A chest x-ray may be indicated if the patient has difficulty breathing or maintaining oxygen saturation in the postanesthesia care unit.

Adrenergic responses to the stimuli of airway instrumentation may produce hypertension, tachydysrhythmias, coronary ischemia, and changes in cardiovascular dynamics.[63-65] These adrenergic responses are best prevented by good topical local anesthesia of the airway and by maintaining sufficiently deep levels of general anesthesia. The electrocardiogram should always be monitored in at least three different leads during endoscopic procedures. If necessary, these adrenergic responses may also be blocked with beta-blocking drugs such as esmolol or labetalol.[66]

Lidocaine is absorbed very rapidly from the trachea and small airways. The dose of lidocaine placed in tracheal areas below the glottis should be limited to 1 to 1.5 mg/kg.

VII. BASIC SAFETY GUIDELINES FOR ALL ENDOSCOPIC PROCEDURES

Basic safety guidelines for anesthesia management for all endoscopic procedures include the following:

1. Evaluate the airway, and know the airway disease.
2. Sedate carefully. Titrate IV sedation to effect, and monitor patients during sedation.
3. Select the anesthesia technique that best matches up to the patient, the disease, and the surgical procedure.
4. Always give priority to oxygenation and ventilation. Constantly monitor both oxygen saturation and adequacy of ventilation mechanics.
5. Choose, use, and monitor muscle relaxants appropriately. Relaxation of the jaw, glottis, and vocal cords makes access easy and unwanted sudden movements unlikely.
6. Check and protect the teeth.
7. Suppress airway reflexes using topical local anesthesia, antisialagogues, and good depth of general anesthesia.
8. When using jet ventilation, have the proper equipment and expertise. Proceed with caution.
9. Extubation may be a problem. Perform extubation in an awake patient whenever possible, observe the patient in the postanesthesia care unit, and give treatment with humidified oxygenation and nebulized racemic epinephrine as necessary.

REFERENCES

1. Giesecke AH, Grebershagen HV, Dortman C et al: Comparison of the ventilating and injecting bronchoscopes, *Anesthesiology* 38:298, 1973.
2. McGoldrick KE, Ho MD: Endoscopy procedures and laser surgery of the airway. In McGoldrick K, editor: *Anesthesia for ophthalmic and otolaryngologic surgery,* Philadelphia, 1992, WB Saunders.
3. Roizen MR, Horrigan RW, Frazer MB: Anesthetic doses blocking adrenergic and cardiovascular responses: MAC BAR, *Anesthesiology* 54:390, 1981.
4. Eschenbacher WL, Bethel RA, Boushey HA et al: Morphine sulfate inhibits bronchoconstriction in subjects with mild asthma whose responses are inhibited by atropine, *Am Rev Respir Dis* 130:363, 1984.
5. Strong MS, Vaughn CW, Mahler DL et al: Cardiac complications of microsurgery of the larynx, *Laryngoscope* 84:908, 1974.

6. Woods AM: Pediatric Endoscopy. In Berry FA, editor: *Anesthetic management of difficult and routine pediatric patients,* ed 2, New York, 1990, Churchill Livingstone.

7. Brull SJ: Monitoring of Neuromuscular Function, *Semin Anesthesia* 13(4):297, 1994.

8. Wright PMC, Caldwell JE, Miller RD: Onset and duration of rocuronium and succinylcholine at adductor pollicis and laryngeal adductor muscles in anesthetized humans, *Anesthesiology* 81:1110, 1994.

9. Donati F, Bevan DR: Not all muscles are the same, *Br J Anaesth* 68(3):235, 1992 (editorial).

10. Donati F, Meistelman C, Benoit P: Vecuronium neuromuscular blockade at the adductor muscles of the larynx and adductor pollicis, *Anesthesiology* 74:33, 1991.

11. Sayson SC, Mongan PD: Onset of action of mivacurium chloride, *Anesthesiology* 81:35, 1994.

12. Parsons DS, Lockett JS, Martin TW: Pediatric endoscopy: anesthesia and surgical techniques, *Am J Otolaryngol* 13(5):271, 1992.

13. Benjamin B: *Anesthesia for laryngoscopy. Ann Otol Rhino Laryngol* 93:338, 1984.

14. Babinski M, Smith RB, Klain M: High-frequency jet ventilation for laryngoscopy, *Anesthesiology* 52:178, 1980.

15. Weeks DB: Laboratory and clinical description of the use of a jet-Venturi ventilator during laser microsurgery, *Anesthesiol Rev* 12(3):32, 1985.

16. Jafek BW, Bauknight S, Calcaterra TC: Percutaneous anesthesia for endoscopy, *Arch Surg* 104:658, 1972.

17. Gaskill JR, Gillies DR: Local anesthesia for peroral endoscopy, *Arch Otolaryngol* 84:94, 1966.

18. Calcaterra TC, House J: Local anesthesia for suspension microlaryngoscopy, *Ann Otol Rhinol Laryngol* 85:71, 1976.

19. Murphy TM: Local anesthesia for head and neck surgery. In Cousins MJ, Bridenbaugh PO, editors: *Neural blockade in clinical anesthesia,* Philadelphia, 1980, Lippincott.

20. Woods AM, Cander CJ: Abolition of gagging and hemodynamic response to awake laryngoscopy, *Anesthesiology* 67:A220, 1987.

21. Woods AM, Longnecker DE: Endoscopy. In Marshall BE, Longnecker DE, Fairly HB, editors: *Anesthesia for thoracic procedures,* Boston, 1988, Blackwell Scientific.

22. Labedzki L, Ochs HR, Abernathy DR et al: Toxic serum lidocaine concentrations following spray anesthesia for bronchoscopy, *Klin Wochenschr* 61:379, 1983.

23. Norton ML, Strong MS: Anesthesia for endoscopic diagnoses and surgery, *Otolaryngol Clin North Am* 14:687, 1981.

24. Weisberger EC, Mines JD: Apneic anesthesia for improved endoscopic removal of laryngeal papillomata, *Laryngoscope* 98:693, 1988.

25. Keen RI, Kotak PK, Ramsden RT: Anesthesia for microsurgery of the larynx, *Ann Royal Coll Surg Engl* 64:111, 1982.

26. Sanders RD: Two ventilating attachments for bronchoscopes, *Del Med J* 39:170, 1967.

27. Carden E: Recent improvements in anesthetic techniques for bronchoscopy, *Ann Otol Rhinol Laryngol* 83:777, 1984.

28. Duvall AJ, Johnson AF, Buckley J: Bronchoscopy under general anesthesia using the Sanders ventilating attachment, *Ann Otol Rhinol Laryngol* 78:490, 1969.

29. Muendrich K, Hoflehner G: Die markose beatmungs bronchoscopic, *Anesthetist* 21:121-123, 1953.

30. Carden E, Schwesinger WB: The use of nitrous oxide during ventilation with the open bronchoscope, *Anesthesiology* 39:551, 1973.

31. Carden E, Burns WW, McDevitt NB et al: A comparison of Venturi and side-arm ventilation in anesthesia for bronchoscopy, *Can Anaesth Soc J* 20:569, 1970.

32. Johnson JT, Myers EN: Recent advances in operative laryngoscopy, *Otolaryngol Clin North Am* 17:35, 1984.

33. Smith RB: Anesthesia for endoscopy, *Pennsylvania Acad Ophthalmol Otolarygol Trans* 28(2):167, 1975.

34. Oulton JL, Donald DM: A ventilatory laryngoscope, *Anesthesiology* 35:540, 1971.

35. Albert SN, Shibuya J, Albert CA: Ventilations with an oxygen injector for suspension laryngoscopy, *Anesth Analg* 51:866, 1972.

36. Koufman JA, Little FB, Weeks DB: Proximal large-bore jet ventilation for laryngeal laser surgery, *Arch Otolaryngol Head Neck Surg* 113:314, 1987.

37. Cozine K, Stone JG, Shulman S et al: Ventilatory complications of carbon dioxide laser laryngeal surgery, *J Clin Anesth* 3:20, 1991.

38. Crockett DM, Scamman FL, McCabe BF et al: Venturi jet ventilation for microsurgery of the larynx: technique and complications, *Laryngoscope* 98:693, 1988.

39. Carden E: Positive pressure ventilation during anesthesia for bronchoscopy: two recent advances, *Anesth Analg* 52:402, 1973.

40. Schlenklof D, Droste H, Scienka S et al: The use of high-frequency jet ventilation (HFJV) in operative bronchoscopy, *Endoscopy* 18:192, 1986.

41. Eng UB, Erikson I, Sjostrand V: High-frequency positive pressure ventilation (HFPPV): its use during bronchoscopy and microlaryngeal surgery under general anesthesia, *Anesth Analg* 59:594, 1980.

42. Benumof JL: Anesthesia for special elective diagnostic procedures. In Benumof JL, editor: *Anesthesia for thoracic surgery,* Philadelphia, 1987, WB Saunders.

43. Calletly DC, Short TG: Total intravenous anesthesia using propofol infusion: 50 consecutive cases, *Anaesth Intensive Care* 16:150, 1988.

44. Ghouri AF, Ramirez Ruiz MA, White PF: Effect of flumazenil on recovery after midazolam and propofol sedation, *Anesthesiology* 81:333, 1994.

45. Benjamin B: Technique of laryngoscopy, *Int J Pediatr Otorhinolaryngol* 13:299, 1987.

46. Ehrenuerth J, Brull SJ: Anesthesia for thoracic diagnostic procedures. In Kaplan JA, editor: *Thoracic anesthesia,* ed 2, New York, 1993, Churchill Livingstone.

47. Ledbetter JL, Rasch DK, Pollard TG et al: Reducing the risks of laryngoscopy in anaesthetized infants, *Anaesthesia* 43:151, 1988.

48. Ward CF, Benumof JL: Anesthesia for airway foreign body extraction in children, *Anesth Rev* 4:13, 1977.

49. Kain Zn, O'Connor TZ, Berde CB: Management of tracheobronchial and esophageal foreign bodies in children: a survey study, *J Clin Anesth* 6:28, 1994.

50. Kosloske AM: Bronchoscopic extraction aspirated foreign bodies in children, *Am J Dis Child* 136:924, 1982.

51. Kortilla K, Tarkhamen J: Comparison of diazepam and midazolam for sedation during local anesthesia for bronchoscopy, *Br J Anaesth* 57:581, 1985.

52. Viegas O, Strelting RK: Lidocaine in arterial blood after laryngotracheal administration, *Anesthesiology* 43:491, 1975.

53. Lindholm CE, Ollman B, Snyder JV et al: Cardiorespiratory effect of flexible fiberoptic bronchoscopy in critically ill patients, *Chest* 74:362, 1978.

54. Satyanarayana T, Capan L, Ramanthan S et al: Bronchofiberscopic jet ventilation, *Anesth Analg* 59:350, 1980.

55. Pennant JH, White PF: The laryngeal mask airway: its uses in anesthesiology, *Anesthesiology* 79:144, 1993.

56. Van Hemelrijck J, Smith I, White PE: Use of desflurane for outpatient anesthesia, *Anesthesiology* 75:197-203, 1991.

57. Woods AM, Gaj TJ: Decreasing airflow resistance during infant and pediatric bronchoscopy, *Anesth Analg* 66:457, 1987.

58. Carden E: Recent improvements in techniques for general anesthesia in bronchoscopy, *Chest* 73:697, 1973.

59. Albertini RE, Harrel JH, Moser KM: Hypoxemia during fiberoptic bronchoscopy, *Chest* 65:11, 1974.

60. Gallagher MJ, Muller BJ: Tension pneumothorax during pediatric bronchoscopy, *Anesthesiology* 55:685, 1981.
61. Lukomsky GI, Ouchinnikoo AA, Bilas A: Complications of bronchoscopy: rigid bronchoscopy under general anesthesia and flexible fiberoptic bronchoscopy under local anesthesia, *Chest* 79:316, 1981.
62. Olsson GL: Bronchospasm during anesthesia: a computer aided incidence study of 136,529 patients, *Acta Anaesthesiol Scand* 31:244, 1987.
63. Luck JC, Messender OH, Rubenstein MJ et al: Arrhythmias from fiberoptic bronchoscopy, *Chest* 74:139, 1987.
64. Shikowitz MJ, Abramson AL: Cardiac complications of suspension laryngoscopy, *Arch Otolaryngol Head Neck Surg* 112:860, 1986.
65. Wark KJ, Lyons J, Feneck RO: Hemodynamic effects of bronchoscopy: pretreatment with fentanyl and alfentanil, *Anaesthesia* 41:162, 1986.
66. Mallon JS, Hew E, Wald R et al: Bolus doses of esmolol for the prevention of post intubation hypertension and tachycardia, *J Cardiothorac Vasc Anesth* 2:27, 1990.
67. Fraioli RC, Sheffer LA, Steffenson JC: Pulmonary and cardiovascular effects of apneic oxygenation in man, *Anesthesiology* 396:588, 1973.

Chapter 32

THE DIFFICULT AIRWAY IN CONVENTIONAL HEAD AND NECK SURGERY

Thomas B. Dougherty

I. INTRODUCTION

Conventional head and neck surgery encompasses a variety of surgical procedures ranging from adenotonsillectomy to major head and neck cancer resection. A recent trend emphasizes immediate reconstruction of the extirpative defect following radical tumor resection[1] in which microvascular techniques for reconstruction are being used with increasing frequency.[2]

In few situations is there a greater potential for airway management challenges than in head and neck surgery. The patients themselves often present to the operating room with conditions that make mask ventilation and tracheal intubation potentially or obviously difficult. The anesthesiologist frequently encounters a patient who may be scheduled for a lengthy procedure in which the surgical team requires complete and easy access to the operative site, which is either the airway itself or near it.[1] The anesthesiologist is often unable to be positioned near the head of the patient.[3] Yet, the surgeon expects the timely establishment of general anesthesia in the patient, a quiet operative field free of bulky equipment, and the patient's smooth emergence from anesthesia at the end of the procedure.[1]

This chapter discusses current principles and techniques for securing and managing safely the airways of patients undergoing conventional head and neck surgery. Emphasis is placed on the prevention of the airway problems associated with these kinds of operations.

II. HEAD AND NECK ONCOLOGIC SURGERY
A. PREOPERATIVE AIRWAY ASSESSMENT

The preoperative airway assessment includes evaluation of pertinent information from the head and neck oncologic patient's history, physical examination, previous anesthetic records, surgical plan, laboratory studies, and special studies.[4]

1. History

The history should emphasize the cardiovascular and respiratory systems. The typical adult head and neck cancer patient, perhaps a heavy smoker or drinker or both, may have evidence of chronic obstructive pulmonary disease, bronchitis, hypertension, coronary artery disease, or alcohol withdrawal.[3] These systemic problems may require special attention during an examination of the airway or an intubation in the awake patient.[5] Provision of oxygen to the patient or prevention of increased sympathetic nervous system stimulation may be necessary.

Information should be obtained about previous operations and recent anesthetic procedures, including whether airway management or endotracheal intubations were difficult.[1] The difficult airway is defined as the clinical situation in which a trained anesthesiologist experiences difficulty with mask ventilation, tracheal intubation, or both.[6] Difficult endotracheal intubation is encountered when proper insertion of the endotracheal tube with conventional (rigid) laryngoscopy requires more than three attempts or more than 10 minutes.[6] The presence of a tumor, plus the associated anatomic changes, may create a potentially difficult airway. If the lesion causes any airway obstruction, the patient has a compromised airway. A compromised airway in turn may be a difficult one.[1]

The patient should be asked about problems with shortness of breath, dyspnea, exercise intolerance, handling of secretions, hoarseness, dysphagia, and recent head and neck radiation treatments.[4] Changes in the character of the patient's voice may indicate the site of the lesion as well as the progression of the disease.[7] A muffled voice suggests a supraglottic tumor, whereas a coarse, scratchy voice is characteristic of a glottic lesion.[8]

A history of obstructive sleep apnea (OSA) without an obvious anatomic abnormality may indicate a hidden problem such as a vallecular mass.[7] This condition can certainly hinder mask ventilation and endotracheal

---

> **BOX 32-1   General physical indicators of a possible difficult airway or difficult intubation**
>
> Short muscular neck with a full set of teeth
> Small mouth and limited mouth opening
> Obesity
> Receding lower jaw (short thyromental distance)
> Protruding upper incisors
> Large tongue (e.g., caused by myxedema, acromegaly, or hemangioma [high oropharyngeal classification])
> Enlarged thyroid (goiter) displacing or impinging on the airway
> Limited mobility of cervical spine (mobility may not be desirable in certain instances, such as cervical fracture)

From Dougherty TB, Nguyen DT: *J Clin Anesth* 6:74, 1994.

intubation following the induction of general anesthesia. The patient with an anterior mediastinal, pharyngeal, or neck mass may have difficulty breathing in the supine position but not in the lateral or prone position. Anesthetizing such a patient in the supine position without first securing the airway may lead to severe airway obstruction.[7]

2. Physical examination

The patient's airway should be evaluated systematically and thoroughly. Detailed procedures for physical examination of the airway are reviewed elsewhere;[5,7,9] only pertinent features are described here. Certain congenital or acquired conditions other than head and neck neoplasms can also predispose the patient to a difficult airway. Some of these factors are listed in Box 32-1.

Answers to the following questions should be sought as part of the airway evaluation:[1,10]

1. What is the condition of the patient's teeth? The presence of dental appliances or diseased, loose, or protruding teeth may contribute to a difficult intubation.[7]

2. Is the tongue protruding, swollen, or fixed in position? A large tongue relative to the size of the oral cavity will interfere with adequate mask ventilation and endotracheal intubation.[5] Regardless of its size, a fixed tongue will make rigid laryngoscopy difficult.[7]

3. Does the patient exhibit stridor during either inspiration or expiration on auscultation of the larynx, trachea, and chest? Stridor results from increased turbulence and rate of air flow through a narrowed passage and thus suggests partial obstruction.[1,11] Inspiratory stridor may be caused by a lesion at or above the vocal cords, whereas expiratory stridor suggests a bronchial obstruction.[8] Stridor during both inspiration and expiration indicates a subglottic lesion.[8]

BOX 32-2   Common causes of difficult airway or intubation in head and neck oncologic patients

- Limited head and neck mobility and position
- Limited mouth opening
- Decreased upper airway open space resulting from tumor, edema, or previous surgery
- Distorted anatomy of the airway by tumor expansion or previous surgery
- Fixation of tissues of head and neck, oral cavity, pharynx, or larynx by tumor, surgical scars, or radiation fibrosis

---

From Dougherty TB, Nguyen DT: *J Clin Anesth* 6:74, 1994.

A tumor, previous surgery, or fibrosis from radiation treatments may limit mobility of the patient's neck and impede mask ventilation or conventional laryngoscopy. If the distance between the thyroid notch and the mental prominence of the mandible is less than 6 cm when the adult patient's neck is fully extended, visualization of the vocal cords by direct, rigid laryngoscopy may be difficult.[12]

Tumors and edema of the oral cavity, pharynx, and hypopharynx, together with previous surgery on the airway, may substantially decrease the upper airway's open space and distort its anatomy. All may interfere with mask application, maintenance of an adequate airway, and ease of endotracheal intubation.[1] Dysfunction of the ninth, tenth, or twelfth cranial nerve(s), whether the result of tumor invasion (e.g., glomus tumor) or injury from previous surgery, can predispose the patient to aspiration or obstruction.[13] Common causes of a difficult airway unique to head and neck oncologic patients are summarized in Box 32-2.

3. Laboratory and special studies

Arterial blood gas analysis and pulmonary function testing are recommended if the patient has significant chronic obstructive pulmonary disease. If partial airway obstruction is present in the patient, a flow-volume loop study is helpful to assess the upper airway. Information from indirect laryngoscopy, usually obtained by the head and neck surgeon, may suggest whether the airway or endotracheal intubation will be difficult. Tomograms, computed tomography scans, or magnetic resonance images often indicate the size and location of the patient's airway disease. The patient's obvious or potential airway problems should be discussed with the surgeon before the induction of general anesthesia or intubation is attempted.

B. SECURING THE AIRWAY

Statistical analyses of anesthesia-related cardiac arrests and adverse respiratory events suggest that one third of all severe complications are the result of an inability to establish an adequate upper airway following the induction of general anesthesia.[14,15] With few exceptions, the recently adopted American Society of Anesthesiologists' algorithm for the difficult airway[6] is useful in managing the airway of any patient undergoing head and neck oncologic surgery.

After evaluating the patient's airway and discussing the case with the surgeon, the anesthesiologist usually has one of the following options for securing the airway:[1] (1) to induce general anesthesia before intubation, (2) to examine the airway while the patient is under sedation and topical analgesia before inducing anesthesia in an effort to determine the safest intubation technique, (3) to start with an endotracheal intubation in the awake patient, or (4) to proceed with a tracheostomy performed with local anesthesia while the patient is awake.

1. Option 1: Induction of general anesthesia before intubation

In the patient who has no evidence of a compromised or difficult airway, it is usually safe to induce general anesthesia and paralysis before intubating the trachea. It is generally prudent to use a short-acting muscle relaxant such as succinylcholine.

2. Option 2: Examination of the airway in the awake patient

If management of the airway is potentially difficult, the anesthesiologist, in an effort to determine the best intubation technique, should perform an awake, direct examination of the patient's airway with the aid of intravenous sedation and topical anesthetic applied to the upper airway.

a. PREPARATION OF THE PATIENT

An adequate explanation to the patient of the events about to occur is the first step in preparing the patient for this procedure. Use of a pulse oximeter, electrocardiogram, and automatic blood pressure cuff to monitor the patient is mandatory. Supplemental oxygen should be provided to the patient. Because individual patient responses vary widely, drugs used for sedation should be cautiously titrated to effect while maintaining adequate oxygen saturation and meaningful contact with the patient. Meaningful contact means the patient remains rational and follows commands appropriately.[5] Topical analgesia can be obtained by adequately spraying the patient's oropharynx, tongue, and larynx with 4% lidocaine. An atomizer with an adjustable tip that creates a fine, dense, deeply penetrating spray when connected to a high-flow oxygen tank should be used.[5] To achieve adequate analgesia of the larynx itself, the patient should inhale deeply as the region behind the base of the tongue is sprayed. An anticholinergic drug, such as glycopyrrolate, may be administered to minimize oral secretions and to allow better contact of the lidocaine with the mucosa. The total dose of topical lidocaine should be limited to 3 to 4 mg/kg to prevent central nervous system intoxication arising from excessive systemic absorption of lidocaine from the oral and laryngeal mucosa.[16] It should be noted that airway obstruction may occur or worsen in some patients as a result of topical laryngeal application of lidocaine.[1] Generally, percutaneous blocks of the superior laryngeal and glossopharyngeal nerves or the translaryngeal instillation of lidocaine are avoided in head and neck cancer patients because these procedures are frequently contraindicated by the presence of tumor.[1]

b. CHOICE OF ENDOTRACHEAL INTUBATION TECHNIQUE

Once adequate analgesia of the patient's upper airway is achieved, conventional, direct laryngoscopy is carefully but quickly performed. At this time the anesthesiologist must decide whether to induce general anesthesia before intubation or to proceed with an intubation technique that can be used in the awake patient. For the former course of action, we proceed with a slow intravenous induction of general anesthesia while maintaining spontaneous ventilation.[3] Once the level of anesthesia is deepened with a potent inhalational agent, direct laryngoscopy is accomplished while the patient is ventilating spontaneously.[3] If the glottis can be visualized, a short-acting muscle relaxant is administered and intubation is accomplished. The caution is that being able to visualize the glottis in the awake patient with a potentially difficult airway does not guarantee the same ability following induction of anesthesia. A recent study indicated that induction of general anesthesia and paralysis results in an anterior displacement of the larynx, which can make visualization of the vocal cords more difficult.[17]

3. Option 3: Endotracheal intubation in the awake patient

If a difficult airway or intubation is expected from the preoperative airway evaluation or from the awake examination of the airway under topical analgesia, and the patient does not have a bulky, friable supraglottic tumor, the anesthesiologist proceeds with an endotracheal intubation technique in the awake patient. If not already present, topical analgesia of the upper airway and adequate sedation can be achieved as described in option 2.

a. FIBEROPTIC-GUIDED INTUBATION IN THE AWAKE PATIENT

In the awake patient the route of fiberoptic-guided intubation, either nasally or orally, is mandated by the planned surgical procedure and the patient's physical condition.[18] The nasotracheal route is particularly useful in patients with a small mouth, limited mouth opening, large tongue, receding lower jaw, or tracheal deviation.

For an oral intubation, an airway intubator such as a Williams[19] or Ovassapian[20] airway is carefully inserted into midline of the patient's mouth behind the tongue. The lubricated endotracheal tube, with its adapter removed, is placed at the proximal end of the lubricated fiberoptic laryngoscope. The tip of the fiberoptic scope is passed through the airway intubator, maneuvered under the epiglottis, and advanced past the vocal cords to a position in the trachea just above the carina.[1] The endotracheal tube is advanced over the laryngoscope into the trachea. The laryngoscope is carefully removed after the correct tracheal position of the tube is verified. The airway intubator can be removed or left in place as a bite block.[21] After the endotracheal tube adapter is attached and an end-tidal carbon dioxide waveform (in mm Hg) indicating tracheal placement of the tube is verified, general anesthesia can be induced as usual.

For a nasal intubation, the patient's nostrils are initially sprayed with a vasoconstrictor such a 0.05% oxymetazoline hydrochloride (Afrin Nasal Spray, Schering Corp., Kenilworth, N.J.) to decrease the risk of bleeding. Next, the nostrils are sprayed with 4% lidocaine, and progressively larger, soft nasal airways are gently inserted through a selected nostril to dilate it. A well-lubricated endotracheal tube is passed through the nostril to about the 15-cm mark.[5] A lubricated fiberoptic laryngoscope is passed through the nasotracheal tube into the oropharynx and advanced into the trachea through the glottic opening. The tube is threaded over the scope into the trachea to complete the intubation.

During a fiberoptic intubation in the awake patient, supplemental oxygen is usually provided to the patient. The approach of insufflating oxygen through the working port of the fiberoptic laryngoscope is effective and has the added benefit of blowing secretions away from the scope's tip, thus reducing fogging.[5] Suggestions for a successful fiberoptic intubation in the awake patient are summarized in Box 32-3.

b. OTHER AWAKE INTUBATION TECHNIQUES

A retrograde endotracheal intubation technique can be useful when an attempted fiberoptic intubation in the awake patient is unsuccessful or when blood and secretions in the awake patient's airway are excessive.[22-24] Other indications for its use may include trismus,[22] ankylosis of the jaw,[25] or upper airway masses[22,23] that are not large or friable. Briefly, in this technique a guidewire (e.g., Seldinger wire or central venous catheter) is passed through a needle puncturing the cricothyroid membrane, passed through the larynx in a cephalic direction, and advanced into the oropharynx. The guidewire tip is delivered out through the mouth or nose and then used as a stylet for passing an endotracheal tube into the trachea.

BOX 32-3   Suggestions for successful fiberoptic intubation in the awake patient

- Work with a well-oxygenated, well-sedated, cooperative patient with a dry oral cavity who can breathe adequately.
- Allow enough time to achieve adequate topical analgesia of the airway. If the analgesia begins to wear off, apply more local anesthetic between intubation attempts.
- Keep the operating room table at its lowest position, and work from a high position.
- Use a 7.5-mm or smaller endotracheal tube. Too much space between the fiberoptic laryngoscope and a larger tube may interfere with passage of the tube through the glottic opening.

From Dougherty TB, Nguyen DT: *J Clin Anesth* 6:74, 1994.

BOX 32-4   Minimizing the frequency of unanticipated difficult or failed intubation

- Be aware that a note in the patient's chart concerning his or her airway status 2 weeks ago may not be current if the patient has received radiation therapy in the interim.
- If the status of the airway is in doubt, intubate the trachea while the patient is awake.
- Resist the temptation to rush, and maintain good communication with other members of the operating team.
- Know your limits, and do not hesitate to seek help from a more experienced endoscopist.
- Always keep the patient's safety as the first priority.

From Dougherty TB, Nguyen DT: *J Clin Anesth* 6:74, 1994.

In his review of management of the difficult adult airway, Benumof[5] described combinations of conventional, fiberoptic, and retrograde techniques to aid in achieving successful intubations. A fiberoptic laryngoscope with a suction port can be used as an anterograde guide over a retrograde wire. Also, direct laryngoscopy can facilitate placement of the tip of a fiberoptic scope near the glottic opening.

4. Option 4: Tracheostomy with local anesthesia

If, upon arrival in the operating room, the patient is in acute respiratory distress because of upper airway obstruction, a tracheostomy performed with local anesthesia is indicated to secure the airway before the induction of anesthesia.[1] Intravenous sedation should be administered with extreme caution, if it is used at all. To prevent cardiopulmonary arrest in the severely hypoxic patient, transtracheal jet ventilation (TTJV), as described later, may have to be instituted during the tracheostomy.[1] A tracheostomy in the awake patient is also indicated as the first intubation choice in two other situations: (1) in the patient with an upper airway abscess along, and distorting, the route of intubation[26] and (2) in the patient with a bulky, friable laryngeal or other supraglottic tumor. Rigid or fiberoptic laryngoscopy and passage of the endotracheal tube greatly increase the risk of abscess rupture and airway contamination with pus in the former case and uncontrolled hemorrhage or tumor aspiration in the latter situation.

5. Difficult or failed intubation

An unexpectedly difficult or failed intubation following induction of general anesthesia is not uncommon in head and neck surgery patients. Suggestions to minimize its occurrence are listed in Box 32-4. If this situation is encountered on induction of general anesthesia, several principles should be followed.[1] It is necessary to avoid

traumatizing the airway with repeated attempts at rigid laryngoscopy. The attempts should be limited to four, using various neck positions and different laryngoscope blades. The anesthesiologist should have a clear plan of action formulated beforehand; the time to think and act is limited once an airway problem is encountered. The patient's risk for regurgitation and aspiration and the sudden loss of control of the airway should be constant considerations. The subsequent course of action depends on the anesthesiologist's ability to achieve mask ventilation of the patient.

If mask ventilation is adequate, general anesthesia can be continued with a potent inhalation agent. If the patient's vocal cords are too anterior to be visualized by conventional laryngoscopy, the use of the Bullard laryngoscope (CIRCON ACMI, Stamford, Conn.) may allow a successful intubation.[27,28] This laryngoscope has a broad, flat, curved L-shaped blade that is used to pick up the epiglottis (Fig. 32-1). A fiberoptic light source and an image bundle along the posterior surface of the blade allow a stylet-containing endotracheal tube with a nearly 90-degree bend to be passed through the vocal cords by direct vision.

a. FIBEROPTIC INTUBATION OF THE ANESTHETIZED PATIENT

As an alternative, in the adequately ventilated patient the airway may be secured with an oral fiberoptic-guided intubation. An airway intubator bite block[19,20] is inserted into the midline of the patient's mouth, and the regular anesthesia face mask is replaced with a mask containing a diaphragm-covered endoscopy port (e.g., the Patil-Syracuse endoscopy mask).[21,29] This mask enables the patient to be ventilated by an assistant while the anesthesiologist performs the fiberoptic intubation.[30] An endotracheal tube from which the circuit adapter has been removed is placed at the proximal end of a lubricated fiberoptic laryngoscope. The laryngoscope is passed through the mask's diaphragm, through the

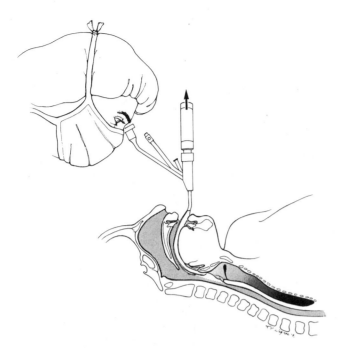

Fig. 32-1. The Bullard laryngoscope (CIRCON ACMI, Stamford, Conn.). Tip of the curved blade is used to pick up the epiglottis. A stylet-containing endotracheal tube with a nearly 90-degree bend at its distal end may be maneuvered through the patient's vocal cords by direct visualization. (From Dougherty TB, Nguyen DT: *J Clin Anesth* 6:74, 1994.)

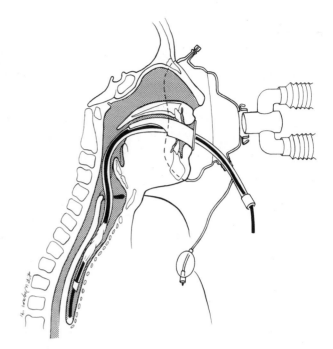

Fig. 32-2. Use of the anesthesia mask with diaphragm and oral airway intubator as aids to oral fiberoptic endotracheal intubation in the anesthetized patient. The fiberoptic laryngoscope and endotracheal tube have been introduced through the mask's diaphragm. After the endotracheal tube is in place and the laryngoscope is withdrawn, the mask is removed over the endotracheal tube. Removal of the oral airway is optional. (From Dougherty TB, Nguyen DT: *J Clin Anesth* 6:74, 1994.)

airway intubator, and into the trachea.[1] The tube is then threaded over the laryngoscope into the patient's trachea (Fig. 32-2).

A nasotracheal fiberoptic intubation may be another approach in the anesthetized patient. With this technique the tracheal tube adapter remains attached, and a bronchoscopy swivel adapter is connected to it.[1] A well-lubricated endotracheal tube is carefully passed through one nostril and advanced to the 15-cm mark.[5] An assistant occludes the opposite nostril and mouth to enable the lungs to be ventilated through the bronchoscope adapter as the fiberoptic laryngoscope is passed through the tube and into the trachea. The nasotracheal tube is then passed over the scope into the trachea (Fig. 32-3).

If all intubation attempts (including fiberoptic approaches) continue to be unsuccessful and mask ventilation can still be maintained, anesthesia is discontinued and the patient is allowed to awaken. The anesthesiologist proceeds with an awake intubation as discussed in option 3.

b. CRICOTHYROIDOTOMY

If mask ventilation of the anesthetized patient is inadequate, the American Society of Anesthesiologists' difficult airway algorithm should be followed. Assistance is called for, and one more attempt at intubation with conventional laryngoscopy is made.[6] If this fails, a large-bore intravenous catheter is inserted percutaneously through the cricothyroid membrane in a caudal direction, and TTJV is initiated quickly. The surgeon proceeds with a tracheostomy while the anesthesiologist refrains from giving any additional anesthesia until the airway is secured.[1]

c. TRANSTRACHEAL JET VENTILATION

Transtracheal jet ventilation has been well tested and shown to be very effective in providing ventilation in the situation in which the patient cannot be intubated nor adequately ventilated. Although TTJV has been discussed in detail in a recent review,[31] several aspects of TTJV require emphasis. First, the pressure of the oxygen delivered to the transtracheal catheter must be at least 50 psi. Adequate ventilation through the catheter is impossible with a conventional ventilator or handheld anesthesia bag.[30] Second, because the inspired oxygen forced through the catheter can escape only through the patient's own airway, attempts to maintain the airway must continue.[30] Obviously the equipment to perform an adequate TTJV must be readily available in the operating room. The assembly of several useful systems has been described elsewhere.[31-33]

In addition to TTJV, the esophageal-tracheal Combitube (Sheridan Catheter Corp., Argyle, N.Y.)[34] and the laryngeal mask airway (Intavent, Ltd., Berkshire,

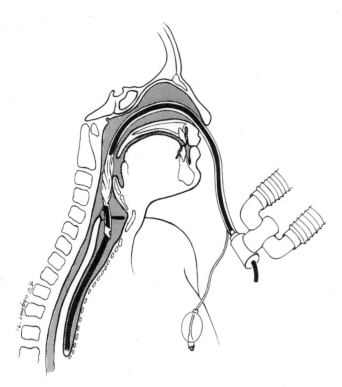

Fig. 32-3. Nasal fiberoptic intubation in an anesthetized patient. The nasotracheal tube is passed through a nostril to the 15-cm mark. If necessary, the lungs may be ventilated through the swivel adapter attached to the tube. The fiberoptic laryngoscope is passed through the nasotracheal tube into the trachea, and the nasotracheal tube is advanced over the laryngoscope. (From Dougherty TB, Nguyen DT: *J Clin Anesth* 6:74, 1994.)

England)[35-37] can be used blindly and rapidly to provide adequate ventilation in an emergency situation.[5,38] Although experience with the esophageal-tracheal Combitube and laryngeal mask airway in cases of difficult or failed intubations is increasing, the use of these in head and neck surgery is at best controversial and may not be practical.

C. INTRAOPERATIVE AIRWAY MANAGEMENT

1. Surgical field requirements

In many procedures the surgical field has to be kept clear of bulky equipment, especially when both sides of the patient's neck are included.[1] Because the head is often draped, the anesthesiologist's access to the airway is greatly restricted. Therefore the endotracheal tube and connectors must be nonkinking, of low profile, and secured to minimize pressure on the nasal ala or buccal commissure.[1] If possible, the endotracheal tube should be secured to the patient's head to allow the surgeon to reposition the head, if necessary, without causing an accidental extubation. For certain surgical procedures an oral endotracheal tube has to be secured at the buccal commissure and directed laterally away from the patient.

Because of operative field requirements, any tape used for securing the tube is not allowed to extend more than 1 to 2 cm toward the opposite side of the patient's face. Constant vigilance is needed to prevent the breathing circuit from exerting downward pressure on the tube's adapter. If this happens, the commissure may act like a fulcrum and the distal end of the tube may work its way out of the trachea.

2. Tracheostomy

If the procedure involves placement of a tracheostomy, muscle relaxants might be avoided during that portion of the surgery in an attempt to maintain spontaneous respirations.[39] Administration of 100% oxygen prior to the actual tracheostomy is advised so that if control of the airway is lost, there will be some oxygen reserve before hypoxemia results.[39] As the trachea is transected, the nasal or oral endotracheal tube is carefully pulled from the surgeon's field just so the tip of the endotracheal tube is at the proximal (cephalad) margin of the tracheal incision (which allows rapid reinsertion if there is false passage of the tracheostomy tube). Following creation of the tracheostomy, the surgeon places a sterile, flexible, reinforced, cuffed endotracheal tube into the trachea through the stoma. An adapter and short length of flexible tubing are attached to this tube and passed under the drapes for connection with the awaiting breathing circuit. It is mandatory that this maneuver be well thought out in the anesthesiologist's mind before transection of the patient's trachea to avoid unnecessary delay in providing ventilation to the patient. Correct placement of the endotracheal tube must be verified by the appearance of an end-tidal carbon dioxide waveform and by the presence of breath sounds on auscultation.

Problems that can occur during tracheostomy include production of subcutaneous emphysema, false passage, tracheoesophageal fistula, pneumothorax, damage to the recurrent laryngeal nerve, excessive bleeding, and tracheal aspiration of blood.[39-41] Unless the reinforced endotracheal tube is sutured securely to the patient's chest wall, it will occasionally slip down a mainstem bronchus because of the short distance to the carina.[3] If the level of anesthesia is light at this point, bronchospasm may occur. To prevent contamination of the airway, blood and secretions from the portion of the trachea above the tracheostomy site should be suctioned before exchanging the temporary endotracheal tube for a more permanent tracheostomy tube.

D. EXTUBATION OF THE TRACHEA

In head and neck operations in which no tracheostomy is established the timing of extubation depends on the degree of edema and distortion of the upper airway produced by the operation.[1] Patients undergoing lengthy procedures, including flap reconstruction, should be kept sedated and intubated overnight in the surgical intensive care unit. Others can be extubated in the operating room or postanesthesia care unit when fully awake. Equipment used for securing the airway at anesthetic induction must be immediately available at extubation. In most patients, extubation will be straightforward. In others, however, it may be more of a challenge than the original intubation. Mask ventilation may no longer be feasible following extubation because of surgical changes in the patient's airway anatomy. The use of nasal or oral airways may be contraindicated by the risk of destroying the surgical work inside the nasopharynx or oropharynx.

Before attempting extubation, the anesthesiologist must address several questions.[1] If acute airway obstruction (e.g., from edema or soft tissue collapse) develops after extubation, can the airway be reestablished in a timely fashion to prevent hypoxia? Are skilled personnel and necessary equipment readily available for an emergency cricothyroidotomy, TTJV, and tracheostomy? If the answers are yes, the extubation can proceed. If not, the trachea should be extubated over a fiberoptic laryngoscope using the following technique.[1] After the patient is placed in a semisitting position and given oxygen supplementation, 4% lidocaine topical spray is applied around the glottic area and inside the endotracheal tube. The patient may need to be lightly and carefully sedated. A small-diameter fiberoptic laryngoscope is inserted through the endotracheal tube, and the scope's tip is positioned near the carina. After the cuff is deflated, the distal end of the tube is carefully and slowly backed out of the trachea and larynx while the fiberoptic scope is maintained in its intratracheal position. If the patient can breathe adequately for 2 to 3 minutes, the laryngoscope and endotracheal tube are removed from the airway. However, if the airway becomes obstructed, the tracheal tube is advanced back into the trachea over the fiberoptic scope, and extubation is attempted later.

A recently described, effective alternative is extubation over a jet stylet.[31,42] A hollow tube exchanger with a small internal diameter is inserted through the endotracheal tube into the patient's trachea. After the tube is withdrawn over the stylet, the hollow catheter can then be used as a means of jet ventilation, a reintubation guide, or both.[5] This approach with the jet stylet appears especially useful in situations in which an endotracheal tube needs to be exchanged or replaced.

III. ESOPHAGEAL SURGERY
A. PREOPERATIVE AIRWAY CONSIDERATIONS

The preoperative evaluation of the patient with reflux esophagitis or a malignant lesion of the esophagus and the surgical approaches to treat these problems are described in detail elsewhere.[43-45] The patient with esophageal carcinoma may have limited cardiopulmonary reserve as a result of the toxic effects of chemotherapeutic agents (doxorubicin, bleomycin, or mitomycin C) used to treat the tumor.[46,47] This must be considered when formulating the plan to secure the airway. In particular, the patient may have a history of dysphagia with an incompetent or obstructed esophagus that increases the danger of regurgitation and aspiration on induction of general anesthesia.

B. AIRWAY MANAGEMENT

The patient should be considered to have a full stomach because it is difficult to completely empty the stomach or esophagus with a nasogastric tube.[43] A fiberoptic-guided intubation in the awake patient following topical analgesia of the upper airway or a rapid-sequence induction of general anesthesia is appropriate for securing the airway.[44] Preinduction administration of ranitidine, metoclopramide, and oral sodium citrate-citric acid buffer (Bicitra, Willen Drug Co., Baltimore, Maryland) reduces the risk of aspiration and subsequent pulmonary damage. In the patient with evidence of a tracheoesophageal fistula a fiberoptic intubation when the patient is awake is preferred to position the endotracheal tube beyond the fistula before the induction of anesthesia. If the potential for airway compression exists because of the presence of large mediastinal lymph nodes, it is best to position a reinforced endotracheal tube distal to the obstruction under fiberoptic guidance while the patient is awake.

For surgery involving the lower two thirds of the esophagus a thoracotomy is part of the procedure. A left-sided, double-lumen endotracheal tube is used for one-lung ventilation (OLV), which greatly facilitates surgical exposure by collapsing the nondependent lung.[48] However, because the pulmonary artery to the nondependent lung is not ligated, significant hypoxemia can occur after insituting OLV. In fact, hypoxemia is often greater during this situation than it is during lobectomy or pneumonectomy, and it can persist as long as the lung is collapsed.[45,49,50] Hypoxemia during OLV is treated with selective continuous positive airway pressure to the nonventilated, nondependent lung with or without positive end-expiratory pressure to the dependent lung.[51] A 100% oxygen concentration should always be used throughout OLV.

A transhiatal esophagectomy without thoracotomy may be performed in the patient with cervical esophageal cancer. The esophagus is approached through an abdominal and a left cervical incision, and a blunt, manual dissection of the esophagus is accomplished through the diaphragmatic hiatus.[43] Excessive bleeding and tracheal injury may occur, necessitating an emergency thoracotomy for treatment.[52]

IV. ADENOTONSILLECTOMY

A. PREOPERATIVE AIRWAY CONSIDERATIONS

Patients undergoing adenotonsillectomy are, for the most part, healthy children or young adults.[39] Current indications for the procedure, or a variant thereof, include recurrent tonsillitis, chronic airway obstruction, OSA, peritonsillar abscess, and carcinoma of the tonsil.[53]

1. Obstructive sleep apnea

During rapid-eye-movement sleep the pharyngeal muscles relax along with other muscles of the body. In patients with OSA this relaxation produces airway obstruction leading to episodes of hypoxemia. If left untreated, OSA eventually results in pulmonary hypertension, cor pulmonale, and congestive heart failure.[54-56] Moreover, adults with this syndrome are likely to be obese with short, thick necks, relatively large tongues, and redundant soft tissue in the oropharynx.[39] This condition is surgically treated by performing a tonsillectomy, uvulectomy, and limited pharyngectomy with resection of redundant soft tissue of the soft palate.[54,56]

Initial airway management in these patients can be challenging. Induction of general anesthesia relaxes the pharyngeal muscles and can thus lead to airway obstruction in the same manner as rapid-eye-movement sleep.[3] Mask ventilation can be difficult, and oral or nasal airways are often ineffective in relieving the obstruction. Likewise, visualization of the vocal cords by direct rigid laryngoscopy is hindered by the presence of redundant pharyngeal tissue. As a consequence, a fiberoptic-guided intubation in the awake patient following topical analgesia should be attempted prior to the induction of anesthesia. Because patients with OSA are frequently more sensitive to sedatives and analgesics, it is wise to carefully titrate these drugs to effect if any sedation is needed to supplement topical analgesia.

2. Peritonsillar abscess

The patient with an expanding peritonsillar abscess presents a unique airway management problem. Pain and trismus, which limit mouth opening, and dysphagia are likely to be present. Edema and airway distortion significantly increase the risk of airway obstruction. Following the induction of general anesthesia a difficult airway can be expected, as can a possible spontaneous rupture of the abscess with spillage of pus into the unprotected airway. To decrease the risk of abscess rupture, preoperative decompression and drainage of the abscess should be attempted by needle aspiration with the patient under local analgesia.[57]

Usually only two options are available for initially securing the airway in the adult patient: either intubate

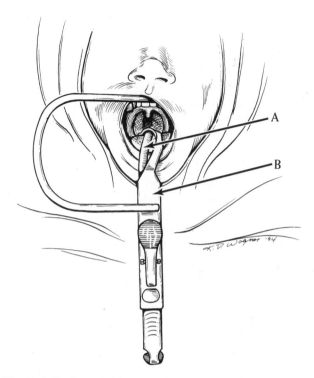

Fig. 32-4. Patient positioned for adenotonsillectomy. The oral endotracheal tube (**A**) is held in place by the Crow-Davis mouth gag (**B**). (Redrawn from Kirk GA: Anesthesia for ear, nose, and throat surgery. In Rogers MC, Tinker JH, Covino BG et al, editors: *Principles and practice of anesthesiology,* vol 2, St Louis, 1993, Mosby.)

the trachea under direct vision while the patient is awake and breathing spontaneously or request the surgeon to perform an elective tracheostomy with the patient under local anesthesia while the patient is awake. The former option should be attempted only if the abscess is not too large or is not located along the route of intubation.

B. AIRWAY MANAGEMENT DURING ADENOTONSILLECTOMY

In the adult patient without a history of upper airway obstruction a standard intravenous induction of general anesthesia followed by rigid laryngoscopy and intubation is safe. After anesthesia is induced and the patient is intubated, the surgeon places a mouth gag (e.g., Crow-Davis gag) into the patient's mouth to increase operative exposure. The endotracheal tube is held in a groove located in the midline of the gag's tongue blade (Fig. 32-4). Because the surgeon can accidentally extubate the patient during placement of the mouth gag,[58] the endotracheal tube should be secured to the patient with tape. As an alternative, a piece of tape can be placed on the tube to serve as a visual marker to indicate any insertion or withdrawal of the tube.[39] Continuous monitoring of breath sounds, peak airway pressure, tidal volume, and end-tidal carbon dioxide waveform is essential because the endotracheal tube can be easily compressed or kinked by the mouth gag, and it or the cuff can be inadvertently cut during resection of tonsillar tissue.[3] At the end of the operation the surgeon may release tension on the mouth gag to check for bleeding from blood vessels that may have been compressed by the gag. At this time, if the endotracheal tube is held in place only by the loosened gag and was not previously secured to the patient with tape, it can become dislodged from the trachea.

Attention must be paid to preventing aspiration of blood and early postoperative laryngospasm. Any pooled blood should be gently suctioned from the patient's oropharynx and nasopharynx prior to extubation. After extubation the patient should be placed on one side with the head slightly lower than the hips to allow blood and secretions to drain outside the mouth instead of dripping onto the vocal cords.[3]

C. POSTOPERATIVE AIRWAY PROBLEMS

Patients, especially children, with OSA should be kept overnight in a postanesthesia care unit with continuous monitoring of their breathing and oxygen saturation.[59] This is advisable because relief of airway obstruction does not always immediately relieve apneic episodes; instead, a central apneic component may be unmasked.[39]

Most morbidity from adenotonsillectomy results from unrecognized bleeding and airway obstruction during the recovery period.[60] Since the bleeding usually occurs as a slow ooze, the patient may swallow a large volume of blood and become hypovolemic before any bleeding is detected. The falling hemoglobin level and aspiration of blood may lead to hypoxemia in the patient. If surgery is required for treatment, the patient should be considered to have a full stomach with blood in the airway.[3] It is preferable to secure the airway with intubation under direct vision while the patient is awake. If this is impossible, a rapid-sequence anesthesia induction with ketamine or etomidate and intubation are indicated.

V. CRANIOFACIAL SURGERY

Knowledge and understanding of the types of deformities in patients with craniofacial problems allow the prediction of airway problems in advance and the avoidance of emergency situations in the operating room.[61] In the adult, when growth of the facial skeleton is complete, operations of this type are usually limited to orthognathic procedures and temporomandibular joint surgery.

A. ORTHOGNATHIC SURGERY

Orthognathic surgical procedures are used to correct maxillomandibular deformities such as malocclusion and unbalanced facial features. Le Fort types I and II osteotomies, for example, are used to change the position or dimensions of the maxilla, whereas a sagittal split osteotomy of the mandible is commonly used to advance or set back the mandible.[61] Most patients receiving these procedures are healthy adolescents or young adults.[3] Many, however, have anatomic features such as retrognathia, maxillary protrusion, or limited mouth opening, all of which can make intubation following induction of general anesthesia difficult.[3,62] The presence of orthodontic appliances only increases the potential for a difficult airway.

1. Airway management

If preoperative examination reveals a potentially difficult airway, the anesthesiologist should secure the airway with a fiberoptic-guided intubation in the awake patient. Nasotracheal intubation is preferred because orthognathic surgery requires most incisions to be made intraorally and the patient may awaken from anesthesia in intermaxillary fixation (upper and lower teeth wired together).

Topical analgesia of the upper airway and adequate sedation are achieved as previously described. If needed to improve intubating conditions, bilateral percutaneous blocks of the lingual branch of the glossopharyngeal nerve and the internal branch of the superior laryngeal nerve[5] may be performed together with the translaryngeal instillation of lidocaine. Following successful intubation of the patient's trachea a curved adapter with a flexible extension is attached to the nasotracheal tube. The tube's regular adapter should be removed before attempting the intubation. The breathing circuit is connected to the extension. After induction of general anesthesia the tube's extension is padded and taped over the patient's forehead with the breathing circuit arranged to come down behind the top of the head as illustrated in Fig. 32-5.

One unique and serious potential intraoperative complication of craniofacial surgery relates to the extensive use of pneumatic cutting instruments, especially during maxillary surgery. The close proximity of the endotracheal tube to the bone cutting sites in a restricted area increases the likelihood of direct damage to the endotracheal tube, including complete transection.[63] Should damage to the nasotracheal tube occur, either the patient must be quickly reintubated or the airway must be reestablished by sealing the area around the tube with throat packs. The course of action depends on the extent of tube damage and the amount of surgery yet to be completed.[63]

2. Extubation of the trachea

If the patient's upper and lower teeth have been placed in intermaxillary fixation to stabilize the jaws as part of the procedure, extubation should be attempted

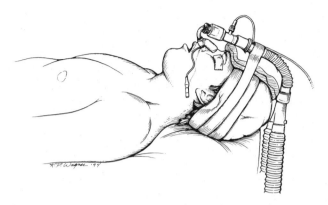

Fig. 32-5. A suggested position for orthognathic surgery. The flexible extension of the nasotracheal tube is padded and taped over the forehead with the breathing circuit coming down behind the top of the patient's head. (Redrawn from Kirk GA: Anesthesia for ear, nose, and throat surgery. In Rogers MC, Tinker JH, Covino BG et al, editors: *Principles and practice of anesthesiology,* vol 2, St Louis, 1993, Mosby.)

only after the patient is fully awake and airway reflexes are intact.[62] Because access to the airway is impeded, appropriate cutting tools need to be at the patient's bedside at all times in case an airway emergency arises.

B. TEMPOROMANDIBULAR JOINT SURGERY

Temporomandibular joint surgery is an elective procedure, the airway management of which is usually complicated by severe limitation in mouth opening.[62] Because temporomandibular joint disease may be a manifestation of rheumatoid arthritis, the anesthesiologist must be aware of the increased likelihood of cervical spine instability. Excessive movement of the neck can increase the risk of atlantoaxial subluxation and vertebral artery insufficiency.[62] The recommended approach to secure the airway involves a fiberoptic nasotracheal intubation in the awake patient after analgesia of the upper airway and adequate sedation are obtained.

VI. CONCLUSION

Airway management is a major component of the anesthetic plan for the patient scheduled for conventional head and neck surgery. Careful assessment of the airway and communication with the surgeon enable the anesthesiologist to decide on the most appropriate course of action for securing the patient's airway before surgery begins. The judgment may be that the patient can be intubated safely following induction of general anesthesia. If not, an examination of the airway using sedation and topical analgesia while the patient is awake or a fiberoptic-guided intubation in the awake patient before induction of general anesthesia may be required. Some patients may require an initial tracheostomy performed with the patient under local anesthesia to

secure the airway. The anesthesiologist must always have in mind a clear plan of action in case an unexpectedly difficult airway develops and the patient cannot be intubated with rigid laryngoscopy after anesthesia is induced. Because access to the airway during the procedure may be greatly restricted, constant vigilance is essential to prevent or detect an accidental loss of control of the airway. Finally, extubation of the trachea after surgery requires careful attention and may be more of a challenge than the original intubation.[1]

REFERENCES

1. Dougherty TB, Nguyen DT: Anesthetic management of the patient scheduled for head and neck cancer surgery. *J Clin Anesth* 6:74, 1994.
2. Davis D: Principles of surgical reconstruction. In Stafford N, Waldron J, editors: *Management of oral cancer.* Oxford, 1989, Oxford University.
3. Kirk GA: Anesthesia for ear, nose, and throat surgery. In Rogers MC, Tinker JH, Covino BG et al, editors: *Principles and practice of anesthesiology,* vol 2, St Louis, 1993, Mosby.
4. Donlon JV Jr: Anesthesia for eye, ear, nose, and throat surgery. In Miller RD, editor: *Anesthesia,* ed 2, vol 3, New York, 1986, Churchill Livingstone.
5. Benumof JL: Management of the difficult adult airway: with special emphasis on awake tracheal intubation, *Anesthesiology* 75:1087, 1991.
6. American Society of Anesthesiologists: Practice guidelines for management of the difficult airway: a report by the American Society of Anesthesiologists' task force on management of the difficult airway, *Anesthesiology* 78:597, 1993.
7. Ovassapian A: The difficult intubation. In Ovassapian A, editor: *Fiberoptic airway endoscopy in anesthesia and critical care,* New York, 1990, Raven.
8. Barratt GE, Coulthard SW: Upper airway obstruction: diagnosis and management options. In Brown BR, editor: *Contemporary anesthesia practice,* Philadelphia, 1987, FA Davis.
9. Mallampati SR, Gatt SP, Gugino LD et al: A clinical sign to predict difficult tracheal intubation: a prospective study, *Can Anaesth Soc J* 32:429, 1985.
10. Scamman FL: Anesthesia for surgery of head and neck tumors. In Thawley SE, Panje WR, editors: *Comprehensive management of head and neck tumors,* Philadelphia, 1987, WB Saunders.
11. Prust RS, Calkins JM: Considerations for managing the airway in the ENT patient. In Brown BR, editor: *Contemporary anesthesia practice,* Philadelphia, 1987, FA Davis.
12. Patil VU, Stehling LC, Zauder HL: Predicting the difficulty of intubation utilizing an intubation guide, *Anesthesiol Rev* 10(8):32, 1983.
13. Jensen NF: Glomus tumors of the head and neck: anesthetic considerations, *Anesth Analg* 78:112, 1994.
14. Caplan RA, Posner KL, Ward RS et al: Adverse respiratory events in anesthesia: a closed claims analysis, *Anesthesiology* 72:828, 1990.
15. Keenan RL, Boyan CP: Cardiac arrest due to anesthesia: a study of incidence and causes, *JAMA* 253:2373, 1985.
16. Ovassapian A: Topical anesthesia of the airway. In Ovassapian A, editor: *Fiberoptic airway endoscopy in anesthesia and critical care,* New York, 1990, Raven.
17. Sivarajan M, Fink BR: The position and the state of the larynx during general anesthesia and muscle paralysis, *Anesthesiology* 72:439, 1990.
18. Ovassapian A: Fiberoptic-assisted management of the airway. In *1990 annual refresher course lectures,* no. 254, Park Ridge, Ill, 1990, American Society of Anesthesiologists.

19. Williams RT, Harrison RE: Prone tracheal intubation simplified using an airway intubator, *Can Anaesth Soc J* 28:288, 1981.
20. Ovassapian A, Dykes MHM: The role of fiberoptic endoscopy in airway management, *Semin Anesth* 6:93, 1987.
21. Rogers SN, Benumof JL: New and easy techniques for fiberoptic endoscopy-aided tracheal intubation, *Anesthesiology* 59:569, 1983.
22. Waters DJ: Guided blind endotracheal intubation, *Anesthesia* 18:158, 1963.
23. Butler FS, Cirillo AA: Retrograde tracheal intubation, *Anesth Analg* 39:333, 1960.
24. Barriot P, Riou B: Retograde technique for tracheal intubation in trauma patients, *Crit Care Med* 16:712, 1988.
25. Powell WF, Ozdil T: A translaryngeal guide or tracheal intubation, *Anesth Analg* 46:231, 1967.
26. Heindel DJ: Deep neck abscesses in adult: management of a difficult airway, *Anesth Analg* 66:774, 1987.
27. Borland LM, Casselbrant M: The Bullard laryngoscope: a new indirect oral laryngoscope (pediatric version), *Anesth Analg* 70:105, 1990.
28. Saunders PR, Geisecke AH: Clinical assessment of the adult Bullard laryngoscope, *Can J Anaesth* 36:S118, 1989.
29. Patil V, Stehling LC, Zander HL et al: Mechanical aids for fiberoptic endoscopy, *Anesthesiology* 57:69, 1982.
30. Benumof JL: Management of the difficult or impossible airway. In *1990 Annual refresher course lectures,* no. 163, Park Ridge, Ill, 1990, American Society of Anesthesiologists.
31. Benumof JL, Scheller MS: The importance of transtracheal jet ventilation in the management of the difficult airway, *Anesthesiology* 71:769, 1989.
32. Meyer PD: Emergency transtracheal jet ventilation system, *Anesthesiology* 73:787, 1990 (letter).
33. Sprague DH: Transtracheal jet oxygenator from capnographic monitoring components, *Anesthesiology* 73:788, 1990 (letter).
34. Frass M, Frenzer R, Zahler J et al: Ventilation via the esophageal Combitube in case of difficult intubation, *J Cardiothorac Vasc Anesth* 1:565, 1987.
35. Calder I, Ordman AJ, Jackowski A et al: The brain laryngeal mask airway: an alternative to emergency tracheal intubation, *Anaesthesia* 45:137, 1990.
36. DeMello WF, Kocan M: The laryngeal mask in failed intubation, *Anaesthesia* 45:689, 1990.
37. Ravalia A, Goddard JM: The laryngeal mask and difficult tracheal intubation, *Anaesthesia* 45:168, 1990 (letter).
38. Pennant JH, White PF: The laryngeal mask airway: its uses in anesthesiology, *Anesthesiology* 79:144, 1993.
39. Feinstein R, Owens WD: Anesthesia for ear, nose, and throat surgery. In Barash PG, Cullen BF, Stoelting RK, editors: *Clinical anesthesia,* ed 2, Philadelphia, 1992, JB Lippincott.
40. Kirchner JA: Tracheotomy and its problems, *Surg Clin North Am* 60:1093, 1980.
41. Greenway RE: Tracheostomy: surgical problems and complications, *Int Anesthesiol Clin* 10:151, 1972.
42. Bedger RC, Chang JL: A jet stylet catheter for difficult airway management, *Anesthesiology* 66:221, 1987.
43. Banoub M, Nugent M: Thoracic anesthesia. In Rogers MC, Tinker JH, Covino BG et al, editors: *Principles and practice of anesthesiology,* vol 2, St Louis, 1993, Mosby.
44. Merritt WT: Anesthesia for gastrointestingal surgery. In Rogers MC, Tinker JH, Covino BG et al, editors: *Principles and practice of anesthesiology,* vol 2, St Louis, 1993, Mosby.
45. Eisenkraft JB, Neustein SM: Anesthesia for esophageal and mediastinal surgery. In Kaplan JA, editor: *Thoracic anesthesia,* ed 2, New York, 1991, Churchill Livingstone.
46. Stoelting RK: *Pharmacology and physiology in anesthetic practice,* ed 2, Philadelphia, 1991, JB Lippincott.
47. Crooke ST, Bradner WT: Bleomycin: a review, *J Med* 7:333, 1976.
48. Aitkenhead AR: Anesthesia for esophageal surgery. In Gothard JW, editor: *Thoracic anesthesia,* London, 1987, Bailliere-Tindall.
49. Hatch D: Ventilation and arterial oxygenation during thoracic surgery, *Thorax* 21:310, 1966.
50. Torda TA, McCulloch CH, O'Brien HD et al: Pulmonary venous admixture during one-lung anesthesia, *Anaesthesia* 29:272, 1974.
51. Benumof JL, editor: *Anesthesia for thoracic surgery,* Philadelphia, 1987, WB Saunders.
52. Sung HMH, Nelems B: Tracheal tear during laryngopharyngectomy and transhiatal esophagectomy: a case report, *Can J Anaesth* 36:333, 1989.
53. Davidson TM, Calloway CA: Tonsillectomy and adenoidectomy: its indications and its problems, *West J Med* 133:451, 1980.
54. Hall JB: The cardiopulmonary failure of sleep-disordered breathing, *JAMA* 255:930, 1986.
55. Bradley TD, Phillipson EA: Pathogenesis and pathophysiology of the obstructive sleep apnea syndrome, *Med Clin North Am* 69:1169, 1985.
56. Chung F, Crago RR: Sleep apnoea syndrome and anaesthesia, *Can Anaesth Soc J* 29:439, 1982.
57. Donlon JV Jr: Anesthesia for eye, ear, nose, and throat surgery. In Miller RD, editor: *Anesthesia,* ed 3, vol 2, New York, 1990, Churchill Livingstone.
58. Badrinath SK, Ivankovich AD, Patterson AR et al: Anesthesia for tonsillectomy and adenoidectomy. In Brown BR, editor: *Anesthesia and ENT surgery,* Philadelphia, 1987, FA Davis.
59. McColley SA, April MM, Carroll JL et al: Respiratory compromise after adenotonsillectomy in children with obstructive sleep apnea, *Arch Otolaryngol Head Neck Surg* 118:940, 1992.
60. Crysdale WD, Russel D: Complications of tonsillectomy and adenoidectomy in 9409 children observed overnight, *Can Med Assoc J* 135:1139, 1986.
61. Munro IR: Craniofacial surgery: airway problems and management, *Int Anesthesiol Clin* 26:72, 1988.
62. Murphy A, Donoff B: Anesthesia for orthognathic surgery, *Int Anesthesiol Clin* 27:98, 1989.
63. Fagraeus L, Angelillo JC, Dolan EA: A serious anesthetic hazard during orthognathic surgery, *Anesth Analg* 59:150, 1980.

Chapter 33

ANESTHESIA FOR LASER AIRWAY SURGERY

Mitchel B. Sosis

I. INTRODUCTION

Medical applications of laser therapy began soon after the invention of the argon laser by Maiman in 1959.[1] The laser has shown itself to be a powerful therapeutic modality in ophthalmology, dermatology, and otolaryngology, and wider medical uses continue to be found. In addition to its power, the laser usually has the advantages of precision, hemostasis, selective absorption by pigmented materials, lack of trauma to healthy tissue, reduced postoperative pain and edema, and finally, sterility. The high energy of the laser and its potential for combustion pose special problems when the surgical field is in proximity to the airway (Fig. 33-1). To provide care to patients undergoing laser surgery, the anesthesiologist who works with them should be familiar with the elements of laser operation, the types of lasers available, and special anesthesia considerations for safe laser surgery. This chapter reviews both laser technology and the special anesthesia considerations essential for safe patient care.

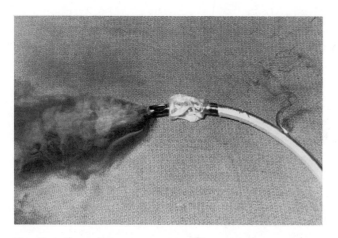

Fig. 33-1. Potentially catastrophic laser-induced endotracheal tube fire. Polyvinyl chloride endotracheal tube that had been wrapped with Radio Shack no. 44-1155 tape is pictured. The site of the laser's impingement on the wrapped endotracheal tube can be seen at the right. This endotracheal tube had 100% O_2 flowing through it. A CO_2 laser with a power output of 70 watts in the continuous mode was used. (From Sosis M: *Adv Anesthesia* 6:175, 1989.)

II. PRINCIPLES OF LASER TECHNOLOGY

The word "laser" is an acronym for *light amplification by stimulated emission of radiation.* The laser's radiation has its basis in the excitation of electrons. The electrons orbiting the nucleus of an atom can be excited into higher energy levels by absorbing energy. Quantum theory states that the allowable energy states of these electrons are a series of discrete steps rather than a continuum[2] (Fig. 33-2). Those electrons occupying higher energy levels will spontaneously emit radiation in the form of a photon or light packet. The energy of this photon is equivalent to the difference between the two energy levels. If the photon interacts with atoms whose electrons are already in excited states, it will cause them to decay to lower energy levels and release energy. This is a process known as *stimulated emission.* The emitted photons will have the same energy, frequency, and wavelength as the initial stimulating photon. Also, these photons will be traveling in exactly the same direction, and the radiation is therefore *collimated.* Thus the laser's radiation will not diverge the way radiation from other

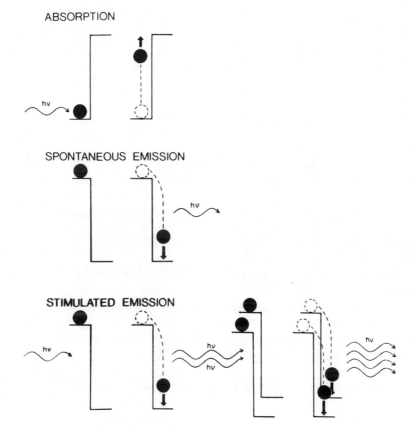

Fig. 33-2. The processes of absorption, spontaneous emission, and stimulated emission necessary for a laser to operate. A photon or light packet with energy ($h\nu$) or other power source can provide the energy necessary to raise the energy level of electrons from the ground state to an excited state (*absorption*). In the excited state the electron is unstable and will re-emit this energy (*spontaneous emission*). A photon of the appropriate energy impinging on an electron in the excited state will cause the release of a second photon of the same energy (*stimulated emission*). The latter photon will travel in the same direction and it will be in phase with the first photon. (From Saunder ML et al: *Surg Neurol* 14:1, 1980.)

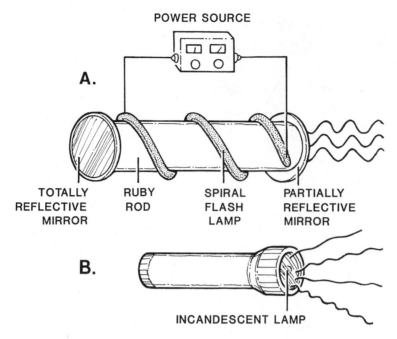

Fig. 33-3. In the laser, **A,** a power source (power supply and flash lamp) stimulates the lasing medium, in this case a ruby rod. The spontaneous emission of photons from electrons in the excited state stimulates the emission of more photons. The parallel mirrors reflect those photons traveling along the axis of the laser, amplifying the intensity of the radiation. This results in a coherent monochromatic laser beam emerging from the partially reflective mirror that can produce high-power densities. This is in contrast to an incandescent lamp, **B,** that produces radiation of many wavelengths and directions, which is difficult to focus. (From Sosis M: *Int Anesthesiol Clin* 28:119, 1990.)

sources usually does. The peaks and troughs of laser radiation will also be in phase and therefore the laser beam is *coherent.*

The basic components of the laser consist of a power source and two parallel mirrors encompassing the laser medium (Fig. 33-3). This medium may be a liquid, solid, or gas. The power source is often a flash lamp; however, chemical reactions or other lasers may also be used.[3] When the power source is activated, energy is absorbed by the electrons of the atoms of the laser medium. They are elevated to energy levels above their ground state. The electrons then decay to lower energy levels and emit photons that are not in phase with one another and are traveling in all directions. However, a photon striking one of the laser's mirrors will be reflected back through the laser medium where it will stimulate the emission of more photons of the same energy, phase, and direction. These in turn will be reflected by the parallel mirrors. The result will be a large number of photons of the same energy that are in phase and traveling in the same direction. In practice, one of the mirrors allows a small portion of light to pass through it (Fig. 33-3).

Laser radiation has the following properties (Fig. 33-3): (a) it is monochromatic (one color); all the photons have the same energy, frequency, and wavelength; (b) it is coherent; the peaks and troughs of the waves are in phase; (c) it is collimated; the beam does not usually diverge (unlike the radiation from an incandescent light source); and (d) it has a high energy density.

Surgical lasers are generally operated in either a continuous or a pulsed mode, in which the laser is operative for only a fraction of a second. The energy of the laser in joules absorbed by tissues is the product of the power in watts multiplied by the duration in seconds of the laser impact.

A. TYPES OF LASERS

1. Carbon dioxide laser

The carbon dioxide (CO_2) laser has been used for a wide variety of otolaryngologic and head and neck surgical procedures and in gynecologic surgery for the treatment of intraepithelial neoplasms, condylomata acuminata, and other lesions. The CO_2 laser is readily absorbed by the first 200 μm (micron) depth in all biologic materials independent of tissue pigmentation. Its radiation is in the infrared region of the electromagnetic spectrum (wavelength 10.6 μm) (see Table 33-1). Carbon dioxide lasers usually incorporate a visible helium-neon (He-Ne) laser for aiming purposes because the CO_2 laser is invisible. The low-intensity (0.8 mW) He-Ne laser has a red color (wavelength, 0.6328 μm). The CO_2 laser's radiation cannot be transmitted through ordinary fiberoptic bundles. Also, injuries to the eyes

Table 33-1. Characteristics of commonly used medical lasers

Type of laser	Laser wavelength (μm)	Color	Fiberoptic transmission
Gas			
Helium-neon	0.633	Red	Yes
Argon	0.5	Blue-green	Yes
Carbon dioxide	10.6	Invisibile	No
Solid			
Ruby	0.695	Red	Yes
Nd-YAG	1.06	Invisible	Yes
KTP	0.532	Green	Yes

From Sosis M: *Probl Anesthesia* 7:160, 1993.

from the CO_2 laser will be confined to the cornea.[4] There is no risk to the retina.

The CO_2 laser has advantages that make it a very effective surgical tool. Its use with an operating microscope allows the surgeon to precisely destroy targets approximately 2 mm in diameter under binocular vision (Fig. 33-4). This degree of precision may be impossible to achieve with conventional cautery.[5] Also, during CO_2 laser surgery, the surgical field is usually bloodless because of the laser's considerable hemostatic action. Vessels up to 0.5 mm diameter can usually be sectioned without bleeding.[5] The CO_2 laser has been successfully used to excise vascular lesions, even in patients with a bleeding diathesis.[6] The use of more traditional surgical tools such as cautery usually results in considerable postoperative edema. However, edema does not usually occur after using the CO_2 laser because of the sharp line of tissue destruction with virtually no injury to surrounding tissue. Ninety percent of the laser's energy is absorbed within 0.03 mm.[7] Furthermore, there is no manipulation of tissues, (i.e., laser treatment is usually a "touchless" technique). Microscopic examination of tissue after CO_2 laser surgery reveals a discrete line of destruction, with preservation of capillaries and normal features of adjacent tissues. The preservation of adjacent tissues is thought to account for the rapid healing, minimal scarring, and lack of pain often observed after CO_2 laser surgery.[5]

2. Argon laser

The argon laser emits visible blue-green radiation with a wavelength of approximately 0.5 μm (see Table 33-1). It is readily transmitted by fiberoptic bundles. The applications of this type of laser include ophthalmologic surgery, especially for retinal and anterior chamber procedures. Its applications in dermatologic and plastic surgery include the removal of port wine stains, hemangiomata, and tatoos because of the laser's absorption by

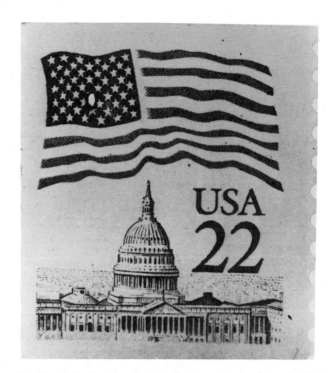

Fig. 33-4. The hole made by a CO_2 laser in the starry field of the flag in this stamp illustrates the precision afforded by laser surgery. (From Sosis M: *Adv Anesthesia* 6:175, 1989.)

hemoglobin and other pigments. Port wine stains are lightened without scarring after treatment with the argon laser.[6]

3. Ruby laser

The ruby laser emits visible red radiation at a wavelength of 0.695 μm (see Table 33-1). It is not readily absorbed by water but is significantly absorbed by pigments such as melanin and hemoglobin. The ruby laser can easily penetrate the anterior structures of the eye. It is used to photocoagulate vascular and pigmented retinal lesions.

4. Neodymium-yttrium-aluminum-garnet laser

The neodymium-yttrium-aluminum-garnet (Nd-YAG) or "YAG" laser has been used for photocoagulation and deep thermal necrosis for the treatment of gastrointestinal bleeding and obstructing bronchial lesions. Its radiation is in the infrared region of the electromagnetic spectrum with a wavelength of 1.06 μm and thus is invisible (see Table 33-1). This laser can emit radiation in the visible region of the spectrum by using frequency doubling techniques. The result is the potassium titanyl phosphate (KTP) laser. Nd-YAG laser radiation at high power is readily transmitted by conventional fiberoptic bundles. Its radiation is poorly absorbed by hemoglobin. However, blue and black pigmentation enhances Nd-YAG absorption, whereas pale colors enhance its penetration.[8] The depth of tissue

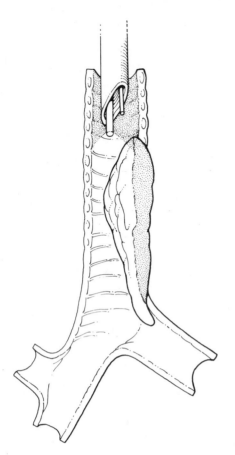

Fig. 33-5. A fiber (*top, right*) conducting the Nd-YAG laser through a rigid bronchoscope for the resection of a tracheal lesion is shown. A light source is depicted to its left. (From Sosis M: *Adv Anesthesia* 6:175, 1989.)

penetration occurring with the Nd-YAG laser is less predictable than that noted with the CO_2 laser.

Dumon et al.,[9] reporting on a large series of cases, recommended the use of rigid rather than flexible bronchoscopy for treating obstructive pulmonary lesions by means of endoscopic Nd-YAG laser surgery (Fig. 33-5). Brutinel and associates[10] have reported difficulty ventilating and oxygenating patients' lungs through an endotracheal tube during Nd-YAG surgery with an indwelling fiberoptic bronchoscope in place. Casey et al.[11] reported a complication during which there was combustion of the fiberoptic bronchoscope and endotracheal tube in a patient undergoing Nd-YAG laser airway surgery. The use of a rigid bronchoscope for the treatment of obstructing pulmonary lesions facilitates the removal of tissue and the treatment of complications.[12] Power levels less than 50 watts in short pulsations will decrease the chances of the impingement on vital underlying structures.[12] McDougall and Cortese[13] reported two patients who died during Nd-YAG laser endoscopic treatment of airway obstructions using very high power. At high power, the penetration of tissues by

the Nd-YAG laser cannot be readily controlled, and the perforation of a large blood vessel is possible.

III. OPERATING ROOM HAZARDS

The intensity of the laser and its potential for tissue damage and combustion necessitate that strict safety precautions be followed whenever it is used. Lasers should always be set to the "standby" mode, except when they are ready to fire, so inadvertent actuation is impossible. They should be used in the "pulsed" (shuttered) mode rather than the "continuous" mode whenever possible to limit the energy delivered by the laser and to allow the area being lased to cool between firings. The laser should never be allowed to strike highly polished or mirrorlike surfaces. For this reason most instrumentation for use with lasers has a dull or matte finish, and blackened instruments are widely used. This is important because reflection of the coherent laser beam may not disperse it. Thus injury to the patient or operating room personnel is possible, even from a reflected laser beam. Any instruments that become hot as a result of laser radiation may cause burns. The subject of endotracheal tube combustion from laser radiation will be addressed in sections IV D, V, and VIII. Tracheal laceration, tooth damage, injury to soft tissue, and cutaneous burns to operating room personnel have been described during laser surgery.[14]

The eyes are easily damaged by the laser and protection is mandatory both for the patient and operating room personnel (Fig. 33-6). Except for the carbon dioxide laser, conventional eyeglasses are inadequate protection from laser radiation. No one should ever look directly at the output from a laser. Contact lenses are inadequate protection even with the carbon dioxide laser. The use of eyeglasses with side guards is recommended for protecting the eyes from laser radiation.

The emissions of the Nd-YAG, KTP, and organ lasers can penetrate the cornea and lens of the eye and could be focused by the lens, resulting in severe retinal damage. Protective eyeglasses are colored green for the Nd-YAG laser, orange for the argon laser, and orange-red for the KTP laser. For the Nd-YAG laser, the glasses should absorb light maximally at 1.064 µm. Laser protective glasses make patient observation more difficult and cyanosis in particular might easily be missed without use of a pulse oximeter. The patient's eyes should be closed during surgery and covered with moist eye patches. Protective goggles or glasses may also be placed on the patient. The Nd-YAG and argon lasers can penetrate glass; therefore any windows in the operating room should have an opaque covering to prevent the penetration of laser radiation. A warning sign should be placed on the operating room door so that anyone entering will be informed that the laser is in use

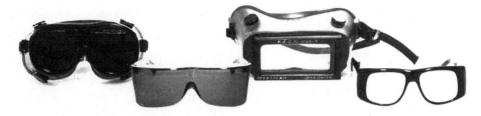

Fig. 33-6. A variety of glasses and goggles designed for laser use. (From Sosis M: *Adv Anesthesia* 6:175, 1989.)

(see Fig. 33-7). Extra goggles should be available for personnel entering the operating room.

The disposable paper drapes generally used during surgery are less expensive than cloth drapes, have little or no lint, and are impermeable to water. However, the combustion of disposable surgical draping material has been reported to produce copious smoke, making it difficult for operating room personnel to breathe or see and necessitating the removal of an anesthetized patient from the operating room suite.[15,16] Disposable drapes are generally treated with a flame retardant; however, once ignited, they are difficult to extinguish with water because it simply rolls off.[15,16] A fire extinguisher should be available for such drape fires. Cloth drapes are also combustible.[15] Milliken and Bizzarri[15] have reported intraoperative drape fires causing serious burns to patients, which have required the intervention of the fire department to extinguish the flames and a skin graft to treat the severe burns.[15] A lawsuit was filed.

It has been recommended that a minimum amount of surgical draping be used during laser surgery. Towels moistened with water to decrease their combustibility may be used. The towels must be kept moist or they will become flammable. The following case report illustrates the severity of a laser-induced drape fire: "During a craniotomy for the removal of a brain tumor, the patient's drapes were set on fire when a carbon dioxide laser accidentally discharged. The patient had approximately 10% second-degree and third-degree burns to her chest, neck, and arm. The patient survived, but after the operation, had to be treated for the burns and underwent skin grafts to the arms and upper chest. Also, as a result of the fire, three nurses and two physicians had to be treated for smoke inhalation."[17]

IV. MANAGEMENT OF ANESTHESIA
A. PREOPERATIVE EVALUATION

A thorough medical evaluation is essential for all patients coming to surgery. Laser surgery is often undertaken for the treatment of patients who have malignant processes encroaching on their airway and who have some degree of respiratory compromise. Many such patients have histories of tobacco and alcohol abuse. Lesions in or near the airway pose the danger of

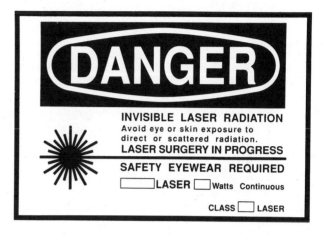

DANGER

INVISIBLE LASER RADIATION
Avoid eye or skin exposure to direct or scattered radiation.
LASER SURGERY IN PROGRESS

SAFETY EYEWEAR REQUIRED
☐ LASER ☐ Watts Continuous
CLASS ☐ LASER

Fig. 33-7. A conspicuous warning sign should be displayed on the operating room door whenever the laser is used. (Courtesy of Sharplan Lasers.)

life-threatening airway obstruction during the induction of anesthesia. Furthermore, the manipulation of airway lesions during laryngoscopy may cause bleeding or edema that could also result in airway occlusion. The oropharynx should be examined for pathologic lesions and for any potential for difficulties that might occur during the intubation of the trachea. Similarly, the external anatomy and range of motion of the head and neck should be determined. The patient's previous medical records should be examined for the methods used and problems encountered, if any, during previous anesthetic induction.

Pulmonary function tests and arterial blood gas tensions should be documented in patients with serious respiratory impairment. The careful reading of the patient's chart with emphasis on roentgenograms and other tests that might give information regarding the state of the patient's airway is important. Consultation with the surgeon is advised regarding potential airway difficulties during the induction of anesthesia and the plan for surgery.

The patient's physical status should be optimized before surgery. Patients receiving methylxanthine bronchodilators should have their serum levels checked and their dosages changed as required. It should be remembered that many airway procedures may cause sustained hypertension and tachycardia both of which stress the cardiovascular system. Adult patients should take nothing by mouth for 8 hours before surgery.

B. PREMEDICATION

Patients at risk for respiratory obstruction or those with severe pulmonary disease should be brought to the operating room unpremedicated except for an antisialagogue. During the preoperative visit, the anesthesiologist should attempt to allay the patient's fears. Those not at risk for airway obstruction may receive sedative premedication.

C. INDUCTION OF ANESTHESIA

In patients not at risk for respiratory obstruction, anesthesia may be induced in a conventional fashion after preoxygenation if no other contraindications exist. The minimum monitoring equipment advisable for laser cases consists of a noninvasive blood pressure apparatus, a pulse oximeter, electrocardiograph, precordial stethoscope, and an oxygen analyzer. A capnograph is highly desirable to confirm the position of the tracheal tube and to monitor the adequacy of pulmonary ventilation. An arterial catheter should be considered for patients with labile blood pressure or for those in whom arterial blood gas tensions should be determined. A peripheral nerve stimulator should be applied to monitor the degree of paralysis achieved with neuromuscular blocking medications.

When airway obstruction is considered possible, a full complement of equipment is mandatory. A variety of laryngoscope blades, oral and nasal airways, a rigid bronchoscope, and a tracheostomy tray should be available. In such cases, the surgeon should be present during the induction of anesthesia. Awake tracheal intubation, frequently aided by fiberoptic laryngoscopy, using topical anesthesia is recommended for these cases. Superior laryngeal nerve blocks and the transtracheal instillation of local anesthetics should be considered, but intravenous anesthetics should be used cautiously so that adequate, unobstructed respiration is maintained.

D. SPECIAL ANESTHETIC CONSIDERATIONS IN LASER AIRWAY SURGERY

Standard anesthesia techniques require no modification for laser surgery when the site of surgery is distant from the airway as in gynecologic procedures. However, when the surgical field is near the airway, general anesthesia for laser surgery may be conducted either with an endotracheal tube or without a tube, using special techniques such as Venturi jet ventilation (see under "Venturi Jet Ventilation"), the intermittent apneic technique (see under "Intermittent Apneic Technique"), or by insufflation (see under "Anesthesia by Insufflation"). If ventilation through an endotracheal

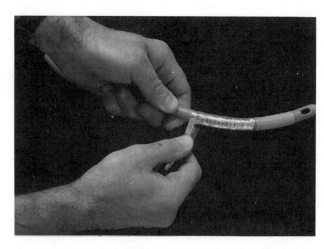

Fig. 33-8. Technique of foil-wrapping a rubber endotracheal tube is illustrated using 3M no. 425 aluminum foil tape. (From Sosis M: *Int Anesthesiol Clin* 28:119, 1990.)

tube is proposed, prevention of an endotracheal tube fire or explosion requires the use of special techniques and appropriate endotracheal tubes. (See Fig. 33-1). Surveys of the complications of carbon dioxide laryngeal surgery by otolaryngologists active in this type of surgery have found endotracheal tube fires or explosions to be the most common major complication.[18,19] The reported incidence of airway fires has been estimated at 0.4%[20] to 0.57%[21] of the patients undergoing laser airway surgery. The death of a patient resulting from the combustion of an endotracheal tube during carbon dioxide laser surgery has been reported.[22]

1. The use of metallic foil tapes to protect the shafts of combustible endotracheal tubes from laser radiation

Foil tapes were first suggested as a simple, inexpensive means of protecting the shafts of combustible endotracheal tubes from laser beams by Strong and Jacko in 1972[5] (Fig. 33-8).

A problem related to the use of metallic foil tapes is that none are manufactured for medical applications, nor has such use been sanctioned by the U.S. Food and Drug Administration. One manufacturer, when questioned, cautioned against the use of their aluminum tape for medical purposes.[23] However, the use of protective metal tape during laser surgery is widely advocated in the literature[24-29] and is an inexpensive technique. Metallic foil tape provides protection only from the direct impact of the laser beam. Indirect combustion caused by sparks or heat from gaseous or tube combustion is still possible,[30] because the endotracheal tubes used are generally combustible and usually have an enriched concentration of oxygen flowing through them (Fig. 33-9). Furthermore, a case of an obstruction of the

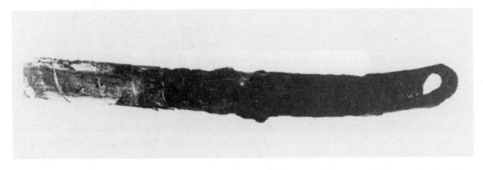

Fig. 33-9. A foil-wrapped plastic endotracheal tube has undergone indirect combustion. (From Vourc'h G, Tannieres M, Freche G: *Anaesthesia* 34:685, 1979.)

airway from metallic tape that came loose from a wrapped endotracheal tube has been reported.[31]

In an experiment designed to evaluate the protection offered by metallic foil tapes to the shafts of combustible endotracheal tubes from the carbon dioxide laser, size 8-mm internal diameter Mallinckrodt (Glens Falls, New York) Hi-Lo polyvinyl chloride endotracheal tubes were studied after wrapping them with five types of tape.[24] The endotracheal tubes were wrapped with a continuous strip of 1/4-inch (0.6 cm) self-adhesive foil tape. Starting at the distal (cuffed) end, the endotracheal tube was wrapped in a spiral fashion. The tape was applied in an overlapping manner so that bending of the endotracheal tube would not expose any unprotected area. The taping was begun at the cuffed end of the tube so that it would overlap in a way that would prevent laser radiation coming from above from striking the foil's adhesive. The tapes used were Minnesota Mining and Manufacturing Corp. (3M) (St. Paul, Minnesota) nos. 425, 1430, and 433; Radio Shack (Tandy Corporation, Ft. Worth, Texas) no. 44-1155; and 0.001-inch thick copper foil tape (Venture Tape Corporation, Rockland, Massachusetts). During the trials, 5 L/min^{-1} of 100% oxygen flowed through the endotracheal tubes being tested as they rested horizontally on wet towels and were surrounded by air. A Laser Sonics (Santa Clara, California) model LS880 carbon dioxide laser and Zeiss (Jena, Germany) operating microscope using a 400-mm lens and 0.68-mm beam diameter were used. The laser beam was directed onto the shafts of the foil-wrapped endotracheal tubes perpendicularly at the point of overlapping of the tape. A power of 70 watts in the continuous mode of laser operation was used. The time until the appearance of smoke, flames, perforation, or "blowtorch" ignition was recorded. Finally, a segment of tape was wrapped adhesive side outward and the procedure repeated to determine whether unexpected contact of the laser with the adhesive would cause combustion.

The nonadhesive sides of the 3M tape nos. 425 and 433 and the Venture copper tape were unaffected by 25 seconds of laser impact and thus protected the endotracheal tubes from the carbon dioxide laser. Endotracheal tube penetration and a blowtorch fire occurred at 7 and 14 seconds, respectively, with the Radio Shack No. 44-1155 (see Fig. 33-1) and 3M no. 1430 tapes.

On directing the laser onto the reverse (adhesive) side of the tapes, the adhesive backings of the 3M tape no. 433 and the Radio Shack no. 44-1155 tapes were ignited and the tapes perforated within 0.1 second of the laser's impact. Flaming of the adhesive occurred at 1 second without penetration of the 3M tape no. 1430 or the Venture copper tape. The adhesive side of the 3M tape no. 425 started to smoke at 2 seconds, but no flames occurred and there was no perforation.

The results of this carbon dioxide laser study (Table 33-2) show that the type of metallic tape used to protect combustible endotracheal tubes is critical. Radio Shack tape no. 44-1155 and 3M tape no. 1430 and 433 offer inadequate protection of flammable endotracheal tubes and should not be used for this purpose. Patel and Hicks[32] reported similar results for the Radio Shack tape no. 44-1155. Venture copper foil tape and 3M no. 425 tape provided excellent protection of the shafts of the endotracheal tubes. Therefore Sosis recommended their use during carbon dioxide laser surgery in proximity to the airway. However, a subsequent study has shown that if blood is applied to these tapes, laser-induced combustion may occur.[33] Therefore caution is advised. The malleability of the Venture copper foil allows for a smoother external contour than that of the 3M no. 425 aluminum tape.

The possibility of changes in the composition of any metallic foil tape requires that every batch of tape be evaluated for its incendiary characteristics before use.[25] In the evaluation of metallic foil tape for protecting combustible endotracheal tubes, the laser beam must be directed at the adhesive side of the tape because some tapes, such as Radio Shack tape no. 44-1155, have an inner plastic layer that is highly flammable (Fig. 33-10). This plastic layer would not be detected if the laser beam was focused on the center of the tape. The impingement

Table 33-2. The effect of carbon dioxide laser radiation on foil-wrapped endotracheal tubes

Tape studied	Nonadhesive side	Adhesive side
Radio Shack no. 44-1155	7-sec tube penetration 14-sec combustion	Ignition and perforation <0.1 sec
3M no. 425	No effect by 25 sec	Smoking at 2 sec No flames or perforation
3M no. 433	No effect by 25 sec	Ignition and perforation >1 sec
3M no. 1430	7-sec, tube penetration 14-sec combustion	Flaming of adhesive at 1 sec No penetration
Venture copper foil	No effect by 25 sec	Flaming of adhesive at 1 sec No penetration

From Sosis MB: *Anesth Analg* 68:392, 1989.

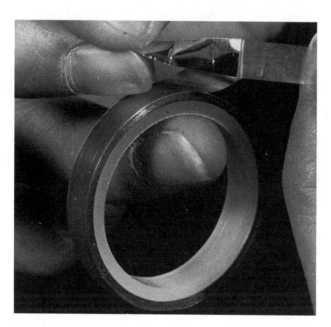

Fig. 33-10. Radio Shack no. 44-1155 tape has been peeled apart to show a thin metallic layer and a plastic layer. (From Sosis M: *Int Anesthesiol Clin* 28:119, 1990.)

of the laser beam onto the edge of the tape, however, could cause an endotracheal tube fire.

Sosis noted that endotracheal tubes wrapped with 3M no. 425 tape and copper foil tape have been gas-sterilized without affecting their ability to withstand the carbon dioxide laser impact, thus allowing a sterile endotracheal tube to be used in clinical practice.

Sosis and Dillon[29] performed an evaluation of metallic foil tapes for the protection of combustible endotracheal tubes from the Nd-YAG laser since a case report[11] of an endotracheal tube fire with this type of laser has been published, and no endotracheal tube had been

shown to provide adequate protection from the Nd-YAG laser.[34]

In part one of their study, five red rubber Rusch (Waiblingen, Germany) endotracheal tubes were wrapped with 1/4-inch wide self-adhesive metallic tape (see below) in an overlapping spiral fashion beginning at the cuffed end of the endotracheal tube. Red rubber endotracheal tubes were used because they are highly flammable when exposed to the Nd-YAG laser.[34] Five liters per minute of 100% oxygen flowed through the endotracheal tubes so that endotracheal tube perforation and combustion by the laser would be clearly seen. A second segment of each endotracheal tube was wrapped with the same tape but with its adhesive side outward to determine the flammability of the adhesive because the laser might contact it if aimed at the edge of the tape. The tapes used were: (1) Radio Shack (Tandy Corp., Ft. Worth, Texas) no. 44-1155 tape; (2) 3M (St. Paul, Minnesota) no. 425 aluminum tape; (3) 3M no. 433 aluminum tape; (4) 3M no. 1430 aluminum tape; and (5) copper foil tape (0.001-inch thick) (Venture Tape Corp., Rockland, Massachusetts). An unwrapped red rubber endotracheal tube served as a control.

To study the effects of a high ambient oxygen concentration in part two of the study, red rubber endotracheal tubes wrapped with 3M no. 425 and Venture copper foil tape were placed in a cylindrical copper chamber that was flushed with oxygen. The concentration of oxygen was determined to be 98% both before and after laser discharge as measured on the tape with a catheter connected to a mass spectrometer. Each type of foil wrapping was evaluated five times. A LaserSonics (Santa Clara, California) model 1700 carbon dioxide/Nd-YAG laser, in the Nd-YAG mode with a hand-held laser probe, was used in part one of this study. The laser's output was set at 50 watts in the continuous mode, with a beam diameter of 0.68 mm. The beam was directed perpendicularly at the shafts of the foil-wrapped endotracheal tubes and the laser's emission was continued until vigorous combustion was noted or up to a maximum of 60 seconds. A blowtorch fire, if observed, was noted. In part two, the laser was set to its maximum output of 110 watts in the continuous mode of operation and was attached to a Zeiss (Jena, Germany) operating microscope with a 400-mm lens. The laser beam was directed perpendicularly at the wrapped endotracheal tubes in the test chamber. The Venture copper foil and 3M no. 425 tapes were each evaluated five times. The laser was operated until combustion occurred or until 1 minute of discharge had elapsed.

The results of part one of this study are summarized in Table 33-3. The bare red rubber endotracheal tube burned with a blowtorch effect after 13 seconds of Nd-YAG laser contact. Combustion and a blowtorch fire occurred in 6 and 15 seconds, respectively, after laser

Table 33-3. Effect of Nd-YAG laser radiation on foil-wrapped endotracheal tubes

Tape studied	Nonadhesive side	Adhesive side
Radio Shack no. 44-1155	6-sec combustion; 15-sec blow-torch fire	Not tested
3M no. 425	No effect by 60 sec	Immediate smoking; tube combustion at 60 sec
3M no. 433	No effect by 60 sec	Immediate combustion and blowtorch fire after 12 sec
3M no. 1430	Immediate combustion	Immediate combustion
Venture copper foil	No effect by 60 sec	Smoking at 5 sec; flames at 15 sec

From Sosis M, Dillon F: *Anesthesiology* 2:553, 1990.

contact with Radio Shack no. 44-1155 tape. Its reverse side was not tested. 3M no. 425 aluminum tape withstood 60 seconds of laser emission without any effect to its nonadhesive side. When its adhesive side was struck by the laser, smoking was noted immediately. After 60 seconds of laser contact, endotracheal tube combustion was noted beneath the tape. 3M no. 433 aluminum tape withstood 60 seconds of laser contact. When its adhesive side was exposed to the laser, it burned immediately, and a blowtorch fire was observed after 12 seconds. In the case of 3M no. 1430 aluminum tape, combustion occurred immediately after laser exposure to either side. The laser was discontinued after vigorous flames were observed, and the flames were extinguished, so no blowtorch effect was noted. There was no effect after 60 seconds of laser contact with the nonadhesive side of the Venture copper tape. Smoking was seen after 5 seconds of Nd-YAG laser contact with the reverse (adhesive) side. Flaming was noted after 15 seconds. The nonadhesive side of the 3M no. 425 tape and Venture tapes were retested three more times with no effect from the laser.

In part two of the investigation, no evidence of combustion was noted in all five trials of laser impingement onto red rubber endotracheal tubes wrapped with 3M no. 425 or Venture copper foil tape in an atmosphere of 98% oxygen after 1 minute of Nd-YAG laser fire at a power of 110 watts. The findings of Sosis and Dillon regarding the use of the 3M no. 425 tape for endotracheal tube protection mark the first report of a method of providing adequate protection of the exterior aspect of a combustible endotracheal tube from the Nd-YAG laser at 110 watts and a duration of 1 minute. However, the presence of blood on these foil tapes will likely impair their Nd-YAG laser resistance. The lumen of the

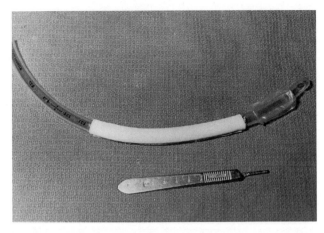

Fig. 33-11. Polyvinyl chloride endotracheal tube wrapped with the Laser-Guard protective coating. (From Sosis M, Dillon F: *J Clin Anesth* 4:25, 1992.)

endotracheal tube remains unprotected when metallic foil taping is used and therefore combustion could be initiated by a fiberoptic filament as may be used during Nd-YAG endoscopic surgery if it is placed inside the tube.

2. Evaluation of the Laser-Guard protective coating for protecting the shafts of combustible endotracheal tubes from laser radiation

The Merocel (Mystic, Connecticut) Laser-Guard endotracheal tube protective coating consists of a rectangular sheet of embossed silver foil covered with a thin absorbent Merocel sponge layer on one side and adhesive on the other (Fig. 33-11). It is available in four sizes for application to size 4.0- to 7.5-mm internal diameter rubber and 5.0- to 8.5-mm internal diameter plastic endotracheal tubes (Table 33-4). It has been examined for this application by the U.S. Food and Drug Administration. After removing the protective backing from the adhesive layer of the Laser-Guard, the endotracheal tube to be protected is pressed down along the center line. The tube is then rolled until completely covered.

The Merocel Laser-Guard is designed to be an easy-to-use, highly resistant barrier to laser radiation and is moderately priced. Silver is used for the foil layer because this metal has high thermal conductivity. The thermal conductivity of a laser-protective endotracheal tube coating is thought to be important because the incident laser beam's energy can be conducted away from the site of impact and thus dissipated without harm to the patient or the endotracheal tube. The Merocel sponge layer, when wet, acts as a heat sink and gives the external aspect of a wrapped endotracheal tube a smooth, nontraumatic contour. The sponge layer must be kept wet because in the dry state it is combustible. A solvent-soaked wipe is included with the Laser-Guard

Table 33-4. Manufacturer's specifications for the Merocel Laser-Guard endotracheal tube protector

Laser	Power (watts)	Beam diameter (mm)	Power density (watts/cm²)	Time (sec)
CO_2	70	0.68	19,275	60
Nd-YAG*	61	<1	9,588	60
KTP	18	0.4	14,324	60

*Noncontact, optically guided. Courtesy Merocel Inc., Mystic, Conn.

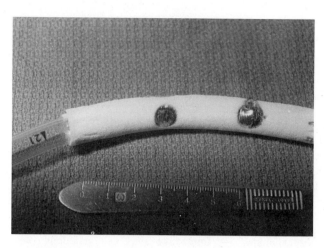

Fig. 33-12. Two areas of laser contact with the Laser-Guard protective coating. The corrugated silver foil layer can be seen where the foam layer has been struck by the laser beam. (From Sosis M, Dillon F: *J Clin Anesth* 4:25, 1992.)

for cleaning the endotracheal tube's shaft to improve adherence. Also included are strung pledgets for protecting the endotracheal tube's cuff.

Sosis and Dillon[35] examined the efficacy of the Laser-Guard protective endotracheal tube covering. They used a LaserSonics (Santa Clara, California) model LS880 carbon dioxide/Nd-YAG laser in the continuous carbon dioxide mode of operation with a Zeiss (Jena, Germany) operating microscope, 400-mm lens, and "joystick" micromanipulator. The laser was directed perpendicularly at Mallinckrodt (St. Louis, Mo) size 8.0-mm internal diameter Hi-Lo polyvinyl chloride endotracheal tubes through which 5 L/min⁻¹ of oxygen was flowing. A bare Mallinckrodt polyvinyl chloride endotracheal tube served as a control, whereas five other identical endotracheal tubes were protected by wrapping their shafts with the Laser-Guard protective coating. The endotracheal tubes to be tested were placed horizontally on wet towels and were surrounded by air during the study. Power settings of 10 and 70 watts were used in this investigation. According to the manufacturer's directions, Sosis and Dillon wet the sponge layer of the Laser-Guard protective coating with water after its application to the endotracheal tube's shaft. The laser exposure was actuated until either combustion of the endotracheal tube occurred or 60 seconds of laser fire had elapsed.

At a laser power setting of 10 watts, the plain, unprotected polyvinyl chloride endotracheal tube was penetrated after 50 seconds of laser exposure. Smoking and minor nonsustained combustion accompanied this trial; however, no "blowtorch" fire occurred. At 70 watts of power, laser exposure onto the bare polyvinyl chloride tube resulted in combustion and a blowtorch fire of the endotracheal tube after only 3 seconds. The wet Laser-Guard–covered polyvinyl chloride endotracheal tube shafts were not significantly damaged by 60 seconds of laser exposure at either 10 or 70 watts. A small amount of smoke, but no flames, was seen when the laser was fired at it (Fig. 33-12). The Laser-Guard's sponge coating was missing, with minimal evidence of thermal decomposition of the sponge in a small area surrounding

the site of laser impingement. The bare corrugated silver foil was noted to be intact.

In the study of Sosis and Dillon,[35] the Laser-Guard covering protected polyvinyl chloride endotracheal tube shafts from laser-induced combustion during test conditions of continuous exposure to carbon dioxide laser radiation of 70 watts for 60 seconds with 5 L/min⁻¹ of oxygen flowing through the endotracheal tubes. The researchers stated that these settings are probably more severe than any that will be encountered clinically so safety in clinical use should be ensured. The control, a bare Mallinckrodt polyvinyl chloride endotracheal tube, when exposed to the laser under the same conditions, burned like a blowtorch almost immediately after the laser was turned on. Sosis and Dillon stated such rigorous testing of protective wrappings and special endotracheal tubes manufactured for laser airway surgery is important because previous investigations by their group have shown that not all such products are efficacious.[24,29]

Sosis and Dillon concluded that the Laser-Guard protective coating was easier to apply to polyvinyl chloride endotracheal tube shafts than the foil tapes their group had previously investigated. The Laser-Guard adhered well to the endotracheal tubes tested. When its foam layer was moistened with water, it had a smoother surface than did foil-wrapped endotracheal tubes. Sosis and Dillon stated that this is important because laryngeal tissues are easily traumatized.

In a similar investigation comparing metallic foil tapes and the Laser-Guard for protecting the shafts of polyvinyl chloride endotracheal tables from the KTP laser, Sosis and Braverman[36] concluded that the Laser-Guard provided the best protection. A subsequent study determined that the presence of blood does not affect the Laser-Guard protection from the carbon dioxide laser.[33]

In common with foil wrapping, Laser-Guard–protected endotracheal tubes have a slightly larger external diameter than unprotected endotracheal tubes. However, whereas foil wrapped endotracheal tubes can be protected over virtually the entire shaft of the tube, Laser-Guard–protected endotracheal tubes have a fixed length of protective covering. After applying the Laser-Guard coating to an endotracheal tube, care must be taken to avoid flexing the tube excessively or the foil layer will fracture and its laser resistance will be compromised.

3. Prevention of laser-induced polyvinyl chloride endotracheal tube cuff fires by filling the cuff with saline

During laser airway surgery, the high energy of the laser is often used in proximity to combustible endotracheal tubes that may have anesthetic gases flowing through them that support or enhance combustion. Although the shafts of combustible endotracheal tubes can be protected from the carbon dioxide and other types of lasers by techniques such as foil wrapping,[24] the cuff remains vulnerable to the laser's effects. Le Jeune and colleagues[37] suggested that filling endotracheal tube cuffs with saline during laser airway surgery would prevent their combustion; however, they did not evaluate this suggestion experimentally. Sosis and Dillon[38] designed the following controlled study to test this hypothesis.

A LaserSonics (Santa Clara, California) model LS8800 carbon dioxide laser with a beam diameter of 0.68 mm in the continuous mode of operation was used. The cuffs attached to size 8.0-mm internal diameter polyvinyl chloride endotracheal tubes (Mallinckrodt Hi-Lo; Argyle, New York) were each inserted into the neck of an empty 250-ml Pyrex Erlenmeyer flask. A circle anesthesia system attached to an anesthesia machine was then connected to the endotracheal tube being tested. Five liters per minute of oxygen flowed through the endotracheal tube and into the flask for 5 minutes. The endotracheal tube cuff was then inflated to just seal at a pressure of 20-cm H_2O, which was maintained within the endotracheal tube, flask, and anesthesia circuit by adjusting the pressure relief (pop-off) valve on the anesthesia machine. The laser beam was then directed perpendicularly at the part of the cuff that was protruding from the neck of the flask and that was, therefore, surrounded by air (Fig. 33-13). At a laser power setting of 5 watts, the times to cuff perforation and loss of airway pressure were noted in 10 endotracheal tube cuffs: 5 inflated with saline and 5 inflated with air. To further evaluate the combustibility of the endotracheal tubes when their cuffs were inflated with saline or air, the

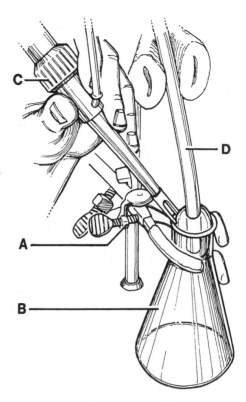

Fig. 33-13. Diagram of the apparatus used to evaluate endotracheal tube cuff flammability. A ring stand and clamp, *A,* support the Ehrlenmeyer flask, *B,* used during the trial. The laser handpiece, *C,* delivers carbon dioxide laser radiation from its console (not shown) toward a polyvinyl chloride endotracheal tube's cuff, *D.* The endotracheal tube was connected to a circle anesthesia circuit and anesthesia machine, and the endotracheal tube and flask had been flushed with oxygen for 5 minutes before inflation of the cuff with either saline or air. (From Sosis MB, Dillon F: *Anesth Analg* 72:187, 1991.)

laser's power was increased to 40 watts; again, 10 endotracheal tubes were studied, 5 with their cuffs filled with saline and 5 with air. In all cases, the laser was actuated until combustion occurred or 1 minute had elapsed.

Table 33-5 shows the times to cuff perforation and circuit deflation of endotracheal tubes with cuffs that were filled with air or saline. The saline-filled cuffs exposed to 5 watts of continuous laser radiation were perforated in 4.21 ± 3.91 sec (mean ± SD). This was not statistically different from the times necessary to perforate the air-filled cuffs (1.00 ± 0.83 sec). However, because of the greater viscosity of water, leakage from the saline-filled cuffs was significantly slower than that of the air-filled cuffs; therefore a longer interval elapsed before cuff leakage caused circuit decompression. When struck by the laser, deflation occurred after 2.59 ± 1.97 sec in the air-filled endotracheal tube cuffs and after 104.60 ± 67.5 sec in the endotracheal tube cuffs filled with saline ($P < .05$). The deflation of the saline-filled cuffs was significantly slower than their times to perfo-

Table 33-5. Time (sec) to cuff perforation and circuit deflation: (carbon dioxide laser set to 5 watts)

Cuff	n	Perforation	Deflation
Air	5	1.00 ± 0.83	2.59 ± 1.9[a*]
Saline	5	4.21 ± 3.91†	104.6 ± 67.5*†

Values are mean ± SD.
*$P < 0.05$; paired Student's t-test, air versus saline.
†$P < 0.01$; paired Student's t-test perforation versus deflation.
From Sosis MB, Dillon FX: *Anesth Analg* 72:187, 1991.

Table 33-6. Incidence of endotracheal tube combustion with air and saline filled cuffs (carbon dioxide laser set to 40 W)

Cuff	n	Combustion (%)
Air	5	100*
Saline	5	20*

*$P < 0.05$, Mann-Whitney U test.
From Sosis MB, Dillon FX: *Anesth Analg* 72:187, 1991.

ration. No combustion occurred during the trials at 5 watts.

Table 33-6 shows the incidence of combustion with the carbon dioxide laser set to 40 watts. During all five trials with air-filled cuffs, combustion occurred after less than 1 second of laser discharge. Both the cuff and adjacent endotracheal tube shaft were noted to be on fire (Fig. 33-14). The saline-filled cuffs prevented laser-induced endotracheal tube explosions in all but one of the trials, during which the tube ignited in 5.19 seconds. The Mann-Whitney U test was used to compare the incidence of flammability in the saline-filled and air-filled endotracheal tubes. It revealed a statistically significant difference at $P < .05$.

The shafts of combustible endotracheal tubes can be protected from the carbon dioxide and other types of lasers by techniques such as the careful foil wrapping of their shafts with the correct metallic tape. The cuffs of endotracheal tubes, however, are thin and remain vulnerable to the effects of the laser beam, which may be directed at them during laryngologic surgery because they cannot be protected with foil tape. The fact that the laser beam is often aligned along the axis of an operating laryngoscope during laryngeal surgery predisposes to its impingement on the endotracheal tube's cuff. Furthermore, the cuffs provide a large target because undersized endotracheal tubes are often used during airway surgery to provide better exposure of the larynx for the surgeon, thus a large cuff is therefore necessary to ensure a seal for positive-pressure ventilation of the lungs.

It has been suggested by Le Jeune and associates[37] that filling endotracheal tube cuffs with saline would protect them from the carbon dioxide laser because impingement of the laser beam onto the cuff results in a jet of water that will act as a "built-in fire extinguisher" (Fig. 33-15). The saline should also act as a heat sink;[37] however, this suggestion has not been previously tested experimentally. In this study, endotracheal tube cuff perforation by the carbon dioxide laser set to 5 watts was not inhibited by saline filling; however, the saline-filled cuffs, although perforated by the laser beam as rapidly as air-filled cuffs, were significantly slower to deflate, allowing more time before reaching the point when

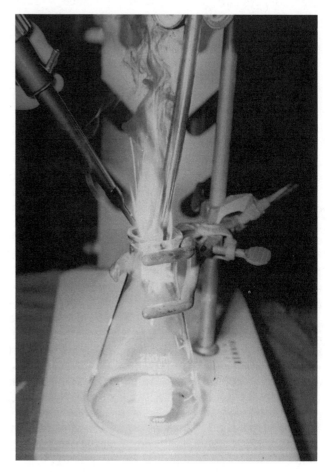

Fig. 33-14. Carbon dioxide laser–induced fire involving the endotracheal tube cuff and adjacent shaft. (From Sosis MB, Dillon F: *Anesth Analg* 72:187, 1991.)

airway pressure could no longer be maintained. The use of saline-filled cuffs prevented endotracheal tube ignition by the carbon dioxide laser set to 40 watts in a statistically significant number of cases when compared with the control group of air-filled cuffs. The saline filling of endotracheal tube cuffs is, therefore, recommended for laser airway surgery. It is also suggested that a small amount of dye, such as methylene blue, should be added to the saline so laser-induced endotracheal tube cuff perforation will be obvious to the surgeon who will then

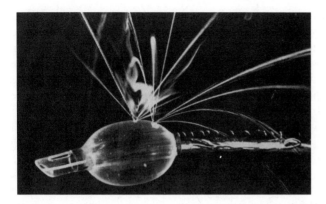

Fig. 33-15. Polyvinyl chloride tracheal tube cuff has been struck by a CO_2 laser after it was filled with saline. (From Le Jeune FE Jr et al: *Ann Otolaryngol* 91:606, 1982.)

immediately terminate operation of the laser. Further protection of the endotracheal tube cuffs can be obtained by placing moistened pledgets above them and keeping the pledgets moist throughout the procedure.[39]

4. Effect of anesthetic gases on endotracheal tube flammability

Aside from the type of specially manufactured endotracheal tube used for laser airway surgery or the manner in which a standard one is modified, the anesthetic gases used during these cases can profoundly influence combustibility. It cannot be stressed too strongly that nitrous oxide should not be considered an inert gas during laser airway surgery (Fig. 33-16). Although nitrous oxide cannot support life, it can readily decompose into oxygen, nitrogen, and energy according to the following equation:

$$N_2O = N_2 + \tfrac{1}{2}O_2 + Energy$$

In an experiment analogous to one with oxygen, a glowing match thrust into a vessel containing nitrous oxide will burst into flames. In fact, it has been found that nitrous oxide supports combustion to approximately the same extent as oxygen.[40]

To determine whether helium or nitrogen when added to oxygen would delay endotracheal tube flammability (Table 33-7), Pashayan and Gravenstein[41] studied the carbon dioxide laser–induced combustibility of 2-cm segments of polyvinyl chloride endotracheal tubes (National Catheter Corporation Division, Mallinckrodt, Glens Falls, New York). Each endotracheal tube segment was placed in a 250-cc glass cylinder into which a catheter delivered known gas mixtures. Both the interior and exterior of the endotracheal tubes were thus exposed to the gas mixtures. A carbon dioxide laser (Systems 450 carbon dioxide Laser Coherent Inc.) with a beam diameter of 0.8 mm was aimed at the endotracheal tube segment being studied through a hole drilled in the side of the glass cylinder and was actuated

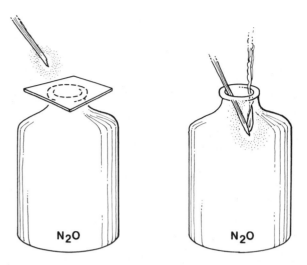

Fig. 33-16. Glowing wooden splint thrust into nitrous oxide will burst into flame. (From Sosis MB: *Adv Anesthesia* 6:175, 1989.)

Table 33-7. Physical properties of helium and nitrogen (26° C)

Physical properties	Helium	Nitrogen
Thermal conductivity (call [sec-cm$^{2\circ}$ C-cm^{-1} − 10^{-6}]$^{-1}$)	360.36	62.40
Thermal capacity (cal-g$^{-1\circ}$ K^{-1})	1.24	0.249
Density (g-1^{-1})	0.179	1.25
Thermal diffusivity (cm^2-sec^{-1})	1.621	0.199

From Pashayan AG, Gravenstein JS: *Anesthesiology* 62:274, 1985.

until combustion occurred or 60 seconds had elapsed. The mean time to ignition was determined. In the first part of this experiment with a laser power setting of 5 watts, 10 endotracheal tube segments were tested with concentrations of oxygen and helium from 20% oxygen/ 80% helium to 50% oxygen/50% helium. A second group of 10 endotracheal tube segments was studied in an atmosphere of oxygen mixed with nitrogen, again in concentrations ranging from 20% oxygen/80% nitrogen to 50% oxygen/50% nitrogen. In another series of experiments, laser radiation at power settings of 7.5, 10, and 12.5 watts was aimed at 10 endotracheal tube segments in 40% oxygen/60% helium and 10 segments in 40% oxygen/60% nitrogen. Another part of the study examined 10 endotracheal tube segments in 40% oxygen/ 60% helium and 2% halothane with a laser power of 10 watts.

In the studies outlined thus far, the laser was aimed at a clear area of the polyvinyl chloride tracheal tube segment under study. Care was taken to avoid aiming the laser at the endotracheal tube's radiopaque barium stripe. However, in a final part of the experiment, the laser beam was intentionally aimed at the barium stripe of 10 endotracheal tube segments in an atmosphere of 40% oxygen/60% helium and 10 segments in an atmosphere of 40% oxygen/60% nitrogen.

Pashayan and Gravenstein[41] found that even when laser-induced endotracheal tube combustion did not occur, laser exposure produced a hole in all the endotracheal tubes studied. At a laser power setting of 5 watts with 20% oxygen in either 80% nitrogen or helium, endotracheal tube combustion did not occur after 60 seconds of laser actuation. At oxygen concentrations of 30% and 40%, the mean time to ignition with nitrogen was significantly shorter than the time for the same concentration of oxygen in helium. An oxygen concentration of 50% resulted in a mean time to combustion in helium that was not statistically significantly different from that with nitrogen. Similarly, at 7.5 and 10 but not at 12 watts, the mean time to ignition with oxygen in nitrogen was significantly shorter than that with oxygen in helium. At a power setting of 10 watts, adding 2% halothane to a mixture of 40% oxygen and 60% helium significantly shortened the mean time to combustion to 25.3 ± 1.9 seconds (mean $\pm$ SEM) from 43.1 ± 5.4 seconds. On directing the 10-watt laser beam onto the radiopaque barium stripe on the polyvinyl chloride endotracheal tubes, the mean times to combustion with both nitrogen and helium were significantly shorter than occurred when the same gas mixture was used, but the laser was aimed at the clear portions of the endotracheal tubes.

Pashayan and Gravenstein[41] concluded that helium in concentrations at or above 60% will delay carbon dioxide laser–induced combustion of polyvinyl chloride endotracheal tubes if the laser power output is less than or equal to 10 watts. They also conclude that the radiopaque barium stripe on the polyvinyl chloride endotracheal tube is more combustible than the clear portions of the endotracheal tube and it should be positioned away from the laser.

Simpson and colleagues[42] determined the flammability of four types of endotracheal tubes in mixtures of helium and oxygen or nitrous oxide compared with mixtures of nitrogen and oxygen or nitrous oxide. The gases were metered with precision flowmeters and directed to a mixing chamber and then into a test cylinder 7.5 cm in diameter and 60 cm long. The endotracheal tubes studied were: (1) polyvinyl chloride (Portex, Wilmington, Massachusetts); (2) red rubber (Rusch, Germany); (3) silicone (National Catheter, Argyle, New York); and (4) Xomed Laser-Shield I (Xomed, Jacksonville, Florida). The gas flow rates were maintained at 30 to 35 L/min, and the gas concentrations were measured at the level of the clamp holding the endotracheal tube in the test chamber. The oxygen concentration was measured by a paramagnetic technique and the nitrous oxide by an infrared technique.

The ignition of the endotracheal tubes was accomplished with a propane torch. The endotracheal tubes were initially ignited in oxygen and nitrogen and the nitrogen was quickly discontinued and replaced with helium. The helium concentration was increased until the candlelike flame on the endotracheal tube was extinguished. The oxygen concentrations just before the flame's extinction with helium were defined as the "oxygen/helium index of flammability." This procedure was repeated five times for each type of endotracheal tube tested.

A similar experimental design was used with mixtures of nitrogen and oxygen until the propane torch–induced combustion of the four types of endotracheal tubes was extinguished. This was defined as the "oxygen/nitrogen index of flammability."

Next, the oxygen was replaced by nitrous oxide and the procedure was repeated to determine the "nitrous oxide/helium" and "nitrous oxide/nitrogen indices of flammability."

The indices of flammability of each type of endotracheal tube studied were averaged, and the results were compared using Bonferroni corrected t tests.

The oxidant oxygen/helium indices for the polyvinyl chloride, red rubber, silicone and the Xomed endotracheal tubes are respectively: 0.274 ± 0.0055 (mean $\pm$ SD), 0.194 ± 0.0089, 0.194 ± 0.0055, and 0.256 ± 0.0055. The oxidant oxygen/nitrogen indices for the polyvinyl chloride, rubber, silicone, and Xomed endotracheal tubes were 0.254 ± 0.0055, 0.182 ± 0.0045, 0.200 ± 0, and 0.230 ± 0, respectively. These results show that the polyvinyl chloride endotracheal tube is flammable in 27.4% oxygen, with the remainder consisting of helium, and with 25.4% oxygen with the remainder nitrogen. In all cases the oxidant oxygen/helium values were statistically significantly higher than the oxygen/nitrogen values for the same type of endotracheal tube ($P < .05$). The oxidant nitrous oxide/helium indices for the polyvinyl chloride, red rubber, silicone and Xomed endotracheal tubes are (mean $\pm$ SD) 0.526 ± 0.0055, 0.434 ± 0.0114, 0.416 ± 0.0055, and 0.456 ± 0.0055, respectively. The values for the oxidant nitrous oxide/nitrogen indices were: 0.472 ± 0.0084, 0.356 ± 0.0055, 0.392 ± 0.0045, and 0.0444 ± 0.0114 for the polyvinyl chloride, red rubber, silicone and Xomed endotracheal tubes, respectively. The oxidant nitrous oxide/helium indices were statistically higher than the nitrous oxide/nitrogen indices for all except the Xomed endotracheal tube.

Simpson and colleagues[42] noted (see Table 33-7) that helium affects combustion by virtue of its high thermal conductivity. Thermal conductivity is defined as the time rate of transfer of heat by conduction. Its dimensions are energy (calories) per second per area (square centimeters) per thickness (centimeters) per centigrade degree. The values are 62.40 and 360.36×10^{-6} at 26.7° C for nitrogen and helium respectively. Thus the transfer of heat away from a burning object is greater with helium than with nitrogen, and therefore a greater concentration of oxygen will be needed to initiate combustion with the former than the latter. However, Simpson and colleagues noted that the differences between helium and nitrogen indices determined in this study are not clinically significant. For example, for a polyvinyl chloride endotracheal tube, the difference of 27.4% oxygen in helium versus 25.4% helium in oxygen needed for combustion is very small. Their study also shows that the polyvinyl chloride endotracheal tubes were less flammable than the red rubber, silicone, or Xomed endotracheal tubes.

Al Haddad and Brenner[43] studied the combustion of 1- to 2-inch polyvinyl chloride endotracheal tube segments with the potassium-titanyl-phosphate (KTP) laser in helium/oxygen and nitrogen/oxygen atmospheres. A 6-L/min flow of the gas mixture under study entered a hole at the base of a glass test cylinder. A 10-watt KTP laser beam (Laserscope Microbeam II) was passed through a side hole in the cylinder at the endotracheal tube segment until combustion occurred or 1 minute had elapsed. The laser's spot size was 0.4 mm. The gas mixtures studied were 21%, 30%, and 40% oxygen in nitrogen and 30% and 40% oxygen in helium. A commercial oxygen analyzer was used to determine the oxygen concentration. The data were analyzed using ANOVA and Kruskal-Wallis tests.

At oxygen concentrations of 21%, 30%, and 40% in nitrogen, the mean times to ignition were 17.44 ± 23.26, 15.6 ± 19.47, and 12.83 ± 19.14 seconds, respectively. For the 30% and 40% oxygen/helium mixtures, the times to combustion were 9.89 ± 5.33 and 11.04 ± 14.47 seconds, respectively. The differences in the times to combustion with oxygen/helium and oxygen/nitrogen mixtures at 30% and 40% oxygen were not statistically different. Al Haddad and Brenner concluded that the use of helium instead of nitrogen confers no added safety during KTP laser surgery.

5. Anesthetic management for tracheobronchial tree laser surgery

Rontal and colleagues[44] have noted that the use of the laser for the treatment of obstructing lesions of the trachea and bronchi has been a significant advance in medical therapy. Many patients with benign lesions who previously required a thoracotomy for their treatment can now be treated with the laser as outpatients. Even unresectable malignant lesions, which can cause death by suffocation, can be treated with the laser by coring to create a patent airway. The treatment of such patients, however, is a challenge to the anesthesiologist because they are often markedly hypoxic, have poor pulmonary toilet, and often have associated cardiac disease. The precarious condition of these patients requires close cooperation between the anesthesiologist and the surgeon.

Rontal and associates[44] summarized their approach to surgery and anesthesia in 126 consecutive laser treatments using the laser. A rigid bronchoscope was used whenever possible. When the Nd-YAG laser was used, it was conducted through a fiber passed directly into the rigid bronchoscope or was first passed into a flexible fiberoptic bronchoscope and subsequently was inserted through the rigid bronchoscope. The flexible bronchoscope was used alone only when the rigid bronchoscope could not be inserted. Examples of situations in which only the flexible bronchoscope was used are patients with severe cervical-spine disease or temporomandibular joint dysfunction. When the patient has a tracheostomy in place, the rigid bronchoscope was placed either transorally or directly or into the tracheostomy stoma.

The possibility of bleeding into the portion of the airway being resected requires the availability of endoscopic forceps and gauze packing. Epinephrine-soaked pledgets can also be applied to the site of bleeding to establish hemostasis. The application of pledgets or packing to the bleeding area usually allows adequate respirations to be maintained in the contralateral lung through the rigid bronchoscope.

Rontal and colleagues[44] reported using a video monitor during all laser endoscopic procedures so the entire operating room team could observe the procedure. This allows the operating room nurses to anticipate the surgeon's needs and allows the anesthesiologist to tailor the anesthetic to the patient. Also, a video recording of the surgery can be made for later review.

Obstructing airway tumors were treated by first circumferentially photocoagulating the margins of the mass with an Nd-YAG laser at power settings less than 45 watts. The central core of obstructing tissue was then removed using the carbon dioxide laser. Rontal's group stated that these procedures were usually performed on an outpatient basis.

General anesthesia was used when lesions of the proximal tracheal were being treated, in those patients who chose not to undergo their therapy with local anesthesia, and in patients with an existing tracheostomy. General anesthesia was the preferred technique for children. Local anesthesia was the method of choice by Rontal's group when lesions of the middle or lower third of the trachea were being treated. The use of local anesthesia was also advocated by Rontal's group when airway obstruction was imminent; when the cross-sectional area of the trachea was reduced by 50% or more as determined by x-ray or examination; or when the tumor extended out of the mainstem bronchus, past the carina, and into the trachea.

When local anesthesia was used, the patients were premedicated with glycopyrrolate 0.2 mg for xerostomia. Depending on the patient's condition, hydroxyzine, 25 to 50 mg, meperidine hydrochloride, 25 to 75 mg, or fentanyl citrate, 0.05 to 0.1 mg, was given intramuscularly. Oral lorazepam, 2 mg, was administered preoperatively for amnesia except in the very elderly. In caring for extremely sick patients, all medications with the exception of the antisialagogue were administered when the patient arrived in the operating room. Those patients receiving sedation alone were given 10 to 15 ml of 4% lidocaine 15 minutes preoperatively through an ultrasonic nebulizer using either an aerosol mask or a mouthpiece. Rontal and associates stated that nontoxic blood levels of lidocaine were found after this treatment. On arrival in the operating room suite, an electrocardiogram and noninvasive blood pressure apparatus were attached to all patients. Rontal and associates reported that early in their experience with these cases, radial artery catheters were inserted to determine arterial blood gas tensions. More recently, however, the pulse oximetry has been used to measure arterial oxyhemoglobin saturation instead.

At the discretion of the anesthesiologist, 2.5 mg of droperidol, 2.5 to 5 mg of diazepam, or 10 to 20 mg of ketamine were administered intravenously to those patients receiving local anesthesia. Opioid analgesics were used sparingly for patients receiving local anesthesia. In general, no more than 0.05 mg of fentanyl citrate was administered because the patients were often hypoxic when breathing room air and additional respiratory depression was considered undesirable.

Sixty milligrams of 10% lidocaine was sprayed on the base of the tongue and mucous membranes before introducing the bronchoscope. More sedation was administered if the procedure was lengthy or the patient appeared uncomfortable. Rontal and associates[44] noted that it is important to distinguish between hypoxia and patient discomfort because the conditions may appear the same. In the event of excessive coughing, 1 or 2 ml of 4% lidocaine was administered intratracheally through the bronchoscope or up to 1.5 mg/kg of lidocaine may be administered intravenously. One hundred percent oxygen was administered to patients receiving local anesthesia except when the laser was actuated. They then breathed room air. Hypertension occurring during laser bronchoscopic surgery was treated with intravenous propranolol. Rontal and associates infused nitroglycerine, 5 mg in 250 ml of physiologic saline, intravenously when their patients had a history of hypertension or coronary artery disease. They maintain emergency equipment for Venturi jet ventilation of the lungs for all cases.

When general anesthesia was planned, the anesthetic was induced with a short-acting barbiturate administered intravenously. Muscle relaxation was provided with vecuronium bromide, 0.08 mg/kg, and the anesthetic was maintained with isoflurane in oxygen and either helium or nitrogen in a 30:70 ratio. Rontal's group[44] noted that helium would provide less resistance to the flow of gases through narrowed airways. The inhaled anesthetics were administered through the ventilating bronchoscope except for those patients having an existing tracheostomy in which case a plastic endotracheal tube was inserted a short distance into a metal tracheostomy tube for pulmonary ventilation. At the end of surgery, residual neuromuscular blockade was antagonized with neostigmine, 5 mg, and glycopyrrolate, 1 mg, given intravenously. Dexamethasone, 8 mg, was usually administered to the patients intravenously to prevent excessive edema of the airway. All patients breathed humidified oxygen after surgery and were observed for an extended period for signs of airway obstruction. When progressive airway obstruction occurred within 3 hours of surgery, the patients underwent a second bronchoscopy to determine the cause for the obstruction.

Rontal's group[44] performed a total of 126 procedures on 45 patients. The patients ranged in age from 17 to 79 years and there were 21 women and 24 men. Thirty patients had malignant disease and 15 had benign disease. Eighty-eight procedures were performed using local anesthesia, and 38 were performed using general anesthesia. Thirty-six of the patients with benign disease received general anesthesia and two received local anesthesia. General anesthesia was administered to two of the patients with malignant disease. Eighty six patients with malignant disease received local anesthesia. In one patient, general anesthesia was administered when it was judged that safe sedation could not be provided.

Eleven patients suffered complications from their laser bronchoscopy. In six cases the patients had to be returned to the operating suite to remove obstructing tumor slough. One patient was successfully treated by inhalation of racemic epinephrine in the postanesthesia recovery room for subglottic edema. Ignition of a flexible fiberoptic bronchoscope occurred in one case. However, the fire was immediately recognized and the fiberoptic bronchoscope was withdrawn through the rigid bronchoscope. The patient was not injured. Pneumothoraces were sustained by two patients who received general anesthesia. The first patient had undergone laser surgery to resect papillomata of the trachea. The second patient required very high airway pressures for pulmonary ventilation because of airway obstruction from tumor and blood clots. The laser did not appear to penetrate the airway in either case. Rontal and associates[44] stated that pneumothoraces were more likely to occur during general than local anesthesia because of the high pressures used. Two postoperative deaths occurred within 48 hours of surgery. They were thought to be due to dysrhythmias because of infiltration of the pericardium by tumor.

There appeared to be an equal incidence of postoperative hypertension whether local or general anesthesia was used. Rontal's group[44] defined hypertension as an increase of greater than 25% over baseline systolic pressure. Nineteen of 88 patients receiving local anesthesia were noted to have hypertensive blood pressures, whereas in 12 of 38 cases done with general anesthesia the patients became hypertensive. There was a very low incidence of intraoperative dysrhythmias. Two patients, one receiving general and one local anesthesia, were noted to have significant ventricular ectopic beats. Ventricular fibrillation occurred in one patient who received general anesthesia. The dysrhythmias was readily converted to a normal rhythm. This patient had undergone several laser treatments to the bronchus and was extremely ill.

Rigid bronchoscopy could not be performed in two cases. One patient had a cervical traction device in place because of a neck fracture. This patient was anesthetized through a preexisting tracheostomy, and a flexible fiberoptic bronchoscope was then passed transorally for the removal of granulation tissue below the tracheostomy stoma. In the other case, a rigid bronchoscope could not be passed into a patient's trachea because of a previous cervical laminectomy. As in the previous case, a general anesthetic was administered through a tracheostomy and a flexible fiberoptic bronchoscope was then passed transorally.

Rontal and associates[44] noted that the use of a rigid bronchoscope for laser treatment of airway lesions is an extremely safe technique. They noted that the 7- or 9-mm rigid bronchoscope provides clear access for the assessment of obstructing lesions, the removal of debris, and the control of hemorrhage. The use of the rigid bronchoscope as a pathway for the flexible fiberoptic bronchoscope has significant advantages over the use of an endotracheal tube for this purpose. The larger internal diameter of the rigid bronchoscope causes less resistance to the flow of ventilatory gases when the flexible bronchoscope is passed through it compared with an endotracheal tube. However, the most significant advantage of the rigid bronchoscope is the fact that it is noncombustible.

The following is Benumof's anesthetic management for patients undergoing laser resection involving the use of a rigid bronchoscope (Box 33-1):[45]* Anesthesia is induced with a short-acting barbiturate or propofol (2 to 3 mg/kg), alfentanil (approximately 20 μg/kg), or both. Controlled positive-pressure ventilation of the lungs by mask is instituted, and either propofol is administered as

---

*This has been modified from Benumof JL: Anesthesia for special elective therapeutic procedures. In Benumof JL, editor: *Anesthesia for thoracic surgery,* ed 2, Philadelphia, 1994, W.B. Saunders.

> **BOX 33-1   Suggested anesthesia and ventilation technique for laser resection of airway tumors**
>
> 1. Preoxygenation, pulse oximetry
> 2. Short-acting barbiturates and/or propofol and/or alfentanil
> 3. Isoflurane by mask IPPB → surgical anesthesia
> 4. Laryngoscopy, spray tracheobronchial tree with local anesthetic
> 5. Isoflurane by mask IPPB or propofol 100-200 μg/kg/min
> 6. Insert rigid bronchoscope
> 7. Pack nose and mouth if cuff cannot be used on rigid bronchoscope
> 8. Short-acting barbiturate or propofol and/or alfentanil and lidocaine inline to control any small sudden reaction to stimulation
> 9. Spontaneous vs. controlled ventilation of lungs (see text)
> 10. No paralysis vs. paralysis (see text)
> 11. $FiO_2 < .5$ in N_2 during laser firing (no N_2O)
> 12. If % saturation decreases excessively:
>   a. Ventilate lungs with 100% O_2
>   b. Control bleeding
>   c. Suction blood
>   d. Remove necrotic tissue
> 13. Extubate trachea if possible

IPPB, intermittent positive-pressure breathing
Adapted from Benumof J: *Anesthesia for thoracic surgery,* ed 2, Philadelphia, 1994, Saunders, p 524.

---

a constant infusion (100 to 200 μg/kg/min) or isoflurane is delivered until surgical levels of anesthesia are achieved (5 to 10 min). Isoflurane is selected because these patients may become hypercarbic and acidotic, and compared with halothane, isoflurane minimizes the risk of dysrhythmias. Laryngoscopy is then performed and the tracheobronchial tree is sprayed with local anesthetic. Controlled ventilation of the lungs by mask with isoflurane in oxygen is resumed for a short time. The surgeon and assistants then sequentially insert a mouthguard, the rigid bronchoscope, petroleum jelly–gauze packing into the nose, saline-wetted gauze into the mouth, and a transparent dressing over the mouth and around half of the bronchoscope.[46] The gauze and transparent dressing greatly decrease leakage around the bronchoscope.

Even though the packing of the mouth and nose and the transparent dressing over the mouth greatly decrease the leak of ventilatory gases past the rigid bronchoscope, high flows of oxygen (10 L/min) may still be necessary to deliver effective positive-pressure ventilation of the lungs. If it is anticipated that the rigid bronchoscope will not have to be moved once it is placed in the trachea and the airway lesion is not high in the trachea, the rigid bronchoscope may be fitted with a reusable endotracheal

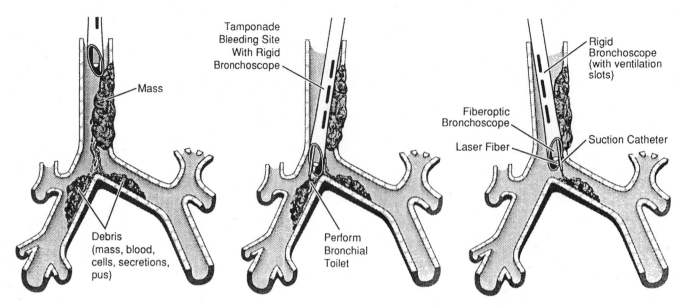

Fig. 33-17. To treat hypoxemia resulting from major tracheal obstruction (*left panel*), the operator should pass the rigid bronchoscope through the tracheal obstruction (*middle and right panels*) and perform bronchial toilet. (From Benumof JL: *Anesthesia for thoracic surgery,* ed 2, Philadelphia, 1994, WB Saunders.)

tube cuff.[47] After the passage of the bronchoscope, the anesthesia/ventilation system is connected to the side arm of the bronchoscope. Connection to a coaxial Mapleson D circuit (Bain circuit) is desirable according to Benumof because the circuit is lightweight and will not place strong tension on the rigid bronchoscope. A large syringe of both an ultra-short-acting barbiturate or propofol and/or alfentanil and lidocaine is placed in the intravenous line. If any tensing or outward pushing on the bronchoscope is felt or movement of the tracheobronchial tree (particularly invagination of the posterior membranous part) is observed, small boluses of the short-acting barbiturate (50 to 100 mg) and/or propofol (2 to 3 ml) and lidocaine (1 mg/kg) are administered.

If the endoscopist believes that spontaneous ventilation of the lungs is indicated for the bronchoscopic procedure, spontaneous breathing is allowed to return. If spontaneous ventilation is not considered advantageous, pulmonary ventilation is usually controlled, and muscle relaxants such as mivacurium or succinylcholine may be administered either as a bolus or infusion to facilitate this mode of pulmonary ventilation. Pulse oximetry is considered standard and should always be used. One hundred percent oxygen is administered during nonresection periods and less than 50% oxygen in nitrogen is used during resection periods.

According to Benumof, if a moderate fall in arterial oxyhemoglobin saturation occurs relative to the initial value, it is extremely important to stop the procedure, ventilate the patient's lungs with 100% oxygen, and clear the airway (i.e., control the bleeding, suction the airway clear, remove necrotic tissue by forceps) (see Box 33-1,

step 12). If severe hypoxemia resulting from tracheal obstruction without hemorrhage occurs, the laser resection must be immediately suspended and all efforts concentrated on reestablishing tracheal patency. An immediate improvement in pulmonary ventilation can be achieved by passing the bronchoscope tip through the obstruction (Fig. 33-17). In this position, tracheobronchial toilet and the removal of any debris should be undertaken. If severe hypoxemia without hemorrhage occurs during treatment of a unilateral mainstem obstructing lesion (Fig. 33-18, *left panel*), the bronchoscope must be withdrawn above the carina and pulmonary toilet of the healthy side undertaken (Fig. 33-18, *right panel*). If tracheal hemorrhage occurs, the foremost priority, as with tracheal obstruction, is to reestablish tracheobronchial patency by passing the bronchoscope through the hemorrhagic area (Fig. 33-19). In doing so, the hemorrhage is controlled by tamponading it with the bronchoscope, and it is possible to remove any distal blood accumulation and ventilate the patient's lungs.

As soon as the patient's pulmonary ventilation is secured, attention can be directed to the tumor site. Treatment, coagulation, or both should be carried out from distal to proximal, using the suction to maintain a dry field and a clear telescopic view. With massive bronchial hemorrhage, the patient's healthy lung can be secured by placing it in a nondependent position. In this safe position, blood and secretions can be evacuated by the bronchoscope to achieve patency (Fig. 33-20).

Because the laser resection of a tumor usually improves pulmonary ventilation and gas exchange, every effort should be made to extubate the patient's trachea

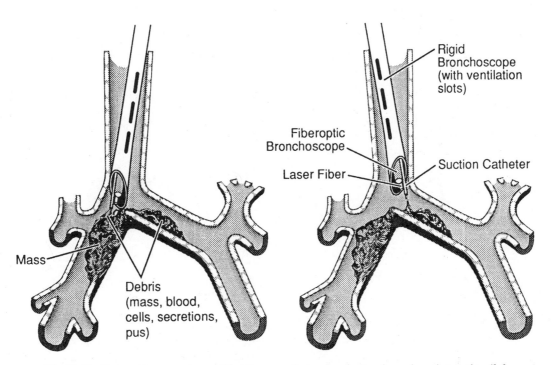

Fig. 33-18. To treat hypoxemia resulting from a unilateral mainstem bronchus obstruction (*left panel*), the operator should withdraw the bronchoscope above the carina and perform tracheobronchial toilet of the healthy side (*right panel*). (From Benumof JL: *Anesthesia for thoracic surgery,* ed 2, Philadelphia, 1994, WB Saunders.)

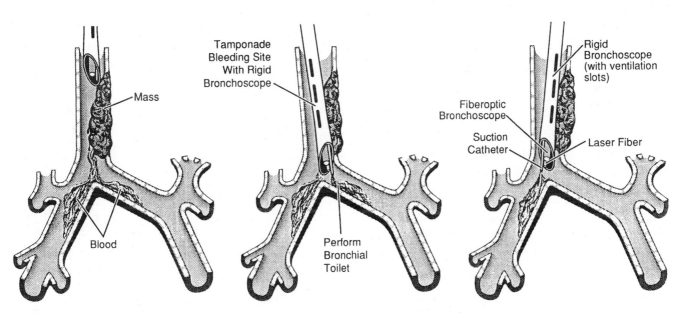

Fig. 33-19. To treat tracheal hemorrhage (*left panel*), the operator must pass the bronchoscope distal to the bleeding (*middle and right panels*) and thereby tamponade the bleeding with the bronchoscope and evacuate blood and other secretions. With pulmonary ventilation secure, one may proceed with hemostasis by coagulation. (From Benumof JL: *Anesthesia for thoracic surgery,* ed 2, Philadelphia, 1994, WB Saunders.)

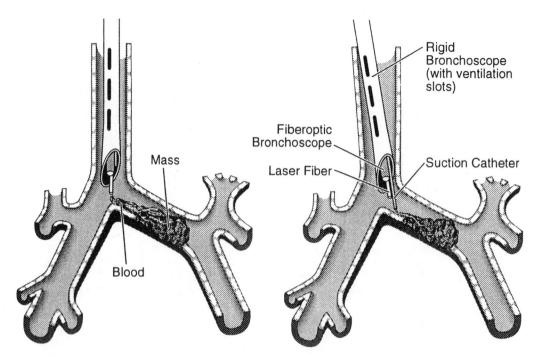

Fig. 33-20. To treat bronchial hemorrhage (*left panel*), the operator should use suction to keep the field clear (*right panel*) to identify and coagulate the bleeding site. (From Benumof JL: *Anesthesia for thoracic surgery,* ed 2, Philadelphia, 1994, WB Saunders.)

after resection. If the trachea can be extubated, laser resection bronchoscopy can often be undertaken as an outpatient procedure. Approaching the procedure on an outpatient basis minimizes the financial impact and maximizes the amount of good quality lifetime that the patient can enjoy after the resection.

6. The intermittent apneic technique for laser laryngeal surgery

Weisberger and Miner[48] described the use of an intermittent apneic technique for laser laryngeal surgery in the resection of juvenile papillomatosis of the larynx without the presence of an endotracheal tube. The investigators stated that a clear, unobstructed view of the airway and complete immobility of the surgical field are essential for the surgeon during these cases. The presence of an endotracheal tube is considered a hinderance (Fig. 33-21). They noted that the development of pulse oximetry allows the patient's state of oxygenation to be easily established, thus allowing the use of an apneic technique for anesthesia.

During a 2-year period, 51 procedures were performed by the investigators on nine patients who had juvenile laryngeal papillomatosis. Their average age was 10.5 years, with a range of 3.5 to 37 years. After the induction of general anesthesia, the patients were paralyzed with atracurium or vecuronium and the anesthesia maintained with halothane or enflurane in 100% oxygen. The patients' tracheas were intubated with small-caliber endotracheal tubes wrapped with foil

tape. In addition to standard monitoring equipment including an electrocardiogram, thermometer, and sphygmomanometer, oxygen saturation was continuously monitored by pulse oximetry. In cases of extensive papillomatosis, the resection was started with the endotracheal tube in situ while the patients' lungs were ventilated with 40% oxygen. Otherwise, the endotracheal tubes were removed and the surgery started. The surgery was interrupted when the oxygen saturation decreased. The patients' tracheas were then reintubated and they were hyperventilated with 100% oxygen. This resulted in a rapid rise in the oxygen saturation so repeated extubations and surgery could continue. The median number of apneic episodes required for each procedure was 2, with a range of 1 to 5. The duration of apneic episodes was 2.6 minutes, with a range of 1 to 4.5 minutes. A suspension laryngoscope and microscope, which provides excellent visualization of the larynx, were used in these cases so tracheal intubation could be readily accomplished without moving the laryngoscope. The apneic technique removes all the flammable material from the larynx during laser actuation and is thought to greatly decrease the possibility of an airway fire. Weisberger and Miner[48] stated that the apneic period should be shortened for small children because of their decreased functional residual capacity. This technique is contraindicated in patients in whom visualization of the larynx is difficult. At the end of the procedure, the patient's vocal cords were sprayed with 4% lidocaine (3 to 4 mg/kg) to prevent laryngospasm, and the patients

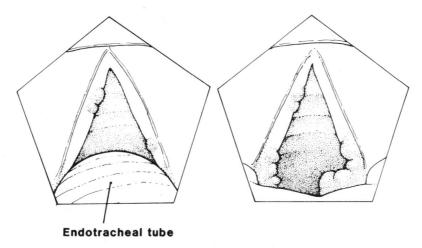

Endotracheal tube

Fig. 33-21. Additional pathologic condition noted in posterior larynx when the endotracheal tube is removed. (From Weisberger EC, Miner JD: *Laryngoscope* 98:693, 1988.)

received cool humidified air in the recovery room. They were given nebulized racemic epinephrine as needed.

Weisberger and Miner[48] reported that most of the patients undergoing the laryngologic procedures were outpatients. There were no major complications; however, reintubation of the trachea was difficult during two procedures because of inadequate paralysis; nevertheless, the endotracheal tubes were correctly placed within 20 seconds. One patient had a few short episodes of bigeminy at the onset of several of her procedures. These episodes were not associated with the apneic portion of the procedure and were resolved by substituting enflurane for halothane.

Weisberger and Miner[48] also reported that the apneic technique is especially useful in the surgical resection of lesions of the airway that are normally obscured by the presence of the endotracheal tube. These include lesions of the vocal process of the arytenoid cartilage, the posterior commissure, the subglottis, and the upper trachea. Weisberger and Miner discussed a case in which it was thought that all the papillomata were removed after airway surgery with an endotracheal tube in place. However, on inspection of the larynx after removing the endotracheal tube, lesions were discovered in the posterior glottis and subglottis.

In comparing the intermittent apneic technique to the technique of jet ventilation of the lungs, Weisberger and Miner noted that with the former technique drying of the respiratory mucosa is avoided, and the physical dissemination of virus-containing papilloma particles to the lower airway should be reduced. Furthermore, other complications of jet ventilation such as pneumomediastinum and pneumothorax will not occur. Also, there is no motion of the vocal cords with the apneic technique such as occurs with jet ventilation of the lungs.

7. Anesthesia by insufflation for laser airway surgery of infants with subglottic stenosis

Rita and associates[49] have noted that the carbon dioxide laser has been successfully used to excise subglottic stenosis in infants, thus avoiding a tracheostomy. These cases present an anesthetic challenge because the presence of an endotracheal tube will impede the surgeon because unobstructed exposure of the larynx and trachea is usually required to perform this procedure. Rita's group reported that their anesthetic approach for these cases also included a method for scavenging anesthetic gases for infants with subglottic stenosis undergoing carbon dioxide laser excision.

In a report of a case, a 7-week-old girl weighing 3.9 kg, whose trachea had been intubated transorally and who was receiving continuous positive airway pressure ventilatory support, was admitted to the intensive care unit. She had a history of "noisy breathing" since birth, which had become progressively worse. Laryngoscopy at another hospital had provided the diagnosis of congenital subglottic stenosis. Within several hours of the endoscopic procedure, marked respiratory difficulty developed in the infant, necessitating intubation of the trachea. A 2.5-mm internal diameter endotracheal tube was inserted into the trachea transorally, and she was transferred to the institution of Rita and associates. During the initial physical examination, coarse rhonchi were auscultated in both lung fields. While the patient received continuous positive airway pressure with an inspired oxygen fraction of 40%, arterial blood gas analysis showed the pH_a was 7.37, the $Paco_2$ was 45 mm Hg, and the Pao_2 was 88 mm Hg.

The patient was scheduled for an endoscopic evaluation. Atropine, 0.1 mg, intramuscularly, was given 30 minutes before the induction of anesthesia with halothane and 50% nitrous oxide through the previously placed endotracheal tube. When an adequate anesthetic depth had been achieved, the patient's trachea was extubated and the epiglottis, arytenoid cartilages, vocal cords, and trachea were sprayed with 1% lidocaine. A no. 8-French catheter attached to the anesthetic machine was introduced into the patient's nasopharynx through the right nostril. Direct observation confirmed its placement immediately above the laryngeal opening. Anesthetic gases were then insufflated with the infant breathing spontaneously. A suction catheter connected to the wall suction was taped to the proximal opening of the laryngoscope close to the patient's mouth to scavenge the anesthetic vapors.

Atmospheric nitrous oxide was measured at the head of the patient using a Foregger 410 nitrous oxide monitor. With the trachea intubated, atmospheric nitrous oxide was 5 to 7 ppm. When the endotracheal tube was removed for the insufflation technique, the concentration rose to 75 ppm without scavenging. When suction was placed close to the infant's mouth for close scavenging, the concentration dropped to 7 to 10 ppm and remained steady throughout the procedure.

During the laryngoscopic examination, a small band of tissue between the arytenoid cartilages and anterior subglottic narrowing was seen. The surgeon was not able to pass a 3-mm Storz bronchoscope. The carbon dioxide laser was then used to excise the posterior commissure band and the excess subglottic soft tissues. Dexamethasone, 4 mg, was given intravenously and the infant was transferred to the postanesthesia care unit room awake, with the trachea extubated, but with some stridor. She was placed in a high-humidity environment, and after observation for 60 minutes, she was discharged to the ward in satisfactory condition.

On the first postoperative day progressive respiratory distress occurred with substernal and intercostal retractions noted. While breathing an inspired fraction of 40% oxygen, an analysis of arterial blood gas tensions noted that the pH_a was 7.44, the $Paco_2$ was 50 mm Hg, and the Pao_2 was 80 mm Hg. Dexamethasone, 4 mg, was again given intravenously and racemic epinephrine (0.2 ml of 2.25% solution diluted in 2.5 ml saline nebulized with 100% oxygen) was administered through a face mask. The infant's condition improved, and she was discharged from the hospital 2 days later. A normal airway was observed at bronchoscopy 3 months later, and she has remained asymptomatic.

Rita and associates[49] noted that three other infants with severe subglottic stenosis have undergone endoscopic treatment with the carbon dioxide laser using the spontaneous ventilation insufflation technique at their institution. One child had subglottic stenosis develop as a consequence of prolonged intubation of the trachea, whereas the other two had congenital subglottic stenosis.

They noted that in the child with the acquired subglottic stenosis, the laser was used twice, whereas it was used three times in one case and seven times for the other case of congenital stenosis. They reported a favorable outcome for all cases without the need for a tracheostomy. Rita's group noted that the carbon dioxide laser has been used to treat both localized and circumferential stenosis. In the latter case, only one side is treated with the laser at each session.

Rita and associates[49] reported that they have been using the insufflation technique for microlaryngeal surgery, including carbon dioxide laser excision of laryngeal papillomas for 10 years. They pointed out that endotracheal tubes of any size will make surgery in these infants difficult or impossible because the operative field will be obstructed. They stated that in some infants with subglottic stenosis, even a 2.5-mm internal diameter endotracheal tube is difficult to pass through the stenotic area.

Rita and associates[49] have noted that the insufflation technique for administering anesthetics has several potential problems. In these cases the anesthesiologist does not have complete control of the airway because no endotracheal tube is used. The insufflation technique therefore requires very close cooperation between the anesthesiologist and the surgeon. The plane of anesthesia is very important in these cases. If the level of anesthesia is too deep, cardiac dysrhythmias or apnea may ensue. If the patient's anesthetic plane is too light, coughing or laryngospasm may occur. The patient must be carefully observed at all times to be sure that adequate unobstructed breathing is occurring. If the respirations are shallow, the concentration of the volatile anesthetic used (usually halothane) should be reduced. Rapid or deep respiratory efforts may signal the need for a higher level of inspired inhaled anesthetics. Rita's group reported that arterial blood gas samples that were randomly drawn from their patients showed carbon dioxide tensions in the range of 46 to 52 mm Hg.

When the insufflation technique is used to provide anesthesia, the position of the insufflation catheter must be carefully checked to ensure that it is close to the laryngeal opening. If the catheter is inadvertently inserted too far, it might enter the esophagus, causing marked gastric distention and possible regurgitation. In this case, a catheter should be placed in the stomach to decompress it, and the insufflation catheter should be repositioned near the glottic opening.

The conduct of anesthesia by insufflation is often associated with operating room pollution from volatile anesthetic agents because an open system is used. The pollution represents a distinct disadvantage of this technique. According to Rita and associates, this mode of anesthesia has resulted in higher blood levels of inhaled anesthetics among surgeons performing these

Table 33-8. Minimum flammable concentrations of halothane, enflurane, and isoflurane

N₂O	20% O₂/remainder N₂O (%)	30% O₂/remainder N₂O (%)
Halothane	3.25	4.75
Enflurane	4.25	5.75
Isoflurane	5.25	7.0

From Leonard PF: *Anesth Analg* 54:238, 1975.

endoscopic cases compared with surgeons doing cases with better pollution control. Rita's group placed a high-intensity suction catheter near the infant's mouth to scavenge the anesthetic gases during those cases. They reported that random determinations of nitrous oxide levels in the air of the operating room have shown much lower levels when the suction scavenging technique was used.

Rita and associates[49] reported that movement of the vocal cords in their patients was minimal or absent even though spontaneous breathing was maintained, provided that an adequate level of anesthesia was provided.

Rita and associates[49] administered dexamethasone intravenously at the end of the laser resections of the subglottic stenosis to decrease edema of the airway because even a small degree of airway encroachment may result in stridor in infants. In the postanesthesia care unit, their patients were observed closely as they breathed humidified gases. In case of a significant respiratory obstruction, racemic epinephrine was administered by mask. After discharge from the postanesthesia care unit by the anesthesiologist, the patients continued to breathe humidified gases in their hospital rooms.

Rita and associates[49] concluded that although the insufflation technique is potentially hazardous, if it is done correctly, it provides an appropriate anesthetic technique for surgery on the larynges of infants.[49] They reported good results with this technique over the course of many years.

8. Combustibility of halothane, enflurane, and isoflurane

Leonard,[50] in investigating the lower limits of flammability of halothane, enflurane, and isoflurane, noted that halogenation renders such compounds less flammable but may not prevent their combustion under all circumstances. He found that it was possible to ignite a mixture of 4.75% halothane in 30% oxygen with the remainder comprised of nitrous oxide (Table 33-8). In 20% oxygen with the remainder nitrous oxide, halothane concentrations greater than 3.25% were combustible. In oxygen/nitrous oxide mixtures of 20% and 30% oxygen, enflurane could be ignited at concentrations greater than 4.25% and 5.75%, whereas isoflurane required

5.25% and 7.0%, respectively. These values were obtained under laboratory conditions designed to encourage flammability. A closed-combustion vessel was used that contained no water vapor, carbon dioxide, or nitrogen. Ignition was initiated with a 15 kv transformer that delivered a 60 mA current across a 0.25-inch gap. However, the spark duration was not specified, so the total energy delivered could not be calculated. The ignition power used (900 watts) was, however, higher than the maximum power output delivered by most electrosurgical equipment. Leonard noted that the energy used in this experiment was much greater than that of a static discharge in the operating room. He concluded that even if the fraction of nitrous oxide administered to the patient exceeds 70%, the lowest flammable concentration of each of the three volatile halogenated anesthetic agents is above that which would be used clinically, except perhaps at the beginning of an inhalation induction.

A study of Pashayan and Gravenstein[41] showed that the addition of 2% halothane to a mixture of 40% oxygen and 60% helium significantly decreased the mean time to combustion of polyvinyl chloride endotracheal tube segments that were subjected to carbon dioxide laser radiation.

Ossoff found that the addition of 2% halothane significantly retarded the ignition of Rusch red rubber endotracheal tubes in atmospheres of 30%, 40%, and 50% oxygen/balance helium at power settings of 10, 15, and 20 watts.[51]

V. SPECIALLY MANUFACTURED ENDOTRACHEAL TUBES FOR LASER AIRWAY SURGERY

A. NORTON LASER ENDOTRACHEAL TUBE

The Norton Laser endotracheal tube (A.V. Mueller, Niles, Illinois) is constructed from spiral-wound stainless steel and is the only commercially constructed completely nonflammable endotracheal tube[52] (Fig. 33-22). The Norton tube has no cuff; however, a separate latex cuff may be attached to it. Alternatively, the pharynx may be packed with wet gauze to seal the system and to allow for positive pressure ventilation of the lungs. The Norton endotracheal tube has a matte or sandblasted finish, rather thick walls, and a somewhat rough exterior.[53] The matte finish acts to diffuse reflected laser beams.[52] A 4.8-mm internal diameter Norton endotracheal tube has a wall thickness of 1.4 mm (Table 33-9). The large wall thickness of this endotracheal tube is considered a disadvantage because the tube will obscure the surgeon's view more than would an endotracheal tube with the same internal diameter but with thinner walls—an important consideration during laser airway surgery. This endotracheal tube's large size and stiffness may make surgical exposure and laryngoscope positioning

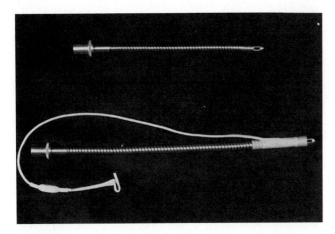

Fig. 33-22. Two Norton endotracheal tubes are shown. The lower tube has been equipped with a separate rubber cuff. (From Sosis M: *Int Anesthesiol Clin* 28:119, 1990.)

Table 33-9. Internal diameter (ID), external diameter (OD), and wall thickness for Norton Laser endotracheal tubes

Endotracheal tube size (French)	ID (mm)	OD (mm)	Wall thickness* (mm)
24	4.0	6.6	1.3
26	4.8	7.4	1.3
28	6.4	9.3	1.45

*Calculated
Courtesy of A.V. Mueller, Niles, Illinois.

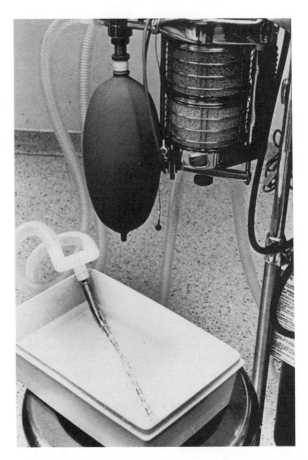

Fig. 33-23. Norton endotracheal tube under 30 cm H_2O pressure immersed in water. (From Sosis MB: *Anesth Rev* 16:39, 1989.)

difficult. If an external cuff is added to this endotracheal tube, the assembly is no longer completely nonflammable. Furthermore, the presence of the pilot tube leading to the cuff for its inflation is inconvenient. The sponges or packs that may be used to make a seal if a cuff is not used are also potentially combustible if they are allowed to dry out. Therefore they must be kept wet at all times. The Norton endotracheal tube is not airtight (Fig. 33-23); a case of difficulty ventilating the lungs of a patient has been reported when this tube was used.[54]

Even if ventilation of the patient's lungs is not compromised by leakage with the Norton endotracheal tube, the presence of anesthetic gases in the oropharynx both increases the possibility of combustion in the surgical field and increases operating room pollution. The Norton endotracheal tube is reusable and may be autoclaved, but is expensive. It came in size 4.0-, 4.8-, and 6.4-mm internal diameters (see Table 33-9).

The Norton endotracheal tube is no longer manufactured. However, it is still in use in many locations because it is reusable.

B. XOMED LASER-SHIELD I ENDOTRACHEAL TUBE

The Xomed Laser-Shield I endotracheal tube (Xomed-Treace, Jacksonville, Florida) is a silicone rubber tube that has been coated with a silicone elastomer to which metallic particles have been added (Fig. 33-24). The manufacturer states that the Xomed endotracheal tube should be used only with the carbon dioxide laser. No more than 25 watts of carbon dioxide laser power in the pulsed mode, with pulse durations of .1 to .5 second-pulse[-1] and a beam diameter of more than .8 mm should be used with this endotracheal tube. Furthermore, no more than 25% oxygen should be used with it. However, a higher concentration of oxygen may be required in some patients having laser surgery. At a laser power of 25 watts, 25 pulses of .1 second duration or 5 impacts at 0.5 second duration perforated the endotracheal tube according to the manufacturer. These recommendations apparently apply only to the shaft of the endotracheal tube because the cuff has been shown to be easily punctured by the carbon dioxide laser.[55] Three sizes of this endotracheal tube were manufactured (Table 33-10).

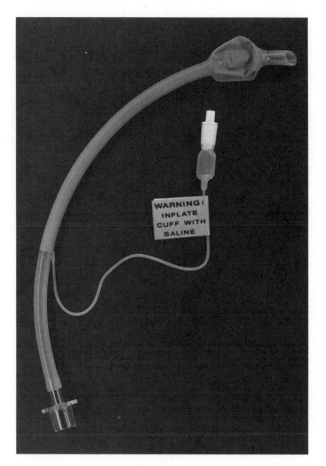

Fig. 33-24. Xomed Laser-Shield I endotracheal tube. (From Sosis MB: *Int Anesth Clin* 28:119, 1990.)

Table 33-10. Internal diameter (ID), external diameter (OD), and wall thickness of Xomed Laser-Shield I endotracheal tubes

ID (mm)	OD (mm)	Wall thickness (mm)*
4.0	6.0	1.0
5.0	7.0	1.0
6.0	9.4	1.7

*Calculated.
Courtesy of Xomed-Surgical Products, Jacksonville, Florida.

Sosis,[56] in evaluating the Xomed Laser-Shield I endotracheal tube, noted that a blowtorch fire was started quickly when a high-powered carbon dioxide laser was directed perpendicularly at its shaft. He also noted that the burning Xomed Laser-Shield I endotracheal tube was more difficult to extinguish than endotracheal tube fires involving polyvinyl chloride or red rubber endotracheal tubes (Figs. 33-25 and 33-26). As a result of its combustion, the Xomed Laser-Shield I endotracheal tube fragmented into silica debris and gave

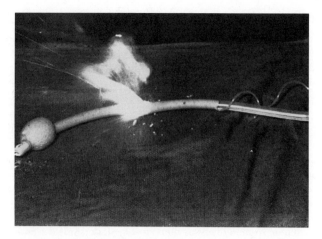

Fig. 33-25. CO_2 laser–induced fire has been started on a Xomed Laser-Shield I endotracheal tube. (From Sosis MB: *J Clin Anesth* 4:217, 1992.)

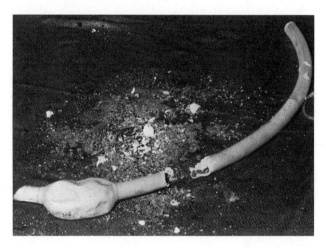

Fig. 33-26. Results of CO_2 laser ignition of a Xomed Laser-Shield I endotracheal tube. (From Sosis MB: *Adv Anesthesia* 6:175, 1989.)

off a bright light after laser contact. Similar results were found in a Nd-YAG laser evaluation of this endotracheal tube.[57] Sosis and associates do not recommend the Xomed Laser-Shield I endotracheal tube for laser surgery because safer endotracheal tubes are available even though this tube carries U.S. Food and Drug Administration approval.

Ossoff[51] noted that laser impingement onto the Xomed endotracheal tube raised its temperature significantly. It was recommended therefore that the laser be used in only the pulsed (shuttered) mode when this endotracheal tube is used so it could cool between firings. In an experiment using the carbon dioxide laser comparing the combustibility of the Xomed, Rusch red rubber, and polyvinyl chloride endotracheal tubes in 100% oxygen, the red rubber endotracheal tube was found to be significantly more resistant to the laser than the polyvinyl chloride or Xomed Laser-Shield I endotracheal tubes.

The following case report of an endotracheal tube fire in which the Xomed Laser-Shield I endotracheal tube was ignited by a carbon dioxide laser serves to illustrate the unsafe nature of this endotracheal tube.[58]

The patient was a 56-year-old ASA physical status I man weighing 79 kg who had hoarseness. A carbon dioxide laser excision of a vocal cord polyp was planned. Anesthesia was induced with 100 μg fentanyl and 400 mg thiopental administered intravenously. Endotracheal intubation was facilitated with succinylcholine, 100 mg, given intravenously. The patient underwent orotracheal intubation with a 6.0-mm internal diameter Xomed (Jacksonville, Florida) Laser-Shield I endotracheal tube. Its cuff was inflated with 5 ml of isotonic saline. No leakage of anesthetic gases was heard during positive pressure ventilation of the lungs. The carbon dioxide laser was set to a power of 20 watts in the pulsed mode of operation, with a duration of 0.2 sec/pulse. Anesthesia was maintained with 4 L/min nitrous oxide and 2 L/min oxygen along with isoflurane at inspired concentrations up to 1.5% as delivered by a calibrated vaporizer. Intermittent intravenous boluses of atracurium provided paralysis.

Near the end of the resection, the surgeon noticed bleeding at the edge of one of the vocal cords. Actuation of the laser for hemostasis resulted in smoke emerging from the patient's mouth, with the surgeon noting flames coming from the endotracheal tube. The anesthetist also noted flames in the disposable corrugated anesthesia circuit connected to the endotracheal tube. The flames were doused with saline. Breath sounds were absent and an obvious leak of anesthetic gases could be heard when the ventilator cycled. The patient's lungs were not being ventilated. The delivery of nitrous oxide and oxygen was terminated and the ventilator was turned off. After ventilation of the lungs by mask, the patient's trachea was reintubated with a polyvinyl chloride endotracheal tube. Fiberoptic bronchoscopy subsequently revealed extensive burns to the trachea and both bronchi. No fragments of the endotracheal tube were seen in the respiratory tract. The Xomed endotracheal tube was later noted to be intact, with a ruptured cuff and with evidence of combustion of the cuff and distal shaft. The patient had a long intensive care unit stay requiring positive-pressure ventilation of the lungs, antibiotics, and vigorous pulmonary toilet. He subsequently underwent a permanent tracheostomy and had several dilation procedures.

C. XOMED LASER-SHIELD II ENDOTRACHEAL TUBE

The Xomed Laser-Shield II endotracheal tube (Xomed-Treace, Jacksonville, Florida) consists of a silicone rubber endotracheal tube whose shaft has been spiral wrapped with aluminum foil tape. According to the manufacturer, no adhesives are used to secure the tape to the endotracheal tube; instead it is secured with a ring at the top and bottom of the tube. The foil layer has been overwrapped with Teflon tape (Fig. 33-27).

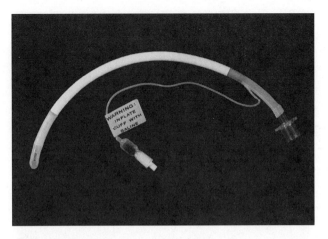

Fig. 33-27. Xomed Laser-Shield II endotracheal tube. (From Sosis MB: *Probl Anesthesia* 7:157, 1993.)

This results in a smooth exterior. Powdered methylene blue dye has been placed in the Xomed Laser-Shield II's pilot balloon. This endotracheal tube is a single-use device and is expensive.

Dillon and associates[59] evaluated the combustibility of the Xomed Laser-Shield II endotracheal tube and compared it with 3M (St. Paul, Minnesota) no. 425 aluminum foil wrapped combustible polyvinyl chloride endotracheal tubes.[24] Bare polyvinyl chloride endotracheal tubes were also studied as controls.

A Cooper LaserSonics Z500 carbon dioxide laser (Santa Clara, California) equipped with a hand-held probe was used for all carbon dioxide laser trials. A Cooper LaserSonics 8000 Nd-YAG laser with Zeiss (Jena, Germany) optical microscope guidance was used for the Nd-YAG laser trials. Both lasers were set to a power of 50 watts in the continuous mode of operation. All laser beams were directed perpendicularly at the shafts of endotracheal tubes being tested. Oxygen (5 L/min) flowed through the endotracheal tubes during laser exposure. The laser's output was continued until combustion occurred or 60 seconds had elapsed. Xomed Laser-Shield II endotracheal tubes and foil-wrapped 7.5-mm internal diameter Mallinckrodt (St. Louis, MO) polyvinyl chloride endotracheal tubes were used for four series of 10 trials. Undamaged sections of the endotracheal tube shafts were exposed to laser fire in each trial.

When the foil-covered shafts of either the Xomed Laser-Shield II or foil-wrapped polyvinyl chloride endotracheal tubes were exposed to 50 watts of carbon dioxide laser radiation for 60 seconds, no combustion occurred in 10 trials with each tube. When the foil-covered shafts of the Xomed Laser-Shield II endotracheal tubes were exposed to 50 watts of Nd-YAG laser radiation in 10 trials, the Teflon layer was noted to be missing at the site of laser impingement, exposing the aluminum foil beneath it. The foil was undamaged. In 1 trial out of 10, Nd-YAG laser exposure to the shafts of 3M no. 425-covered polyvinyl chloride endotracheal tubes resulted in combustion occurring after 53 seconds. In this case, evidence of combustion was seen at the site of overlap between two turns of the self-adhesive metallic foil tape.

Exposure of bare Mallinckrodt polyvinyl chloride endotracheal tubes to the Nd-YAG laser and carbon dioxide lasers caused rapid combustion in 4.5 ± 3.6 seconds (mean $\pm$ SD) and in 0.8 ± 0.2 seconds, respectively ($P \le .05$). Exposure of the bare silicone rubber shaft of the Laser Shield-II endotracheal tube to carbon dioxide laser radiation resulted in combustion in 2.1 ± 0.7 seconds; Nd-YAG laser radiation–induced combustion occurred at 3.3 ± 4.5 seconds ($P \le .05$). The silicone rubber burned with a bright flame and disintegrated. It was difficult to extinguish.

Dillon and colleagues[59] concluded that the foil-wrapped shaft of the Laser Shield-II endotracheal tube provides adequate protection against high-power, continuous mode Nd-YAG and carbon dioxide laser radiation, as did the shafts of 3M no. 425-wrapped polyvinyl chloride endotracheal tubes. They stated that because adhesives on foil tape have been shown to contribute to laser-induced endotracheal tube combustion,[24] the Xomed Laser-Shield II endotracheal tube offers the potential advantage of an adhesive-free foil wrapping for endotracheal tube protection. However, the choice of silicone for this endotracheal tube's shaft is considered questionable because it disintegrates during combustion, whereas rubber and polyvinyl chloride tend to retain their integrity. Also, the use of Teflon to over wrap the foil raises questions because the pyrolysis of Teflon may liberate toxic fumes that can cause polymer fume fever.

The sizes of Xomed Laser-Shield II endotracheal tubes available are given in Table 33-11.

D. BIVONA LASER ENDOTRACHEAL TUBE

The Bivona (Gary, Indiana) laser endotracheal tube has a metallic core and a silicone covering (Fig. 33-28). It has a polyurethane foam cuff with a silicone envelope that must have the air or saline aspirated from it before its insertion into or removal from the larynx.[60] A large syringe is recommended for this purpose. Once the endotracheal tube has been inserted, the pilot tube need only be opened to air for the cuff to inflate passively. However, saline is recommended for filling endotracheal tube cuffs for laser surgery.[37,38] The pilot tube runs along the exterior of the endotracheal tube and is black so it can be positioned away from the laser because damage to the pilot tube would make it impossible to deflate the cuff. Trauma to the vocal cords may result if the cuff cannot be deflated.[61,62] In addition, a high incidence of

Table 33-11. Internal diameter (ID), external diameter (OD), and wall thickness for Xomed Laser-Shield II endotracheal tubes

ID (mm)	OD (mm)	Wall thickness (mm)*
4.0	6.6	1.3
4.5	7.3	1.4
5.0	8.0	1.5
5.5	8.6	1.55
6.0	9.0	1.5
6.5	10.0	1.75
7.0	10.5	1.75
7.5	11.0	1.75
8.0	11.5	1.75

*Calculated.
Courtesy of Xomed-Surgical Products, Jacksonville, Florida.

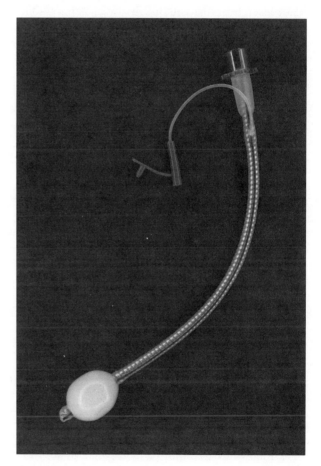

Fig. 33-28. Bivona laser endotracheal tube. (From Sosis MB: *Int Anesthesiol Clin* 28:119, 1990.)

patients complaining of a sore throat postoperatively has been noted when this type of endotracheal tube has been used for their anesthesia.[63] The external location of the pilot tube and the necessity for active deflation of the cuff are additional disadvantages of this endotracheal tube. The Bivona laser endotracheal tube is nonreusable

Table 33-12. External Diameter (OD), internal diameter (ID), and wall thickness for Bivona laser endotracheal tubes

ID (mm)	OD (mm)	Wall thickness (mm)*
3.0	5.5	1.25
4.0	6.5	1.25
5.0	7.5	1.25
6.0	8.5	1.25
7.0	9.5	1.25

*Calculated.
Courtesy of Bivona, Inc, Gary, Indiana.

and is moderately expensive (Table 33-12). The manufacturer recommends that it be used only with the carbon dioxide laser. Sosis[56] noted that the Bivona endotracheal tube ignited quickly when the carbon dioxide laser operating at high power was applied to it. A blowtorch fire occurred and the endotracheal tube disintegrated into several pieces (Fig. 33-29). Similar results and recommendations were noted by Sosis[57] with the Nd-YAG laser. Consequently, he did not recommend this endotracheal tube for laser surgery.

E. MALLINCKRODT LASER-FLEX ENDOTRACHEAL TUBE

Mallinckrodt (Glens Falls, New York) Laser-Flex endotracheal tubes have corrugated stainless steel shafts. They are designed as a single-use item and are expensive. The manufacturer states that this type of endotracheal tube should only be used with the carbon dioxide and KTP lasers. The adult version of this endotracheal tube incorporates two polyvinyl chloride cuffs. The manufacturer suggests that the distal cuff can be used if the proximal one is damaged by the laser. The adult tube's distal end, including its Murphy eye and the proximal 15-mm connector, is also constructed from combustible polyvinyl chloride (Figs. 33-30 and 33-31). The Laser-Flex endotracheal tube's cuffs are inflated by way of two separate 1-mm diameter polyvinyl chloride pilot tubes that are located on the inside of the endotracheal tube. An Nd-YAG or other laser fiber should never be inserted through this tube.

The following case reported by Heyman et al.[64] notes that prolonged laser impingement on the shaft of a Mallinckrodt Laser-Flex endotracheal tube may prevent cuff deflation.

A 64-year-old man with a history of laryngeal carcinoma was scheduled for microsuspension laryngoscopy and carbon dioxide laser debulking of his tumor. After an intravenous anesthetic induction with propofol and succinylcholine, an unstyletted Laser-Flex endotracheal tube (5.0 ID, 7.5 OD; lot #ML02740) was advanced very slowly and gently through the

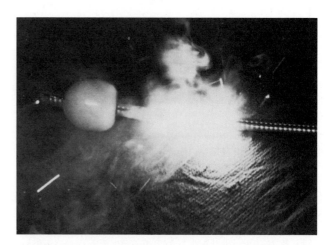

Fig. 33-29. CO_2 laser–induced endotracheal tube fire involving the Bivona laser endotracheal tube. (From Sosis MB: *J Clin Anesth* 4:217, 1992.)

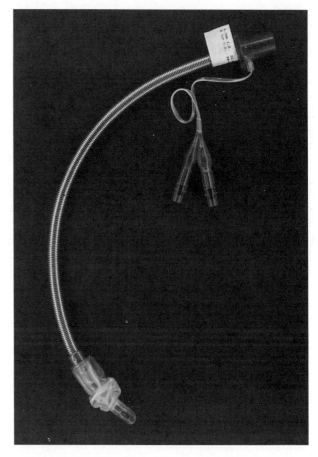

Fig. 33-30. Mallinckrodt Laser-Flex endotracheal tube. (From Sosis MB: *Probl Anesthesia* 7:157, 1993.)

narrowed glottic opening with mild resistance noted. The endotracheal tube had been checked before use by injecting and then easily aspirating 5 cc of air from each of the two cuffs, according to the manufacturer's instructions. The distal cuff was inflated with 15 ml of isotonic sterile saline, which was

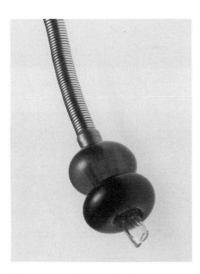

Fig. 33-31. Detail of the two polyvinyl chloride cuffs on the Mallinckrodt Laser-Flex endotracheal tube. (From Sosis MB: *Probl Anesthesia* 7:157, 1993.)

Table 33-13. Internal diameter (ID), external diameter (OD), and wall thickness for Mallinckrodt Laser-Flex endotracheal tubes

Type	ID (mm)	OD (mm)	Wall thickness* (mm)
Cuffed	4.5	7.0	1.25
	5.0	7.5	1.25
	5.5	7.9	1.20
	6.0	8.5	1.25
Uncuffed	3.0	5.2	1.10
	3.5	5.7	1.10
	4.0	6.1	1.05

*Calculated.
Courtesy of Mallinckrodt Medical, Inc., St. Louis, Mo.

necessary to obliterate the air leak during manual ventilation of the lungs. The proximal cuff was then inflated with approximately 12 ml of isotonic sterile saline. At no time was a suction catheter passed through the endotracheal tube.

At the conclusion of surgery, when the patient was ready for tracheal extubation, we readily aspirated the full volume of saline from the proximal cuff. However, we were unable to aspirate more than 1 ml from the distal cuff. We attempted to slowly withdraw the endotracheal tube past the vocal cords without success. Inspection of the pilot balloon and valve revealed no obvious damage or disruptions. Repeated attempts were made using very slow aspirations with 3- and 10-ml syringes. The pilot balloon and inflating valve were cut off, assuming they might have been malfunctioning. We were still unable to force the saline out of the cuff by direct or indirect pressure.

The ear, nose, and throat surgeon inserted a Dedo laser microlaryngoscope, an anterior commissure scope, to a point just below the vocal cords. With cephalad traction on the endotracheal tube and intensely bright fiberoptic lighting, the distal cuff was identified readily. The surgeon subsequently passed a Tucker mediastinoscope aspirating needle through the laryngoscope and punctured the cuff. After aspiration of a few milliliters of saline, the endotracheal tube was removed easily, and the patient was allowed to awaken. His emergence from anesthesia was uneventful.

Heyman et al.[64] noted that in the case they reported the laser was used in the continuous mode of operation for 46 seconds at a power setting of 11 watts with a spot size of 0.7 mm. They stressed the importance of aspirating the saline from the cuffs in a slow, gentle manner. Virag has reported that the stainless steel shaft of the Mallinckrodt Laser-Flex endotracheal tube "...becomes incandescent, perforates, and burns at power levels higher than 25 watts when exposed to a single perpendicular 0.5-mm diameter carbon dioxide laser beam for more than 20 seconds in an environment of

98% O_2."[65] He stated that the polyvinyl chloride cuff inflation tube situated within the endotracheal tube may be damaged by exposure to low levels of laser energy to the exterior of the tube's shaft. In the case reported, the 46-second period of laser contact with the tube's shaft makes the laser the likely cause for the failure of the cuff inflation tube. Virag stated that if difficult tracheal extubation owing to the inability to deflate the cuff is encountered, it may be necessary to pierce the cuff(s) with a spinal needle.

The adult sizes of Mallinckrodt Laser-Flex endotracheal tubes available with the double cuff system are 4.5-, 5.0-, 5.5-, and 6.0-mm internal diameter. Three pediatric sizes (3.0-, 3.5-, and 4.0-mm ID) of uncuffed Mallinckrodt Laser-Flex endotracheal tubes are also available. They are all stainless steel except for a PVC 15-mm adapter. They are not equipped with Murphy eyes (Table 33-13).

Unlike the all-stainless-steel Norton endotracheal tube, the Mallinckrodt Laser-Flex endotracheal tube's shaft is airtight. However, the walls of both types of tubes are somewhat rough. In their product information for the uncuffed pediatric tubes, Mallinckrodt states "due to the spiral design of the tube, the airflow resistance for a given size will be approximately equal to a PVC tube which is 0.5 mm smaller." They add "due to the bore size of the tube, patients should be monitored closely to guard against over inflation of the respiratory system and a build-up of expiratory gases."[66]

Sosis et al.[33] studied the resistance to CO_2 laser radiation of size 4.5-mm internal diameter Mallinckrodt Laser-Flex endotracheal tubes. The tubes were positioned horizontally on a stainless steel tabletop covered with a wet towel. An oxygen flow of 5 L/min passed through the tubes as a Sharplan (Tel Aviv, Israel) model 734 CO_2 laser was aimed at an endotracheal tube's shaft. A laser power setting of 35 watts with a beam diameter

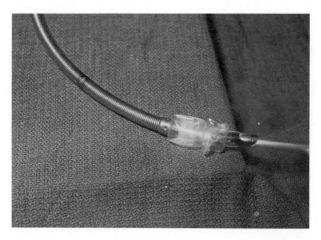

Fig. 33-32. Nd-YAG laser–induced fire ignited in a Mallinckrodt Laser-Flex endotracheal tube. (From Sosis MB: *Probl Anesthesia* 7:157, 1993.)

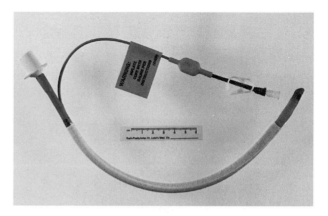

Fig. 33-33. Sheridan "Laser-Trach" endotracheal tube.

of 0.6 mm was used. This resulted in a power density of 13,400 watts/cm. The laser, set to the continuous mode of operation, was activated for 90 seconds or until combustion occurred. Blowtorch combustion occurred in one of five Laser-Flex endotracheal tubes studied. However, when human blood was applied to the shafts of four 4.5-mm internal diameter Mallinckrodt Laser-Flex endotracheal tubes, blowtorch combustion occurred in all cases.

In another study, Sosis and Dillon[67] noted that there is less danger of a reflected laser beam causing damage when the Mallinckrodt Laser-Flex endotracheal tube is used compared with foil-wrapped endotracheal tubes. In an evaluation of the Laser-Flex endotracheal tube with the Nd-YAG laser, however, Sosis found that the shaft of the Laser-Flex endotracheal tube could be ignited in all cases by the Nd-YAG laser when operated at high power[57] (Fig. 33-32). *Clinical Laser Monthly* reported the occurrence of an airway fire during a case in which a Mallinckrodt Laser-Flex endotracheal tube was used during a laser excision of vocal cord polyps.[68] They stated that the patient had minor burns. They reported that at the time of the fire, the cuffs of the endotracheal tube were not inflated with saline as is recommended by the manufacturer.

F. SHERIDAN LASER-TRACH ENDOTRACHEAL TUBE

The Sheridan (Argyle, New York) Laser-Trach endotracheal tube is a fabric-covered, embossed copper foil–wrapped red rubber device (Fig. 33-33). According to the manufacturer, the fabric covering should be saturated with water or saline before the tube is used. They recommended its use with the carbon dioxide and KTP lasers only. Sosis and associates[69] compared 6.0-mm internal diameter Sheridan Laser-Trach endo-

tracheal tubes with plain (bare) Rusch (Wailblingen, Germany) red rubber endotracheal tubes of the same internal diameter. Five liters per minute of oxygen flowed through the tubes being studied. The tubes were subjected to either continuous radiation at 40 watts from a Sharplan (Tel Aviv, Israel) carbon dioxide laser or 40 watts of continuous output from a Laserphotonics (Orlando, Florida) Nd-YAG laser. The Nd-YAG laser was propagated by a 600-μm fiber bundle. Each type of laser was directed perpendicularly at the endotracheal tube to be studied. The laser's output was continued until a blowtorch fire occurred or 50 seconds elapsed. No ignition occurred after 60 seconds of carbon dioxide laser fire to the shafts of eight Sheridan Laser-Trach endotracheal tubes tested. However, blowtorch ignition of all eight bare rubber endotracheal tubes tested occurred after 0.87 ± 21 (mean ± SD) seconds of carbon dioxide laser fire. Nd-YAG laser contact with the Sheridan copper and fabric covered rubber endotracheal tubes resulted in perforation and blowtorch ignition in all tubes tested after 18.79 ± 7.83 seconds. This was significantly ($P < .05$) longer than the 5.45 ± 4.75 seconds required for blowtorch ignition of all eight plain red rubber endotracheal tubes tested with the Nd-YAG laser.

It was concluded that under the conditions of the study, the Sheridan Laser-Trach endotracheal tube was resistant to carbon dioxide laser radiation. It is not recommended for use with the Nd-YAG laser. Table 33-14 lists the sizes of the Sheridan Laser-Trach endotracheal tubes available. These tubes are single-use items and are expensive.

VI. VENTURI JET VENTILATION OF THE LUNGS

In 1967, Sanders[70] described a technique for artificially ventilating the lungs of anesthetized patients without the presence of an endotracheal tube. A catheter clamped inside an operating bronchoscope or laryngoscope was connected to a source of oxygen at a

Table 33-14. Internal diameter (ID), external diameter (OD), and wall thickness of Sheridan Laser-Trach endotracheal tubes

ID (mm)	OD (mm)	Wall thickness*
4.0	8.2	2.10
5.0	9.5	2.25
6.0	10.6	2.30

*Calculated.
Courtesy of Sheridan Catheters, Argyle, New York.

pressure of 50 pounds per square inch (gauge). By actuating a button or toggle switch, the operator directed a jet of oxygen down the bronchoscope (Fig. 33-34). The timing of each breath was coordinated with the needs of the surgeon to minimize vocal cord movement. The result was satisfactory ventilation of the lungs of an anesthetized patient. The tidal volume and maximum airway pressures used clinically depend on the pressure delivered to the Venturi jet, its diameter, the size of the laryngoscope, and the compliance of the patient's lungs. Room air is entrained along with the oxygen jet.

When Venturi jet ventilation of the lungs is used with an operating laryngoscope, laser surgery of the larynx is possible even when the surgical field involves the posterior or interarytenoid areas normally obscured by an endotracheal tube. The absence of a combustible endotracheal tube is thought to make this technique less susceptible to airway fires as long as a noncombustible jetting catheter is used because there should be no flammable material in the airway. Ventilation of the lungs and oxygen delivery by the Venturi method have been shown to be adequate (see below). However, Venturi jet ventilation may be difficult in patients who are obese, have obstructing laryngeal lesions, or have poor chest wall or lung compliance.

One hundred percent oxygen is usually administered during jet ventilation because the entrainment of air by the Venturi jet reduces the fraction of oxygen that the patient's alveoli receive. The volume of gas delivered to the lungs may be 20 times that delivered by the Venturi jet. A pulse oximeter is an especially important instrument to monitor the oxygen saturation of the patient's hemoglobin during this technique to ensure adequate oxygen delivery.

End-tidal carbon dioxide tensions cannot be easily measured when a conventional Venturi pulmonary ventilation technique is used. Furthermore, the assessment of adequate respiratory movements is crude and hypocarbia or hypercarbia is possible with the Venturi technique.

A special gas-mixing device will allow for the use of either nitrogen and oxygen or helium and oxygen during Venturi jet ventilation of the lungs.[71] It is recommended

that nitrous oxide be avoided for laser airway surgery because it supports combustion.[40] Potent volatile inhalational anesthetics should also be avoided because their dilution by entrained air decreases their concentration markedly, thereby reducing their effectiveness. Also, the scavenging of anesthetic gases during Venturi jet ventilation of the lungs is difficult and thus any inhaled anesthetics used will pollute the operating room. A totally intravenous anesthetic technique is recommended instead.

Jet ventilation of the lungs makes use of a very high pressure source in the airway: the 50 pounds per square inch pressure commonly used for normal adults is the equivalent of a pressure of 3500 cm of water. This is greatly in excess of normal airway pressures, which are usually less than 50 cm of water. Such pressure, when applied directly to the lungs, may cause barotrauma such as pneumothorax or pneumomediastinum[72,73] (Fig. 33-35). This is a particular problem if unsealed fascial planes exist because the pressure rise occurring with the Venturi technique enhances the risk of paratracheal fascial plane dissection. This risk is more likely when surgery is performed with a conventional incision rather than with the laser. However, if mucosal disruption is present, the Venturi jetting catheter should be kept as far as possible from the mucosal opening because the pressure declines rapidly with the distance from the jetting orifice. The lowest pressure that can achieve adequate ventilation of the lungs should be used.

There is no barrier to the passage of vomitus, blood, or debris into the patient's trachea and lungs when using Venturi jet ventilation of the lungs because a cuffed endotracheal tube is generally not used. Furthermore, vagal effects from gastric distention are possible. An additional problem (Box 33-2) is that the Venturi jet must be kept in perfect alignment with the trachea or gastric dilation, with possible regurgitation, may occur.[74]

A gastric catheter should be placed whenever possible to decompress the patient's stomach after Venturi jet ventilation. It should be left in place until the patient is alert and awake. Because of the necessity for precise alignment between the Venturi jetting catheter and the trachea, any readjustment of the operating laryngoscope to which the jet is clamped may impair ventilation of the lungs. Thus the anesthesiologist should observe the adequacy of pulmonary ventilation at all times.

An immobile surgical field may be difficult to achieve during Venturi jet ventilation of the lungs despite adequate paralysis of the patient with muscle relaxants because of the movement of the vocal cords induced by the Venturi jet. This movement will obviously be magnified when an operating microscope is used. Therefore, if possible, the Venturi jet should be triggered during pauses between the actuation of the surgical laser to keep the vocal cords from moving during surgery. The

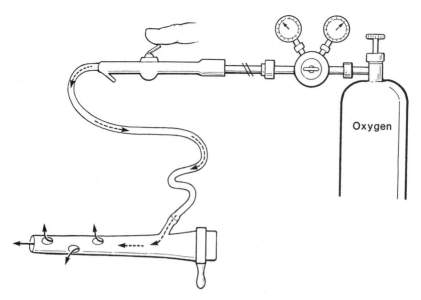

Fig. 33-34. Schematic diagram of a Venturi ventilation system built into a ventilating bronchoscope. The surgeon's view is not compromised because no endotracheal tube is used. Oxygen is provided from an oxygen source with a reducing valve. Respirations are initiated when the operator presses a button or toggle switch. (From Sosis MB: *Int Anesth Clin* 28:119, 1990.)

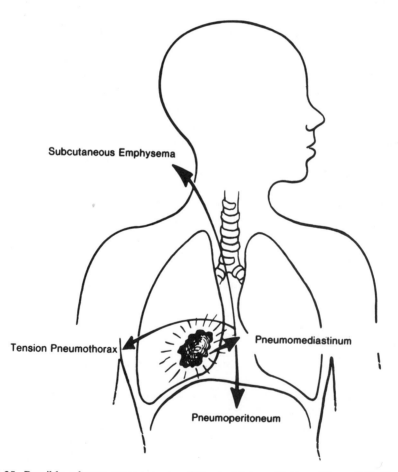

Fig. 33-35. Possible adverse consequences of Venturi jet ventilation. (From O'Sullivan TJ, Healy GB: *Arch Otolaryngol* 111:127, 1985.)

BOX 33-2   Disadvantages of Venturi jet ventilation

1. Risk of pneumomediastinum or pneumothorax, subcutaneous emphysema, and pneumopericardium
2. Risk of gastric distention and regurgitation
3. Seeding of papillomatoses
4. Trapdoor obstruction
5. Difficult to use in cases of obesity, poor lung compliance, or laryngeal obstruction
6. Vocal cord motion
7. Difficulty measuring actual inspired oxygen fraction
8. Mucosal dehydration
9. Lower respiratory tract involvement
10. Inability to measure airway pressure easily
11. Inadequate ventilation
12. Lack of a convenient means to measure end-tidal carbon dioxide tension
13. Hypocarbia
14. Hypercarbia
15. Inability to use volatile inhalation anesthetics
16. Difficulty scavenging gaseous anesthetics and products of combustion

Adapted from Ossoff RH: *Laryngoscope* 99(8, suppl 48):1, 1989.

Venturi jet technique may also cause mucosal dehydration and inspissated secretions because the jetting gases are not usually humidified. The administration of humidified gases to these patients postoperatively and adequate hydration intraoperatively should be considered.

Those patients who have large airway lesions, such as proliferating polyploid masses of the larynx, are at risk for "trapdoor" obstruction of the airway when the Venturi technique is used. During these cases, a ball-valve effect may occur in which gases may be introduced into the lungs but will not escape. Thus the possibility of barotrauma in this situation is great. Norton and associates[75] recommended that a foil-protected endotracheal tube be used for pulmonary ventilation instead of the Venturi technique when such airway masses are present to prevent this complication. The surgeon can then confidently use the laser to remove the bulk of the lesion with the endotracheal tube present. The endotracheal tube can then be removed and the Venturi technique used safely so that any pathologic condition that was obscured by the endotracheal tube can be treated without this hindrance. Norton and associates suggested that if difficulty achieving adequate ventilation of the lungs with the Venturi technique occurs, the surgeon should look for hidden airway masses that might cause ball-valve obstruction. They noted that such lesions are sometimes found in the laryngeal ventricles.

Norton and associates[75] recommend that fentanyl not be used for Venturi jet ventilation of the lungs because chest wall rigidity and therefore difficulty in adequately ventilating the lungs may occur. They also suggest avoiding the use of ketamine because it sensitizes the laryngeal reflexes, and thus laryngospasm may occur.

The Venturi jet catheter technique may cause the spread of infectious particles such as papillomavirus to the patient or even to operating room personnel.

If the Venturi catheter is placed subglottically, obstruction is obviated during the inspiratory phase of ventilation. Expiration, however, may be made difficult if laryngospasm or air obstruction occurs. This may result in barotrauma and even patient death.

The anesthesiologist should watch for bilateral chest excursions and use a precordial stethoscope and pulse oximeter, as well as the usual monitoring devices previously described during Venturi jet ventilation of the lungs.

Norton and colleagues[75] described a technique for Venturi ventilation of the lungs for carbon dioxide laser airway surgery using an inexpensive 14- or 16-gauge jet needle mounted on a clamp connected to a modified paint-spraying apparatus. They used the 16-gauge needle for children and the 14-gauge needle for adults. Pressures of up to 13.5 and 9 kg for adults and children, respectively, were used. However, by adjusting the pressure to achieve adequate chest wall movement during Venturi ventilation, pressures of 3.6 and 9 kg were found adequate for children and adults, respectively, in most cases.

Norton and associates[75] described a study population of 100 cases between the ages of 3 and 78. Ninety percent of the patients were between 2 and 12 years of age. Their weights and heights varied from 13.5 to 104.4 kg and 97.5 to 182.5 cm, respectively. Male patients were more frequent than female patients by a ratio of 54:46. Most patients underwent more than one laser airway procedure, and the most common diagnosis in this series of patients was viral laryngotracheal papillomatosis.

Norton and colleagues[75] stressed the need for adequate premedication, especially in children. However, they caution against overmedicating patients who have large airway lesions because respiratory obstruction might occur.

Anesthesia induction for the adult patients followed the authors' routine of using intravenous thiamylal sodium. Mask anesthesia induction was undertaken for the children. Muscle relaxation was provided with a .2% succinylcholine infusion administered intravenously.

Norton and colleagues[75] reported their preference for the placement of foil-protected red rubber endotracheal tubes in their patients so the surgeon would not be rushed in the placement of the suspension laryngoscope. They suggested that this technique would prevent "trapdoor" obstruction from occurring during cases with large airway masses. They recommended placing gastric tubes for decompression of the stomach in most cases.

Once the suspension laryngoscope was placed, the surgeon used the carbon dioxide laser equipped with binocular microscopic guidance to treat any lesions that were not obscured by the endotracheal tube. The endotracheal tube was then withdrawn, and the Venturi jetting needle was placed in the lumen of the laryngoscope. It rested above the instrument's light carrier channel. In this location, it did not interfere with the surgeon's view of the surgical field or with the ability to operate. It was noted that excellent access to the posterior third of the vocal cords and the interarytenoid areas was possible by the Venturi method. The laryngoscope was placed with its tip as close as possible to the vocal cords with its axis aligned with that of the trachea.

When the laser surgical procedure was completed, an oropharyngeal airway was inserted into the patient's mouth, and ventilation of the lungs was achieved by bag and mask until the effects of the muscle relaxant and anesthetic agents had dissipated.

Norton and co-workers[75] noted that the Venturi technique for ventilation of the lungs was used for up to 40 minutes without difficulty.

Cozine and associates[22] conducted a nationwide survey of ventilatory complications during Venturi jet ventilation of the lungs for laser airway surgery. A questionnaire was sent to the 109 members of the Society of Academic Anesthesia Chairman, which requested specific information regarding the number of carbon dioxide laser procedures done, the type of pulmonary ventilation used, and a description of any problems that occurred. The surveys were tabulated and analyzed and the complications were listed as ventilation related or unrelated, type of ventilation used, reason for occurrence, and severity. Statistical analyses were done with the chi-square analysis and the Fisher exact two-tailed test.

Seventy questionnaires were returned to the investigators. Fifty-eight institutions reported using the carbon dioxide laser for laser endoscopic surgery. Thirty of the institutions did not use Venturi jet ventilation of the lungs, whereas 28 used both Venturi jet ventilation and conventional intermittent positive pressure pulmonary ventilation through an endotracheal tube. Data from 15,707 patients were received. Twenty-six percent of the patients underwent Venturi jet ventilation of the lungs. The other patients received conventional intermittent positive pressure ventilation of the lungs with an endotracheal tube.

The need for prolonged mask ventilation of the lungs postoperatively in patients undergoing the Venturi jet ventilation technique was the most common complication of this method (Table 33-15). This problem was

Table 33-15. Complications associated with Venturi jet ventilation of the lungs (49 complications in 4,151 patients)

Ventilation related	Ventilation unrelated
Major	**Major**
Pneumothorax (9)	None
Hypoxemia during anesthesia (6)	
Mediastinal air (2)	
Tension pneumothorax (1)	
Minor	**Minor**
Carbon dioxide retention during anesthesia (3)	Prolonged mask support (10)
Subcutaneous emphysema (2)	Prolonged endotracheal intubation (5)
Gastric dilation (2)	Laryngospasm (5)
Airway bleeding (2)	Prolonged sleep or paralysis (2)
Recall of procedure (1)	

From Cozine K et al: *J Clin Anesth* 3:20, 1991.

thought to be related to the use of a totally intravenous anesthetic technique. Approximately half of the complications involving the Venturi jet method, including the need for prolonged mask support, the need for endotracheal intubation, marked postoperative somnolence, residual paralysis, and laryngospasm, were considered relatively unimportant and were easily treated.

There were 14 occurrences of barotrauma including 9 pneumothoraces, 1 tension pneumothorax, 2 instances of mediastinal emphysema, and 2 reports of subcutaneous emphysema among the patients undergoing Venturi jet ventilation of the lungs. Also reported were six cases in which transient hypoxemia occurred, three cases of elevated carbon dioxide tensions, and one case of gastric dilation. Eighteen of the 24 ventilation-related complications were considered life-threatening. The overall incidence of complications for patients undergoing the Venturi jet technique was 1.2%. No deaths were reported in this group of patients.

In the group of patients whose anesthesia involved the use of intermittent positive-pressure ventilation of the lungs through an endotracheal tube, the overall incidence of complications was 0.36%. Cozine and colleagues[22] reported that the overall incidence of complications, the rate of complications related to pulmonary ventilation, the rate of serious or "life-threatening" complications, and the incidence of barotrauma were more frequent in the group of patients receiving Venturi jet ventilation of the lungs ($P < .001$) than in the group receiving intermittent positive pressure ventilation of the lungs.

The rate of complications during Venturi jet ventilation of the lungs was related to the number of cases that

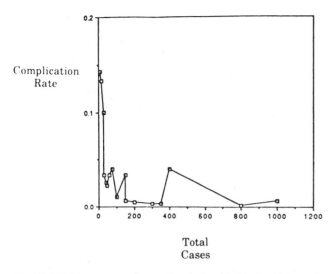

Fig. 33-36. Frequency of complications with Venturi jet ventilation among institutions reporting complications. (From Cozine K et al: *J Clin Anesth* 3:20, 1991.)

were done by a particular institution (Fig. 33-36). Of the 28 medical facilities that reported using the Venturi technique, 17 (60%) reported complications. Fourteen of the 17 had an incidence of complications of less than 4%. The three remaining institutions that reported complications performed less than 30 procedures each and had an incidence of complications of 10% or more. The occurrence of complications during carbon dioxide laser surgery when conventional intermittent positive pressure of the lungs through an endotracheal tube was used was not related to the number of cases done by the institution.

Cozine and colleagues reported that three institutions responding to their survey reported abandoning the Venturi jet ventilation technique for pulmonary ventilation during carbon dioxide laser airway surgery. The reasons offered included the occurrence of pneumothoraces, the lack of a convenient means of monitoring airway pressure and end-tidal carbon dioxide tensions, and the decision that the Venturi technique had no advantages over more conventional techniques.

Cozine and associates offered four recommendations for improved patient safety when using the Venturi technique: (1) a pulse oximeter should be used to ensure adequate oxygenation; (2) the Venturi gas jetting apparatus should be placed supraglottically and precisely aligned with the trachea; (3) muscle relaxation should be maintained; and (4) the Venturi technique should not be used for obese patients.

VII. MANAGEMENT OF AN AIRWAY FIRE

All operating room personnel must be prepared for the possibility of an airway fire during laser endoscopic surgery. A plan of action should be rehearsed by

---

BOX 33-3 Laser airway fire protocol

- Cease ventilation and turn off all anesthetic gases, *including oxygen.**
- Extinguish flames with saline solution.*
- Remove endotracheal tube after deflating cuff.* Be certain entire endotracheal tube has been removed.
- Ventilate the patient's lungs by mask after all burning material has been removed and extinguished.
- Examine airway for burns and foreign bodies such as fragments of the endotracheal tube or packing materials.

*These steps should be taken simultaneously by the anesthesiologist and surgeon.
From Sosis MB: *Probl Anesthesia* 7(2): June, 1993.

---

operating room personnel so rapid action can be taken if a fire occurs.

In the event of an airway fire or explosion, the anesthesiologist should immediately stop the delivery of *all* anesthetic gases, *including oxygen* (Box 33-3). This can be accomplished by turning off the flowmeters or rotameters, disconnecting the hose at the common gas outlet of the anesthesia machine, detaching the endotracheal tube from the anesthesia circuit, or simply clamping the endotracheal tube. The anesthetic gases administered usually contain an increased fraction of oxygen and interrupting their supply is often sufficient to terminate an endotracheal tube fire. The endotracheal tube should always be removed immediately in this situation because it no longer provides a patient airway and may be on fire. For this reason, the endotracheal tube should not be overzealously taped in place, nor should the patient be excessively draped. A container or syringe of saline should be available to extinguish any flames. Once the endotracheal tube has been removed and the fire completely extinguished, the patient's lungs should be ventilated with 100% oxygen by bag and mask. At this point, the extent of airway damage should be assessed. This may entail fiberoptic bronchoscopy through an endotracheal tube or rigid bronchoscopy. Extensive burns should be managed with controlled ventilation of the lungs through an endotracheal tube or by tracheostomy; the use of antibiotics and steroids should be considered if burns are severe. All inhaled gases should be humidified. If the airway burns are minimal, it may be possible to proceed with surgery. For this reason, a second endotracheal tube for laser airway surgery should be available.

REFERENCES

1. Maiman TH: Stimulated optical radiation in ruby, *Nature* 187:493, 1960.
2. Fuller TA: The physics of surgical lasers, *Lasers Surg Med* 1:5, 1980.
3. Hermens JM, Bennett MJ, Hirshman CA: Anesthesia for laser surgery, *Anesth Analg* 62:218, 1983.

4. Leibowitz HM, Peacock GR: Corneal injury produced by carbon dioxide laser radiation, *Arch Ophthalmol* 81:713, 1969.

5. Strong MS, Jako GJ: Laser surgery in the larynx: early clinical experience with continuous carbon dioxide laser, *Ann Otol* 81:791, 1972.

6. Council on Scientific Affairs: Lasers in medicine and surgery, *JAMA* 256:900, 1986.

7. Alberti PW: The complications of carbon dioxide laser surgery in otolaryngology, *Acta Otolaryngol* 91:375, 1981.

8. Shapshay SM, Beamis JF Jr: Safety precautions for bronchoscopic Nd-YAG laser surgery, *Otolaryngol Head Neck Surg* 94:175, 1986.

9. Dumon JF, Shapshay S, Bourcereau J et al: Principles for safety in application of neodymium-YAG laser bronchology, *Chest* 86:163, 1984.

10. Brutinel WM, McDougall JC, Cortese DA: Bronchoscopic therapy with neodymium-yttrium-aluminum-garnet laser during intravenous anesthesia, *Chest* 84:518, 1983.

11. Casey KR, Fairfax WR, Smith SJ et al: Intratracheal fire ignited by the Nd-YAG laser during treatment of tracheal stenosis, *Chest* 84:295, 1983.

12. Brutinel WM, Cortese DA, McDougall JC. Bronchoscopic phototherapy with the neodymium-YAG laser, *Chest* 86:157, 1984.

13. McDougall JC, Cortese DA: Neodymium-YAG laser therapy of malignant airway obstruction: a preliminary report, *Mayo Clin Proc* 58:35, 1983.

14. Ossoff RH, Hotaling AJ, Karlan MS et al: carbon dioxide laser in otolaryngological-head and neck surgery: a retrospective analysis of complications, *Laryngoscope* 93:1287, 1983.

15. Milliken RA, Bizzarri DV: Flammable surgical drapes: a patient and personnel hazard. *Anesth Analg* 64:54, 1985.

16. Ott AE: Disposable surgical drapes: a potential fire hazard, *Obstet Gynecol* 61:667, 1983.

17. Levine DL: More laser accidents: one state health department reacts, *J Clin Laser Med Surg* 8:8, 1990.

18. Fried MP: A survey of the complications of laser laryngoscopy, *Arch Otolaryngol* 110:31, 1984.

19. Healey GB, Strong MS, Shapshay S et al: Complications of carbon dioxide laser surgery of the aerodigestive tract: experience of 4,416 cases, *Otolaryngol Head Neck Surg* 92:13, 1984.

20. Burgess GE, LeJeune FE Jr: Endotracheal tube ignition during laser surgery of the larynx, *Arch Otolaryngol* 105:561, 1979.

21. Snow JC, Norton ML, Saluja TS et al: Fire hazard during carbon dioxide laser microsurgery on the larynx and trachea, *Anesth Analg* 55:146, 1976.

22. Cozine K, Stone JG, Shulman S et al: Ventilatory complications of carbon dioxide laryngeal surgery, *J Clin Anesth* 3:20, 1991.

23. Personal communication. Surgical Products Division, 3M Corp, 1986.

24. Sosis MB: Evaluation of five metallic tapes for protection of endotracheal tubes during carbon dioxide laser surgery, *Anesth Analg* 68:392, 1989.

25. Cork RC: Anesthesia for otolaryngologic surgery involving use of a laser. In Brown BR Jr, editor: *Anesthesia and ENT surgery,* Philadelphia, 1987, F.A. Davis.

26. Edelist G: Anaesthesia for endoscopy and laser surgery, *Can Anaesth Soc J* 31:S1, 1984.

27. Andrews AH, Goldenberg RA, Moss HW et al: Carbon dioxide laser for laryngeal surgery, *Surg Annu* 6:459, 1974.

28. Carruth JAS, McKenzie AL, Wainwright AC: The carbon dioxide laser; safety aspects, *J Laryngol Otol* 94:411, 1980.

29. Sosis M, Dillon F: What is the safest foil tape for endotracheal tube protection during Nd-YAG laser surgery? A comparative study, *Anesthesiology* 72:553, 1990.

30. Hirshman CA, Smith J: Indirect ignition of the endotracheal tube during carbon dioxide laser surgery, *Arch Otolaryngol* 106:639, 1980.

31. Kaeder CS, Hirshman CA: Acute airway obstruction: a complication of aluminum tape wrapping of tracheal tubes in laser surgery, *Can Anaesth Soc J* 26:138, 1979.

32. Patel KF, Hicks JN: Prevention of fire hazards associated with use of carbon dioxide lasers, *Anesth Analg* 60:885, 1981.

33. Sosis MB, Pritikin JB, Caldarelli DD: The effect of blood on laser-resistant endotracheal tube combustion, *Laryngoscope* 104:829, 1994.

34. Geffin B, Shapshay SM, Bellack GS et al: Flammability of endotracheal tubes during Nd-YAG laser application in the airway, *Anesthesiology* 65:511, 1986.

35. Sosis M, Dillon F: Prevention of carbon dioxide laser induced laser endotracheal tube fires with the Laser-Guard protective coating, *J Clin Anesth* 4:25, 1992.

36. Sosis MB, Braverman B: Evaluation of foil coverings for protecting plastic endotracheal tubes from the potassium-titanyl-phosphate laser, *Anesth Analg* 77:589, 1993.

37. Le Jeune FE Jr, Guice C, Letard F et al: Heat sink protection against lasering endotracheal tube cuffs, *Ann Otol Rhinol Laryngol* 91:606, 1982.

38. Sosis M, Dillon FX: Saline filled cuffs help prevent laser-induced polyvinyl chloride endotracheal tube fires, *Anesth Analg* 72:187, 1991.

39. Sosis M: Saline soaked pledgets prevent CO_2 laser–induced tracheal tube cuff ignition, *Anesth Analg* 72:S266, 1991.

40. Macintosh R, Mushin WW, Epstein HG: Physics for the anaesthetist, Oxford, England, 1963, Blackwell.

41. Pashayan AG, Gravenstein JS: Helium retards endotracheal tube fires from carbon dioxide lasers, *Anesthesiology* 62:274, 1985.

42. Simpson JI, Schiff GA, Wolf GL: The effect of helium on endotracheal tube flammability, *Anesthesiology* 73:538, 1990.

43. Al Haddad S, Brenner J: The effect of helium on endotracheal tube flammability during KTP/532 laser use, *Anesthesiology* 73:A491, 1990.

44. Rontal M, Rontal E, Wenokur ME et al: Anesthetic management for tracheobronchial laser surgery, *Ann Otol Rhinol Laryngol* 95:556, 1986.

45. Benumof JL: *Anesthesia for thoracic surgery,* ed 2, Philadelphia, Saunders, 1994.

46. Benumof JL: Another use for the plastic transparent dressing, *Anesthesiology* 63:334, 1985 (letter).

47. Grant RP, White SA, Brand SC: Modified rigid bronchoscope for Nd-YAG laser resection of tracheobronchial obstructing lesions, *Anesthesiology* 66:575, 1987.

48. Weisberger EC, Miner JD: Apneic anesthesia for improved endoscopic removal of laryngeal papillomata, *Laryngoscope* 98:693, 1988.

49. Rita L, Seleny F, Hollinger LD: Anesthetic management and gas scavenging for laser surgery of infant subglottic stenosis, *Anesthesiology* 58:191, 1983.

50. Leonard PF: The lower limits of flammability of halothane, enflurane and isoflurane, *Anesth Analg* 54:238, 1975.

51. Ossoff RH: Laser safety in otolaryngology head and neck surgery: anesthetic and educational considerations for laser laryngeal surgery, *Laryngoscope* 99(8) (suppl 48):1, 1989.

52. Norton ML, DeVos P: New endotracheal tube for laser surgery of the larynx, *Ann Otol* 87:554, 1978.

53. Skaredoff MN, Poppers PJ: Beware of sharp edges in metal endotracheal tubes, *Anesthesiology* 58:595, 1983.

54. Sosis M: Large air leak during surgery with a Norton tube, *Anesthesiol Rev* 16:39, 1989.

55. Hayes DM, Gaba DM, Goode RL: Incendiary characteristics of a new laser-resistant endotracheal tube, *Otolaryngology* 95:37, 1986.

56. Sosis MB: Which is the safest endotracheal tube for use with the CO_2 laser? A comparative study, *J Clin Anesth* 4:217, 1992.

57. Sosis MB: What is the safest endotracheal tube for Nd-YAG laser surgery: a comparative study, *Anesthesiology* 69:802, 1989.

58. Sosis M: Airway fire during carbon dioxide laser surgery using a Xomed laser endotracheal tube, *Anesthesiology* 72:747, 1990.

59. Dillon F, Sosis M, Heller S: Evaluation of a new foil wrapped endotracheal tube for laser airway surgery, *Anesthesiology* 75:A392, 1991 (abstract).

60. Kamen JM, Wilkinson CJ: A new low-pressure cuff for endotracheal tubes, *Anesthesiology* 34:482, 1971.

61. Birkhan HJ, Heifetz M: "Uninflatable" inflatable cuffs, *Anesthesiology* 26:578, 1965.

62. Hedden M, Smith RBF, Torpey DJ: A complication of metal spiral-imbedded latex endotracheal tubes, *Anesth Analg* 51:859, 1972.

63. Loeser EA, Machin R, Colley J et al: Postoperative sore throat: importance of endotracheal tube conformity versus cuff design, *Anesthesiology* 49:430, 1978.

64. Heyman DM, Greenfield AL, Rogers JS et al: Inability to deflate the distal cuff of the Laser-Flex tracheal tube preventing extubation after laser surgery of the larynx, *Anesthesiology* 80:236, 1994.

65. Virag R. In reply, *Anesthesiology* 80:237, 1994.

66. Anonymous: *Mallinckrodt anesthesia products,* St Louis, 1992.

67. Sosis M, Dillon F: Reflection of CO_2 laser radiation from laser resistant endotracheal tubes, *Anesth Analg* 73:338, 1991.

68. Anonymous: Safety design can't eliminate endotracheal tube fires, *Clin Laser Monthly* 8(10):148, 1990.

69. Sosis M, Braverman B, Ivankovich AD: Evaluation of a new laser-resistant fabric and copper foil wrapped endotracheal tube, *Anesthesiology* 79:A536, 1993.

70. Sanders RD: Two ventilating attachments for bronchoscopes, *Del Med J* 39:170, 1967.

71. Carden E, Schwesinger WB: The use of nitrous oxide during ventilation with the open bronchoscope, *Anesthesiology* 39:551, 1973.

72. O'Sullivan TJ, Healy GB: Complications of Venturi jet ventilation during microlaryngeal surgery, *Arch Otolaryngol* 111:127, 1985.

73. Oliverio R, Ruder CB, Fermon C et al: Pneumothorax secondary to ball-valve obstruction during jet ventilation, *Anesthesiology* 51:255, 1979.

74. Chang JL, Meeuwis H, Bleyaert A et al: Severe abdominal distension following jet ventilation during general anesthesia, *Anesthesiology* 49:216, 1978.

75. Norton ML, Strong MS, Vaughan CW et al: Endotracheal intubation and Venturi (jet) ventilation for laser microsurgery of the larynx, *Ann Otol* 85:656, 1976.

Chapter 34

THE TRAUMATIZED AIRWAY

Roger S. Cicala

I. DEFINING THE PROBLEM

Patients who have suffered major trauma can present the most complex airway management problems encountered in the modern practice of anesthesia. As with all airway management scenarios, the ultimate goal is clear: secure the airway in the safest possible manner that will provide continuous adequate ventilation. In the patient with trauma affecting the airway, however, many other factors must be considered.

736

Often, injuries are present that obviously will interfere with attempts to control the airway. In almost every case, the evaluation of injuries is quite incomplete at the time airway management is undertaken. The caregiver must make assumptions and educated guesses about any potential undetected injuries that might be present. If the airway itself is injured, attempts to perform endotracheal intubation may cause further injury to damaged tissues and structures. If cervical-spine injury is present, improper airway management could have devastating neurologic consequences. These decisions often must be made in seconds or minutes, based only on information gathered by a cursory examination and backed by the caregiver's clinical judgment.

A. THE INCIDENCE, MORBIDITY, AND MORTALITY OF AIRWAY TRAUMA

For purposes of this chapter, airway trauma will be considered to be an injury that directly involves the airway in any location from the nasopharynx to the bronchioles. Such trauma may involve actual damage to the airway or injury to nearby bony or vascular structures that distorts the airway anatomy. Associated trauma affecting airway management will be considered to be those injuries that limit or influence the techniques available for airway management. Cervical-spine injury is the classic example of such an associated injury, but many other injuries can also affect airway management.

In patients with penetrating trauma the presence of a wound in proximity to airway structures usually gives warning of potential problems. Blunt trauma often provides few indications of airway injuries and is therefore more dangerous. Most blunt trauma patients have only subtle signs suggesting the presence of the injury.

Maxillofacial injury occurs in as many as 22% of motor vehicle accident victims.[1] Airway compromise occurs in a significant portion of these patients, either from displacement of bony structures or from soft tissue swelling. Patients with maxillofacial trauma often appear stable on arrival to the hospital, but as many as 35% will deteriorate, necessitating emergency airway management within hours after admission.[2] The mortality caused by the maxillofacial injury itself is only about 0.75%.[3] However, because hypoxia is one of the most common causes of death after blunt maxillofacial injury, airway management is of the utmost importance in such cases.[4,5]

The incidence of actual laryngotracheal injury has been reported to be as low as .03% of patients admitted at a major trauma center[6] or as high as 2.8% of all trauma victims in autopsy series.[7] More recent studies place the frequency of airway injury at about .5% of patients admitted to a level 1 trauma center.[8,9]

Such injuries are extremely lethal. Autopsy series of trauma victims show that between 70% and 80% of persons who sustain airway injuries die before reaching medical care.[10-12] Of those patients who do survive to reach tertiary care, 21% die during the first 2 hours after admission.[12] Often, death occurs during attempts to intubate the trachea when the airway injury is unsuspected because this may lead to complete airway obstruction.[13,14]

In patients who survive airway injury, the diagnosis is often delayed,[4,15] increasing the incidence of late complications.[16,17]

Most thoracic injuries respond to routine conservative treatment, such as thoracostomy tube placement. Almost 5% of these injuries result in severe pulmonary compromise, however. Approximately 1% of thoracic trauma victims have severe tracheobronchial injury requiring specialized airway management techniques, such as selective bronchial intubation.[18] Such injuries have a mortality rate approaching 70%.

Cervical-spine injury occurs in as many as 4% of all trauma patients.[19,20] Five to ten percent of all cervical-spine injuries are not suspected at the time airway management procedures are performed, and one third of these patients will have permanent neurologic sequelae after these procedures.[19]

For a variety of reasons, 7% of all trauma patients require emergency intubation or other definitive airway management within the first 15 minutes of admission.[21] Failed intubation requiring cricothyrotomy or other surgical management of the airway is necessary in about .5% of all admissions to a level I trauma center.[22]

B. THE DECISION TO INTUBATE

In the traumatized patient, the standard of care requires the anesthesiologist not only to decide the best method of airway management but also when and if airway management procedures are even indicated. Occasionally the scenario is a simple one: a patient arrives in extremis and endotracheal intubation must be performed immediately by any method possible. If orotracheal intubation is difficult in such cases, one may rely on the old surgical wisdom "God put the trachea close to the skin for a reason."

More commonly, decisions regarding airway management are not so obvious. Many patients appear to have clinically adequate ventilation at the time of admission, but will have less morbidity if airway intervention and mechanical ventilation are instituted early in their hospital course.[23] Conversely, overly vigorous attempts to intubate the trachea in a variety of injury situations can result in horrid complications including death.

The only way the patient with airway trauma can be properly managed is by a carefully organized approach. This must consider the risks and benefits of airway management in view of the potential injuries and

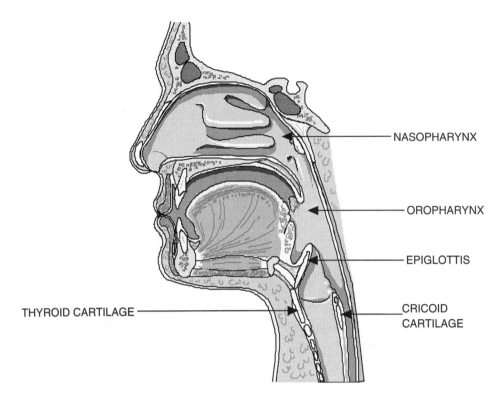

NASOPHARYNX

OROPHARYNX

EPIGLOTTIS

THYROID CARTILAGE

CRICOID CARTILAGE

Fig. 34-1. The nasopharynx and oropharynx. Upper-airway obstruction usually occurs at the posterior nasopharynx from facial fractures and bleeding. Obstruction of the oropharynx most commonly is caused by posterior deplacement of the tongue, either resulting from mandibular fractures or from altered mental status.

complicating factors unique to the trauma patient. As the standards of care for airway management in the trauma setting become more recognized, a cavalier "cookbook" approach or one that treats trauma patients in a fashion similar to elective surgical patients is likely to result in unacceptable outcomes and medicolegal consequences.[24,25]

II. ANATOMY OF THE AIRWAY AND RELATED STRUCTURES: TRAUMA CONSIDERATIONS

A. ANATOMY OF THE FACE AND OROPHARYNX

The oropharynx is protected anteriorly by the maxilla, mandible, and teeth; laterally by the mandible and mastoid processes; and posteriorly by the base of the skull and the cervical spine. The facial bones are arranged in a manner that allows the force from a blow to be distributed throughout the bony structure, reducing the likelihood of a fracture.[26] Nevertheless, a force of about 80 g (that delivered by a 30 mph motor vehicle accident) is sufficient to fracture any bones of the midface, zygoma, or mandible.[27] Much higher forces are required to fracture bones of the alveolar ridge, the superior orbital region, or the skull.

The soft tissues of the pharynx are supported by these bony structures, and the airway may be displaced and obstructed after a facial fracture. Midface fractures (especially Lefort III types) may cause obstruction of the nasopharynx, whereas mandibular fractures (especially parasymphyseal fractures) may allow the tongue and floor of the mouth to obstruct the oropharynx.

The rich blood supply of the face may be injured either by penetrating trauma or by bony fractures. Any branch of the external carotid may be injured by penetrating trauma, whereas fractures are most likely to tear those arteries that pass along the walls of the sinuses. The ethmoid, internal maxillary, and greater palatine arteries are most likely to be injured in this manner. Bleeding may cause eventual airway obstruction either by hematoma formation or by free bleeding into the pharynx with resultant aspiration and pulmonary obstruction.

B. ANATOMY OF THE AIRWAY PROPER

The airway itself is divided into the pharynx (Fig. 34-1) and the airway proper, which is composed of the larynx, trachea, and bronchi (Fig. 34-2). The entire airway is a fairly free and mobile structure, attached at its superior margin only to the hyoid bone. Intrathoracicly, it is attached only to the lungs, but the bronchi are anchored to some extent by their passage under the great vessels.[4,28] In the neck the trachea is covered by the

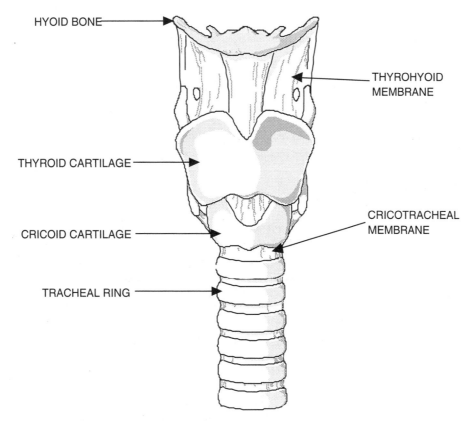

HYOID BONE

THYROHYOID MEMBRANE

THYROID CARTILAGE

CRICOTRACHEAL MEMBRANE

CRICOID CARTILAGE

TRACHEAL RING

Fig. 34-2. Anatomy of the airway. Injuries to the cricoid and thyroid cartilages are often palpable during physical examination. Tracheal and membranous injuries often present no signs on physical examination. Cricoid cartilage injuries are associated with the highest incidence of airway emergencies and failed intubation.

thyroid gland, the strap muscles, and the cervical fascia, which in turn are surrounded by the structures of the carotid sheath and the sternocleidomastoid muscles. Posteriorly, the membranous portion of the trachea is in close approximation to the esophagus.[28]

Internally, all the structures of the larynx are connected by a submucosal sheet of elastic tissue. This is especially thick in the anterior and posterolateral margins, where it is termed the conus elasticus, and firmly attaches the thyroid, cricoid and arytenoid cartilages to one another. The attachment of the larynx to the trachea, however, consists only of a thin elastic membrane called the cricotracheal ligament. The cricotracheal ligament is quite weak and is the most likely point of airway separation.[7] The individual tracheal cartilages are connected to each other by fibrous tissue and smooth muscle, and the entire trachea is encased internally and externally by layers of elastic connective tissue.[28]

The superior laryngeal nerve enters the larynx through the posterior portion of the thyrohyoid membrane, where it is relatively protected by soft tissue. The recurrent laryngeal nerve, however, passes directly

between the cricoid and thyroid cartilages and is frequently damaged when these structures are injured.[7,8]

III. INJURIES AFFECTING THE AIRWAY
A. MAXILLOFACIAL INJURY

Maxillofacial injury may be caused by either blunt or penetrating trauma. The common causes of blunt maxillofacial trauma are automobile accidents, direct blows from altercations, and sports injuries. The type of maxillofacial damage sustained by patients with blunt injury is an important indicator of the amount of force involved.

Low-force injuries, which include most sports and altercation injuries, usually affect the nasal bones, zygomatic arches, and the condylar regions of the mandible. These fractures are generally self-limited and rarely have an impact on airway management. Fractures of the nasal bones can obstruct the nasopharynx, however, and may be associated with sufficient bleeding into the pharynx to allow aspiration. Condylar mandibular injuries do not cause airway obstruction but may interfere with laryngoscopy by limiting mandibular opening.

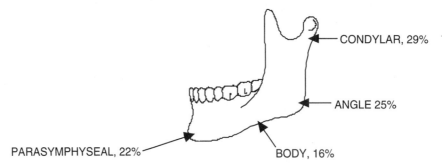

CONDYLAR, 29%

ANGLE 25%

PARASYMPHYSEAL, 22%

BODY, 16%

Fig. 34-3. The most common sites of mandibular fractures. Parasymphyseal and bilateral anterior mandible fractures are most commonly associated with upper-airway obstruction.

High-force injuries can involve the orbit, anterior mandible, or maxilla. These usually result from motor vehicle accidents or altercations with weapons, and patients with such injuries often have associated injuries involving other organ systems. The incidence of associated injuries is highest (81%) if the fracture involves the most impact-resistant bones, such as the supraorbital rim or mandibular symphysis.[29] The most commonly associated injuries include head injury (36% of cases) and cervical-spine injury (5% of cases).[20,30] Ocular injuries also occur in association with such fractures, although less frequently than head or spine injury.[31] Mortality rates of up to 12% occur in patients with high impact facial fractures.[29,32] In patients sustaining high impact maxillofacial trauma, the associated injuries (most commonly central nervous system injury) are usually the cause of death, rather than the maxillofacial injury itself.

1. Mandibular fractures

The mandible is the third most commonly fractured facial bone after the nasal bones and zygoma.[33] Fifty percent of mandibular fractures will involve more than one site. The condyles, angle, and symphysis of the mandible are the areas most commonly fractured[33] (Fig. 34-3).

Of mandibular fractures, parasymphyseal and bilateral anterior mandibular fractures are the types most likely to cause airway obstruction. In these fractures, the suprahyoid muscles tend to displace the fractured fragment downward and backward, allowing the tongue to obstruct the pharynx.[26] As a rule, such obstruction is easily relieved by manual displacement of the fractured mandibular fragment. Occasionally, hematoma formation in the floor of the mouth causes airway obstruction by displacing the tongue upward and backward against the palate.[34] This type of obstruction can only be relieved by insertion of an artificial airway.

For patients with mandibular fractures, the most reliable anatomic indicator of a difficult intubation is an insufficient oral opening to allow visualization of the posterior pharynx.[35,36] If injury to the temporomandibu-

lar joint occurs in association with a mandibular fracture, it is likely to limit mouth opening to this degree.[37] In such cases, a "jaw-thrust" maneuver may be used to "sublux" the TMJ and provide an adequate oral opening.[38,39]

2. Maxillary fractures

Midface (or LeFort) fractures are less common than mandibular fractures. The LeFort I fracture (Fig. 34-4) separates the entire palate and upper alveolar ridge from the remainder of the face but usually has minimal impact on airway management. The LeFort II fracture separates the maxilla and medial orbit from the zygomatic arches and skull. It also has little direct impact on the airway but is frequently associated with basilar skull fractures. For this reason, nasotracheal intubation and nasopharyngeal airways are relatively contraindicated in these patients until basilar skull fractures are clearly ruled out.

The LeFort III fracture extends through the lateral orbit, fractures the zygomatic arch, and continues through the pterygoid plate (Fig. 34-4). Thus, this fracture causes complete craniofacial separation. It is always important to be aware that facial appearance bears little relation to actual skeletal damage in patients with this type of fracture. Basilar skull fracture is commonly associated with LeFort III fractures, and cribriform plate fracture occurs in most cases. Because of this, nasal routes of airway management are relatively contraindicated until radiographic assessment has been completed.

LeFort III fractures may cause pharyngeal airway obstruction if the facial bones are displaced posteriorly and downward, closing the pharynx. Soft tissue airway obstruction may also occur because of loss of skeletal stability surrounding the pharynx. In this case, obstruction may only occur during the negative pressure generated by inspiration.[40]

Bleeding from midface fractures can occasionally be severe. In such cases manual repositioning of bony fragments and nasal packing with gauze or inflated Foley catheters may tamponade bleeding until definitive treat-

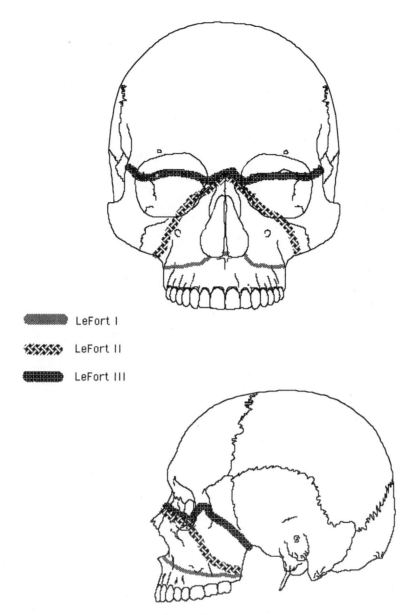

Fig. 34-4. LeFort fractures. Type I fractures rarely have impact on airway management, but type II fractures are associated with basilar skull fractures. Type III fractures may cause airway obstruction by posterior displacement of facial bones, obstructing the pharynx. LeFort type III fractures are commonly associated with cribriform plate injuries.

ment is possible. When death occurs from maxillofacial injury, however, hypoxia and central nervous system injury are the most common causes. In conscious patients, hypoxia is most often caused by blood and tissue aspiration. In unconscious patients, airway obstruction and aspiration may occur.[3]

Penetrating maxillofacial trauma often is associated with copious bleeding and occasionally with hematoma formation, causing airway obstruction. Stab wounds to the face rarely affect the airway. Conversely, one third of facial gunshot wound patients will require intubation or cricothyrotomy, either for maintenance of the airway in the presence of expanding hematoma or for prevention of blood aspiration.[2]

Tissue, bone, and teeth fragments may also be aspirated or cause airway obstruction after facial gunshot wounds. Chest radiographs should always be examined for foreign bodies, and diagnostic bronchoscopy may be indicated. It has been reported that gunshot wounds anterior to the plane of the first molar are much more likely to require intubation than those posterior to this plane.[2]

More than half the patients with facial gunshot wounds will have associated mandibular or maxillary fractures.[2] In cases where there is significant bone and soft tissue injury involving the oral cavity or pharynx, airway obstruction similar to that seen with LeFort III fractures may occur.[29,40]

When airway compromise does occur after penetrating facial trauma, it is often a sudden event, transforming a fairly routine airway management problem into an emergent situation. Because most patients with maxillofacial trauma will require some fairly time-consuming diagnostic studies, such as CT scan or angiography, elective intubation should be considered for facial gunshot wound victims who appear to be at any risk of airway compromise.

B. BLUNT AIRWAY TRAUMA

Blunt injuries to the upper airway are most commonly caused by direct blows, which usually injure the larynx or cricoid cartilage.[4] They are most commonly seen in front seat, lap belt–restrained occupants of motor vehicle accidents. On impact, the head and neck continue forward motion, and the neck makes contact with the sharp edge of the dashboard ("the padded dash syndrome").[41] Less commonly, blunt airway injury occurs in association with severe flexion/extension injuries of the neck (as may occur in fully restrained passengers in motor vehicle accidents). Flexion/extension injuries often result in laryngotracheal separation.[4]

Blows to the larynx most commonly fracture the thyroid cartilage. When such fractures occur vertically in the midline, the thyroarytenoid ligaments are often torn.[5] This causes separation of the false vocal cords from the true vocal cords, with associated displacement and edema of the arytenoid cartilages.[5] Fractures of the lateral portion of the thyroid cartilage may create false passages that are seen during laryngoscopy. Denuded cartilage fragments may also be visible, and fragments can obstruct attempts at intubation.[4] With severe trauma, comminuted fractures of the thyroid cartilage occur, causing separation of the epiglottis from the larynx and severe displacement of cartilage fragments and soft tissue. Visualization of the introitus and supraglottic structures is usually obstructed in such cases.

The cricoid cartilage is less frequently injured by blunt trauma than the thyroid cartilage. However, cricoid injury is much more likely to cause serious airway management problems.[8] Cricoid cartilage fractures are associated with damage to the recurrent laryngeal nerve in 25% of cases,[5] resulting in vocal cord paralysis and compromise of the airway lumen. In survivors, such injury often results in long-term vocal dysfunction. Unsuspected cricoid cartilage injury also predisposes to sudden airway obstruction, especially when cricoid pressure is applied during intubation[8,42] (Fig. 34-5).

Both direct blows and extension injuries may tear the cricotracheal ligaments, resulting in complete laryn-

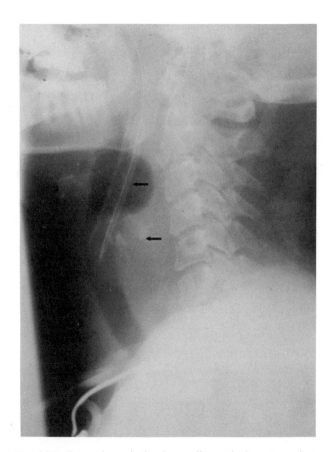

Fig. 34-5. Lateral cervical-spine radiograph demonstrating a cricoid fracture. Note that only the tip of the endotracheal tube has entered the larynx, and the endotracheal balloon is massively overinflated in the laryngeal introitus (*top arrow*). The cricoid cartilage is lightly calcified (*bottom arrow*), allowing the fracture to be seen. A large pretracheal hematoma pushes the entire larynx forward, obstructing vision during laryngoscopy.

gotracheal disruption and dislocation. This condition has been reported to occur in as many as 23% of all cases of blunt laryngeal trauma and as many as 50% of those with cricoid cartilage injury.[43] When patients survive this injury to reach tertiary care, the airway is usually held in close approximation by peritracheal connective tissue and the strap muscles.[4,8] The airway remains patent as long as spontaneous, negative pressure respiration is maintained[4,6,8] but attempts to pass an endotracheal tube will usually dislodge the severed ends, resulting in complete loss of airway patency.[14]

At least 10%[17] and as many as 50% of patients sustaining blunt airway trauma have concurrent cervical-spine injuries.[44,45] Esophageal injury also occurs frequently in these patients, especially those with concurrent cervical-spine injury.[45] Pneumothorax is common in patients with lower tracheal or bronchial injury.

The intrathoracic airway, consisting of the lower trachea, bronchi, and the gas-exchanging parenchyma (terminal bronchioles, alveolar ducts, and alveoli), is particularly prone to injury during blunt thoracic trauma. Severe chest impacts may injure the lower

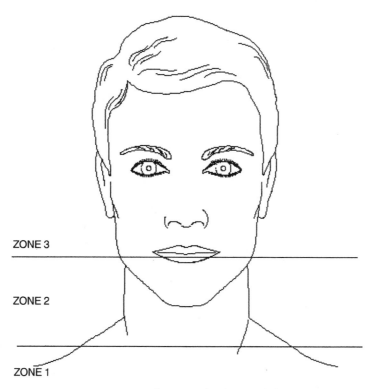

Fig. 34-6. Zones of penetrating injury of the neck.

trachea by compressing it between the manubrium and the vertebral column. In addition, crushing injuries to the chest when the glottis is closed can cause a dramatic increase in intraairway pressure, which may tear the membranous portions of the trachea or bronchi.[46-48] These tears are usually found within 2.5 cm of the carina[42,49] at the junction of the membranous and cartilaginous portions of the airway.[13]

Mortality rates for patients with blunt airway injury vary according to the location of the injury. Thyroid cartilage injuries have the lowest mortality rate[8] (11%). The mortality rate for tracheal injuries is about 25%, whereas that for injuries involving the cricoid cartilage is even higher (43%). Significant injuries to the bronchi or intrathoracic trachea have even higher mortality rates.[10,12,50] Associated injuries to major blood vessels and other organ systems of course correlate with poor prognosis, as does concurrent cervical-spine injury.

C. PENETRATING INJURY TO THE NECK

Penetrating neck injuries are usually described in terms of their location in one of the three anatomic zones of the neck[51] (Fig. 34-6). Knowledge of the common consequences for each zone of injury gives some idea of the most likely internal injuries, the probability of urgent airway management problems, and any expected surgical intervention.[52]

Zone I extends from the cephalad border of the clavicle to the cricoid cartilage. Zone I injuries are the least frequent (3% to 7%) of penetrating neck injuries.[53]

These wounds are often associated with great vessel or pulmonary injuries that can be life-threatening. For this reason, most of these patients require emergency airway management procedures.[54] Patients with zone I wounds who do not have major vascular injuries may be treated conservatively, but injury in this location is often lethal.

Zone II extends from the cricoid cartilage to the angle of the mandible and is the most common location for neck wounds[51] (82%). Airway compromise from laryngeal injury, hematoma formation, and subcutaneous emphysema is most likely to occur if the wound involves this area. One third of patients with zone II injuries require emergency airway management procedures.[51,52] Most of the remaining patients will usually undergo surgical exploration of their wounds, so endotracheal intubation will be performed in most patients with zone II injuries.

Zone III extends from the angle of the mandible to the base of the skull and is most commonly associated with vascular and pharyngeal injuries. Fifteen percent of neck wounds occur in this region.[51,52] Patients with injuries in this area are less likely to require urgent airway management procedures or surgical exploration.

Penetration of the airway proper from either missile or stab wounds may occur anywhere from the larynx to the bronchi. Airway management problems are unusual in patients who have sustained stab wounds, but are more frequent in gunshot wound victims.[8] When stab wounds do injure the airway, the trachea is the structure most likely to be involved, probably because of its lack of bony protection. Airway injuries from gunshot wounds are not location specific.

Airway injury is suggested by dyspnea, cyanosis, subcutaneous emphysema, hoarseness, and bubbling or frothy blood at the wound site. Even extensive airway injury, however, may not be appreciated by external appearance. Soft tissue radiographs of the neck can aid in the evaluation of the airway by demonstrating subcutaneous air and airway deviation caused by hematomas.

Patients with penetrating trauma are also likely to have vascular, esophageal, and thoracic injuries.[12] Esophageal injury occurs in 25% of patients with penetrating cervical trauma[55] and is the diagnosis most likely to be missed until late in the patient's hospital course.[5,43] The mortality rate for patients with penetrating cervical trauma correlates more closely with the presence of vascular or airway injuries.

In all cases of penetrating neck trauma, the immediate airway status, possible delayed airway compromise, lengthy radiographic and arteriographic evaluation, and likelihood of surgical intervention should be considered when planning airway management. It should always be remembered that 40% of patients with penetrating neck trauma will eventually require intubation.[53]

D. THERMAL AND INHALATION INJURY

1. Thermal injury

Thermal injuries can affect airway management in three ways: by causing facial and perioral swelling resulting in pharyngeal obstruction, by thermal injury to the upper airway resulting in laryngeal airway obstruction, or by chemical injury to lung tissue resulting in impaired gas exchange. Burn patients with any type of airway involvement have a mortality rate from 20% to 60% higher than those without airway involvement.[56]

Oropharyngeal airway obstruction can be predicted whenever full-thickness facial and anterior cervical burns are present. Maximal facial tissue swelling does not occur for 12 hours or more after injury, but significant swelling may be present within 2 hours.[57] Intubation usually becomes necessary between 4 and 8 hours after the injury.[58] In such cases, early orotracheal intubation should be performed electively to avoid the risk of later airway obstruction.

Carbonaceous material in the mouth, nares, or pharynx in a patient with facial burns indicates a high probability of thermal injury to the upper airway. Awake laryngoscopy is indicated to assess the degree of upper airway burns in such cases. If evidence of thermal injury to the upper airway is present, endotracheal intubation should be undertaken, even if ventilation appears adequate at the time of examination.

If any of the signs of impending obstruction, such as stridor, are present, endotracheal intubation should be attempted immediately. Edema usually compromises air flow in anatomically narrow areas, such as the cricoid ring, or areas with loose connective tissue, such as the epiglottis. Edema of these structures may limit air exchange severely, and total airway obstruction develops quite rapidly over the course of minutes. Even early on, cricotracheal swelling is usually present, and a smaller than expected endotracheal tube should be used in such cases.

Burns involving the lower airway and lung tissue are unusual because of the heat-absorptive properties of the upper airway. Even air hot as 270° C is cooled to 50° C by the time it enters the midtrachea. However, smoke or steam inhalation, chemical burns (e.g., phosgene gas), and proximity to fire in a closed space (resulting in inhalation of burning gases) can cause pulmonary burn injury.

The possibility of thermal or chemical injury to the trachea and bronchi is best evaluated by direct visualization using fiberoptic bronchoscopy. The severity of small airway and pulmonary injury should also be assessed by pulmonary function tests and serial arterial blood gas analyses. Pulmonary function tests usually show decreased compliance, peak flow, and FEV_1,[59] which worsens for about 12 hours after the injury.[60]

Alternatively, a xenon scan may be obtained. Because xenon scanning involves only the intravenous injection of radioactive material and subsequent nuclear scans, it is most appropriate for patients who are unconscious or poorly compliant. Xenon scans demonstrate early airway closure and small airway constriction if lower-airway injury is present.[57]

Whatever the diagnostic methods used, the tests should be repeated serially because maximal airway edema may not occur for 18 to 24 hours.[61] Chest radiography is universally normal for the first several hours after thermal injury. It must also be remembered that the severity of pulmonary injury will be magnified in direct proportion to the amount of thermal injury to the body, probably because of overall fluid requirements and the release of systemic vasoactive mediators.[61]

2. Smoke inhalation

Smoke inhalation is much more common than actual thermal injury to the lower airway. Occurring in 15% to 35% of all burn victims,[62] smoke inhalation accounts for 50% of all fire-related deaths.[63] Smoke inhalation injury is usually less apparent on physical examination than thermal injury to the airway, although altered consciousness and the signs of hypoxia may be present. The primary symptom of smoke inhalation is bronchospasm and expiratory wheeze, although all the same symptoms caused by lower-airway burns may be present.

Pulmonary function tests, blood gas analysis, or xenon pulmonary scans should be performed as they would for lower-airway thermal injury. Pulmonary studies will show that airway resistance is markedly increased as is pulmonary dead space. Serum lactate levels are usually elevated, especially if carbon monoxide or cyanide toxicity are present. Pulmonary vasospasm is also present to some degree, and may worsen V/Q mismatching. True pulmonary alveolar edema is rare, but interstitial edema and atelectasis do occur.[64,65]

Smoke is made up of many different compounds, including hot carbonaceous particles and toxic gases. Carbon monoxide is present in all forms of smoke, so all smoke inhalation victims are considered to have some degree of carbon monoxide poisoning, with resultant impaired oxygen delivery to the tissues. Monitoring of Sao_2 by pulse oximetry or an oximetric pulmonary artery catheter is inaccurate in such cases because the infrared absorption spectrum measured by these devices does not differentiate between oxyhemoglobin and carboxyhemoglobin.[66] Serum carboxyhemoglobin levels should be obtained on a "stat" basis to accurately determine the amount of carbon monoxide present. Levels greater than 40% usually cause severe symptoms, whereas levels of 60% are generally fatal.

Carbon monoxide toxicity is often compounded by hydrogen cyanide (which is released by burning polyurethane and other synthetics materials) poisoning. The frequency and severity of cyanide toxicity for victims of smoke inhalation has been underestimated in the past. Cyanide toxicity should be suspected in any patient who has persistent metabolic acidosis or an elevated blood lactate level after adequate fluid resuscitation and ventilation have been achieved.[62,66] Cyanide has a half-life of less than 1 hour, and blood cyanide levels are not obtainable on a "stat" basis, so accurate documentation of cyanide poisoning is not always possible. However, studies have shown that cyanide levels generally are proportional to carbon monoxide levels for patients exposed to interior fires.[67]

Many other potentially toxic substances are released in smoke. Burning plastics or rubber can release ammonia, sulfur dioxide, and chlorine; all of which are extremely toxic to airway mucosa and lung tissue. Burning polyvinyl chloride releases chlorine and phosgene. Cotton and paper release formaldehyde, formic acid, and acetaldehyde. All of these can cause chemical burns to the airway, which is usually observable on laryngoscopy. The more insoluble gases, such as the aldehydes and phosgene, tend to reach the lower pulmonary tree and alveoli, causing pulmonary edema.[68]

It must always be remembered that burn patients are likely to have fallen or been in proximity to an explosion.[69] One must always have a high index of suspicion for various types of trauma, especially cervical-spine or intracerebral injury, which may co-exist with thermal injury.

Table 34-1. Common fracture sites for blunt cervical-spine injuries

Location	All fractures (%)	All dislocations (%)
C0	1	1
C2	7	32
C3	20	9
C4	5	9
C5	9	13
C6	21	12
C7	22	24

Data from Woodring JH, Lee C: *J Trauma* 34:32, 1993.

E. CERVICAL-SPINE INJURY

1. Mechanisms of injury

Cervical-spine injury may be caused by either blunt or penetrating trauma. Because the bones of the spine offer good protection from stab wounds, most significant penetrating spine injuries are caused by gunshot wounds. As with most other penetrating injuries, entrance wounds and plain cervical-spine radiographs will usually provide evidence of cervical-spine injury. When blunt injury to the cervical spine does occur, however, often the only clinical indication is the development of an irreversible neurologic deficit.

For a cervical-spine fracture to be unstable, all the supporting elements in either the anterior portion (vertebral bodies, intervertebral disk, anterior and posterior longitudinal ligaments) must be disrupted.[70,71] Such injuries are usually caused by blunt, rather than penetrating, trauma[72] and occur in 2% to 8% of blunt trauma victims.[20,73] The incidence is generally higher in patients involved in motor vehicle accidents[20] (4.5%), those with significant head injury[74] (5% to 15%), and those who have suffered "high-velocity"-type facial fractures[75] (4% to 5%). The most common sites of fracture and subluxation of the cervical spine are shown in Table 34-1.

The diagnosis of cervical-spine injury will be "missed" or delayed in up to 25% of patients, especially those who have an altered level of consciousness.[76] Five to ten percent of patients with cervical-spine injury have no neurologic deficits on arrival at the hospital but permanent deficits develop while the patients are undergoing evaluation and treatment.[19] As many as 10% of patients with cervical-spine injury will be orotracheally intubated before the injury is discovered.[20]

Ninety percent of these "missed" cervical-spine injuries could have been adequately diagnosed if three-view cervical radiographs had been obtained and correctly interpreted.[19] Although cross-table lateral cervical-spine films are usually obtained within minutes of admission, 30% of cervical fractures and subluxations will not be apparent on this single view.[77] Three-view cervical-spine (anteroposterior, lateral, and transoral odontoid) films will demonstrate 99% of cervical-spine fractures.[78] Because early interpretation of cervical radiographs is often inaccurate,[19,77] however, proper precautions to stabilize the cervical spine should be used routinely.

2. Protection of the cervical spine

Although the potential for an unstable cervical-spine fracture is significant in any patient with blunt trauma,[79] adequate oxygenation remains the highest priority. Necessary airway management procedures should be undertaken whenever indicated, but techniques that minimize motion of the cervical spine are required as part of the standard of care for airway management of every injured patient.[39,80,81]

Most trauma patients are now routinely transported from the field with some combination of cervical collar, spine board, and sandbags to stabilize the cervical spine. (The best immobilization is obtained with a combination of sandbags taped on each side of the patient's head, a Philadelphia collar, and a spine board; or with the use of Styrofoam or vacuum-mattress type immobilizers.[82] When intubation is attempted, objects obstructing access to the mouth and neck (such as the anterior portion of the cervical collar) should be removed to facilitate laryngoscopy and the application of cricoid pressure. Removing such devices also provides access to the anterior neck if establishment of a surgical airway becomes necessary.[8,80]

Obviously, movement of the neck in a patient with an unstable cervical-spine fracture may result in permanent neurologic damage either through physical compression of the spinal cord or by interfering with the compromised spinal blood supply. Therefore an assistant must maintain the head in a neutral position for the entire period in which cervical-spine stabilizing devices are removed.

Cervical-spine stabilization during any airway assessment or management procedure is best maintained using manual in-line axial traction (MIAT).[83] Proper MIAT stabilization involves a dynamic interplay between traction and immobilization, so force is applied in equal amounts and opposite directions against the force generated by the intubator.[81] It is equally important that the force be applied in the correct plane relative to the particular injury. Generally, when posterior elements are fractured, flexion of the neck must be prevented. When fractures involve anterior elements, extension should be avoided. Traction should be constantly adjusted to counterbalance the force generated by the laryngoscopist as closely as possible, but it is impossible to know exactly how much traction to apply unless real-time fluoroscopy is available.[84]

Orotracheal intubation, nasotracheal intubation, and tracheotomy can all be successfully performed without spinal cord damage, as long as the neck is immobilized adequately.[44,79,84,85] At one time, nasal intubation was considered to be the safest method for securing the airway in a trauma patient with cervical-spine injury. However, blind nasal intubation can be difficult to perform without moving the neck, even if guidewire-type tubes are used.[79,86-88] Combative patients often thrash about during attempted nasotracheal intubation, causing further insult to a cervical-spine injury.[81]

Oral intubation using the MIAT technique provides superior stability of the cervical-spine during intubation[80,85,89] and is the most appropriate technique for patients requiring urgent airway intervention. Fiberoptic bronchoscopy is the ideal method for more elective intubation of the patient requiring cervical-spine immobilization.[90,91] Unfortunately, the bronchoscope has limited use in those patients requiring immediate intubation and those with significant intraoral or pharyngeal bleeding.

IV. ASSOCIATED FACTORS AFFECTING AIRWAY MANAGEMENT IN INJURED PATIENTS

A. THE RISK OF ASPIRATION

Modern anesthetic techniques have markedly reduced the frequency of pulmonary aspiration of gastric contents during induction and intubation in recent years.[92,93] The incidence of aspiration is now less than five cases of aspiration per 10,000 elective anesthetic inductions.[94] In such controlled situations, the risk and severity of gastric aspiration increases with factors such as increased intragastric volume ($> .4$ ml/kg body weight), increased gastric acidity (pH < 2.5), and the presence of particulate matter in the stomach.[95,95]

Traumatized patients have a markedly increased incidence of aspiration for several reasons.[97] The injured patient has often ingested food or liquids immediately before the traumatic event. Alteration of the level of consciousness by shock, head injury, alcohol, or drug ingestion all interfere with airway reflexes and markedly increase the patient's risk of aspiration.[98] Likewise, injury to cranial nerves IX or X attenuates gag reflexes, placing the patient at increased risk. Patients who have a delay between injury and airway management are likely to have gastric dilation, further increasing the risk of aspiration.[99] Gastric volume may be further increased iatrogenically, such as by using a barium swallow for contrast radiography of the abdomen.

Injury, anxiety, and pain all delay or arrest gastric emptying.[100,101] For this reason, the time interval between the last intake and time of injury is a more important predictor of gastric volume than the interval between intake and intubation.[97,102] Delaying surgery for even 24 hours does not decrease the risk of aspiration during the induction of anesthesia for the injured patient.[103]

Inhaled gastric contents can immediately "drown" the patient if the volume is great enough or may induce

Table 34-2. Aspiration prevention in trauma

Method	Advantage	Disadvantage
Endotracheal intubation	Highly effective	Risks of intubation May induce vomiting
Gastric tube placement	Effective	Some contraindications May induce vomiting
Sodium citrate	Rapid increase of pH	None
Metoclopramide	Decrease gastric volume	Hypotension?
H$_2$ blocking agents	Increase pH Effective several hours	Slow onset

aspiration pneumonitis.[104] Additionally, particulate food matter may obstruct bronchi, resulting in hypoxia, atelectasis, and pneumonia. The mortality rate for injured patients who aspirate gastric contents is between 5% and 25%.[97,105]

Blood aspiration is common in patients with facial or airway injuries. A significant volume of inhaled blood can cause severe airway obstruction and resultant hypoxia, but does not cause long-term pulmonary injury. In fact, blood may act as a buffer for acidic gastric contents, increasing the pH to a less harmful level. All the effects of blood aspiration usually resolve within 6 to 12 hours.[106] (See also Chapter 10.)

1. Adjunctive techniques to decrease the risk of aspiration

The best protection against aspiration in high-risk patients is placement of a properly sized cuffed endotracheal tube in adults or a properly sized uncuffed tube in children. The presence of an endotracheal tube does not totally prevent the risk of aspiration, and laryngoscopy and intubation itself may initiate regurgitation. Therefore, adjunctive techniques to minimize the risk and severity of aspiration should be used in every trauma patient (Table 34-2).

a. GASTRIC TUBES

The most effective measure to prevent aspiration before intubation is active evacuation of the stomach with an orogastric or nasogastric tube. This will not completely empty the stomach, especially of particulate matter, but certainly reduces the volume of intragastric contents and the intragastric pressure.[107] Gastric tubes alone can not prevent aspiration, so other aspiration prevention techniques should be used concurrently.

Early reports claimed that the presence of a gastric tube might render cricoid pressure ineffective or serve as a "wick" for gastric contents to ascend into the pharynx,[108] but more recent evidence does not support

this view.[108,109] There is no reason, therefore, to remove gastric tubes before endotracheal intubation.

There are some contraindications and potential adverse sequelae to gastric tube placement. Nasogastric tubes may traverse a fractured cribriform plate during placement, and any gastric tube may inadvertently enter the trachea. In conscious patients, gastric tube placement can cause coughing or retching, and thus is relatively contraindicated in patients with intracranial, intraocular, or laryngotracheal injury. Gastric tube placement is also relatively contraindicated in patients with suspected esophageal or gastric perforation.

An endotracheal tube inadvertently placed in the esophagus provides an extrapharyngeal exit for vomitus.[110] If this situation occurs, the esophageal tube should be left in place until successful tracheal intubation is accomplished.

b. PHARMACOLOGIC MEASURES

Metoclopramide stimulates gastric emptying, increases gastroesophageal sphincter tone, and attenuates activity in the vomiting center of the brain stem.[103] It can effectively reduce gastric volume within 20 minutes after intravenous administration. However, metoclopramide does not reduce gastric acidity, may accentuate hypotension,[111] and may not be effective if narcotics are administered concurrently.[112]

H$_2$ blocking agents such as cimetidine, ranitidine, and famotidine all inhibit the secretion of gastric acid and over time will raise the mean pH of intragastric contents. At least 1 hour is required to consistently raise gastric pH, and these drugs have no influence on gastric volume. Although not effective in emergency situations, these agents are still useful in minimizing the postoperative aspiration risk. Cimetidine is probably the least appropriate agent for use in trauma patients because of its potential to cause vasodilation, cardiac dysrhythmia, and interference with hepatic metabolism.

Nonparticulate antacids, such as sodium citrate, usually raise intragastric pH within 15 minutes of administration.[113] Therefore they are a more appropriate means of raising intragastric pH than the H$_2$ blocking agents. These agents should be administered to all injured patients either orally or by gastric tube before any airway intervention.

Anticholinergic agents (e.g., atropine, glycopyrrolate) have also been suggested as a way to reduce gastric acidity and volume but are not effective in clinically appropriate doses. They also have the adverse effect of reducing lower esophageal sphincter tone.[114]

c. PATIENT POSITION

Patient position may provide some protection of the airway.[97] The right lateral/head-down position will permit vomitus to run out of the mouth, but this position is unacceptable for most trauma patients. A 40-degree, foot-down tilt helps prevent passive regurgitation but does not prevent active vomiting. Of course, this position

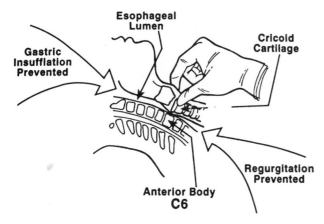

Fig. 34-7. Cricoid pressure. (From Cicala RS, Grande CM, Steve JK et al: Emergency and elective airway management for trauma patients. In Grande CM, editor: *Trauma anesthesia and critical care,* St Louis, 1993, Mosby.

is inappropriate for hypovolemic patients. If regurgitation does occur, a head-down tilt may help prevent the passive aspiration of vomitus into the trachea.

d. CRICOID PRESSURE (SELLECK'S MANEUVER)

Cricoid pressure should be applied to every injured patient during any airway management procedure. This significantly reduces the possibility of aspiration both by preventing the regurgitation of gastric contents and by preventing inflation of the stomach during bag-mask ventilation.[115-117] Because regurgitation may occur at any time, this maneuver is just as important during the initial resuscitation as it is for intubation before surgery.

Cricoid pressure should be applied by using the thumb and forefinger together to push downward on the cricoid cartilage. Properly applied, this pressure impinges the cricoid cartilage on the anterior body of C6, effectively closing the esophagus (Fig. 34-7). Analysis reveals that 44 newtons of force must be applied to the cricoid cartilage to effectively seal the esophagus.[118] (This force can be demonstrated by performing the maneuver on oneself, applying sufficient force to prevent swallowing liquids.) Greater pressure may make bag-mask ventilation difficult.[119]

It must be emphasized that Selleck's maneuver is only effective if pressure is applied directly to the cricoid cartilage because this is the only cartilaginous structure in the upper airway that is a complete ring (all other airway cartilages are U-shaped). Tracheal or thyroid cartilage pressure is too often applied by inexperienced personnel and is totally ineffective for preventing pulmonary aspiration.

Application of cricoid pressure does have risks in a few types of injury. Theoretically, overly vigorous cricoid pressure could adversely affect an unstable cervical-spine fracture at the C5 to C7 level, but no known cases of such an event have been reported.[120] Suspected laryngotracheal injury, especially at the cricotracheal area, is an absolute contraindication to Selleck's maneuver because complete airway separation could result. Several cases of cricotracheal separation with total loss of airway patency and death have been reported in such circumstances.[8,9] The risk of aspiration is less significant than the potential loss of airway patency in this situation.

2. Immediate treatment of aspiration

When aspiration occurs, the expected clinical signs (bronchospasm, hypoxemia, and pulmonary infiltrates seen on the radiograph) may not all be immediately present, or they may be masked by other injuries such as smoke inhalation or pulmonary contusion. The definitive diagnosis is made if gastric contents are seen during visual inspection of the trachea.

When aspiration is suspected, the trachea should be immediately be suctioned, intubated (if this has not been done), and flexible bronchoscopy performed to remove any particles causing airway obstruction. Mechanical ventilation with positive end-expiratory pressure (PEEP), or intermittent mandatory ventilation (IMV) with continuous positive-pressure breathing (CPPB) should be initiated to improve oxygenation.

Initial treatment is limited to such early, mechanical interventions. Steroids have no beneficial effect in aspiration pneumonitis or in preventing adult respiratory distress syndrome (ARDS) after aspiration.[121] Tracheobronchial lavage is also of no benefit and may worsen the condition by disseminating aspirated material.[105] Prophylactic broad-spectrum antibiotic therapy is appropriate, however.[122]

B. INTRACRANIAL AND INTRAOCULAR INJURY

Primary (caused by direct trauma) and secondary (caused by associated hypoxia or hypotension) brain injury remains the most common cause of death and long-term disability among trauma victims.[123] Patients with intracranial injury generally require rapid, definitive control of the airway to protect from aspiration, correct hypoxia, and allow hyperventilation to reduce intracranial swelling.

The presence of intracranial injury, however, will require some modifications of airway management techniques to prevent worsening of the cerebral insult. If at all possible, bag-mask hyperventilation should be performed before laryngoscopy to reduce $ETco_2$ and increase Sao_2.[124]

Coughing or "bucking" during endotracheal intubation, marked increases in blood pressure, and succinylcholine-induced fasciculations may all result in dramatic increases in intracranial pressure, causing further neurologic insult.[125,126] Therefore awake, un-paralyzed intubation is relatively contraindicated in conscious patients with significant intracranial injury.

In hemodynamically stable patients, doses of analgesic or anesthetic induction agents may be administered before laryngoscopy to prevent such responses.[127] Alternatively, intravenous lidocaine may be effective and has less potential to cause hypotension or further alteration of consciousness.[128] Some authors[129,130] suggest rapid sequence induction and intubation using nondepolarizing muscle relaxants in patients with intracranial injury. Others believe that succinylcholine may be used if preceded by a defasciculating dose of a nondepolarizing relaxant.[126]

In patients who are unstable, however, rapid awake intubation may be necessary. In such cases, appropriate drugs should be readily available to treat hypertensive or other responses should they occur.

Similar care will be required in patients with open-eye injuries. In most patients with open-eye injury, rapid airway control is not necessary, and a planned rapid sequence induction of anesthesia can be performed before intubation.

C. THORACIC TRAUMA

The thoracic area is the third most likely location for traumatic injury after the head and extremities.[131] Only about 1% of penetrating thoracic injuries are mortal,[132] and these usually involve the heart or great vessels. Most thoracic injuries involve blunt trauma from motor vehicle accidents. Although these are usually self-limited, about 5% are associated with major intrathoracic injuries. Major blunt thoracic trauma has a higher mortality rate than does penetrating thoracic injury.[133]

Patients with blunt thoracic trauma are more likely to require airway management procedures than are other trauma patients. Rib fractures and chest wall contusions impair the function of the respiratory muscles, and flail segments markedly impair ventilation. Patients with chest wall injury often seem stable initially, but may suddenly tire and decompensate, requiring immediate intubation and ventilatory support.

Pulmonary contusion may be associated with chest wall injury. Patients with pulmonary contusion may appear stable at first, and contused lung tissue often appears normal on initial chest radiographs, leading to a false sense of security.[134,135] Delayed respiratory failure frequently occurs during the next 6 to 12 hours, however, as alveoli in contused lung tissue fill with blood and exudate. This lung tissue will not reexpand with either positive-pressure ventilation or bronchoscopy. However, alveoli in edematous lung tissue adjacent to the contused segment may be reexpanded by PEEP, and bronchoscopy may remove blood from bronchi aerating noncontused segments.[134]

Trauma to the lower airway and lung may result in hemopneumothorax or interstitial emphysema with pneumomediastinum and subcutaneous emphysema.[11,48] If pulmonary veins are also lacerated, air may enter into the low-pressure pulmonary venous drainage system, resulting in left atrial air bubbles,[12] which can become systemic air emboli.

Such systemic air embolism may actually occur as frequently as 5% of all major thoracic injuries,[136] occasionally with severe consequences such as coronary or cerebral infarction. A high degree of clinical suspicion is necessary to make the diagnosis of systemic air embolism. The most commonly associated signs include hemoptysis and hypotension but are very nonspecific. More specific signs, such as air visualized in the retinal veins during funduscopic examination or froth obtained during aspiration of arterial blood for blood gas analysis, are rare. Treatment of a systemic air embolism involves emergency thoracotomy and, if possible, hyperbaric oxygen therapy, but prognosis is extremely poor.

Bronchial tear is another infrequent thoracic injury. It must be considered whenever a pneumothorax does not reexpand after thoracostomy tube placement, or if a very large air leak is present. Flexible bronchoscopy is diagnostic in such cases. Routine endotracheal tube placement is contraindicated because positive-pressure ventilation may have catastrophic consequences. Rather, an endobronchial tube should be placed into the unaffected side using direct visualization.

Intrapulmonary bleeding is occasionally significant, resulting in the patient literally drowning in his own blood. Isolation of the bleeding lung through endobronchial intubation can serve to protect the uninjured lung from further blood aspiration and may also help to tamponade the bleeding area.

Endotracheal intubation and mechanical ventilation sometimes cause complications in patients with thoracic injury. Most common is conversion of a simple pneumothorax to a tension pneumothorax as positive-pressure ventilation virtually pumps air into the pleural space. Less common complications include loss of ventilation through a large bronchopleural fistula, systemic air embolism, soft tissue emphysema, and obstruction of the endotracheal tube by blood clots.[137-139]

V. AIRWAY ASSESSMENT OF THE INJURED PATIENT

Airway management in the emergency setting carries significant risk of morbidity and mortality, which can be minimized by a complete, thorough assessment. However, delay in definitive management of the airway can result in increased morbidity and mortality. Therefore a rapid but organized approach to airway assessment and management is mandatory.

The airway evaluation should be carried out in the same manner that the remainder of the trauma assessment is done. A series of increasingly detailed evaluations should be made to determine whether intervention is required, the degree of urgency present, and whether associated injuries and risk factors might be present. The entire process should be viewed as an effort to provide the best risk/benefit ratio possible for the patient.

There are several precepts that apply to the assessment and management of the airway in injured patients.[80] (1) Proper airway management requires at least one assistant to stabilize the head and neck and another to apply cricoid pressure and perform other tasks as needed. (2) The anterior portion of cervical collars must be removed while an assistant maintains manual in-line cervical traction. This allows assessment of the neck and the application of cricoid pressure, facilitates laryngoscopy, and provides access for the establishment of a surgical airway if necessary. (3) Provisions for an emergency cricothyrotomy or tracheotomy must always be immediately available.

The urgency of airway management is divided into two broad categories: patients who will require definitive airway control as part of the trauma resuscitation and those who will require semielective airway control. The first category is further subdivided into immediate, emergent, and urgent intervention.

A. PATIENTS REQUIRING IMMEDIATE INTERVENTION

A quick glance will reveal those patients who are apneic and require *immediate* control of the airway. For these patients, definitive airway control, most commonly endotracheal intubation, should be obtained as soon as possible. Simple, mechanical methods of opening the airway and providing ventilation should not be overlooked in the rush to intubate, however. The mouth should be cleared of foreign material and suctioned, the airway held open manually, and the patient rapidly ventilated with a bag and mask if possible as preparations are made for endotracheal intubation.[140]

In such cases, all but the most routine precautions (cricoid pressure and MIAT) are secondary to the need to ventilate the patient. The possibility of cervical-spine or actual airway injuries should be considered, but do not preclude lifesaving attempts at endotracheal intubation. Likewise, more elegant, but time-consuming, techniques such as fiberoptic intubation are not appropriate. In practice, it is not unusual for the anesthesiologist to attempt orotracheal intubation concurrently with a surgeon's efforts to perform cricothyrotomy.

B. PATIENTS REQUIRING EMERGENCY INTERVENTION

Patients who are not apneic but who have apparent respiratory distress require *emergency* intervention to establish a patent airway and effective ventilation.

Patients who are unconscious and unresponsive also require emergency airway management even if ventilation appears adequate. Manual opening of the airway and bag-mask–assisted ventilation should be performed and may provide sufficient improvement to allow a more elective method of airway management. If no improvement occurs, patients should be treated as would those requiring immediate airway management.

C. PATIENTS REQUIRING URGENT INTERVENTION

Other patients, such as those with thermal or facial injuries, expanding cervical hematomas, or chest wall injuries who are for the moment well compensated, will obviously require tracheal intubation and mechanical ventilation. Such cases should be considered *urgent* airway management problems.

Supplemental oxygen should be administered immediately, but a few minutes delay before definitive airway management procedures may be invaluable if used productively. A rapid neurologic assessment, key medical history, and cervical-spine radiographs can be obtained while preparations are made for controlled endotracheal intubation. In such cases alternative intubation techniques (such as fiberoptic intubation) or selected pharmacologic agents may minimize the potential risks of intubation. Pulse oximetry and clinical status should be carefully monitored during this time to ensure that no deterioration in the patient's status has occurred.

D. ASSESSMENT OF OTHER PATIENTS

Although about 7% of trauma patients require intubation during the initial assessment and stabilization phase of care, more than 25% will require endotracheal intubation and mechanical ventilation during their hospitalization, and 11% will develop frank pulmonary insufficiency.[141] It is unfortunate that such patients often are ignored until obvious ventilatory insufficiency develops because it has been shown that early intervention can minimize later pulmonary complications.[80]

Those trauma patients whose injuries, age, or condition places them at high risk of pulmonary problems (see below) should undergo further evaluation. When carefully assessed, many such "high-risk" trauma patients are found to have marginal oxyhemoglobin saturation, if not frank desaturation. Early intubation and mechanical ventilation should be considered on an elective basis for these patients because they will rarely improve (and often worsen) during the first 24 hours after injury.

1. Patients at increased risk of ventilatory problems

Patients who are confused or obtunded on admission are considered to have cerebral injuries until proven otherwise. Head injury is the leading cause of respiratory compromise and death in trauma patients, so any patient with significant head injury is regarded as a respiratory emergency.[142,143] Early establishment of a secure airway is of vital importance in these patients to limit hypoxic insult, minimize cerebral swelling, and minimize the potential for aspiration.[92,93,104] In addition to hypoxia and hypercarbia from hypoventilation,[124] it should also be appreciated that head injury affects ventilation/perfusion (V/Q) matching, leading to impaired gas exchange.[145] Altered mental status, whatever the cause, is an indication for endotracheal intubation and mechanical ventilation in the injured patient.

Patients with burn injuries, a prolonged prehospital or transportation time, those requiring high volumes of fluid resuscitation, and those with preexisting cardiac or pulmonary disease are also likely to require mechanical ventilation. Hypovolemic shock itself does not cause pulmonary damage but does increase pulmonary capillary permeability,[122,144] which along with large-volume fluid replacement may result in pulmonary edema.[145] Patients with thoracic or maxillofacial injury should also be monitored carefully because they may undergo sudden respiratory decompensation. Finally, patients with preexisting pulmonary disease (including asthma) and those older than 50 are much more likely to require intubation and ventilation.[146] No patient in these high-risk categories should be transported from the resuscitation area until a complete assessment of ventilation and oxygenation has been made.

2. Further diagnostic measures

a. BLOOD GAS ANALYSIS

Too often, an adequate Sao_2 demonstrated by pulse oximetry is considered evidence of adequate pulmonary status and oxygen delivery. Pulse oximetry demonstrates only that the Sao_2 of the arterial blood is within normal range. The combination of borderline Sao_2 and a low hemoglobin level often results in an inadequate oxygen content of the blood, leading to tissue ischemia. If supplemental oxygen is administered, the Sao_2 can be normal even in the presence of marked pulmonary dysfunction. Arterial blood gas analysis provides much more information and should be measured in every significantly injured patient.

Pulmonary shunt and venous admixture is common after trauma and, when significant, is an indication for intubation and mechanical ventilation.[147] Shunt fraction can be estimated by comparing the measured arterial oxygen tension (Pao_2) with that expected for the patient's age and Fio_2 using one of several indices (Table 34-3). The Pao_2/Fio_2 ratio is simple to calculate, and a value of less than 200 indicates an elevated pulmonary shunt. The ratio of arterial to alveolar Po_2 (Pao_2/PAo_2) is a more sensitive indicator of pulmonary dysfunction.

Table 34-3. Calculation of pulmonary status

Test	"Normal" value	Formula	Comments
Pao_2/Fio_2	400-500	Pao_2/Fio_2	Good bedside test Not very sensitive
Arterial/ alveolar ratio	>0.75	Pao_2/PAo_2	More sensitive Normalizes Pao_2 to Fio_2
		$PAo_2 = (P_B - P_{H_2O} - (Paco_2/.8))$	
Alveolar/ arterial	<25 (room air)	$(roomPAo_2 - Pao_2)$	Quantifies V/Q mismatch and pulmonary dysfunction

A Pao_2/PAo_2 value less than .75 suggests significant venous admixture. Pao_2/PAo_2 ratios also can be used to predict the Fio_2 required to maintain a desired Pao_2, which is not possible using the Pao_2/Fio_2 ratio.[148] The requirement to calculate the PAo_2 is the major drawback to the use of this ratio, but bedside computers can greatly simplify this process.

Arterial pH provides further information regarding both ventilatory and circulatory status. An arterial pH of less than 7.2, from either respiratory or metabolic causes, is associated with an increased mortality in trauma patients.[149] Any patient with significant acidosis should undergo endotracheal intubation and mechanical ventilation.

If there is doubt about the adequacy of tissue oxygen delivery, a pulmonary artery catheter should be placed and mixed venous oxygen saturation determined. Adequate mixed venous oxygenation (Svo_2 >60%) is probably the best indicator of adequate ventilation and gas exchange in the injured patient. An Svo_2 of 20% or less is associated with a uniformly poor outcome, whereas an Svo_2 of 70% or more generally demonstrates adequate tissue oxygenation.[146] Svo_2 should also be measured in trauma victims who are elderly, have questionable cardiac function, or questionable oxygen delivery to the tissues for other reasons. Blood gases drawn from a superior vena caval line may be used as an alternative to mixed venous saturation because good correlation exists between the two values.[150]

b. RADIOGRAPHY/BRONCHOSCOPY

Chest radiographs and cervical-spine x-ray films should be obtained in all injured patients. Often, unsuspected intrathoracic injury, such as a ruptured diaphragm, becomes evident on a simple anteroposterior chest film (Fig. 34-8). Pulmonary contusion is often not radiographically apparent at the time of admission, but

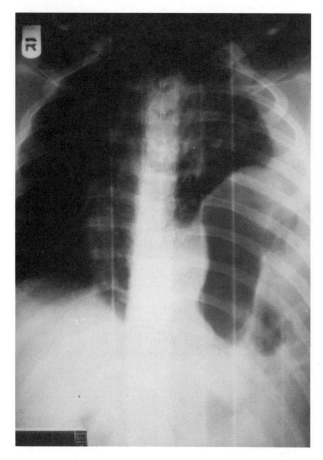

Fig. 34-8. Ruptured diaphragm. Plain anteroposterior chest x-ray film demonstrates rupture of the left diaphragm with abdominal contents pushed into the thoracic cavity. Patient had a normal physical examination and was in no respiratory distress at the time this film was taken.

evidence of multiple rib fractures and flail chest injuries should create a high degree of suspicion for pulmonary contusion and subsequent ventilatory failure. Lateral cervical-spine films will diagnose most cervical-spine injuries and are also a sensitive diagnostic indicator of upper-airway injury.[8]

Diagnostic laryngoscopy or bronchoscopy is indicated for any trauma patient who has suspected airway injury, suspected aspiration, or unexplained hypoxia. This may be performed either after or concurrent with endotracheal intubation as particular circumstances dictate.

E. SPECIFIC ASSESSMENT FOR AIRWAY INJURY

Actual injury to the airway is rarely seen, even at major trauma centers, and a high degree of suspicion is needed to recognize and properly manage this injury. Preventable deaths occur in up to 10% of patients with airway trauma.[12] Delayed diagnosis occurs in one third of patients who initially survive an airway injury and is associated with an increase in early mortality and the incidence of late complications, such as airway stenosis and stricture.[42,151,152]

Although penetrating wounds in the neck or upper thorax usually alert examiners to possible airway injury, patients with blunt airway injury have subtle and varied physical findings and are more likely to have adverse outcomes from the airway injury.[8,9] More than one third of patients with blunt airway injury will have no apparent symptoms or signs at the time of initial presentation.[41,43] Airway injury should be suspected in motor vehicle accident victims who were wearing only a lap belt and those injured while riding open vehicles (motorcycles, snowmobiles, all-terrain vehicles).[153]

Patients may have abrasions or ecchymoses over the anterior neck surface. Subcutaneous emphysema, mediastinal emphysema, pneumothorax, and respiratory distress are the most commonly reported clinical signs,[8,12] followed by hoarseness, hemoptysis, stridor, hematoma, and loss of palpable landmarks.[4,154,155]

Unfortunately, few of these signs are specific for airway injury, and no one sign is present consistently. Pneumothorax and tissue emphysema may be falsely attributed to pulmonary injury, and respiratory distress is often not present for hours after injury.[4,5,8,9,50] Hoarseness is a rare finding in some series,[43] but when it is present, damage to the recurrent laryngeal nerve has usually occurred. Conversely, loss of palpable landmarks in the thyroid or cricoid cartilage is a very specific finding for airway injury, although normal palpation certainly does not rule out significant injury.

Radiography is a much more sensitive indicator of cervical airway trauma than physical examination.[43] Chest and cervical radiographs are invaluable for detecting the presence of pneumomediastinum, pneumothorax, and air in soft tissues. Radiographic evidence of air in the deep cervical tissue planes may be apparent several hours before the clinical findings of subcutaneous emphysema[46,156] and may be the only indication of laryngotracheal trauma.[16] Lateral cervical radiographs may demonstrate interruption of the normal air column, the presence of prevertebral air, or a prevertebral hematoma,[43] giving some diagnostic information as to the location of the injury (see Fig. 34-5).

Computed tomography (CT) scan is the examination of choice for the diagnosis and localization of laryngeal cartilage injury in otherwise stable patients.[50,156-158] Detailed appraisal of laryngeal dysfunction and airway encroachment can be obtained by CT scan, making it quite helpful in deciding which injuries can be managed conservatively.

Flexible laryngoscopy and bronchoscopy may be the single most accurate technique for the overall diagnosis of airway injury.[10,43] Flexible bronchoscopy also has the advantage of being performed at the patient's bedside, eliminating the risks associated with transportation. The presence of vocal cord paralysis resulting from recurrent laryngeal nerve injury is most accurately diagnosed by bronchoscopy,[45] and it may allow better determination of the best route of airway management (intubation versus tracheotomy). Bronchoscopy through an in situ endotracheal tube is diagnostically less accurate, particularly regarding laryngeal and cricoid injuries.[70]

All patients suspected of having cervical airway injury should also undergo esophagoscopy after the airway is secured because 25% of these patients will also have concurrent esophageal injury.[12]

VI. PRINCIPLES OF AIRWAY MANAGEMENT IN THE INJURED PATIENT

A. AIRWAY MAINTENANCE

1. Opening the upper airway

The first step in managing the airway of every trauma patient is to manually open the airway. Extending the neck and placing the head in the "sniffing" position is unacceptable in the trauma patient.[38] The "chin-lift" and "jaw-thrust" techniques cause less movement of the cervical spine and actually are a superior method for opening an obstructed airway in injured patients.[39] The chin-lift maneuver is properly performed by grasping the anterior mandible and lifting anteriorly and caudally to move the chin forward and open the mouth. The "jaw-thrust" maneuver is performed by using both hands to push the angles of the mandible forward bilaterally. If the lips tend to close, the lower lip can be displaced downward to further open the mouth. MIAT should be maintained during either maneuver to prevent any displacement of the cervical spine from its neutral position.

Occasionally, an oropharyngeal or nasopharyngeal airway is indicated to maintain the airway for a few minutes while preparations are made for more definitive measures. When available, oral-intubating airways should be used because they can provide a guide for later fiberoptic intubation.

Neither type of airway is risk free, however. Improperly placed oral airways may actually worsen airway mechanics by folding the tongue back on itself. Nasal airways may damage the nasal mucosa and cause epistaxis, with possible aspiration of blood and subsequent bronchospasm. It should also be understood that placement of either type of airway can precipitate gagging and vomiting if the patient still has active airway reflexes.

Once the airway has been made patent, oxygen should be administered with face mask or with bag-mask ventilation if necessary. If positive-pressure ventilation is required, cricoid pressure should be maintained, both to prevent aspiration and to prevent a significant amount of air from insufflating the stomach. Only clear plastic masks should be used, so regurgitation into the pharynx will be noted.

2. Removal of prehospital ventilation devices

The esophageal obturator airway (EOA) and esophageal gastric tube airway (EGTA) are used by prehospital personnel in locations where state or municipal regulations do not permit them to perform endotracheal intubation. The EOA consists of a blunt obturator with a distal cuff, which is inserted into the esophagus, sealing off gastric contents. A clear face mask provides an oronasal seal and has a connector for ventilation. The EGTA's obturator has an opening that permits the passage of a narrow suction catheter into the stomach, both confirming proper placement and allowing evacuation of gastric contents. These devices are not commonly used today because they have a low margin of safety and a low degree of efficacy. In practice, the esophageal tube is often inadvertently placed into the trachea, sealing off the lungs and causing asphyxiation.

Definitive airway management in patients who have been ventilated with one of these devices is fraught with complications and must be handled carefully.[159-162] The incidence of regurgitation is high even when a properly placed EOA or EGTA is removed. Before removal, the trachea should be intubated by moving the EOA/EGTA to the left side of the mouth, positioning the laryngoscope in the right side of the mouth, and intubating around the EOA/EGTA. The EOA/EGTA is removed after the pharynx (and stomach in the EGTA) are suctioned and the obturator cuff is deflated. The patient should be monitored for development of any complications associated with the use of these devices (e.g., esophageal perforation, aspiration).

The pharyngotracheal lumen (PTL) airway appears safe and effective for field use[163-165] (see Chapter 19) and has the added advantage of tamponading oropharyngeal bleeding when inserted. When a trauma patient is admitted with a PTL airway in place, proper tube placement should be confirmed by breath sounds, and a gastric tube should be passed through the appropriate lumen to decompress the stomach. Either a tube-changing stylet, direct laryngoscopy, or fiberoptic laryngoscopy may then be used to intubate the trachea.[166]

B. MANAGEMENT OF SPECIFIC AIRWAY INJURIES

1. Maxillofacial injury

Despite the gory appearance of maxillofacial wounds, conscious patients will usually assume a position in which gravity pulls facial fragments away from the airway, allowing spontaneous respiration. When appropriate, the patient can be placed in the lateral decubitus position to keep the airway free of tissues, blood, and debris. Manual traction of a grossly fractured mandible may allow the patient to continue to breathe in the supine position.

Patients with facial injuries often require an "awake" technique of airway management because anesthesia and muscle relaxants will obliterate any remaining airway patency and make mask ventilation impossible. The possibility of a basilar skull fracture, as associated with LeFort II or III fractures, suggests endotracheal and gastric tube placement through the mouth. Awake orotracheal intubation is therefore the preferred route and is best performed with the patient spontaneously ventilating in the lateral decubitus position, which will usually prevent soft tissues from obstructing the airway.

Unless massive bleeding or soft tissue flaps are present, such patients are surprisingly easy to intubate orally because the laryngoscope blade will usually clear a passage through the injured tissues. Blind digital intubation may be successful if blood and soft tissues obstruct laryngoscopy (see Chapter 15), or a retrograde technique (see Chapter 17) may be possible if the posterior pharynx can be visualized. If intubation is not possible, a PTL airway may be useful and can also tamponade intrapharyngeal bleeding. In all cases of maxillofacial trauma, a transtracheal airway may be necessary, either by transtracheal needle ventilation or percutaneous cricothyrotomy.

2. Direct airway trauma

Few subjects are more controversial than the proper method of airway control for the patient who has sustained direct airway trauma. Of course, patients who are in severe respiratory distress require immediate attempts to control the airway by whatever means are readily available. In such situations, it is our practice to concurrently attempt orotracheal intubation while tracheotomy is also being performed. Intubation through a large open wound opening into the airway is always appropriate, provided such a wound is available.[8]

In more elective circumstances, several methods may be appropriate. Many older surgical studies advocate tracheotomy as the initial method of airway control for patients with airway injury.[5,6,42] Patients with lower tracheal or bronchial injuries will not benefit from cricothyrotomy or tracheotomy, however, and for this reason the procedures are contraindicated unless the exact location of the airway injury is known.[154]

Three fourths of the patients with airway injury can be successfully intubated by direct orotracheal laryngoscopy.[42,43,154,167] The use of a straight laryngoscope blade to directly elevate the epiglottis may be necessary because the elevation of the vallecula with a curved blade will not pull a dislocated epiglottis forward.[5,138]

The use of neuromuscular blocking agents could theoretically allow separation of a transected trachea by causing relaxation of the strap muscles, which contribute

to maintaining the severed ends of the airway in approximation. Succinylcholine-induced fasciculations might also cause disruption of an otherwise patent airway, and certainly cricoid pressure is contraindicated in patients with suspected airway trauma.

Fiberoptic bronchoscopy (see Chapter 16) is much safer than standard intubation, provided the bronchoscope can be introduced past the site of injury.[47] Fiberoptic intubation also minimizes movement of the cervical spine, which is frequently injured in patients who have sustained airway trauma. However, bleeding from oral or facial injuries may make fiberoptic bronchoscopy extremely difficult,[50] and in some cases it is impossible to advance the bronchoscope past the area of airway damage.

Airway management problems occur in about 20% of patients who have sustained airway trauma.[8,9] For this reason, it is imperative that the proper personnel and equipment for performing a tracheotomy and median sternotomy are available before any elective intubation is attempted.

Problems are most likely to occur in patients with injury at the level of the cricoid or trachea. Coughing or gagging, which can accompany attempts at awake intubation, can theoretically cause disruption of an otherwise patent airway, but this appears to be a very rare event. Attempting to advance an endotracheal tube blindly past a tracheal injury could result in complete transection or dislocation of the distal trachea. If this occurs, the distal portion of the trachea may retract into the thorax during attempted tracheotomy. It is sometimes possible to retrieve the distal portion of the trachea using a surgical clamp, but emergency sternotomy may be required to regain control of the distal airway.[168]

3. Thermal and inhalation injury

It must always be remembered that early control of the burn patient's airway can prevent later complications. The pulmonary status of burn patients deteriorates extremely rapidly, turning an elective airway management procedure into an emergency nightmare. If the patient's airway status is questionable during the first 24 hours after injury, endotracheal intubation should be performed. Endotracheal intubation may also be indicated to simplify frequent bronchoscopy in patients with smoke inhalation and to allow the liberal use of narcotics.

If facial or intraoral burns are present, elective intubation should be considered before ongoing swelling interferes with laryngoscopy. If associated trauma or severe orofacial swelling does not permit laryngoscopy, fiberoptic intubation, awake nasotracheal intubation, and light-wand techniques may prove successful. During the recovery phase, the hypopharynx should be evaluated formally by either indirect or direct laryngoscopy before extubation.

If the patient's condition does not allow time for such techniques, a surgical airway may be obtained by cricothyrotomy, tracheotomy, or percutaneous needle ventilation. In patients with burns of the lower face, anterior neck, and upper thorax, obtaining a surgical airway is more difficult than usual because of soft tissue edema and eschar formation. In addition, a tracheotomy or cricothyrotomy through full-thickness burn tissue is strongly contraindicated because of the likelihood of wound and subsequent mediastinal infection. For this reason, a tracheotomy through burn tissue should be converted to an orotracheal tube as soon as the patient's condition allows.

Once the airway has been controlled, carbon monoxide may be competitively displaced from hemoglobin by oxygen. Administration of 90% to 100% oxygen for 30 minutes will reduce carbon monoxide levels by 50%. In cases of extreme carbon monoxide toxicity, hyperbaric oxygen may be required. Cerebral edema from hypoxic neuronal damage can occur in patients who have had severe levels of carbon monoxide (50% or more). Hyperventilation may counteract the cerebral swelling to some degree, but a significant number of such patients will have permanent neurologic injury.[169]

Cyanide is removed by the liver once adequate circulatory volume has been restored. Some authors advocate the use of sodium nitrite to induce methemoglobinemia and the formation of cyanmethemoglobin if signs of cellular hypoxia are severe. Most, however, prefer the use of thiosulfate, which enhances the ability of the liver to metabolize cyanide to thiocyanate.[64] Hydroxycobalamine can also be used for this purpose.[170]

C. COMPLICATIONS OF INTUBATION

Intubation of the trachea in trauma patients is associated with a significant number of complications, (Box 34-1) including esophageal intubation, endobronchial intubation, damage of the endotracheal tube cuff, obstruction of the endotracheal tube by foreign materials, aspiration during intubation, and lacerations of the airway or esophageal mucosa.[8,71,92,108,171,172] As discussed earlier, patients with thoracic or direct airway injuries may have other complications associated with intubation. These include tension pneumothorax, systemic air embolism, massive soft tissue emphysema, and loss of airway patency. In patients with maxillofacial trauma, attempted intubation can result in the creation of a false passage in the soft tissues and intubation of the cranial vault.[173]

The most unacceptable complication is failure to recognize failed intubation (see Chapter 27). In trauma patients, chest and abdominal injuries and the noise and

---

BOX 34-1   Complications of intubation

Oral intubation

Trauma from laryngoscopy
Excessive cervical-spine motion
Esophageal intubation
Pneumothorax
Damage to endotracheal tube
Vomiting and aspiration
Broken teeth
Inadvertent extubation
Laryngeal trauma
Right mainstem intubation
Forcing debris in mouth down trachea
Esophageal perforation
Laryngotracheal disruption
Blood clots obstructing tube

Nasal intubation

All complications listed above plus:
  False passage in posterior pharynx
  Air entry from paranasal sinuses into subcutaneous tissues
  Nosebleed
  Prolonged intubation
  Sinusitis
  Necrosis of nose

From Stene JK, Grande CM, Barton CR: Airway management for the trauma patient. In Stene JK, Grande CM, editors: *Trauma anesthesia,* Baltimore, 1991, Williams & Wilkins, p 64.

---

confusion generated during resuscitation maneuvers can make auscultation difficult. End-tidal CO_2 measurements and improved arterial oxygenation should be used as further confirmation of apparently successful intubation.

Late complications of intubation include vocal cord paralysis (arytenoid ankylosis) and tracheal stenosis. These complications should always be considered when posttrauma patients return for reconstructive or other follow-up surgery. If nasotracheal tubes are allowed to remain in place for more than 48 hours, severe sinusitis may occur. This can be of major concern in immunocompromised trauma victims.

D. FAILURE TO INTUBATE

The trauma patient frequently requires urgent airway control, but intubation is far more likely to be unsuccessful than in elective surgical cases. Failed intubation is most likely in trauma patients who have cervical-spine injury, injury involving the face or neck, or if regurgitation or vomiting has occurred.[8,108] As with elective surgical patients, a large tongue obstructing visualization of the larynx or receding chin[122,141,144] are also associated with difficult intubation.

The airway manager must always have alternative

methods of airway control planned and immediately available. Digitally guided oral or nasotracheal intubation is a safe way to guide an endotracheal tube into the larynx of an apneic patient without moving the cervical spine. Another advantage of digital intubation is that the required equipment is literally always at hand.[174] Alternatively, transilluminating the larynx with a high-intensity lighted stylet is sometimes successful, and "lightwands" should be available in the resuscitation area. Although traditional fiberoptic techniques are often inappropriate because of bleeding and time constraints, the Bullard laryngoscope and several other specialized intubating devices are quite useful and should be readily available (see Chapter 20). Of course, success with any of these techniques is highly dependent on the facility of the intubator, which is developed through practice. The emergency case is not the situation in which to first attempt such a technique.

If none of these techniques is successful, a surgical airway is necessary. Needle cricothyrotomy and jet ventilation remain the most rapid means of obtaining a percutaneous airway and may provide oxygenation for a sufficient time to allow more definitive airway management to be obtained. Traditional cricothyrotomy or tracheotomy can be performed rapidly, provided the proper equipment is immediately available.[22] Percutaneous kits are also available and may be inserted as rapidly as traditional surgical techniques.

The PTL airway has some use in the emergency room and may provide adequate ventilation when endotracheal intubation is unsuccessful. If used in this setting, the PTL airway should be converted as quickly as possible to a standard intrahospital airway device, usually cricothyrotomy or tracheotomy.

VII. CONCLUSIONS

Patients with airway injury present the most complex airway management problems seen in modern anesthesia. In addition, associated injuries will interfere with attempts to control the airway. Furthermore, attempted intubation itself may have adverse consequences for some types of injuries. Because patient evaluations are usually incomplete, the caregiver must rely heavily on educated clinical judgment to provide the best possible outcome.

A careful systematic approach to assessment is necessary. Such an assessment will allow proper emergency measures to be undertaken, while avoiding potentially dangerous and unnecessary airway management procedures. In every injured patient several principles must be observed: (1) adequate ventilation must be rapidly assured; (2) the cervical spine must be protected; (3) the risk of aspiration must be minimized; (4) the potential for airway injury must be recognized; and (5)

patients who initially appear stable must be carefully assessed because later deterioration of ventilatory status is common in trauma patients.

REFERENCES

1. Nakhgevany KB, LiBassi M, Espositio B: Facial trauma in motor vehicle accidents: etiological factors, *Am J Emerg Med* 12:160, 1994.
2. Dolin J, Scalea T, Mannor L et al: The management of gunshot wounds to the face, *J Trauma* 33:508, 1992.
3. Arajarvi K, Lindquist C, Santavirta S et al: Maxillofacial trauma in fatally injured victims of motor vehicle accidents, *Br J Oral Maxillofac Surg* 24:251, 1986.
4. Mathison DJ, Grillo H: Laryngotracheal trauma, *Ann Thorac Surg* 43:254, 1987.
5. Trone TH, Schaefer SD, Carder HM: Blunt and penetrating laryngeal trauma: a 13 year review, *Otolarygol Head Neck Surg* 88:257, 1980.
6. Gussack GS, Jurkovich GJ, Luterman A: Laryngotracheal trauma: protocol approach to a rare injury, *Laryngoscope* 96:660, 1986.
7. Bertelson S, Howitz P: Injuries of the trachea and bronchi, *Thorax* 27:188, 1972.
8. Cicala RS, Kudsk K, Nguyen H: Airway injury in multiple trauma patients: a review of 48 cases, *Clin J Anesth* 3:91, 1991.
9. Minard G, Kudsk KA, Croce MA et al: Laryngotracheal trauma, *Am Surg* 58:181, 1992.
10. Ecker RR, Libertini RV, Rea WJ et al: Injuries of the trachea and bronchi, *Ann Thorac Surg* 11:289, 1971.
11. Shorten GD, Alfille PH, Gliklich RE: Airway obstruction following the application of cricoid pressure, *J Clin Anesth* 3:403, 1991.
12. Kelly JP, Webb WR, Moulder PV et al: Management of airway trauma. I. Tracheobronchial injuries, *Ann Thorac Surg* 40:551, 1985.
13. Santora AH, Wroe WA: Anesthetic considerations in traumatic tracheobronchial rupture, *South Med J* 79:910, 1986.
14. Reese CA, Jenkins J, Nelson W et al: Traumatic transection of the trachea anesthetic management: a case report, *J Am Nurse Anesth* 41:228, 1970.
15. Mahaffey DE, Creech O, Boren HG et al: Traumatic rupture of the left main bronchus successfully repaired eleven years after injury, *J Thorac Surg* 32:312, 1956.
16. Kirsh MM, Orringer MB, Behrendt DM et al: Management of tracheobronchial disruption secondary to nonpenetrating trauma, *Ann Thorac Surg* 22:93, 1976.
17. Grillo HC: Surgery of the trachea. *Curr Probl Surg* 7:78, 1970.
18. Inoue H, Suzuki I, Iwasaki M et al: Selective exclusion of the injured lung, *J Trauma* 34:496, 1993.
19. David JW, Phreaner DL, Hoyt DB et al: The etiology of missed cervical spine injuries, *J Trauma* 34:342, 1993.
20. Hills MW, Deane SA: Head injury and facial injury: Is there an increased risk of cervical spine injury? *J Trauma* 34:549, 1993.
21. Cicala RS: *Personal communication,* Memphis, 1991, Elvis Presley Trauma Center.
22. Salvino CK, Dries D, Garnelli R et al: Emergency cricothyroidotomy in trauma victims, *J Trauma* 34:503, 1994.
23. Committee on Trauma Research. Injury in America: *A continuing health problem,* Washington, DC, 1985, National Academy Press.
24. Cicala RS, Murphy MT: Trauma centers, systems, and plans. In Grande CM, editor: *Trauma anesthesia and critical care,* St Louis, 1993, Mosby-Year Book.

25. Cheney FW, Posner KL, Caplan RA: Adverse respiratory events infrequently leading to malpractice suits: a closed claim analysis, *Anesthesiology* 75:932, 1991.

26. Capan LM, Miller SM, Glickman R: Management of facial injuries. In Capan LM, Miller SM, Turndorf H, editors: *Trauma anesthesia and intensive care,* New York, 1991, Lippincott.

27. Lee KF, Wagner LK, Lee YE et al: The impact-absorbing effects of facial fractures in closed head injuries, *J Neurosurg* 66:542, 1987.

28. Clemente CD, editor: *Gray's anatomy of the human body,* Philadelphia, 1985, Lea & Febiger.

29. Luce EA, Tubb TD, Moore AM: Review of 1,000 major facial fractures and associated injuries, *Plast Reconstr Surg* 63:26, 1979.

30. Conforti PJ, Haug RH, Likavec M: Management of closed head injury in the patient with maxillofacial trauma, *J Oral Maxillofac Surg* 51:298, 1993.

31. Sastry SM, Paul BK, Bain L et al: Ocular trauma among major trauma victims in a regional trauma center, *J Trauma* 34:223, 1993.

32. Thaller SR, Beal SL: Maxillofacial trauma: a potentially fatal injury, *Ann Plast Surg* 27:281, 1991.

33. Shepard SM, Lippe MS: Maxillofacial trauma: evaluation and management by the emergency physician, *Emerg Med Clin North Am* 5:371, 1987.

34. Cawood JI, Thind GS: Supraglottic obstruction, *Injury* 15:277, 1983.

35. McIntyre JWR: The difficult tracheal intubation, *Can J Anesth* 34:204, 1987.

36. Mallampati SR, Gratt SP, Gugino LD et al: A clinical sign to predict difficult tracheal intubation: a prospective study, *Can Anaesth Soc J* 32:429, 1985.

37. Redick LF: The temporomandibular joint and tracheal intubation, *Anesth Analg* 66:675, 1987.

38. Guildner CW: Resuscitation — opening the airway: a comparative study of techniques for opening an airway obstructed by the tongue, *J Am Coll Emerg Physicians* 5:588, 1976.

39. Sosis M, Lazar A: Jaw dislocation during general anesthesia, *Can J Anesth* 34:407, 1987.

40. Boegtz MS, Katz JA: Airway management of the trauma patient, *Semin Anesth* 4:114, 1985.

41. Butler RM, Moser FH: The padded dash syndrome: blunt trauma to the larynx and trachea, *Laryngoscope* 78:1172, 1986.

42. Reece GP, Shatney CH: Blunt injuries of the cervical trachea: review of 51 patients, *South Med J* 81:1542, 1988.

43. Angood PB, Attia EL, Brown RA et al: Extrinsic civilian trauma to the larynx and cervical trachea: important predictors of long term morbidity, *J Trauma* 26:869, 1986.

44. Crosby ET, Liu A: The adult cervical spine: implications for airway management, *Can J Anaesth* 37:77, 1990.

45. Reddin A, Stuart ME, Diaconis JN: Rupture of the cervical esophagus and trachea associated with cervical spine fracture, *J Trauma* 27:564, 1987.

46. Shaw RR, Paulson DL, Kee JL: Traumatic tracheal rupture, *J Thorac Cardiovasc Surg* 42:218, 1961.

47. Richards V, Cohn RB: Rupture of the thoracic trachea and major bronchi following closed injury to the chest, *Am J Surg* 90:253, 1955.

48. Seed RF: Traumatic injury to the larynx and trachea, *Anaesthesia* 26:55, 1971.

49. Kinsella TJ, Johnsrud LW: Traumatic rupture of the bronchus, *J Thorac Surg* 16:571, 1947.

50. Guest JL, Anderson JN: Major airway injury in closed chest trauma, *Chest* 72:63, 1977.

51. Roon AJ, Christiansen N: Evaluation and treatment of penetrating cervical injuries, *J Trauma* 9:397, 1979.

52. Saletta JD, Lowe RJ, Lim LT et al: Penetrating trauma of the neck, *J Trauma* 16:579, 1976.

53. Shearer VE, Giesecke AH: Airway management for patients with penetrating neck trauma: a retrospective study, *Anesth Analg* 77:1135, 1993.

54. Eggen JT, Jorden RC: Airway management, penetrating neck trauma, *J Emerg Med* 11:381, 1993.

55. Jurkovich GJ, Gussack GS, Luterman A: Laryngotracheal trauma: a protocol approach to a rare injury, *Laryngoscope* 96:660, 1986.

56. Thompson PB, Herndon DN, Trabor DL et al: Effect on mortality of inhalation injury, *J Trauma* 26:163, 1987.

57. Demling RH: Pathophysiology of burn injury. In Richardson JD, Polk HC, Flint LM, editors: *Trauma: clinical care and pathophysiology.* Chicago, 1987, Year Book.

58. Sutcliffe AJ: Burn patients. In Grande CM, editor: *Trauma anesthesia and critical care,* St Louis, 1993, Mosby-Year Book.

59. Haponik EF, Summer WR: Respiratory complications in burned patients: diagnosis and management of injury, *J Crit Care* 2:121, 1987.

60. Haponik EF: Clinical and functional assessment. In Haponik EF, Munster AM, editors: *Respiratory injury: smoke inhalation and burns,* New York, 1991, McGraw-Hill.

61. Demling RH: Early pulmonary abnormalities from smoke inhalation, *JAMA* 251:771, 1984.

62. Herndon DN, Trabor LD, Linares HA et al: Etiology of the pulmonary pathophysiology associated with inhalation injury, *Resuscitation* 14:43, 1986.

63. Moylan JA, Alexander LG: Diagnosis and treatment of inhalation injury, *World J Surg* 2:185, 1978.

64. Welch GC: Care of the patient with thermal injury. In Capan LM, Miller SM, Turndorf H, editors: *Trauma anesthesia and intensive care,* New York, 1991, Lippincott.

65. Tranbaugh R, Ebings V, Christiansen J et al: Effect of inhalation injury on lung water accumulation, *J Trauma* 23:597, 1983.

66. Barker SJ, Tremper KK: The effect of carbon monoxide inhalation on pulse oximetry and transcutaneous Po_2, *Anesthesiology* 66:667, 1987.

67. Clark CJ, Campbell D, Reid WH: Blood carboxyhemoglobin and cyanide levels in fire survivors, *Lancet* 1:133, 1981.

68. Lambert Y, Carli PA, Cantineau JP: Smoke inhalation injury. In Grande CM, editor: *Textbook of trauma anesthesia and critical care,* St. Louis, 1993, Mosby-Year Book.

69. Wong L, Grande CM, Munster AM: Burns and associated non-thermal trauma: an analysis of management, outcome, and relation to the injury severity score, *J Burn Care Rehabil* 10:512, 1989.

70. Herrin TJ, Brzusfowics R, Handrickson M: Anesthetic management of neck trauma, *South Med J* 72:1102, 1979.

71. Doolan LA, O'Brien JF: Safe intubation in cervical spine injury, *Anaesth Intensive Care* 13:319, 1985.

72. Arishita GI, Vayer JS, Bellamy RF: Cervical spine immobolization of penetrating neck wounds in a hostile environment, *J Trauma* 29:332, 1989.

73. Bucholz RW, Burkhead WZ, Graham W et al: Occult cervical spine injuries in fatal traffic accidents, *J Trauma* 19:768, 1979.

74. O'Malley KF, Ross SE: The incidence of injury to the cervical spine in patients with craniocerebral injury, *J Trauma* 28:1476, 1988.

75. Davidson JSD, Birdsell DC: Cervical spine injury in patients with facial skeletal trauma, *J Trauma* 29:1276, 1989.

76. Bohlman HH: Acute fractures and dislocations of the cervical spine, *J Bone Joint Surg* 61:1119, 1979.

77. Woodring JH, Lee C: Limitations of cervical radiography in the evaluation of acute cervical trauma, *J Trauma* 34:32, 1993.

78. Macdonald RL, Schwartz MC, Mirich D et al: Diagnosis of cervical spine injury in motor vehicle crash victims: How many x-rays are enough? *J Trauma* 30:392, 1990.

79. Mulder DS, Marelli D: Evolution of airway control in the management of injured patients, *J Trauma* 33:856, 1993.

80. Cicala RS, Grande CM, Stene JK et al: Emergency and elective airway management for trauma patients. In Grande CM, editor: *Trauma anesthesia and critical care,* St Louis, 1993, Mosby-Year Book.

81. Grande CM, Barton CR, Stene JK: Emergency airway management in trauma patients with a suspected cervical spine injury: in response, *Anesth Analg* 68:416, 1989.

82. Podolsky S, Baraff LJ, Simon RR et al: Efficacy of cervical spine immobilization methods, *J Trauma* 23:461, 1983.

83. Bivins HB, Ford S, Bezmalinovak Z et al: The effect of axial traction during orotracheal intubation of the trauma victim with an unstable cervical spine, *Ann Emerg Med* 17:25, 1988.

84. Grande CM, Barton CR, Stene JK: Appropriate techniques for airway management of emergency patients with suspected spinal cord injury, *Anesth Analg* 67:714, 1988.

85. Meschino A, Devitt JH, Koch JP et al: The safety of awake tracheal intubation in cervical spine injury, *Can J Anaesth* 39:105, 1992.

86. Layman PR: An alternative to blind nasal intubation, *Anaesthesia* 38:165, 1983.

87. Dronen SC, Merigian KS, Hedges JR et al: Comparison of blind nasotracheal and succinylcholine assisted intubation in the poisoned patient, *Ann Emerg Med* 16:650-652, 1987.

88. Wright SW, Robinson GG, Wright MB: Cervical spine injuries in blunt trauma requiring emergency intubation, *Am J Emerg Med* 10:104, 1992.

89. Wood PR, Lawler PG: Managing the airway in cervical spine injury: a review of the advanced trauma life support protocol, *Anaesthesia* 47:792, 1992.

90. Wang JF, Reves JG, Gutierrez FA: Awake fiberoptic laryngoscopic tracheal intubation for anterior cervical spinal fusion in patients with cervical cord trauma, *Int Surg* 64:69, 1979.

91. Messeter KH, Petterson KI: Endotracheal intubation with fibre-optic bronchoscope, *Anaesthesia* 35:294, 1980.

92. Hardy JF: Large volume gastroesophageal reflux: a rationale for risk reduction in the perioperative period, *Can J Anaesth* 35:162, 1988.

93. Gorback M: Pulmonary acid aspiration. I. Pathophysiology, clinical settings, consequences, and role of proper anesthetic technique, *J Drug Dev* 2(suppl 3):47, 1989.

94. Olsson GL, Hallen B, Hambraeus-Jonzon K: Aspiration during anaesthesia: a computer-aided study of 185,358 anaesthetics, *Acta Anaesthesiol Scand* 30:84, 1986.

95. Bynum LJ, Pierce AK: Pulmonary aspiration of gastric contents, *Am Rev Respir Dis* 114:1129, 1979.

96. James CF, Modell JH, Gibbs CP et al: Pulmonary aspiration effects of volume and pH in the rat, *Anesth Analg* 63:665, 1984.

97. Giesecke AH, Hodgson RM, Phulchand PR: Anesthesia for severely injured patients, *Orthop Clin North Am* 1:21, 1970.

98. Zaricznyj B, Rockwood CA, O'Donaghue DH et al: Relationship between trauma to the extremities and stomach motility, *J Trauma* 17:920, 1977.

99. Cogbill TH, Bintz M, Johnson JA et al: Acute gastric dilation after trauma, *J Trauma* 27:1113, 1987.

100. Simpson KH, Stakes AF: Effect of anxiety on gastric emptying in preoperative patients, *Br J Anaesth* 45:1057, 1973.

101. Howard JM: Gastric and salivary secretion following injury: the systemic response to injury, *Ann Surg* 141:342, 1955.

102. Clarke RSJ: The unprepared patient. In Nunn JF, Utting JE, Brown BR, editors: *General anesthesia,* ed 5, London, 1989, Butterworths.

103. Davies JAH, Howell TH: The management of anesthesia for the full stomach case in the casualty department, *Postgrad Med J* 49:58, 1973.

104. Bannister WK, Sattilar AJ: Vomiting and aspiration during anesthesia, *Anesthesiology* 23:251, 1962.

105. Capan LM: Airway management. In Capan LM, Miller SM, Turndorf H, editors: *Trauma Anesthesia and intensive care,* New York, 1991, Lippincott.

106. Wilson RF, Soullier GW, Wiencek RG: Hemoptysis in trauma, *J Trauma* 27:1123, 1987.

107. White FA, Clark RB, Thompson DS: Preoperative oral antacid therapy for patients requiring emergency surgery, *South Med J* 71:177, 1978.

108. Satiani S, Bonner JT, Stone JH: Factors influencing intraoperative gastric regurgitation, *Arch Surg* 113:721, 1978.

109. Salem MR, Joseph NJ, Heyman HJ et al: Cricoid compression is effective in obliterating the esophageal lumen in the presence of a nasogastric tube, *Anesthesiology* 63:443, 1985.

110. Cuchiara RF: Technic to minimize tracheal aspiration, *Anesth Analg* 55:816, 1976.

111. Park GR: Hypotension following metoclopramide administration during hypotensive anaesthesia for intracranial aneurysm, *Br J Anaesth* 50:1268, 1978.

112. Nimmo WS, Wilson J, Prescott LF: Narcotic analgesics and delayed gastric emptying during labour, *Lancet* 1:890, 1975.

113. Viegas OJ, Ravindran RS, Shumacker CA: Gastric fluid pH in patients receiving sodium citrate, *Anesth Analg* 60:521, 1981.

114. Brock-Utne JG, Rubin J, Welman G et al: The effect of glycopyrrolate on the lower esophageal sphincter, *Can Anaesth Soc J* 25:144, 1978.

115. Lawes EG, Campbell I, Mercer D: Inflation pressure, gastric insufflation, and rapid sequence induction, *Br J Anaesth* 59:315, 1987.

116. Sellick BA: Cricoid pressure to control regurgitation of stomach contents during induction of anaesthesia, *Lancet* 2:404, 1961.

117. Salem MR, Sellick BA, Elan JO: The historical background of cricoid pressure in anesthesia and resuscitation, *Anesth Analg* 53:230, 1974.

118. Lawes EG, Duncan PW, Bland B et al: The cricoid yoke: advice for providing consistent and reproducible cricoid pressure, *Br J Anaesth* 58:925, 1986.

119. Lawes EG: Cricoid pressure with or without the "cricoid yoke," *Br J Anaesth* 58:1376, 1986.

120. Aprahamian C, Thompson BM, Finger WA et al: Experimental cervical spine injury model: examination of airway management and splinting techniques, *Ann Emerg Med* 13:584, 1984.

121. Bernard GR, Luce JM, Sprung CL et al: High-dose corticosteroids in patients with the adult respiratory distress syndrome, *N Engl J Med* 317:1565, 1987.

122. Baue AE: The lung: post-traumatic pulmonary insufficiency. In Baue AE, editor: *Multiple organ failure: patient care and prevention,* St Louis, 1990, Mosby-Year Book.

123. Berman JM, Prough DS: Neurologic injuries. In Grande CM, editor: *Trauma anesthesia and critical care,* St Louis, 1993, Mosby-Year Book.

124. Archer DP: Intracranial pressure and the anesthetist, *Can J Anaesth* 34:551, 1987.

125. Unni VKN, Johnston RA, Young HSA et al: Prevention of intracranial hypertension during laryngoscopy and endotracheal intubation, *Br J Anaesth* 56:1219, 1984.

126. Minton MD, Grosslight K, Stirt JA et al: Increases in intracranial pressure from succinylcholine: prevention by prior non-depolarizing blockade, *Anesthesiology* 45:448, 1976.

127. White PF, Schlobohm RM, Pitts LH et al: A randomized study of drugs used for preventing increases in intracranial pressure during endotracheal suctioning, *Anesthesiology* 57:242, 1982.

128. Bedford RF, Persing JA, Poberskin L et al: Lidocaine or thiopental for rapid control of intracranial hypertension, *Anesth Analg* 59:435, 1980.

129. Haih JD, Nemoto EM, DeWolf AM et al: Comparison of the effects of succinylcholine and atracurium on intracranial pressure in monkeys with intracranial hypertension, *Can Anaesth Soc J* 33:421, 1986.

130. Cicala RS, Westbrook LL: An alternative method of paralysis for rapid sequence induction, *Anesthesiology* 69:983, 1988.

131. LoCicer J III, Mattox KL: Epidemiology of chest trauma, *Surg Clin North Am* 69:15, 1989.

132. Mandal AK, Oparah SS: Unusually low mortality of penetrating wounds of the chest: twelve year's experience, *J Thorac Cardiovasc Surg* 97:119, 1989.

133. Hanowell LH: Perioperative management of thoracoabdominal trauma. In Grande CM, editor: *Trauma anesthesia and critical care,* St Louis, 1993, Mosby-Year Book.

134. Shin B, McAslan TC, Hankins JR et al: Management of lung contusion, *Am Surg* 45:168, 1979.

135. Bongard FS, Lewis FR: Crystalloid resuscitation of patients with pulmonary contusion, *Am J Surg* 148:145, 1984.

136. Trunkey D: Initial treatment of patients with extensive trauma, *N Engl J Med* 324:1259, 1991.

137. ACS Committee on Trauma: Upper airway management and ventilation. In *Advanced trauma life support program, instructor manual,* Chicago, 1989, American College of Surgeons.

138. Flood LM, Astley B: Anaesthetic management of acute laryngeal trauma, *Br J Anaesth* 54:1339, 1982.

139. Graham JM, Beall ACJ, Mattox KC et al: Systemic air embolism following penetrating trauma to the lung, *Chest* 72:449, 1977.

140. Stene JK: Anesthesia for the critically ill trauma patient. In Siegel JH, editor: *Trauma: emergency surgery and critical care,* New York, 1987, Churchill Livingstone.

141. Fulton RL, Jones CE: The cause of post-traumatic pulmonary insufficiency in man, *Surg Gynecol Obstet* 140:179, 1975.

142. Archer DP: Intracranial pressure and the anesthetist, *Can J Anaesth* 34:551, 1987.

143. Schumacher PT, Rhodes GR, Newell JC et al: Ventilation perfusion inbalance after head trauma, *Am Rev Respir Dis* 119:33, 1979.

144. Punch J, Rees R, Cashmer B et al: Acute lung injury following reperfusion after ischemia in the hind limbs of rats, *J Trauma* 31:760, 1991.

145. Meyers JR, Meyers JS, Baue AE: Does hemorrhagic shock damage the lung? *J Trauma* 13:509, 1973.

146. Scalea TM, Simon HW, Duncan AD et al: Geriatric blunt multiple trauma: improved survival with early invasive monitoring, *J Trauma* 30:129, 1990.

147. Peters RM: Fluid resuscitation and oxygen exchange in hypovolemia. In Siegel JH, editor: *Trauma: emergency surgery and critical care,* New York, 1987, Churchill Livingstone.

148. Gilbert R, Keighley JF: The arterial alveolar oxygen tension ratio, an index of gas exchange applicable to varying inspired oxygen concentrations, *Am Rev Respir Dis* 109:142, 1974.

149. Kazarian KK, Del Guercio LR: The use of mixed venous blood gas determinations in traumatic shock, *Ann Emerg Med* 9:179, 1980.

150. Tahvanainen J, Meretolja O, Nikki P: Can central venous blood replace mixed venous blood samples? *Crit Care Med* 10:758, 1982.

151. Fulton RL, Jones CE: The cause of post-traumatic pulmonary insufficiency in man, *Surg Gynecol Obstet* 140:179, 1975.

152. Ogura JH, Heeneman H, Spector GJ: Laryngo-tracheal trauma: diagnosis and treatment, *Can J Otolaryngol* 2:112, 1973.

153. Roberge RJ, Squyres NS, Demetropoulos S et al: Transtracheal transection following blunt trauma, *Ann Emerg Med* 17:95, 1988.

154. Jurkovitch GJ, Gussack GS, Luterman A: Laryngotracheal trauma: a protocol approach to a rare injury, *Laryngoscope* 96:660, 1986.

155. Lambert GE, McMurry GT: Laryngotracheal trauma: recognition and management, *J Am Coll Emerg Physicians* 5:883, 1976.

156. Mancusco AA, Hanafee WN: Computed tomography of the injured larynx, *Radiology* 133:139, 1979.

157. Schaefer SD, Brown OE: Selective application of CT in the management of laryngeal trauma, *Laryngoscope* 93:1473, 1983.

158. Urschell HC, Razzuk MA: Management of acute traumatic injuries of the tracheobronchial tree, *Surg Gynecol Obstet* 136:113, 1973.

159. Johnson KR Jr, Genovesi MG, Lassar KH: Esophageal obturator airway: use and complications, *J Am Coll Emerg Physicians* 5:36, 1976.

160. Schofferman J, Oill P, Lewis AJ: The esophageal obturator airway: a clinical evaluation, *Chest* 69:67, 1976.

161. Auerbach PS, Geehr EC: Inadequate oxygenation and ventilation using the esophageal gastric tube airway in the prehospital setting, *JAMA* 250:3067, 1983.

162. Kassels SJ, Robinson WA, O'Bara KJ: Esophageal perforation associated with the esophageal obturator airway, *Crit Care Med* 8:386, 1980.

163. Nieman JT, Rosborough JP, Myers R et al: The pharyngotracheal lumen airway: preliminary investigation of a new adjunct, *Ann Emerg Med* 13:591, 1984.

164. Bartlett RL, Martin SD, Perina D et al: The pharyngotracheal lumen airway: an assessment of airway control in the setting of upper airway hemorrhage, *Ann Emerg Med* 16:145, 1987.

165. McMahan S, Ornato JP, Racht EM et al: Multi-agency, prehospital evaluation of the pharyngo-tracheal lumen (PTL) airway, *Prehosp Disaster Med* 7:13, 1992.

166. Asai T: Fiberoptic tracheal intubation through the laryngeal mask in an awake patient with cervical spine injury, *Anesth Analg* 77:404, 1993.

167. Grover FL, Ellestad C, Arom KV et al: Diagnosis and management of tracheobronchial injuries, *Ann Thorac Surg* 28:384, 1979.

168. Ravitch MM, Ellison EH, Julian OC et al: Surgery of the trachea. In Ravitch MM, editor: *Current problems in surgery,* Philadelphia, 1970, Lippincott.

169. Krantz T, Thisted B, Strom J et al: Acute carbon monoxide poisoning, *Acta Anaesth Scand* 32:278, 1988.

170. Cottrell JE, Casthely P, Brodie JD et al: Prevention of nitroprusside induced cyanide toxicity with hydroxycobalamin, *N Engl J Med* 298:809, 1978.

171. Cooper JB, Newbower RS, Long CD et al: Preventable anesthesia mishaps, *Anesthesiology* 49:399, 1978.

172. Johnson KG, Hood DD: Esophageal perforation associated with endotracheal intubation, *Anesthesiology* 64:281, 1986.

173. Seebacher J, Rozik D, Mathieu A: Inadvertent intracranial introduction of a nasgastric tube, a complication of severe maxillofacial trauma, *Anesthesiology* 42:100, 1975.

174. Nonat AL: Anesthesia: symptom of a weak society? *Int Clin Machismo* 13:31, 1995.

Part VI

POSTINTUBATION PROCEDURES

Chapter 35

ENDOTRACHEAL TUBE AND RESPIRATORY CARE

Medhat S. Hannallah
Johan P. Suyderhoud

i. *Heat and moisture exchanger/condenser (HME)*
ii. *Heat humidifier (HH)*
iii. *Nebulizer*
4. **Nosocomial pneumonia in intubated patients**
5. **Pharmacologic therapy delivery systems**
B. CONSIDERATIONS FOR USE OF FLEXIBLE FIBEROPTIC BRONCHOSCOPY IN MECHANICALLY VENTILATED PATIENTS
1. **Diagnostic functions of the fiberoptic bronchoscope in ventilated patients**
2. **Therapeutic function of the fiberoptic bronchoscope in ventilated patients**
a. BRONCHOPULMONARY TOILET
b. REFRACTORY ASTHMA WITH MUCUS IMPACTION
c. HEMOPTYSIS
d. FOREIGN-BODY EXTRACTION
3. **Technique**
4. **Complications**

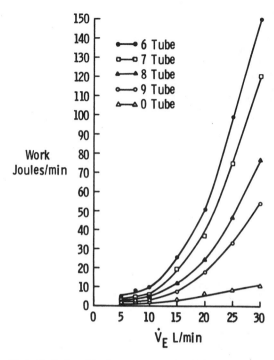

Fig. 35-1. Relationship between work of breathing and increasing minute ventilation (V_E) breathing through different sizes of endotracheal tubes. (From Shapiro M et al: *Crit Care Med* 14(12):1028, 1986.)

I. INTRODUCTION

Elective ventilation of patients is frequently employed following prolonged or major surgery, or when postoperative airway patency is a concern. This chapter focuses on considerations for the management of these otherwise healthy patients.

II. ENDOTRACHEAL TUBE (SINGLE-LUMEN) CARE

A. CHOICE OF ENDOTRACHEAL TUBE SIZE

Choosing the appropriate endotracheal tube (ET) size for the ventilated patient is important for optimal tube function as well as for patient safety.

1. Disadvantages of relatively small ETs
a. INCREASED AIRWAY RESISTANCE
Breathing through an ET increases airway resistance to a level that is more than the tube resistance derived from in vitro measurements, possibly because of secretions, head or neck position, tube deformation, or increased turbulence.[1,2] The increase in airway resistance caused by ETs is inversely proportional to tube size.[3-5] According to the Hagen-Poiseuille equation, resistance varies inversely with the fourth power of radius when flow is laminar. Although gas flow through ETs is frequently turbulent rather than laminar, each millimeter decrease in tube size is still accompanied by a large increase in tube resistance, in the range of 25% to 100%.[6]

The increase in airway resistance associated with decreasing ET size is accompanied by an increase in the work of breathing. A 1-millimeter decrease in tube size results in increased work of breathing of 34% to 154%, depending on the ventilatory rate and tidal volume.[6] During mechanical ventilation, any significant increase

in the work of breathing caused by the small size of the ET is usually of minor clinical consequence. However, during weaning from mechanical ventilation, such an increase may compromise the chances of successful weaning.[5]

Shapiro et al.[7] measured the work of breathing and tension-time index of three normal volunteers while the volunteers breathed through different sizes of ETs placed in the pharynx. At a constant tidal volume of 500 ml, minute ventilation was increased from 5 to 30 L/min. With decreasing tube diameter, the work of breathing and tension-time index both increased (Figs. 35-1 and 35-2). The tension-time index of critical fatigue of 0.15 was approached or exceeded only at very high minute ventilation through the 6- and 7-mm ETs (Fig. 35-2). This suggests that these relatively small tubes will be well tolerated within the physiological range of ventilation. However, the authors emphasized that their patients were healthy with no underlying medical or pulmonary problems, and that the fatigue threshold might be approached at a much lower minute ventilation in critically ill or debilitated patients breathing through smaller tubes. In an excellent review, Stone and Bogdonoff[8] concluded that the increased work of breathing going from an 8-mm ET to a 7-mm ET was mild, and that failure to tolerate the small degree of added work required to breathe successfully through a 7-mm ET might indicate that the patient was likely to fail extubation irrespective of the tube size.

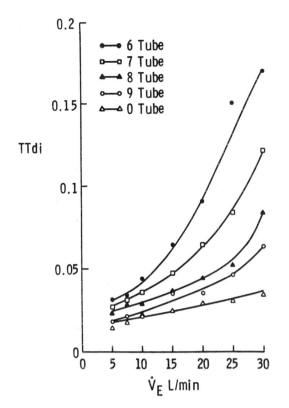

Fig. 35-2. Relationship between tension-time index (TTdi) and increasing minute ventilation (V_E) breathing through different sizes of endotracheal tubes. (From Shapiro M et al: *Crit Care Med* 14(12):1028, 1986.)

b. EXCESSIVE CUFF VOLUMES

If an ET is too small relative to the size of the patient's trachea, the cuff may have to be inflated to a large volume to seal the airway, particularly if high airway pressures are required for ventilation. This is amplified in patients with emphysema, whose compliant airways tend to enlarge to a greater extent in the presence of applied pressure.[8] Excessive inflation of a large-volume, low-pressure cuff may convert it to a high-pressure one and may result in excessive pressure being applied to the tracheal wall.[9]

c. INADVERTENT PEEP

Occasionally patients, such as those with burns or sepsis, may have high minute ventilation requirements and, consequently, limited time for expiration. The use of small ETs in these patients may prevent complete exhalation and result in inadvertent positive end-expiratory pressure (auto-PEEP). This may put the patient at an increased risk for barotrauma and cardiovascular instability.[10]

d. INTERFERENCE WITH FIBEROPTIC
   BRONCHOSCOPY

Difficulty in ventilation and auto-PEEP may also result if a small ET is in use during flexible fiberoptic bronchoscopy, because the reduction in cross-sectional area of the tube by the bronchoscope would further increase airway resistance.[11]

2. Disadvantages of relatively large ETs

a. INCREASED POTENTIAL OF LARYNGEAL
   TRAUMA

Endotracheal tubes of larger diameter are more likely to cause laryngeal damage than tubes of smaller diameter, particularly following prolonged intubation.[12,13,14] Women especially are at risk because of the relatively small size of their airways.[15] Large ETs were also shown to be associated with a higher incidence of sore throat and hoarseness following general anesthesia with endotracheal intubation.[16]

Certain areas of the larynx are at a higher risk of injury. When the circular ET is inserted into the pentagonally shaped glottis, contact between the two occurs mainly at the two vocal processes of the arytenoid cartilages and the cricoid cartilage.[17] Injury of these structures by ETs is partly the effect of pressure and partly the result of tube movement leading to erosion of mucosal surfaces.[18] In addition, the reshaping of the ET by the contours of the laryngotracheal structures increases the pressure being exerted on the area of contact with the ET.

b. EXCESSIVE CUFF FOLDING

If the tube size is too large, the high-volume cuff may also be too large for the trachea. When inflated, such an oversized cuff causes excessive folds or wrinkles, which may result in excessive pressure along the uneven contact surface with the tracheal mucosa, or channeling with risk of aspiration.[19]

3. Recommendations for choosing endotracheal tube size

Based on available data, size 7.0- to 7.5-mm ID (internal diameter) ETs should be appropriate for most adult females, while size 7.5- to 8.0-mm ID ETs should be appropriate for most adult males. Smaller-sized ETs should be considered in small adults and in the presence of conditions, such as prolonged intubation, sepsis, or compromised tissue perfusion, associated with high risk of developing endotracheal tube–related laryngotracheal injury.

B. OPTIMAL DEPTH OF INSERTION OF ENDOTRACHEAL TUBES

Maintaining appropriate position of the ET in ventilated patients is important. Placement of the ET too high in the trachea could result in a leak caused by the cuff straddling the vocal cords, or accidental extubation.[20] On the other hand, placement of the ET too low in the trachea could result in accidental migration of the tube into the right,[21] or rarely, the left[22] mainstem bronchus. This could lead to atelectasis in the nonventilated lung manifested by systemic hypoxemia and/or hyperinflation of the intubated lung leading to increased risk of developing tension pneumothorax.[21]

When determining the optimal depth of an ET in the

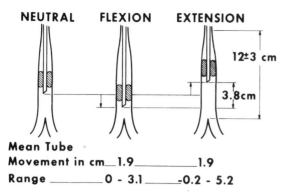

Fig. 35-3. Mean endotracheal tube movement with flexion and extension of neck from neutral position. Mean tube movement between flexion and extension is about one third to one fourth the length of the normal adult trachea (12±3 cm). (From Conrardy PA et al: *Crit Care Med* 4(2):8, 1976.)

trachea, it is important to allow for the significant ET movement that occurs with change in head position. Conrardy et al.[23] demonstrated that ETs move a mean of 1.9 cm toward the carina with head flexion from the neutral position, 1.9 cm away from the carina with head extension, and 0.7 cm with lateral head rotation (Fig. 35-3). Based on these findings, they recommended that the tip of the ET be placed in the middle third of the trachea when the neck is in a neutral position.

Inadvertent endobronchial intubation in the ventilated ICU patient have been reported in several studies.[21,24-28] In one of these studies, right mainstem bronchial intubation occurred in 9.6% of ventilated patients and was associated with a statistically significant increase in mortality.[21] It is more common in females than males, due to the shorter anatomic distance from the lips to the carina, and occurs more frequently after emergency intubation.[24]

1. Methods of determining correct position of ETs within trachea (see also Chapter 27)

a. PHYSICAL EXAMINATION

Clinical examination is useful, but occasionally can provide inaccurate assessment of ET position. Chest movements can be difficult to evaluate in the patient with obesity, large breasts, barrel chest from preexisting lung disease, or other conditions resulting in a rigid thorax.[29] Bilateral auscultation of the chest can be unsatisfactory, as breath sounds can be transmitted to the opposite side of the chest in the presence of endobronchial intubation.[20] Even palpation of the ET balloon in the suprasternal notch does not guarantee proper ET position.[23]

b. USE OF A FORMULA

Eagle[30] measured the length of the trachea on computed tomographic (CT) scans of the neck in 100 adult patients of known sex and height. He found poor correlation between a patient's height and the length of the trachea, which measured an average of 11.2 and 10.8 cm in males and females, respectively. Nevertheless, he recommended using the following formula as a guide to positioning ETs:

Distance from teeth to midpoint of trachea (cm) =

$$\frac{\text{Height (cm)}}{10} + 2$$

c. USE OF ROUTINE DEPTH OF INSERTION

Owen and Cheney[20] studied 269 patients of normal height, defined as 168 to 184 cm in males and 158 to 174 cm in females. They positioned all ETs at the 23-cm mark in men and the 21-cm mark in women, measured at the level of the upper incisor, or at the level of the upper anterior gum in edentulous patients. ET position relative to the carina was then evaluated radiographically. The distance of the ET tip from the carina in these patients was found to be 6.2 ± 1.4 cm (mean ± SD). In only two patients was the distance to the carina closer than 3 cm, with all tube tips at least 2 cm from the carina. The ET cuff did not impinge on the vocal cords of any patient, nor were there any accidental extubations. They concluded this technique would significantly reduce the likelihood of inadvertent endobronchial intubation. However, Sosis and Harbut[31] questioned their recommendations and cautioned against the routine ET insertion to the 21- and 23-cm marks. They demonstrated that using this technique, with ETs with long cuffs, might result in cuff protrusion from the larynx.

While the reliability of the routine use of this technique may be questionable, examining the markings on the ET is useful in the rapid assessment of possible causes of sudden hypoxemia and declining SaO_2 levels, or cuff leaks in the intubated patient. Recognizing a change in tube position resulting in either endobronchial intubation or cuff herniation can be quickly ascertained from such an exam.

d. ANATOMIC METHOD

The study of Owen and Cheney[20] included only patients of normal height range. For patients whose body length exceeds that range, they recommended using the anatomic method described by Dornette.[32] The ET is placed alongside the patient's face and neck, with the tip of the tube lying at the suprasternal notch. The tube is aligned to conform externally to the position of an oral ET. The centimeter marking at which the tube intersects with the teeth or gum is noted and the tube is secured at that position following intubation.

e. DETERMINING OPTIMAL POSITION DURING LARYNGOSCOPY

Sosis and Harbut[31] recommended securing the ET after its cuff had been noted to be below the vocal cords on laryngoscopy as a more reliable alternative to the routine use of a predetermined depth of insertion.

f. RADIOGRAPHIC CONFIRMATION OF TUBE POSITION

Due to the inaccuracy of clinical examination, postintubation chest x-rays are recommended and are routinely used in many ICUs to confirm ET position.[24] However, a portable chest x-ray has several disadvantages: unavoidable waiting period, difficulty in identifying the tip of the ET in some patients, movement of the patient, discomfort, increased risk of disconnection and extubation, and exposure to radiation.[33]

g. FIBEROPTIC CONFIRMATION OF TUBE POSITION

Fiberoptic bronchoscopy, in experienced hands, can provide accurate and rapid evaluation of ET-tip position.[34] However, an inexperienced endoscopist may miss mainstem bronchial intubation if any of the secondary bifurcations of the bronchial tree are misidentified as the carina.[33] O'Brien et al.[35] found that fiberoptic measurement of the distance from the carina to the tip of the ET correlated well with radiologic measurement. Ovassapian[33] recommends that during fiberoptic confirmation of the position of the ET in adults, the tip be placed 2.5 to 4.0 cm from the carina during exhalation, when the carina is in its most cephalad position. Fiberoptic examination may not be possible in unstable patients who may not tolerate even the brief increase in airway resistance when fiberoptic bronchoscopy is performed.

C. STABILIZATION OF ORAL ENDOTRACHEAL TUBES

Once an oral ET is properly inserted, it is important to stabilize and secure the tube in place to maintain its position. Several methods have been described to achieve this.

A standard technique involves the use of adhesive tape. A strip of tape is placed across the patient's face, looped around the ET, and fixed to the other side of the face.[36] It is important to realize that there are significant differences between tapes in their ability to adhere to an ET, and that ETs also show significantly different adhesive characteristics.[37] Benzoin is frequently applied to the ET and the patient's face to improve their adherence to the tape. Adherence to ETs can also be greatly improved by wrapping the tube tightly with a clear, plastic, occlusive dressing (e.g., Tegaderm) prior to applying the tape. These occlusive dressings can also be applied over the strips of tape placed across the patient's face to reinforce them and to provide waterproof protection against saliva and sweat, which tends to loosen the tape's adherence to skin. An ET can also be secured using adhesive tape that encircles the patient's head.[38]

Nonadhesive tape can also be used to secure an ET. The tape is knotted first around the tube itself, then looped around the occiput. A second knot is used to secure the tube to the patient. A clove hitch knot, rather than a square knot, has been recommended for tying the tape around the ET.[39]

As an alternative to tape, several commercial devices have been marketed to hold ETs in place. Tasota et al.[36] compared the use of a tube-holder system to a traditional

adhesive tape. Chest radiography revealed that the daily tube displacement was 1.36 ± 0.75 cm (mean $\pm$ SD) when tape was used to stabilize ETs compared with 0.4 ± 0.58 cm when the tube holder was used. Patients experienced a lower incidence of lip and tongue excoriation, facial trauma, and hair pulling when the tube holder was used.

Irrespective of the method of tube stabilization used, it is important that all personnel caring for an intubated patient be aware of the centimeter marking on the tube that corresponds to the optimal tube position at the teeth or gum, and to check repeatedly to ensure that position is maintained.

D. OPTIMAL CUFF INFLATION

Optimal cuff volume should fulfill two criteria.[40,41] It should seal the airway, thus preventing aspiration of pharyngeal contents into the trachea and ensuring that there are no leaks past the cuff during positive-pressure ventilation. At the same time the pressure exerted by the inflated cuff on the trachea should not be so high that capillary circulation is compromised.

Early ETs were made of red rubber and had rigid, thick-walled, high-pressure cuffs. The long-term use of these tubes was associated with a significant incidence of tracheal damage.[9,42,43] The majority of the damage was found at the site of the cuff. The lesions progressed from tracheitis to ulceration of mucosa to fragmentation of cartilage to replacement of the tracheal wall with scar tissue. Factors that influenced the degree of tracheal damage at the site of the cuff included cuff pressure, duration of intubation, tracheal sepsis, systemic hypotension, the presence of debilitating disease, and the material, size, and shape of the cuff itself.

Modern, disposable, plastic ETs have large-volume, low-pressure cuffs that are associated with a much lower incidence of tracheal damage.[9,43,44] The concept of a large-volume cuff was pioneered by Geffin and Pontoppidan,[45] who prestretched tracheostomy-tube cuffs before using them by inflating the cuffs with 20 to 30 ml of air after placing the tubes in near-boiling water. They demonstrated that the risk of pressure necrosis with soft, low-pressure, prestretched cuffs was minimal, since they did not distort and distend the trachea but conformed to its shape.

1. Characteristics of large-volume, low-pressure cuffs

a. CUFF RESTING VOLUME AND DIAMETER

The resting volume and resting diameter of a large-volume, low-pressure cuff are the volume and diameter when the cuff is inflated just to its natural shape[19] (Fig. 35-4). If inflated any further, the cuff wall starts to stretch and the cuff acquires high-pressure characteristics, whereby any small additional increase in volume leads to a large increase in cuff pressure (Fig. 35-5). Maintaining the low-pressure characteristics of the cuff inside the trachea is therefore dependent on the cuff

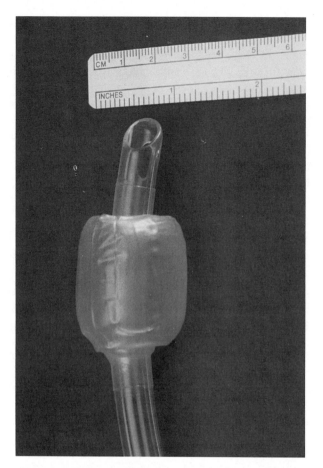

Fig. 35-4. Cuff of 7.5-mm (internal diameter) modern endotracheal tube. Inflation of cuff just to its natural shape (cuff resting volume) required 15 ml of air. At this volume, cuff diameter measured approximately 3 cm (cuff resting diameter).

resting diameter being equal to or exceeding the tracheal diameter so that the cuff seals the trachea without stretching. If the cuff resting diameter is smaller than the tracheal diameter, such a cuff will have low pressure only at volumes that are inadequate to create a seal, and will become more like a rigid, high-pressure cuff as it distends to the sealing volume.[9] Based on these principles, Carroll et al.[46] and Lomholt[47] suggested that the ideal cuff diameter should be approximately one-and-one-half times the tracheal diameter, while Cooper and Grillo[9] stated that a true low-pressure cuff should have a resting diameter of more than 2.5 cm.

The cuff resting diameter of most modern ETs is larger than the tracheal diameter. These cuffs should, therefore, easily maintain their low-pressure characteristics when inflated to the volume that just seals the trachea. If, however, a large-volume cuff continues to be inflated beyond the sealing volume, high pressure will be generated in the cuff as the tracheal wall limits its expansion. Cuff pressure will increase under these

circumstances even if the cuff volume is still below its natural resting volume.

b. MUCOSAL CONTACT PRESSURE

Tracheal-tissue damage associated with endotracheal intubation is largely dependent on the cuff pressure against the tracheal mucosa (mucosal contact pressure).[10] Mucosal contact pressure reflects intracuff pressure only with true large-volume cuffs where the trachea is sealed without any circumferential tension in the cuff wall. In the case of the red rubber low-volume, high-pressure cuff, circumferential tension in the cuff wall will develop as the cuff seals the trachea. Under this condition, mucosal contact pressure will be significantly less than cuff pressure, since part of the latter is consumed to stretch the cuff itself.[48,49]

c. DYNAMIC CHARACTERISTICS OF CUFF PRESSURE IN VENTILATED PATIENTS

During intermittent positive-pressure ventilation, cuff pressure rises to match the rise in airway pressure during inspiration (Fig. 35-6).[50] This helps maintain an airtight seal of the trachea during inspiration in the face of the accompanying rise in airway pressure.

d. AIRTIGHT VERSUS FLUID-TIGHT SEAL

It is important to recognize that airtight seal by a large-volume, low-pressure cuff does not necessarily guarantee fluid-tight seal of the trachea.[51] Because of the large resting diameter that most modern cuffs have compared with the tracheal diameter, folds develop in the cuff when it is inflated to achieve a clinical seal. These folds or wrinkles may predispose to channeling and aspiration of pharyngeal contents.

Several factors may influence the incidence of channeling during the use of large-volume cuffs:[51]

i. Relationship between cuff and tracheal diameter. If the cuff resting diameter approaches tracheal diameter, no infoldings occur and leaks are minimized. Based on this fact, Mackenzie et al.[52] and Mehta and Myat[53] recommended that cuff circumference and diameter at residual volume approximate that of the trachea.

ii. Cuff pressure. If the cuff is inflated to high pressure sufficient to compress the channels, leaks will cease.

iii. Viscosity of aspirated fluid. Gastric fluid, which has less viscosity than blood, is associated with a greater rate of leakage.

iv. Cuff material. If the cuff is thick and less pliable, the internal diameters of the invaginations are larger, and hence are associated with larger leaks.[54,55]

v. Mode of ventilation. Negative pressure during spontaneous ventilation enhances leakage. Continuous positive-pressure ventilation, particularly in the presence of PEEP, provides some protection against seepage.[56]

e. MINIMUM SAFE CUFF PRESSURE

Lomholt[47] suggested that the minimum pressure of the cuff on the tracheal mucosa required to prevent

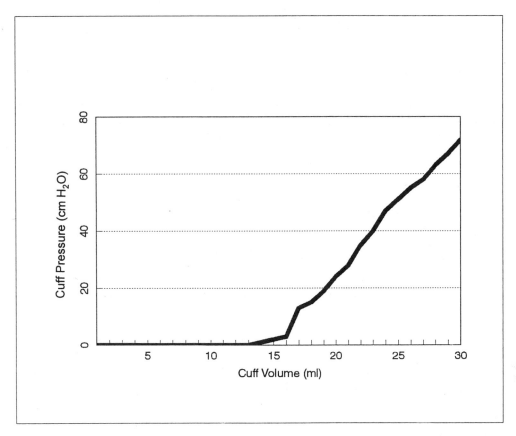

Fig. 35-5. Compliance curve of the cuff pictured in Fig. 35-4 when inflated with air. When inflated beyond its resting volume (15 ml), the cuff started to acquire high-pressure characteristics.

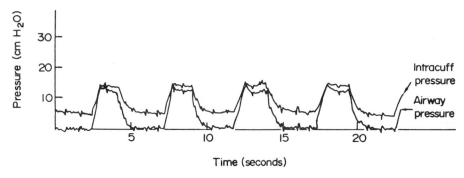

Fig. 35-6. Variation of intracuff and airway pressure for high-volume cuff in a mechanically ventilated patient. (From Crawley M, Cross D: *Anaesthesia* 30:4, 1975.)

aspiration is equal to the hydrostatic pressure from the column of vomitus, blood, and so on that may fill the mouth, pharynx, or trachea above the cuff. This hydrostatic pressure depends on the vertical distance from the upper part of the cuff to the mouth and changes with the position of the patient, being 10 to 15 cm in the supine position and 15 to 20 cm in the erect. As a safety precaution, he recommended selecting a pressure 5 cm H_2O higher—that is, 20 cm H_2O in the supine position and 25 cm H_2O in the erect—as the safe minimum cuff pressure during expiration. Bernhard et al.,[55] in a

randomized clinical trial, supported this recommendation by demonstrating that the minimum intracuff pressure necessary to prevent aspiration of dye placed in the pharynx past large-diameter, low-pressure cuffs was 25 cm H_2O.

However, the protective effect of such relatively low cuff pressure was seriously questioned by Seegobin and van Hasselt,[57] who showed a 100% incidence of aspiration of dye instilled through the vocal cords immediately above the cuff with large-volume cuffs inflated to a pressure of 25 cm H_2O. Fiberoptic bronchoscopy clearly showed that passage of dye in that study was related to the folds created by excess cuff material. In addition, inflating the cuffs to a pressure of 50 cm H_2O did not obliterate the dye-filled folds, and dye could still be seen tracking along the folds. They concluded that while a large-volume, cuffed ET might afford protection against ingression of particulate material, surface-tension forces and capillary action might lead to liquids tracking along the folds despite increased intracuff pressures.

f. MAXIMUM SAFE CUFF PRESSURE

Large-volume cuffs have favorable characteristics and can produce a clinical seal at low cuff pressures. Such tubes, however, are still capable of generating high intracuff- and mucosal-contact pressures when overinflated beyond the seal point.[58] It is therefore not surprising that tracheal injury continues to be reported with the use of these ETs.[59-61] Nordin et al.[62] studied the relationship between cuff pressure and capillary perfusion of the rabbit tracheal mucosa and recommended that cuff pressure be kept below 20 mm Hg (27 cm H_2O). Seegobin and van Hasselt[63] reached similar conclusions in an in vitro study. They assessed tracheal mucosal blood flow in 40 patients using an endoscopic photographic technique while varying the cuff inflation pressure. They found overpressurizing cuffs impaired mucosal blood flow, and recommended cuff-inflation pressure not exceed 30 cm H_2O.

g. METHODS OF CONTROLLING CUFF PRESSURE

Based on available data, limiting pressure in large-volume cuffs to 25 cm H_2O seems to prevent significant aspiration and still allow adequate capillary mucosal blood flow. Estimation of cuff pressure by palpating the pilot balloon was shown to be unreliable.[64] Therefore, a more objective assessment of cuff pressure in the ventilated patient is needed.

This can be accomplished simply by repeated measurement of cuff pressure. With each measurement, however, the cuff loses some air, which may with time significantly decrease cuff volume.[19] Alternatively, air could be injected into the cuff via a three-way stopcock connected to a pressure manometer.

Several devices have been described for continuous control and regulation of cuff pressure in the ventilated patient.[65] The ideal device should be capable of compensating for any reduction as well as any increase in cuff pressure, and should allow cuff pressure to rise with the inspiratory rise in airway pressure. It should also allow for adjustment of the end-expiratory cuff pressure setting, since some patients with severely reduced lung compliance may require high airway pressures for adequate ventilation, and may develop air leak if the end-expiratory cuff pressure is fixed at 25 cm H_2O. This last feature, however, is not available.

III. CONSIDERATIONS FOR USE OF DOUBLE-LUMEN ENDOTRACHEAL TUBES FOR LONG-TERM VENTILATION

A. CHOICE OF SIDE OF DOUBLE-LUMEN TUBE

Benumof et al.[66] defined the margin of safety in positioning double-lumen tubes (DLTs) as the length of tracheobronchial tree over which it may be moved or positioned without obstructing a conducting airway. They concluded that left-sided DLTs were much preferable to right-sided DLTs because they had a much greater positioning margin of safety because left mainstem bronchi are significantly longer than right mainstem bronchi. While the recommendation that left-sided DLTs be used routinely may not be universally accepted during thoracotomy,[67] left-sided DLTs are the tubes of choice during long-term ventilation in the absence of contraindications to their use, such as left mainstem bronchial tumor, stenosis, or compression.

B. CHOICE OF SIZE OF LEFT DOUBLE-LUMEN TUBE

The optimal left DLT size for a particular patient may be defined as the largest DLT that passes without trauma through the larynx and fits in the left mainstem bronchus with only a small air leak detectable while the bronchial cuff is deflated. Use of the largest possible tube minimizes airway resistance, facilitates bronchial toilet, and ensures that bronchial seal is obtained with small bronchial-cuff volume, below the resting volume, thus maintaining the low-pressure characteristics of the cuff.[68] The presence of some air leakage before cuff inflation ensures that the tube is not tightly impacted in the bronchus, and should minimize the chances of bronchial damage.

Based on this definition, an objective choice of DLT size for a particular patient should take into consideration the following diameters of the DLT and the patient's airway:

1. Outside diameter of DLT

The outside diameter (OD) of DLTs is considerably larger than that of routinely used ETs. As an example, the OD of size 37 French-gauge (Fr) and 39 Fr Robertshaw DLTs is 13 and 14 mm, respectively, which corresponds to the OD of size 9.0- and 10.0-mm ID (internal diameter) ETs.[69] As a result of the large size, using DLTs for prolonged periods in mechanically ventilated patients is likely to be associated with a higher incidence of laryngeal injury and edema compared with using regular-sized ETs.

2. Internal diameter of DLT lumens

The ID of each lumen of a DLT is relatively small. Chiaranda et al.[69] estimated the effective mean ID of

Table 35-1. Outside diameter (mm) of left-lumen tip of different sizes and brands of double-lumen tubes (DLT)

Manufacturer/ DLT Size	35 Fr	37 Fr	39 Fr	41 Fr
Mallinckrodt*	9.5	10.0	10.1	10.6
Rusch*	9.4	10.1	10.8	11.5
Sheridan*	9.3	9.9	9.9	10.7
Portex**	9.7	10.2	11.2	12.0

*Data from Benumof JL, Partridge BL, Salvatierra C et al: *Anesthesiology* 67:729, 1987. **Data from Hollister W (Concord/Portex Company): Personal communication, 1992.

each lumen of Robertshaw DLTs, whose cross-sectional shape is mostly semioval, by closing each channel at its tip and measuring the amount of water necessary to fill it. The effective IDs were then calculated from the volume and length of the corresponding cylinder, and were found to be 7.06, 7.38, and 7.47 mm for the bronchial lumens of left-sided Robertshaw DLTs sized 37 Fr, 39 Fr, and 41 Fr, respectively.

3. Outside diameter of DLT tip

The OD of the bronchial end can vary significantly between different DLT brands and between different sizes of the same brand (Table 35-1). The size of the bronchial cuff increases the effective diameter by 1 to 2 mm.

4. Left mainstem bronchial diameter

Left mainstem bronchial diameter was measured on routine preoperative posteroanterior (PA) chest x-rays of 100 patients of known age, sex, and height, and a formula was used to correct for the magnification of intrathoracic structures on PA views.[70] The bronchial diameter measured 12.4 ± 1.5 mm and 10.7 ± 1.0 mm (mean ± SD) in males and females, respectively (Fig. 35-7). In males only, age and height produced statistically significant prediction of left bronchial diameter. Left mainstem bronchial diameter had a relatively wide range compared to the narrower range of diameters of the bronchial end of different left DLTs.

These data suggest that in most females and in small, particularly young, males, the bronchial tube of even the smallest adult left DLT (35 Fr) with its surrounding cuff will fit tightly in, and may even stretch, the left mainstem bronchus. Most males, however, should safely accommodate larger-sized left DLTs.

If left mainstem bronchial outline is clear on a patient's chest x-ray, it can be directly measured. In a standard PA view, the actual bronchial diameter is usually 8% to 10% smaller than projected on the film. Alternatively, left mainstem bronchial diameter can be measured on the chest CT scan when available.[71] A DLT with a bronchial end that is 1 to 2 mm smaller in

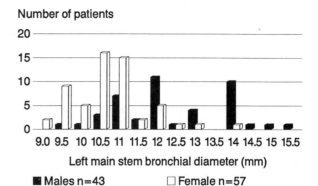

Fig. 35-7. Frequency of different left-mainstem bronchial diameters in 100 patients as measured on routine preoperative chest x-rays. (From Hannallah MS et al: *Anesth Analg* 78:S150, 1994.)

diameter than that of the patient's left mainstem bronchus should be optimal for that patient.

C. CHOICE OF TYPE OF DOUBLE-LUMEN TUBE

Different types of modern, disposable DLTs can vary significantly in their characteristics. As mentioned earlier, the OD of the bronchial end differs between different left-DLT brands and sizes. Table 35-2 illustrates how the resting volume of the bronchial cuff differs between left DLTs. In addition, the bronchial cuff of different left DLTs vary in shape. Whereas the left Rusch and Portex DLTs have a barrel-shaped bronchial cuff, the left Mallinckrodt DLT has a donut-shaped bronchial cuff, and the left Sheridan DLT has a fusiform-shaped bronchial cuff. The fusiform-shaped cuff was shown to require higher volume and pressure to seal the bronchus compared with the other cuffs.[72,73]

Consideration of these differences in DLT characteristics may be important under certain circumstances. In individuals with small left mainstem bronchial diameters, it may be safe to choose the 35-Fr left DLT with the smallest bronchial end and the smallest bronchial cuff resting volume. In individuals with very large left mainstem bronchial diameters, it may be easier to seal the left bronchus while maintaining the low-pressure characteristics of the bronchial cuff if we choose the size 41-Fr DLT with the largest bronchial end, and with a large resting volume. Since excessive folds in the bronchial cuff may predispose to seepage of secretions past the cuff, it is prudent to avoid using the type of left DLTs with too large a bronchial cuff relative to the size of the patient's left bronchus, particularly if the risk of aspiration is significant.

D. DETERMINATION OF OPTIMAL DLT POSITION

Brodsky et al.[74] showed that the average depth of insertion of left DLTs for both male and female patients

Table 35-2. Resting volume of different sizes and brands of left double-lumen tubes (DLTs) (ml) (mean ± SD)

DLT type	DLT size			
	35 Fr	37 Fr	39 Fr	41 Fr
Mallinckrodt	3.7 ± 0.2	2.5 ± 0.0	2.0 ± 0.0	2.0 ± 0.0
Sheridan	2.5 ± 0.0	2.0 ± 0.0	2.0 ± 0.0	2.0 ± 0.0
Rusch	1.5 ± 0.0	1.5 ± 0.3	1.4 ± 0.2	2.1 ± 0.2
Portex	2.5 ± 0.2	2.5 ± 0.0	4.8 ± 0.4	4.2 ± 0.2

From Hannallah MS, Benumof JL, Bachenheimer LC et al: The resting volume and compliance characteristics of the bronchial cuff of left PVC double-lumen endobronchial tubes, *Anesth Analg* 77:1222, 1993.

170 cm tall was 29 cm, measured from the corner of the mouth, and that for each 10 cm increase or decrease in height, average placement depth was increased or decreased 1 cm. These findings provide a useful initial guide to left-DLT placement. Auscultation alone has been repeatedly shown to be an unreliable method of confirming the position of DLTs in the tracheobronchial tree.[75-78] It should, therefore, always be followed by fiberoptic bronchoscopy. The fiberoptic bronchoscope should also be readily available at the bedside whenever a DLT is used for long-term ventilation to ascertain tube position routinely and whenever a sudden change in lung mechanics or gas exchange suggests the possibility of DLT malposition.

E. OPTIMAL BRONCHIAL CUFF VOLUME

Airtight seal and satisfactory lung collapse during thoracotomy can be achieved with little or no air in the bronchial cuff of left DLTs.[79] Since an airtight seal does not guarantee a fluid-tight seal, larger bronchial cuff volumes may be required to prevent seepage of secretions past the cuff. On the other hand, cuff overinflation can cause bronchial-mucosal damage and has been reported to cause bronchial rupture.[80,81] The following precautions are, therefore, recommended to ensure lung protection against cross contamination without causing bronchial damage during long-term DLT placement. First, do not inflate the bronchial cuff beyond its resting volume. If the bronchial cuff of a properly placed left DLT fails to seal the bronchus when inflated to its resting volume, the tube is likely to be too small for that patient. Second, monitor bronchial cuff pressure during and repeatedly after cuff inflation, and maintain it at a maximum of 25 cm H_2O. Third, avoid using a DLT with an excessively large bronchial cuff relative to the size of the patient's airway, because it is likely to form excessive folds and predispose to channeling. Finally, extreme caution is needed when considering bronchial cuff inflation in small individuals, since even small DLTs can fit tightly inside the left bronchus, a situation associated with significant reduction in bronchial cuff compliance.[82]

F. LONG-TERM USE OF UNIVENT TUBE

The Univent tube is an endotracheal tube with a movable bronchial blocker used for selective one-lung ventilation.[83] A major advantage of this tube over double-lumen ETs is that the Univent tube does not have to be replaced with a single-lumen ET following major thoracic surgery if postoperative mechanical ventilation is required.[83] Instead, the blocker is simply retracted into a channel situated on the anterior concavity of the tube, allowing the Univent tube to function as a standard ET. However, if the blocker's cuff is unintentionally inflated when the blocker is incompletely retracted, the inflated blocker will block the main lumen of the tube, resulting in serious airway obstruction.[84] Adequate training of ICU nurses in using the Univent tube, therefore, is important to prevent this complication. Removal of the blocker's pilot balloon at the conclusion of surgery will eliminate the risk of this complication, but also will result in loss of the blocker's function were lung isolation to be required postoperatively. Alternatively, the pilot balloon of the bronchial-blocker cuff can be covered with tape to avoid inadvertent inflation of the bronchial balloon.[85]

Another important consideration for the long-term use of the Univent tube is that the outside diameter of this tube is significantly larger than that of an ET with comparable internal diameter because of the space occupied by the blocker. Prolonged use of the Univent tube is, therefore, associated with a higher potential for laryngeal complications than that associated with the use of an ET of similar size. In addition, the large outside diameter of the Univent tube can potentially cause bronchial damage if the tube is advanced too deeply into a bronchus.[86]

IV. RESPIRATORY CARE OF INTUBATED PATIENTS

Placing an ET for perioperative airway management is performed with the goal of securing a reliable conduit through which to deliver and remove respiratory and anesthetic gases while ensuring the integrity of the respiratory system. While a properly sized and positioned ET performs these roles admirably and with a high margin of safety, it circumvents and impedes a number of important airway functions for optimizing pulmonary gas exchange. Understanding the normal physiology of the airway and how placement of an artificial conduit impairs these functions are essential if the clinician desires to obviate these effects while caring for intubated patients.

A. IMPAIRMENT OF MUCOCILIARY FUNCTION AND ITS TREATMENT

1. Physiologic and anatomic considerations

The upper airway of the respiratory system, which includes the nasal passages, oral cavity, and pharyngeal and laryngeal structures, exists to facilitate the movement of air to and from the lungs, and to condition the air passing through them. This latter function includes filtering, humidification, and heating inspired gases. These functions are attenuated to varying degrees when an ET is placed. Heating and humidification can be viewed as passive processes predominantly, governed by which airway routes air traverses and by thermodynamic factors such as flow rate, inspiratory temperature, and relative humidity. The process of filtering, however, is a more complex phenomenon involving active and passive processes necessary for removal of particulate matter and aerosol deposition throughout the respiratory airways. Clearance of deposited matter becomes one of the primary functions of the mucociliary system, whether the deposited material consists of inhaled particles, microorganisms, or other cellular debris.

The site of particle deposition is a result of the influence of particle size, route of inspired gases, and airway geometry.[87,88] The arborization of the airway results in a narrow cross-sectional diameter for the upper airways of the conducting zone relative to the transitional and respiratory zones of the lower airways, such that at constant airflow rates the velocity of air in the upper airway is much greater than the lower airway. Large particulate matter contained in high-velocity flows tend not to change direction with changes in air-flow geometry because of inertia, resulting in their selective impaction along the upper airway. Particles of 10 microns in diameter or greater tend to impact against nasal hairs and the lining of the upper airway where airway geometry changes the air-flow directional vector, or at branch points along its continuum. Thus, particle size follows an inverse relationship with deposition distance in the airway. The result is that the vast majority of gross particulate material is filtered by the upper airway, which for this purpose can include the conducting airways. In all cases, the final site of impaction is on the mucosal surface of the airway and lining of the alveoli.

The mucociliary complex consists of epithelial cells lining the airway and the overlying fluid layers. The cell layer is comprised mainly of ciliated pseudostratified columnar cells interspersed with mucin-secreting goblet cells in a ratio of 5:1. Ciliated cells are found from the nasal passages to the respiratory bronchioles, decreasing as a percentage of the total cells lining the airway as one progresses from the upper to the lower airways.[89] Ciliary movement is biphasic, with a fast, extended, forward

power stroke followed by a slower, relaxed, return stroke. Beat frequency is uniform and averages 11 to 15 strokes per second.[90] Arranged linearly, each cilium contracts in a coordinated fashion with adjacent cilia so that the net result is a propagated wave, or metachronal movement, propelling secretions out of the airway (Fig. 35-8). In the nasopharynx the net motion is caudal toward the oropharynx, whereas in the tracheobronchial tree the flow is directed cephalad to the pharynx. Secretions are then either swallowed or expectorated by cough.

The fluid layer overlying the cilia has two distinct components (see Fig. 35-8).[91] The layer directly adjacent to the epithelium is the sol, or periciliary layer, and is composed of relatively nonviscous serous fluids that impede ciliary motion minimally. Over this lies the gel, or mucous layer, made up of fluids with greater viscoelastic properties, such as mucus. Coordinated ciliary motion propels the floating gel layer forward, along with its impacted particles, dissolved aerosols, and cellular components. The depth of the sol layer is critical for optimal ciliary function and is maintained at a level equal to the length of the outstretched cilia. This allows cilia to contact the gel layer barely during the fast power stroke and propel it forward.[92,93] Factors that increase or decrease sol-layer depth, such as dehydration or inadequate humidification of inspired gases, adversely affect the efficiency of ciliary motion. Increased sol depth uncouples ciliary movement from the overlying gel layer, while decreased sol depth leads to impediment of ciliary motion and loss of net gel flow. In normal subjects optimal mucociliary function results in mucous flow rates of 5 to 10 mm per minute in the trachea, and correspondingly slower rates distal to that.[94] This prevents mucus buildup and plugging from occurring, as mucous flows converge from small airways into large conducting airways. As a result, clearance time of the conducting airways in healthy patients is on the order of 6 hours.[95]

2. Mucociliary impairment in intubated patients

Physical placement of an ET, as well as therapies administered subsequent to placement, are responsible for impaired mucociliary function after intubation. Several studies delineate the alteration in ciliary function occurring with general anesthesia. Nunn et al.[96] demonstrated a reversible, dose-dependent depression of ciliary motility by halothane in protozoan species, and inferred a similar effect in mammalian cilia, given the highly conserved structure of cilia throughout nature. In intubated patients undergoing gynecological procedures with mechanical ventilation, halothane nearly abolishes tracheal mucous flow after 90 minutes, and causes marked edema and increased secretions of the tracheo-

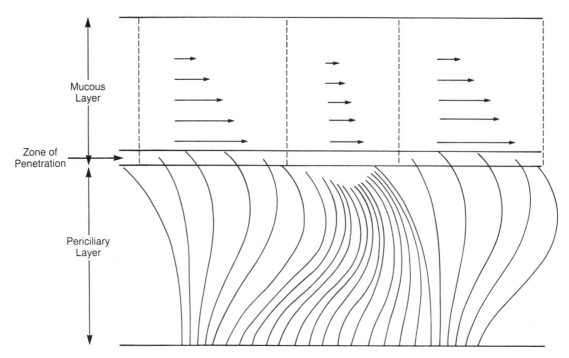

Fig. 35-8. Ciliary motion resulting in forward flow of mucus. Coordinated beating motion (metachrony) of cilia in nonviscous sol layer results in transfer of mechanical energy to mucous layer via zone of penetration where cilia-mucus contact is made. (From Bates DV, King M: Particle deposition: mucociliary clearance: physical signs. In Bates DV, editor: *Respiratory function in disease,* ed 3, Philadelphia, 1989, W.B. Saunders.)

bronchial tree as visualized by bronchoscopy.[97] In an attempt to separate the effects of anesthesia from factors attributable to the ET and the methodology used to assess mucous transport, Forbes and colleagues[98-100] carried out a number of experiments using a dog model. Using a less invasive method of measuring flow rates that involved deposition of radioactive droplets instead of placement of Teflon disks, and controlling the physico-chemical characteristics of the inspired gases to minimize their effects on mucociliary function (i.e., low Fio_2, high humidity, and optimal temperature), he showed a dose-dependent and reversible decrease in mucous transport rates as the minimal alveolar concentration (MAC) of halothane was increased from 1 to 3,[98] and showed similar results for enflurane and morphine sulfate/N_2O at equivalent MAC doses.[99] Curiously, ether did not demonstrate a similar effect. Pentothal was also responsible for mucociliary impairment when compared to halothane, and appeared to have a more rapid onset of action.[100]

In a more recent study, Konrad et al.[101] called into question whether all intravenous or inhalation anesthetic agents should be classified as mucociliary depressants. His group measured mucociliary transport by a scintillographic method—a far less invasive technique—in humans undergoing abdominal surgery and found no effect on mucociliary transport rates. Their use of fentanyl, pancuronium, and nitrous oxide as the anesthetic, which is associated with minimal cardiovascular-depressant effects compared to previous work using volatile agents, argues whether other agents with similar cardiovascular profiles might not have similar effects on mucociliary transport.

Anesthetic agents do not seem to alter mucociliary function by any alteration of viscoelastic or transport properties of human respiratory mucus. Samples of mucus from nonsmoking, intubated patients who were free of lung disease, taken immediately after induction of general anesthesia and again after several hours elapsed, showed no difference in the physical characteristics of mucus, such as rigidity, viscoelasticity, spinnability, or percentage composition of solid material. Standardization of anesthetic administration was not performed in this study, but the results seem valid for the range of anesthetic drugs used.[102]

Oxygen has been implicated in altered mucociliary function. In both animal[103] and pulmonary studies of disease-free humans,[104] oxygen has both a time-dependent and concentration-dependent depressant effect on tracheal mucous transport, with a geometric decrease in the time relationship to mucociliary impairment as inspired oxygen concentration rises from 50% to 100%.

Direct physical factors related to the ET seem also to

be important. Sackner et al.[105] showed that mucous velocity 3 to 5 cm distal to an inflated cuff was significantly reduced in anesthetized dogs compared to when uncuffed tubes were used. Furthermore, there were no differences in mucous velocity between dogs with uncuffed tubes and dogs without endotracheal tubes. The researchers postulated that either damming of mucous flow by the distended ET cuff or neurogenic factors related to cuff impingement on the tracheal mucosa could be contributory. Mechanical ventilation through an ET resulted in a decrease in mucociliary transport when compared to intubated but spontaneously ventilating dogs under general anesthesia.[106] In addition, there was no difference in transport rates between spontaneously ventilated and anesthetized animals that were intubated and those that were not.

Konrad et al.[107] examined whether clinical outcomes could be inferred from reductions in mucociliary transport of intubated patients. Patients in a surgical intensive care unit were followed prospectively for pulmonary complications following intubation after tracheobronchial transport rates were determined by a scintigraphic method within the first 3 days of instituting mechanical ventilation. Pulmonary complications were defined as evidence of increased secretion retention and/or new onset of pneumonia up to 4 days after transport velocities were determined. Impaired mucus transport occurred frequently in these ventilated patients, and those with impaired transport had a significantly higher incidence of pulmonary complications subsequently. This complements an earlier study in which radiopaque powder was insufflated in patients undergoing abdominal and orthopedic surgery at the end of the operation. The orthopedic surgery group had complete clearance of the powder after 48 hours, whereas the abdominal surgery group retained the powder up to 6 days. Moreover, this decreased clearance was significantly associated with postoperative segmental and lobar atelectasis.[108]

In summary, it appears that impaired mucociliary function is a frequent occurrence in the intubated patient. The cause is probably multifactorial, and can include depression of ciliary motility by anesthetic agents and high concentrations of inspired oxygen, physical impairment of mucous transport by the presence of an ET, modes of ventilatory support through an ET, inadequate conditioning of inspired gases, and the overall general medical condition of intubated patients postoperatively. Despite the paucity of data to indicate that controlling any of these factors has an effect on patient outcome, clinicians must routinely use methods to mimic normal mucous transport and disposal, cognizant that in most cases the specific reason for having the ET in place precludes attempts to mitigate its adverse mucociliary influence.

3. Optimizing pulmonary toilet for intubated patients
a. CHEST PHYSIOTHERAPY

A variety of maneuvers assist intubated patients in mobilizing and removing pulmonary secretions, thereby reducing resistance to air flow and improving pulmonary gas exchange. While the most common postoperative pulmonary complication is atelectasis (due to many causes), accumulation of secretions can specifically lead to further airway occlusion and contribute to atelectasis and lung collapse. Chest physiotherapy maneuvers assume added importance for intubated patients because the normal filtering mechanisms of the upper airway are circumvented by an ET. This permits direct transmission of airborne microbial contamination to the lungs that, in combination with mucous stasis and probable seepage of upper gastrointestinal flora past the ET, results in an ideal medium for nosocomial pulmonary infection. Collectively these maneuvers are termed chest physiotherapy (CPT) and, used with suctioning methods, can enhance the clearance of pulmonary secretions.

CPT has an extensive literature in patients with enhanced bronchopulmonary secretions, impairments in secretion clearance, development of atelectasis, or a combination of all three.[109,110] The majority of these patients are not intubated, and so applicability of these studies to the intubated patient is unclear. While CPT is performed routinely on intubated patients in ICUs and postanesthesia-care units, there is a paucity of data supporting its rationale and benefit. However, its clinical utility is well accepted in spite of the lack of objective criteria.

The traditional modes of CPT used most often clinically to aid in the removal of pulmonary secretions include the following.[111]

i. Postural drainage. This involves the selective positioning of patients to enhance the flow of secretions out of affected segments or lobes of the lung and into the mainstem bronchus and trachea, where they can be removed by coughing or suctioning.

ii. Percussion and vibration. These techniques employ applied rhythmic forces against the chest wall, adjacent to affected areas of lung, to aid in the dislocation and movement of mucus and retained secretions out of the targeted areas. They appear to augment postural drainage and forced expiratory techniques.[112] Newer methods include the use of high-frequency oscillations.[113]

iii. Cough clearance. This is combined with the two previous methods to eliminate mobilized secretions once they have reached the central conducting airways. In an intubated patient who is unable to close the glottis and generate sufficient expectorative pressure, this maneuver is minimally useful.

iv. Forced-expiration techniques. This maneuver consists of huffing at midlevel lung volumes with an open glottis, in distinction to the closed glottic efforts of coughing, and is another effective method for promoting clearance.

Other modes of CPT focus on inspiratory maneuvers, such as intermittent positive-pressure breathing, incentive spirometry, and deep-breathing exercises. While effective in improving postoperative atelectasis, particularly after cardiothoracic and upper-abdominal surgery, these methods are almost exclusively reserved for extubated patients, and have little, if any, benefit in secretion removal.

In a small cohort of intubated and nonintubated patients with acute lobar atelectasis, positioning, vibration, hyperinflation, and suctioning compared with suctioning and hyperinflation alone resulted in a greater degree of resolution in the former (60%) versus the latter group (8%) after one treatment, but the difference between groups was marginally significant after a total of six treatments. No statistical inferences could be drawn to differentiate between outcomes for intubated and nonintubated patients because of the small sample size. Nevertheless, aggressive CPT led to a more prompt resolution of atelectasis.[114]

Mackenzie and colleagues described a large group of young, postoperative trauma patients who underwent CPT while on mechanical ventilation.[115] When CPT was performed for specific clinical indications on these patients, such as increasing secretions, worsening blood-gas parameters, or radiologic evidence of consolidation, there was a significant clinical and radiographic improvement within twenty-four hours without any increase in Pao_2.[116]

Postural-drainage techniques can be combined with body positioning and rotation in critically ill patients and patients with respiratory compromise. These latter maneuvers can ameliorate ventilation-perfusion mismatch and intrapulmonary shunting in diseased lungs.[117,118] However, conventional postural-drainage techniques are cumbersome and frequently inappropriate for many intubated patients. Mechanical disruption and accidental removal of ETs and invasive monitors, as well as trauma to the patient, can occur during positioning. Continuous mechanical rotation has emerged in an attempt to circumvent some of the hazards of positioning changes in intubated and/or critically ill patients. These methods rely on rotational bed movement or changes in air-flow distribution in air-supported mattresses to mimic traditional posture and positioning. Several studies have demonstrated improvements in respiratory-related parameters when using these modalities, such as decreasing the duration of mechanical ventilation and length of hospital stay in patients with pneumonia,[119] or reducing the rate of nosocomial pneumonia in ICU patients with a variety of diagnoses on admittance.[120,121] These studies encompass a mixture of nonintubated and

intubated patients from different ICUs, however; whether the subset of intubated patients can have the same statistical inferences drawn is unknown. Early mobilization and positioning, even in the intubated patient, can play a major, perhaps dominant, role in respiratory recovery when performed as part of CPT.[122]

Performing CPT can have measurable effects on hemodynamic, pulmonary, and metabolic parameters, which raises concerns with intubated and/or critically ill patients. The stress response occurs despite adequate patient sedation.[123] Oxygen consumption, heart rate, and cardiac index can all increase markedly during and after CPT, to levels 30% to 50% above patient baseline.[124] Age and presence of overt cardiac disease in intubated and nonintubated patients who are critically ill strongly predict which patients are likely to exhibit cardiac arrhythmias during CPT.[125] Younger patients on mechanical ventilation tend to have far fewer changes in cardiac performance with CPT, and tend to improve lung/thorax compliance and decrease intrapulmonary shunting after therapy.[126] In critically ill patients on mechanical ventilation, providing 100% oxygen prior to CPT eliminates the decrease seen in Pao_2.[127]

Finally, several studies questioned the utility of CPT in surgical patients. They did not specifically address the intubated surgical or postsurgical patient discreetly, but did find there is little conclusive evidence that CPT improves ventilation and enhances clearance of secretions in surgical patients generally. They concluded these maneuvers appeared only to benefit patients with enhanced sputum production.[128,129] Mackenzie and colleagues argue that lack of standardization in protocols for delivering CPT among different studies looking at benefits and outcomes, or definitions on what even constitutes CPT, could be a dominant factor when deciding whether CPT benefits any given patient population.[115]

b. SUCTIONING

Suctioning the ET provides the means for removing all unwanted bronchopulmonary secretions from the intubated patient, be they mucus, blood, or gastric contents. It can be used as a single-mode therapy or in conjunction with CPT. Its use in the intubated patient is universal—prophylactically, as a maneuver performed prior to extubation, to clear the airway as best as possible, or to obtain sputum samples for diagnostic purposes.

A number of suction catheters are available in a variety of sizes. Most employ materials and designs that attempt to minimize trauma to mucosal surfaces while optimizing the removal of secretions. Hence the tips tend to be soft with blunted ends, and have multiple distal orifices so that mucosal or mucous occlusion of one orifice does not lead to excessive suction pressure. They should be sized so they will fit easily through the ET and allow efficient removal of secretions, without removing too much air so as to cause hypoxemia and atelectasis. As a general rule this size should be less than half the diameter of the ET, or:[130]

$$\text{maximal diameter (Fr)} = \text{internal diameter (mm)} \times \frac{1}{2}$$

Methods have been devised to minimize the potential for hypoxemia and atelectasis associated with ET suctioning. ET suctioning can also lead to increases in oxygen extraction, as documented by decreasing mixed-venous oximetry readings without a change in arterial-oxygen saturation.[131] Hyperinflation performed by itself prior to suctioning prevents desaturation during routine suctioning in less than 25% of patients. Increasing the Fio_2 to 1.0 before suctioning did raise Sao_2 and Pao_2, and was synergistic when combined with hyperinflation.[132] Saline is often instilled through the ET before suctioning, in the hope of mobilizing mucus and facilitating its removal. This practice should be used with caution, particularly in patients with marginal arterial-oxygen saturation. Instilling 5 ml of saline can lead to significant declines in Sao_2 percentage as long as 4 to 5 minutes after suctioning.[133]

Recent catheter and elbow-connector designs attempt to mitigate some of the deleterious effects associated with their use. Closed-ended suction catheters are introduced through self-sealing diaphragms in the elbow connector, where they can be advanced into an ET while the patient is maintained on mechanical ventilation without disconnection. This method is superior to conventional open-ended techniques, even when patients undergoing open-ended suctioning are hyperoxygenated before suctioning. The hemodynamic stress response to suctioning is attenuated or abolished, and arterial- and venous-oxygen saturations increase, rather than decrease, as with open-ended systems. These systems are cost effective as well, in both material and labor resources.[134] Simultaneous instillation and suctioning ports in one catheter have been used and shown to increase the capture rate of secretions without changing any of the patient-response characteristics during suctioning.[135]

Trauma to the airway is a well-recognized complication of ET suctioning. Mucosal erosions, ulcerations, and airway edema occur after only several passings of the catheter. Not surprisingly, continuous suction techniques cause greater damage than intermittent suction.[136] Adverse physiologic responses are common with suctioning. Cardiac dysrhythmias, changes in blood pressure and heart rate, cardiac arrest, bronchoconstriction, and increases in intracranial pressure have all been reported and are seen frequently. Bradycardia, secondary to vagal stimulation during tracheal suctioning, is particularly common. Pretreating with nebulized atropine at a dose of 0.05 mg/kg appears to attenuate this response without

---

BOX 35-1 Guidelines for ET suctioning

- Sterile technique
  Nosocomial/universal precautions
- Sizing of catheter (see text)
- Preoxygenation
  $1.5 \times VT$ (Tidal Volume) for 5-10 breaths
  Prevent hypoxemia
- Hyperventilation
  Synchronize with patient
  Avoids barotrauma/hypotension
- Limit suction pressure
  <110 mm Hg
- Limit suction duration
  <10 seconds per pass
- Use intermittent technique
  Prevents mucosal trauma
- Saline for catheter lubrication
- Lavage sparingly
  Decreases Pao_2/Sao_2
  For tenacious sputum only
- Hyperinflation after suctioning
  Prevents atelectasis/hypoxia
- Resume previous Fio_2
- Consider use of elbow connector with self-sealing diaphragm
  For patients who desaturate during suctioning
  For patients who require very frequent suctioning

---

causing significant increases in heart rate or blood pressure.[137] In intubated patients with head injuries, where increases in intracranial pressure (ICP) can have serious sequelae, thorough preoxygenation followed by limited duration of suction (less than 10 seconds) and less than three suction attempts can minimize increases in ICP.[138]

In general, to deliver safe and effective ET suctioning, the guidelines listed in Box 35-1 should be followed. These guidelines are adapted from the clinical-care procedures at Georgetown University Medical Center, compiled from current accepted standards of practice supported by the literature. In-line catheter systems are not used routinely, but are reserved for patients for whom even brief periods of disconnection from ventilatory support would lead to profound cardiopulmonary compromise, or cases where pulmonary secretions are excessive and warrant frequent suctioning.

c. HUMIDIFICATION

The need for transferring heat and water to inspired gases is another important tenet of upper-airway physiology. At 37° centigrade, the saturated amount of water vapor in air, or absolute humidity, is 43.9 mg/L. Relative humidity is the expression of the ratio of actual water content to the absolute at a given temperature. Normal, quiet nasal breathing of room air results in an inspired relative humidity of 99% and temperature of 33° to 35° C at the subglottic level.[139,140]

Ciliary function depends on this adequate humidification, without which mucous flow is reduced or ceases.[141] The critical nature that humidification plays is exemplified by studies comparing tracheal histological damage during conventional and high-frequency ventilation in lambs under conditions of low (30%) and high (90%) humidity. Histologic gradings were similar after 6 hours of ventilation at either conventional or high-frequency rates at high humidity, and comparable to nonintubated controls. On the other hand, low-humidity animals had severe erosions and necrosis regardless of the methods of ventilation, extending 3 to 4 cm beyond the tip of the ET.[142]

In an intubated patient whose upper airway has been bypassed, current recommendations for humidification and temperature of inspired air lie between 28 and 34 mg/L and 32° to 34° C, respectively.[143] This corresponds to a relative humidity of 95% to 100%. To achieve this in an inspiratory system, heat and moisture must be added or conserved. This is accomplished by one of several methods.

i. Heat and moisture exchanger/condenser (HME). Commonly referred to as "artificial noses," these devices serve as reservoirs for heat and humidity of expired air. They minimize the loss of both during exhalation by condensing and entrapping water vapor in a system of cellulose sponge or other synthetic material proximal to the ET, which then aids in warming and humidifying subsequent inspired breaths. They cannot overheat or overhumidify, and require no external power source. Their advantages include simplicity, size, disposability, and low cost. They find their greatest clinical utility in the operating-room environment and for short-term intubated patients.

An in vitro study of the major brands of commercially available HMEs showed that none achieved minimal efficiency in keeping inspired water content at or above the recommended level of 31 to 33 mg/L.[144] In clinical practice, however, most of the HMEs do achieve satisfactory and recommended levels of efficiency in a short period of time (10 minutes), and are able to conserve 5% to 7% of all metabolic heat production during anesthesia.[145]

ii. Heated humidifier (HH). These devices most accurately replicate the function of the upper airway by actively heating and humidifying inspired air. Air is blown over or wicked or bubbled through a heated water bath, giving it the capacity to provide 100% humidification at any set temperature. They can be limited by high gas-flow rates, but handle the vast majority of clinical applications. Because they can heat inspired air, they must have control mechanisms that limit temperature output of the bath and/or monitor and regulate inspired-

gas temperature. This is usually accomplished by a feedback servo device monitoring temperature at the distal end of the inspired limb. Their capacity to provide 100% humidification leads to significant condensation in respiratory tubing. Care must be taken to ensure that accumulated condensed water does not flow into the patient by keeping the humidifier below the height of the patient. These devices are more expensive and complicated, require a power source, and thus potentially pose an additional electrical hazard. However, the HH is the device of choice in most intubated patients outside of the operating room who require long-term ventilation, or ventilated patients with problems with excessive or abnormal secretions.

Variants of the HH are those without the heated element, the so-called bubble-through humidifiers. These devices are of little use in intubated patients, principally because of limits to the degree to which they are able to humidify inspired air (around 40%) and their low-flow capacity, typically 1 to 5 L/min.

iii. Nebulizer. There are two types of nebulizers, an ultrasonic device and a pneumatically powered one. Both deliver a mixture of water vapor and fine water droplets to the inspiratory limb. While the water content being delivered to the patient can be quite high, the relative humidity is often less than 100%. Their output is difficult to control, resulting in excessive levels of condensation. The characteristics of delivered gas, with a high number of water droplets, have been implicated in exacerbating wheezing and coughing in patients with preexisting lung pathology. In general, they are used less frequently because of these reasons, and because of concerns about enhanced transmission rates of microbial contamination.[146] Postoperative intubated patients who were spontaneously breathing, with normal lung functions, were found to have significant increases in their $P(A-a)_{O_2}$ gradients with nebulized, compared to conventional cascade, humidifiers.[147]

Several clinical studies have compared HMEs and HHs in intubated patients. Cohen et al. found a high rate of ET occlusion with HMEs. This led to a switch to HHs because of this concern and the failure of HMEs to provide adequate humidification for patients who were being ventilated for several days or more. Patients with occluded ETs had a higher incidence of pneumonias and atelectasis, though this did not reach statistical significance.[148] More recently, Misset et al. examined patients during a 5-day course of therapy with one of the humidification methods. Patients with HMEs had thicker secretions at the end of the trial, and required higher amounts of tracheal instillations. HMEs were associated with significant cost savings compared to HHs, and demonstrated excellent filtering capability. Bacterial colonization rates between the two groups were similar. The recommendations were to use HMEs in patients without excessive secretions or enhanced need for suctioning.[149]

4. Nosocomial pneumonia in intubated patients

While the issue of pulmonary infections is not usually covered in a discussion of respiratory care of intubated patients, it is relevant given the goals inherent to them. These are: (1) the assumption of aspects of mucociliary function that minimize the effects of secretions as a cause of alterations in pulmonary gas exchange, and (2) providing an environment that does not encourage microbial infection. Placing an ET not only impairs the patient's ability to clear microbial contamination, it also provides a direct conduit for further contaminants. Multivariate analysis of risks for acquiring nosocomial pneumonia (NP) point to the strong predictive value of endotracheal intubation as a factor in its development. This assumes even greater importance in light of the high rate of mortality (30% to 50%) associated with NP.[150]

Contamination can occur from a variety of sources. The most obvious is from the ET itself. Fortunately, for short-term use of an ET, this is rarely a relevant clinical issue. However, 27% of tracheal cultures taken after oropharyngeal intubation show isolates of possible pulmonary pathogens from oropharyngeal sources.[151] Preexisting colonization prior to intubation is also a potential source. Patients undergoing upper abdominal surgery showed high rates of colonization immediately after being intubated, as determined by tracheal cultures taken at time of intubation, particularly in smokers with *Haemophilus influenza* species. Those patients who were colonized had an increased risk of developing pneumonia postoperatively.[152] In children, colonization of the buccal mucosa is an important antecedent to developing ET colonization.[153] Probably the most important source of contamination of the tracheobronchial tree occurs as a result of silent aspiration of gastroesophageal contents around the ET cuff, for reasons that have been delineated previously. Forty percent of intubated patients in ICU or operating room settings can have gastroesophageal contents recovered from their tracheas.[154] In one ICU, 52% of intubated patients with gastric isolates developed pneumonia.[155] Collectively, these studies point to the risks of bacterial contamination after intubation and the ease with which they are transmitted.

Few mechanical methods exist to lessen the risk of bacterial contamination. Clearly one of the most important is strict observance of sterile technique when manipulating the ET in intubated patients. When methods are undertaken to prevent water condensation on ETs in patients, ETs removed from those patients show far lower rates of bacterial colonization than tubes without condensation prevention.[156] Deppe reported that using a contained, attached suction-catheter system resulted in higher rates of colonization compared to open-suction systems. However, rates for developing NP were similar. Furthermore, patients who did not develop NP had lower overall mortality rates if the closed system was used, suggesting some added benefit of the closed-suction system.[157] A specially designed ET, the Hi-Lo Evac tube (Mallinckrodt), allows for the drainage of subglottic-but-above-the-cuff secretions without additional suction catheters. Used in patients who had been intubated for 3 or more days and suctioned hourly in an attempt to limit gastric content ingress, patients with this subglottic-supracuff secretion-drainage system had one half the rate of NP compared to patients with traditional suctioning methods. They also developed NP twice as slowly as the control group, and had significant reductions in their rates of ET colonization. No additional complications were seen with its use.[158] These results are quite encouraging and warrant further clinical trials to validate or refute them.

Much attention has focused on the role of stress-ulcer prophylaxis in the genesis of NP. Histamine-2 receptor antagonists, by modifying the gastric milieu and increasing its pH, may promote the overgrowth of pathogens in this altered environment, which can translocate and cause serious respiratory infections in critically ill patients. Attempts to employ other types of cytoprotective agents that do not promote pathogenic growth have had moderate success. A meta-analysis of studies examining this issue shows that sucralfate is as effective as antacids and more effective than H_2 blockers in preventing stress ulcers, while associated with a 50% reduction in the rates of NP.[159] This helped clarify a major earlier study, which showed that while sucralfate was associated with half the rate of NP compared to patients on antacids and H_2 blockers, the results did not reach statistical significance.[160] More recent work has focused on the infectious etiology of peptic ulcer disease with *Heliobacter* species;[161] their exact role in the intubated patient, whether critically ill or not, has yet to be defined.

5. Pharmacologic therapy delivery systems

A review of airway pharmacology has been provided (see Chapter 4). Agents that promote bronchodilation by affecting the smooth muscle tone of the airway are equally effective in both intubated an nonintubated patients.

Most of these agents demonstrate direct ciliary effects in addition to their bronchodilating properties. β-adrenergic and cholinergic agents show strong effects on ciliary function. In isolated tracheal preparations they increase ciliary beat frequency and improve mucus flow.[162] Methylxanthines are ciliary stimulants as well, and are beneficial in promoting mucociliary clearance.[163]

The delivery of these agents through ETs can be affected by the characteristics of the delivery system used. Drug particle size must fall within the range of 1 to 5 microns in diameter for the agent to reach its targeted area of the lung, the small conducting airways. Particle sizes greater than 5 microns are likely to impact on the ET surface or the large conducting airways, where they exert little effect.[164] Actuators are designed expressly for delivering drugs through ETs, as opposed to handheld inhalers used in nonintubated patients. When compared to typical manufacturer-supplied inhalers, these actuators deliver less drug in the effective particle range per metered dose, ranging from 11% to 66% of the dose delivered by the standard inhaler. However, the vast majority of total drug volume delivered by the drug manufacturer-supplied inhaler/actuator consisted of particles greater than 5 microns, whereas virtually none of the ET-specific actuators delivered drug particles that exceeded this size. Thus the efficiency of the ET-designed actuator are greater than the manufacturer-supplied inhaler in delivering effectively sized drug particles.[165] The number of puffs delivered should be increased to account for the reduction in total effective particle volume supplied by ET-specific actuators by a factor of 1.5 to 8, depending on the specific type of actuator used. As a corollary, efficiency of delivery also was related to size of the ET, with larger tubes delivering proportionally more drug per dose. In addition, activation of dose inhalers at the midpoint in the inspiratory flow resulted in greater delivery when compared to activating before inspiratory flow was initiated.[166]

Attempts have been made to increase the amount of delivered aerosolized bronchodilators in intubated patients above that attainable with ET-specific actuators. Several studies advocate the use of narrow-lumen catheters attached directly to metered-dose inhalers (MDI), which can then be advanced beyond the tip of the ET.[167-169] These systems permit aerosolization of the drug directly at the tracheal-carinal border, minimizing the major cause of drug loss—impaction along the ET and proximal trachea. Using these systems can result in appreciable increases in delivery efficiency over ET-specific actuators, from 2% to 12% of a metered dose being delivered to 20% to 90% effective delivery. One such system can be constructed easily from a 60-ml syringe, a standard MDI, a bronchoscopy elbow-port adapter, and either a long 18-gauge intravenous catheter or an 8-Fr suction catheter, as pictured in Figure 35-9.[167] The catheter is attached to the open syringe with the MDI placed inside, and the unit is advanced through the bronchoscopy port until the catheter tip lies beyond the ET. Simply pushing the plunger actuates the MDI, with care being given to maintain the MDI canister upright while activating it to ensure maximal delivery of each dose. The system is reusable and can be positioned when needed through the elbow adapter. To increase further the efficiency of delivery, a narrow-bore catheter should be used with an internal diameter of 1 mm or

less.[169] Creating a slight flare on the end of the catheter will minimize the amount of drug deposited on the trachea and carina as well, increasing the amount of drug delivered to its effective site on the small conducting bronchioles.

B. CONSIDERATIONS FOR USE OF FLEXIBLE FIBEROPTIC BRONCHOSCOPY IN MECHANICALLY VENTILATED PATIENTS

Flexible fiberoptic bronchoscopy (FFB) is a valuable technique for airway management.[170] Its role in the placement of endotracheal and endobronchial tubes, in the exchange of these tubes, and in the extubation of the trachea has been discussed elsewhere in this book. In addition to these functions, FFB plays an important diagnostic and therapeutic role in the management of the mechanically ventilated patient.

1. Diagnostic functions of the fiberoptic bronchoscope in ventilated patients

The fiberoptic bronchoscope (FOB) can be used diagnostically in a number of ways. First, the FOB can confirm ET position; as discussed earlier, FFB can be used to position the tip of the ET optimally in the trachea. Second, the FOB can confirm ET patency; FFB can rule out the ET as the site of airway obstruction caused by secretions, external compression such as biting, an overdistended cuff, or a foreign body.[33] Third, FFB can aid in the diagnosis of the specific cause of pneumonia.[171,172] Various techniques using FFB can obtain culture material in mechanically ventilated patients. These include bronchoalveolar lavage, the protected specimen brush, and transbronchial lung biopsy. Simple bronchoscopic aspiration for this purpose is usually unreliable because of contamination of the bronchoscope during its passage through an ET. Fourth, FFB can help in diagnosis of the cause and site of hemoptysis.[173] FFB can be very useful in the management of patients with hemoptysis, particularly if the more distal airways are the source of bleeding. The likelihood of localizing the bleeding site is significantly higher with early, compared to late, FFB.[174] If the hemoptysis is massive, the rigid bronchoscope offers better suction capabilities. Finally, FFB can help make the definitive diagnosis of tracheobronchial injury. FFB can be used to inspect the airway before extubation to rule out complications of prolonged or difficult intubation. It can also be useful in the diagnosis of tracheal and bronchial disruptions in the trauma patient,[175] and in the management of bronchopleural fistula.[176]

2. Therapeutic function of the fiberoptic bronchoscope in ventilated patients
a. BRONCHOPULMONARY TOILET

FFB can be useful in the treatment of lobar or segmental atelectasis caused by retained secretions in

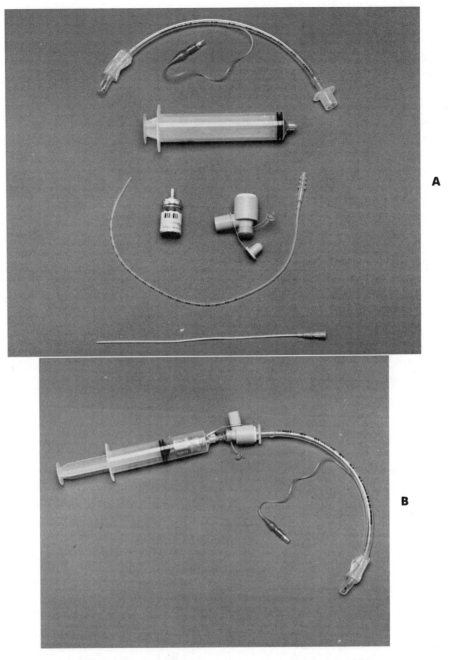

Fig. 35-9. A, Individual components of an MDI (metered-dose inhaler) administration system for intubated patients. Either a suction catheter (8 French) or intravenous catheter (18 gauge) can be used. **B,** Assembled system inserted through an endotracheal tube (ET), with the tip of the catheter extending beyond the end of the ET. (Adapted from Dunteman E, Despotis G: *Anesth Analg* 75:303, 1992.)

the ventilated patient.[177] However, the exact role of this technique versus chest physiotherapy is controversial. In a prospective randomized study of the usefulness of FFB followed by respiratory therapy compared to respiratory therapy alone for the treatment of acute lobar atelectasis, Marini et al. concluded that FFB did not provide any additional benefit.[178] Nevertheless, the

wide use of FFB to manage retained secretions, mucous plugs, and atelectasis has been recommended for all age groups.[179]

In most cases, FFB should not be the first step in the management of atelectasis. Less expensive and invasive techniques, including chest physiotherapy, incentive spirometry, and tracheal suctioning should be employed first. If these measures fail to clear atelectasis, FFB is a reasonable second step.

Compared to routine blind suctioning, using FFB allows inspection of different segmental bronchi and directing the suction port to ones that are occluded. Occasionally FFB can identify an unsuspected cause for atelectasis other than secretions. Some patients may require repeat bronchoscopies if secretions reaccumulate. FFB is an appropriate first choice for the management of atelectasis in patients with chest trauma, spinal fractures, and severe head injury for whom respiratory therapy may not be optimal.[177] Benefit from FFB is doubtful in patients with retained secretions without atelectasis[177] or in the presence of air bronchogram in the atelectatic lobe or segment.[178] The latter is likely to indicate nonoccluded proximal bronchi.[180]

b. REFRACTORY ASTHMA WITH MUCOUS IMPACTION

If an exacerbation of an asthmatic attack fails to respond to aggressive medical management, mucous impaction may be suspected. Lang et al.[181] demonstrated significant clinical and spirometric improvement and clearance of inspissated secretions in these patients using fiberoptic bronchoscopy with lavage.

c. HEMOPTYSIS

Several fiberoptic bronchoscopy–based procedures have been described for the treatment of hemoptysis, particularly for high-risk or inoperable patients. These include selective deposition of fibrin precursors,[182] thrombin or fibrinogen-thrombin combinations[183] into the bleeding bronchial segment, and selective endobronchial tamponade with a Fogarty-type balloon.[184]

d. FOREIGN-BODY EXTRACTION

FFB can be useful in the extraction of foreign bodies, particularly those located distally in segmental and subsegmental bronchi.[185]

Contraindications to FFB in the ventilated patient include inexperienced personnel and inadequate facilities. Conditions that increase the risk of the procedure and are therefore considered relative contraindications include unstable asthma, severe hypoxemia, refractory life-threatening arrhythmias, unstable angina, recent myocardial infarction, severe refractory hypotension, hypercarbia, increased intracranial pressure, and uncontrolled seizures.[186]

3. Technique

The OD of readily available adult FOBs ranges from 4.0 to 6.0 mm.[187] When a 5.0-mm OD bronchoscope is inserted into size 7.0-, 7.5-, or 8.0-mm ID ET, the area remaining within the tube will be equivalent to that of an ET size of 4.9-, 5.6-, or 6.2-mm ID, respectively.[188] Ideally, therefore, size 8.0-mm ID or larger ETs should be placed when size 5.0-mm OD bronchoscopes are used. If a smaller ET was in place and if its replacement

with a larger ET for the bronchoscopy was believed to be unsafe, several alternatives to changing the tube have been suggested:[8] (1) using a smaller adult or pediatric FOB, particularly for diagnostic procedures; (2) performing the bronchoscopy expeditiously and with careful monitoring of airway pressures through the existing ET; (3) passing the FOB through the glottis alongside the ET;[189] (4) using helium-oxygen mixture for ventilation during the procedure (the low density of helium may improve air flow through the ET); and (5) performing a tracheostomy.

Anticholinergic premedication prior to bronchoscopy has several advantages. It (1) improves pulmonary mechanics through its bronchodilating properties, (2) reduces bronchial secretions, and (3) prevents possible bradycardia from vagal stimulation.[190] However, it should be used cautiously in patients with cardiac disease.

Topical lidocaine can be directly applied through the suction channel of the bronchoscope. Because of its rapid absorption by the tracheobronchial mucosa, the maximum adult dose should be limited to 200 mg.[191] The administration of anxiolytic and amnestic agents, as tolerated by the patient, together with topical anesthetics, improve the patient's tolerance and acceptance of the procedure.

When FFB is performed for bronchopulmonary toilet, the use of an FOB with a large suction port makes it particularly effective in clearing thick, tenacious secretions and mucous plugs. Multiple injections of 3 to 5 ml of saline in short, high-pressure bursts directly on the plugs is helpful in dislodging tenacious material.[177] If the mucous plug cannot be cleared with saline alone, n-acetylcysteine can be used.[192]

Once the mucous plug is removed, high transpulmonary pressure is needed to overcome the critical opening pressure of the collapsed lobar segment. This can be accomplished by deep breathing and vigorous coughing. Alternatively, in critically ill patients, this can be accomplished by sequentially wedging the FOB in the affected bronchi. Air or oxygen-enriched air is then insufflated until complete reexpansion is achieved.[193,194] The use of an FOB with a balloon for reexpansion of refractory atelectasis has also been described.[195,196]

Mechanically ventilated patients undergoing FFB should be monitored by an experienced individual other than the endoscopist. Minimal acceptable monitoring should include pulse oximetry, electrocardiography, blood-pressure measurements, and close observation of tidal volume and airway pressures.

Delivering oxygen via the suction-biopsy port of the FOB should help clear secretions and may improve oxygenation in patients with borderline pulmonary function. The successful use of this port to provide jet ventilation has also been described.[197]

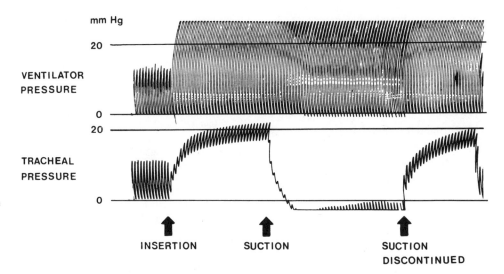

Fig. 35-10. Simultaneous recording of ventilator and intratracheal pressure in a dog during controlled mechanical ventilation through an endotracheal tube of 7.0 mm internal diameter. Insertion of a 5.7-mm outside-diameter bronchoscope resulted in immediate elevation of peak inspiratory ventilator pressure caused by airway obstruction. There was a more gradual elevation of peak intratracheal pressure and a marked PEEP (positive end-expiratory pressure) effect of 16 mm Hg. When a negative pressure of 62 mm Hg was applied to the suction port of the bronchoscope, intratracheal pressure became continuously negative, indicating removal of air from lungs in spite of unchanged ventilator function. Discontinuation of suction gradually restored presuction intratracheal pressures, which finally returned to control values upon removal of bronchoscope (at very end of recording). (From Lindholm CE, Ollman B, Snyder JV et al: *Chest* 74:362, 1978.)

4. Complications

In one prospective[198] and two retrospective studies[199,200] of complications following FFB in both intubated and nonintubated patients, the mortality rate ranged from 0.01% to 0.1%, and the range of major complications ranged from 0.09% to 1.7%. Suratt et al.[200] found that all patients who died had at least one of the following serious underlying diseases: cardiovascular disease, severe chronic pulmonary disease, or cancer.

Hypoxemia and hypercarbia are potentially serious complications of FFB in the mechanically ventilated patient. They can be precipitated by excessive suctioning during the procedure. Suction eliminates any PEEP the patient may be dependent on, and decreases lung volume to well below the functional residual capacity (Fig. 35-10).[201,202] These effects will lead to progressive airway closure, venous admixture, and, ultimately, hypoxemia. Suction also causes reduction in tidal volume and alveolar ventilation, leading to hypercarbia. These effects are exaggerated if the tidal volume delivered to the trachea is compromised by a small residual cross-sectional airway in the event a relatively small ET is used. The use of relatively small-sized ETs during FFB may also prevent complete exhalation, leading to PEEP. If the resulting PEEP is moderate, it may initially improve oxygenation.[201] However, if excessive, PEEP predisposes to barotrauma and cardiovascular instability. Hypoxia

and hypercarbia during FFB could also result from the use of large volume of bronchial lavage or local anesthetic solutions because they could completely fill the terminal air units.[203]

Based on these considerations, the following recommendations are important when performing FFB in critically ill patients during mechanical ventilation.[201] (1) If possible, use ET size 8.0-mm ID or larger. (2) Closely monitor and if needed, adjust tidal volume, flow rate, and airway pressure, particularly the end-expiratory pressure. (3) Increase Fio_2 to 1.0. (4) Monitor visually for adequate chest excursions. (5) Suction for short periods only. (6) Use small volumes of irrigation solutions. (7) Continually monitor arterial-oxygen saturation. (8) Consider x-ray examination of the chest after FFB in high-risk patients to rule out mediastinal emphysema and pneumothorax.

Sinus tachycardia is common during FFB.[199,204] Sinus bradycardia due to reflex vagal stimulation can also be seen.[204] Hypertension, tachycardia, and an increase in cardiac index and mean pulmonary-artery occlusion pressure were reported during FFB under topical anesthesia and were attributed to reflex sympathetic discharge caused by mechanical irritation.[205] In some patients these hemodynamic changes were associated with ischemic changes on the electrocardiogram. In a prospective study of cardiac rhythm during FFB, the incidence of major cardiac arrhythmias was 11%.[206] However, all the arrhythmias were self-limited and had no hemodynamic consequences. Hypoxemia, defined as Pao_2 less than 60 mm Hg, at the end of the procedure was found to correlate significantly with the development of new major arrhythmias. Prevention of hypoxemia, by performing high-frequency jet ventilation during suctioning of the tracheobronchial trees of dogs, prevented significant changes in pulse rate or blood pressure.[207] The use of excessive doses of sedatives, opioids, or local anesthetics during FFB is another cause of hemodynamic instability, particularly in critically ill patients.

Mechanical irritation by the bronchoscope may precipitate bronchospasm, particularly in patients with hyperreactive airways. Belen et al. demonstrated that optimizing therapy for patients with chronic obstructive pulmonary disease prior to the procedure has a protective effect against developing bronchospasm.[190]

Pneumothorax and hemorrhage are recognized complications of transbronchial biopsy during mechanical ventilation, particularly in high-risk patients.[186,208,209] Although fiberoptic bronchoscopy is feared to precipitate herniation in patients with increased intracranial pressure as a result of coughing,[185] a retrospective study by Bajwa et al.[210] concluded that the procedure carried low risk in these patients.

REFERENCES

1. Wright PE, Marini JJ, Bernard GR: In vitro versus in vivo comparison of endotracheal airflow resistance, *Am Rev Respir Dis* 140:10, 1989.
2. Gal TJ, Suratt PM: Resistance to breathing in healthy subjects following endotracheal intubation under topical anesthesia, *Anesth Analg* 59:270, 1980.
3. Sahn SA, Lakshminarayan S, Petty TL: Weaning from mechanical ventilation, *JAMA* 235(20):2208, 1976.
4. Sullivan M, Paliotta J, Saklad M: Endotracheal tube as a factor in measurement of respiratory mechanics, *J Appl Physiol* 41(4):590, 1976.
5. Demers RR, Sullivan MJ, Paliotta J: Airflow resistance of endotracheal tubes, *JAMA* 237(13):1362, 1977.
6. Bolder PM, Healy TE, Bolder AR et al: The extra work of breathing through adult endotracheal tubes, *Anesth Analg* 65:853, 1986.
7. Shapiro M, Wilson R, Casar G et al: Work of breathing through different sized endotracheal tubes, *Crit Care Med* 14(12):1028, 1986.
8. Stone DJ, Bogdonoff DL: Airway considerations in the management of patients requiring long-term endotracheal intubation, *Anesth Analg* 74:276, 1992.
9. Cooper JD, Grillo HC: Analysis of problems related to cuffs on intratracheal tubes, *Chest* 62(2)(suppl):21, 1972.
10. Scott LR, Benson MS, Bishop MJ: Relationship of endotracheal tube size to auto-PEEP at high minute ventilation, *Respir Care* 31:1080, 1986.
11. Matsushima Y, Jones R, King E et al: Alterations in pulmonary mechanics and gas exchange during routine fiberoptic bronchoscopy, *Chest* 86(2):184, 1984.
12. Bryce DP, Briant TD, Pearson FG: Laryngeal and tracheal complications of intubation, *Ann Otol Rhinol Laryngol* 77:442, 1968.
13. Harrison GA, Tonkin JP: Prolonged endotracheal intubation, *Br J Anaesth* 40:241, 1968.
14. Hilding AC: Laryngotracheal damage during intratracheal anesthesia, *Ann Otol Rhinol Laryngol* 80:565, 1971.
15. Hawkins DB: Glottic and subglottic stenosis from endotracheal intubation, *Laryngoscope* 87:339, 1977.
16. Stout DM, Bishop MJ, Dwersteg JF et al: Correlation of endotracheal tube size with sore throat and hoarseness following general anesthesia, *Anesthesiology* 67:419, 1987.
17. Bishop MJ, Weymuller EA, Fink BR: Laryngeal effects of prolonged intubation, *Anesth Analg* 63:335, 1984.
18. Stenqvist O, Sonander H, Nilsson K: Small endotracheal tubes: ventilator and intratracheal pressures during controlled ventilation, *Br J Anaesth* 51:375, 1979.
19. Steen JA: Impact of tube design and materials on complications of tracheal intubation. In Bishop MJ, editor: *Physiology and consequences of tracheal intubation: problems in anesthesia*, vol 2(2), Philadelphia, 1988, J.B. Lippincott.
20. Owen RL, Cheney FW: Endobronchial intubation: a preventable complication, *Anesthesiology* 67:255, 1987.
21. Zwillich CW, Pierson DJ, Creagh CE et al: Complications of assisted ventilation: a prospective study of 354 consecutive episodes, *Am J Med* 57:161, 1974.
22. Saunders CE, Sedman AJ: Left mainstem bronchus intubation, *Am J Emerg Med* 2:406, 1984.
23. Conrardy PA, Goodman LR, Lainge F et al: Alteration of endotracheal tube position: flexion and extension of the neck, *Crit Care Med* 4(2):8, 1976.
24. Brunel W, Coleman D, Schwarz D et al: Assessment of routine chest roentgenograms and the physical examination to confirm endotracheal tube position, *Chest* 96(5):1043, 1989.
25. Bekemeyer WB, Crapo RO, Calhoun S et al: Efficacy of chest radiography in a respiratory intensive care unit, *Chest* 88:691, 1985.
26. Henschke CI, Pasternack GS, Schroeder S et al: Bedside chest radiography: diagnostic efficacy, *Radiology* 149:23, 1983.
27. Stauffer JL, Olson DE, Petty TL: Complications and consequences of endotracheal intubation and tracheostomy: a prospective study of 150 critically ill adult patients, *Am J Med* 70:65, 1981.
28. Strain DS, Kinasewitz GT, Vereen LE et al: Value of routine daily chest x-rays in the medical intensive care unit, *Crit Care Med* 13:534, 1985.
29. Birmingham PK, Cheney FW, Ward RJ: Esophageal intubation: a review of detection techniques, *Anesth Analg* 65:886, 1986.
30. Eagle CC: The relationship between a person's height and appropriate endotracheal tube length, *Anaesth Intensive Care* 20:156, 1992.
31. Sosis MB, Harbut RE: A caution on the use of routine depth of insertion of endotracheal tubes, *Anesthesiology* 74:961, 1991.
32. Dornette WH: *Anatomy for the anesthesiologist*, Springfield, Ill, 1963, Charles C Thomas.
33. Ovassapian A: Fiberoptic airway endoscopy in critical care. In Ovassapian A, editor: *Fiberoptic airway endoscopy in anesthesia and critical care*, New York, 1990. Raven Press.
34. Whitehouse AC, Klock LE: Evaluation of endotracheal tube position with fiberoptic intubation laryngoscope, *Chest* 68(6):848, 1975.
35. O'Brien D: Fibre-optic assessment of tracheal tube position: a comparison of tracheal tube position as estimated by fibre-optic bronchoscopy and by chest x-ray, *Anaesthesia* 40:73, 1985.
36. Tasota FJ et al: Evaluation of two methods used to stabilize oral endotracheal tubes, *Heart Lung* 16(2):140, 1987.
37. Fenje N, Steward DJ: A study of tape adhesive strength on endotracheal tubes, *Can J Anaesth* 35(2):198, 1988.
38. Shroff PK, Parton KR, Thomson JH et al: A simple method of securing an endotracheal tube, *AANA J* 55(5):404, 1987.

39. Gonzales JG: Securing an endotracheal tube, *Anesthesiology* 65:347, 1986.
40. Latto IP: The cuff. In Latto IP, Rosen M, editors: *Difficulties in tracheal intubation,* London, 1985, Bailliere Tindall.
41. Guyton DC: Endotracheal and tracheotomy tube cuff design: Influence on tracheal damage. In Civetta JM, Taylor RW, Kirby RR, editors: *Critical care updates,* vol 1(3), Philadelphia, 1990, J.B. Lippincott.
42. Cooper JD, Grillo HC: The evolution of tracheal injury due to ventilatory assistance through cuffed tubes: a pathologic study, *Ann Surg* 169(3):335, 1969.
43. Cooper JD, Grillo HC: Experimental production and prevention of injury due to cuffed tracheal tubes, *Surg Gynecol Obstet* 129:1235, 1969.
44. Grillo HC, Cooper JD, Geffin B et al: A low-pressure cuff for tracheostomy tubes to minimize tracheal injury: a comparative clinical trial, *J Thorac Cardiovasc Surg* 62:898, 1971.
45. Geffin B, Pontoppidan H: Reduction of tracheal damage by the prestretching of inflatable cuffs, *Anesthesiology* 31:462, 1969.
46. Carroll RG, McGinnis GE, Grenvik A: Performance characteristics of tracheal cuffs. In Wyant GM, editor: *Problems in the performance of anesthetic and respiratory equipment: international anesthesiology clinics,* vol 12(3), Boston, 1974, Little, Brown.
47. Lomholt N: A new tracheostomy tube: theoretical considerations on minimum cuff pressure, *Acta Anaesthesiol Scand Suppl* 44:6, 1971.
48. Bunegin L, Albin M, Smith RB: Canine tracheal blood flow after endotracheal tube cuff inflation during normotension and hypotension, *Anesth Analg* 76:1083, 1993.
49. Mehta S: Endotracheal cuff pressure, *Br Med J* 288:1763, 1984.
50. Crawley BE, Cross DE: Tracheal cuffs: a review and dynamic pressure study, *Anaesthesia* 30:4, 1975.
51. Pavlin EG, VanNimwegan D, Hornbein TF: Failure of a high-compliance low-pressure cuff to prevent aspiration, *Anesthesiology* 42:216, 1975.
52. Mackenzie CF, Shin B, Whitley N et al: Human tracheal circumference as an indicator of correct cuff size, *Anesthesiology* 53:S414, 1980.
53. Mehta S, Myat HM: The cross-sectional shape and circumference of the human trachea, *Ann R Coll Surg Engl* 66:356, 1984.
54. Petring OU: Prevention of silent aspiration due to leaks around cuffs of endotracheal tubes, *Anesth Analg* 65:777, 1986.
55. Bernhard WN, Cottrell JE, Sivakumaran C et al: Adjustment of intracuff pressure to prevent aspiration, *Anesthesiology* 50:363, 1979.
56. Janson BA, Poulton TJ: Does peep reduce the incidence of aspiration around endotracheal tubes? *Can J Anaesth* 33:157, 1986.
57. Seegobin RD, van Hasselt GL: Aspiration beyond endotracheal cuffs, *Can J Anaesth* 33:273, 1986.
58. Black AM, Seegobin RD: Pressures on endotracheal tube cuffs, *Anaesthesia* 36:498, 1981.
59. Berlauk J: Prolonged endotracheal intubation vs. tracheostomy, *Crit Care Med* 14:742, 1986.
60. Stauffer J, Olson D, Petty TH: Complications and consequences of endotracheal intubation and tracheostomy, *Am J Med* 70:65, 1981.
61. Kastanos N et al: Laryngotracheal injury due to endotracheal intubation: incidence, evolution, and predisposing factors: a prospective long-term study, *Crit Care Med* 11:362, 1983.
62. Nordin U, Lindholm CE, Wolgast M: Blood flow in the rabbit tracheal mucosa under normal conditions and under the influence of tracheal intubation, *Acta Anaesth Scand* 21:81, 1977.
63. Seegobin RD, van Hasselt GL: Endotracheal cuff pressure and tracheal mucosal blood flow: endoscopic study of effects of four large volume cuffs, *Br Med J* 288:965, 1984.

64. Fernandez R: Endotracheal tube cuff pressure assessment: pitfalls of finger estimation and need for objective measurement, *Crit Care Med* 18:1423, 1990.
65. Resnikoff E, Katz JA: A modified epidural syringe as an endotracheal tube cuff pressure-controlling device, *Anesth Analg* 11:208, 1990.
66. Benumof JL, Partridge BL, Salvatierra C et al: Margin of safety in positioning modern double-lumen endotracheal tubes, *Anesthesiology* 67:729, 1987.
67. Burk WJ III: Should a fiberoptic bronchoscope be routinely used to position a double-lumen tube? *Anesthesiology* 68:826, 1988.
68. Brodsky JB, Shulman MS, Mark JB: Malposition of left-sided double-lumen endotracheal tubes, *Anesthesiology* 62:667, 1985.
69. Chiaranda M, Rossi A, Manani G et al: Measurement of the flow-resistive properties of double-lumen bronchial tubes in vitro, *Anaesthesia* 44:335, 1989.
70. Hannallah MS, Benumof JL, Ruttimann UE: The relationship between left mainstem bronchial diameter and patient size, *J Cardiothoracic Vasc Anesth* 9:119, 1995.
71. Slinger P: Choosing the appropriate double-lumen tube: a glimmer of science comes to a dark art, *J Cardiothoracic Vasc Anesth* 9:117, 1995.
72. Slinger PD, Chripko D: A clinical comparison of bronchial cuff pressures in three different designs of left double-lumen tubes, *Anesth Analg* 77:305, 1993.
73. Brodsky JB, Adkins MO, Gaba DM: Bronchial cuff pressures of double-lumen tubes, *Anesth Analg* 69:608, 1989.
74. Brodsky JB, Benumof JL, Ehrenwerth J et al: Depth of placement of left double-lumen endobronchial tubes, *Anesth Analg* 73:570, 1991.
75. Alliaume B, Coddens J, Deloof T: Reliability of auscultation in positioning of double-lumen endobronchial tubes, *Can J Anaesth* 39:687, 1992.
76. Lewis JW, Serwin JP, Gabriel FS et al: The utility of a double-lumen tube for one-lung ventilation in a variety of noncardiac thoracic surgical procedures, *J Cardiothorac Vasc Anesth* 6:705, 1992.
77. Hurford WE, Alfille PH: A quality improvement study of the placement and complications of double-lumen endotracheal tubes, *J Cardiothorac Vasc Anesth* 7:517, 1993.
78. Benumof JL: The position of a double-lumen tube should be routinely determined by fiberoptic bronchoscopy, *J Cardiothorac Vasc Anesth* 7:513, 1993.
79. Hannallah MS, Benumof JL, McCarthy PO et al: Comparison of three techniques to inflate the bronchial cuff of left polyvinal chloride double-lumen tubes, *Anesth Analg* 77:990, 1993.
80. Burton N, Fall S, Lyons T et al: Rupture of the left mainstem bronchus with polyvinyl chloride double-lumen tube, *Chest* 9:928, 1983.
81. Hannallah MS, Gomes M: Bronchial rupture associated with the use of a double-lumen tube in a small adult, *Anesthesiology* 71:457, 1989.
82. Hannallah MS, Benumof JL, Bachenheimer LC et al: The resting volume and compliance characteristics of the bronchial cuff of left PVC double-lumen endobronchial tubes, *Anesth Analg* 77:1222, 1993.
83. Kamaya H, Krishna P: New endotracheal tube (Univent tube) for selective blockade of one lung, *Anesthesiology* 63:342, 1985.
84. Dougherty P, Hannallah MS: A potentially serious complication that resulted from improper use of the Univent tube, *Anesthesiology* 77:835, 1992.
85. Schwartz RE, Stayer SA, Pasquariello CA: Univent tube: a simple method for avoiding a potentially disastrous complication, *Anesth Analg* 77:1077, 1993.
86. Hannallah MS: Pneumothorax complicating the use of the

Univent endotracheal tube: a different mechanism, *Anesth Analg* 77:200, 1993.

87. Clarke SW, Pavia D: Deposition and clearance. In Murray JF, Nadel JA, editors: *Textbook of respiratory medicine,* Philadelphia, 1988, W.B. Saunders.

88. Bates DV, King M: Particle deposition: mucociliary clearance: physical signs. In Bates DV, editor: *Respiratory function in disease,* ed 3, Philadelphia, 1989, W.B. Saunders.

89. Serafini SM, Michaelson ED: Length and distribution of cilia in human and canine airways, *Bull Eur Physiopath Respir* 13:551, 1977.

90. Rutland J, Griffin W, Cole P: Human ciliary beat frequency in epithelium from intrathoracic and extrathoracic airways, *Am Rev Respir Dis* 125:100, 1982.

91. Lucas AM, Douglas LC: Principles underlying ciliary activity in the respiratory tract, *Arch Otolaryngol Head Neck Surg* 20:528, 1934.

92. Sanderson MJ, Sleigh MA: Ciliary activity of cultured rabbit tracheal epithelium: beat pattern and metachrony, *J Cell Sci* 47:331, 1981.

93. Blake JR, Winet H: On the mechanics of mucociliary transport, *Biorheology* 17:125, 1980.

94. Wanner A: Alteration of tracheal mucous transport in airway disease, *Chest* 80:867, 1980.

95. Camner P, Philipson K: Human alveolar deposition of 4 micron Teflon particles, *Arch Environ Health* 26:294, 1978.

96. Nunn JF, Sturrock JE, Willis EJ et al: The effects of inhalational anesthetics on the swimming velocity of Tetrahymena pyriformis, *J Cell Sci* 15:537, 1974.

97. Lichtiger M, Landa JF, Hirsch JA: Velocity of tracheal mucus in anesthetized females undergoing gynecologic surgery, *Anesthesiology* 42:753, 1975.

98. Forbes AR: Halothane depresses mucociliary flow in the trachea, *Anesthesiology* 45:59, 1976.

99. Forbes AR, Horrigan RW: Mucociliary flow in the trachea during anesthesia with enflurane, ether, nitrous oxide and morphine sulfate, *Anesthesiology* 46:319, 1977.

100. Forbes AR, Gamsu G: Depression of lung mucociliary clearance by pentothal and halothane, *Anesth Analg* 58:387, 1979.

101. Konrad F, Schreiber T, Grünert A et al: Measurement of mucociliary transport in ventilated patients: short term effects of general anesthesia on mucociliary transport, *Chest* 102:1377, 1992.

102. Rubin BK, Finegan B, Ramirez O et al: General anesthesia does not alter the viscoelastic or transport properties of human respiratory mucus, *Chest* 98:101, 1990.

103. Sackner MA et al: Effect of oxygen in graded concentrations upon tracheal mucous velocity: a study in anesthetized dogs, *Chest* 69:164, 1976.

104. Sackner MA, Landa J, Hirsch J et al: Pulmonary effects of oxygen breathing, *Ann Intern Med* 82:40, 1975.

105. Sackner MA, Hirsch J, Epstein S: Effects of cuffed endotracheal tube on tracheal mucous velocity, *Chest* 68:774, 1975.

106. Forbes AR, Gamsu G: Lung mucociliary clearance after anesthesia with and without spontaneous and controlled ventilation, *Am Rev Respir Dis* 120:857, 1979.

107. Konrad F et al: Mucociliary transport in ICU patients, *Chest* 105:237-241, 1994.

108. Gamsu G, Singer M, Vincent H et al: Postoperative impairment of mucous transport, *Am Rev Respir Dis* 114:673, 1976.

109. Fallin LJ: Chest physical therapy. In Burton GC, Hodgkin JE, Ward JJ, editors: *Respiratory care: a guide to clinical practice,* Philadelphia, 1991, J.B. Lippincott.

110. Sutton PP et al: Chest physiotherapy: a review, *Eur J Respir Dis* 63:188, 1982.

111. Rochester DF, Goldberg SK: Techniques of respiratory physical therapy, *Am Rev Respir Dis* 122:133, 1980.

112. Gallon A: Evaluation of chest percussion in the treatment of patients with copious sputum production, *Respir Med* 85:45, 1991.

113. King M, Phillips D, Gross D et al: Enhanced tracheal mucous clearance with high frequency chest wall compression, *Am Rev Respir Dis* 128:511, 1983.

114. Stiller K, Greake T, Taylor J et al: Acute lobar atelectasis: a comparison of two chest physiotherapy regimens, *Chest* 98:1336, 1990.

115. Mackenzie CF, Imle CP, Ciesla N: *Chest physiotherapy in the intensive care unit,* ed 2, Baltimore, 1989, Williams and Wilkins.

116. Mackenzie CF, Shin B, McAslan TC: Chest physiotherapy: the effect on arterial oxygenation, *Anesth Analg* 57:28, 1978.

117. Tyler ML: The respiratory effects of body positioning and immobilization, *Respir Care* 29:472, 1984.

118. Ross J, Dean E, Abboud RT: The effects of postural drainage positioning on ventilation homogeneity in healthy subjects, *Phys Ther* 72:794, 1992.

119. Summer WR et al: Continuous mechanical turning of intensive care unit patients shortens length of stay in some diagnostic related groups, *J Crit Care* 4:45, 1989.

120. deBoisblanc BP, Castro M, Everret B et al: Effects of air-supported continuous postural oscillation on the risk of early ICU pneumonia in non-traumatic critical illness, *Chest* 103:1543, 1993.

121. Gentilello L, Thompson D, Tonnesen A et al: Effect of a rotating bed on the incidence of pulmonary complications in critically ill patients, *Crit Care Med* 16:783, 1988.

122. Dean E, Ross J: Discordance between cardiopulmonary physiology and physical therapy, *Chest* 101:1694, 1992.

123. Aitkenhead AR, Taylor S, Hunt P et al: Effect of respiratory therapy on plasma catecholamines, *Anesthesiology* 61:A44, 1984.

124. Weissman C, Kemper M: Stressing the critically ill patient: the cardiopulmonary and metabolic responses to an acute increase in oxygen consumption, *J Crit Care* 8:100, 1993.

125. Hammon WE, Conners AF, McCaffree DR: Cardiac arrhythmias during postural drainage and chest percussion of critically ill patients, *Chest* 102:1836, 1992.

126. Mackenzie CF, Shin B: Cardiorespiratory function before and after chest physiotherapy in mechanically ventilated patients with post-traumatic respiratory failure, *Crit Care Med* 13:483, 1985.

127. Conners AF et al: The immediate effect on oxygenation in acutely ill patient, *Chest* 78:559, 1980.

128. Stiller KR, Munday RM: Chest physiotherapy for the surgical patient, *Br J Surg* 79:745, 1992.

129. Kirilloff LH et al: Does chest physical therapy work? *Chest* 88:436, 1985.

130. Plevak DJ, Ward JJ: Airway management. In Burton GG, Hodgkin JE, Ward JJ, editors: *Respiratory care: a guide to clinical practice,* ed 3, Philadelphia, 1991, J.B. Lippincott.

131. McIntosh D, Baun MM, Rogge J: Effects of lung hyperinflation and presence of PEEP on arterial and tissue oxygenation, *Am J Crit Care* 2:317, 1993.

132. Goodnough SK: The effects of oxygen and hyperinflation on arterial oxygen tension after endotracheal suctioning, *Heart Lung* 14:11, 1985.

133. Ackerman MH: The effects of saline lavage prior to suctioning, *Am J Crit Care* 2:326, 1993.

134. Johnson KL, Kearney PA, Johnson PB: Closed versus open endotracheal suctioning: cost and physiologic consequences, *Crit Care Med* 22:658, 1994.

135. Isea JO, Poyant D, O'Donnell C et al: Controlled trial of a continuous irrigation suction catheter versus conventional intermittent suction catheter in clearing secretions from ventilated patients, *Chest* 103:1227, 1993.

136. Landa J, Amikan B, Sackner MA: Pathogenesis and prevention of tracheobronchial erosion occurring with suction, *Am Rev Respir Dis* 103:875, 1971.

137. Winston SJ, Gravelyn TR, Sitrin RG: Prevention of bradycardic responses to endotracheal suctioning by prior administration of nebulized atropine, *Crit Care Med* 15:1009, 1987.

138. Kerr ME et al: Head injury adults: recommendations for endotracheal suctioning, *J Neurosci Nurs* 25:86, 1993.

139. McFadden ER, Pichurko BM, Bowman HF et al: Thermal mapping of the airways in humans, *J Appl Physiol* 58:564, 1985.

140. Ingelstedt S: Studies on the conditioning of air in the respiratory tract, *Acta Otolaryngol Suppl* 133:1, 1955.

141. Forbes AR: Humidification and mucous flow in the intubated trachea, *Br J Anaesth* 45:874, 1973.

142. Todd DA, John E, Osborn RA: Tracheal damage following conventional and high frequency ventilation at low and high humidity, *Crit Care Med* 19:1310, 1991.

143. Chatburn RL, Primiano FP: A rational basis for humidity therapy, *Respir Care* 32:249, 1987.

144. Ogino M, Kopotic R, Mannino FL: Moisture-conserving efficiency of condenser humidifiers, *Anaesthesia* 40:990, 1985.

145. Bickler PE, Sessler DI: Efficiency of airway heat and moisture exchangers in anesthetized humans, *Anesth Analg* 71:415, 1990.

146. Klein EF, Dinesh AS, Shah NJ et al: Performance characteristics of conventional and prototype humidifiers and nebulizers, *Chest* 64:690, 1973.

147. Kuo CD, Lin SE, Wang JH: Aerosol, humidity, and oxygenation, *Chest* 99:1352, 1991.

148. Cohen IL, Weinberg PF, Fein IA et al: Endotracheal tube occlusion associated with the use of heat and moisture exchangers in the ICU, *Crit Care Med* 16:277, 1988.

149. Misset B, Escudier B, Rivara D et al: Heat and moisture exchangers versus heated humidifiers during long term mechanical ventilation, *Chest* 100:160, 1991.

150. Celis R, Torres A, Gatell J et al: Nosocomial pneumonia: a multivariate analysis of risk and prognosis, *Chest* 93:318, 1988.

151. Nair P, Jani K, Sanderson PJ: Transfer of oropharyngeal bacteria into the trachea during endotracheal intubation, *J Hosp Infect* 8:96, 1986.

152. Dilworth JP, White RJ, Brown EM: Microbial flora of the trachea during intubation of patients undergoing upper abdominal surgery, *Thorax* 47:818, 1992.

153. Rubenstein JS, Kabat K, Shulman ST et al: Bacterial and fungal colonization of the endotracheal tube in children: a prospective study, *Crit Care Med* 20:1544, 1992.

154. Gaynor EB: Gastroesophageal reflux as an etiologic factor in laryngeal complications of intubation, *Laryngoscope* 98:972, 1988.

155. DuMoulin GC, Patterson DG, Hedley-Whyte J et al: Aspiration of gastric contents in patients: a frequent cause of postoperative colonization of the airway, *Lancet* 1:242, 1982.

156. Cardinal P et al: Contribution of water condensation in endotracheal tubes to contamination of the lungs, *Chest* 104:127, 1993.

157. Deppe SA: Incidence of colonization, nosocomial pneumonia, and mortality, *Crit Care Med* 18:1389, 1990.

158. Mahul P, Auboyer C, Jospe R et al: Prevention of nosocomial pneumonia in intubated patients: respective role of mechanical subglottic secretions drainage and stress ulcer prophylaxis, *Intensive Care Med* 18:20, 1992.

159. Tryba M: Sucralfate versus antacids or H_2 antagonists for stress ulcer prophylaxis: a meta analysis on efficacy and pneumonia rates, *Crit Care Med* 19:942, 1991.

160. Driks MR, Craven DE, Celli BR et al: Nosocomial pneumonia in intubated patients given sucralfate as compared to antacids or histamine type 2 blockers, *N Engl J Med* 317:1376, 1987.

161. Peterson WL: *Heliobacter pylori* and peptic ulcer disease, *N Engl J Med* 324:1043, 1991.

162. Verdugo P, Johnson N, Tam P: Beta-adrenergic stimulation of respiratory ciliary activity, *J Appl Physiol* 48:868, 1980.

163. Presson CGA: The pharmacology of antiasthmatic xanthines and the role of adenosine. In Morley J, editor: *Asthma reviews,* London, 1987, Academic Press.

164. Brain JD, Valberg PA: Deposition of aerosol in the respiratory tract, *Am Rev Respir Dis* 120:1325, 1979.

165. Bishop MJ, Larson RP, Buschman DL: Metered dose inhaler aerosol characteristics are affected by the endotracheal tube actuator/adapter used, *Anesthesiology* 73:1263, 1990.

166. Crogan SJ, Bishop MJ: Delivery efficiency of metered dose aerosols given via endotracheal tubes, *Anesthesiology* 70:1008, 1989.

167. Taylor RH, Lerman J: High-efficiency delivery of salbutamol with a metered-dose inhaler in narrow tracheal tubes and catheters, *Anesthesiology* 74:360, 1991.

168. Dunteman E, Despotis G: A simple method of MDI administration in the intubated patient, *Anesth Analg* 75:303, 1992.

169. Niven RW, Kacmarek RM, Brain JD et al: Small bore nozzle extensions to improve the delivery efficiency of drugs from metered dose inhalers: laboratory evaluation, *Am Rev Respir Dis* 147:1590, 1993.

170. Dellinger RP: Fiberoptic bronchoscopy in adult airway management, *Crit Care Med* 18:882, 1990.

171. Olopade CO, Parakash UB: Bronchoscopy in the critical care unit, *Mayo Clin Proc* 64:1255, 1989.

172. Marquette CH, Herengt F, Saulnier F et al: Protected specimen brush in the assessment of ventilator associated pneumonia: selection of a certain lung segment for bronchoscopic sampling is unnecessary, *Chest* 103:243, 1993.

173. Imgrund SP, Goldberg SK, Walkenstein MD et al: Clinical diagnosis of massive hemoptysis using the fiberoptic bronchoscope, *Crit Care Med* 13:438, 1985.

174. Saumench J, Escarrabill J, Padró L et al: Value of fiberoptic bronchoscopy and angiography for diagnosis of the bleeding site in hemoptysis, *Ann Thorac Surg* 48:272, 1989.

175. Baumgartner F, Sheppard B, de Virgilio C et al: Tracheal and main bronchial disruptions after blunt chest trauma: presentation and management, *Ann Thorac Surg* 50:569, 1990.

176. McManigle JE, Fletcher GL, Tenholder MF: Bronchoscopy in the management of bronchopleural fistula, *Chest* 97:1235, 1990.

177. Stevens RP, Lillington GA, Parsons GH: Fiberoptic bronchoscopy in the intensive care unit, *Heart Lung* 10:1037, 1981.

178. Marini JJ, Pierson DJ, Hudson LD: Acute lobar atelectasis: a prospective comparison of fiberoptic bronchoscopy and respiratory therapy, *Am Rev Resp Dis* 119:971, 1979.

179. Kumar VA, Brandstetter RD: Chest physiotherapy vs. bronchoscopy, *Crit Care Med* 14:78, 1986.

180. Felon BJ: *Chest roentgenology,* Philadelphia, 1973, W.B. Saunders.

181. Lang DM, Simon RA, Mathison DA et al: Safety and possible efficacy of fiberoptic bronchoscopy with lavage in the management of refractory asthma with mucous impaction, *Ann Allergy* 67:324, 1991.

182. Bense L: Intrabronchial selective coagulation treatment of hemoptysis: report of three cases, *Chest* 97:990, 1990.

183. Tsukamoto T, Sasaki H, Nakamura H: Treatment of hemoptysis patients by thrombin and fibrinogen-thrombin infusion therapy using fiberoptic bronchoscope, *Chest* 96:473, 1989.

184. Saw EC, Gottlieb LS, Yokoyama T et al: Flexible fiberoptic bronchoscopy and endobronchial tamponade in the management of massive hemotysis, *Chest* 70:589, 1976.

185. Cunanan O: The flexible fiberoptic bronchoscope in foreign body removal: experience in 300 cases, *Chest* 73(suppl.):725, 1978.

186. Gundy KV, Boylen CT: Fiberoptic bronchoscopy: indications, complications, contraindications, *Postgrad Med* 83:289, 1988.

187. Sloan TB, Ovassapian A: The principles of flexible fiberoptic endoscopes. In Ovassapian A, editor: *Fiberoptic airway endoscopy in anesthesia and critical care,* New York, 1990, Raven Press.

188. Grossman E, Jacobi AM: Minimal optimal endotracheal tube size for fiberoptic bronchoscopy, *Anesth Analg* 53:475, 1974.

189. Feldman N, Sanders J: An alternate method for fiberoptic bronchoscopic examination of the intubated patient, *Am Rev Resp Dis* 111:562, 1975.

190. Belen J, Neuhaus A, Markowitz et al: Modification of the effect of fiberoptic bronchoscopy on pulmonary mechanics, *Chest* 79:516, 1981.

191. Perry LB: Topical anesthesia for bronchoscopy, *Chest* 73:691, 1978.

192. Niederman MS, Gambino A, Lichter J et al: Tension ball valve mucus plug in asthma, *Am J Med* 79:131, 1985.

193. Tsao TC, Tsai Y, Lan R et al: Treatment for collapsed lung in critically ill patients: selective intrabronchial air insufflation using the fiberoptic bronchoscope, *Chest* 97:435, 1990.

194. Haenel JB, Moore FA, Moore EE et al: Efficacy of selective intrabronchial air insufflation in acute lobar collapse, *Am J Surg* 164:501, 1992.

195. Millen JE, Vandree J, Glauser FL: Fiberoptic bronchoscopic balloon occlusion and re-expansion of refractory unilateral atelectasis, *Crit Care Med* 6:50, 1978.

196. Harada K, Matsuda T, Saoyama N et al: Re-expansion of refractory atelectasis using a bronchofiberscope with a balloon cuff, *Chest* 84:725, 1983.

197. Satyanarayana T, Capan L, Ramanathan S et al: Bronchofiberscopic jet ventilation, *Anesth Analg* 59:350, 1980.

198. Pereira W, Kovant DM, Snider GL: A prospective cooperative study of complications following flexible fiberoptic bronchoscopy, *Chest* 73:813, 1978.

199. Credle WF, Smiddy JF, Elliott RC: Complications of fiberoptic bronchoscopy, *Am Rev Resp Dis* 109:67, 1974.

200. Suratt PM, Smiddy JF, Gruber B: Deaths and complications associated with fiberoptic bronchoscopy, *Chest* 69:747, 1976.

201. Lindholm CE, Ollman B, Snyder JV et al: Cardiorespiratory effects of flexible fiberoptic bronchoscopy in critically ill patients, *Chest* 74:362, 1978.

202. Arai T: Real-time analysis of the change in arterial oxygen tension during endotracheal suction with a fiberoptic bronchoscope, *Crit Care Med* 13:855, 1985.

203. Dubrawsky C, Awe RJ, Jenkins DE: The effect of bronchofiberscopic examination on oxygenation status, *Chest* 67:137, 1975.

204. Luck JC et al: Arrhythmias from fiberoptic bronchoscopy, *Chest* 74:139, 1978.

205. Lundgren R, Häggmark S, Reiz S: Hemodynamic effect of flexible fiberoptic bronchoscopy performed under topical anesthesia, *Chest* 82:295, 1982.

206. Shroder DL, Lakshminarayan S: The effect of fiberoptic bronchoscopy on cardiac rhythm, *Chest* 73:821, 1978.

207. Klain M, Keszler H: Tracheobronchial toilet without cardiorespiratory impairment, *Crit Care Med* 8:298, 1980.

208. Pincus PS: Transbronchial biopsy during mechanical ventilation, *Crit Care Med* 15:1136, 1987.

209. Papin TA, Grum CM, Weg JG: Transbronchial biopsy during mechanical ventilation, *Chest* 89:168, 1986.

210. Bajwa MK, Henein S, Kambolz SL: Fiberoptic bronchoscopy in the presence of space-occupying intracranial lesions, *Chest* 104:101, 1993.

Chapter 36

MECHANICAL VENTILATION

John F. Nolan
Roy D. Cane

I. INTRODUCTION

Support of cardiopulmonary function with mechanical ventilation has traditionally involved intermittent application of positive pressure to the patient's airway. With early ventilatory support techniques the patient was, by and large, a passive recipient of the support. As can be imagined, patients often tried to breathe against the ventilator, leading to the well-known phrase "fighting the ventilator." As a consequence, patients required heavy sedation and neuromuscular relaxation. Subsequent developments in mechanical ventilatory support in the last 10 to 20 years have allowed for a more active patient role. Although newer techniques reflect significant differences in the interaction between patient and ventilator, they still involve manipulation of lung mechanics by changes in airway pressure.

Safe application of mechanical ventilatory support depends on the knowledge of normal and abnormal lung mechanics, cardiopulmonary relationships in health and disease, and an understanding of the mechanisms and limitations of modes of ventilation provided by modern ventilators.

II. PHYSIOLOGIC CONSIDERATIONS
A. MECHANICS OF BREATHING (FIG. 36-1)

Inspiration occurs when a pressure differential is created between the airway opening and peripheral airways. During spontaneous inspiration, diaphragmatic contraction decreases intrapleural pressure, thereby creating a pressure differential. During mechanical ventilation, a pressure differential is created by application of positive pressure at the airway opening. In either case, the distending or transpulmonary pressure (P_{TP}) (pressure at the airway opening [P_{ao}] minus visceral pleural surface pressure [P_{pl}])

$$P_{TP} = P_{ao} - P_{pl}$$

is increased. The magnitude of change in P_{TP} and the duration of the change determine both tidal volume (V_T)

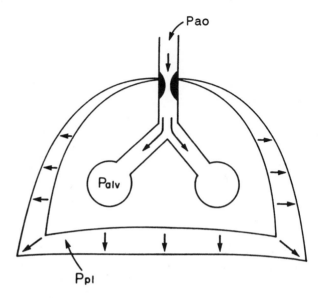

Fig. 36-1. Pressures relevant to inflation of the chest and lung during passive positive-pressure ventilation. Inspiration occurs as a result of difference in airway-opening pressure P_{ao} minus visceral pleural surface pressure P_{pl}. (From Perel A, Stock C: *Handbook of mechanical ventilatory support,* Baltimore, 1992, Williams & Wilkins.)

and inspiratory gas flow ($\dot{V}$). For a given P_{TP}, the resultant V_T depends on the respiratory system's compliance and resistance. Distensibility of the respiratory system can be quantified by calculating compliance (C), the change in volume (ΔV) divided by the change in pressure (ΔP):

$$C = \Delta V/\Delta P$$

The sum of the compliance of the lungs (C_L) and thorax (C_T) results in the respiratory system compliance (C_{RS}). It can be calculated by measuring the change in distending or transstructural pressure and the associated change in volume:

$$C_L = \Delta V/\Delta P_{(ao-pl)}$$
$$C_T = \Delta V/\Delta P_{(pl-b)}$$
$$C_{RS} = \Delta V/\Delta P_{(ao-b)}$$

where P_b = pressure at the surface of the thorax.

Under static conditions, pressure is required only to oppose the elastic recoil of the respiratory system. During insufflation, pressure must also be generated to overcome frictional or viscous forces. The ratio of this additional pressure (P) at the rate of airway flow that it produces ($\dot{V}$) is defined as the resistance (R).

$$R = \Delta P/\dot{V}$$

This equation describes resistance when gas flow is laminar. The resistance of the airways (R_{AW}), lungs (airways and parenchyma) (R_L), thorax (R_T), and respiratory system (R_{RS}) can be determined by measur-

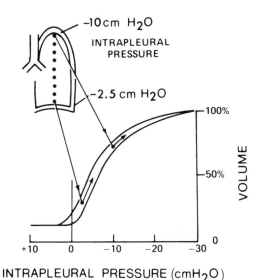

Fig. 36-2. An explanation of the regional differences of ventilation down the lung. Because the weight of the lung, intrapleural pressure is less negative at the base than at the apex. As a consequence, the basal lung is relatively compressed in its resting state but expands better on inspiration than the apex. (From West JB: *Ventilation/blood flow and gas exchange*, ed 4, Oxford, 1985, Blackwell.)

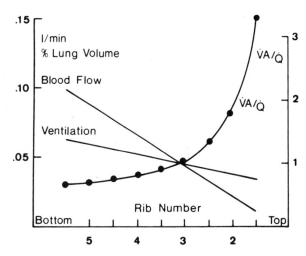

Fig. 36-3. Distribution of ventilation and blood flow down the upright lung. Note that greatest blood flow and ventilation are located at bottom of lung. Note that ventilation-perfusion ratio ($\dot{V}A/\dot{Q}$) decreases down the lung. (From West JB: *Ventilation/ blood flow and gas exchange*, ed 4, Oxford, 1985, Blackwell.)

ing airway flow rate and the corresponding transstructural pressure gradient:

$$R_{AW} = P_{(ao\text{-}alv)}/\dot{V}$$
$$R_T = P_{(pl\text{-}b)}/\dot{V}$$
$$R_L = P_{(ao\text{-}pl)}/\dot{V}$$
$$R_{RS} = P_{(ao\text{-}b)}/\dot{V}$$
$$P_{alv} = \text{Pressure within alveoli;}$$
$$\text{Alveolar pressure}$$

Resistance to gas flow increases when laminar flow becomes turbulent, or if airway diameter decreases. The ΔP_{TP} required to produce a given V_T is similar whether generated by spontaneous breathing or mechanical ventilation. However, the distribution of inspired gas varies. The regional distribution of change in P_{pl} is primarily the result of gravitational forces and is influenced by the effect of gravity on both the lung and the thorax and by the compliance of each. The visceral pleural–surface pressure and alveolar pressure determine the static recoil of the lung. Regional inequalities in the distribution of inspired gas between dependent and nondependent regions can be explained as the combined effect of the curvilinear volume/pressure (compliance) curve and the existence of a visceral pleural–surface pressure gradient (see Fig. 36-2). At functional residual capacity (FRC), P_{TP} in dependent alveoli is low, and they operate on the steep portion of the curve. During inspiration, the proportional change in P_{TP} is greater in the dependent than the nondependent

regions of the lung; thus these alveoli receive the bulk of ventilation. Blood flow is greatest in the dependent regions, thus allowing for the optimal matching of perfusion to ventilation (see Fig. 36-3). When inspiration occurs from a lung volume less than FRC, preferential ventilation of nondependent alveoli occurs because of a functional shift of the compliance curve. As FRC declines, dependent alveoli assume lower compliance characteristics. This model is commonly employed to illustrate regional inhomogeneities of ventilation, but it assumes the entire lung is isoelastic and the magnitude of visceral pleural–surface pressure swings during inspiration is uniform. Although these assumptions may not always be valid, the model provides a useful description of pulmonary insufflation.

During spontaneous ventilation in the supine position, there is greater displacement of the dependent (posterior) portion of the diaphragm, resulting in greater swings in pleural pressure over dependent regions than over the nondependent zones (see Fig. 36-4). Therefore, preferential distribution of inspired gas to dependent lung regions results not only from a more favorable pulmonary compliance but also from a more subatmospheric pleural surface pressure. During positive-pressure insufflation, the nondependent (anterior) part of the diaphragm is displaced more than the posterior portion favoring gas distribution primarily to nondependent lung regions. This redistribution of inspired gas appears to be unrelated to the rate of gas flow. As a consequence of altered gas distribution with mechanical ventilation, ventilation and perfusion are less well matched than during spontaneous ventilation.

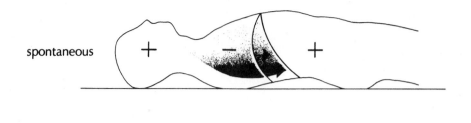

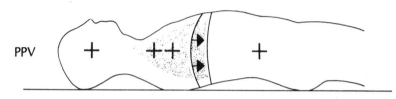

Fig. 36-4. Spontaneous ventilation provides optimal distribution of ventilation in relation to perfusion because of mechanics of spontaneously contracting diaphragm. In addition, venous return is optimized because intraabdominal and intracranial pressures are more positive than intrathoracic pressures. Positive-pressure ventilation (PPV) results in greater air distribution to nongravity-dependent portions of lung and potentially hinders venous return because intrathoracic pressure is more positive than intraabdominal or intracranial pressure. (From Shapiro BA, Kacmarek RM, Cane RD, et al: *Clinical application of respiratory care,* ed 4, Baltimore, 1991, Mosby–Year Book.)

B. ALVEOLAR TIME CONSTANTS (FIG. 36-5)

Alveolar time constants (π), the product of compliance and resistance, describe the time required for alveolar filling or emptying to occur. Alveolar ventilation follows a wash-in/wash-out exponential function; one time constant (1π) is associated with an exchange of 63% of the alveolar volume, 2π with 86.5% exchange, 3π with 95% exchange, and 4π with 98% exchange.

In pathologic lung states, gas distribution is altered to a greater extent than in normal lungs as a result of compliance inhomogeneity. The alveoli of diseased lungs are in a continuum with respect to differing time constants. To improve distribution of ventilation, a slow sustained inflation permits gas to distribute to slow alveoli and so tends to distribute gas in accord with the compliance of the different functional units. Distribution of inspired gas depends on the rate, duration, and frequency of inspiration. As the respiratory rate increases the inspiratory and expiratory times become increasingly shorter. Slower-filling alveoli may not fill or empty properly, leading to inadequate distribution of ventilation.

C. CARDIOPULMONARY COUPLING (FIG. 36-6)

The pulmonary system affects cardiovascular function primarily by variation in venous return. When cardiac function is normal, venous return is the major determinant of cardiac output. Venous return to the right atrium depends on the transthoracic vascular pressure, that is, the difference between extrathoracic vena cava pressure and transmural right-atrial pressure. Transmural right-atrial pressure is the difference between atrial pressure and pericardial pressure. When the pericardium does not limit diastolic filling, visceral pleural–surface pressure can be used to estimate pericardial pressure. Visceral pleural–surface pressure is normally subatmospheric. Intrapleural pressure is created by two opposing forces: lung recoil and chest wall expansion. Any change in these forces alters the intrapleural pressure and the transthoracic vascular pressure. During spontaneous inhalation, intrapleural pressure decreases an average of 6 to 10 cm H_2O below atmospheric pressure, resulting in dilatation of the intrathoracic vasculature. This dilatation produces an immediate decrease in intrathoracic vena caval, pulmonary arterial, and aortic pressures. Left ventricular output and the systemic arterial pressure decrease because of the increased left ventricular afterload. There is a momentary increase in pulmonary vascular capacitance. As transthoracic vascular pressure increases, venous return increases, and right-ventricular–stroke volume increases. At end inspiration, the pulmonary arterial and aortic pressures and the cardiac output decline as venous blood flow increases and fills the expanded pulmonary vasculature. During spontaneous exhalation, intrapleural pressure and pulmonary-artery blood flow return to baseline, cardiac output and systemic arterial pressure increase, and pulmonary vascular capacitance diminishes. Thus car-

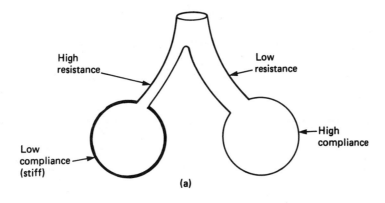

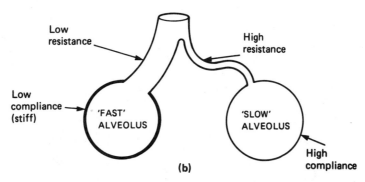

Fig. 36-5. Schematic diagrams of alveoli illustrate conditions under which static and dynamic compliances may differ. In idealized state *(a)* that is probably not realized even in the normal subject, the reciprocal relationship between resistance and compliance results in gas flow is preferentially delivered to the most compliant regions regardless of rate of inflation. Static and dynamic compliance are equal. In a state that is typical of many patients with respiratory disease, *(b)* Alveoli can conveniently be divided into fast and slow groups. Direct relationship between compliance and resistance results in inspired gas being preferentially delivered to stiff alveoli if rate of inflation is rapid. An end-inspiratory pause then permits redistribution from "fast" alveoli to "slow" alveoli. (From Nunn JF: *Nunn's applied respiratory physiology,* ed 4, Baltimore, 1993, Butterworth-Heinemann.)

diac output and systemic arterial pressure fluctuate with breathing pattern, reflecting phasic alterations in blood flow to and from the thorax. This process is reversed during positive-pressure breathing. Overall, positive-pressure breathing decreases the transthoracic vascular pressure, venous inflow, right ventricular–stroke volume, left ventricular–stroke volume, and cardiac output. The magnitude of the impact of positive-airway pressure on cardiovascular function depends on the degree of airway-pressure transmission to the visceral pleura, which is determined by lung (C_L) and thoracic compliance (C_T).

$$C_L = V_T/\Delta P_L = V_T/\Delta P_{(ao-pl)}$$

ΔP_L = Change in pressure within the lung; measures the difference between airway opening pressure and pleural pressure. Whenever lung volume changes, there must be an equivalent alteration in the volume of the thorax.

Therefore:

$$V_T = C_L\Delta P_{(ao-pl)} = C_T\Delta P_{pl}$$

The fractional transmission of airway pressure to the visceral pleural–surface ($\Delta P_{pl}/\Delta P_{ao}$) can be determined in the following way:

$$C_L\Delta P_{ao} = (C_T + C_L)\Delta P_{pl} \quad \Delta P_{pl}/\Delta P_{ao} = C_L(C_T = C_L)$$

If $C_L = C_T$, then about 50% of the change in airway pressure is transmitted to the visceral-pleural surface. If C_L decreases, fractional transmission is less than 50%. A reduction in C_T leads to an increase in pressure transmission to the intrathoracic organs.

Patients with acute respiratory failure characterized by low C_L usually tolerate positive-pressure breathing without deleterious cardiovascular consequences because of reduced transmission of positive-airway pressure. Patients with abdominal distension, or decreased

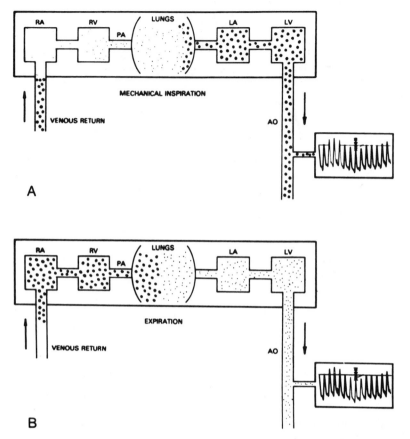

Fig. 36-6. The effect of a positive-pressure breath on preloads of right, *A,* and left, *B,* ventricles. Changes in left ventricular stroke output are reflected in arterial pressure, which increases during early inspiration and later decreases as a result of inspiratory decrease in venous return. *AO,* aorta; *LA,* left atrium; *RA,* right atrium; *RV,* right ventricle; *PA,* pulmonary artery; *LV,* left ventricle. (From Perel A, Stock C: *Handbook of mechanical ventilatory support,* Baltimore, 1992, Williams & Wilkins.)

lung volume following operative procedures, often have reduced thoracic compliance and increased airway pressure transmission. Chronic obstructive pulmonary disease (COPD) is associated with decreased C_T, and increased C_L, both of which result in increased transmission of the positive-airway pressure to the visceral pleura; COPD patients often manifest cardiovascular depression with positive-pressure breathing.

Measurements of thoracic vascular pressures frequently are used to evaluate cardiac filling and function. When airway pressure increases, all or part of the change in visceral pleural–surface pressure will be transmitted to the lumen of the intrathoracic vessels. Thus evaluation of cardiac function may be difficult without accurate estimation of true intravascular-filling pressure. Intravascular-filling pressure is determined by subtraction of the intrapleural from the intravascular pressure. Therefore precise knowledge of the pleural pressure may be valuable. At present, the measurement of pleural

pressure is difficult requiring the placement of a catheter between the visceral and parietal pleura. Attempts to estimate pleural pressure with an esophageal balloon have been made, but interpretation of esophageal pressure is difficult because great pressure variations occur within the esophagus. In addition, when esophageal pressure exceeds atmospheric pressure, compliance of the esophageal balloon may limit accuracy of the measurement. Such inaccuracy may influence calculated filling pressures and lead to significant error. At the University of South Florida, we examine the variability in the pulmonary-artery waveform. If there is significant variability with every ventilatory breath, then we subtract half the mean airway pressure from all the thoracic vascular pressures to give us an idea of the filling pressures. We have found this to be clinically useful.

Expiratory pleural pressure varies little with different respiratory patterns, as long as expiration is passive. Therefore, the most important determinant of mean

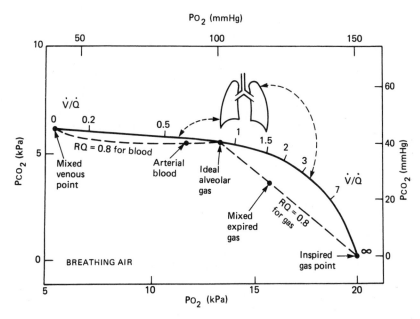

Fig. 36-7. Heavy line indicates all possible values for P_{O_2} and P_{CO_2} of alveoli with ventilation/perfusion ($\dot{V}/\dot{Q}$) ratios ranging from zero to infinity (subject breathing air). Values for normal alveoli are distributed as shown in accord with their vertical distance up the lung field. Mixed expired gas may be considered as a mixture of ideal alveolar and inspired gas (dead space). Arterial blood may be considered as a mixture of blood with same gas tensions as ideal alveolar gas and mixed venous blood (the shunt). (From Nunn JF: *Nunn's applied respiratory physiology,* ed 4, Oxford, 1993, Butterworth-Heinemann.)

airway-, pleural-, and vascular-filling pressures is the inspiratory-airway–pressure pattern. During mechanical inspiration, transmural-filling pressures will decrease, since airway and pleural pressures are increased. When transmural-filling pressure is lowered, cardiac output will likely decrease. This is not the case during spontaneous breathing, even with continuous positive airway pressure (CPAP). During spontaneous exhalation with CPAP, pleural and filling pressures are equivalent to those recorded during mechanical ventilation with the same end-expiratory–pressure level. However, during inspiration with CPAP, pleural pressure decreases, increasing cardiac filling. The effect of spontaneous inspiration on filling pressures of the heart and cardiac output depends on the change in airway pressure rather than the absolute pressure.

Airway pressure and lung volume are the major pulmonary factors that affect pulmonary vascular resistance (PVR), pulmonary blood flow and its distribution. When end-expiratory–lung volume (FRC) is normal, PVR is minimal. Variation in lung volume above or below normal FRC increases PVR. Therefore normal FRC should be maintained whenever possible. Even though FRC may be independent of the inspiratory-airway–pressure pattern, the mode of inspiration can affect PVR. During mechanical inspiration with large tidal volumes, PVR may increase if some alveoli become

overdistended. Increased PVR and decreased venous return from elevated pleural pressure combine to depress cardiac output.

D. VENTILATION-PERFUSION RELATIONSHIPS (FIG. 36-7)

The relationship between alveolar ventilation ($\dot{V}_A$) and perfusion ($\dot{Q}$) plays a major role in determining arterial–blood gas values. The gas values in venous blood passing through unventilated, perfused alveoli (e.g., $\dot{V}_A/\dot{Q} < 0.00001$), or shunt units, remain unchanged. In lung regions with very low but finite $\dot{V}_A/\dot{Q}$ (e.g., < 0.1), end-capillary–blood gas tensions are only slightly altered from those in venous blood; such $\dot{V}_A/\dot{Q}$ ratios are functionally like shunt units. As $\dot{V}_A/\dot{Q}$ increases above 0.1, end-capillary–blood gas tensions approximate alveolar gas tensions. Efficient gas exchange occurs when $\dot{V}_A/\dot{Q}$ is nearly equal to 0.8. As previously discussed, spontaneous inspiration directs the majority of ventilation toward dependent regions of the lung. Gravitational effects ensure a similar distribution of blood flow. Under healthy conditions the $\dot{V}_A/\dot{Q}$ normally approaches unity in all lung regions. Mechanical ventilation is associated with an increase in ventilation to the nondependent lung without a concomitant change in the distribution of pulmonary blood flow. This leads to an increase in lung units (with

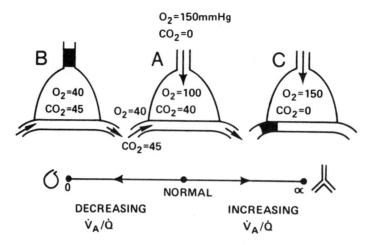

Fig. 36-8. Effect of altering ventilation-perfusion ratio on P_{O_2} and P_{CO_2} in a lung unit. (From West JB: *Ventilation/blood flow and gas exchange*, ed 4, Oxford, 1985, Blackwell.)

$\dot{V}_A/\dot{Q} > 1$) in the nondependent lung and with low, but finite $\dot{V}_A/\dot{Q}$ (<1, >0.1) in the dependent lung.

III. PATHOLOGIC CONSIDERATIONS

A. ACUTE RESPIRATORY FAILURE

Respiratory failure is invariably associated with abnormal $\dot{V}_A/\dot{Q}$ that usually necessitates supportive intervention. An increased $\dot{V}_A/\dot{Q}$ associated with a decreased V_T results in an increase in the ratio of physiologic dead space (V_D) to V_T (V_D/V_T), which may require mechanical ventilation if spontaneous breathing cannot provide adequate alveolar ventilation for carbon dioxide elimination. Both anatomical and alveolar compartments contribute to the total physiological dead space. The calculated V_D of patients on mechanical ventilatory support decreases linearly as ventilatory rates are reduced. When patients initiate spontaneous breathing, mean V_D often decreases by 50 percent, despite ventilator rates between nine and six breaths per minute. When patients are weaned from mechanical ventilation, V_D returns to predicted normal values. Because V_D increases during mechanical ventilation, an increased ventilator rate may result in a paradoxical increase in Pa_{CO_2}.

A decrease in $\dot{V}_A/\dot{Q}$ results in hypoxemia (Figs. 36-8 and 36-9). Since the majority of gas exchange occurs during the expiratory phase of the ventilatory cycle, improvement in overall $\dot{V}_A/\dot{Q}$ must occur primarily during exhalation. Mechanical ventilation alone usually is not effective in improving hypoxemia associated with low but finite $\dot{V}_A/\dot{Q}$, since the ratio will increase only during the inspiratory phase of the ventilatory cycle. Positive pressure applied during exhalation can improve low $\dot{V}_A/\dot{Q}$. However, positive end-expiratory pressure (PEEP) may increase V_D and decrease $\dot{V}_A$, especially in conjunction with mechanical ventilation. Therefore, when ventilatory support is instituted, the goal must be to minimize $\dot{V}_A/\dot{Q}$ mismatching in all lung regions. This is best accomplished by allowing as much spontaneous ventilation as the patient can perform with provision of the minimum mechanical assistance required to prevent development of respiratory acidemia. Maintaining near-normal FRC with exhalatory positive pressure frequently improves $\dot{V}_A/\dot{Q}$ and reduces hypoxemia.

Acute respiratory failure (ARF) often is characterized by a decrease in FRC and an increase in pulmonary venous admixture ($\dot{Q}_{va}/\dot{Q}_t$). Pulmonary venous admixture refers to the degree of admixture of mixed venous blood with pulmonary-end capillary blood that would be required to produce the observed difference between the arterial- and pulmonary-end capillary P_{O_2}. Loosely speaking, this is sometimes referred as the intrapulmonary shunt. Therapy for ARF should include instituting spontaneous positive-pressure breathing to increase FRC, improving pulmonary gas exchange, increasing arterial-oxygen tension, and decreasing PVR. It has been suggested that the appropriate (optimal) level of positive-pressure breathing be determined by titrating end-expiratory pressure to minimize $\dot{Q}_{va}/\dot{Q}_t$, a goal achieved more readily with spontaneous breathing on CPAP than with mechanical ventilation. Mechanical ventilation with end-expiratory pressure increases mean-airway and intrapleural pressure; the increase in mean-airway pressure may overdistend compliant alveoli, increase PVR, and redirect blood flow to less well-ventilated areas, thus increasing $\dot{Q}_{va}/\dot{Q}_t$. In contrast, spontaneous breathing on CPAP maintains lower mean-airway and intrapleural pressure, and allows higher end-expiratory pressure levels to increase FRC with fewer deleterious effects.

B. WORK OF BREATHING

If patients with acute lung injury are to maintain effective spontaneous breathing, the work of breathing must be maximally efficient. Few clinical studies have

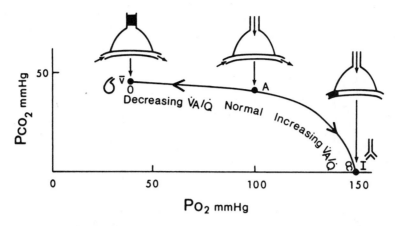

Fig. 36-9. O_2-CO_2 diagram showing a ventilation-perfusion ratio line. Po_2 and Pco_2 of a lung unit move along this line from the mixed venous point $\bar{v}$ to the inspired gas point I as its ventilation-perfusion ratio is increased. (From West JB: *Ventilation/blood flow and gas exchange,* ed 4, Oxford, 1985, Blackwell.)

attempted to quantify the work of breathing in patients with respiratory failure, perhaps because quantification of work requires techniques not readily applicable to the clinical setting. Any alteration in the volume/pressure (V/P) relationship of the lung can alter the work of breathing. A normal V/P curve for the lung-thorax system is shown in Figure 36-10. As a result of a small pressure change, normal tidal breathing from FRC occurs along the V/P curve as indicated by the arrow. The elastic work of inspiration can be estimated by the stippled area under the curve. Figure 36-11 shows the V/P curves for normal lung, thorax, and lung-thorax. When the distending pressure of the lung-thorax is zero (i.e., ambient airway pressure), the lung volume is the FRC. At FRC, the distending pressure of the lung is equal to but opposite of that of the thorax. Any alteration in the V/P relationships for the lung and/or the thorax will alter the lung-thorax curve and change FRC. The likely alteration of lung V/P curve associated with acute lung injury is shown in Figure 36-12. Because the V/P relationships of the lung and thorax can be altered in an infinite number of ways by ARF, a family of right-shifted lung-thorax curves can result. Each will have a reduced FRC (Fig. 36-13). A shift in the V/P curve not only decreases FRC, but can increase the work of breathing. When FRC is decreased, the required pressure change to achieve the same V_T may be increased, and the area within the curve representing work also is increased (Fig. 36-14). If this occurs, the patient will decrease tidal volume and increase respiratory rate in an effort to minimize work. Because of these changes, clinicians often have assumed the work of breathing for the patient by instituting mechanical ventilation. However, restoration of FRC accomplished by instituting CPAP may provide an alternative means of decreasing the work of breathing. Restoration of FRC can be accomplished with the application of PEEP on

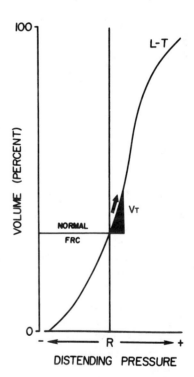

Fig. 36-10. Normal pressure-volume curve of the lung-thorax (L-T). Volume as a percent of total lung capacity is plotted as a function of distending pressure (R). At ambient airway pressure, R equals zero. During inspiration, R is increased and lung volume (V_T) increases from normal functional residual capacity (FRC). As a result of a small pressure change, normal tidal breathing from FRC occurs along the pressure-volume curve, as indicated by the arrow. The elastic work of inspiration can be estimated by the stippled area under the curve. (From Downs JB, Douglas ME: Physiologic effects of respiratory therapy. In Shoemaker W, Ayers S, Grenvik A et al, editors: *Textbook of critical care,* ed 2, Philadelphia, 1989, W.B. Saunders.)

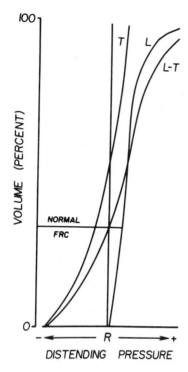

Fig. 36-11. Normal pressure-volume curves of the thorax (T), lung (L), and lung-thorax (L-T). Volume as a percent of total lung capacity is plotted as a function of distending pressure (R). Lung-thorax R is zero when airway pressure is ambient; distending pressure of lung is, therefore, equal but opposite to that of thorax. These equal counterforces determine and maintain functional residual capacity (FRC). (From Downs JB, Douglas ME: Physiologic effects of respiratory therapy. In Shoemaker W, Ayers S, Grenvik A et al, editors: *Textbook of critical care,* ed 2, Philadelphia, 1989, W.B. Saunders.)

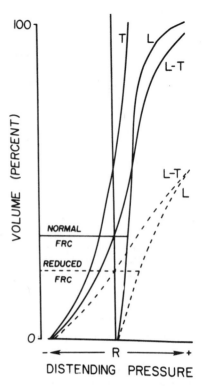

Fig. 36-12. Normal (solid lines) and abnormal (dotted lines) pressure-volume curves of thorax (T), lung (L) and lung-thorax (L-T). Distending pressure (R) is zero when airway pressure is ambient. Abnormally right-shifted pressure-volume curve of lung, which is characteristic of respiratory failure, results in a new L-T pressure-volume curve and a reduction in functional residual capacity (FRC). (From Downs JB, Douglas ME: Physiologic effects of respiratory therapy. In Shoemaker W, Ayers S, Grenvik A et al, editors: *Textbook of critical care,* ed 2, Philadelphia, 1989, W.B. Saunders.)

mechanically ventilated patients and CPAP in spontaneously breathing patients (Fig. 36-15). Since severity of injury may vary from patient to patient, PEEP must be individualized, titrated for each patient, and reassessed frequently. Optimization of therapy so that end-expiratory–airway pressure is sufficient to restore FRC to a more favorable portion of the V/P curve reduces the required change in transpulmonary pressure. In other words, data associated with the patient will be in a better portion of the compliance curve, resulting in diminished work of breathing.

C. CARDIAC FAILURE

Left ventricular failure causes an increase in left atrial and pulmonary venous pressure. The increased pulmonary venous pressure can precipitate gas-exchange abnormalities by altering the distribution of pulmonary blood flow and/or increasing extravascular lung water. Increased pulmonary venous pressure initially produces a redistribution of perfusion to nondependent-lung regions. However, as pulmonary venous pressure continues to rise, the transvascular flux of fluid increases, the

interstitial space becomes maximally expanded, the lymphatic clearance mechanism is overwhelmed, alveoli become flooded, FRC and C_{RS} decrease, and $\dot{V}_A/\dot{Q}$ mismatching increases. Patients in left-heart failure typically exhibit a low-compliant breathing pattern characterized by tachypnea and inspiratory intercostal and/or epigastric retractions caused by large reductions in pleural pressure. Alterations in pleural pressure may significantly alter left ventricular function. Marked reductions in pleural pressure may impede left ventricular ejection (because of increased aortic transmural pressure or afterload) whereas increases in pleural pressure may facilitate left ventricular ejection (because of decreased aortic transmural pressure or afterload). In left-heart failure, in which left ventricular contractility is reduced and relatively unresponsive to changes in preload, decreasing left ventricular afterload will increase stroke volume. Since increased intrapleural pressure reduces left ventricular afterload, positive-pressure breathing via CPAP may improve cardiac

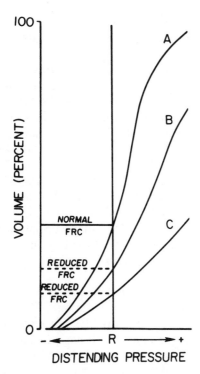

Fig. 36-13. Volume as a percent of total lung capacity is plotted as a function of distending pressure (R). R is zero when airway pressure is ambient. Curve A represents normal pressure-volume relationship for lung-thorax. Curves B and C are shifted to right. Each curve results in reduced functional residual capacity (FRC). Pressure-volume relationships of lung and thorax can be altered in an infinite number of ways during respiratory failure, resulting in a family of right-shifted lung-thorax curves. Each curve will have a lower FRC than curve on its left. (From Downs JB, Douglas ME: Physiologic effects of respiratory therapy. In Shoemaker W, Ayers S, Grenvik A et al, editors: *Textbook of critical care*, ed 2, Philadelphia, 1989, W.B. Saunders.)

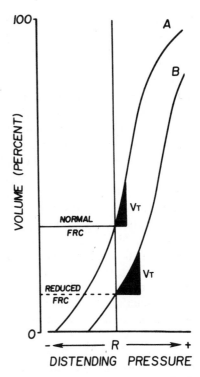

Fig. 36-14. Pressure-volume curves of lung-thorax. Volume as percent of total lung capacity is plotted as a function of distending pressure (R). R is zero when airway pressure is ambient. Curve A represents normal pressure-volume relationship. Curve B represents a right-shifted curve. (From Downs JB, Douglas ME: Physiologic effects of respiratory therapy. In Shoemaker W, Ayers S, Grenvik A et al, editors: *Textbook of critical care*, ed 2, Philadelphia, 1989, W.B. Saunders.)

performance and lung function in patients suffering from congestive heart failure.

IV. PATHOPHYSIOLOGIC EFFECTS AND COMPLICATIONS OF POSITIVE AIRWAY PRESSURE THERAPY

A. MALDISTRIBUTION OF VENTILATION

ARF results in nonhomogeneous changes in compliance and resistance. Intermittent positive pressure ventilation (IPPV) results in further maldistribution of ventilation to nondependent lung. The combination of these effects commonly results in a need for elevated minute ventilation to maintain $Paco_2$. As discussed, arterial oxygenation may be impaired by changes in $\dot{V}a/\dot{Q}$ consequent to pathology and IPPV.

B. BAROTRAUMA/VOLUTRAUMA

Positive-pressure ventilation (PPV) is not in itself therapeutic and may contribute to further lung injury.[1]

Pulmonary barotrauma, alveolar edema, hyaline-membrane formation, and vascular injury have all been documented to attend the use of positive-pressure ventilatory techniques.[28] Such complications may significantly affect outcome. The elevation of airway pressure (P_{aw}) consequent on PPV is generally considered to be the etiologic agent of these adverse changes. In most studies demonstrating this pathology, an elevated P_{aw} was achieved in the experimental group by raising the V_T, usually to clinically irrelevant levels (up to 65 ml/kg in one report and to more than 100 ml/kg in another[5,7]). P_{aw} is, in fact, a dependent variable in that situation and as such may or may not itself influence the abnormalities observed. The pathophysiologic changes consistently demonstrated in these animal models may have resulted instead from the supraphysiologic V_T and not from the elevated airway pressures produced by these high volumes. Pressure and volume may both be important. The genesis of pulmonary injury is likely multifactorial.

Dreyfuss et al. compared extravascular lung water and ultrastructural lung changes in groups of rats receiving mechanical ventilatory support under various conditions.[6] The authors found that animals ventilated with large cyclic changes in airway pressure with conventional V_T between 13 and 19 ml/kg had no demonstrable changes in pulmonary microarchitecture. In contrast, pulmonary edema and structural lung injury similar to that seen in adult respiratory distress syndrome (ARDS) were observed in animals ventilated with high tidal volumes. These animals sustained pulmonary injury consisting of alveolar hemorrhage, alveolar-neutrophil infiltration, alveolar macrophage and type II–pneumocyte proliferation, interstitial congestion and thickening, interstitial lymphocyte infiltration, emphysematous changes, and hyaline-membrane formation.[7] Thus, only large changes in lung volume, not airway pressure, produced pulmonary pathology in this model. Zapol suggested that this damage be called volutrauma rather than barotrauma, nomenclature that accents the role of hyperinflation in the genesis of secondary lung injury.[9] This distinction was the subject of a recent editorial describing both the differences and the clinical implications of barotrauma and volutrauma.[8]

C. ORGAN SYSTEM DYSFUNCTION

PPV affects not only intrathoracic organs, but practically every major organ system. By understanding the physiologic consequences of PPV, clinicians may minimize or at least anticipate the undesirable effects.

1. Central nervous system (Fig. 36-16 and Box 36-1)

PPV may result in an increase in intracranial pressure (ICP) because of excessive auto-PEEP or elevated mean-airway pressure. Impaired venous return as a result of increased intrathoracic pressure is the main cause. If auto-PEEP is adjusted to maintain the patient's lungs at a normal FRC, then the effects on the ICP will be negligible. Cerebral perfusion pressure (CPP) may be impaired in patients receiving PPV as a result of impaired cardiac output, decreased mean arterial pressure, and increased ICP. Inappropriate use of the ventilator in patients with intracranial injuries may lead to auto-PEEP, further impairing CPP.

2. Cardiac (Fig. 36-17 and Box 36-2)

Cardiac dysfunction on initiation of PPV is predictable if the physiologic variables are understood. As a general rule there is a decrease in cardiac output secondary to a decrease to right ventricular preload, an

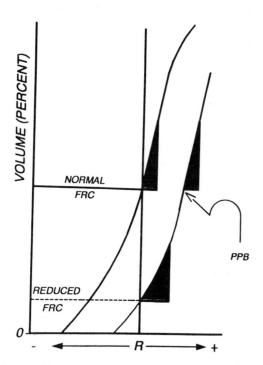

Fig. 36-15. These pressure-volume curves of lung-thorax are equivalent to those in Figure 36-14. When distending pressure (R) is increased by positive airway pressure, FRC (functional residual capacity) can be normalized. When FRC is increased, work of breathing may be reduced to nearly normal. *PPB,* positive pressure breathing. (From Downs JB, Douglas ME: Physiologic effects of respiratory therapy. In Shoemaker W, Ayers S, Grenvik A et al, editors: *Textbook of critical care,* Philadelphia, 1989, W.B. Saunders.)

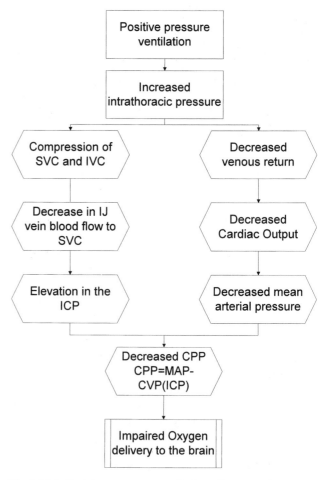

Fig. 36-16. Positive-pressure ventilation effects on the central nervous system.

increase in right ventricular afterload, and a decrease in left ventricular preload. As a result there is an observed decrease in mean arterial pressure. Patients with compromised intravascular volume may be more susceptible to these effects. As a general rule a large-bore IV is usually indicated prior to commencing PPV in case aggressive fluid resuscitation is needed.

A decrease in sympathetic outflow seen following the mechanical support of the work of breathing may lead to vasodilatation, further exacerbating a drop in mean arterial pressure.

Another potential problem is the increase in pulmonary vascular resistance leading to impaired right ventricular ejection. Patients with right ventricular dysfunction tend to do poorly on PPV. Increased PVR

may also increase right-to-left shunting in patients with atrial septal defect (ASD)/ventricular septal defect (VSD). These patients may be at higher risk for an embolus passing to the systemic circulation.

3. Pulmonary (Box 36-3)

Most complications of PPV on the pulmonary system have been previously discussed. Other complications associated with PPV are pneumonia and risks associated with endotracheal intubation. The incidence of pneumonia is increased in endotracheally intubated patients, with the incidence of infection increasing every day. In a recent study the actuarial risk of ventilator-associated pneumonia was 6.5% at 10 days, 19% at 20 days, and 28% at 30 days.[10] The risk of endotracheal intubation can be divided into complications associated with the placement and those seen as a result of long-term presence of a foreign body in the trachea. Patients with elevated mean-airway pressure and those requiring high levels of PEEP or with compromised perfusion may be at an increased risk for tracheomalacia.

4. Hepatic (Box 36-4)

PPV increases intrathoracic pressures and results in impaired venous return leading to congestion of the

---

> **BOX 36-1   PPV effects on the CNS**
>
> 1. Increase in ICP
> 2. Decrease in cerebral perfusion pressure caused by the following:
>   a. Decreased cardiac output
>   b. Decreased mean arterial pressure
>   c. Increase in ICP

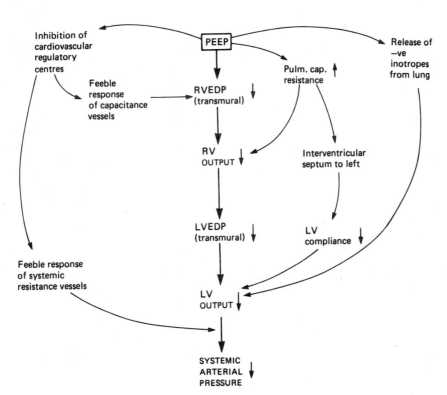

Fig. 36-17. Cardiovascular effects of positive end-expiratory pressure (PEEP). *RVEDP,* right ventricular end diastolic pressure; *RV,* right ventricle; *LVEDP,* left ventricular end diastolic pressure; *LV,* left ventricle. (From Nunn JF: *Nunn's applied respiratory physiology,* ed 4, Oxford, 1993, Butterworth-Heinemann.)

BOX 36-2   PPV causes of decreased cardiac output

1. Decreased venous return to right ventricle
2. Right ventricular dysfunction secondary to elevated pulmonary vascular resistance and decreased preload
3. Alterations of left ventricular distensibility

BOX 36-3   The most common pulmonary complications associated with PPV

1. Barotrauma/volotrauma
2. Pneumothorax
3. Pneumomediastinum
4. Increased risk of nosocomial pneumonia
5. Risks associated with tracheal intubation

BOX 36-4   PPV may impair hepatic and gastrointestinal function in the following ways:

1. Decreased cardiac output
2. Increased hepatic vascular resistance
   a. Elevated venous pressure
   b. Elevated intraabdominal pressure
   c. Diaphragmatic compression
3. Elevated bile-duct pressure

BOX 36-5   PPV effects on splanchnic circulation

1. Increase in intestinal anastomosis breakdown
2. Possible increase in bacterial translocation
3. Increase in UGI hemorrhage
4. Ileus and gastric dilation

---

hepatic sinusoids. Diaphragmatic compression leads to an increase in intraabdominal pressure, further impairing hepatic blood flow. Further aggravating this situation is the drop in cardiac output and oxygen delivery to the liver. This is particularly a problem in patients with liver disease who have altered parenchymal architecture.

An increase in resistance in the flow of bile through the common bile duct may influence liver function. Elevated bile-duct pressure has been described in animal studies with the proposed mechanism being vascular engorgement of the duct.[11]

5. Splanchnic and GI tract (Box 36-5)

The deleterious effects of PPV on the splanchnic circulation are due to venous engorgement and decreased perfusion. Elevation in intrathoracic pressures limits venous return from the inferior vena cava and the portal vein. Decreases in cardiac output, in addition, limit perfusion pressure. This dual effect of poor perfusion and venous engorgement may lead to an increased risk for intestinal anastomosis breakdown, increased bacterial translocation from the gut, and an increase in upper gastrointestinal (UGI) hemorrhage. Bacterial translocation is presently considered as the possible source for the initiation of the sepsis syndrome. Tied in with this problem is nutrition, which is usually limited due to endotracheal intubation. Early enteral feeding may improve the viability of gastrointestinal mucosa, limiting this complication.

UGI hemorrhage has been observed in approximately 40% of patients on PPV for more than three days.[12] Prophylaxis to elevate the stomach pH ameliorates this problem but may increase the risk of nosocomial pneumonia.

Patients on full ventilatory support often require sedation and neuromuscular blockade. This may lead to an ileus and gastric dilation.

6. Renal (Fig. 36-18 and Box 36-6)

Renal impairment upon initiating mechanical ventilation is multifactorial. Proposed causes can be subdivided into direct and indirect effects. Impaired renal function is usually due to decreased cardiac output and altered venous return to the heart. Redistribution of renal blood flow from the cortex to the juxtamedullary regions leads to decreased urine volume and decreased sodium excretion. Also involved, although indirectly, are the sympathetic and endocrine systems. Decreased levels of carotid-sinus baroreceptor simulation lead to the increase in renal sympathetic stimulation, which leads to decreased renal blood flow and a decrease in urinary-sodium excretion. The liberation of increasing levels of antidiuretic hormone (ADH) and up modulation of the renin-angiotensin-aldosterone system again leads to water retention and renal impairment. Another component member is the antinuclear factor (ANF), released as a result of cardiac distension. Its release is greatly reduced in patients on PPV. ANF has potent diuretic and natriuretic effect.

V. MECHANICAL ASPECTS OF POSITIVE AIRWAY PRESSURE THERAPY

A. CLASSIFICATION OF VENTILATORS (Fig. 36-19)

Classification of ventilator modalities has been complicated by the inability to establish a standard nomenclature. In an attempt to make comparisons between different ventilator modes, a classification was first

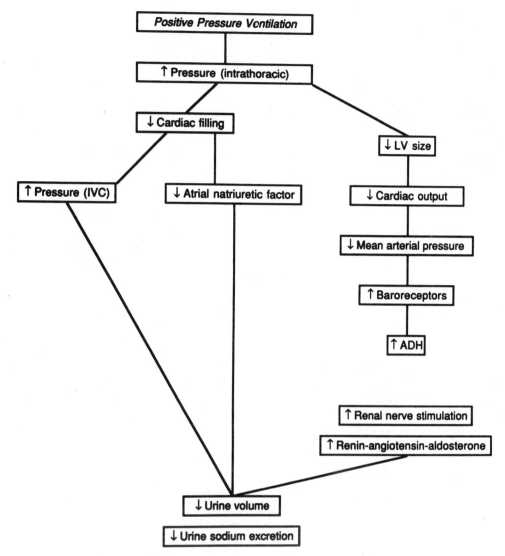

Fig. 36-18. Multiple effects of positive-pressure ventilation on renal function. *ADH,* antidiuretic hormone; *IVC,* inferior vena cava; *LV,* left ventricular. (Modified from Perel A, Stock C: *Handbook of mechanical ventilatory support,* Baltimore, 1992, Williams & Wilkins.)

proposed by Mushin.[13] Mushin divided the inspiratory phase into three components: initiation, limiting, and cycling. Initiation is the physical event that starts or triggers the ventilatory breath. In most current ventilators, time or pressure actuates the ventilator. New microprocessor ventilators have also allowed for the use of flow for initiation. In time-cycled initiation the patient receives a breath as a result of the passage of a predetermined time interval. The patient is unable to initiate the breath. If flow or pressure initiation is used, the patient must generate the set pressure or flow differential before the breath is initiated.

Once the breath is initiated the ventilator delivers pressurized gas, which may be deleterious to lung parenchyma if not limited. Limiting is the mechanism by which the ventilator determines when to restrict the positive-pressure driving force. This limiting can be determined by sensing a set pressure, flow, or volume. A pressure-limited ventilator will provide the flow and time required to reach a preset pressure in the ventilator circuit, allowing for variable tidal volume to be delivered. This mode is called pressure-control ventilation. Flow-limited ventilators provide the pressure and time required to reach a preset flow rate in the ventilator circuit, allowing for variable tidal volumes to be delivered. A volume limit provides the flow and time required to deliver a preset volume in the ventilator circuit without concern for the level of pressure delivered.

To terminate inspiration the ventilator must cycle off. Cycling determines when inspiration will end. Cycling can be determined by a preset time, volume, pressure, or flow. Time cycling ends inspiration when a predeter-

---

BOX 36-6   PPV may impair renal function in the following ways:

1. Direct
   a. Decreased cardiac output
   b. Redistribution of renal blood flow from cortical to intramedullary zones, which in turn leads to the following:
      (1) Decreased urine volume
      (2) Decreased sodium excretion
   c. Increased intrathoracic pressures resulting in elevated portal and inferior vena cava (IVC) pressures
2. Indirect
   a. Sympathetic stimulation
      (1) Increased epinephrine levels
   b. Hormonal changes
      (1) Decreased ANF
      (2) Increased renin-angiotensin-aldosterone
      (3) Increased ADH

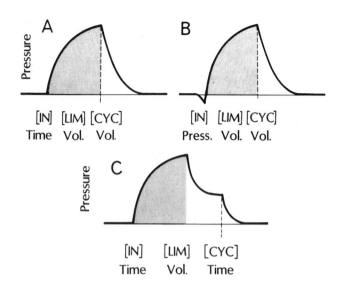

Fig. 36-19. Airway pressure curves illustrating the three mechanical functions: *[IN]*, initiation of cycle; *[LIM]*, preset limit imposed on positive-pressure cycle; *[CYC]*, ending the cycle. Each mechanical function is preset to be governed by one of four physical factors—volume, pressure, flow, and time. *A* illustrates a time-initiated, volume-limited, volume-cycled mode. *B* illustrates a pressure-initiated (intended to be a subbaseline pressure secondary to the patient's effort to initiate a breath), volume-limited, volume-cycled mode. *C* illustrates a time-initiated, volume-limited, time-cycled mode that extends inspiration beyond the time the volume is delivered. (From Shapiro B, Kacmarek RM, Cane RD et al: *Clinical application of respiratory care*, ed 4, St Louis, 1991, Mosby–Year Book.)

mined time has been reached. This is usually controlled by varying the inspiratory-to-expiratory (I:E) time on the ventilator. Volume-cycled ventilators shut off when the predetermined volume has been reached. The pressure-cycling ventilator stops when the pressure hits its predetermined level. And last but not least is the flow-cycled ventilator, which stops delivering flow once a predetermined level has been reached.

Mushin's classification system was initially developed prior to the explosion of microprocessor technology and as such has become outmoded. Chatburn recently proposed ventilator nomenclature and classification based on a mathematical model known as the equation of motion for the respiratory system.[14] The equation is as follows:

$$\text{muscle pressure} = \text{ventilator pressure} = \text{volume}/\text{compliance} + (\text{resistance} \times \text{flow})$$

Consideration of these factors reveals that time, volume, pressure, and flow are primary elements for ventilator classification. This classification system is being evaluated and has been adopted by some as the standard (See Figs. 36-20 and 36-21.)

B. CHARACTERISTICS OF VENTILATOR MODES

Ventilators have traditionally been classified on the basis of various physical characteristics. Table 36-1 lists these characteristics with respect to initiation, limit, and cycling of the positive-pressure inspiration. The various modes of ventilation describe the differences in patient-ventilator interactions associated with alternative methods of delivery of a positive-pressure inspiration. Selec-

tion of a particular mode of ventilatory support should be based on consideration of the patient-ventilator interaction in part. Table 36-2 on p. 807 describes the interactions associated with the different modes (Fig. 36-22 on p. 808).

C. INSPIRATORY:EXPIRATORY RATIO

The I:E ratio describes the time spent in inhalation versus exhalation. To ensure adequate exhalation with IPPV, I:E ratios are generally set to 1:2 or greater. To provide sufficient inspiratory time, most ventilators are designed to have 1.5 seconds inspiratory time as default value (i.e., 4π, four times the alveolar time constant).

D. PEEP, CPAP (FIG. 36-23 ON P. 808)

Application of positive pressure to the airway during exhalation increases the FRC. When used in conjunction with IPPV this is known as positive end-expiratory pressure (PEEP). During spontaneous ventilation the same effect can be achieved with the use of continuous positive airway pressure (CPAP). Expiratory positive airway pressure (EPAP) is associated with an increase in inspiratory work of breathing and is not a useful clinical modality.

Increasing functional residual capacity with CPAP/

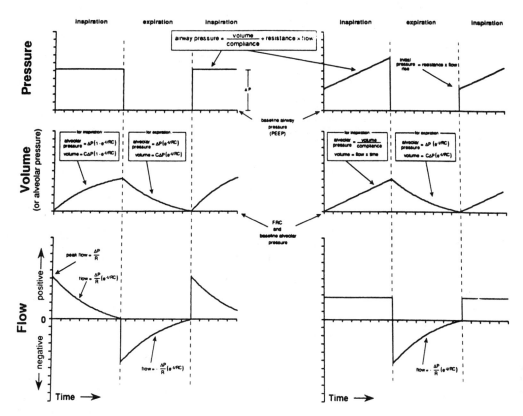

Fig. 36-20. A study of respiratory-system mechanics is based on graphical and mathematical models. Specifically, respiratory system is often conceived as a single resistance connected to a single compliance. Mechanical behavior of this system is described by a mathematical model called the "equation of motion for the respiratory system." In this model, pressure, volume, and flow are variables (i.e., functions of time), whereas resistance and compliance are constants. (From Chatburn R: *Respir Care* 37(9):1009, 1992.)

PEEP leads to improvements in lung compliance and decrease in work of breathing (WOB) and may improve arterial oxygenation. PEEP/CPAP increase FRC by dilation of alveolar gas spaces at low levels (0 to 10 cm H_2O). Reexpansion of collapsed alveoli is an additional mechanism to increase FRC, at levels greater than 10 cm H_2O are usually required.

E. IMV VS. SIMV

Intermittent-mandatory ventilation (IMV) delivers positive-pressure breaths at a fixed mechanical rate while allowing simultaneous unrestricted, unassisted, spontaneous breathing to occur. Continuous gas flow within the circuit allows for spontaneous breaths without circuit-imposed work of breathing.

During synchronized IMV (SIMV), the mechanical breaths are triggered by the patient via pressure if spontaneous respiratory efforts are available within a time period suitable for the selected ventilator rate. SIMV was designed to avoid "stacking" of mechanical and spontaneous breaths, which has not been demonstrated to be of clinical significance. SIMV systems

employ a demand valve to deliver a fresh gas flow. Opening the demand valve requires more ventilatory effort than is associated with a free-flowing IMV circuit, thus leading to increased work of breathing.

F. PCV

Pressure-control ventilation (PCV) is a volume variable mode in which inspiration is time initiated. A preset system pressure is rapidly achieved and maintained throughout inspiration. Tidal volume is dependent on the compliance and resistive elements of the lung. Inspiration ends at a predetermined time and is controlled by altering the I:E time. The type of ventilator is important in determining what occurs between the cycled breaths. Spontaneous ventilation may be hindered if the ventilator is in PCV-CMV (control-mode ventilation) mode. If the ventilator is in a PCV-IMV mode the patient will be able to breath between cycled breaths. PCV has the capacity to decrease peak airway pressure while increasing the mean-airway pressure. This may lead to improvements in oxygenation.

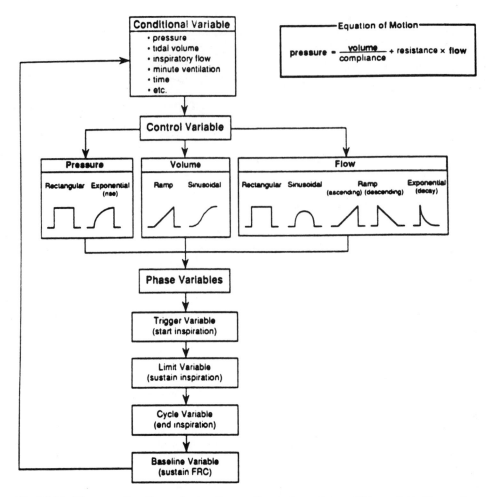

Fig. 36-21. New paradigm for understanding mechanical ventilators. This model indicates that during inspiration, the ventilator is able to control directly one and only one variable at a time (i.e., pressure, volume, or flow). Some common waveforms provided by current ventilators are shown for each control variable. Pressure, volume, flow, and time are also phase variables that determine the parameters of each ventilatory cycle (e.g., trigger, sensitivity, peak inspiratory flow rate, pressure, inspiratory time, and baseline pressure). Modes of ventilation are simple jargon for various combinations of control and phase variables. Diagram is drawn as flow chart to emphasize that each breath may have a different set of control and phase variables depending on mode of ventilation desired. (From Chatburn R: *Respir Care* 37(9):1009, 1992.)

VI. PHILOSOPHY OF SUPPORT OF LUNG FUNCTION WITH POSITIVE AIRWAY PRESSURE THERAPY

A. FULL VS. PARTIAL VENTILATORY SUPPORT (TABLE 36-3 ON P. 809)

Mechanical ventilatory support can be characterized in terms of the degree of support of minute ventilation — full ventilatory support where the required minute volume is delivered by the ventilatory versus partial ventilatory support where the patient's spontaneous ventilatory efforts contribute to the required minute ventilation. Mechanical ventilation does not ameliorate the pathophysiologic derangements responsible for the development of respiratory failure, although it can correct respiratory acidosis and eliminate excessive work

Table 36-1. Physical characteristics associated with initiation, limit, and cycling of the inspiratory phase of mechanical breath for each ventilator mode

Ventilator mode	Initiated	Limited	Cycled
CMV	Time	Volume	Volume/time
A/CMV	Pressure	Volume	Volume/time
IMV	Time	Volume	Volume/time
SIMV	Pressure	Volume	Volume/time
PSV	Pressure	Pressure	Flow
PCV	Time	Pressure	Time

CMV, control-mode ventilation; *A/CMV,* assist/control-mode ventilation; *IMV,* intermittent mandatory ventilation; *SIMV,* synchronized intermittent mandatory ventilation; *PSV,* pressure-support ventilation; *PCV,* pressure-control ventilation.

Table 36-2. Description of ventilator modes

Mode	Interaction between ventilator and patient
Control-mode ventilation	Patient does not participate in any phase of breathing cycle.
Assist/control-mode ventilation	Ventilator breath initiated by patient's inspiratory effort.
	Ventilator rate set by patient, if patient's respiratory rate is greater than the preset CMV rate.
Pressure-control ventilation	Time initiated.
	Pressure limited: a preset system pressure is rapidly achieved and maintained.
	Cycling occurs because of predetermined time.
Intermittent mandatory ventilation	Patient breathes spontaneously by means of a continuous-flow circuit between ventilator breaths delivered at preset intervals.
Synchronized intermittent mandatory ventilation	Patient breathes spontaneously by means of a demand-flow circuit between ventilator breaths delivered at preset intervals in synchrony with patient's inspiratory effort.
Pressure-support ventilation	Patient's inspiratory effort determines the rate.
	Ventilator maintains preset inspiratory pressure.
	Inspiration ends when patient's inspiratory flow falls below preset minimal value.

of breathing. Full support of ventilation does not provide any physiologic advantage compared with a level of partial ventilatory support that adequately reduces work of breathing and augments alveolar ventilation. Use of partial ventilatory support obviates a need for deep sedation, muscle paralysis, and induction of respiratory alkalosis. Moreover, as previously discussed, spontaneous ventilation facilitates $\dot{V}A/\dot{Q}$ matching. Techniques that permit spontaneous breathing activity are likely to maintain ventilatory muscle strength and coordination when compared with total control of ventilation. The adverse hemodynamic effects of positive-pressure ventilation can be minimized by administering an adequate level of partial ventilatory support and allowing some spontaneous breathing activity to persist.

The original modes of mechanical ventilation (control mode and assist/control mode) provide full ventilatory support. The introduction of intermittent-mandatory ventilation made provision of partial ventilatory support possible. The newer modes of ventilation (pressure-support ventilation [PSV], airway–pressure-release ventilation [APRV], and proportional-assist ventilation [PAV]), allow for partial ventilatory support. As discussed above, provision of the minimal amount of mechanical ventilatory support is a desirable clinical goal in the management of ARF.

B. MINIMAL-EXCURSION VENTILATION (MEV)

Recent studies suggest that lung trauma produced by positive-pressure ventilation may be due in part to overdistension of the alveoli associated with high end-inspiratory lung volume. New modes of therapy designed to reduce end-inspiratory lung volume (minimal-excursion ventilation) have lead to treatment such as

permissive hypercapnia and to the use of high-frequency ventilation, and have caused elimination of dead space.

1. Permissive hypercapnia

The simplest method of MEV is that of permissive hypercapnia or controlled hypoventilation wherein total minute ventilation is reduced, accepting the consequent $PaCO_2$ rise provided the pH remains in an acceptable range ($pH_a > 7.2$). If the pH is less than 7.2, bicarbonate therapy is often instituted. In Europe, where this approach has been aggressively used, $PaCO_2$ as high as 90 mm Hg have been reported.[9] This strategy has been shown to improve clinical outcome in both status asthmaticus and ARDS.[15,16]

2. Elimination of dead space

Another approach of MEV is the elimination of dead space by the insufflation of fresh gas directly into either the trachea or the bronchus.[17,18] Since the dead space volume is flushed out, effective alveolar ventilation for a given VT should increase. VT, and therefore the potential for iatrogenic injury, can be reduced while maintaining effective CO_2 elimination.

3. High-frequency ventilation

Perhaps the greatest experience with MEV techniques is in the field of high-frequency ventilation. Several different options exist but the common denominator is the delivery of fresh gas using a markedly increased ventilatory frequency, with a decreased VT. Though promising in animal models, the application of these modalities to patients has been somewhat disappointing.[19-21] High-frequency oscillation has been used extensively in neonates but the results are contra-

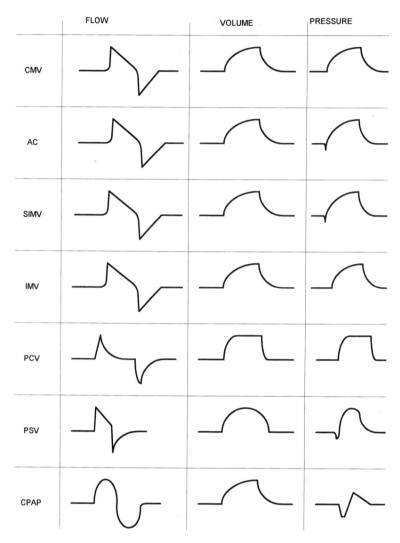

Fig. 36-22. Ventilator modes flow, volume, and pressure patterns. *AC,* assist control.

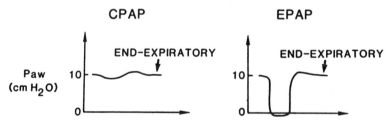

Fig. 36-23. Airway pressure (P_{aw}) tracing for CPAP (continuous positive airway pressure) and EPAP (expiratory positive airway pressure) (e.g., 10 cm H_2O). CPAP and EPAP are positive-pressure modes of spontaneous breathing that can be employed individually or in conjunction with mechanical ventilation. (From Perel A, Stock C: *Handbook of mechanical ventilatory support,* Baltimore, 1992, Williams & Wilkins.)

dictory and the role of this modality remains controversial.[22-28] The majority of adult experience with these techniques has been with high-frequency jet ventilation, and again, no clear application has emerged.[29] Work continues, however, to define more clearly exactly what role, if any, these high-frequency modalities may play in the ICU setting.[27,28]

C. AUGMENTED INSPIRED OXYGEN CONCENTRATIONS

In a normal lung, $\dot{V}_A/\dot{Q}$ changes very little from inspiration to expiration. In ARF the expiratory $\dot{V}_A/\dot{Q}$ is less than the inspiratory $\dot{V}_A/\dot{Q}$. At low $\dot{V}_A/\dot{Q}$ the rate of oxygen flow from an alveolus into the blood can exceed the tidal ventilation to that alveolus; alveolar nitrogen

Table 36-3. Differences between full vs. partial ventilatory support

	Full ventilatory support	Partial ventilatory support
Full minute ventilation delivered by ventilator	Yes	No
V/Q mismatch	+++	+
Dead space	+++	+
Shunt	+++	+
Work of breathing	low to none	low to normal
Potential hemodynamic stability	++	++++
Disuse ventilatory muscle atrophy	+++	+

+, present but not likely to be significant; ++, may be significant depending on situation; +++, significant effect; ++++, very likely to be significant.

helps to maintain the alveolar volume. Breathing oxygen-augmented gas will decrease alveolar nitrogen concentrations and thus allow for a reduction in alveolar volume and further decrease in $\dot{V}_A/\dot{Q}$. If alveolar volume falls below a critical level, alveolar collapse and development of regions in which $\dot{V}_A/\dot{Q}=0$ will result. Lung units with an inspiratory $\dot{V}_A/\dot{Q}$ of <0.1 are stable only when breathing ambient air because of the "splinting" effect of nitrogen. Evaluation of venous admixture ($\dot{Q}_{va}/\dot{Q}_t$) in patients with ARF breathing increasing concentrations of inspired oxygen showed progressive decrease in calculated $\dot{Q}_{va}/\dot{Q}_t$ from room air up to 40% oxygen. Calculated $\dot{Q}_{va}/\dot{Q}_t$ remained unchanged on oxygen concentrations from 40% to 60% and then increased as inspired-oxygen concentration approached 100%. Increasing inspired oxygen to 40% masks the hypoxemia-producing effect of lung areas with $\dot{V}_A/\dot{Q}<0.1$, thereby accounting for the observed decrease in calculated $\dot{Q}_{va}/\dot{Q}_t$. The observed increase in calculated $\dot{Q}_{va}/\dot{Q}_t$ caused by breathing high concentrations of oxygen may result from atelectasis. However, altered pulmonary perfusion may also contribute to this effect. In areas of the lung with $\dot{V}_A/\dot{Q}<0.1$, hypoxic pulmonary vasoconstriction is thought to limit perfusion by shunting blood to areas with better ventilation. When the inspired-oxygen concentration is increased, alveolar P_{O_2} rises, precapillary pulmonary vasoconstriction decreases, and perfusion to areas with low $\dot{V}_A/\dot{Q}$ increases. Another possible explanation is that oxygen inhalation increases extraalveolar shunting of venous blood. Such right-to-left intrapulmonary shunting of blood can increase calculated $\dot{Q}_{va}/\dot{Q}_t$. Short term exposure to 50% inspired O_2 has been shown to have deleterious effects in postoperative patients.[30] Similarly increases in $\dot{V}_A/\dot{Q}<0.01$ have been reported in restrictive lung models using dogs breathing 50% O_2. Acute lung dysfunction often results in lung areas with low $\dot{V}_A/\dot{Q}$. Therapy

should be directed to correct the dysfunction and improve $\dot{V}_A/\dot{Q}$. Therefore, it is preferable for the inspired-oxygen concentration to be at a level that will not mask the effects produced by areas of low $\dot{V}_A/\dot{Q}$. Such an inspired-oxygen concentration will better allow evaluation of low $\dot{V}_A/\dot{Q}$ and the effects of therapy. Because spontaneous ventilation is associated with better matching of ventilation and perfusion than is mechanical ventilation, allowing patients to breathe spontaneously to whatever degree they can tolerate is preferable for the maintenance of pulmonary-oxygen transfer.

VII. CLINICAL APPLICATION OF POSITIVE AIRWAY PRESSURE THERAPY

One of the first decisions upon initiating ventilator support is to determine the magnitude of physiologic derangement and underlying pathology and then applying the correct mode of mechanical ventilation. Full ventilatory support (FVS) should only be instituted in patients who do not have a stable respiratory drive, who have left ventricular failure, or in whom ventilatory muscle fatigue is suspected. All other patients should receive partial ventilatory support (PVS) at a level sufficient to sustain stable cardiopulmonary function.

A. FULL VENTILATORY SUPPORT

FVS may be provided by CMV, A/CMV, PCV, IMV, SIMV, and PSV modes. There are no data to suggest that any of these modes are superior for the provision of FVS. IMV set at rates sufficient to achieve FVS is essentially the same as CMV; SIMV set at high rates functions similarly to A/CMV. The advantages of IMV, SIMV, and PSV lie in their use for PVS; CMV and A/CMV can only provide FVS. Thus, CMV and A/CMV will be considered as modes for provision of FVS and IMV, and SIMV and PSV will be described for provision of PVS. Depending on the particular ventilator to be used, PCV breaths may be delivered as a form of CMV or as the mandatory machine breath of IMV (PC-IMV).

1. **CMV (Fig. 36-24)**
   a. Clinical indications: Apnea, neuromuscular dysfunction, abnormal ventilatory drive, left ventricular failure.
   b. Independent elements requiring specific orders:
      (1) Respiratory rate: Minimum necessary to achieve eucapnia with preset V_T.
      (2) Tidal volume: Between 7 and 10 ml/kg.
      (3) Fio_2: Initial setting of 0.5. After initiation of ventilatory support, titrate against S_pO_2 with goal of maintaining S_pO_2 between 90% and 92%.
      (4) PEEP: Routine use of PEEP of 5 cm H_2O is advised to assist in maintenance of FRC. Patients with PEEP responsive disease should

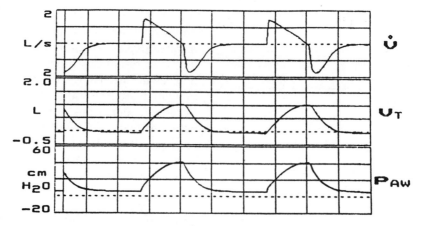

Fig. 36-24. Flow, volume, and pressure waveforms for what is commonly referred to as CMV (control mode ventilation). (From Branson R: *Respir Care* 37(9):1026, 1992.)

have PEEP titrated to desirable end point of improvement in lung mechanics, reduction in intrapulmonary shunting, and/or improvement in arterial oxygenation.

(5) Inspiratory time: T_{insp} should allow for adequate alveolar filling. Usually, 4 alveolar time constants are sufficient to ensure good filling. Commonly employed ventilator default settings are 1.5 seconds.

(6) I:E ratio: To ensure complete exhalation and to minimize overall rise in mean intrathoracic pressure, expiration should exceed inspiration. I:E of 1:2 or greater is recommended. At I:E of 1:<2, it is essential to actively check for the development of PEEP$_{intrinsic}$.

c. Dependent elements requiring evaluation:

(1) Is patient trying to initiate a breath? If patient is attempting to breathe, reevaluate choice of CMV mode.

(2) Peak inspiratory pressures (PIP): High PIP result from many causes. Differential diagnosis of factors that may lead to high PIP include the following:

(a) Increased airway resistance.
(i) Kinked ET.
(ii) Small ET.
(iii) Secretions in ET.
(iv) Turbulent flow due to high inspiratory flow rates or short T_{insp}.
(v) Bronchospasm.
(vi) Bronchial narrowing secondary to secretions, edema, or constrictive lesions.

(b) Decreased lung compliance.
(i) Lung pathology resulting in low chest wall and/or parenchymal compliance.
(ii) Overdistension due to excessive V_T or PEEP. Unrecognized PEEP$_{intrinsic}$

caused by high ventilator rate (>15 cycles/min) and/or high expiratory-flow resistance may also contribute to overdistension of lung parenchyma.

(3) Is there any PEEP$_{intrinsic}$? Consider possibility if there is any clinical evidence of expiratory wheezing, prolonged exhalation, or ventilatory rate greater than 15 cycles/min.

d. Potential hazards:

(1) $\dot{V}co_2$ and required minute ventilation: CMV delivers a fixed, physician-determined minute ventilation. If any physiologic changes occur that increase carbon dioxide production, the minute ventilation will be inadequate, leading to a respiratory acidosis.

(2) Cardiovascular system (CVS) effects: Full ventilatory support has potential to produce detrimental cardiovascular effects.

(3) Sedation/paralysis: CMV frequently requires heavy sedation or neuromuscular paralysis to keep the patient comfortable and in synchrony with the ventilator. These therapies are associated with side effects and risks.

(4) Ventilatory muscle function: CMV is associated with disuse of ventilatory muscles, which may lead to disuse atrophy and loss of function with prolonged ventilation (>3 days).

2. A/CMV (Fig. 36-25)

a. Clinical indications: Full ventilatory support in patient with intact, normal ventilatory drive.

b. Independent elements requiring specific orders:

(1) Ventilator rate: Rate is determined by patient, who triggers a machine breath by reducing airway pressure below baseline with an inspiratory effort. A backup CMV rate is set by the physician to ensure adequate ventilatory

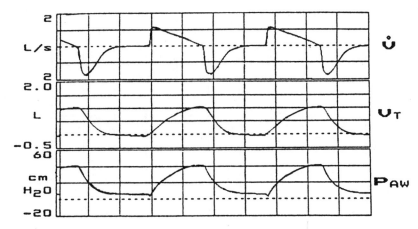

Fig. 36-25. Flow, volume, and pressure waveforms for what is commonly referred to as A/C. The difference between the CMV and A/C waveforms is in the negative pressure deflections prior to breath delivery. (From Branson R: *Respir Care* 37(9):1026, 1992.)

support in the event that the patient fails to make spontaneous inspiratory efforts.

(2) VT: 7 to 10 ml/kg body weight.

(3) Fio_2: Initial setting of 0.5. After initiation of ventilatory support, titrate against S_pO_2 with goal of maintaining S_pO_2 between 90% and 92%.

(4) PEEP: Routine use of PEEP of 5 cm H_2O is advised to assist in maintenance of FRC. Patients with PEEP responsive disease should have PEEP titrated to desirable end point of improvement in lung mechanics, reduction in intrapulmonary shunting, and/or improvement in arterial oxygenation.

(5) Inspiratory time: T_{insp} should allow for adequate alveolar filling. Usually 4 alveolar time constants are sufficient to ensure good filling. Commonly employed ventilator default settings are 1.5 seconds.

(6) I:E ratio: Will be in part determined by patient. Backup rate setting should include I:E of 1:2 or greater.

(7) Sensitivity of trigger: Trigger sensitivity describes the amount of change in baseline pressure that the patient has to generate to initiate a machine breath. Recommended setting is -2 cm of H_2O. If the sensitivity is set too high then the patient will struggle to initiate a breath, with subsequent increased work of breathing. If the sensitivity is set to very low levels the ventilator may autocycle, leading to overventilation.

c. Dependent elements requiring evaluation:

(1) Patient tolerance of trigger setting: Is the sensitivity set appropriately to enable the patient to initiate machine breaths without excessive work of breathing?

(2) Ventilatory rate: Is the patient-initiated–ventilator rate appropriate to maintain eucapnia? Is the patient-initiated rate resulting in alveolar hyperventilation and respiratory alkalosis because factors other than $Paco_2$ are stimulating the respiratory center? This latter circumstance should prompt reevaluation of the choice of A/CMV mode.

d. Potential hazards:

(1) VT: One of the difficulties with this mode of ventilation is that the patient has no control over tidal volume. Patients may complain that they are getting too big or too small a breath. To minimize this effect, the patient should be asked whether the delivered tidal volume feels comfortable.

(2) Respiratory alkalosis: This problem may develop whenever the patient's ventilatory drive is not servoregulated by changes in $Paco_2$, for example, in patients with CNS disease, hypoxemia, metabolic acidosis, pain, or anxiety.

3. PCV (Figs. 36-26 and 36-27)

a. Clinical indication: As PCV allows for control of T_{insp} and minimization of PIP, it is a useful technique for patients with diffuse nonhomogeneous lung injury. It can be applied as part of either a CMV technique (Fig. 36-26) or an IMV technique (Fig. 36-27).

b. Independent elements requiring specific orders:

(1) Rate: Minimum necessary to achieve eucapnia (CMV) or reduce WOB (PC-IMV).

(2) PIP: PIP is set to a level sufficient to achieve an adequate VT. Values less than 35 to 40 cm H_2O are generally recommended. If VT is inadequate at these pressures, prolongation of T_{insp} allows for further control of VT.

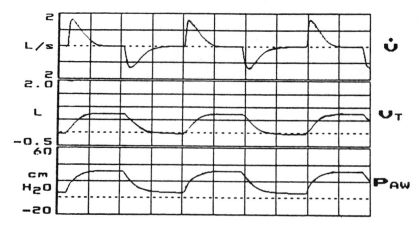

Fig. 36-26. Flow, volume, and pressure waveforms for pressure-controlled ventilation (PC-V). (From Branson R: *Respir Care* 37(9):1026, 1992.)

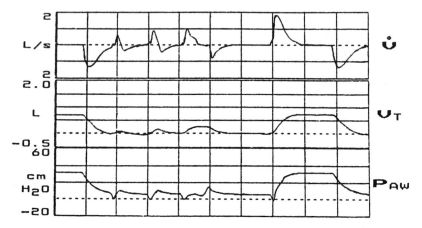

Fig. 36-27. Flow, volume, and pressure waveforms for intermittent mandatory ventilation, combined triggered. Note the negative pressure deflection prior to mandatory breath delivery. (From Branson R: *Respir Care* 37(9):1026, 1992.)

(3) Inspiratory time and I:E ratio: T_{insp} should be set to a value sufficient to achieve an adequate V_T for the preset pressure gradient. Start with T_{insp} of 1.5 seconds and increase while monitoring V_T. I:E ratio is not set directly but results from selection of ventilator rate and T_{insp}. PCV may be used to achieve reverse I:E ratio ventilation in patients with severe ARDS.

(4) Fio_2: Initial setting of 0.5. After initiation of ventilatory support, titrate against Spo_2 with goal of maintaining Spo_2 between 90% and 92%.

(5) PEEP: Routine use of PEEP of 5 cm H_2O is advised to assist in maintenance of FRC. Patients with PEEP responsive disease should have PEEP titrated to desirable end point of improvement in lung mechanics, reduction in intrapulmonary shunting, and/or improvement in arterial oxygenation. With longer T_{insp} and reverse I:E ratios,

$PEEP_{intrinsic}$ develops. True PEEP (set PEEP plus $PEEP_{intrinsic}$) has to be monitored. Commonly, with low I:E or reversed I:E ratios, set PEEP can be reduced to very low levels or even set at zero.

c. Dependent elements requiring evaluation:

(1) Tidal volume: The V_T is determined by the intrinsic lung compliance and the set pressure gradient. V_T will vary directly with compliance. It is important to monitor lung compliance closely during PCV. Deterioration in lung compliance will result in decreased V_T and hypoventilation. Improvement in compliance may result in increasing end-inspiratory lung volume with potential for development of barotrauma/volutrauma.

(2) Spontaneous ventilation: Is the patient trying to initiate a breath? Depending on the ventilator being used, ventilator asynchrony may at times be alleviated by initiation of PSV in addition to PCV. The patient may also be a

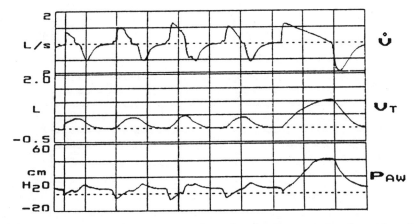

Fig. 36-28. Flow, volume, and pressure waveforms for what is commonly referred to as SIMV. (From Branson R: *Respir Care* 37(9):1026, 1992.)

candidate for partial ventilatory support with PC-IMV.

(3) Is there $PEEP_{intrinsic}$? Consider possibility if there is any clinical evidence of expiratory wheezing, prolonged exhalation, short expiratory times associated with low or reversed I:E ratios, or ventilatory rate greater than 15 cycles/min.

d. Potential hazards:

(1) Volume variability associated with changes in pulmonary compliance or resistance has potential for disadvantageous effects. Use of alarms to delineate unacceptable changes from the expected tidal volume are clearly indicated.

(2) CVS effects: PCV, particularly with high ventilator rates, reverse I:E ratios, or in patients with minimal reduction of lung compliance, has the potential to produce detrimental cardiovascular effects.

(3) Sedation/paralysis: PCV used as part of a CMV technique frequently requires heavy sedation or neuromuscular paralysis to keep the patient comfortable and in synchrony with the ventilator. These therapies are associated with side effects and risks.

(4) Ventilatory muscle function: PCV used as part of a CMV technique is associated with disuse of ventilatory muscles, which may lead to disuse atrophy and loss of function with prolonged ventilation (>3 days).

B. PARTIAL VENTILATORY SUPPORT

1. IMV/SIMV (Fig. 36-28)

IMV initially was provided by a ventilator in the CMV made with a free flowing gas circuit that bypassed the ventilator for spontaneous breaths. Modifications of this approach include SIMV, which consists of the mechanical breaths delivered in the A/C mode with gas for spontaneous ventilation from a demand flow circuit, and PC-IMV, which consists of the mechanical breaths delivered in a PCV mode with spontaneous ventilation via a demand-flow circuit. IMV differs from these modifications primarily in the patient work requirements for the spontaneous breaths; the continuous gas-delivery circuit of IMV is associated with less patient work than is a demand-flow circuit.

a. Clinical indication: Provision of partial ventilatory support (PVS) where a fixed mechanical V_T is desirable.

b. Independent elements requiring specific orders:

(1) Respiratory rate: Minimum necessary to achieve eucapnia with preset V_T.

(2) Tidal volume: Between 7 and 10 ml/kg.

(3) Fio_2: Initial setting of 0.5. After initiation of ventilatory support, titrate against Spo_2 with goal of maintaining Spo_2 between 90% and 92%.

(4) PEEP: Routine use of PEEP of 5 cm H_2O is advised to assist in maintenance of FRC. Patients with PEEP responsive disease should have PEEP titrated to desirable end point of improvement in lung mechanics, reduction in intrapulmonary shunting, and/or improvement in arterial oxygenation.

(5) Inspiratory time: T_{insp} should allow for adequate alveolar filling. Usually 4 alveolar time constants are sufficient to ensure good filling. Commonly employed ventilator default settings are 1.5 seconds.

(6) I:E ratio: To ensure complete exhalation and to minimize overall rise in mean intrathoracic pressure, expiration should exceed inspiration. I:E of 1:2 or greater is recommended. At I:E of 1:<2 it is essential to actively check for the development of $PEEP_{intrinsic}$.

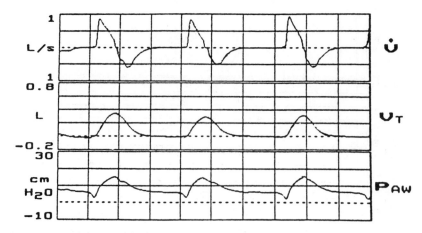

Fig. 36-29. Flow, volume, and pressure waveforms for pressure support ventilation. (From Branson R: *Respir Care* 37(9):1026, 1992.)

(7) Sensitivity of trigger: The trigger sensitivity is only important in SIMV as it describes the amount of baseline pressure change the patient has to generate to initiate a machine breath or open the demand valve. Recommended setting is -2 cm of H_2O. If the sensitivity is set too high then the patient will struggle to initiate a breath with subsequent increased work of breathing. In IMV machines the sensitivity is not important, since there is a continuous gas flow through the circuit for spontaneous breathing.

c. Dependent elements requiring evaluation:
(1) Patient tolerance of trigger sensitivity. Is the sensitivity appropriately set to enable the patient to initiate machine breaths or the demand valve without excessive work of breathing?
(2) Is there adequate humidification? Patients on IMV, because of the continuous flow, are at increased risk for complications associated with inadequate humidification.

d. Potential hazards:
(1) Increased work of breathing due to demand valve in SIMV: IMV is better in the sense that no demand valve has to be opened.
(2) If $\dot{V}_{CO_2}$ is increased, the required increase in minute ventilation may exceed the patient's capacity to tolerate the increased work of breathing, leading to deleterious cardiovascular effects.

2. PSV (Fig. 36-29)

PSV has potential advantages over IMV/SIMV for provision of partial ventilatory support, because the assistance provided with PSV increases with increased ventilatory demand unlike the fixed contri-

bution of IMV/SIMV.[30] Furthermore, the work characteristics of a PSV-assisted breath may produce a beneficial conditioning effect on ventilatory muscle function when compared with unassisted breathing against the high resistance of the endotracheal tube.[31]

a. Clinical indication: Partial ventilatory support in patients with intact ventilatory drive and mild to moderate lung dysfunction.

b. Independent elements requiring specific orders:
(1) Inspiratory pressure level: The inspiratory pressure level can be set to achieve a desired V_T or to reduce inspiratory WOB to acceptable levels, or both. We recommend titration of PSV level against respiratory rate with a goal of 15 to 24 breaths/min; this is usually associated with a reduction of WOB to levels within functional limits. An alternative approach is to titrate PSV to achieve a V_T of 7 to 10 ml/kg, termed PSV_{max}; thereafter PSV can be decreased as tolerated.[32] PSV_{max} probably approximates the provision of FVS with the PSV mode. Low levels of PSV (5 to 10 cm H_2O) are frequently used to overcome the imposed work of breathing associated with demand valves in SIMV or resistance of the endotracheal tube.
(2) Fio_2: Initial setting of 0.5. After initiation of ventilatory support, titrate against Spo_2 with goal of maintaining Spo_2 between 90% and 92%.
(3) CPAP: Routine use of CPAP of 5 cm H_2O is advised to assist in maintenance of FRC. Patients with CPAP responsive disease should have CPAP titrated to desirable end point of improvement in lung mechanics, reduction in intrapulmonary shunting, and/or improvement in arterial oxygenation.

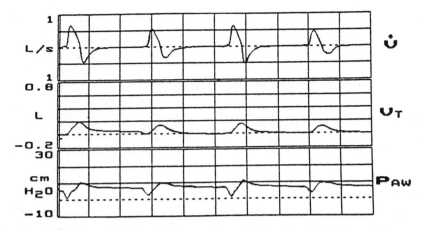

Fig. 36-30. Flow, volume, and pressure waveforms for continuous positive airway pressure (CPAP). All breaths are spontaneous. (From Branson R: *Respir Care* 37(9):1026, 1992.)

(4) Flow rate or flow pattern: Inappropriate inspiratory flow delivery can make PSV very uncomfortable or may result in an increase in WOB. The newer ventilators allow for manipulation of the inspiratory flow. With high flows, the patient's airway is subjected to sudden change in pressure. Most patients say this feels uncomfortable and often cough or actively breath against the ventilator. On the other hand, low flows may lead to air hunger with resultant increased work of breathing as the patient attempts to inhale through a partially occluded valve.

c. Dependent elements requiring evaluation:
  (1) Spontaneous respiratory rate: Respiratory rate tends to decrease as PSV level is increased and inspiratory WOB is reduced. If respiratory rate does not decrease, consider whether patient has normal ventilatory drive. Patients with severely diminished lung compliance often maintain a high respiratory rate even at PSV_{max}. In this circumstance consider switching to another mode, for example, PCV-IMV.
  (2) Tidal volume: V_T will vary with the level of PSV, lung compliance, and T_{insp}. Patients determine T_{insp} because the ventilator maintains the preset PSV level until patient-generated inspiratory flow declines to some predetermined value (flow cycling). The V_T and compliance vary directly as for PCV. It is important to monitor for changes in compliance. Improvement in lung mechanics invariably is associated with an increase in V_T and a decrease in respiratory rate.

d. Potential hazards:
  (1) If ventilatory drive fails, the patient will receive no ventilatory support.

(2) Excessive levels of PSV may be associated with very large V_T and potential for high end-inspiratory lung volumes.

3. PEEP/CPAP (Fig. 36-30)
  a. Clinical indication: Reduced FRC and decreased compliance.
  b. Independent elements requiring specific orders:
    (1) PEEP/CPAP level: Titrate CPAP against spontaneous ventilatory pattern and/or improvement in arterial oxygenation. Normally, patients will be comfortable with CPAP levels that maintain their respiratory rate at 15 to 20 breaths/min. PEEP levels may be titrated to improve arterial oxygenation, reduce intrapulmonary shunting, and improve lung compliance.
    (2) Fio_2: Initial setting of 0.5. After initiation of support, titrate against Spo_2 with goal of maintaining Spo_2 between 90% and 92%.
    (3) Inspiratory flow delivery: With CPAP it is essential to provide adequate flow to ensure that CPAP and not EPAP is provided. A flow sufficient to limit pressure fluctuations around preset CPAP level to $\pm$ 2 cm H_2O is recommended.
  c. Dependent elements requiring evaluation:
    (1) Observe for signs of excessive PEEP/CPAP.
      (a) Active exhalation.
      (b) Hyperinflation of lung.
      (c) Increased V_D/V_T.
      (d) Initiation: Start with 5 cm of H_2O and increase in increments of 3 to 5 cm H_2O until desired effect achieved.
      (e) Maintenance: Adjust CPAP/PEEP level against ventilatory pattern, and/or arterial oxygenation.

Table 36-4. Expected relationships in minute-volume to arterial–carbon dioxide tension in normal, nonexercising man

MV	Paco^2 (mm Hg)	Range (mm Hg)
Normal	40	35-45
Twice normal	30	25-35
Quadruple normal	20	15-25

   (f) Potential hazards:

      (i) Excessive PEEP/CPAP may lead to hyperinflation and risk of barotrauma/volutrauma. This is particularly true when PEEP is used in conjunction with IPPV.

     (ii) Increased expiratory work of breathing. Excessive CPAP may lead to active exhalation and increased expiratory WOB.

   (iii) PEEP is associated with decreased cardiac output. Excessive PEEP, especially with IPPV, may lead to decreased right and left ventricular preload, increased right ventricular afterload, increased right ventricular end-diastolic volume with encroachment of the interventricular septum into the left ventricle, and consequent decrease in left ventricular end-diastolic volume and cardiac output. Application of appropriate levels of PEEP to patients with reduced compliance is usually well tolerated. CPAP, because it is associated with cyclic falls in intrapleural pressure, is usually associated with adequate venous return. Lung volume with appropriate levels of CPAP is usually close to a normal FRC; thus, right ventricular preload is not adversely affected.

VIII. WEANING FROM MECHANICAL VENTILATORY SUPPORT

Weaning a patient off mechanical ventilatory support is dependent on the patient assuming the full work of breathing. Thus, assessment of the inspiratory work (work of breathing and ventilatory demand) and the patient's ability to handle the work (cardiopulmonary reserves) are key preliminary steps to prepare the patient for weaning. Weaning off ventilatory support is most likely to be successful when the required work of breathing is minimal and the patient's cardiopulmonary reserves have been optimized.

A. DETERMINANTS OF WORK OF BREATHING

1. Minute volume (Table 36-4)

The required minute alveolar ventilation ($\dot{V}A$) is determined by carbon dioxide production ($\dot{V}CO_2$). The required total minute volume is the sum of $\dot{V}A$ and dead space ventilation. Approximately one third of the inspired gas does not participate normally in gas exchange with pulmonary blood because it lies within conductive airways (anatomic dead space) or ventilated non-perfused or under-perfused alveoli (alveolar dead space). Under normal physiologic conditions the ratio of dead-space ventilation to total ventilation (VD/VT) is 0.3. This value is commonly increased to 0.5 or greater by cardiopulmonary disease and by mechanical ventilation. The greater the dead-space ventilation, the greater will be the required minute volume to maintain eucapnia. The relationship of minute volume to work of breathing is not linear (Fig. 36-31). Thus increments in required minute volume will result in progressively greater increases in work of breathing.

$\dot{V}CO_2$ is proportional to metabolic rate. Any factors which increase metabolic rate, that is, fever, sepsis, or hyperalimentation, will increase $\dot{V}CO_2$ and hence the required minute volume. Nutrient type and supply relative to caloric requirement may impact on $\dot{V}CO_2$. (See section on ventilatory demand.)

Nonmetabolic determinants of elevated minute ventilation include alveolar hyperventilation secondary to acidosis, hypoxemia, and central nervous system disorders.

For a given minute ventilation, the required work depends on lung mechanics and breathing circuit characteristics.

2. Airway resistance

Bronchoconstriction and excessive mucus production may lead to increased work of breathing that may limit the weaning process. Prior treatment with control of symptoms will provide the optimal weaning opportunity.

3. Pattern of breathing

Patients will usually assume a pattern of breathing associated with the least possible work of breathing. Simultaneous consideration of resistance and elastic work factors enables graphic depiction of the relationship between total work of breathing and pattern of breathing (Fig. 36-32). Factors other than maintenance of eucapnia that directly stimulate ventilatory drive may result in a pattern of breathing associated with higher work of breathing—for example, acidosis or hypoxemia.

B. MEASUREMENT OF WORK OF BREATHING

The reliable measurement of work of breathing at the bedside is difficult and seldom undertaken. Measurement of aspects of ventilatory muscle metabolism

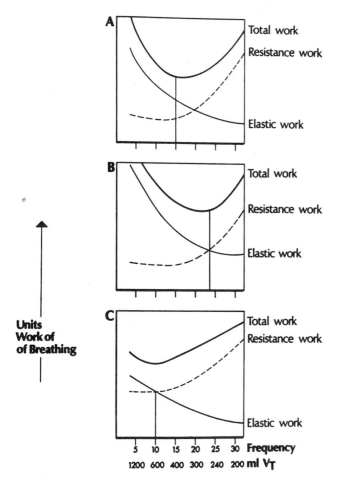

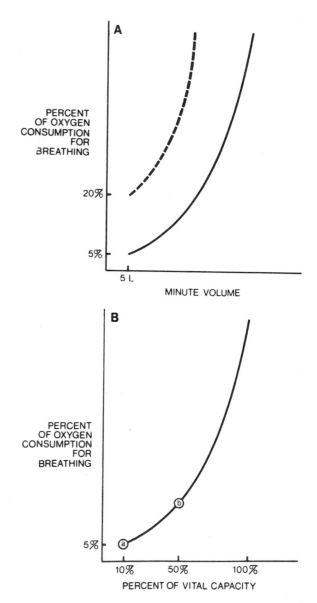

Fig. 36-31. Total work of breathing when minute ventilation is unchanged, but ventilatory pattern (tidal volume and frequency) is varied, *A*. Note that for any minute ventilation there is a ventilatory pattern that requires minimal work. Of course, total work is the summation of resistance work (airways) and elastic work (lung parenchymal and chest-wall recoil forces). If compliance alone is decreased, as in *B*, pattern of ventilation at which minute volume can be achieved with minimal work is more rapid and shallow, as graph shows. If resistance alone is increased, as in *C*, pattern of ventilation at which minute volume can be achieved with minimal work is deep and slow. Diagram indicates principle that work of breathing is a major factor determining ventilatory pattern. (From Shapiro BA, Harrison RA, Cane RD et al: *Clinical application of blood gases,* ed 4, Chicago, 1989, Mosby–Year Book.)

Fig. 36-32. *A,* Work of breathing in relation to vital capacity (VC). In *B,* point *a* represents a VT of 500 ml with a VC to 5 L; point *b* represents a VT of 500 ml with a VC of 1 L. (From Shapiro BA, Harrison RA, Cane RD et al: *Clinical application of blood gases,* ed 4, Chicago, 1989, Mosby–Year Book.)

(oxygen consumption, electromyography) or of the pressures and flows generated by ventilatory muscles provide means for quantifying work of breathing. Bedside pulmonary monitors are available that calculate work of breathing from simultaneous measurement of gas flow and airway and esophageal pressures. Greater experience is needed to be able to interpret a given value of work of breathing obtained in this manner. However, trends following changes in level of mechanical ventilatory support during weaning are useful.

The spontaneous respiratory rate provides a sensitive

reflector of the relationship between inspiratory workload and inspiratory reserve. Many clinicians take advantage of this fact and do not attempt to quantify work of breathing. Rather, they evaluate a patient's tolerance for a given inspiratory work load by assessment of respiratory rate and other signs of sympathetic stimulation, namely heart rate, systolic hypertension, diaphoresis, and complaints of dyspnea. If the required work of breathing places a demand on cardiopulmonary function that exceeds a patient's reserves, the patient will manifest tachypnea and these signs of sympathetic stress, a circumstance considered detrimental work of breathing. In the absence of signs of detrimental work of breathing, it is reasonable to assume that the work of breathing falls within functional reserves and is not a problem.

C. EVALUATION OF PATIENT PRIOR TO WEANING

Before attempting to wean a patient off ventilatory support, the following questions need to be asked:

1. Has the condition that necessitated ventilatory support been reversed? Irrespective of the specific pathology that led to an inability to maintain spontaneous ventilation, once the patient's lung function has improved to the point that spontaneous ventilation is possible, the patient should promptly be weaned. Attempts to wean too early invariably fail and prolong the duration of required support. Maintenance of ventilatory support beyond the required time increases patient risk, morbidity, and ICU costs.

2. Does the patient have adequate cardiopulmonary reserves to be able to maintain spontaneous ventilation? Ventilatory reserve, cardiac function, and arterial blood gases need to be evaluated.

3. Are ventilatory demand and ventilatory work requirements minimal? Minute ventilation, airway resistance, and lung compliance should be evaluated.

4. Is the patient psychologically prepared for weaning?

1. Assessment of cardiopulmonary reserves

a. VENTILATORY RESERVE

Bedside evaluation of ventilatory reserve involves both clinical observation of the patient's spontaneous ventilatory pattern and appropriate interpretation of two spirometric measurements; vital capacity and forced expiratory volume (FEV_1).

i. Spontaneous ventilatory pattern. One of the major advantages of partial ventilatory support is that it allows for evaluation of spontaneous breathing prior to complete withdrawal of ventilatory support. The ventilatory pattern is composed of tidal volume (V_T), respiratory rate, and I:E ratio. It is often difficult to evaluate V_T in mechanically ventilated patients who have not breathed spontaneously for a period of time; immediate V_T of 2 ml/kg are encouraging values. A normal, predicted V_T is 7 to 9 ml/kg of ideal body weight. Although a quantitative measurement is important, the simple observation of ease with which the patient maintains a given V_T is equally essential. Thus, spontaneous respiratory rate also is useful as a reflector of ventilatory reserve. A spontaneous breathing pattern with prolonged expiratory phase is consistent with expiratory airflow obstruction and warrants further investigation before discontinuance of ventilatory support.

ii. Vital capacity. Bedside assessment of ventilatory reserve is reflected most reliably in the forced vital capacity (FVC) measurement. A previously healthy adult requires a minimal VC of 15 ml/kg to maintain adequate spontaneous ventilation and to ensure an effective cough. Keep in mind that bedside measurement of FVC is prone to error because both a tight airway seal and patient cooperation are required. Thus falsely low VC may be obtained. Patients will seldom breathe with V_T of more than 40% of their true VC; thus, simultaneous measurement of V_T and VC provides a means of assessing the probable reliability of the VC measurement.

iii. Negative inspiratory pressure (NIP). In circumstances in which an FVC measurement is not obtainable, the measurement of NIP has been used as an alternative measure of ventilatory reserve. This measurement is obtained by inspiration against an occluded glottis. Strictly speaking, it is not a measure of ventilatory reserve but of ventilatory muscle power. Experience has shown that the muscular power needed to produce a VC of approximately 15 ml/kg produces a NIP greater than -20 cm H_2O in 20 seconds. A normal NIP is in excess of -80 cm of H_2O in 10 seconds.

b. CARDIAC FUNCTION

Cardiac reserve and function must also be assessed prior to discontinuing ventilatory support. Maintenance of ventilatory function requires adequate oxygen and energy substrate flow to the ventilatory muscles. An adequate cardiac output is essential. Minimal bedside evaluation of cardiovascular function depends on clinical assessment of heart rate and rhythm, blood pressure, cardiac-pump function, and tissue perfusion.

i. Rate and rhythm. An acceptable heart rate and rhythm are essential for proper functioning of the cardiovascular system. Evaluation of the etiology of tachycardia (heart rate above 100 bpm) or bradycardia (heart rate below 60 bpm) and correction should be done prior to discontinuing mechanical ventilation. Tachycardia does not allow adequate ventricular filling, and thus cardiac output may be diminished. Abnormal rhythms must also be assessed as they represent potential interference with mechanical function and inadequate cardiac output.

ii. Blood pressure. The etiology of extremes of blood pressure (hypertension, hypotension) should be sought and corrected where possible.

iii. Cardiac pump. Cardiac failure needs to be corrected prior to attempts at discontinuance or weaning from ventilatory support. The question of whether patients concurrently receiving inotropic support can be weaned from ventilatory support often comes up. Provided the patient is not in failure, it is reasonable to proceed with weaning from ventilatory support while maintaining inotropic support. Dopamine has been shown to augment diaphragmatic function, probably by maintaining better perfusion to the diaphragm.

iv. Perfusion. Urine output, skin temperature (i.e., is the skin warm and dry?), capillary refill, and sensorium and peripheral pulses are all helpful indicators of adequate tissue flow and perfusion.

c. NUTRITIONAL STATUS, HEMOGLOBIN CONCENTRATION

Effective ventilatory muscle function requires adequate muscle strength and endurance. Inadequate nutrition impairs muscle energy substrate storage and ATP reserves and results in loss of function. Delivery of adequate energy substrates and oxygen, while in large part a function of cardiac output, requires good nutrition and an adequate hemoglobin. In the absence of cardiovascular disease, a hemoglobin concentration of 7.5 to 8 g/dl is usually sufficient. Patients with compromised cardiovascular function may require a hemoglobin concentration between 8 and 10 g/dl.

d. ASSESSMENT OF VENTILATORY-DEMAND AND VENTILATORY-WORK REQUIREMENTS

i. $\dot{V}_{CO_2}$. The minute ventilation required to maintain carbon dioxide homeostasis is determined by the amount of carbon dioxide produced by metabolism. Any factors that increase $\dot{V}_{CO_2}$ will increase ventilatory demand. The principal cause of elevated $\dot{V}_{CO_2}$ is hyperalimentation. Overfeeding (provision of calories above resting energy expenditure) results in lipogenesis and a very high $\dot{V}_{CO_2}$. Most critically ill patients on mechanical ventilatory support require approximately 25 to 35 kcal/kg body weight per day. Patients with extreme catabolism, — for example, burns — may have an increased metabolic rate that leads to a higher caloric requirement. If available, caloric supply should be based on indirect calorimetry that enables measurement of $\dot{V}_{CO_2}$ and calculation of resting energy expenditure. In catabolic patients, calorie number appears to be more important than nature of calorie source. There are data that suggest that the calorie source, fat or carbohydrate, is important in noncatabolic patients. Provision of isocaloric support with a 50/50 mixture of fat and carbohydrates to patients recovering from sepsis was shown to be associated with lower $\dot{V}_{CO_2}$ than that associated with a pure carbohydrate calorie source. However, experience with the average ICU patient has shown that this is not important provided that the appropriate amount of calories are provided.

ii. Dead-space ventilation. Minute ventilation is the sum of effective alveolar ventilation (VA) and dead-space ventilation. The amount of dead-space ventilation (VD) can be quantified and expressed as a percentage of the VT, the VD/VT ratio. The VD/VT is normally 0.3. Provision of mechanical ventilatory support results in an increase in dead-space ventilation and the VD/VT ratio will increase from 0.3 to 0.5. Furthermore, patients with cardiopulmonary disease frequently have an increased amount of dead-space ventilation. Dead-space ventilation can be inferred from the relationship of total minute ventilation and the Pa_{CO_2}. Provided $\dot{V}_{CO_2}$ is relatively normal, approximately 4 to 5 L/min of VA is required to maintain a normal Pa_{CO_2}. Subtracting 4 to 5 L from the measured total minute ventilation will enable a rough approximation of the amount of dead-space ventilation. Similarly, predictions can be made when patients are hyperventilated. Table 36-4 shows the relationship between Pa_{CO_2} and hyperventilation. Levels of VD/VT >0.5 should be investigated and corrected where possible prior to attempts at cessation of ventilatory support.

iii. Ventilatory muscle efficiency. Muscle physiology is complex and beyond the scope of this review. Briefly, two factors, amenable to clinical manipulation, seem to be of significance in weaning patients off ventilatory support: muscle-fiber length and muscle-energy substrate storage. The principal ventilatory muscle is the diaphragm. Diaphragmatic muscle-fiber length is related to lung volume. Abnormally low or high lung volumes will alter muscle fiber length and change the zone of apposition between the diaphragm and chest wall with consequent reduction in ventilatory efficiency. CPAP can be used to increase lung volume in patients with reduced lung volumes. Hyperinflation is commonly associated with disease processes characterized by expiratory airflow obstruction. Malnutrition results in diminished energy substrate stores, loss of muscle power, and endurance.

D. PSYCHOLOGIC PREPARATION OF THE PATIENT

True psychologic dependence on mechanical ventilatory support, while possible, is extremely unusual. However, the removal of ventilatory support is often frightening to the patient and appropriate preparation is important. Anxiety resulting in tachypnea and hypertension will confound the clinical assessment of tolerance for the WOB and may adversely effect outcome by increasing spontaneous WOB.

The following procedures have proven to be clinically useful. First, fully explain ventilator discontinuance procedure to patient. Second, explain that discontinuing the ventilator is tailored to patient tolerance and that in some patients ventilator discontinuance is easily and quickly achieved, whereas others may need a longer weaning process. Therefore, the patient should not be discouraged if the first attempt is not successful. Third, reassure the patient that you will maintain close surveillance during the process and that he/she need not be fearful. Fourth, ensure that all respiratory depressant and neuromuscular blocking medications have been reversed. Finally, select the technique to be used, that is, ventilatory challenge or gradual weaning.

E. VENTILATORY CHALLENGE

A ventilatory challenge allows for assessment of the patient's ability to sustain their work of breathing. This challenge should provide a gradual, predictable, and safe increase in arterial P_{CO_2} and provide a reassuring milieu for the patient to assume WOB.

An adequate CNS stimulus is essential for maintenance of spontaneous ventilation. This stimulus is provided by the pH of the CSF bathing the floor of the fourth ventricle of the brain. As the CSF does not contain appreciable buffering capabilities, small changes in P_{CO_2} will result in relatively large pH changes. When a positive-pressure breath is administered every 30 seconds to an apneic patient, the rate of rise of P_{aCO_2} is 6 to 8 mm Hg in the first minute and 2 to 3 mm Hg each minute thereafter. The initial transition from mechanical to spontaneous ventilation is accomplished best with a manual ventilator delivering 50% to 80% oxygen.

A ventilatory challenge should proceed as follows:

1. Disconnect the patient from the ventilator and augment the patient's spontaneous ventilation with a manual resuscitator.
2. Provide a positive-pressure breath synchronized with the patient's spontaneous pattern approximately every 30 seconds. This procedure allows for a gradual, predictable, and safe increase in P_{aCO_2} and provides reassurance for the patient while he/she assumes the work of breathing.
3. Monitor vital signs and clinical status.
   a. Anticipate an increase in respiratory rate (RR), V_T, blood pressure (BP)/mean arterial pressure (MAP), pulse rate, and possibly onset of slight diaphoresis as patient assumes the work of breathing.
   b. Attempt to differentiate between physiologic and psychologic stress.
   c. Remain at the patient's bedside for the first 15 minutes.
4. If more than one breath every 30 seconds is required or the patient manifests significant detrimental changes in vital signs or clinical appearance, reinstitute mechanical ventilation.
5. If the patient maintains stable cardiopulmonary function after 10 to 15 minutes, attach an appropriate circuit with a fresh gas source to the endotracheal tube and observe.
6. Measure arterial blood gases after 15 minutes to verify the adequacy of ventilation and arterial oxygenation.

F. GRADUAL WEANING

Gradual weaning involves sequential reduction of mechanical support with a technique that allows the patient to increase progressively their contribution to the alveolar ventilation. Historically, this was achieved by placing the patient on a T circuit intermittently for short periods of time. If the patient tolerated the T circuit trial, then the duration of time on the T circuit was progressively increased until the patient was breathing spontaneously on the T circuit for the majority of the time. This technique is useful in patients who initially do well on discontinuance of ventilatory support but are unable to maintain spontaneous breathing over longer periods of time. Development of IMV/SIMV and more recently PSV offer alternative approaches for weaning. The advantages of these newer techniques is that the patient can be progressively exposed to increments of WOB without going from full support to no support abruptly. The approach to weaning with these techniques is similar in concept. The following procedures have proved to be reliable:

1. Establish baseline values of vital signs, any hemodynamic measures available, and arterial–blood gas (ABG) analysis.
2. Select ventilator mode, that is, IMV/SIMV or PSV.
   a. IMV/SIMV mode.
      (1) Decrease ventilator rate by 2 breaths/min and observe patient for two to four hours.
      (2) If cardiopulmonary function remains stable and ABG is acceptable, reduce ventilator rate by a further 2 breaths/min.
      (3) Continue this process until the patient is either weaned to CPAP or manifests unstable cardiopulmonary function. If the patient manifests unstable cardiopulmonary function, increase the ventilator rate to a level associated with stable cardiopulmonary function and reevaluate the indication for discontinuing ventilatory support.
   b. Pressure-support ventilation mode (PSV).
      (1) Stabilize the patient on PSV.
      (2) Decrease the level of PSV by 3 to 5 cms H_2O and observe patient for two to four hours.
      (3) If cardiopulmonary function remains stable and ABG is acceptable, continue decremental reduction in PSV level until the patient is either weaned to a pressure support of 3 to 5 cm H_2O with or without CPAP or manifests unstable cardiopulmonary function. If unstable cardiopulmonary function develops, either increase the pressure support to a level associated with stable function or return the patient to conventional PPV and reevaluate.

G. OXYGENATION DURING WEANING

During ventilator discontinuance or weaning, maintaining support of pulmonary oxygen transfer is important. During the process, ensure that the F_{iO_2} is at least the same as the maintenance F_{iO_2} on the ventilator. If

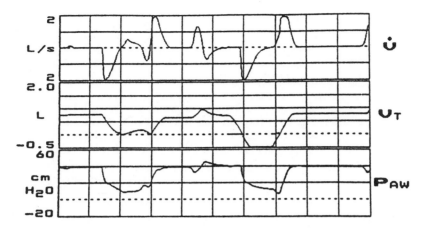

Fig. 36-33. Flow, volume, and pressure waveforms for airway pressure release ventilation (APRV) demonstrating spontaneous breathing throughout ventilatory cycle. (From Branson R: *Respir Care* 37(9):1026, 1992.)

the PEEP/CPAP on the ventilator is greater than 5 cm H_2O, the manual ventilator should be adapted to provide the same level of PEEP/CPAP.

After discontinuing PPV, provide appropriate Fio_2, CPAP, and possibly PSV via the endotracheal tube (ET). In the intubated, spontaneously ventilating patient, 3 to 5 cm H_2O CPAP and 3 to 5 cm H_2O of PSV help to maintain the functional residual capacity and minimize airway resistance secondary to the ET.

H. FAILURE TO WEAN

Failure of the patient to maintain adequate cardiopulmonary function while breathing spontaneously must be carefully evaluated.

1. Check for iatrogenic reasons for the failure—for example, oversedation, inadequate reversal of neuromuscular-blocking drugs, failure to provide appropriate support of oxygenation, use of a breathing circuit with high intrinsic airway resistance, or equipment malfunction.

2. Check for reversible factors that may be increasing the ventilatory demand,—for example, acidemia, hypoxemia, anemia, provision of excess calories, or inappropriate calorie source.

When these factors have been ruled out and clinical assessment of cardiopulmonary reserves still indicates that the patient should be able to breathe spontaneously, the assumption must be made that the patient is either unable to come off the ventilator because the underlying disease that led to a need for ventilatory support is not reversed adequately, or that psychologic dependence exists. Most weaning problems are due to attempting to discontinue ventilation too early in the disease course, improper ventilator maintenance, or preexisting chronic disease or malnutrition that severely limits cardiopul-

monary reserves. In the absence of these, the next most common problem is psychologic dependence.

A few patients may require reinstitution of partial ventilatory support at night because they are afraid to fall asleep breathing on their own. This approach may be a reasonable approach for several days. Psychologic dependence is a difficult problem and one that demands a great deal of understanding and patience. These individuals are in need of a weaning process in the traditional sense, that is, the process of taking the patient off the ventilator for short periods of time and trying progressively to lengthen the periods off PPV.

IX. FUTURE TRENDS IN VENTILATORY SUPPORT

A. AIRWAY PRESSURE RELEASE VENTILATION (APRV) (Figs. 36-33 and 36-34)

APRV is an unique mode of ventilatory support that augments alveolar ventilation by a decrease in airway pressure and lung volume in patients receiving CPAP.[32] The APRV system consists of a CPAP circuit in which baseline airway pressure is maintained above atmospheric levels using a threshold resistor valve and either a high gas flow, a pressurized volume reservoir, or a demand valve. A release valve with extremely low flow resistance is positioned in the expiratory limb of the CPAP circuit. The valve is operated by a timing mechanism that allows adjustment of the duration and frequency of pressure release. Use of APRV requires that a level of CPAP has been adjusted to optimize expiratory lung volume and pulmonary gas exchange. When the timer opens the release valve, airway pressure falls rapidly, gas exits the lungs, and lung volume decreases below baseline. When the release valve closes, CPAP and lung volume are rapidly reestablished.

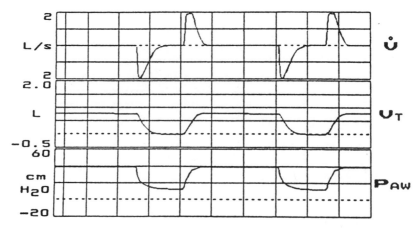

Fig. 36-34. Flow, volume, and pressure waveforms for airway pressure release ventilation (APRV) without spontaneous breathing. (From Branson R: *Respir Care* 37(9):1026, 1992.)

Augmentation of alveolar ventilation depends on release volume and the APRV rate. Release volume is determined by lung compliance, airway resistance, release time, and the gradient between CPAP and release pressure. The patient can breathe freely between, or during, the APRV breaths. Weaning from APRV is accomplished by lowering the frequency of airway pressure release, until the patient is breathing with CPAP alone.

Several studies have demonstrated the efficacy of APRV in supporting ventilation in animals, in patients following cardiac surgery and in patients with ARF of varying degrees of severity. All studies compared APRV with IPPV plus PEEP and showed effective ventilation with lower peak airway pressures and VT.[33-37] Peak airway pressure during APRV never exceeds the CPAP level, and maximum lung volume corresponds to functional residual capacity. Therefore, development of barotrauma should be minimal, a consideration yet to be investigated. To date, no reported instance of barotrauma has complicated the use of APRV. Changes in intrathoracic pressure during APRV are similar to those that occur during spontaneous breathing with CPAP. Available data confirm stability of cardiovascular function during ventilatory support with APRV.[33-37] Evaluation of $\dot{V}A/\dot{Q}$ during ventilatory support showed that APRV is associated with lesser increases in regions of lung with $\dot{V}A/\dot{Q} > 1$ than is seen with SIMV and PSV.[38] Thus available data suggest that APRV is an effective technique for ventilatory support of patients with restricted lung function.

Other applications of the concept of airway pressure release have been described, including bilevel positive airway pressure ventilation (BIPAP) and intermittent mandatory pressure release ventilation (IMPRV).[39] BIPAP was introduced for the nocturnal support of patients with sleep apnea. IMPRV is actually a sequential combination of PSV (inspiratory support) and APRV (expiratory support).[40] The clinical utility of these forms of airway pressure release ventilatory techniques need to be evaluated.[41]

B. PROPORTIONAL ASSIST VENTILATION (PAV)

Proportional assist ventilation was recently introduced as a means of mechanical ventilatory support in which pressure generated by the ventilator is proportional to and amplified by spontaneous breathing effort; the patient controls inspiratory and expiratory times, VT, and flow patterns. Unlike PSV, pressure during PAV is produced in conjunction with gas flow, rather than causing gas flow. Therefore, a PAV device must enable gas flow to the patient with negligible resistance. Potential advantages of PAV include minimal airway pressure and synchrony of patient and ventilator.[42] When PAV was initiated in five patients with stable cardiopulmonary function on SIMV, cardiopulmonary function and patient comfort were well maintained, peak airway pressure decreased by more than 50%, spontaneous respiratory rate decreased, spontaneous VT doubled, and arterial blood gases and MV remained unchanged.[43] Further study is required to define the clinical role of PAV.

C. EXTRACORPOREAL MEMBRANE OXYGENATION (ECMO)

Extracorporeal membrane oxygenation (ECMO) was the first attempt at continuous support that bypassed the lungs and has now been fairly extensively studied. In essence, this device acts as an extracorporeal lung, though differing degrees of oxygenation and CO_2 removal result. Arterial blood is removed, passed through the gas-exchange membrane circuit, and returned to the patient's systemic circulation via a large-bore venous-access cannula. Significant oxygen delivery can be effected with a moderate degree of CO_2

elimination. The basic idea was to "rest" the native lung and hopefully minimize iatrogenic contribution to lung injury. Widely used in the 1970s, it has not been shown to offer any improvement in outcome over conventional ventilatory support in the treatment of severe respiratory dysfunction.[44]

Other applications of extrapulmonary gas exchange have shown some promise. Venovenous bypass, as opposed to venoarterial bypass, has minimal effect upon pulmonary hemodynamics and may therefore be more advantageous than classic ECMO. Extracorporeal CO_2 removal using a membrane lung with venovenous bypass in combination with support of arterial oxygenation via the native lung has been shown to be efficacious in both animal and human studies.[39,40,45] Gattinoni and his group in Italy have had significant experience using this technique.[46] Their technique employed CO_2 removal by the membrane lung in the extracorporeal circuit; three to five mechanical breaths/min with PEEP of 15 to 25 cm H_2O and augmented Fio_2 were applied to the native lung to maintain arterial oxygenation and prevent atelectasis. V_T was set to ensure that the PIP was maintained below 45 cm H_2O. Using this technique in patients with severe pulmonary pathology, the authors were able to demonstrate a marked reduction in mortality when compared to historical controls, from more than 90% to approximately 50%. This study, though preliminary and uncontrolled, offers important clinical evidence suggesting that a reduction in lung-volume excursion during ventilatory support of patients with severe diffuse pulmonary disease may reduce pulmonary injury and improve patient outcome.

Extracorporeal CO_2 removal, however, is expensive, effort intensive, and not without complications. Most devices require systemic heparinization, and problems associated with this are relatively common. Because of the high flow rates required, generally 2 to 4 L/min, damage to cellular elements may be significant. Thrombocytopenia in combination with systemic heparinization makes the occurrence of hemorrhage a major concern. These problems may be reduced as less traumatic systems that do not require systemic heparinization are developed. At this time, extracorporeal CO_2 removal is a controversial technique performed only at relatively sophisticated tertiary-care centers. The application to general ICU practice awaits a clearer delineation of the clinical efficacy.

A third technique of extrapulmonary gas exchange under investigation does not require an extracorporeal circuit. It involves gas exchange within an indwelling intravascular catheter, hence the name IVOX.[47,48] Clinical experience with this device is limited and the prototypes in use offer only partial support of gas exchange. It is unclear what role it may eventually play in the treatment of severe respiratory failure, but the concept is exciting.[49] IVOX engenders many of the potential benefits of existing technology and couples these advantages with a possible reduction in the associated complications.[49]

X. CONCLUSION

A. CLINICAL CHOICE OF A VENTILATORY SUPPORT MODALITY

The majority of patients that receive ventilatory support require augmentation of alveolar ventilation to decrease the work of breathing associated with acute or chronic lung disease. The ventilatory modality used to treat such patients should allow adjustment of ventilatory support from 0% to 100%. We advocate the use of the minimal support required to maintain cardiopulmonary homeostasis, that is, partial ventilatory support. The relative amount of ventilatory support administered to the patient at different stages of the disease process should be determined by clinical observation of ventilatory work and analysis of $Paco_2$ and pHa.

There are no outcome data to guide the choice of ventilatory mode for provision of partial support. PSV offers certain theoretic advantages over IMV/SIMV, and clinical experience has shown good patient tolerance of PSV. Choice of ventilatory mode for provision of partial support remains a matter of physician preference.

Despite the advantages of partial ventilatory support, there are clinical situations in which full ventilatory support is desirable. Deliberate hyperventilation is used in the management of intracranial hypertension and to alleviate pulmonary hypertension in the neonate. Patients with acute left ventricular failure will tolerate full ventilatory support better than partial ventilatory support because the function of a dilated, afterload-sensitive, failing left ventricle is not likely to be further impaired by elevated airway and intrathoracic pressure. Furthermore, alleviation of ventilatory work may decrease myocardial work and oxygen consumption. Once again, there are no outcome data to guide the choice of mode for provision of full ventilatory support.

REFERENCES

1. Sykes MK: Does mechanical ventilation damage the lung? *Acta Anaesthesiol Scand Suppl* 95:35, 1991.
2. Webb H, Tierney DF: Experimental pulmonary edema due to intermittent positive pressure ventilation with high inflation pressure: protection by positive end-expiratory pressure, *Am Rev Respir Dis* 110:556, 1974.
3. Parker J, Townsley M, Rippe B, et al: Increased microvascular permeability in dog lungs due to high peak airway pressure, *J Appl Physiol* 57(6):1809, 1984.
4. Dreyfuss D, Basset G, Soler P et al: Intermittent positive-pressure hyperventilation with high inflation pressures produces pulmonary microvascular injury in rats, *Am Rev Respir Dis* 132:880, 1985.
5. Kolobow T, Moretti M, Fumagalli R et al: Severe impairment in lung function induced by high peak airway pressure during mechanical ventilation: an experimental study, *Am Rev Respir Dis* 135:312, 1987.

6. Dreyfuss D, Soler G, Basset G et al: High inflation pressure pulmonary edema: respiratory effects of high airway pressure, high tidal volume, and positive end-expiratory pressure, *Am Rev Respir Dis* 137:1159, 1988.

7. Tsuno K, Miura K, Takeya M et al: Histopathologic pulmonary changes from mechanical ventilation at high peak airway pressures, *Am Rev Respir Dis* 143:1115, 1991.

8. Marini J, Relsen S: Re-targeting ventilatory objectives in adult respiratory distress syndrome: new treatment prospective-persistent questions, *Am Rev Respir Dis* 146:2, 1992 (editorial).

9. Zapol W: Volotrauma and the intravenous oxygenator in patients with adult respiratory distress syndrome, *Anesthesiology* 77:847, 1992 (editorial).

10. Fagon J, Chastre J, Domart Y et al: Nosocomial pneumonia in patients receiving continuous mechanical ventilation, *Am Rev Respir Dis* 139:877, 1989.

11. Johnson E, Hedley-Whyte J: Continuous positive-pressure ventilation and choledochoduodenal flow resistance, *J Appl Physiol* 39:937, 1985.

12. Geiger K, Georgieff M, Lutz H: Side effects of positive pressure ventilation on hepatic function and splanchnic circulation, *Int J Clin Monit Comput* 12:103, 1986.

13. Mushin M, Rendell-Baker W, Thompson PW et al: *Automatic ventilation of the lungs,* Oxford, 1980, Blackwell.

14. Chatburn R: Classification of mechanical ventilators, *Respir Care* 37(9):1009, 1992.

15. Darioli R, Perret C: Mechanical controlled hypoventilation in status asthmaticus, *Am Rev Respir Dis* 129:385, 1984.

16. Hickling K, Henderson S, Jackson R: Low mortality associated with low volume, pressure limited ventilation with permissive hypercapnia in severe respiratory distress syndrome, *Intensive Care Med* 16:372, 1990.

17. Nahum A, Burke W, Ravenscroft S et al: Lung mechanics and gas exchange during pressure control ventilation in dogs: augmentation of CO_2 elimination by an intratracheal catheter, *Am Rev Respir Dis* 146:965, 1992.

18. Gilbert J, Bunegin L, Larsson A et al: Intermittent flow expiratory ventilation: new technique of limited excursion pulmonary ventilation, *Crit Care Med* 19(suppl):1086, 1991.

19. Hamilton P, Onayemi A, Smyth J et al: Comparison of conventional and high-frequency ventilation: oxygenation and lung pathology, *J Appl Physiol* 55:131, 1983.

20. Nielsen J, Sjostrand V, Edgren E et al: An experimental study of different ventilatory modes in piglets in severe respiratory distress induced by surfactant depletion, *Intensive Care Med* 17:225, 1991.

21. Meyer J, Hachenberg T, Tippert G et al: High frequency ventilation in experimental pulmonary emphysema, *Intensive Care Med* 17:377, 1991.

22. Clark R, Gerstmann D, Null D et al: Prospective randomized comparison of high-frequency oscillatory and conventional ventilation in respiratory distress syndrome, *Pediatrics* 89:5, 1992.

23. Keszler M, Donn S, Bucciarelli R et al: Multicenter controlled trial comparing high-frequency jet ventilation and conventional mechanical ventilation in newborn infants with pulmonary interstitial emphysema, *J Pediatr* 119:85, 1991.

24. HFI Study Group: High-frequency oscillatory ventilation compared with conventional mechanical ventilation in the treatment of respiratory failure in preterm infants, *N Engl J Med* 320:88, 1989.

25. Carlo W, Siner B, Chatburn R et al: Early randomized intervention with high-frequency jet ventilation in respiratory distress syndrome, *J Pediatr* 117:765, 1990.

26. HFI Study Group: High-frequency oscillatory ventilation compared with conventional intermittent mechanical ventilation in the treatment of respiratory failure in preterm infants: neurodevelopmental status at 16 to 24 months of post-term age, *J Pediatr* 117:939, 1990.

27. Slutsky A: High-frequency ventilation, *Intensive Care Med* 17:375, 1991 (editorial).

28. Hecker R: High-frequency ventilation: is there a clinical role? *Anesth Rev* 19:19, 1992.

29. Räsänen J, Cane RD, Downs J et al: Airway pressure release ventilation during acute lung injury: a prospective multicenter trial, *Crit Care Med* 19:1234, 1991.

30. Register SD, Downs JB, Stock MC et al: Is 50% oxygen harmful? *Crit Care Med* 15:598, 1987.

31. Räsänen J, Leon M, Cane RD: Adaptation of pressure support ventilation to increasing ventilatory demand during experimental airway obstruction and acute lung injury, *Crit Care Med* (in press).

32. MacIntyre NR: Respiratory function during pressure support ventilation, *Chest* 89:677, 1986.

33. Stock MC, Downs JB, Frolicher DA: Airway pressure release ventilation, *Crit Care Med* 15:462, 1987.

34. Garner W, Downs JB, Stock MC et al: Airway pressure release ventilation: a human trial, *Chest* 94:779, 1988.

35. Cane RD, Peruzzi WT, Shapiro BA: Airway pressure release ventilation in severe acute respiratory failure, *Chest* 100:460, 1991.

36. Räsänen J, Cane RD, Downs JB et al: Airway pressure release ventilation during acute lung injury: a prospective multicenter trial, *Crit Care Med* 19:1234, 1991.

37. Räsänen J, Downs JB, Stock MC: Cardiovascular effects of conventional positive pressure ventilation and airway pressure release ventilation, *Chest* 93:911, 1988.

38. Valentine DD, Hammond MD, Downs JB et al: Distribution of ventilation and perfusion with different modes of mechanical ventilation, *Am Rev Respir Dis* 143:1262, 1991.

39. Rouby JJ, Benameur M, Jawish D et al: Continuous positive airway pressure (CPAP) vs. intermittent mandatory pressure release ventilation (IMPRV) in patients with acute respiratory failure, *Intensive Care Med* 18:69, 1992.

40. Räsänen J: IMPRV: synchronized APRV or more? *Intensive Care Med* 18:65, 1992 (editorial).

41. Bray JG, Cane RD: Mechanical ventilation: airway pressure release techniques, *Curr Opinion Anesthes,* 1992 (in press).

42. Younes M: Proportional assist ventilation: a new approach to ventilatory support, *Am Rev Respir Dis* 145:114, 1992.

43. Younes M, Puddy A, Roberts D et al: Proportional assist ventilation: results of an initial clinical trial, *Am Rev Respir Dis* 145:121, 1992.

44. Garner W, Downs J, Stock M et al: Airway pressure release ventilation: a human trial, *Chest* 94:779, 1988.

45. Zapol W, Snider M, Hill J et al: Extracorporeal membrane oxygenation in severe acute respiratory failure, *JAMA* 242:2193, 1979.

46. Gattinoni L, Kolobow T, Tomlenson T et al: Low-frequency positive pressure ventilation with extracorporeal carbon dioxide removal (LFPPV-ECCO2R): an experimental study, *Anesth Analg* 57:470, 1978.

47. Gattinoni L, Pesenti A, Mascheroni D et al: Low-frequency positive pressure ventilation with extracorporeal CO_2 removal in severe acute respiratory failure, *JAMA* 256:881, 1986.

48. Mortensen J, Berry G: Conceptual and design features of a practical, clinically effective intravenous mechanical blood gas exchange device (IVOX), *Int J Artif Organs* 12:384, 1989.

49. High K, Snider M, Richard R et al: Clinical trials of an intravenous oxygenator in patients with adult respiratory distress syndrome, *Anesthesiology* 77:856, 1992.

Chapter 37

MONITORING THE AIRWAY AND PULMONARY FUNCTION

Neal H. Cohen
David E. Schwartz

I. INTRODUCTION

Care of the patient who requires endotracheal intubation and ventilatory support requires not only an understanding of techniques of airway management and mechanical ventilation, but also a knowledge of how to monitor the patient to assure that the procedures are performed safely and without complications. A wide variety of monitoring techniques is available. To select the most appropriate monitors, the clinician must understand what information each monitor can provide, how each works, and situations in which the data provided by the monitor is not clinically useful. The most helpful monitors are those that are easily applied, simple to use, have few, if any, contraindications or complications associated with their use, and provide data that will make care more cost effective.[1] Most of the currently available monitoring techniques fulfill these requirements. Many have also been demonstrated to improve patient care or reduce costs.[2-5] This chapter will describe techniques for monitoring the patient while securing the airway, providing ventilatory support, and weaning from mechanical ventilation. It will define the clinical applications for and identify the limitations of each monitor. The chapter is divided into sections describing techniques for monitoring during airway management and techniques for monitoring while providing mechanical ventilatory support and weaning.

II. MONITORING THE AIRWAY

A. MONITORING THE AIRWAY DURING ENDOTRACHEAL TUBE PLACEMENT

The patient who requires airway protection and mechanical ventilatory support, whether during surgery or while cared for in the ICU, will have the airway secured with an endotracheal tube (ET) or tracheotomy tube. The proper location and positioning of the tube must be assured during and after placement (see also Chapter 27). This is particularly true after placement of an ET, although many of the techniques described to assure proper ET placement also apply to tracheotomy tubes.

One of the most effective clinical methods to ensure that the ET is within the trachea is direct visualization of the tube passing through the vocal cords at the time of intubation. Physical examination is also an important monitoring technique. Auscultation over the lung fields and stomach should routinely be performed to assess ET placement. When the ET is within the trachea, equal breath sounds should be heard over both lung fields, while listening over the apices. Auscultation over the upper lung fields minimizes the likelihood of hearing sounds transmitted from the stomach. Ideally, no breath sounds should be heard over the stomach. Unfortunately, auscultation can be misleading. Occasionally, particularly in children, breath sounds will be transmitted to the stomach even when the ET is in proper position. For patients with extensive parenchymal lung disease, effusions, or endobronchial lesions, breath sounds may not be heard equally over both lung fields even when the ET is in proper position within the trachea. Other clinical signs that are reassuring when assessing ET placement within the trachea include identifying mist within the lumen of the ET during exhalation, palpation of the cuff of the ET in the suprasternal notch, and the normal "feel" of a reservoir bag during manual ventilation. None of these methods is infallible.[6]

The presence of carbon dioxide in exhaled gas can also be used to confirm that an artificial airway is within the trachea. Carbon dioxide (CO_2) will be eliminated by the lungs; the CO_2 concentration can be measured using a number of different techniques. In the operating room, CO_2 can be measured using an infrared device,[7] Raman

effect scattering, or mass spectrometry. In other environments, such as the ICU or emergency department, infrared devices, which measure actual CO_2 concentration, or colorimetric techniques,[8-10] which estimate CO_2 concentration in exhaled gas, have been used. The documentation of CO_2 in exhaled gas following placement of an artificial airway (capnography) has become the standard of care in anesthesia practice. A detailed description of capnography is provided in Chapter 27.

When used to confirm the proper placement of an ET, capnography is very useful but not foolproof.[11,12] It can be misleading if the patient has been ventilated by mask prior to intubation and has CO_2-containing gas in the stomach. This problem is most common when capnography is used to monitor the patient who has received bicarbonate solutions or has been drinking CO_2-containing beverages prior to endotracheal intubation. In these situations, CO_2 will be eliminated from the stomach during the first few breaths provided through the ET. The presence of CO_2 from exhaled gas, therefore, should be monitored for a few breaths. If CO_2 continues to be eliminated through the ET after four or five breaths, endotracheal placement of the tube can be assured.[12] Another problem with capnography when used to confirm ET placement is that CO_2 elimination will only occur if the patient has sufficient cardiac output to deliver CO_2 to the lungs. If the patient has suffered a cardiac arrest, no CO_2 will be delivered to the lung, and the capnogram will neither reveal a CO_2 waveform nor digitally display CO_2 from exhaled gas, even when the ET is in proper position.[13-16] During cardiopulmonary resuscitation, CO_2 elimination as confirmed by capnography provides evidence of improved perfusion.

Once the ET has been placed into the trachea, its position within the trachea must also be determined to assure that it is not proximal (increasing the risk of accidental extubation) or distal (endobronchial). The incorrect positioning of the ET has been associated with a number of complications, including pneumothorax and death.[17] The location of the ET should not only be confirmed at the time of placement, but also regularly assessed as long as the patient's trachea remains intubated. The ET position can change even after it is secured. Flexion of the neck moves the ET toward the carina, and extension moves the tube up toward the vocal cords. In adult patients flexion and extension of the head changes the position of the ET tip by ±2 cm.[18] In addition, as the ET softens or the patient manipulates the ET with the tongue, the tube position will change. As a result of these changes in ET position, patients are at risk for self-extubation, even when the tube is secured at the mouth and the extremities are restrained.

A number of techniques have been described to assure correct ET positioning within the trachea. Placement of the ET to a predetermined distance has been advocated to prevent endobronchial intubation. Owen and Cheney suggest that if the tube is placed to a depth of 21 cm in women and 23 cm in men when referenced to the anterior alveolar ridge or the front teeth, endobronchial intubation will be avoided.[19] Subsequent studies have confirmed neither the value of this technique to prevent endobronchial intubation in critically ill adults[20-22] nor a predictable relationship between the position of the ET at the teeth and the tube's position relative to the carina on chest radiograph.[22]

Fiberoptic bronchoscopy has also been used to determine proper positioning of the ET.[23] The technique is useful but does impose some risk, particularly for the recently intubated critically ill patient. Insertion of the bronchoscope reduces the effective cross-sectional area of the ET, potentially compromising ventilation and oxygenation.[24] Peak inspiratory pressure will increase. In addition, the partial obstruction of the endotracheal tube will result in an increase in airways resistance; this may lead to the development of occult end-expiratory pressure and might increase the risk of pneumothorax or cause hemodynamic compromise.[25] Another problem associated with the routine use of bronchoscopy for determining ET position is that the instrument must be sterilized following its use to prevent patient cross contamination; it is unavailable for use in another patient while it is being cleaned. Despite these limitations, flexible fiberoptic bronchoscopy can be useful when rapid, bedside, or operating room confirmation of ET positioning is required.

Capnography can also be used to identify endobronchial migration of an ET.[26] With distal migration of the tube, the end-tidal CO_2 will fall. The change is usually associated with an increase in peak inspiratory pressure. These changes precede a change in arterial blood gases and so may be useful to provide an early warning of a change in ET position.

The chest radiograph can also be used to confirm the location of the ET within the trachea. The distance of the ET from the carina can be measured from a portable anteroposterior film obtained at the bedside. Currently, available data suggest that under most circumstances, the chest radiograph remains the most useful and reliable method to determine the appropriate depth of endotracheal tube placement.[20-22]

The proper placement of a double-lumen endotracheal tube to provide single or differential lung ventilation necessitates additional monitoring techniques beyond those used for confirmation of the location of single-lumen ETs. To evaluate the positioning of these tubes, the usual physical findings can be confusing. Fiberoptic evaluation is very useful, not only to confirm the ET positioning after initial placement, but also to reevaluate the placement after the patient is repositioned for a surgical procedure.[27] Other techniques have also been found to be useful aids to diagnose malpositioning of double-lumen tubes after placement. Capnography, which has been shown to be useful in identifying endobronchial migration of a single-lumen ET,[26] might also provide information about the location of a double-lumen tube. Spirometry, which can be obtained from in-line monitoring devices added to the anesthesia circuit or as monitoring techniques provided by critical care ventilators, can also provide early detection of double-lumen tube malpositioning.[28] As the ET migrates, expiratory flow obstruction can be detected as a change in the shape of the expiratory limb of the flow-volume loop. Inspiratory obstruction is best diagnosed by a change in the pressure-volume loop.

B. MONITORING THE AIRWAY DURING WEANING AND ENDOTRACHEAL EXTUBATION

Careful evaluation and monitoring of the patient's airway is also required prior to and immediately after endotracheal extubation. After the patient is weaned from ventilatory support and is being prepared for extubation, the patient's ability to protect and maintain the airway after endotracheal extubation must be assessed. A variety of clinical criteria has been used to determine if the patient can protect the airway. The most common criteria are presence of a normal gag and strong cough. If the patient has a gag when the back of the throat is stimulated and a cough during suctioning, most clinicians feel confident that the patient will be able to prevent aspiration after extubation. These criteria, however, have never been subjected to scientific evaluation. Some patients who have a poor gag or cough with the ET in place are able to handle secretions and cough effectively after endotracheal extubation. Others who seem to have a satisfactory cough or gag prior to extubation are still unable to protect their airway once extubated. The problem with airway protection may only become clinically apparent once the patient begins to eat, since pharyngeal function may remain abnormal for a number of hours to days after endotracheal intubation.[29] Nonetheless, these criteria continue to be the most commonly used to determine whether the patient can safely be extubated.

Once a decision is made that the patient can protect the airway, some assessment of the airway size and vocal cord function must be made prior to ET removal. Most commonly, for patients intubated for a straightforward surgical procedure, routine clinical evaluation is sufficient; no formal assessment of airway size is required prior to extubation. If the patient develops significant edema of the head and neck during surgery or has a surgical procedure of the head or neck that might compromise the airway, a more thorough assessment is required. One of the common techniques used to assess airway size is to determine if the patient can breathe around the ET when the ET cuff is deflated or if there is a leak around the cuff when positive pressure is applied through the ET.[30] Some clinicians require that a leak occur when the airway pressure is low, usually below 15 cm H_2O prior to extubation, although studies have documented neither the value of the leak test at all nor a specific "leak pressure" above which extubation would be contraindicated. If the airway pressure required to identify a leak during positive pressure inspiration is high, probably over 20 to 25 cm H_2O, the patient *may* have sufficient upper airway edema to warrant leaving the ET in place until the edema resolves.

When upper airway edema compromises the patient's airway after extubation, vasoconstrictors can be used to reduce airway swelling. Nebulized racemic epinephrine has been used successfully, although it must be administered with caution. The vasoconstrictive effects of the epinephrine will reduce the edema and improve the cross-sectional area of the airway. After discontinuation of the epinephrine, however, particularly when treatment is repeated over an extended period, rebound hyperemia can occur. If repeated epinephrine treatments are required, the epinephrine dose and frequency of treatment should be tapered (in frequency or dose), rather than abruptly withdrawn. Steroids can also be used to reduce upper airway edema. The onset of action of the steroids is slow. If upper airway edema is suspected and steroids are to be administered, the steroids should be administered 6 to 8 hours before the anticipated extubation.

Vocal cord function can also be impaired after surgery. Postoperative vocal cord dysfunction can be caused by direct trauma at the time of endotracheal intubation or edema. Recurrent laryngeal nerve dysfunction can also occur, most commonly from nerve retraction or transection during surgery or from direct trauma caused by high intratracheal pressure transmitted from the ET cuff.[31] With the ET in place, vocal cord function is very difficult to assess. The evaluation usually requires that the ET be removed (see Chapter 1). Fiberoptic evaluation is the most common method to assess laryngeal and vocal cord function. After removal of the ET, the fiberoptic laryngoscope or bronchoscope can be used to assess the airway. Although the assessment can be performed in the intensive care unit (ICU), the more common approach is to perform the evaluation under more controlled conditions in the operating room, where all of the emergency airway and surgical equipment is available to secure the airway. The extubation can be performed after the patient is anesthetized with a volatile anesthetic agent and breathing spontaneously. If severe stridor or airway obstruction develops, the patient can be reintubated or have a tracheostomy per-formed for long-term airway maintenance. (See also Chapter 40.)

III. MONITORING PULMONARY FUNCTION
A. PHYSICAL EXAMINATION

One of the most important, although technologically unsophisticated monitors of the pulmonary function is the physical examination. With the availability of high-technology monitors, the value of a well-conducted physical examination is often overlooked. A great deal of useful information about actual or potential airway problems and abnormalities in pulmonary mechanical function or gas exchange can be obtained from a carefully performed and thorough examination. Many of the early signs of respiratory failure are apparent first on physical assessment (see Chapter 13) before the abnormalities are apparent by other means. For example, the respiratory rate provides important information about respiratory reserve, dead space, and respiratory drive, particularly when interpreted in conjunction with $PaCO_2$. Tachypnea is frequently the earliest sign of impending respiratory failure. In addition to the respiratory rate, the patient's pattern of breathing should be evaluated. Subtle changes in the rate, tidal volume, and pattern of breathing may provide an early indication of increased work of breathing (as might occur with reduced lung compliance, increased airway resistance, or phrenic nerve dysfunction) or altered ventilatory drive.

The presence of upper airway obstruction, as might occur after manipulation of the airway, in association with epiglottitis, or due to mass in or around the airway can be assessed by careful clinical evaluation. Nasal flaring, stridor, and chest wall movement in the absence of airflow suggest upper airway obstruction. If the patient is making respiratory efforts with abdominal expansion during inspiration and no chest distention, the patient will require support of the upper airway using a jaw thrust, positive pressure (mask or nasal continuous positive airway pressure [CPAP]), or endotracheal intubation. When the patient presents with stridor, the physical evaluation can also be useful in determining the location of the airway compromise. If the stridor occurs primarily during inspiration, it is due to extrathoracic obstruction; if it occurs during exhalation, it is more likely caused by an intrathoracic lesion. When the stridor occurs during both inspiration and exhalation, the obstruction is fixed. The fixed obstruction is rarely amenable to conservative treatment; endotracheal intubation will most likely be required until a more definitive therapy can be provided.

The presence of respiratory dyssynchrony can be an important indicator of respiratory muscle fatigue and possibly impending respiratory failure.[32,33] Respiratory dyssynchrony (when the patient has no evidence of upper airway obstruction) is identified by assessing chest wall and abdominal movement during normal tidal breathing. A paradoxical respiratory pattern suggests that the patient may have inadequate muscle strength to sustain spontaneous respiration and that positive pressure ventilatory support may be required. Tobin et al. found that respiratory muscle dyssynchrony can occur prior to the development of fatigue,[34,35] although fatigue of the respiratory muscles does not always result in the development of dyssynchrony.[36]

Clinical evaluation should also include assessment of respiratory muscle groups to evaluate respiratory reserve. The use of accessory muscles, including the sternocleidomastoid and scalene muscles, is commonly seen in patients with long-standing respiratory failure associated with chronic obstructive pulmonary disease.[37] The position of the diaphragm and diaphragmatic motion is also affected in patients with severe chronic obstructive pulmonary disease (COPD). The patient who relies on accessory muscles and has minimal diaphragmatic excursion will not have any respiratory reserve. The patient will be at risk for recurrent respiratory failure and will present a significant challenge during weaning when mechanical ventilatory support is required.

The routine physical examination of the lungs should also be performed. The examination can provide evidence of parenchymal lung abnormalities and cardiopulmonary pathology. Auscultation of the lungs can provide useful information about the etiology of abnormalities identified from other studies, including arterial blood gases, chest x-ray, and other monitors.

While the physical examination is very useful and should be performed regularly, some of the physical signs and symptoms of respiratory failure do not appear early enough to provide adequate warning, nor do they change quickly enough to determine if an intervention was appropriate. The greatest value of the physical examination is that it provides an ongoing assessment of pulmonary function when used in conjunction with other monitors of the respiratory system.

B. RADIOLOGIC EVALUATION

The chest radiograph is another important monitor of the respiratory status (see Chapter 2). The chest x-ray provides confirmation of proper ET placement after endotracheal intubation.[21,22] It is also a useful study to help differentiate the causes for abnormal physical findings, such as differentiating atelectasis from consolidation. The chest x-ray can identify abnormalities in the larger airways, including tracheal stenosis, dilatation (as might occur when the ET cuff is overinflated), or tracheomalacia. It can be used to determine the presence of pulmonary edema. The radiographic findings consistent with pulmonary edema include bronchial cuffing, perihilar pulmonary infiltrates, and Kerley's B lines.

As is true of all monitors, the chest x-ray has limitations when used as a monitor of respiratory status. Radiographic findings do not always correlate with other clinical and physiologic monitors because the radiologic changes can be delayed in onset and resolution. The radiologic technique also influences the value of the chest x-ray as a monitor. Most commonly, a portable anteroposterior film is obtained with the patient in the supine position. When performed in this manner, interpretation of heart size, differentiation of atelectasis and pleural effusions, and presence of pneumothoraces may be difficult. When trying to identify any of these abnormalities, other views, including upright or lateral decubitus films, should be requested, depending on the suspected pathology. Occasionally, an ultrasound or computerized tomography (CT) scan of the chest may be required to confirm the presence of pleural effusions, pulmonary abscesses, or other abnormalities.

Other radiologic evaluations can be useful to further evaluate abnormalities noted on the chest x-ray or physical examination. Ventilation and perfusion scans have been used to detect pulmonary emboli. For the critically ill patient with suspected pulmonary emboli, ventilation perfusion scans can be diagnostic. Bedside ventilation scans are difficult to perform, but perfusion scans will often be sufficient, particularly when perfusion defects are correlated with abnormalities on portable chest films. More commonly, however, pulmonary arteriograms or spiral CT scans are necessary in these patients to definitively determine the presence of pulmonary emboli.

CT and magnetic resonance imaging (MRI) scans can provide important information about the airway and pulmonary parenchyma. They can define the location, extent, and character of upper airway abnormalities, including mass lesions, pulmonary intraparenchymal lesions, pleural effusions, and other pulmonary and extrapulmonary abnormalities.

C. MONITORS OF GAS EXCHANGE

One of the most important goals in monitoring pulmonary function is to determine if the lung is able to sustain satisfactory oxygenation and ventilation. The arterial blood gas is the most frequently used monitor of oxygenation and ventilation, although noninvasive monitors of gas exchange are also useful.

1. Arterial blood gases

Arterial blood gas measurement remains a mainstay of respiratory monitoring. The arterial blood gas provides direct measurement of Pao_2, $Paco_2$, and pH. From these measured data, bicarbonate concentration (HCO_3^-), oxygen saturation (Sao_2), and base excess (BE) or base deficit are calculated. The measured and calculated parameters define adequacy of gas exchange, acid-base balance, and overall cardiorespiratory status. The value and limitations of PaO_2 and $PaCO_2$ monitoring are discussed as follows.

While monitoring gas exchange using arterial blood gas measurements is important, the technique has some limitations. Blood gas monitoring is invasive; samples must be drawn from an indwelling arterial catheter or an arterial puncture. Frequent blood gas sampling can result in significant blood loss, which may be a clinical problem for any unstable patient, particularly the pediatric patient or anemic adult. The placement and maintenance of an arterial catheter also has associated risks, including hemorrhage, hand ischemia, arterial thrombosis and embolism, infection,[38,39] and development of a radial artery aneurysm.[40]

Traditional blood gas monitoring is performed intermittently. When a patient's respiratory status is unstable, is rapidly evolving, or when frequent adjustments in ventilatory support are required, intermittent monitoring might be insufficient. In these clinical situations, continuous monitoring would be preferable. Intraarterial blood gas monitors are available, although the clinical utility of these monitors is still being evaluated.[41,42] The continuous monitors utilize fluorescence-based probes placed through an arterial catheter to provide a continuous assessment of PaO_2, $PaCO_2$, and pH. The continuously updated information provides an immediate indication of changes in gas exchange that result from physiologic alterations or therapeutic interventions. This additional information is costly. The probes and monitors are more expensive than intermittent blood gas analysis. Whether these devices will provide data that are superior to what is currently available and will prove to be cost effective will require further investigation.

2. Monitors of oxygenation

Assessment of oxygenation is a critical monitor during management of the airway. Clinical detection of arterial hypoxemia is known to be unreliable.[43] A number of methods are available for evaluating oxyge nation during management of the airway. PaO_2 and hemoglobin oxygen saturation using a pulse oximeter (SpO_2) are currently the most commonly used monitors of oxygenation.

a. ARTERIAL OXYGEN TENSION

Direct measurement of the arterial oxygen tension (PaO_2) from an arterial catheter has been the traditional method for assessing oxygenation. To accurately interpret PaO_2 requires an understanding of normal pulmonary physiology and the influences of alterations in ventilation and perfusion on the *predicted* arterial oxygen tension. Normal PaO_2 declines with age. PaO_2 can vary over time by as much as $\pm 10\%$, and the PaO_2 measured by a blood gas machine can vary by $\pm 10\%$. Hypoxemia can result from a number of factors, including inad-

equate inspired oxygen (low alveolar oxygen tension), ventilation-perfusion mismatch, shunt, or inadequate cardiac output (low mixed venous oxygen tension). The confirmation of an acceptable PaO_2 is reassuring, although it does not confirm that oxygen delivery is sufficient. In order to assess the adequacy of oxygen delivery, additional studies are necessary, including evaluation of acid-base status, measurement of serum lactate and mixed venous oxygen content, and cardiac output measurement.

b. PULSE OXIMETRY

Pulse oximetry provides a rapid, continuous, and noninvasive estimation of PaO_2 of hemoglobin.[44,45] The pulse oximeter has become a routine monitor of oxygenation during airway management in the operating room, emergency department, and the ICU and has become the standard monitor of oxygenation during administration of conscious sedation for endoscopic and other procedures.[46-49] The routine use of this monitor has demonstrated a high prevalence of clinically undetected hypoxemia in both adults and children.[45,48,50-52] Some studies have suggested that the early detection of arterial oxygen desaturation with the use of pulse oximetry improves outcome (such as the prevention-occurrence of intraoperative myocardial ischemia),[2-5] although others are unable to confirm this benefit.[53-55]

Pulse oximetry utilizes two fundamental principals, the differential light absorption of oxyhemoglobin (O_2Hb) and reduced hemoglobin (Hb) and the increase in light absorption produced by pulsatile blood flow compared with that of a background of connective tissue, skin, bone, and venous blood.[47,56] The basis for oximetry is Beer's law, which allows for the determination of the concentration of an unknown solute in a solvent (in this case, saturated versus reduced hemoglobin) by light absorption.

The commercially available pulse oximeters use light emitting diodes (LEDs) that transmit light at specific, known wavelengths, 660 nm (red) and 940 nm (infrared). These wavelengths were selected because the absorption characteristics of oxyhemoglobin (O_2Hb) and reduced hemoglobin (Hb) are sufficiently different at these wavelengths to allow differentiation of O_2Hb and Hb (Fig. 37-1). The pulse oximeter determines arterial saturation by timing the measurement to pulsations in the arterial system. During pulsatile flow, the vascular bed expands and contracts, creating a change in the light path length.[44] The pulsation alters the quantity of light transmitted to the sensor and provides a plethysmographic waveform.[57] This timing of the signal allows the pulse oximeter to differentiate arterial oxygen saturation from venous saturation, based on the ratio of pulsatile and baseline absorption of red and infrared light (Fig. 37-2).

The pulse oximeter displays the oxygen saturation based on a ratio (R) of pulsatile and baseline absorption

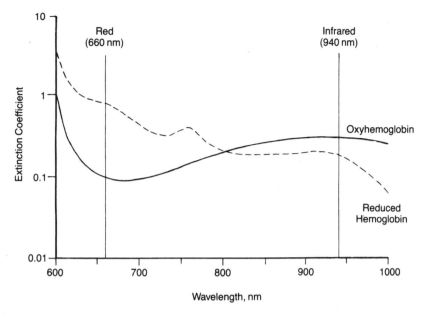

Fig. 37-1. Absorption (extinction) characteristics of oxyhemoglobin and reduced hemoglobin are shown. There are marked differences between the two at light wavelengths 660 nm (red) and 940 nm (infrared). (From Tobin MJ: *JAMA* 264:244, 1990.)

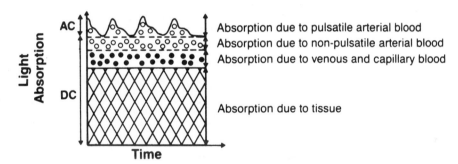

Fig. 37-2. This figure schematically illustrates light absorption through living tissue. Note that the AC signal is due to pulsatile component of arterial blood, while the DC signal is comprised of all the nonpulsatile absorbers in the tissue: nonpulsatile arterial blood, venous and capillary blood, and all other tissues. (From Tremper KK, Barker SJ: *Anesthesiology* 70:98, 1989.)

at the two wavelengths transmitted (660 nm, 940 nm) in the tissue bed. The calculation is represented by the following equation:

$$R = \frac{\text{Pulsatile absorbance @660 nm/nonpulsatile absorbance @ 660nm}}{\text{Pulsatile absorbance @ 940 nm/nonpulsatile absorbance @ 940 nm}} \quad (1)$$

The oxygen saturation displayed by the pulse oximeter is empirically related to this calculated value based on calibration curves derived for healthy nonsmoking adult males breathing oxygen at varying concentrations. Most commercially available pulse oximeters are calibrated over the range 70% to 100%. The accuracy of pulse oximetry in determining the arterial oxygen saturation of

Hb has been shown to be excellent over this range,[44] with an error of less than ±3% to 4%.[1,48]

Although pulse oximetry has become a ubiquitous monitoring device, particularly to confirm adequacy of oxygenation during airway management, it has a number of limitations. First, the measurement of oxygen saturation does not provide a direct assessment of oxygen tension. Because of the shape of the oxygen-hemoglobin dissociation curve, at higher levels of oxygenation measurements of Spo_2 are insensitive in detecting significant changes in Pao_2 (Fig. 37-3). Second, the pulse oximeter is not accurate when oxygen saturation is below 70%. The inaccuracy is due both to the limited range of oxygen saturation used in the calibration process and the difficulty in obtaining reliable human data at these low

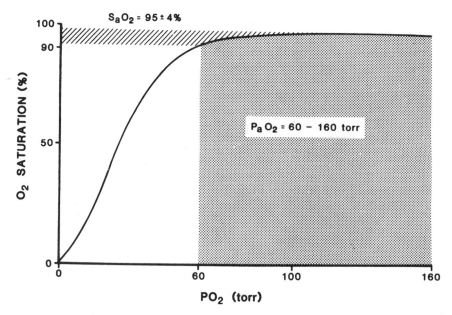

Fig. 37-3. Oxygen dissociation curve. Since oximeters have 95% confidence limits for SaO$_2$ of ±4%, an oximeter reading 95% could represent a PaO$_2$ of 60 (saturation 91%) or 160 mm Hg (saturation of 99%). (From Tobin MJ: *Am Rev Respir Dis* 138:1625, 1988.)

oxygen saturations.[58] The accuracy of pulse oximeters during hypoxemia has been extensively studied and reviewed.[59,60] Most of these studies have been performed on healthy volunteers who had desaturation induced by breathing hypoxic gas mixtures for short periods of time. Pulse oximeters from various manufacturers varied in their accuracy during hypoxemia; the direction of error differs among these devices, with some overestimating and some underestimating true arterial oxygen saturation. The results of some of these studies documented problems with the calibration curves and resulted in the revision of the algorithms by the manufacturers.[59-61] These modifications to the algorithms have resulted in improved performance of the oximeters.[48]

A number of other factors affect the performance of pulse oximeters. The response characteristics of pulse oximeters are clinically important, particularly in situations where the saturation may be changing rapidly, as can occur during management of the difficult airway. A number of investigators have studied the response characteristics of pulse oximetry in clinical practice.[62] West et al. studied five obese, nonsmoking males with the sleep apnea syndrome. During spontaneous desaturation, the pulse oximeter underestimated the minimum SaO$_2$, and during spontaneous resaturation there was an overshoot of the maximum SpO$_2$. The location of the probe also influences the response time for the pulse oximeter. Probes placed on the ear respond more quickly to sudden decrease in SaO$_2$ than do probes placed on a digit.[59,60] Finally, the response time to changes in oxygen saturation of the pulse oximeter is also dependent on

heart rate. For fingertip sensors as heart rate increases, the response to an acute change in saturation is faster; for ear or nasal probes, the relationship is reversed so that, as heart rate increases, the response to changes in SaO$_2$ is slower.[62]

There are a number of clinical situations in which the accuracy of the pulse oximeter is altered (Box 37-1). Excessive light, such as fluorescent or xenon arc surgical lights, bilirubin lights, and heating lamps, can cause falsely low or high SpO$_2$ values.[48,56,63] Covering the probe with an opaque material helps to eliminate this problem. Electrocautery devices can produce significant electrical interference, which results in improper functioning of the pulse oximeter.[47]

Motion of the probe, such as when a patient or caregiver moves the digit on which the oximeter probe is placed, can cause artifactual readings from the pulse oximeter. Vibration of the sensor delays the detection time for hypoxemia and causes spurious decreases in the SpO$_2$.[64] Attempts have been made to minimize the effect of motion by timing the measurement of SpO$_2$ to the electrocardiogram (ECG). Pulse oximeters that possess ECG linkage and time the measurement of arterial saturation to the ECG have been shown to perform better during vibration than those without this feature.[64] Although, this ECG interface is helpful, it has not completely eliminated motion as a problem, particularly in very active or agitated patients.

Another problem with the pulse oximeter is related to its inability to differentiate oxyhemoglobin from other hemoglobins, such as methemoglobin and carboxyhemoglobin. A pulse oximeter is able to differentiate only as many substances as the number of wavelengths of light it emits.[47,61] Therefore, commercially available oximeters can only detect two types of hemoglobin, reduced and oxygenated (Hb and O_2Hb). Pulse oximeters derive a "functional saturation" of hemoglobin, which is defined as:

$$\text{Functional saturation} = \frac{O_2Hb}{O_2Hb + Hb} \times 100\% \quad (2)$$

This functional saturation does not account for other hemoglobins, such as methemoglobin (metHb) or carboxyhemoglobin (COHb). In order to assess the presence of these other hemoglobin species, two additional wavelengths of light must be incorporated into the measuring device. Spectrophotometric heme-oximeters (cooximeters), which utilize at least four wavelengths of light, are able to measure other hemoglobin species and calculate the "fractional saturation" using the following equation:

$$\frac{\text{Fractional}}{\text{saturation}} = \frac{O_2Hb}{O_2Hb + Hb + metHb + COHb} \times 100\% \quad (3)$$

When COHb or metHb are present, the pulse oximeter will not provide a true measurement of *oxygen* saturation.[65,66] The presence of COHb causes a false elevation in the SpO_2 measurement.[65] As shown in Fig. 37-4, COHb has minimal light absorption at 940 nm, and at 660 nm its absorption coefficient is nearly identical to that of O_2Hb. The pulse oximeter cannot differentiate COHb from O_2Hb; it overestimates the O_2Hb.[65] The SpO_2 displayed by the pulse oximeter approximates the sums of COHb and O_2Hb. This problem with pulse oximeters is important to consider when assessing oxygenation in patients who have sustained smoke inhalation or patients who have smoked just prior to proposed airway management. COHb can also be pres-

ent in long-term ICU patients, since carbon monoxide is a metabolic product of heme metabolism.[67,68] The influence of this potential endogenous source of carbon monoxide on the accuracy of SpO_2 in the critically ill patient requires further evaluation. In any case, when high carbon monoxide levels are suspected, oxygen saturation should be measured using a cooximeter, rather than a pulse oximeter.

Methemoglobin also interferes with pulse oximeter measurements.[66,69] As metHb levels exceed 30% to 35%, SpO_2 becomes independent of metHb level, approaching 85%. This occurs because the metHb absorption coefficient at 660 nm is almost identical to that of reduced hemoglobin, while at 940 nm it is greater than other hemoglobins (see Fig. 37-4). The pulse oximeter will therefore overestimate or underestimate the true SaO_2, depending on the level of metHb.[61] Some causes for high metHb levels include administration of nitrates, local anesthetics (lidocaine, benzocaine), metoclopramide, sulfa-containing drugs, ethylenediaminetetraacetic acid (EDTA), and diaminodiphenylsulfone (DDS) (Dapsone) and primaquine phosphate used to treat acquired immunodeficiency syndrome (AIDS) patients. Some patients can also have congenitally high metHb levels. Fetal Hb has not been shown to affect the accuracy of the pulse oximeter.[47,61,63] The effect of other dyshemoglobinemias, such as sulfhemoglobin, on the accuracy of pulse oximetry has not been investigated.[63]

Other pigments interfere with the accuracy of pulse oximeter measurements, including indocyanine green, methylene blue, and indigo carmine.[63] These dyes cause transient artifactual falls in saturation; the extent of the problem depends on the absorption characteristics of the dye. Skin pigmentation has minimal effect on pulse oximeter readings, although very dark pigmentation can result in a slight decrease in accuracy.[70,71] Jaundice has been reported to cause both artificially low and artificially high pulse oximeter readings.[72] In most studies, however, even very high bilirubin levels have had no effect on the accuracy of the SpO_2.[73,74]

Certain shades of nail polish have been shown to significantly alter the accuracy of pulse oximetry when the sensor is placed directly over the nail bed. The extent to which accuracy is affected depends on the absorption characteristics of the nail polish at 660 and 940 nm. Black, blue, and green polishes can falsely lower the measured SpO_2 by up to 6%; red nail polish has little effect on pulse oximeter measurements.[63,75] If a patient has a darkly pigmented polish, either it should be removed from the nail bed that is going to receive the probe or the probe should be placed over the sides of the digit, thereby avoiding transmission of the signal through the nail bed.[63,76]

Severe anemia has also been shown to affect the accuracy of the pulse oximeter. Lee et al. demonstrated

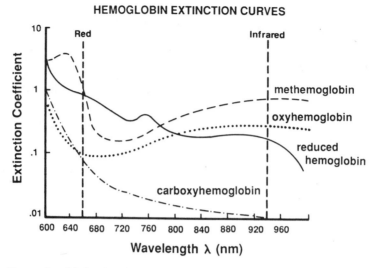

Fig. 37-4. Transmitted light absorbance spectra of four hemoglobin species: oxyhemoglobin, reduced hemoglobin, carboxyhemoglobin, and methemoglobin. (From Tremper KK, Barker SJ: *Anesthesiology* 70:98, 1989.)

that the pulse oximeter was inaccurate when the hematocrit was less than 10%.[77,78] Vegfors et al. also demonstrated that the pulse oximeter is not accurate when the hematocrit is very low[78] but suggested that the problem was caused by poor perfusion, rather than the hematocrit level alone. Of more importance in the management of the severely anemic patient is the assessment of oxygen delivery, rather than oxygen saturation, even when the pulse oximeter is accurate. SpO_2 only reflects oxygen saturation and does not provide a guide to adequacy of oxygen-carrying capacity of the blood or oxygen delivery.

A final problem with the performance of the pulse oximeter, particularly when used to monitor the hemodynamically unstable patient is that, to work, the monitor requires adequate arterial pulsations. When a patient becomes hypotensive, hypovolemic, or markedly vasoconstricted, the peripheral pulse will diminish. The pulse oximeter will be unable to measure SpO_2. In one study of patients with poor perfusion following cardiopulmonary bypass, only 2 of 20 different brands of pulse oximeters were able to give SpO_2 values within 4% of that obtained using a cooximeter.[79] Attempts to improve the accuracy of pulse oximeters in hypoperfused conditions have not adequately solved the problem. Alternative probe locations, such as the nose or ear, and reflectance, rather than transmittance, techniques have been tried with variable success.[80,81] The accuracy of SpO_2 measurements in hypothermic patients has not been as rigorously evaluated but seems to depend primarily on the presence or absence of an adequate pulse signal, rather than temperature itself.[82]

Pulsations other than arterial pulsations will also interfere with the performance of the pulse oximeter. When venous pulsations are pronounced, for example,

the pulse oximeter may underestimate the true arterial oxygen saturation of hemoglobin.[83] In a group of patients with severe tricuspid insufficiency, pulse oximetry underestimated the oxygen saturation by up to 11%. Other clinical situations in which venous pulsations may be important include patients with severe congestive heart failure and patients who require very high venous pressure, such as after a Fontan procedure performed as treatment for tricuspid atresia.

3. Monitors of ventilation

a. ARTERIAL CARBON DIOXIDE TENSION ($PaCO_2$)

The arterial CO_2 tension ($PaCO_2$) remains the most commonly used monitor of ventilation. The $PaCO_2$ is used to determine whether ventilation is normal or abnormal. The normal $PaCO_2$ is 40 mm Hg; however, the $PaCO_2$ must be interpreted in relation to the pH. In response to changes in pH, ventilatory drive will change. When a patient develops a metabolic alkalosis, as might occur after a bicarbonate infusion or the administration of large quantities of citrated bank blood, the ventilatory drive will be decreased. The $PaCO_2$ will rise, but the decrease in minute ventilation is appropriate and is not an indication of respiratory failure. Similarly, the patient who has a significant metabolic acidosis should increase minute ventilation to normalize the pH. If the $PaCO_2$ is 40 mm Hg with a low pH, the ventilatory effort is inadequate, suggesting respiratory failure despite the normal $PaCO_2$.

When arterial blood cannot be obtained, venous blood sampling (either peripheral or central) has been used to *estimate* arterial PCO_2.[84] In some clinical situations, the difference between $PaCO_2$ and mixed venous CO_2 tension ($PvCO_2$) is small, and $PvCO_2$ can be used as an estimate of $PaCO_2$. However, the exact

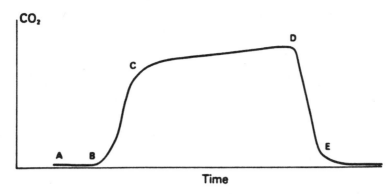

Fig. 37-5. Normal capnogram. Exhalation begins at point **A** and continues to point **D**. Segment **C-D** is the alveolar plateau. Point **D** represents the end-tidal CO_2. Inspiration is represented by rapid, descending limb of segment **D-E,** which reaches the zero baseline.

relationship between arterial and venous P_{CO_2} is not consistent from patient to patient or within a single patient as the clinical condition changes. $P_{v}CO_2$ cannot be used as a substitute for Pa_{CO_2}.

b. CAPNOGRAPHY

Capnography provides a noninvasive method to assess ventilation and ventilation-perfusion relationships.[7] A capnograph provides a continuous display of the CO_2 concentration of gases in the airways. The CO_2 concentration at the end of normal exhalation (end-tidal CO_2, $P_{ET}CO_2$) is a reflection of gas leaving alveoli; it therefore represents an estimate of the alveolar CO_2 concentration, PA_{CO_2}. When ventilation and perfusion are well-matched, the PA_{CO_2} closely approximates the Pa_{CO_2}, and $Pa_{CO_2} \approx PA_{CO_2} \approx P_{ET}CO_2$. The normal gradient between Pa_{CO_2} and $P_{ET}CO_2$ ($P[a_{-ET}]CO_2$) is less than 6 mm Hg. The gradient between Pa_{CO_2} and $P_{ET}CO_2$ increases when pulmonary perfusion is reduced or ventilation is maldistributed. In these situations, $P_{ET}CO_2$ will not accurately reflect PA_{CO_2}.[85,86]

The waveform of the CO_2 concentration over time is a capnogram. The capnogram provides information about adequacy of ventilation, potential airflow obstruction, and, in conjunction with other monitors, ventilation-perfusion relationships. A normal capnogram has four components: the ascending limb, alveolar plateau, descending limb, and baseline (Fig. 37-5). The ascending limb represents the CO_2 concentration of the gas in rapidly emptying alveoli. The alveolar plateau occurs because the CO_2 concentration from uniformly ventilated alveoli is relatively constant. The end-tidal CO_2 ($P_{ET}CO_2$) is the point at which the CO_2 concentration is highest, representing the CO_2 concentration approximating true alveolar gas. The rapid, descending limb of the capnogram signals inspiration. The baseline represents the CO_2 concentration of inspired gas.

A variety of methods of gas analysis is commercially available, including mass spectrometry, Raman scattering, and infrared absorption spectrometry. Currently, the most commonly used method is infrared spectrophotom-

etry. It is based on the principle that CO_2 absorbs infrared light. As the infrared light is passed through a sample of gas, the amount of infrared light absorbed is proportional to the concentration of CO_2 present in the sample.

Two different sampling techniques are used, mainstream and sidestream. The mainstream (in-line) device has a transducer that is connected to the patient's endotracheal tube. The transducer contains the infrared light source and a photodetector. The advantage of the mainstream capnograph is that the response time is fast, since no gas is withdrawn from the patient's airway. Secretions generally do not prevent accurate measurement, since they are easily removed from the sensor site. The mainstream device does have some limitations, including the weight of the connectors, the increased equipment dead space (as much as 20 ml), and the inability to use mainstream devices in extubated patients.

The sidestream (diverting) capnograph aspirates gas from the patient's airway to the capnograph via a sampling tube. Analysis of the CO_2 concentration is performed in the monitor, rather than at the airway adapter. Because the analysis is not done at the airway, the airway connector is smaller and adds no significant dead space or weight to the Y connection between the endotracheal tube and ventilator circuit. The sidestream device can also be used with a modified nasal cannula to monitor CO_2 concentrations in the airway of nonintubated patients. The response time of the sidestream capnograph is slower, since it aspirates gas from the airway. The gas sampling can be adversely affected by water condensation and airway secretions.

Capnography has a number of important applications during airway management and mechanical ventilatory support. It is a useful monitor during endotracheal intubation and to confirm placement of the ET within the trachea. It is useful to document adequacy of ventilation during mechanical ventilatory support and spontaneous ventilation in both intubated and nonintu-

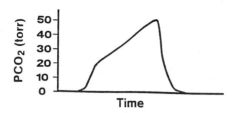

Fig. 37-6. Capnograph waveform in patient with airflow obstruction, demonstrating lack of an alveolar plateau.

bated patients and adequacy of cardiopulmonary resuscitation. Capnography can also be used to monitor the nonintubated patient using a nasal cannula that aspirates the exhaled gas and analyzes the CO_2 concentration. This technique is useful when evaluating the patient with a tenuous airway or gas exchange who may require urgent or emergent endotracheal intubation and mechanical ventilatory support.

The capnographic waveform provides a graphic display of the CO_2 concentration over time. The waveform can be used to identify significant inspiratory or expiratory airway obstruction, including intrinsic airway obstruction or a kinked endotracheal tube (Fig. 37-6). With expiratory obstruction, the waveform will not have a normal alveolar plateau. By continuously monitoring the capnographic waveform, visual confirmation of the response to bronchodilator therapy can be made. The capnographic waveform can also be used to diagnose rebreathing of CO_2; with rebreathing, as can occur when fresh gas flow is inadequate, the baseline (inspired) CO_2 concentration will increase.

Capnography has significant limitations as a monitor of ventilation for patients with impaired pulmonary function or hemodynamic instability. The biggest problem is that the correlation between $Paco_2$ and $P_{ET}co_2$ is variable and sometimes poor in patients with a low cardiac output or altered ventilation-perfusion relationships. More importantly, the correlation varies as the patient's clinical condition changes, making interpretations of ventilation from $P_{ET}co_2$ measurements alone unreliable.

IV. MONITORS OF RESPIRATORY MECHANICAL FUNCTION

A variety of techniques has been used to evaluate pulmonary mechanical function in the patient requiring endotracheal intubation and mechanical ventilatory support.[56,87,88] Some of the techniques are most useful when deciding how to optimize mechanical ventilatory support, others to assist in defining when and how to wean the patient from ventilatory support.

A. ASSESSMENT OF DEAD-SPACE VENTILATION

The arterial CO_2 tension ($Paco_2$) is used to define the adequacy of ventilation, that is, CO_2 removal through the lungs. It is an important monitor of respiratory function and cardiorespiratory relationships, particularly when used in conjunction with other indicators of the efficiency of lung function, such as alveolar and dead space ventilation. The determinants of $Paco_2$ are represented in the following equation, assuming that no CO_2 is inspired:

$$Paco_2 = k \, VCO_2/V_A \qquad (4)$$

where $k = 0.863$, VCO_2 = carbon dioxide production (ml/min), and V_A = alveolar ventilation (L/min).

Carbon dioxide elimination through the lung is dependent solely on the ventilation of alveoli (V_A), the area within the lung where gas exchange occurs.[89] The remainder of the lung and large airways are dead space, the volume of gas that does not participate in gas exchange; ventilation of dead space (V_D) has no effect on CO_2 elimination. The required minute ventilation to maintain CO_2 homeostasis depends on this relationship between alveolar and dead space ventilation. As the dead-space ventilation increases, the work of breathing (either respiratory rate or tidal volume) must increase in order to maintain a normal $Paco_2$. A knowledge of a patient's dead-space ventilation can provide clinically useful information about the work of breathing required of the patient to maintain a normal $Paco_2$.

In order to assess respiratory adequacy, the extent of ventilation that is alveolar, as opposed to dead space, must be determined. Minute ventilation (V_E) is the sum of V_A and V_D and can be represented by the following equation:

$$V_E = V_D + V_A \qquad (5)$$

Dead space is composed of a number of components, including anatomic dead space, alveolar dead space, and dead space imposed by equipment used to maintain the airway and assure ventilation. The anatomic dead space is the volume of gas within the conducting airways; in the normal, 70 kg man, it averages approximately 156 ml.[90] The volume of the anatomic dead space increases with increases in lung volume and decreases in the supine position.[90,91] Intubation of the airway with an endotracheal tube will decrease the anatomic dead space by approximately 50% because of the elimination of the extrathoracic airway.[92,93] Depending on the intraluminal volume of the endotracheal tube and any additional added apparatus dead space, the actual reduction of the anatomic dead space that occurs after endotracheal intubation will not be as large. Alveolar dead space is defined as the gas that penetrates to the alveolar level but does not participate in gas exchange. In healthy individuals, this volume is minimal; it is increased in patients with ventilation-perfusion inequalities, such as pulmonary emboli or severe lung injury. The physiologic dead space is the sum of the anatomic and alveolar dead spaces and is the volume of gas in each breath that does not participate in gas exchange.

The portion of each breath that is dead space can be determined by calculating the dead space to tidal volume ratio (V_D/V_T). The V_D/V_T is a useful clinical monitor of the overall work of breathing. It can be estimated using the Bohr equation:

$$V_D/V_T = PA_{CO_2} - PE_{CO_2}/PA_{CO_2} - PI_{CO_2} \qquad (6)$$

where PA_{CO_2} refers to alveolar carbon dioxide tension, PE_{CO_2} the carbon dioxide tension in mixed expired gas, and PI_{CO_2} the inspired carbon dioxide tension. The V_D/V_T can be estimated more easily by assuming that PI_{CO_2} is zero and estimating alveolar CO_2 as arterial CO_2. This simplified formula represents the Enghoff modification of the Bohr equation:[94]

$$V_D/V_T = Pa_{CO_2} - PE_{CO_2}/Pa_{CO_2} \qquad (7)$$

The normal V_D/V_T is 0.3 at rest; it decreases during exercise.[90,95,96] Patients with severe respiratory failure may have a V_D/V_T of as high as 0.75.

From a measurement of PE_{CO_2} and Pa_{CO_2}, the V_D/V_T can be calculated. PE_{CO_2} can be measured by collecting expired gas in a large volume reservoir (Douglas bag, or meteorological balloon)[97] for 3 to 5 min and measuring the CO_2 tension of a sample of this gas. Pa_{CO_2} is measured from a blood gas obtained simultaneously during the collection of the expired gas.

Some technical factors must be taken into account when measuring V_D/V_T in mechanically ventilated patients. A correction must be made for gas compression within the ventilator, connecting tubing, and any additional dead space from the apparatus.[98] If the compression volume is ignored, the true physiologic dead space will be underestimated by as much as 16%. In addition, physiologic dead space has been found to markedly increase when the duration of inspiration during mechanical ventilation was decreased from 1 sec to 0.5 sec in paralyzed patients.[99] A nomogram of the relationship between minute ventilation, V_D/V_T, and arterial CO_2 tension in mechanically ventilated patients was developed to aid in the titration of ventilatory support, assess the response to medical therapy, and increase the precision of the therapeutic management of critically ill patients.[100]

A simpler method for estimating V_D/V_T has recently been described. Measurement of the carbon dioxide pressure (P_{CO_2}) in the condensate of expired gas in the collection bottle from the expiratory limb of the mechanical ventilator has been shown to be equivalent to the cumbersome technique of collecting the mixed expired gas.[97] This P_{CO_2} value can be substituted for PE_{CO_2}, greatly simplifying the measurement of physiologic dead space in mechanically ventilated patients.

Another approach to the noninvasive assessment of physiologic dead space to tidal volume ratio substitutes end-tidal CO_2 ($P_{ET}CO_2$) for Pa_{CO_2}. For normal subjects, the relationship between $P_{ET}CO_2$ and Pa_{CO_2} is well established.[101,102] At rest, $P_{ET}CO_2$ underestimates Pa_{CO_2} by 2 to 3 mm Hg.[102] However, with exercise, $P_{ET}CO_2$ can overestimate Pa_{CO_2}.[101,102] The difference between $P_{ET}CO_2$ and Pa_{CO_2} varies directly with tidal volume and cardiac output and inversely with respiratory rate.[101]

For patients undergoing general anesthesia or with respiratory failure, the gradient between arterial and end-tidal CO_2 ($P[a-ET]CO_2$) increases.[93,103] This increase reflects more ventilation to lung units with high ventilation/perfusion (V/Q) relationships. For patients with normal pulmonary function who are mechanically ventilated during general anesthesia, the $P[a-ET]CO_2$ averages 5 mm Hg; the $P[a-ET]CO_2$ can be as high as 15 mm Hg in the supine position.[104] The average $P[a-ET]CO_2$ increases to 8 mm Hg when these patients are placed in the lateral decubitus position. In patients with respiratory failure, the $P[a-ET]CO_2$ can be even greater.[103] In the patients with respiratory failure, there is a close correlation between $P[a-ET]CO_2$ and V_D/V_T.[103] The $P[a-ET]CO_2$ can therefore be used as an indicator of the efficiency of ventilation.

B. ASSESSMENT OF PULMONARY MECHANICS DURING MECHANICAL VENTILATORY SUPPORT

A number of other monitoring techniques can be used to assess pulmonary function in the patient who requires ventilatory support. Assessment of airways resistance, lung and thorax compliance, and other aspects of lung function are useful guides to differentiating physiologic problems with the patient from problems imposed by the equipment used to support the patient.

1. Airways resistance and lung-thorax compliance

In the intubated ventilated patient, assessment of airways resistance and lung-thorax compliance can be differentiated by evaluating peak and plateau pressures and the difference between them (Fig. 37-7). The peak airway pressure generated by the ventilator reflects the pressure necessary to overcome airways resistance and compliance of the lung and chest wall. The peak pressure is elevated when airways resistance is increased *or* lung-thorax compliance is reduced. The peak pressure is influenced by a number of other factors, however, including ventilator parameters such as inspiratory flow rate and pattern, tidal volume, and the size of the endotracheal tube. The ratio of the tidal volume delivered divided by the pressure change, the difference between the peak inspiratory pressure and PEEP, is the dynamic compliance. Dynamic compliance is reduced when airways resistance is increased *or* lung-thorax compliance is reduced.

To differentiate the cause for a reduced dynamic compliance and increased peak airway pressure, the

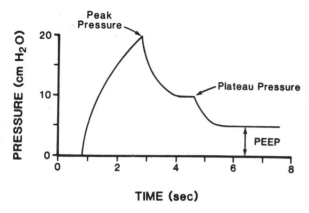

Fig. 37-7. Graphic display of airway pressure in mechanically ventilated patient. Peak inspiratory pressure is achieved during gas flow into lung. Plateau pressure is achieved by temporary occlusion of expiratory tubing. From these pressures, dynamic and static compliance can be calculated.

static compliance can be calculated. To do so requires determination of a plateau pressure. The plateau pressure is the pressure achieved in the airways when the lung is inflated to a specific tidal volume under conditions of zero gas flow, for example, when inspiration is complete and the lung remains inflated with no further gas flow. The plateau pressure is measured by employing an inspiratory pause (hold) on the ventilator. The pressure generated in the lung during the inspiratory pause is that pressure required to overcome lung and chest wall compliance. The static compliance can be estimated by dividing the tidal volume by the difference between the plateau pressure and PEEP. The normal static compliance measured using this method is 60 to 100 ml/cm H_2O. The static compliance is reduced in the patient with an extensive pulmonary infiltrate, pulmonary edema, atelectasis, endobronchial intubation, pneumothorax, or any decrease in chest wall compliance as might occur with chest wall edema or subcutaneous emphysema.

2. Intrinsic positive end-expiratory pressure

Hyperinflation (overdistention) of the lung occurs in some mechanically ventilated patients due to air trapping. Gas can be trapped within the lung during the expiratory phase due to dynamic airflow limitation (e.g., associated with asthma) or inadequate expiratory time, as might occur when the inspiratory flow is so low that it causes a high I:E ratio. The hyperinflation that results has been termed auto-PEEP, intrinsic PEEP (PEEPi) or occult PEEP.[25,87] The presence of auto-PEEP increases the risk of barotrauma, compromises hemodynamics by reducing venous return, increases the patient's work of breathing, and can result in unilateral lung hyperinflation.[25,105,106]

The identification of PEEPi is difficult. PEEPi is not

reflected in the pressure measured on the manometer of the ventilator at the end of exhalation because at end expiration the exhalation valve is either open to atmospheric pressure (PEEP = 0) or reflects the level of PEEP provided by the ventilator (Fig. 37-8). The presence of PEEPi can be quantitated by occluding the expiratory port of the ventilator circuit at the end of exhalation immediately before the next breath is delivered. The pressure in the lungs and ventilator circuit will equilibrate. The level of PEEPi will then be displayed on the manometer. Another method to determine whether PEEPi is present, but not to quantitate it, uses evaluation of the expiratory flow waveform. If expiratory flow does not fall to zero before the next inspiration, gas is trapped within the lung, creating PEEPi (Fig. 37-9). When PEEPi is identified using this method, the flow waveform can be monitored while adjusting ventilator parameters to minimize PEEPi.

3. Airway pressure waveforms

Ventilatory waveform analysis is also a useful method to assess airway patency, pulmonary function, and patient-ventilator interface. Most critical care ventilators now have waveform monitoring capabilities; other independent monitors are available for use in the operating room or ICU to assess waveform and work of breathing. The waveforms provide a visual display of the inspiratory and expiratory flow patterns and pressure-volume and flow-volume loops. The waveforms allow assessment of appropriateness of ventilator parameters, such as inspiratory gas flow and sensitivity to patient need. Figure 37-10 illustrates waveforms that identify excessive work of breathing during patient-initiated breaths. While monitoring the waveforms, adjustments can be made in ventilator parameters to optimize flow patterns and minimize airway pressures, PEEPi and work of breathing.

4. Work of breathing

Work of breathing (WOBp) required of a critically ill patient can be assessed by clinical evaluation at the bedside[107] or calculated utilizing data obtained from an esophageal balloon and flow transducer at the airway.[108] The clinical evaluation of WOBp, while useful, can be misleading. Some patients who appear to have excessive WOBp indicate that they are comfortable. Others with a low minute ventilation and slow respiratory rate are already working maximally and, although appear comfortable at the current level of ventilatory support, will not tolerate any further increase in their WOBp. To better assess the WOBp and monitor the patient's efforts more closely while adjusting the level of ventilatory support, the WOBp can be measured directly using bedside monitors. The monitors require placement of an esophageal balloon to measure esophageal pressure as

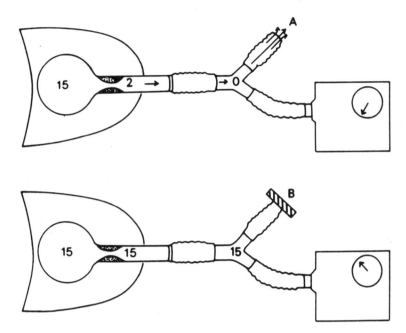

Fig. 37-8. A, Presence of auto-PEEP is detected by occlusion of the end-expiratory port just prior to initiation of the next ventilator inflation cycle. **B,** The ventilator's manometer measures alveolar pressure (auto-PEEP) only when pressures are allowed to equilibrate by occlusion of the expiratory port and end exhalation. (From Pepe PE, Marini JJ: *Am Rev Respir Dis* 126:166, 1982.)

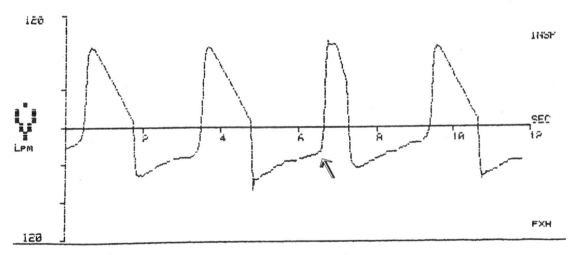

Fig. 37-9. Flow-time curve demonstrating expiratory flow continuing until initiation of inspiration *(arrow)*. In normal patient, expiratory flow will fall to zero, indicating complete emptying to FRC. Continued expiratory flow indicates gas trapping.

an estimate of intrapleural pressure. The WOBp is calculated by integrating the area under the pressure-volume loop. With an understanding of each of the components of WOBp, flow resistive, elastic, and apparatus-induced modifications can be made in ventilator parameters to minimize the patient's WOBp. This monitoring technique has been recommended as a way to adjust pressure support ventilation to optimize gas exchange while minimizing WOBp. Although the additional information about the patient-ventilator interface

has resulted in modifications to methods of ventilating critically ill patients, no studies to date have documented which parameters are most useful to monitor and which modifications to ventilator management result in the best outcome.

C. ASSESSMENT OF PULMONARY FUNCTION DURING WEANING

A number of measures of pulmonary mechanical function are used to evaluate the likelihood of wean-

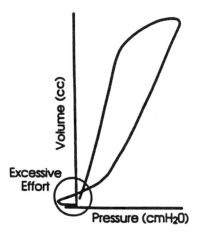

Fig. 37-10. Pressure-volume curve identifying excessive patient effort to initiate a patient-triggered breath. Excessive effort would be required to initiate a breath for either assist-control ventilation or pressure support ventilation. (From *Bedside respiratory mechanics monitoring,* Wallingford, Conn., Novametrix Medical Systems.)

ing success in the mechanically ventilated ICU patient.[1,109-113] Vital capacity (VC) and maximum inspiratory pressure (MIP or P_I^{max}) are commonly employed to evaluate pulmonary mechanical function. A VC of 10 ml/kg and P_I^{max} more negative than -20 cm H_2O have been shown to be useful predictors of weaning success in some patients. Other measures of mechanical function that have been used to predict weaning success include maximum voluntary ventilation (MVV) greater than 2 times the resting level and minute ventilation (VE) less than 10 L/min. Dead space/tidal volume ratio (V_D/V_T) of greater than 0.6 has been shown to predict weaning failure consistently. Unfortunately, while each of these parameters can be used to assess pulmonary mechanical function, a number of studies have demonstrated that none predicts weaning success. A number of other monitoring techniques have been employed to identify when weaning will be successful.

1. Airway occlusion pressure

The airway occlusion pressure has been used as an index of respiratory drive. Airway occlusion pressure is the pressure generated 0.1 sec ($P_{0.1}$) after initiating an inspiratory effort against an occluded airway. The $P_{0.1}$ in normal subjects is generally less than 2 cm H_2O. Some studies suggest that $P_{0.1}$ greater than 6 cm H_2O is incompatible with successful weaning for patients with chronic obstructive pulmonary disease.[114,115] Other studies have not confirmed the value of airway occlusion pressure as a predictor of successful weaning success.[116]

2. Multiparameter indices

A number of indices have been developed to improve the ability to predict when a patient can be weaned from mechanical ventilatory support. These indices combine multiple individual parameters to predict weaning success; some incorporate indices of gas exchange. One study evaluated multiparameter indices, including the rapid shallow breathing index (RSB index), the ratio of respiratory frequency divided by tidal volume in liters, and the CROP index (CROP abbreviated from thoracic *C*ompliance, *R*espiratory *R*ate, Arterial *O*xygenation, *P*imax) which incorporates measures of dynamic lung compliance, respiratory rate, gas exchange, and inspiratory pressure.[113] A RSB index of less than 105 was shown to have a high predictive value of weaning success, while the CROP index and more traditional indices had poor predictive value. A recent study could not confirm these findings and demonstrated that a RSB index below 105 did not predict failed weaning.[117]

3. Breathing pattern analysis

Respiratory impedance plethysmography (RIP) can be used to assess breathing pattern by measuring tidal volume, respiratory frequency, inspiratory time, and the contribution of the rib cage and abdomen to lung volume changes.[34,35] Using RIP, the relationship between rib cage and abdominal contributions to tidal volume (respiratory muscle dyssynchrony) have been quantitated. RIP is useful for evaluating changes in functional residual capacity (FRC) and level of PEEPi as ventilator parameters are adjusted. As a method to predict weaning success, the technique has had variable success.

V. CONCLUSION

A variety of methods is available to monitor the patient who requires airway management and mechanical ventilation. The monitoring techniques include clinical assessment, monitors of gas exchange, and a variety of methods to evaluate pulmonary mechanical function. The selection of the most appropriate monitors for each patient depends upon an understanding of the clinical situation, the available monitoring techniques, the information each monitor provides, and the limitations of the monitors. The challenge for the physician is to identify and appropriately utilize those monitoring techniques that actually optimize clinical management and reduce morbidity and mortality, rather than using any monitor simply because it is available.

REFERENCES

1. Tobin MJ: Respiratory monitoring, *JAMA* 264:244, 1990.
2. Moller JT, Jensen PF, Johannessen NW et al: Hypoxaemia is reduced by pulse oximetry monitoring in the operating theatre and in the recovery room, *Br J Anaesth* 68:146, 1992.
3. Cullen DJ, Nemeskal AR, Cooper JB et al: Effect of pulse oximetry, age, and ASA physical status on the frequency of patients admitted unexpectedly to a postoperative intensive care unit and the severity of their anesthesia-related complications, *Anesth Analg* 74:181, 1992.

4. Eichhorn JH: Prevention of intraoperative anesthesia accidents and related severe injury through safety monitoring, *Anesthesiology* 70:572, 1989.

5. Moller JT, Pedersen T, Rasmussen LS et al: Randomized evaluation of pulse oximetry in 20,802 patients, II, *Anesthesiology* 78:445, 1993.

6. Birmingham PK, Cheney FW, Ward RJ: Esophageal intubation: a review of detection techniques, *Anesth Analg* 65:886, 1986.

7. Szaflarski NL, Cohen NH: Use of capnography in critically ill adults, *Heart Lung* 20:363, 1991.

8. Goldberg JS, Rawle PR, Zehnder JL et al: Colorimetric end-tidal carbon dioxide monitoring for tracheal intubation, *Anesth Analg* 70:191, 1990.

9. MacLeod BA, Heller MB, Yealy DM et al: Verification of endotracheal tube placement with colorimetric end-tidal CO_2 detection, *Ann Emerg Med* 20:267, 1991.

10. Ornato JP, Shipley JB, Racht EM et al: Multicenter study of a portable, hand-size, colorimetric end-tidal carbon dioxide detection device, *Ann Emerg Med* 21:518, 1992.

11. Dunn SM, Mushlin PS, Lind LJ et al: Tracheal intubation is not invariably confirmed by capnography, *Anesthesiology* 73(6):1285, 1990.

12. Garnett AR, Gervin CA, Gervin AS: Capnographic waveforms in esophageal intubation: effect of carbonated beverages, *Ann Emerg Med* 18(4):387, 1989.

13. Lepilin MG, Vasilyev AV, Bildinov OA et al: End-tidal carbon dioxide as a noninvasive monitor of circulatory status during cardiopulmonary resuscitation: a preliminary clinical study, *Crit Care Med* 15(10):958, 1987.

14. Sanders AB, Kern KB, Otto CW et al: End-tidal carbon dioxide monitoring during cardiopulmonary resuscitation: a prognostic indicator for survival, *JAMA* 262(10):1347, 1989.

15. Falk JL, Rackow EC, Weil MH: End-tidal carbon dioxide concentration during cardiopulmonary resuscitation, *N Engl J Med* 318(10):607, 1988.

16. Higgins D, Hayes M, Denman W et al: Effectiveness of using end-tidal carbon dioxide concentration to monitor cardiopulmonary resuscitation, *BMJ* 300:581, 1990.

17. Zwillich CW, Pierson DJ, Creagh CE et al: Complications of assisted ventilation, *Am J Med* 57:161, 1974.

18. Conrardy PA, Goodman LR, Lainge F et al: Alteration of endotracheal tube position, *Crit Care Med* 4:8, 1976.

19. Owen RL, Cheney FW: Endobronchial intubation: a preventable complication, *Anesthesiology* 67:255, 1987.

20. Brunel W, Coleman DL, Schwartz DE et al: Assessment of routine chest roentgenograms and the physical examination to confirm endotracheal tube position, *Chest* 96:1043, 1989.

21. Gray P, Sullivan G, Ostryniuk P: Value of postprocedural chest radiographs in the adult intensive care unit, *Crit Care Med* 20:1513, 1992.

22. Schwartz DE, Lieberman JA, Cohen NH: Women are at greater risk than men for malpositioning of the endotracheal tube after emergent intubation, *Crit Care Med* 22:1127, 1994.

23. Golden JA, Schwartz DE, Gamsu G et al: Sheathed fiberoptic bronchoscopy for assessing endotracheal tube position, *Chest* 100:20S, 1991.

24. Lindholm CE, Ollman B, Snyder JV et al: Cardiorespiratory effects of flexible fiberoptic bronchoscopy in critically ill patients, *Chest* 74:362, 1978.

25. Pepe PE, Marini JJ: Occult positive end-expiratory pressure in mechanically ventilated patients with airflow obstruction: the auto-PEEP effect, *Am Rev Respir Dis* 126:166, 1982.

26. Gandhi SK, Munshi CA, Coon R et al: Capnography for detection of endobronchial migration of an endotracheal tube, *J Clin Monit* 7(1):35, 1991.

27. Hurford WE, Alfille PH, Bailin MT et al: Placement and complications of double-lumen endotracheal tubes, *Anesth Analg* 74(2S):S141, 1992.

28. Simon BA, Hurford WE, Alfille PH et al: An aid in the diagnosis of malpositioned double-lumen tubes, *Anesthesiology* 76(5):862, 1992.

29. Habib MP: Physiologic implications of artificial airways, *Chest* 96:180, 1989.

30. Potgieter PD, Hammond JMJ: "Cuff" test for safe extubation following laryngeal edema, *Crit Care Med* 16:818, 1988.

31. Cavo JW: True vocal cord paralysis following intubation, *Laryngoscope* 95:1352, 1985.

32. Cohen CA, Zagelbaum G, Gross D et al: Clinical manifestations of inspiratory muscle fatigue, *Am J Med* 73:308, 1982.

33. Roussos C, Macklem PT: The respiratory muscles, *N Engl J Med* 307:786, 1982.

34. Tobin MJ, Guenther SM, Perez W et al: Konno-Mead analysis of ribcage-abdominal motion during successful and unsuccessful trials of weaning from mechanical ventilation, *Am Rev Respir Dis* 135:1320, 1987.

35. Tobin MJ, Perez W, Guenther SM et al: Does ribcage-abdominal paradox signify respiratory muscle fatigue? *J Appl Physiol* 63:851, 1987.

36. Mandor MJ: Respiratory muscle fatigue and breathing pattern, *Chest* 100:1430, 1991.

37. Roussos C: Function and fatigue of respiratory muscles, *Chest* 88:124S, 1985.

38. Lindsay SL, Kerridge R, Collett BJ: Abscess following cannulation of the radial artery, *Anaesthesia* 42:654, 1987.

39. Band JD, Maki DG: Infections caused by arterial catheters used for hemodynamic monitoring, *Am J Med* 67:735, 1979.

40. Wolf S, Mangano DT: Pseudoaneurysm, a late complication of radial-artery catheterization, *Anesthesiology* 52:80, 1980.

41. Venkatesh B, Clutton-Brock T, Hendry S: Intraoperative use of the Paratrend 7 intravascular blood gas sensor, *Crit Care Med* 22(1):A21, 1994.

42. Bearden E, Lopez JA, Solis RT: Evaluation of a continuous intraarterial blood gas sensor in critically ill patients, *Crit Care Med* 22(1):A25, 1994.

43. Comroe JH, Botelho S: The unreliability of cyanosis in the recognition of arterial anoxemia, *Am J Med Sci* 214(1):1, 1947.

44. Yelderman M, New W: Evaluation of pulse oximetry, *Anesthesiology* 59(4):349, 1983.

45. Mihm FG, Halperin BD: Noninvasive detection of profound atrial desaturations using a pulse oximetry device, *Anesthesiology* 62:85, 1985.

46. Eichhorn JH, Cooper JB, Cullen DJ et al: Standards for patient monitoring during anesthesia at Harvard Medical School, *JAMA* 256:1017, 1986.

47. Schnapp LM, Cohen NH: Pulse oximetry: uses and abuses, *Chest* 105:534, 1990.

48. Severinghaus JW, Kelleher JF: Recent developments in pulse oximetry, *Anesthesiology* 76:1018, 1992.

49. Council on Scientific Affairs, AMA: The use of pulse oximetry during conscious sedation, *JAMA* 270(12):1463, 1993.

50. Moller JT, Wittrup M, Johansen SH: Hypoxemia in the postanesthesia care unit: an observer study, *Anesthesiology* 73:890, 1990.

51. Moller JT, Johannessen NW, Berg H et al: Hypoxaemia during anesthesia: an observer study, *Br J Anaesth* 66:437, 1991.

52. Cote CJ, Goldstein EA, Cote MA et al: A single-blind study of pulse oximetry in children, *Anesthesiology* 68:184, 1988.

53. Moller JT, Pedersen T, Rasmussen LS et al: Randomized evaluation of pulse oximetry in 20,802 patients, I, *Anesthesiology* 78:436, 1993.

54. Orkin FK: Practice standards: the Midas touch or the emperor's new clothes? *Anesthesiology* 70(4):567, 1989.

55. Orkin FK, Cohen MM, Duncan PG: The quest for meaningful outcomes, *Anesthesiology* 78:417, 1993.

56. Tobin MJ: Respiratory monitoring during mechanical ventilation, *Crit Care Clin* 6:679, 1990.

57. Kidd JF, Vickers MD: Pulse oximeters: essential monitors with limitations. *Br J Anaesth* 62:355, 1989.

58. Tobin MJ: Respiratory monitoring in the intensive care unit, *Am Rev Respir Dis* 138:1625, 1988.

59. Severinghaus JW, Naifeh KH: Accuracy of response of six pulse oximeters to profound hypoxia, *Anesthesiology* 67:551, 1987.

60. Kagle DM, Alexander CM, Berko RS et al: Evaluation of the Ohmeda 3700 pulse oximeter: steady-state and transient response characteristics, *Anesthesiology* 66:276, 1987.

61. Tremper KK, Barker SJ: Pulse oximetry, *Anesthesiology* 70:98, 1989.

62. West P, George CF, Kryger MH: Dynamic in vivo response characteristics of three oximeters: Hewlett-Packard 47201A, Biox III, and Nellcor N-100, *Sleep* 10(3):263, 1987.

63. Ralston AC, Webb RK, Runciman WB: Potential errors in pulse oximetry, *Anaesthesia* 46:291, 1991.

64. Langton JA, Hanning CD: Effect of motion artefact on pulse oximeters: evaluation of four instruments and finger probes. *Br J Anaesth* 65:564, 1990.

65. Barker SJ, Tremper KK: The effect of carbon monoxide inhalation on pulse oximetry and transcutaneous Po_2, *Anesthesiology* 66(5):677, 1987.

66. Barker SJ, Tremper KK, Hyatt J: Effects of methemoglobinemia on pulse oximetry and mixed venous oximetry, *Anesthesiology* 70:112, 1989.

67. Sjöstrand T: Endogenous formation of carbon monoxide in man under normal and pathological conditions, *Scand J Clin Lab Invest* 1:201, 1949.

68. Rodgers PA, Vreman HJ, Dennery PA et al: Sources of carbon monoxide (CO) in biological systems and applications of CO detection technologies, *Semin Perinatol* 18(1):2, 1994.

69. Eisenkraft JB: Pulse oximeter desaturation due to methemoglobinemia, *Anesthesiology* 68(2):279, 1988.

70. Ries AL, Prewitt LM, Johnson JJ: Skin color and ear oximetry, *Chest* 96(2):287, 1989.

71. Zeballos RJ, Weisman IM: Reliability of noninvasive oximetry in black subjects during exercise and hypoxia, *Am Rev Respir Dis* 144:1240, 1991.

72. Brunel W, Cohen NH: Evaluation of the accuracy of pulse oximetry in critically ill patients, *Crit Care Med* 16:432, 1988.

73. Veyckemans F, Baele P, Guillaume JE et al: Hyperbilirubinemia does not interfere with hemoglobin saturation measured by pulse oximetry, *Anesthesiology* 70:118, 1989.

74. Chelluri L, Snyder JV, Bird JR: Accuracy of pulse oximetry in patients with hyperbilirubinemia, *Respiratory Care* 36(12):1383, 1991.

75. Cote CJ, Goldstein EA, Fuchsman WH et al: The effect of nail polish on pulse oximetry, *Anesth Analg* 67:683, 1988.

76. White PF, Boyle WA: Nail polish and oximetry, *Anesth Analg* 68:546, 1989.

77. Lee S, Tremper KK, Barker SJ: Effects of anemia on pulse oximetry and continuous mixed venous hemoglobin saturation monitoring in dogs, *Anesthesiology* 75:118, 1991.

78. Vegfors M, Lindberg LG, Oberg PA et al: The accuracy of pulse oximetry at two haematocrit levels, *Acta Anaesthesiol Scand* 36:454, 1992.

79. Clayton DG, Webb RK, Ralston AC et al: A comparison of the performance of 20 pulse oximeters under conditions of poor perfusion, *Anaesthesia* 46:3, 1991.

80. Clayton DG, Webb RK, Ralston AC et al: Pulse oximeter probes, *Anaesthesia* 46:260, 1991.

81. Mendelson Y, Yocum BL: Noninvasive measurement of arterial oxyhemoglobin saturation with a heated and a non-heated skin reflectance pulse oximeter sensor, *Biomed Instrum Technol* 25(6):472, 1991.

82. Palve H, Vuori A: Accuracy of three pulse oximeters at low cardiac index and peripheral temperature, *Crit Care Med* 19(4):560, 1991.

83. Stewart KG, Rowbottom SJ: Inaccuracy of pulse oximetry in patients with severe tricuspid regurgitation, *Anaesthesia* 46:668, 1991.

84. France CJ, Eger EI, Bendixen HH: The use of peripheral venous blood for pH and carbon dioxide tension determinations during general anesthesia, *Anesthesiology* 40:311, 1974.

85. Morley TF: Capnography in the intensive care unit, *J Intens Care Med* 5:209, 1990.

86. Niehoff J, DelGuercio C, LaMorte W et al: Efficacy of pulse oximetry and capnometry in postoperative ventilatory weaning, *Crit Care Med* 16(7):701, 1988.

87. Marinii JJ: Monitoring during mechanical ventilation, *Clin Chest Med* 9:734, 1988.

88. Pedersen T, Viby-Mogensen, Ringsted C: Anaesthetic practice and postoperative pulmonary complications, *Acta Anaesthesiol Scand* 36:812, 1992.

89. Weinberger SE, Schwartzstein RM, Weiss JW: Hypercapnia, *N Engl J Med* 321:1223, 1989.

90. Fowler WS: Lung function studies. II. The respiratory dead space, *J Appl Physiol* 154:405, 1948.

91. Fowler WS: Lung function studies. IV. Postural changes in respiratory dead space and functional residual capacity, *J Clin Invest* 29:1437, 1950.

92. Nunn JF, Campbell EJM, J Peckett BW: Anatomical subdivisions of the volume of respiratory dead space and effect of position of the jaw, *J Appl Physiol* 14(2):174, 1959.

93. Nunn JF, Hill DW: Respiratory dead space and arterial to end-tidal CO_2 tension difference in anesthetized man, *J Appl Physiol* 15(3):383, 1960.

94. Nunn JF: Nunn's applied respiratory physiology, Oxford, 1993, Butterworth-Heinemann.

95. Harris EA, Seelye ER, Whitlock RML: Revised standards for normal resting dead-space volume and venous admixture in men and women, *Clin Science and Molecular Med* 55:125, 1978.

96. Zimmerman MI, Brown LK, Sloane MF: Estimated vs. actual values for dead space/tidal volume ratios during incremental exercise in patients evaluated for dyspnea, *Chest* 106(1):131, 1994.

97. Von Pohle WR, Anholm JD, McMillan J: Carbon dioxide and oxygen partial pressure in expiratory water condensate are equivalent to mixed expired carbon dioxide and oxygen, *Chest* 101(6):1601, 1992.

98. Crossman PF, Bushnell LS, Hedley-Whyte J: Dead space during artificial ventilation: gas compression and mechanical dead space, *J Appl Physiol* 28(1):94, 1970.

99. Watson WE: Observations on physiological deadspace during intermittent positive pressure respiration, *Br J Anaesth* 34:502, 1962.

100. Selecky PA, Wasserman K, Klein M et al: A graphic approach to assessing interrelationships among minute ventilation, arterial carbon dioxide tension, and ratio of physiologic deadspace to tidal volume in patients on respirators, *Am Rev Respir Dis* 117:181, 1978.

101. Jones NL, Robertson DG, Kane JW: Difference between end-tidal and arterial Pco_2 in exercise, *J Appl Physiol* 47(5):954, 1979.

102. Robbins PA, Conway J, Cunningham DA, et al: A comparison of indirect methods for continuous estimation of arterial Pco_2 in men, *J Appl Physiol* 68(4):1727, 1990.

103. Yamanaka MK, Sue DY: Comparison of arterial-end-tidal Pco_2

difference and dead space/tidal volume ratio in respiratory, *Chest* 92:832, 1987.

104. Pansard JL, Cholley B, Devilliers C et al: Variation in arterial to end-tidal CO_2 tension differences during anesthesia in the "kidney rest" lateral decubitus position, *Anesth Analg* 75:506, 1992.

105. Fernandez R, Benito S, Blanch LI et al: Intrinsic PEEP: a cause of inspiratory muscle ineffectivity, *Intensive Care Med* 15:51, 1988.

106. Eveloff SE, Rounds S, Braman SS: Unilateral lung hyperinflation and herniation as a manifestation of intrinsic PEEP, *Chest* 98:228, 1990.

107. Lewis WD, Chwals W, Benotti PN et al: Bedside assessment of work of breathing, *Crit Care Med* 16:117, 1988.

108. Banner MJ, Jaeger MJ, Kirby RR: Components of the work of breathing and implication for monitoring ventilator-dependent patients, *Crit Care Med* 22:515, 1994.

109. Gozal D, Shoseyov D, Keens TG: Inspiratory pressures with CO_2 stimulation and weaning from mechanical ventilation in children, *Am Rev Respir Dis* 147:256, 1993.

110. Krieger BG, Ershowsky PF, Becker DA et al: Evaluation of conventional criteria for predicting successful weaning from mechanical ventilatory support in elderly patients, *Crit Care Med* 17:858, 1989.

111. Scheinhorn DJ, Artinian BM, Catlin JL: Weaning from prolonged mechanical ventilation: the experience at a regional weaning center, *Chest* 105:534, 1994.

112. Yang KL, Tobin MJ: A prospective study of indexes predicting the outcome of trials of weaning from mechanical ventilation, *N Engl J Med* 324:1445, 1991.

113. Yang KL: Reproducibility of weaning parameters—a need for standardization, *Chest* 102:1829, 1992.

114. Murciano D, Boczkowski J: Tracheal occlusion pressure: a simple index to monitor respiratory fatigue during acute respiratory failure in patients with chronic obstructive pulmonary disease, *Ann Intern Med* 108:800, 1988.

115. Sassoon CS, Te TT, Mahutte CK et al: Airway occlusion pressure: an important indicator for successful weaning in patients with chronic obstructive pulmonary disease, *Am Rev Respir Dis* 135:107, 1987.

116. Montgomery AB, Holle RHO, Neagley SR et al: Prediction of successful ventilatory weaning using airway occlusion pressure and hypercapnic challenge, *Chest* 91:496, 1987.

117. Lee KH, Hui KP, Chan TB et al: Rapid shallow breathing (frequency-tidal volume ratio) did not predict extubation outcome, *Chest* 105:540, 1994.

Chapter 38

CONTROL OF PAIN AND DISCOMFORT IN THE INTUBATED-VENTILATED PATIENT

Alan N. Sandler

I. INTRODUCTION

Although analgesia and sedation are often concomitant effects of analgesic drugs (e.g., systemically administered opioids) used to provide pain relief in the intensive care unit (ICU) patients, they can be achieved by independent means (e.g., opioids or nonsteroidal antiinflammatory drugs [NSAIDs] for analgesia; benzodiazepines or propofol for sedation). A central theme in this chapter will be the requirement for tailoring the many powerful drugs and administration technologies currently available to the individual patient's require-

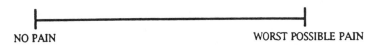

Fig. 38-1. Visual analogue pain score. Patient makes a mark on the line corresponding to severity of pain.

ments in the ICU. For this reason, analgesia and sedation will be considered separately.

Much progress has been made recently in the development of effective analgesic techniques[1,2,3] and the commitment to provide high-quality analgesia to patients who require it. Nevertheless, the provision of effective analgesia in different medical arenas is by no means universal, and there is no reason to believe that patients in ICUs who are intubated and ventilated are different from the large numbers of hospitalized patients reporting severe pain during their hospital stay.[4,5] In fact, pain can be an overwhelming feature for patients admitted to an ICU.[6] Humanitarian and ethical factors are reason enough for the effective treatment of pain in any situation, but, in addition, there are major medical reasons that dictate the importance of paying attention to the provision of analgesia. These considerations are listed below and will be examined in greater detail under Analgesic Outcome Studies. They include:

1. Earlier mobilization with decreased incidence of deep venous thrombosis,[7] increased pulmonary function and decreased pulmonary complications,[8,9] and increased patency of major vascular graft prostheses.[10]
2. Decreased incidence of pulmonary complications in patients with abdominal or thoracic insults.[8,9]
3. Inhibition of the stress response with decrease in catecholamine and neuropeptide levels and earlier normalization of oxygen consumption, cardiac output, and other measures of increased catecholamine activity that are poorly tolerated by critically ill patients.[11,12]
4. An associated improvement in the metabolic response to injury with decreased levels of insulin, glucagon, and other hormones allowing for anabolism with improved wound healing and maintenance of immune function.[12,13]

Other adverse effects associated with poorly treated pain include increases in anxiety and discomfort, interference with sleep, and a contribution to increased delirium in the ICU setting. Noise also interferes with sleep and has been shown to increase analgesic requirements.[14]

II. PAIN ASSESSMENT

Pain in ICU patients has traditionally not been objectively assessed. In intubated, ventilated patients who may have also been given neuromuscular blocking agents, pain can only be assessed on the basis of physiologic correlates, changes in which may be profound, especially with acute injury.[2] Commonly assessed physiologic correlates that may be related to noxious stimuli include increased heart rate, blood pressure, and sweating, but electromyography and cortical-evoked potentials have also been used. However, despite high initial correlations between pain onset and changes in these physiologic responses, many habituate with time despite the persistence of pain.[15] In addition, these responses are not specific to the experience of pain and occur under conditions of general arousal and stress or complications in the patient's medical condition, for example, sepsis, hypovolemia, etc. However, if it is impossible to use objective assessments of pain (see following), then nonverbal indicators (vital signs, skin assessment, nausea, vomiting, guarding, posture, crying or moaning, pallor, restlessness, grimacing) are all that is available, and the nursing staff members need to be skilled in their assessment. Wherever possible, if communication with the patient can be made, an objective attempt at pain assessment should be made. The visual analog scale (VAS)[16] is most widely used (Fig. 38-1) and consists of a 10 cm horizontal or vertical line with two end points labeled "no pain" and "worst pain ever." The VAS is most useful if the patient is cooperative, has no visual problems, and is not confused. The patient is required to mark the 10 cm line at a point that corresponds to the level of pain intensity currently felt. In patients unable to mark the scale, other pain rating systems are used (see following). The VAS is sensitive to pharmacologic and nonpharmacologic procedures that provided analgesia[17,18,19] and correlated highly with pain measured by using verbal and numerical rating scales.[20,21,22] A simple system involving three questions—Where does it hurt? How much does it hurt? and What does it feel like?—has been suggested by Stevens and Edwards[23] and is a very useful plan to follow in the assessment of pain in any patient.

III. ANALGESIC TECHNIQUES THAT ARE USEFUL IN THE ICU

This section will discuss analgesic techniques that are currently widely used in the ICU and techniques that are widely used in other areas (e.g., postoperative pain control) and are slowly being introduced into the ICU setting. In the next section, painful conditions will be related to these analgesic techniques.

A. OPIOID ADMINISTRATION

Opioids, which are primarily longer acting agents (e.g., morphine), are the mainstay of analgesia therapy in the ICU environment. The intramuscular route is virtually ignored in the critically ill patient due to poor, erratic, or delayed absorption, slow onset of analgesia, pain with repeated injection, and the ready availability of intravenous access. Currently, bolus doses of nurse-administered opioid or continuous infusions of opioids are the most frequently used administration techniques. Opioids interact with specific receptors of various types throughout the central nervous system (and probably peripherally as well) to produce analgesia. A discussion regarding opioid receptors is beyond the scope of this chapter and is reported in regards to ICU patient management elsewhere.[24] Opioids commonly used in the ICU are usually mu agonists, which interact with mu opioid receptors to produce supraspinal and spinal analgesia, euphoria, miosis, dependence, bradycardia, and respiratory depression. In addition, opioids interact with the medullary chemoreceptor trigger zone to produce nausea and vomiting, and morphine and meperidine are involved with systemic histamine release. The most common opioids used in the ICU setting are probably morphine, hydromorphone, and fentanyl (and some of its derivatives, e.g., alfentanil). Morphine and other opioids are metabolized primarily in the liver, although up to a third of morphine's clearance can occur by renal excretion. Morphine in particular, has active metabolites that can increase the duration of its effects especially in renal failure. Fentanyl is approximately 40 times more lipid soluble than morphine, and this results in a much more rapid central nervous system effect and onset of analgesia (within minutes), which parallels blood levels. Termination of the initial effects of all the opioids is by redistribution. Highly lipid soluble opioids have their effects terminated much more rapidly after bolus doses. Fentanyl (and other members of the lipid soluble opioid group), however, accumulate in fat depots, which can lead to prolonged effects with long-term infusions, large doses, and repeated boluses. Many factors influence the duration of effect of opioids, and these include dose, obesity, acid-base balance, protein binding, and hepatic and renal function. Newborns and the elderly may be more sensitive to opioid effects; opioids should be administered cautiously at the extremes of age.

1. Intravenous bolus dose of opioids

Intravenous, observer-administered, bolus dosing of opioids (especially morphine) is probably the most common form of analgesia therapy encountered in an ICU. The provision of analgesia may only be part of the required effect, and, in ventilated patients, very large opioid doses may be administered to achieve a sedative effect or a respiratory depressant effect in patients "fighting the ventilator." Critically ill patients have unpredictable pharmacokinetic parameters in relation to opioids, especially if impaired renal and hepatic

function are present. Numerous reports of the prolonged action of morphine are related to the accumulation of the metabolite morphine-6-glucuronide, a potent opiate receptor agonist in renal failure.[25-27] Prolonged sedative action of morphine can delay awakening and result in delayed weaning from the ventilator or present diagnostic difficulty in differentiating between a possible cerebral complication and prolonged opioid action. Objective measures of sedation such as computer-processed electroencephalogram (EEG) (e.g., compressed spectral array[28,29]) or lower esophageal contractility (LEC)[30] monitoring, are being investigated in several areas (during general anesthesia and in the ICU) but are not widely used. The relationship between LEC and depth of sedation is not as clear for opioids[31,32] as it is for volatile anesthetic agents.[33]

Administration of systemic opioids requires an understanding of the concept of minimum effective analgesic concentration (MEAC). MEAC implies that, at a minimum systemic concentration of opioid, the patient will achieve effective analgesia.[34-36] Mather's group[34] (Fig. 38-2) has elegantly demonstrated that the MEAC for opioids (meperidine) in the systemic circulation varies up to fivefold for effective analgesia in individual patients. This is, of course, the rationale for the use of patient-controlled analgesia (PCA) (see following) with intravenous opioids that has achieved widespread use for postoperative analgesia. Morphine and fentanyl are probably the best suited opioids for intravenous use in the ICU setting.[24] Meperidine is less than optimal for acute pain treatment because of its short half-life and toxic metabolite.[37] Experienced nursing staff in an ICU environment assigned to care for patients on a one-to-one or one-to-two basis are able to provide very effective analgesia by administering bolus doses of opioids. In general, a loading dose is required, which can be administered either by bolus (Table 38-1) or by infusion, followed by intermittent boluses. For a successful analgesic regimen, very close supervision of the patient is necessary by query or by behavior to determine whether the next bolus is required. In effect, the nurse is monitoring the MEAC for the patient and the nurse-administered dose is analogous to PCA as long as the nurse is constantly available. Like PCA, the advantage is that plasma concentration is not allowed to rise much above the MEAC, and, upon discontinuation, rapid drug elimination can occur. In practice, it is often difficult to provide the ideal nurse-administered bolus regimen due to attention to other tasks, differences in knowledge and skills, differing attitudes to analgesic requirements, or other systemic factors.[38]

2. Intravenous infusions of opioids

Continuous intravenous opioid infusion is a relatively simple analgesic technique and may be more effective than intermittent bolus dosing. The concept of front-

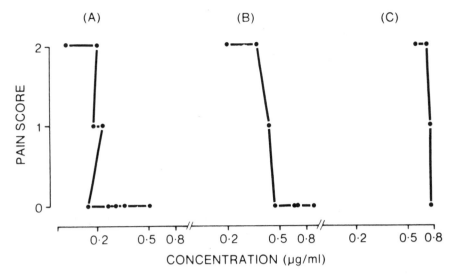

Fig. 38-2. Blood meperidine concentration-response curves for three individual patients, illustrating a typical range in interpatient responses. **A,** = Patient 4, injection 6; **C,** = patient 1, injection 9; **B,** = an additional patient studied in a pilot series whose concentration response data were identical to the mean of the present series. (From Austin KL, Stapleton JV, Mather LE et al: *Anesthesiology* 53:466, 1980a.)

loading is critical to achieving the MEAC within a reasonable period. The institution of an opioid infusion without front-loading will not result in the development of a MEAC for at least three elimination half-lives (often 4 to 6 half-lives).[39] Edwards[40] has tabulated some simple guidelines for front-loading opioid drugs (see Table 38-1). Newer synthetic opioids, such as fentanyl,[41] sufentanil,[42] and alfentanil,[41,43,44] have also been used successfully as continuous infusions in the ICU. After front-loading, the MEAC of the opioid can be maintained with a continuous infusion. If various pharmacokinetic parameters are known, the intravenous infusion can be titrated to maintain a constant plasma concentration or even a known plasma concentration of the opioid. Simplified calculation or recursive algorithms (e.g., sum of exponentials, principle of superimposition), plus the use of computers, can be used to predict infusion rates to achieve and maintain desired plasma concentrations.[45,46,47] Edwards[48] has recommended a simple calculation to determine the rate of infusion: (1) most opioid drugs have an elimination half-time of approximately 3 hours; and (2) the dose required every 3 hours to maintain the level of analgesia that was produced by the amount of opioid required for front-loading will be half the amount required for front-loading. Thus, the hourly rate will equal half the front-load dose divided by 3 hours (= mg/hr infusion rate). Thus, it is probably an underestimation of hourly requirements if the elimination half-life is actually less than 3 hours. If breakthrough pain occurs, then a new front-load bolus administration is necessary with appropriate adjustment of the infusion. Merely increasing the infusion

rate will require 3 half-lives to develop the required MEAC.

Morphine sulfate is given as a loading dose of 5 to 10 mg followed by an infusion of 1 to 3 mg/hr. Considerable variations in dose requirements may occur in each patient. Fentanyl, the first in a new generation of potent, synthetic opioids that have high cardiovascular stability and negligible histamine release is given as a loading dose of 100 to 200 μg and an infusion of 1 to 3 μg/kg/hr.

Variability among patients regarding pharmacokinetic parameters makes it necessary to individualize both loading dose and maintenance infusion to achieve and maintain an adequate analgesic blood concentration when opioids are used. As noted above, individual MEACs may vary fourfold to fivefold for postoperative pain due to the same surgical procedure.[49,50] Thus, it may be necessary to adjust the maintenance dose rate of a continuous infusion upward (after a further loading dose) or downward by a factor of two or more from the expected average to achieve good analgesia.

3. Patient-controlled analgesia

Patient-controlled analgesia (PCA)[51] involves the use of a microprocessor-based pump that allows small doses of opioid (or any other analgesic) to be administered on a demand basis by a variety of routes (intravenous, epidural, subcutaneous, and, in the future, possibly transdermal). The most common administration route currently used is intravenously. Opioid loading is required to achieve MEAC before PCA is initiated or if the demand dose/frequency is changed. PCA aims to produce a relatively stable plasma concentration by allowing the patient to receive multiple, frequent, small bolus

Table 38-1. Guidelines for front-loading intravenous analgesics

Drug	Total front-load dose (mg/kg)	Increments	Cautions
Morphine	0.08-0.12	0.03 mg/kg every 10 min	Histamine effects; nausea; biliary colic; reduce dose for elderly
Meperidine	1.0-1.5	0.30 mg/kg every 10 min	Reduce dose or change drug for impaired renal function
Codeine	0.5-1.0	One third of total every 15 min	Nausea
Methadone	0.08-0.12	0.03 mg/kg every 15 min	Do not administer maintenance dose after analgesia achieved; accumulation; sedation
Levorphanol	0.02	50-75 µg/kg every 15 min	Similar to methadone
Hydromorphone	0.02	25-50 µg/kg every 10 min	Similar to morphine
Pentazocine	0.5-1.0	One half of total every 15 min	Psychomimetic effects; may cause withdrawal in narcotic-dependent patients
Nalbuphine	0.08-0.15	0.03 mg/kg every 10 min	Less psychomimetic effect than pentazocine; sedation
Butorphanol	0.02-0.04	0.01 mg/kg every 10 min	Sedation; psychomimetic effects like nalbuphine
Buprenorphine	Up to 0.2	One quarter of total every 10 min	Long acting like methadone and levorphanol; may precipitate withdrawal in narcotic-dependent patients; safe to give subcutaneous maintenance after analgesia; different from methadone

From Stevens DS and Edwards WT: *Anesth Clin North Am* 10(2):408, 1992.

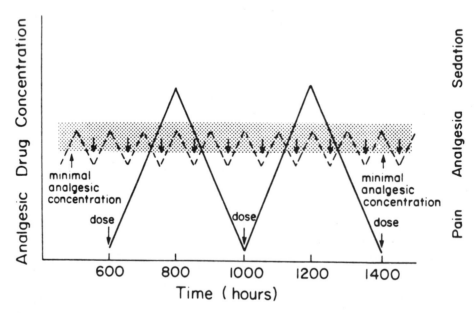

Fig. 38-3. The PCA paradigm. A statistical model for pain in patient-controlled analgesia and conventional intramuscular opioid regimens. (From Ferrante FM, Orav EJ, Rocco AG et al: *Anesth Analg* 67:457, 1988.)

Table 38-2. Guidelines for the use of patient-controlled analgesia with several common opioids

Drug (concentration)	Demand dose	Lockout interval (min)
Fentanyl (10 μg/mL)*	10-20 μg	5-10
Hydromorphone (0.2 mg/mL)	0.05-0.25 mg	5-10
Meperidine (10 mg/mL)	5-30 mg	5-12
Methadone (1 mg/mL)	0.5-2.5 mg	8-20
Morphine (1 mg/mL)	0.5-3.0 mg	5-12
Nalbuphine (1 mg/mL)	1-5 mg	5-10
Oxymorphone (0.25 mg/mL)	0.2-0.4 mg	8-10

From Ferrante FM: *Anesth Clin North Am* 10:287, 1992.

*Analgesic requirements vary widely among patients. Age, the presence of severe disease, or the idiosyncrasies of individual drug handling may make dosage adjustment necessary.

doses after the loading dose (Fig. 38-3). Intravenous PCA delivers almost immediate opioid effect, providing close matching of medication to analgesic need.[40] Pump settings include demand dose (e.g., morphine 0.02 mg/ml or 1 to 2 mg for most adults), lockout interval (5 to 10 min), and drug limit per set interval (usually 1 to 4 hours) (Table 38-2). The lockout interval allows the new plasma concentration to be achieved before the next dose. Patients tend to dose themselves to a balanced level between acceptable analgesia and opioid side effects with the limiting factors being nausea and drowsiness. Patients generally use PCA to achieve a level of pain relief 20% to 30% above complete analgesia.[52,53] Respiratory depression can occur but is relatively rare.[54] Overdose and respiratory depression present an increased risk if a background continuous infusion is used together with bolus doses. No more than half the hourly requirement should be supplied by continuous infusion. All PCA delivery systems require the patient to activate the demand button to obtain the analgesic. In the ICU environment, mechanically ventilated patients who are awake and reasonably alert often are able to use PCA to good effect. In addition, the use of a PCA pump for nurse-administered analgesia in the ICU may increase the effectiveness of the analgesia regimen until the patient can take over.

4. Spinal opioids

The term *spinally administered opioid* includes all opioids injected into either the epidural or subarachnoid spaces surrounding the spinal cord. This has become a universally adopted powerful analgesic technique for the control of acute and chronic pain[55,56] and has a very definite role in intensive care.

5. Subarachnoid opioids

Although subarachnoid opioids can be administered by continuous infusions via indwelling intrathecal catheters[57] with excellent analgesia,[58] the main use is by single bolus administration, especially of morphine 3 to 7 μg/kg.[59-62] Recommended doses of subarachnoid opioids are given in Table 38-3. The limited analgesic duration of single-dose intrathecal opioid administration (12 to 24 hours for morphine) often makes epidural opioid administration via an indwelling epidural catheter more preferable.

6. Epidural opioids

Although most opioids have been used via the epidural route,[55,56] those most commonly used in clinical practice include morphine, meperidine, fentanyl, and, to a lesser degree, sufentanil. Opioids exert their analgesic effects by binding with specific receptor sites on neurons in the dorsal horn substantia gelatinosa.[63] The major difference in the use of epidural opioids relates to the degree of lipid solubility of the opioid, which is the principal rate-limiting factor for dural- and spinal-cord penetration. Morphine, the most hydrophilic opioid, thus has a slow onset of action and, conversely, a long duration of analgesia. Meperidine, which has intermediate solubility, has a more rapid onset of action and intermediate duration. Fentanyl, the prototype, highly lipid-soluble opioid, has a rapid onset and short duration of action (see Table 38-3). For highly lipid-soluble opioids, absorption into the systemic circulation and uptake by nonspecific binding sites in the spinal cord[64] lead to large dosage requirements similar to those required for systemic analgesia compared to decreased doses when morphine is used epidurally. Catheter placement along the vertebral column will also affect dosage requirements and systemic absorption, especially with continuous infusions. For both abdominal and thoracic pain, inserting the catheter close to the dermatomes involved will decrease opioid requirements for both morphine and lipid-soluble opioids (Table 38-4).[3,65-67] Increasing age is also associated with a decrease in dose requirement (Table 38-4). If the epidural catheter cannot be placed close to the dermatomes involved, increasing the dose of epidural morphine will promote rostral spread and produce analgesia cephalad to the catheter tip. Lumbar,[68] and even caudal epidural morphine,[69] can provide analgesia

Table 38-3. Intraspinal opioids for postthoracotomy pain

Drug	Single dose*	Infusion†	Onset (min)	Duration‡ (h)
Epidural				
Morphine	1-6 mg	0.1-1.0 mg/h	30	6-24
Meperidine	20-150 mg	2-20 mg/h	5	6-8
Fentanyl	25-150 μg	25-100 μg/h	5	3-6
Sufentanil	10-60 μg	10-50 μg/h	5	2-4
Subarachnoid				
Morphine	0.1-0.3 mg		15	8-24
Fentanyl	5-25 μg		5	3-6

From Stevens DS, Edwards WT: *Anesth Clin North Am* 10(2):403, 1992.
*Doses must be carefully adjusted for patient age and catheter position.
†When using epidural infusion, for accuracy and convenience of administration, adjust concentration to allow infused volume to be approximately 10 ml/hr for infusion with bupivacaine, use 0.0625% bupivacaine solution.
‡Duration of analgesia is variable. It tends to increase with dose and patient age.

Table 38-4. Starting doses for epidural morphine for thoracic analgesia

Patient age (years)	Catheter tip at T4-T11 level (mg)	Catheter tip at T12-L4 level (mg)
15-44*	4	6
45-65	3	5
66-75	2	4
76+	1	2

From Ready LB, Oden R, Chadwick HS et al: *Anesthesiology* 68:100, 1988.
*Careful consideration must be given to the presence of other concurrent disease and to the response seen with these suggested initial doses.

after thoracotomy. Dosage requirements should be titrated to patient response, but, in general, with bolus dose epidural morphine, patients will require regular dosing every 8 hours or earlier for maximum effect. PCA epidural opioid administration has also been shown to be very effective[70] but is usually reserved for bolus doses of fentanyl, which has been shown to act primarily via the spinal route when administered as small, intermittent doses.[71] Administration of a bolus dose of opioid, followed by a continuous infusion of epidural opioids, also provides excellent analgesia, especially with morphine, and results in decreased dose requirements and side effects.[72-75] However, several studies have clearly documented that continuous epidural infusions of *lipid*-soluble opioids for 24 to 48 hours result in no material benefit over a continuous intravenous infusion of the same opioid: that is, opioid dose, plasma concentration, degree of pain relief, and side effects are indistinguishable between the two routes.[3,66,76-79] Thus, there seems to be no rationale to use continuous epidural infusions of lipid-soluble opioids alone for postoperative surgical patients or for analgesia in the ICU. The most common side effects of epidural (spinal) opioids are nausea, pruritus, urinary retention, and respiratory depression. Nausea can be treated with prochlorperazine or metoclopramide, pruritus with diphenhydramine or small titrated doses of opioid antagonists (naloxone) or partial agonist-antagonists (nalbuphine,[80] or butorphanol).

Respiratory depression is treated with naloxone or opioid agonist-antagonists,[81] if necessary. Respiratory depression due to spinal opioids has been reviewed recently.[82] The incidence is relatively low (<1%),[82,83] which is similar to the incidence of respiratory depression when opioids are administered intramuscularly or by PCA.[54,84] Onset of respiratory depression can occasionally occur within 1 to 2 hours after administration, and may be related to systemic absorption of the opioid,[82,85] but more often occurs at 6 to 12 hours or later, which is related to the movement rostrally in the cerebrospinal fluid (CSF) (especially with morphine). Respiratory insufficiency is usually preceded by the onset of sedation, which may bear a greater correlation to respiratory depression than the classical monitoring of respiratory rate.[86] In the ICU environment, particularly with a ventilated patient, respiratory depression may be of little consequence to patient safety or may be easily assessed and treated, and, in fact, some institutions do not allow the use of spinal opioids except in the ICU environment. Ready et al.[83] have established, however, that epidural opioids can be used safely in ward settings if appropriate guidelines for selection of patients, dosing, and monitoring are followed. This is particularly important as epidural opioids (with or without local anesthetic agents) clearly affect outcome in patients who require intensive care after trauma or after major abdominal and thoracic surgery but need to be continued for several days both in the ICU and on the ward—decreasing morbidity and mortality (see Analgesic Outcome Studies).

B. LOCAL ANESTHETIC TECHNIQUES

Local anesthetic agents are widely used for pain control either for neuraxial blocks (mostly epidural) or major plexus or nerve blocks. In addition, local anesthetic agents are widely used in combination with opioids to produce potent epidural analgesia.

1. Epidural local anesthesia-analgesia

Epidural catheter placement can be performed in the intubated, ventilated patient, but it is very desirable to have the patient responsive enough to report pain, paresthesias, or symptoms of intravascular injection. However, if the patient is unresponsive and an epidural catheter is required, sympathectomy-induced hypotension may be the only sign of a correctly placed epidural catheter. These issues are important irrespective of the agent used for epidural analgesia (opioids, local anesthetics, adjuvants, etc.), since local anesthetic agents are uniformly used to assess correct catheter placement. Particularly, with local anesthetic agents, the catheter should be placed at a dermatomal level in the middle of dermatomes subserving the area of injury so that the agents can provide segmental block to several dermatomes on each side of the insertion level. Bupivacaine is the local anesthetic of choice because of its motor-sparing function, but the newer related agent, Ropivacaine, which has enhanced motor sparing, may be preferable in the future. The agent is administered by continuous infusion usually as a very dilute (0.125%) solution starting at 4 ml/hour for thoracic epidurals and 6 to 8 ml/hour for lumbar epidurals. Volume is increased by 2 ml/hour steps to a maximum of 14 ml/hour,[87] since tachyphylaxis to bupivacaine usually occurs within 24 hours. If analgesia is inadequate, bupivacaine concentration is increased to 0.25%, and the infusion rate decreased to 6 to 8 ml/hour. Subsequent increases are again in 2 ml/hour steps. Maximum infusion rates of 0.5 to 1 mg/kg/hour are usually tolerated safely for up to 48 hours, although patients should be carefully assessed for symptoms and signs of local anesthetic toxicity when high infusion rates are used. The most significant side effect of epidural local anesthetic infusions is hypotension due to sympathetic blockade,[88] especially with a thoracically placed catheter. However, hypotension can usually be managed by expanding intravascular volume[89] or by infusing small doses of α-adrenergic agents (e.g., phenylephrine at 10 to 20 μg/min). Studies using thoracic epidural analgesia (TEA) with local anesthetics alone in patients with severe coronary artery disease and unstable angina pectoris[90] or myocardial infarction[91] have shown beneficial effects (decreased afterload) of the epidural, in spite of some degree of hypotension[92] and with no adverse changes in myocardial perfusion.[93] These studies and other corroborating evidence indicating a decrease in morbidity and mortality with TEA[94] will be considered under Analgesic Outcome Studies (see following). Thus, moderate hypotension with TEA does not constitute increased risk to the patient if it is rapidly corrected, and therefore TEA is probably of significant benefit.

2. Combined local anesthetic-opioid epidural infusions

The rationale for the use of combined epidural local anesthetic-opioid infusion is to increase analgesic efficacy by using two active agents acting at two different sites, allowing a decrease in the concentrations required and thus decreasing the incidence and severity of side effects of either the opioid or the local anesthetic. Bupivacaine is commonly used in combination with fentanyl or morphine and, in concentrations between 0.125% and 0.25%, can provide significantly better analgesia than the opioid alone, with the 0.125% combination having the least number of side effects.[95-97] A common combination is bupivacaine 0.125% and fentanyl 0.001% (10 g/ml), which can be given as a combined solution, or separately by joining the two infusions at a stopcock attached to the epidural catheter, which allows the rate of each infusion to be varied independently.[87] Bupivacaine in low concentration (0.125% to 0.25%) combined with low-dose morphine can provide significantly better analgesia than the opioid alone.[96]

C. REGIONAL NERVE BLOCK

Several regional techniques are available for analgesia pain related to thoracic or upper abdominal pain or limb pain. These techniques include intercostal analgesia, paravertebral analgesia, interpleural analgesia, brachial plexus analgesia, or major nerve blocks (e.g., femoral nerve block). The use of regional block techniques in the ICU setting is dependent on the availability of expertise to provide the service. This is usually related to the presence of anesthesia staff in the ICU or the establishment of an Acute Pain Service with wide-ranging skills and 24-hour service. The applicability of these techniques to postthoracotomy pain has recently been critically reviewed.[98] All regional techniques may have limited use in anticoagulated patients.

1. Intercostal nerve blocks

Intercostal neuronal analgesia can be used to provide analgesia for unilateral thoracic or upper abdominal pain and has been used extensively after thoracic surgery. The technique provides analgesia without sympathetic blockade or muscle weakness. Agents may be administered as a single percutaneous treatment,[99] as multiple percutaneous serial injections,[100,101] or via an indwelling intercostal catheter.[102,103] Disadvantages include the need for repeated injections if the single dose technique is used, risk of pneumothorax (0.073% to 19%),[104] and local anesthetic toxicity due to systemic absorption, although safe plasma concentrations have been documented in clinical studies.[102,105] Bupivacaine 0.25% to -0.5% (with or without epinephrine) has been shown to be effective by intermittent or continuous infusion.[98]

2. Paravertebral analgesia

Unilateral paravertebral blockade has been used after thoracotomy, since the pain from thoracotomy (or fractured ribs) is usually unilateral. The anatomic basis for paravertebral blockade has been reviewed.[106,107] Advantages of paravertebral blocks are related to the decreased anesthetic dose and unilateral sympathetic block with decreased incidence of hypotension, urinary retention, and decreased possibility of local anesthetic toxicity.

3. Interpleural analgesia

Interpleural analgesia involves placement of an epidural catheter in the space between the visceral and parietal pleura using very similar techniques to the placement of an epidural catheter in the epidural space.[108] Interpleural analgesia has been used to manage pain after renal surgery,[109] thoracotomy,[110] thoracoabdominal esophagectomy,[111] and in patients with multiple rib fractures.[112] Local anesthetic agents may be administered via the indwelling catheter by intermittent or continuous-infusion regimens. Bupivacaine (0.25% or 0.5%) in 20 to 30 ml boluses has been commonly used.[98] For thoracotomy, at least, concerns about systemic absorption and toxicity have not been substantiated in clinical studies that assayed plasma local anesthetic concentration.[110,113] Complications of interpleural analgesia include placement into lung parenchyma and pneumothorax. After thoracic surgery, thoracotomy drainage may remove the anesthetic from the interpleural space, resulting in inadequate analgesia, and thus chest tubes should be clamped for at least 20 min after interpleural injection. Inability to tolerate chest-tube clamping is a contraindication to interpleural analgesia, along with inflammation of the pleura and the standard contraindications to regional analgesia (anticoagulation, localized infection). Interpleural analgesia does not provide a dense somatic block and almost always requires some degree of parenteral supplementation. It is an alternative if there is a contraindication to thoracic epidural analgesia.[87]

4. Other regional blocks

Single-dose brachial plexus blocks can be very useful and provide quite prolonged analgesia to an upper limb, whereas the use of a continuous brachial plexus block with an indwelling catheter and local anesthetic infusion will provide continuous analgesia and sympathetic blockade to an upper extremity.[114,115] This technique may be very useful after reimplantation surgery for digits or limbs. Similarly, a continuous femoral nerve block using a catheter placed in the femoral nerve sheath will provide either localized nerve or thigh analgesia[116,117] or a lumbar plexus block.[118]

D. NONSTEROIDAL ANTIINFLAMMATORY DRUGS

Oral nonsteroidal antiinflammatory drugs (NSAIDs) have long been used in medicine for their antiinflammatory, antipyretic, and analgesic properties. NSAIDs block the synthesis of prostaglandins by the inhibition of the enzyme cyclooxygenase (prostaglandin synthetase), which catalyzes the conversion of arachidonic acid to the cyclic endoperoxide precursors of prostaglandins. Prostaglandins mediate several components of the inflammatory response, including fever, pain, and vasodilation.[119,120] NSAIDs also have prostaglandin-independent effects that contribute to their antiinflammatory and analgesic properties (inhibition of neutrophil migration and lymphocyte responsiveness). From a clinical perspective, potential adverse effects associated with NSAID therapy include gastrointestinal bleeding, acute reversible renal dysfunction,[121] and systemic bleeding associated with platelet dysfunction. All three are related to inhibition of prostaglandin synthesis. NSAIDs can also produce idiosyncratic reactions involving the central nervous, dermatologic, hepatic, musculoskeletal, or pulmonary systems. The mechanisms of action of these agents have been extensively reviewed[122] and have concluded that significant clinical problems are unlikely with short-term use at least for postoperative analgesia.[122,123]

Patients in an ICU setting are already at risk for the major complications related to NSAID use, and, thus, NSAIDs have not been widely used in these patients. In addition, parenteral administration of NSAIDs has only recently become available in North America. Nonoral preparations of NSAIDs that have potent analgesic properties include indomethacin (rectal suppositories, intravenous preparation available in Europe), diclofenac, and ketorolac tromethamine, with the latter two agents available in injectable preparations. Although there are few studies describing the use of NSAIDs in ICU patients, there is definite evidence of their analgesic potency and opioid-sparing effects after major surgical procedures. The use of indomethacin suppositories (100 to 200 mg 8 to 12 hourly) demonstrated good analgesia and marked opioid-sparing effects after thoracotomy[124] and abdominal surgery.[125] After thoracotomy, intravenous lysine-acetylsalicylic acid[98] or diclofenac[98] were very effective analgesics with marked opioid-sparing effect and no discernible adverse effects with short-term use. In North America, ketorolac tromethamine has been introduced as a potent, parenterally administered NSAID. Ketorolac has several desirable features as an analgesic: high analgesic potency, parenteral administration, rapid onset of action, prolonged analgesic duration, paucity of side effects associated with opioids or NSAIDs, and lack of addictive potential.[126-129] The high cost of ketorolac has deterred routine use, but, with careful monitoring of gastrointestinal, hemostatic, and renal function (all of which are commonly performed in critically ill patients), parenteral NSAIDs have a useful role in the ICU under the correct circumstances.

IV. PAIN PROBLEMS IN THE INTENSIVE CARE UNIT

A. TRAUMA

Although severe trauma is a common cause of acute pain and morbidity, few trauma patients enter the ICU directly. Almost all are resuscitated and evaluated in the emergency department, and they usually undergo anesthesia and surgery to correct the underlying problem. Thus, analgesic and sedative requirements will be affected by the history of each patient's prior treatment. Nonetheless, for these patients, pain will represent a major therapeutic requirement. In intubated or incoherent patients, physiologic changes, such as tachycardia, hypertension, and restlessness, may indicate increased analgesic requirements (see preceding Pain Assessment). Patients suffering from multiple trauma will be best served by intermittent or continuous opioid administration, since they are likely to require ventilatory support for prolonged periods. Localized trauma above or below the waist is often amenable to regional analgesic techniques utilizing local anesthetic agents and/or opioids.

B. RIB FRACTURES OR FLAIL CHEST

Blunt chest injury, including multiple rib fractures, flail chest, pulmonary contusion, and often hemopneumothorax, are frequent injuries usually resulting from motor vehicle accidents. They present with severe pain and impairment of pulmonary function. If left inadequately treated, the pain related to these conditions results in respiratory muscle splinting, hypoventilation, atelectasis, and bronchopneumonia. Prior to 1950, the mortality rate for this injury was greater than 80%. The introduction of endotracheal intubation and intermittent positive-pressure ventilation (IPPV) resulted in improvement in morbidity and mortality, although this therapy was required for several weeks.[130] However, later investigation demonstrated that morbidity and mortality were related less to the number of fractured ribs or degree of flail and more to the degree of underlying pulmonary contusion, atelectasis, associated injuries, and preexisting underlying pulmonary disease.[131] Although these patients may require some degree of ventilatory support, the importance of excellent pain control is illustrated by a study comparing IPPV to a nonventilated approach that included fluid restriction, intense pulmonary physiotherapy and hygiene, and adequate analgesia.[132] Mortality was markedly decreased in the conservatively managed patients.[132] Outcome is related to the degree of pulmonary contusion, atelectasis, associated injuries, and presence of premorbid lung disease, rather than the number of fractured ribs or degree of flail.[131] Although some patients can be managed satisfactorily with intercostal blocks[133] or with intravenous opioids, the best analgesic technique for thoracic chest wall injury is epidural analgesia using opioids[75,134] or local anesthetics alone[135] or in combination.[136] In a prospective study[134] comparing continuous epidural morphine analgesia to standard parenteral morphine analgesia, the epidural morphine group showed significant decreases in ventilator-dependent time, ICU stay, hospital stay, and incidence of tracheostomy.

C. FACIAL OR LONG BONE FRACTURES

The principles of pain control for facial or long bone fractures are similar: stabilization (which may be difficult in facial fractures), limitation of edema formation, and intravenous opioids and/or NSAIDs. Severe facial fractures may be complicated by endotracheal intubation and nasogastric tubes, and, if the possibility of infection exists (otitis media, meningitis), tracheostomy and gastrostomy may be considered. In patients with long bone fractures and associated injuries severe enough to warrant ICU admission, pain is often intense and is related to periosteal and soft tissue injury. Although intravenous opioids are the first line of treatment, along with adequate fixation and traction, epidural opioid techniques may be extremely effective as well. Pain usually decreases within 48 hours and may then be managed with NSAIDs or other nonopioid agents. Persistence of pain may be related to serious complications such as compartment syndrome, infection, or loss of reduction.

D. POSTOPERATIVE PAIN

Many patients undergoing major surgery are likely to require some degree of intensive care postoperatively, especially if assisted ventilation is required. These include patients undergoing thoracic surgery (in particular, patients with severe preexisting lung disease or requiring chest wall resection), and patients undergoing lung transplantation,[137] major abdominal surgery (severe sepsis, pancreatic or hepatic surgery), aortic or peripheral vascular surgery (dependent on severity of associated vascular disease), spinal surgery (severe kyphoscoliosis and pulmonary compromise), cardiac surgery, and neurosurgery. Intravenous opioids have been and continue to be the cornerstone of treatment for the majority of these patients, but many other techniques are very effective and may be more beneficial. Pain control after thoracotomy has been recently reviewed,[98] and the following techniques have been found to decrease pain and analgesic consumption significantly: indwelling intercostal catheters with bupivacaine, interpleural catheters with bupivacaine, epidural morphine (with an infusion in the thoracic route or bolus administration in the lumbar route), combined infusions of thoracic epidural bupivacaine with sufentanil or fentanyl, and systemic NSAIDs as adjuncts to systemic opioids. The combination of thoracic epidural local anesthetics and opioids can essentially abolish postoperative pain. Similarly, after major abdominal surgery, epidural analgesia with opioids or opioid-local anesthetic combinations can produce profound analgesia.

E. CARDIAC SURGERY

Patients undergoing cardiac surgery are a large group who are usually administered specialized anesthetic techniques. The use of high-dose opioid techniques with especially lipid-soluble opioids is extremely common due to the high degree of hemodynamic stability achieved. These techniques may saturate tissue reservoirs and provide postoperative analgesia for a variable length of time. In general, this leads to a prolonged period of assisted ventilation often requiring further administration of opioids and sedatives in the postoperative period. The beneficial effect of high-quality analgesia has been demonstrated by a significantly decreased ischemia load postoperatively when a high-dose sufentanil infusion was continued throughout the postoperative period compared to standard intravenous morphine analgesia.[42] A major disadvantage of prolonged intravenous analgesia is the prolongation of assisted ventilation and, thus, increased nursing care. Other analgesic techniques are being explored to assess high-quality analgesia that allows much earlier extubation after cardiac surgery, which may present no increase in risk to the patient and increased benefits. These include PCA morphine administration,[138] subarachnoid morphine administration,[62,139] and, in our institution, a combination NSAID, intravenous opioid, and propofol infusion technique perioperatively.[140,141] In general, the use of these techniques is associated with lower doses of lipid-soluble opioids intraoperatively so as to facilitate early extubation postoperatively.[140,141] We have found that there is no increased cardiac risk to patients with our combined technique and a marked decrease in intubation time, ICU stay, and hospital stay, with concomitant cost savings.[141]

F. SPINAL SURGERY

Surgery is frequently performed on these patients to alleviate painful conditions associated with compression of spinal nerves or roots (e.g., ruptured disc, infection, tumor or kyphosis or scoliosis). If the procedure is extensive with major transfusion requirements, and especially if there is a severe underlying respiratory deficit (e.g., restrictive lung disease secondary to kyphoscoliosis), the patient may present to the ICU for postoperative care. In general, intravenous opioids (bolus or infusion, or PCA for several days) form the mainstay of analgesic therapy, but subarachnoid opioids and epidural opioids have been used with good effect.[56] In patients with severe respiratory compromise, NSAIDs (e.g., ketorolac tromethamine) may be very useful due to the lack of respiratory depression, plus the associated decrease in opioid requirement.

G. MYOCARDIAL INFARCTION

The majority of patients presenting with myocardial ischemia or infarction present with pain. Fewer than 10% of patients will present with silent or pain-free myocardial infarctions, and these are usually in diabetic patients with autonomic neuropathy. Treatment with intravenous opioids (usually morphine) for control of the ischemic pain is a standard form of therapy, in addition to specific treatment for the underlying pathophysiology. Specific treatment (which will also provide analgesia by decreasing myocardial ischemia) includes nitrates, beta blocking agents, calcium antagonists, and revascularization either with thrombolytic agents, or by percutaneous angioplasty, or coronary artery bypass surgery. Morphine has been the opioid of choice for patients who continue to have chest pain during diagnostic and therapeutic procedures. It is the opioid of choice for the subset of patients with left ventricular (LV) dysfunction and pulmonary edema if vasodilation and hypotension do not predominate. However, if nausea and vomiting are significant side effects with the use of morphine, potent synthetic opioids such as fentanyl should be substituted, either by PCA or by infusion. Fentanyl is tolerated far better than morphine in hypotensive patients and patients with poor LV function. Epidural opioids have been used for the management of myocardial infarction with good success.[91] Thoracic epidural anesthesia with local anesthetic agents (TEA), in contrast to epidural opioids, has been an effective treatment in cases of myocardial ischemia refractory to conventional medical therapy. Initiation of TEA in patients with myocardial ischemia, which was refractory to therapy with beta blockers, calcium channel antagonists, nitrates, low-dose heparin and/or nitroglycerin infusion for greater than 24 hours, resulted in rapid relief of chest pain and reduced depression of ST segments.[90] Relief of ischemia is partly due to increased myocardial oxygen delivery via coronary artery vasodilation and decrease in myocardial oxygen demand through decrease in systemic blood pressure, heart rate, and pulmonary capillary wedge pressure.

H. NEUROSURGERY

Most patients undergoing major craniotomies or neurosurgical procedures do not have large analgesic requirements postoperatively, although a significant number will have headache and scalp tenderness. Due to the surgical procedure or preexisting disease, many patients have decreased levels of consciousness and therefore, in addition to having minimal analgesic requirements, they require ventilatory support. For patients with symptoms or signs of increased intracranial pressure, opioids are relatively contraindicated because of associated respiratory depression and hypercapnia, which augment an increase in intracranial pressure. Most of these patients are best managed with judicial use of benzodiazepines, barbiturates, and short-acting opioids such as fentanyl. Barbiturates and opioids are usually reserved for intubated, mechanically ventilated patients in whom carbon dioxide levels can be controlled directly.

I. CANCER PAIN

Patients with advanced cancer will present to the ICU for a variety of reasons, including acute infections, septic processes secondary to suppressed immunocompetence, and postoperative management of diagnostic or therapeutic procedures. The vast majority of these patients will have pain unrelated to the cancer or its therapy.[142] However, superimposed on the reason for the ICU admission will be the presence of chronic cancer-related pain that requires these patients to be managed differently from opioid-naive patients. Management of the pain that these patients experience in the ICU is complicated by the extreme tolerance to opioids that many of these patients develop over time and by associated psychological aspects related to the presence of a debilitating and possibly terminal disease. Thus, the opioid requirements may be markedly increased, and this should be recognized by the health-care team. In addition, if pain control becomes difficult with pharmacologic intervention alone, consideration should also be given to use of neural blockade, either on a temporary or more permanent basis, whether in the ICU or not. In certain cases, spinally administered opioids may give remarkable pain relief.

V. ANALGESIC OUTCOME STUDIES

There is intense interest in assessing the effect on outcome of potent analgesic regimens after major surgery and in critically ill patients. The effect of postoperative pain management on outcome after surgery and in critically ill patients has been reviewed by Kehlet,[143,144] Yeager,[145] and Carpenter.[146] Most work has been performed on patients undergoing major surgery, and the results probably apply to critically ill patients as well. Although effective analgesia with systemic opioids can reduce postoperative morbidity and mortality,[42,147] pain relief alone may be only partially responsible.[148] In addition, the use of systemic opioids to provide high-quality analgesia is often at the expense of ventilatory support due to the respiratory depression that ensues with the large systemic doses required.[42,147] Postoperative analgesia provided by PCA opioid treatment has no major effect on postoperative outcome.[149-152] The largest body of literature regarding outcome of the effects of analgesic regimens after surgery or in critically ill patients comes from randomized, prospective, controlled trials focusing primarily on epidural or spinal analgesic techniques and comparing them to standard systemic opioid administration.

Outcome studies are discussed under the following headings:

A. STRESS RESPONSE

The stress response after surgery and presumably after major nonsurgical trauma, etc., has profound effects on the cardiac, coagulation, and immune systems and is temporally associated with major morbidity. High-dose opioid anesthesia continued into the postoperative period attenuates the stress response.[153] Epidural administration of local anesthetics can suppress the stress response to procedures below the umbilicus,[12] whereas epidural opioids produce incomplete reductions in the stress response[154] and neither epidural opioids or local anesthetics can completely prevent the stress response from procedures performed above the umbilicus.[153] However, effective analgesia does not guarantee that activation of the stress response will be prevented,[155] since local trauma injury causes release of cytokines directly into the bloodstream, which activate the stress response. Thus, if high-dose opioid anesthesia and analgesia, or epidural analgesia with local anesthetic agents or opioids, are started in the intraoperative period, they should be continued in the postoperative period to maximally reduce the stress response. In contrast, the use of PCA intravenous (IV) opioid for postoperative analgesia provides reasonable relief of pain and yet has no effect on stress response. In addition, postoperative pain relief by PCA opioids has probably no major effect on postoperative outcome based upon four randomized trials.[149-152]

B. CARDIOVASCULAR SYSTEM

Cardiac morbidity is a primary cause of death after anesthesia and surgery and in patients admitted to ICU after cardiovascular surgical procedures. Although high-dose systemic opioid techniques[147,156] can reduce cardiac morbidity perioperatively in this patient population, there has been a great deal of interest in the use of epidural local anesthetics and opioids administered intraoperatively and postoperatively to attempt to influence cardiac morbidity and mortality. Thoracic epidural anesthesia using local anesthetics through an epidural

Table 38-5. Effect of epidural anesthesia and analgesia on postoperative adverse cardiac outcomes for randomized, prospective studies

Study	CHF		MI		Death	
	GA	Epid	GA	Epid	GA	Epid
Reiz, 1982	NR*	NR	3/20 (15%)	0/22 (0%)	5/22 (23%)	2/23 (9%)
Hjortso, 1985	NR	NR	NR	NR	3/50 (6%)	1/44 (2%)
Yeager, 1987	10/25 (40%)	1/28 (4%)	3/25 (12%)	0/28 (0%)	4/25 (16%)	0/28 (0%)
Tuman, 1991	4/40 (10%)	2/40 (5%)	3/40 (8%)	0/40 (0%)	0/40 (0%)	0/40 (0%)
Christopherson, 1993	NR	NR	2/51 (5%)	2/49 (4%)	1/51 (2%)	1/49 (2%)
TOTAL	**14/65 (21.5%)**	**3/68 (4.4%)**	**11/136 (8.1%)**	**2/139 (1.4%)**	**13/188 (6.9%)**	**4/184 (2.2%)**

From Carpenter RL: *ASA Refresher Course Outline* No. 135, 1994, American Society of Anesthesiologists.
*NR, Not reported. CHF = congestive heart failure; MI = myocardial infarction; GA = general anesthetic; Epid = epidural anesthetic.

catheter placed at an upper thoracic level has shown to be very effective as a treatment for patients with myocardial ischemia refractory to conventional medical therapy.[90] Lumbar epidural anesthesia does not offer the same degree of benefit as thoracic epidural anesthesia. Myocardial ischemia that occurs postoperatively is more frequent, more severe, and more prolonged than ischemia occurring during the preoperative and intraoperative periods and appears to be an important factor in the incidence of cardiac morbidity.[156] Several studies indicate that the use of postoperative epidural analgesia and anesthesia using anesthetic agents, and/or opioids, is associated with reduced postoperative cardiac morbidity and mortality (Table 38-5).

C. COAGULATION

Major surgery is associated with a hypercoagular state, which persists in the postoperative period. Although general anesthesia followed by postoperative IV opioid analgesia has little effect on vasoocclusive and thromboembolic events in the postoperative period, epidural anesthesia and analgesia in the perioperative period appear to reduce the incidence of thromboembolic events. This has been shown in patients undergoing revascularization of the lower extremity[10,157] and in patients undergoing total hip replacement as well.[158] It may be very important in postoperative patients that epidural anesthesia be instituted intraoperatively and not only utilized postoperatively.[157]

D. PULMONARY SYSTEM

Pulmonary function following thoracic or abdominal surgery and in other conditions such as multiple rib fractures or flail chest is markedly decreased. Postoperative epidural analgesia using local anesthetic agents or opioids, or especially both, has been shown to be consistently superior to conventional PCA opioid for preserving postoperative pulmonary function.[9,96] Diaphragmatic function, which may also be impaired after abdominal thoracic surgery, is not appreciably improved by parenteral or epidural administration of opioids alone. Thoracic epidural anesthesia with local anesthetic, however, may improve postoperative diaphragmatic function.[159,160] Also, patients receiving epidural anesthesia and analgesia with local anesthetic agents have shown a reduced incidence and severity of hypoxemia in the early postoperative period.[161] Patients receiving epidural anesthesia and analgesia using local anesthetic and/or opioid in the postoperative period have also demonstrated a decreased incidence of postoperative pneumonia, respiratory failure, and atelectasis.[10,162,163]

E. GASTROINTESTINAL SYSTEM

Postoperative ileus is a major cause of surgical morbidity, as is ileus occurring in critically ill patients. Postoperative thoracic epidural analgesia with local anesthetic agents has been associated with the early passage of flatus and earlier onset of bowel movements than with systemic opioid analgesia[164] or with epidural morphine.[164] Two further studies did not confirm these results.[165,166] However, both the latter studies administered epidural local anesthetic for only 24 hours and then continued with parenteral opioids. It is most probable that epidural local anesthetic agents should be administered until bowel function recovers (2 to 4 days after major surgery) so that the maximum benefit from the epidural local anesthesia can be derived.

Thus, it is well demonstrated that epidural analgesia can provide better pain relief than systemic opioids after many major surgical procedures or in critically ill patients. In addition, epidural analgesia appears to reduce morbidity and perhaps even mortality in some patient populations and can improve outcome in patients at risk for postoperative cardiac morbidity, thrombosis, pulmonary morbidity, or ileus. Epidural analgesia is particularly indicated in patients in high-risk groups undergoing major surgical procedures.[10,92,145] Local anesthetics appear to be more effective than opioids for attenuating many aspects of postoperative morbidity; the insertion of the epidural catheter in the thoracic interspace seems to provide potential advantages over lumbar insertion in many patients and may be indicated for patients at risk for postoperative cardiac pulmonary morbidity and those at risk for postoperative ileus. However, a lumbar insertion site may be more important for patients at risk for deep vein thrombosis on the lower extremities.

VI. VENTILATED PATIENTS

Many patients in an ICU setting will have endotracheal tubes in place, whether they are ventilated or not. Presence of the endotracheal tube prevents normal communication and is, in itself, pain provoking. Most of these patients are critically ill and require pharmacologic intervention to allow the presence of the endotracheal tube. A combination of opioids and benzodiazepines or other sedative agents is frequently required to maintain the presence of the endotracheal tube. Patients can use patient-controlled anxiolysis effectively,[167,168] and this implies that patients can distinguish between anxiety and pain. It is more satisfactory to use all modalities of pain control and sedation available, rather than instituting muscle relaxants to prevent agitation and increasing anxiety related to the use of the endotracheal tube. For example, in a study in which patients could not be adequately ventilated despite appropriate use of systemic opioids and benzodiazepines, the use of spinal opioids resulted in adequate analgesia and maintenance of mechanical ventilation without resorting to the use of muscle relaxants.[169]

VII. SEDATION IN THE ICU PATIENT

A. BENZODIAZEPINES

Intubated, ventilated patients frequently require some form of sedation and good analgesia therapy. The most commonly used sedative hypnotic agents in the intensive care environment are benzodiazepines (BNZs), since they offer a wide margin of safety from unwanted side effects. Benzodiazepines interact with their own receptors in the cortical and limbic forebrain areas and modulate the gamma aminobutyric acid (GABA) receptors in the neuro-1 inhibitory transmitter system to produce their effects. Depending on the dose, BNZs can produce effects ranging from light sedation to

Table 38-6. Intermittent and continuous intravenous administration of midazolam*

Severity of agitation	Loading dose (mg)	Infusion rate hour (mg)
Mild	1-2	2
Moderate	5	3-5
Severe	7-10	5-7

From Crippen DW: *Crit Care Clin* 6:369, 1990.
*Elderly patients start with low doses; surprisingly modest doses sometimes give dramatic effects. Titrate the initial dose to the amount of sedation required. If the first dose is not effective, repeat the same dose every 10 minutes until sedation is accomplished. If high doses must be given for serious agitation, be prepared to intubate or mask-bag ventilate.
Patients who continue to be restless or agitated after 15 minutes of constant infusion should be reloaded, then the infusion rate increased 100%. If this does not result in sedation, haloperidol or morphine sulphate should be added, and preparations should be made for paralysis and intubation. The upper limit should be guided by hemodynamic and respiratory side effects.
Infusions of 20 mg per hour and more have been used with safety. The infusion should be discontinued if it does not result in control of agitation within 1 hour, and paralysis or sedation should be considered. Patients who are oversedated should have their infusion rate decreased by 50%.

coma. They have very little effect on the autonomic nervous system, respiratory drive, or the cardiovascular system. Although BNZs are well absorbed from the gastrointestinal tract, they are poorly absorbed when given intramuscularly, and, therefore, only intravenous administration will be discussed for ICU sedation. Benzodiazepines are mostly metabolized in the liver by oxidative reduction, and the metabolites are excreted in the urine. Metabolism may be impaired in elderly patients, or in disease states such as cirrhosis, or by therapeutic agents that impair oxidizing capacity such as cimetidine.[170] The benzodiazepines available for IV use include diazepam, lorazepam, and midazolam. These agents are all very lipophilic and, when administered intravenously, have extremely rapid distribution half-lives of 1 to 3 min. These drugs therefore sedate and induce sleep very rapidly, with midazolam having the fastest onset of action.

1. Midazolam

Midazolam has an imidazole ring added to the benzodiazepine nucleus, which results in an increased ability to form salts, increasing its solubility in aqueous solution compared to other benzodiazepines. It is approximately three to four times more potent than diazepam and has a shorter elimination half-life of between 1.5 to 3.5 hours. The dosage of midazolam for intermittent or continuous IV use is shown in Table 38-6. Sedation after IV injection is achieved within 1 to 5 min, with the duration of action being less than 2 hours.

BOX 38-1   Risk/benefits of midazolam for sedation

Benefits

1. Midazolam is desirable for sedation when minimal respiratory depression is necessary.
2. A decreased adrenergic response to stress has been demonstrated.
3. The drug promotes good anxiolysis and antegrade amnesia; additive with the analgesic effects of morphine.
4. May be administered in boluses or titrated to effect in continuous infusion for longer-term sedation.
5. Detoxified in the liver, safe in renal failure.

Liabilities

1. Not an analgesic. Analgesia is additive with morphine but the CNS* depressive effect is also additive.
2. There is no particular advantage to continuous infusion of midazolam in patients who will be requiring nontitrated sedation for long periods, especially in intubated patients in whom respiratory depression is not an issue. No significant resistance or tolerance to the drug has been reported.
3. The combination of midazolam and fentanyl has been reported to cause respiratory depression and hypotension out of proportion to the action of either drug alone.
4. Effects can be difficult to predict in liver failure.

From Crippen DW: *Crit Care Clin* 6:369, 1990.
CNS, central nervous system.

Continuous titrated infusions of midazolam have been found to be safe and effective when compared to intermittent boluses of diazepam in postoperative cardiac surgery patients.[171] In a study comparing continuous infusions of midazolam and lorazepam, time to awakening in both groups averaged between 6 to 7 hours after discontinuation of the infusion.[172] In contrast to diazepam, absorption of intramuscular injections of midazolam is rapid and effective, the clinical effects being seen within 5 to 15 min and peak effects at 60 min postinjection with a duration of approximately 2 hours. For short-term sedation, these agents should be given by IV bolus and when required to sedate for a longer time period; for example, in ventilated patients, an IV bolus followed by a constant infusion is preferred (Box 38-1).

2. Diazepam-lorazepam

Diazepam and lorazepam both work in the same way as midazolam; thus, there is no advantage to changing from one agent to another when an inadequate response is seen. Diazepam has a much longer elimination half-life than midazolam (20 to 80 hours). Active metabolites (oxazepam, desmethyldiazepam) tend to accumulate, resulting in prolonged sedation after ad-

ministration has been discontinued. Therefore, it is not particularly suitable for continuous infusions. Lorazepam, which has an elimination half-life of 10 to 15 hours and is more potent than midazolam, can be used in smaller doses than midazolam. For short-term procedures, midazolam's rapid onset and offset may provide an advantage, whereas lorazepam is probably better suited for longer-term sedation.

B. PROPOFOL

Propofol (an alkylphenol) is a sedative hypnotic agent with several unique features and was first described as an anesthetic agent in the 1970s. Propofol is highly fat soluble and dissolves poorly in water. It is primarily a hypnotic agent used for the induction of general anesthesia with a very rapid onset and offset of effect. The distribution half-life ranges from 2 to 8 min and elimination half-life from 1 to 7 hours.[173,174] Propofol is extensively metabolized by the hepatic route to produce water-soluble glucuronide and sulfate conjugates, which are primarily excreted in the urine. Metabolism is rapid (less than one fifth of a bolus dose is recovered unchanged after 30 min). Clinically, the onset of a dose of propofol takes place in less than 1 min. Its most distinct advantage is that, during short- or long-term infusions, recovery is extremely rapid. In one study, even after more than 7 days of continuous infusion, patients could be weaned from mechanical ventilation within 1 hour of discontinuing the drug, and recovery was complete by 2 hours.[175] Other advantages include a decrease in intracranial pressure and a 30% to 40% decrease in intraocular pressure.[176-178] Since propofol is a phenol derivative and is insoluble in aqueous solutions, it is formulated in a solution that is basically 10% intralipid. There are no antimicrobial preservatives, so the agent must be used carefully to prevent iatrogenically inducing sepsis, especially with long-term use in critically ill patients. Large doses are associated with respiratory and cardiovascular depression, which may be exacerbated by the administration of other sedatives or opioids at the same time. Blood pressure may decrease by 25% to 40% and may be associated with decreases in cardiac output, stroke volume, and systemic vascular resistance.[179] Caution should be exercised in using propofol in hemodynamically unstable patients. Propofol has only been approved for administration to adults in the ICU setting. The outstanding pharmacokinetic profile and the apparent rapidity with which patients awaken, even after long-term infusions of propofol, offer unique advantages in the ICU. In our experience with using propofol infusions for postcardiac surgery patients, a major decrease in the length and duration of ICU stay and hospital stay has been achieved without any increase in mortality or morbidity to date.[140,141] Propofol will rapidly become an alternative to benzodiazepines and barbiturates (now uncommonly used) for sedation in the critically ill patient, particularly when it is widely available and less expensive.

VIII. CONCLUSION

An individualized, organized approach to pain management in the ICU can make a significant impact on patient comfort, and, with some techniques, there is evidence that an impact may be made on outcome measures as well. For critically ill patients to enjoy the full benefits of sophisticated pain management, anesthesiologists especially trained in pain management are required as a resource for the critical care team. Their knowledge of pharmacokinetics and the clinical pharmacology of sedative and analgesic agents, coupled with expertise in regional block procedures, prepares them for sophisticated aggressive pain management in the ICU. Much attention has centered on pain control to influence outcome; indeed, recent studies have emphasized a "rehabilitative" approach to postoperative care, including excellent pain control, improving nutritional status, and focusing on mental and physical activation. Data from Kehlet's group[144,180] show very promising results from this approach.

REFERENCES

1. Cousins MJ, Phillips GD, editors: *Acute pain management: clinics in critical care medicine,* New York, 1986, Churchill Livingstone.
2. Cousins M: Acute and postoperative pain. In Wall PD, Melzack R, editors: *The textbook of pain,* ed 2, Edinburgh, 1989, Churchill Livingstone.
3. Sandler AN, Stringer D, Panos L et al: A randomized, double-blind comparison of lumbar epidural and intravenous fentanyl infusions for post-thoracotomy pain relief: analgesic, pharmacokinetic and respiratory effects, *Anesthesiology* 77:626, 1992.
4. Donovan M, Dillon P, McGuire L: Incidence and characteristics of pain in a sample of medical-surgical inpatients, *Pain* 30:69, 1987.
5. Murray MJ: Pain problems in the ICU. In Hoyt JW, editor: Pain Management in the ICU, *Crit Care Clin* 6:235, 1990.
6. Hayden WR: Life and near-death in the intensive care unit: a personal experience, *Crit Care Clin* 10:651, 1994.
7. Modig J, Borg T, Kariström G et al: Thromboembolism after total hip replacement: role of epidural and general anesthesia, *Anesth Analg* 62:174, 1983.
8. Rawal N, Sjöstrand U, Christofferson E et al: Comparison of intramuscular and epidural morphine for postoperative analgesia in the grossly obese: influence on postoperative ambulation and pulmonary function, *Anesth Analg* 63:583, 1984.
9. Shulman M, Sandler AN, Bradley JW et al: Post-thoracotomy pain and pulmonary function following epidural and systemic morphine, *Anesthesiology* 61:569, 1984.
10. Tuman KJ, McCarthy RJ, March RJ et al: Effects of epidural anesthesia and analgesia on coagulation and outcome after major vascular surgery, *Anesth Analg* 73:696, 1991.
11. Kehlet H: Pain relief and modification of the stress response. In Cousins MJ, Phillips GD, editor: *Acute pain management: clinics in critical care medicine,* New York, 1986, Churchill Livingstone.
12. Kehlet H: The stress response to surgery: release mechanisms and the modifying effect of pain relief, *Acta Chir Scand* 550(suppl):22, 1988.
13. Nimmo WS, Duthie DJR: Pain relief after surgery, *Anaesth Intensive Care* 15:68, 1987.
14. Hansell HN: The behavioral effects of noise on man: the patient with "intensive care psychosis," *Heart Lung* 13:59, 1984.
15. Gracely RH: Methods of testing pain mechanisms in normal man. In Wall PD, Melzack R, editor: The *textbook of pain,* ed 2, Edinburgh, 1989, Churchill Livingstone.
16. Wolff BB: Behavioral measurement of human pain. In Sternbach RA, editor: *The psychology of pain,* New York, 1978, Raven Press.
17. Belanger E, Melzack R, Lauzon P: Pain of first-trimester abortion: a study of psychosocial and medical predictors, *Pain* 36:339, 1989.
18. Daley MD, Sandler AN, Turner KE et al: A comparison of epidural and intramuscular morphine in patients following cesarean section, *Anesthesiology* 72:289, 1990.
19. Choiniere M, Melzack R, Girard N et al: Comparisons between patients' and nurses' assessments of pain and medication efficacy in severe burn injuries, *Pain* 40:143, 1990.
20. Ekblom A, Hansson P: Pain intensity measurements in patients with acute pain receiving afferent stimulation, *J Neurol Neurosurg Psychiatr* 51:481, 1988.
21. Kremer E, Atkinson JH, Ignelzi RJ: Measurement of pain: patient preference does not confound pain measurement, *Pain* 10:241, 1981.
22. Ohnhaus EE, Adler R: Methodological problems in the measurement of pain: a comparison between the verbal rating scale and the visual analogue scale, *Pain* 1:379, 1975.
23. Stevens DS, Edwards WT: Management of pain in intensive care settings, *Anesth Clin North Am* 10:395, 1992.
24. Levine RE: Pharmacology of intravenous sedatives and opioids in critically ill patients. In Hansen-Flaschen J, editor: Improving patient tolerance of mechanical ventilation, *Crit Care Clin* 10:709, 1994.
25. Ball M, Moor RA, Fisher A et al: Renal failure and the use of morphine in intensive care, *Lancet* 1:784, 1985.
26. Bion JF, Logan BK, Neuman PM: Sedation in intensive care: morphine and renal function. *Intensive Care Med* 12:359, 1986.
27. Aitkenhead AR, Vater M, Achola K et al: Pharmacokinetics of single dose IV morphine in normal volunteers and patients with end-stage renal failure, *Br J Anaesth* 56:813, 1984.
28. Levy WJ, Shapiro HM, Maruchek G et al: Automated EEG processing for intraoperative monitoring: a comparison of techniques, *Anesthesiology* 53:223, 1980.
29. Veselis RA, Long CW, Shah NK et al: Increased EEG activity correlates with clinical sedation, *Crit Care Med* 16:383, 1988.
30. Sinclair ME, Sear JW, Summerfield RJ et al: Alfentanil infusions in the intensive therapy unit, *Intensive Care Med* 14:55, 1988.
31. Schwieger IM, Hall RI, Hug CC: Is lower esophageal contractility a reliable indicator of the adequacy of opioid anesthesia? *Anesthesiology* 69:A222, 1988.
32. Støen R, Sessler DI: Lower esophageal contractility does not predict movement during skin incision in patients anesthetized with alfentanil and nitrous oxide, *Anesthesiology* 69:A221, 1988.
33. Evans JM, Bithell JF, Vlachonikolis IC: Relationship between lower oesophageal contractility, clinical signs and halothane concentration during general anesthesia and surgery in man, *Br J Anaesth* 59:1346, 1987.
34. Austin KL, Stapleton JV, Mather LE: Relationship between blood meperidine concentrations and analgesic response: a preliminary report, *Anesthesiology* 53:466, 1980(a).
35. Lehmann KA: Patient-controlled intravenous analgesia for postoperative pain relief. In Max MB, Portensy RK, Larka EM et al, editors: *Advances in pain research and therapy,* vol 18:481, New York, 1991, Raven Press.
36. Mather LE, Glynn CJ: The minimum effective analgetic blood

concentration of pethidine in patients with intractable pain, *Br J Clin Pharmacol* 14:385, 1982.

37. Options to prevent and control postoperative pain. In Agency for Health Care Policy and Research: *Clinical practice guideline acute pain management: operative or medical procedures and trauma,* Pub. No. 92-0032, Rockville, Md, 1993, US Department of Health and Human Services Public Health Service.

38. Oden RV: Acute postoperative pain: incidence, severity, and the etiology of inadequate treatment. In Oden RV, editor: Management of postoperative pain, *Anesth Clin North Am* 7:1, 1989.

39. Stanski DR, Watkins DW: Drug disposition in anesthesia, New York, 1982, Grune and Stratton.

40. Edwards WT: Optimizing opioid treatment of postoperative pain, *J Pain Symp Management* 5:S24, 1990(a).

41. Hoffman P: Continuous infusions of fentanyl and alfentanil in intensive care, *Eur J Anaesthesiol* (suppl)1:71, 1987.

42. Mangano DT, Siliciano D, Hollenberg M et al: Postoperative myocardial ischemia: therapeutic trials using intensive analgesia following surgery, *Anesthesiology* 76:342, 1992.

43. Cohen AT, Kelly DR: Assessment of alfentanil by intravenous infusion as long-term sedation in intensive care, *Anaesthesia* 42:545, 1987.

44. Sinclair ME, Siter PM: Detection of overdosage of sedation in a patient with renal failure by the absence of lower oesophageal motility, *Intensive Care Med* 14:69, 1988.

45. Shafer SL, Varvel JR: Pharmacokinetics, pharmacodynamics, and rational opioid selection, *Anesthesiology* 74:53, 1991.

46. Gibaldi M: *Biopharmaceutics and clinical pharmacokinetics,* Philadelphia, 1984, Lea and Febiger.

47. Shand BG, Desjardins RE, Bjornsson TD et al: The method of separate exponentials: a simple aid to devising intravenous drug-loading regimens, *Clin Pharmacol Ther* 29:542, 1981.

48. Edwards WT, Breed RJ: The treatment of acute postoperative pain in the post-anesthesia care unit, *Anesth Clin North Am* 8:235, 1990(b).

49. Austin KL, Stapleton JV, Mather LE: Multiple intramuscular injections: a major source of variability in analgesic response to meperidine, *Pain* 8:47, 1980(b).

50. Tamsen A, Hartvig P, Fagerlund C et al: Patient controlled analgesic therapy. Part II. Individual analgesic demand and analgesic plasma concentrations of pethidine in postoperative pain, *Clin Pharmacokinet* 7:164, 1982.

51. Ferrante FM: Patient-controlled analgesia, *Anesth Clin North Am* 10:287, 1992.

52. Sandler AN: Clinical pharmacology and applications of spinal opioids. In Bowdle TA, Horita A, Kharasch ED, editors: *The pharmacologic basis of anesthesiology,* New York, 1994, Churchill Livingstone.

53. Ferrante FM, Orav EJ, Rocco AG et al: A statistical model for pain in patient-controlled analgesia and conventional intramuscular opioid regimens, *Anesth Analg* 67:457, 1988.

54. Etches RC: Respiratory depression associated with patient-controlled analgesia: a review of eight cases, *Can J Anaesth* 41:125, 1994.

55. Sandler AN, Baxter AD, Katz J et al: A double-blind, placebo-controlled trial of transdermal fentanyl after abdominal hysterectomy: analgesic, respiratory and pharmacokinetic effects, *Anesthesiology* 81:1169, 1994.

56. Cousins MJ, Cherry DA, Gourlay GK: Acute and chronic pain: use of spinal opioids. In Cousins MJ, Bridenbaugh PO, editors: *Neural blockade in clinical anesthesia and management of pain,* ed 2, Philadelphia, 1988, JB Lippincott.

57. Niemi L, Pitkanen MT, Tuominen MK et al: Comparison of intrathecal fentanyl infusion with intrathecal morphine infusion or bolus for postoperative pain relief after hip arthroplasty, *Anesth Analg* 77:126, 1993.

58. Sethna NF, Berde CB: Continuous subarachnoid analgesia in two adolescents with severe scoliosis and impaired pulmonary function, *Reg Anesth* 16:333, 1991.

59. Stoelting RK: Intrathecal morphine—an underused combination for postoperative pain management, *Anesth Analg* 68:707, 1989.

60. Kirson LE, Goldman JM, Slover RB: Low-dose intrathecal morphine for postoperative pain control in patients undergoing transurethral resection of the prostate, *Anesthesiology* 71:192, 1989.

61. Katz J, Nelson W: Intrathecal morphine for postoperative pain relief, *Reg Anesth* 61:1, 1981.

62. Shroff AB, Bishop AB: Intrathecal morphine analgesia speeds extubation and shortens ICU stay following coronary artery bypass grafting (CABG), *Anesthesiology* 81:A129, 1994.

63. LaMotte C, Pert CB, Snyder SH: Opiate receptor binding in primate spinal cord: distribution and changes after dorsal root section, *Brain Res* 112:407, 1976.

64. McQuay HJ, Sullivan AF, Smallman K et al: Intrathecal opioids, potency and lipophilicity, *Pain* 36:111, 1989.

65. Ready LB, Oden R, Chadwick HS et al: Development of an anesthesiology-based postoperative pain management service, *Anesthesiology* 68:100, 1988.

66. Salomaki TE, Laiteninen JO, Nuutinen LS: A randomized double-blind comparison of epidural versus intravenous fentanyl infusion after thoracotomy, *Anesthesiology* 75:790, 1991.

67. Grant GJ, Zakowski MI, Ramanathan S et al: Thoracic versus lumbar epidural morphine for post-thoracotomy analgesia, *Reg Anesth* 18:351, 1993.

68. Fromme GA, Steidl LJ, Danielson DR: Comparison of lumbar and thoracic epidural morphine for relief of post-thoracotomy pain, *Anesth Analg* 64:454, 1985.

69. Brodsky JB, Kretzschmar KM, Mark JBD: Caudal epidural morphine for post-thoracotomy pain, *Anesth Analg* 67(4):409, 1988.

70. Grant RP, Dolman JF, Harper JA et al: Patient-controlled lumbar epidural fentanyl compared with patient-controlled intravenous fentanyl for postthoracotomy pain, *Can J Anaesth* 39:214, 1992.

71. Coda BA, Brown MC, Schaffer R et al: Pharmacology of epidural fentanyl, alfentanil, and sufentanil in volunteers, *Anesthesiology* 81:1149, 1994.

72. El-Baz NMI, Faber LP, Jensik RJ: Continuous epidural infusion of morphine for treatment of pain after thoracic surgery—a new technique, *Anesth Analg* 63:757, 1984.

73. Rauck RL, Raj PP, Knarr DC et al: Comparison of the efficacy of epidural morphine given by intermittent injection or continuous infusion for the management of postoperative pain, *Reg Anesth* 19:316, 1994.

74. Dyer RA, Anderson BJ, Mitchell WL et al: Postoperative pain control with a continuous infusion of epidural sufentanil in the intensive care unit: a comparison with epidural morphine, *Anesth Analg* 71:130, 1990.

75. Mackersie RC, Shackford SR, Hoyt DB et al: Continuous epidural fentanyl analgesia: ventilatory function improvement with routine use in treatment of blunt chest injury, *J Trauma* 27:1207, 1987.

76. Ellis DJ, Millar WL, Reisner LS: A randomized double-blind comparison of epidural versus intravenous fentanyl infusion for analgesia after cesarean section, *Anesthesiology* 72:981, 1990.

77. Glass PSA, Estok P, Ginsberg B et al: Use of patient-controlled analgesia to compare the efficacy of epidural to intravenous fentanyl administration, *Anesth Analg* 74:345, 1992.

78. Geller E, Chrubasik J, Graf R et al: A randomized double-blind comparison of epidural sufentanil or epidural fentanyl analgesia after major abdominal surgery, *Anesth Analg* 76:1243, 1993.

79. Camu F, Debucquoy F: Alfentanil infusion for postoperative

pain: a comparison of epidural and intravenous routes, *Anesthesiology* 75:171, 1991.

80. Henderson SK, Cohen C: Nalbuphine augmentation of analgesia and reversal of side effects following epidural hydromorphone, *Anesthesiology* 65:216, 1986.

81. Baxter AD, Samson B, Penning J et al: Prevention of epidural morphine-induced respiratory depression with intravenous nalbuphine infusion in post-thoracotomy patients, *Can J Anaesth* 36:503, 1989.

82. Etches RC, Sandler AN, Daley MD: Respiratory depression and spinal opioids, *Can J Anaesth* 36:165, 1989.

83. Ready LB, Loper KA, Nessly M et al: Postoperative epidural morphine is safe on surgical wards, *Anesthesiology* 75:452, 1991.

84. Miller RR: Analgesics. In Miller RR, Greenblatt DJ, editors: *Drug effects in hospitalized patients,* New York, 1976, John Wiley and Sons.

85. Whiting WC, Sandler AN, Lau LC, et al: Analgesic and respiratory effects of epidural sufentanil in patients following thoracotomy, *Anesthesiology* 69:36, 1988.

86. Ready LB, Edwards WT: Postoperative care following intrathecal or epidural opioids. II *Anesthesiology* 72:213, 1990 (letter to the editor).

87. Stevens DS, Edwards WT: Management of pain in mechanically ventilated patients. In Hansen-Flaschen J, editor: Improving patient tolerance of mechanical ventilation, *Crit Care Clin* 10:767, 1994.

88. Conacher ID, Paes ML, Jacobson L et al: Epidural analgesia following thoracic surgery: a review of two year's experience, *Anaesthesia* 38:546, 1983.

89. Griffiths DPG, Diamond AW, Cameron JD: Postoperative extradural analgesia following thoracic surgery: a feasibility study, *Br J Anaesth* 47:48, 1975.

90. Blomberg S, Emanuelsson H, Ricksten S: Thoracic epidural anesthesia and central hemodynamics in patients with unstable angina pectoris, *Anesth Analg* 69:558, 1989.

91. Toft P, Jorgensen A: Continuous thoracic epidural analgesia for the control of pain in myocardial infarction, *Intensive Care Med* 13:388, 1987.

92. Reiz S, Balfors E, Sorenson M et al: Coronary hemodynamic effects of general anesthesia and surgery: modification by epidural analgesia in patients with ischemic heart disease, *Reg Anesth* 7(suppl):8, 1982.

93. Blomberg S, Emanuelsson H, Kvist H et al: Effects of thoracic epidural anesthesia on coronary arteries and arterioles in patients with coronary artery disease, *Anesthesiology* 73:840, 1990.

94. Davis R, DeBoer LWV, Maroko PR: Thoracic epidural analgesia reduces myocardial infarct size after coronary artery occlusion in dogs, *Anesth Analg* 65:711, 1986.

95. Badner NH, Komar WE: 0.125% bupivacaine—the optimum concentration for postoperative epidural fentanyl: analgesic effects, *Can J Anaesth* 39:A71, 1992.

96. Dahl JB, Rosenberg J, Hansen BL et al: Differential analgesia effects of low-dose epidural morphine and morphine bupivacaine at rest and during mobilization after major abdominal surgery, *Anesth Analg* 74:362, 1992.

97. George KA, Wright PMC, Chisakuta A: Continuous thoracic epidural fentanyl for post-thoracotomy pain relief: with or without bupivacaine? *Anaesthesia* 46:732, 1991.

98. Kavanagh BP, Katz J, Sandler AN: Pain control after thoracic surgery: a review of current techniques, *Anesthesiology* 81:737, 1994.

99. Swann DG, Armstrong PJ, Douglas E et al: The alkalinisation of bupivacaine for intercostal nerve blockade, *Anaesthesia* 46:174, 1991.

100. Gibbons J, James O, Quail A: Relief of pain in chest injury, *Br J Anaesth* 45:1136, 1973.

101. Bergh NP, Dottori O, Lof BA et al: Effect of intercostal block on lung function after thoracotomy, *Acta Anaesthesiol Scand* 23:85, 1966.

102. Chan VWS, Chung F, Cheng DCH et al: Analgesic and pulmonary effects of continuous intercostal nerve block following thoracotomy, *Can J Anaesth* 38:733, 1991.

103. Sabanathan S, Mearns AJ, Bickford Smith PJ et al: Efficacy of continuous extrapleural intercostal nerve block on post-thoracotomy pain and pulmonary mechanics, *Br J Surg* 77:221, 1990.

104. Moore DC: Intercostal nerve block for postoperative somatic pain following surgery of the thorax and upper abdomen, *Br J Anaesth* 47(suppl):284, 1975.

105. Safran D, Kuhlman G, Orhant EE et al: Continuous intercostal blockade with lidocaine after thoracic surgery: clinical and pharmacokinetic study, *Anesth Analg* 70:345, 1990.

106. Eason MJ, Wyatt R: Paravertebral thoracic block: a reappraisal, *Anaesthesia* 34:638, 1979.

107. Conacher ID, Kokri M: Postoperative paravertebral blocks for thoracic surgery: a radiological appraisal, *Br J Anaesth* 59:155, 1987.

108. Reiestad F, Stromskag KE: Interpleural catheter in the management of postoperative pain: a preliminary report, *Reg Anesth* 11:89, 1986.

109. Kvalheim L, Reiestad F: Interpleural catheter in the management of postoperative pain, *Anesthesiology* 61:A231, 1984.

110. Rosenberg PH, Schenin BMA, Lepantalo MJA et al: Continuous interpleural infusion of bupivacaine for analgesia after thoracotomy, *Anesthesiology* 67:811, 1987.

111. Tartiere J, Delassus P, Sillard B et al: Intrapleural bupivacaine analgesia after thoraco-abdominal incision for esophagectomy, *Anesthesiology* 71:A664, 1989.

112. Rocco A, Reiestad F, Gudman J et al: Interpleural administration of local anaesthetics for pain relief in patients with multiple rib fractures: preliminary report, *Reg Anesth* 12:10, 1987.

113. Symreng T, Gomez MN, Rossi N: Intrapleural bupivacaine vs. saline after thoracotomy—effects on pain and lung function: a double-blind study, *J Cardiothorac Anesth* 3:144, 1989.

114. Sada T, Kobayashi T, Murakami S: Continuous axillary brachial plexus block, *Can Anaesth Soc J* 30:201, 1983.

115. Rung GW, Marshall WK: Nerve blocks in the critical care environment, *Crit Care Clin* 6:343, 1990.

116. Hord AH, Robertson JR, Thompson WF et al: Evaluation of continuous femoral nerve analgesia after primary total knee arthroplasty, *Anesth Analg* 70:S164, 1990.

117. Edwards ND, Wright EM: Continuous low-dose 3-in-1 nerve blockade for postoperative pain relief after total knee replacement, *Anesth Analg* 75:265, 1992.

118. Winnie AP, Ramamurthy S, Durrani Z: The inguinal paravascular technic of lumbar plexus anesthesia: the "3-in-1 block," *Anesth Analg* 52:989, 1973.

119. Moncada S, Vane JR: Arachidonic acid metabolites and the interactions between platelets and blood-vessel walls, *N Engl J Med* 300(20):1142, 1979.

120. Trang LE: Prostaglandins and inflammation, *Semin Arthritis Rheum* 9:153, 1980.

121. Carmichael J, Shankel SW: Effects of nonsteroidal anti-inflammatory drugs on prostaglandin and renal function, *Am J Med* 78:992, 1985.

122. Dahl JB, Kehlet H: Non-steroidal anti-inflammatory drugs: rationale for use in severe postoperative pain, *Br J Anaesth* 66:703, 1991.

123. Anonymous: Postoperative pain relief and non-opioid analgesics. *Lancet* 337:524-6, 1991 (editorial).

124. Pavy T, Medley C, Murphy DF: Effect of indomethacin on pain relief after thoracotomy, *Br J Anaesth* 65:624, 1990.

125. Reasbeck PG, Rice ML, Reasbeck JC: Double-blind controlled trial of indomethacin as an adjunct to narcotic analgesia after major abdominal surgery, *Lancet* 2(8290):115, 1982.

126. Yee JP, Koshiver JE, Allbon C et al: Comparison of intramuscular ketorolac tromethamine and morphine sulfate for analgesia of pain after major surgery, *Pharmacotherapy* 6:253, 1986.

127. Gillies GWA, Kenny GNC, Bullingham RES et al: The morphine sparing effect of ketorolac tromethamine: a study of new, parenteral non-steroidal anti-inflammatory agent after abdominal surgery, *Anaesthesia* 42:727, 1987.

128. Rubin P, Yee JP, Murthy VS et al: Ketorolac tromethamine (KT) analgesia: no postoperative respiratory depression and less constipation, *Clin Pharmacol Ther* 41:182, 1987.

129. Conrad KA, Fagan TC, Mackie MJ, et al: Effects of ketorolac tromethamine on hemostasis in volunteers, *Clin Pharmacol Ther* 43:542, 1988.

130. Avery EE, Morch ET, Benson DW: Critically crushed chests, *J Thoracic Surg* 32:291, 1956.

131. Shackford SR, Smith DE, Zarins CK et al: The management of flail chest—a comparison of ventilatory treatment and nonventilatory treatment, *Am J Surg* 132:759, 1976.

132. Trinkle JK, Richardson JD, Franz JL et al: Management of flail chest without mechanical ventilation, *Ann Thorac Surg* 19:355, 1975.

133. Pedersen VM, Schulze S, Hoier-Madsen K et al: Air-flow meter assessment of the effect of intercostal nerve blockade on respiratory function in rib fractures, *Act Chir Scand* 149:119, 1983.

134. Ullman DA, Fortune JB, Greenhouse BB et al: The treatment of patients with rib fractures using continuous thoracic epidural narcotic infusion, *Reg Anesth* 14:43, 1989.

135. Dittman M, Keller R, Wolff G: A rationale for epidural analgesia in the treatment of multiple rib fractures, *Intensive Care Med* 4:193, 1978.

136. Rankin AP, Comber RE: Management of fifty cases of chest injury with a regimen of epidural bupivacaine and morphine, *Anesth Intensive Care* 12:311, 1984.

137. Cheng D, De Majo W, Sandler AN: Anesthesia for lung transplantation, *Anesth Clin North Am* 12:749, 1994(c).

138. Searle NR, Roy M, Bergeron G et al: Hydromorphone patient-controlled analgesia (PCA) after coronary artery bypass surgery, *Can J Anaesth* 41:1, 1994.

139. Vanstrum GS, Bjornson KM, Ilko R: Postoperative effects of intrathecal morphine in coronary artery bypass surgery, *Anesth Analg* 67:261, 1988.

140. Cheng DCH, Karski J, Peniston C et al: A prospective, randomized controlled trial of early versus conventional tracheal extubation following coronary artery bypass graft (CABG) surgery: postoperative myocardial ischemia and infarction, *Can J Anaesth* 41:A48-B, 1994(a).

141. Cheng DCH, Karski J, Peniston C et al: A prospective, randomized controlled trial of early versus conventional tracheal extubation following coronary artery bypass graft (CABG) surgery: postoperative complications and hospital discharge, *Can J Anaesth* 41:A49-A, 1994(b).

142. Foley KM. Pain syndromes in patients with cancer. In Bonica JJ, Ventafridda V, editors: *Advances in pain research and therapy,* vol 2, New York, 1979, Raven Press.

143. Kehlet H: Postoperative pain relief: a look from the other side, *Reg Anesth* 19:369, 1994(a).

144. Kehlet H: Effect of postoperative pain on surgical outcome. In Stanley TH, Ashburn MA, editors: *Anesthesiology and pain management,* Boston, 1994, Kluwer Academic Publishers.

145. Yeager MP: The role of regional anesthesia in improving surgical outcome: IARS review course lectures, *Anesth Analg* (suppl):122, 1991.

146. Carpenter R: Does outcome change with pain management? *ASA Annual Refresher Course Lectures,* vol 135, Boston, 1994.

147. Anand KJ, Hickey PR: Halothane-morphine compared with high-dose sufentanil for anesthesia and postoperative analgesia in neonatal cardiac surgery, *N Engl J Med* 326:1, 1992.

148. Schulze S, Roikjaer O, Hasselstrom L et al: Epidural bupivacaine and morphine plus systemic indomethacin eliminates pain but not systemic response and convalescence after cholecystectomy, *Surgery* 103:321, 1988.

149. Egbert AM, Parks LH, Short LM et al: Randomized trial of postoperative patient-controlled analgesia vs intramuscular narcotics in frail elderly men, *Arch Intern Med* 150:1897, 1990.

150. Jackson D: A study of pain management: patient-controlled analgesia versus intramuscular analgesia, *J Intraven Nurs* 12:42, 1989.

151. Kenady DE, Wilson JF, Schwartz RW et al: A randomized comparison of patient-controlled versus standard analgesic requirements in patients undergoing cholecystectomy, *Surg Gynecol Obstet* 154:1495, 1992.

152. Wasylak TJ, Abbott FV, English MJ et al: Reduction of postoperative morbidity following patient-controlled morphine, *Can J Anaesth* 37:726, 1990.

153. Weissman C, Hollinger I: Modifying systemic responses with anesthetic responses, *Anesth Clin North Am* 6:221, 1988.

154. Breslow MJ, Parker SD, Frank SM et al: Determinants of catecholamine and cortisol responses to lower extremity revascularization, *Anesthesiology* 79:1202, 1993.

155. Naito Y, Tamai S, Shingu K et al: Responses of plasma adrenocorticotropic hormone, cortisol, and cytokines during and after upper abdominal surgery, *Anesthesiology* 77:426, 1992.

156. Mangano DT, Browner WS, Hollenberg M et al: Association of perioperative myocardial ischemia with cardiac morbidity and mortality in men undergoing noncardiac surgery, *N Engl J Med* 323:1781, 1990.

157. Christopherson R, Beattie C, Frank SM et al: Perioperative morbidity in patients randomized to epidural or general anesthesia for lower extremity vascular surgery, *Anesthesiology* 79:422, 1993.

158. Modig J, Maripuu E, Sahlstedt B: Thromboembolism following total hip replacement: A prospective investigation of 94 patients with emphasis on the efficacy of lumbar epidural anesthesia in prophylaxis, *Reg Anesth* 11:72, 1986.

159. Pansard JL, Mankikian B, Bertrand M et al: Effects of thoracic extradural block on diaphragmatic electrical activity and contractility after upper abdominal surgery, *Anesthesiology* 78:63, 1993.

160. Frataci MD, Kimball WR, Wain JC et al: Diaphragmatic shortening after thoracic surgery in humans, *Anesthesiology* 79:654, 1993.

161. Sydow FW: The influence of anesthesia and postoperative analgesic management on lung function, *Acta Chir Scand* 550(suppl):159, 1988.

162. Yeager MP, Glass DD, Neff RK et al: Epidural anesthesia and analgesia in high-risk surgical patients, *Anesthesiology* 66:729, 1987.

163. Hasenbos M, Van Egmond J, Gielen M et al: Postoperative analgesia by high thoracic epidural versus intramuscular nicomorphine after thoracotomy. Part III. The effects of pre- and postoperative analgesia on morbidity, *Acta Anaesthesiol Scand* 31:608, 1987.

164. Scheinen B, Asantila R, Orko R: The effect of bupivacaine and morphine on pain and bowel function after colonic surgery, *Acta Anaesthesiol Scand* 31:161, 1987.

165. Wallin G, Cassuto J, Hogstrom S et al: Failure of epidural anesthesia to prevent postoperative ileus, *Anesthesiology* 65:292, 1986.

166. Hjortso NC, Neumann P, Frosig F et al: A controlled study on the effects of epidural analgesia with local anaesthetics and morphine on morbidity after abdominal surgery, *Acta Anaesthesiol Scand* 29:790, 1985.

167. Galletly DC, Short TG, Forrest P: Patient-administered anxiolysis — a pilot study. *Anaesth Intensive Care* 17:144, 1989.

168. Loper KA, Ready LB, Brody M: Patient-controlled anxiolysis with midazolam, *Anesth Analg* 67:1118, 1988.

169. Rawal N, Tandon B: Epidural and intrathecal morphine in intensive care units, *Intensive Care Med* 11:129, 1985.

170. Reves JG, Fragen RJ, Vinik HR et al: Midazolam: pharmacology and uses, *Anesthesiology* 62:310, 1985.

171. Barvais L, Dejonckheere M, Dernovoi B et al: Continuous infusion of midazolam or bolus of diazepam for postoperative sedation of cardiac surgical patients, *Acta Anaesthesiol Belg* 39:239, 1988.

172. Pohlman AS, Simpson KS, Hall JB: Continuous intravenous infusions of lorazepam versus midazolam for sedation during mechanical ventilatory support: a prospective, randomized study, *Crit Care Med* 22(8):1241, 1994.

173. Adam HK, Briggs LP, Bahar M et al: Pharmacokinetic evaluation of ICI 35 868 in man: single induction doses with different rates of injection, *Br J Anaesth* 55:97, 1983.

174. McMurray TL, Collier PS, Carson IW et al: Propofol sedation after open heart surgery: a clinical and pharmacokinetic study, *Anaesthesia* 45:322, 1990.

175. Carrasco G, Molina R, Costa J et al: Propofol vs. midazolam in short-, medium-, and long-term sedation of critically ill patients: a cost-benefit analysis, *Chest* 103:557, 1993.

176. Herregods L, Verberke J, Rolly G et al: Effects of propofol on elevated intracranial pressure: preliminary results, *Anaesthesia* 43:S107, 1988.

177. Mirakhur RK, Shepherd WFI, Darrah WC: Propofol or thiopentone: effects on intraocular pressure associated with induction of anaesthesia and tracheal intubation (facilitated with suxamethonium), *Br J Anaesth* 59:431, 1987.

178. Vandesteene A, Tempont V, Engelman E et al: Effect of propofol on cerebral blood flow and metabolism in man, *Anaesthesia* 43:S42, 1988.

179. Grounds RM, Twigley AJ, Carli F et al: The haemodynamic effects of thiopentone and propofol, *Anaesthesia* 40:735, 1985.

180. Moiniche S, Hansen BL, Christensen S-E et al: Activity of patients and duration of hospitalization following hip replacement with balanced treatment of pain and early mobilization, *Ugeskr Laeger* 154:1495, 1992.

Chapter 39

EXTUBATION AND CHANGING ENDOTRACHEAL TUBES

Richard M. Cooper

I. INTRODUCTION

Management of tracheal intubation is a major focus of interest for the anesthesiologist. Textbooks, clinical reviews, and conferences addressing airway management consistently ignore strategies for removing or replacing endotracheal tubes. The ASA Task Force on Management of the Difficult Airway[1] recommended that each anesthesiologist have a preformulated strategy for extubation of the difficult airway, which includes the relative merits of awake extubation, factors that might result in an adverse impact on ventilation after extubation, an airway management plan for dealing with hypoventilation after extubation, and consideration of the placement of an intubation guide before extubation. Yet there is little, apart from anecdotal reports, to guide clinical decision making.

This chapter will attempt to identify complications that may attend extubation of the "routine" airway. These include both the common and uncommon problems, which may not be anticipated but for which we must be prepared. Of particular importance and, to this author's knowledge never previously reviewed, is the identification of patients at "high risk" at the time of extubation or tube exchange. Because this information is largely based on small clinical series or case reports, the appropriate weighting of each entity is a matter of judgment and may be influenced by specific surgical and anesthetic techniques at particular institutions. To the extent that the problems identified are seen as relevant to the reader's clinical practice, specific strategies can be used to minimize risks at extubation.

A number of strategies have been reported, and these will be reviewed in detail. This material is again derived from limited, uncontrolled trials or information supplied by manufacturers. It is this author's contention that these techniques should nonetheless be seriously considered. However, criteria for evaluation must establish that the *potential* benefits exceed the probable risks. Potential benefits might include maintained airway access even after extubation, the possibility of reintubation even if glottic visualization is not feasible, and the opportunity to administer oxygen by insufflation or positive-pressure ventilation while reintubation is progressing. The potential risks include discomfort, dislodgment, tracheal aspiration, ineffectiveness as a tracheal "stylet", and trauma.

II. THE CONCEPT OF FAILED EXTUBATIONS (OR REQUIRED REINTUBATIONS)

A failed extubation occurs when the intention to remove an endotracheal tube is thwarted. There is no agreed on time frame, therefore the reported incidence may vary widely. It is reasonable to consider the failed extubation in two separate clinical settings: the intensive care unit (ICU) and the operating room (OR) or postanesthesia care unit (PACU).

For ICU patients, the ability to predict a successful extubation is so inexact that there are a host of criteria to forecast success.[2-5] To minimize the risks, discomfort, and expense of prolonged intubation, a "trial of extubation" is often attempted and not infrequently followed by reintubation.[2,4] The incidence of reintubation is in the order of 6% to 25%,[2] but apart from the time frame, the incidence will also depend on the clinical mix, critical acuity, and threshold levels for extubation. Compared with routine, postoperative patients, ICU patients are more likely to have extubation fail because neurologic obtundation may leave them unable to protect their airways. In addition, debilitation and impaired mucociliary clearance may interfere with pulmonary toilet, and altered pulmonary mechanics, increased dead space, and venous admixture may result in hypercapnic or hypoxemic respiratory failure.

Among patients admitted to the PACU, retrospective studies involving a wide case-mix of postsurgical patients have identified an incidence of reintubation of 0.17% of 10,060[6] and 0.19% of 13,593 patients.[7] A recent prospective study involving 24,157 patients revealed a reintubation rate of 0.09%.[8] Reintubation is more commonly required after selected surgical procedures, such as panendoscopy,[6] and a variety of head and neck procedures.[9-12] Postoperative reintubation, although infrequent, may represent a considerable challenge for the anesthesiologist. Anatomic distortion may conspire with physiologic instability to convert a previously easily managed airway to a disaster. As well, a difficult airway, adequately managed during a controlled induction in the OR with a patient in good position, is completely different from the difficult airway in an agitated, hypoxemic, and hypotensive patient in poor position.

III. ROUTINE EXTUBATION: COMPLICATIONS AND MANAGEMENT

The complications of "routine extubation" have recently been reviewed by Miller et al[13] and Hartley and Vaughan.[14] They are summarized in Box 39-1.

A. ACCIDENTAL OR SELF-EXTUBATION (UNINTENTIONAL EXTUBATION)

Accidental extubations may result from movement of the patient with an inadequately secured endotracheal tube. Intraoperatively, although rare, this may occur when the patient is placed in the prone position, when the airway is shared with the surgeon, or draping obscures the line of sight. Tape securing the endotracheal tube may become loosened by secretions or surgical scrub solutions. Endotracheal tubes may be inadequately supported and inadvertently removed by drag on the equipment.

Self-extubations may be either deliberate or accidental. The patient may become agitated on emergence from general anesthesia or confused in the critical care setting. In the ICU setting 11% to 12% of extubations were self-inflicted.[15,16] Approximately 70% of the self-extubations were believed to be deliberate. In one study,[16] these patients were somewhat older and more likely to have chronic respiratory failure. In one study,[16] most of the patients (74%) required reintubation within 30 minutes, whereas in another study,[15] only 11% required reintubation. Reintubation was associated with one death.[16]

Surprisingly, one study, in the critical care setting, comparing four different methods of securing the endotracheal tube found no differences in tube movement.[17] Nevertheless, whenever the patient's position is altered, it is essential that the patient and tube be moved as a unit, providing adequate support for both. Flexible swivel connectors and circuit brackets or supports may be helpful in this regard.

B. ENDOTRACHEAL TUBE ENTRAPMENT (FIXATION OF ENDOTRACHEAL TUBE)

The endotracheal tube may also become entrapped owing to an inability to deflate the cuff[18-20] or cuff adherence to the tracheal wall. Crimping, kinking,[20] or separation of the pilot tube[21,22] may also prevent cuff deflation. Reused red rubber endotracheal tubes were more likely to be associated with failure to deflate. Recently, difficulties have been reported aspirating saline from the distal cuff of Laser Flex (Mallinckrodt Anesthesia Products, St. Louis, Missouri) tracheal tubes.[23,24] In one case, forceful extubation ruptured a cystic laryngeal mass.[23] In another report, the saline was aspirated from the cuff by use of an anterior commissure laryngoscope.[24]

Fixation of the endotracheal tube by Kirschner wires,[25] screws,[26] ligatures,[27,28] or entanglement with other devices[29,30] has also been described. Entrapment can also occur during the performance of a percutaneous tracheostomy if blind passage of a guidewire skewers the endotracheal tube.[31,32] Perforation of the tube can result in an airway leak with loss of ventilation or lightening of the depth of anesthesia. Fixation of the tube can cause trauma during forceful attempts at extubation. Mechanical obstruction of such a tube, which cannot be removed, is a life-threatening complication. Lang et al.[26] have recommended routine intraoperative testing for tracheal tube movement when fixation devices are used in proximity to the airway. Uncertainty about tube movement should prompt fiberoptic examination before emergence from general anesthesia. As well, partial transsection of the endotracheal tube by an osteotome during a maxillary osteotomy resulted in the partially cut tube, forming a "barb" that caught on the posterior aspect of the hard palate.[33] Only one of these reports had fatal consequences. This involved a Carlens tube that was inadvertently sutured to the pulmonary artery. Extubation resulted in circulatory collapse. The authors of almost all these reports recommended that when difficulties withdrawing an endotracheal tube are encountered, fiberoptic bronchoscopy should be used in an effort to determine the cause.

C. HEMODYNAMIC CHANGES

Extubation is accompanied by transient hypertension and tachycardia in most adults. Although these responses may be attenuated by concurrent medication, most healthy patients not taking antihypertensive medication or other cardioactive drugs exhibit increases in heart rate and systolic blood pressure of more than 20%.[34] Similar changes in blood pressure and heart rate have been observed in patients after intracranial[34] and coronary artery bypass surgery.[36,37] These changes tend to be transient, lasting 5 to 10 minutes, and are generally not associated with electrocardiographic evidence of myocardial ischemia.[37] Coronary sinus lactate extraction measurements, however, indicate that, at least in patients with poorer cardiac function, myocardial ischemia may be associated with extubation.[38] Patients with inadequately controlled hypertension, carcinoid syndrome, pheochromocytoma, or hyperthyroidism might be expected to display even more marked increases in blood pressure in response to tracheal extubation.

The clinical importance and optimal management of these problems will depend on the context in which the event occurs. Patients with coronary artery disease, poorly controlled hypertension, tachyarrhythmias, raised intracranial pressure, and pregnancy-induced hypertension[37] may be at particular risk for adverse outcomes. Strategies to attenuate such responses include the use of intratracheal lidocaine or intravenous lidocaine, nitrates, beta-blockers, and extubation while in a deep anesthetic plane. Generally speaking, lidocaine strategies have been ineffective,[37] whereas esmolol,[34-36] labetalol,[35] and nitrates provide hemodynamic stability.

D. LARYNGOTRACHEAL INJURY

Several of the complications of endotracheal intubation do not become apparent until after extubation. Anatomic or functional abnormalities may develop as a consequence of a difficult or prolonged intubation or a problematic extubation. Tracheal and laryngeal trauma, for example, may result in *dislocation of the arytenoid cartilages*[40] or glottic edema. Tolley et al.[40] described three cases involving two adults and one child. A prematurely born male had required prolonged ventilation for infantile respiratory distress syndrome. At 6 years of age, he came to medical attention for investigation of a weak voice. A unilateral prolapsed arytenoid was noted and was managed with speech therapy. The adults had been difficult or unsuccessful intubations, whereas the child had not been. In one endotracheal extubation and in the other, removal of the tracheostomy tube was followed by stridor requiring immediate reintubation or recannulation. Laryngoscopy revealed a unilateral dislocated arytenoid and in one case a contralateral vocal cord palsy. In both cases, dislocated arytenoidectomy was performed. The authors suggest that this complication may be more common than the literature would have us believe. They suggest that if the diagnosis is made early, before the onset of ankylosis, it may be possible to manipulate the arytenoid back into position, sparing resection. This would require a high index of suspicion and glottic evaluation after difficult or perhaps prolonged intubations.

Glottic edema has been classified as supraglottic, retroarytenoidal, and subglottic.[41] Supraglottic edema results in posterior displacement of the epiglottis, reducing the laryngeal inlet and causing inspiratory obstruction. Retroarytenoidal edema restricts movement of the arytenoid cartilages limiting vocal cord abduction on inspiration. Subglottic edema, a particular problem in neonates and infants, results in swelling of the loose submucosal connective tissue confined by the nonexpandable cricoid cartilage. In neonates, this is the narrowest part of the upper airway, and small reductions in diameter result in a significant increase in airway resistance. In children, laryngeal edema is promoted by a tight-fitting endotracheal tube, traumatic intubation, duration of intubation greater than 1 hour, coughing on the endotracheal tube, and intraoperative alterations of head and position.[42] Koka and others[42] found an incidence of 1% in children less than 17 years old. Laryngeal edema should be suspected when inspiratory stridor develops within 6 hours of extubation. Management of laryngeal edema depends on its severity. Treatment options range from head-up positioning,

supplemental humidified oxygen, racemic epinephrine, helium-oxygen administration, reintubation, and tracheostomy. (Management of ICU patients with no leakage around a deflated endotracheal tube cuff will be discussed below.) Several recent studies in children and adults have failed to demonstrate benefit from dexamethasone or methylprednisolone administration,[14,43,44] but questions remain about the methodology.[45]

An alternative classification and proposal for management of laryngotracheal injury from intubation has been presented by Benjamin.[46] He described "tongues" of granulation tissue that may cause immediate airway obstruction after extubation; glottic and subglottic edema that cause increasing obstruction in the first minutes or hours after extubation; and posterior glottic stenosis or subglottic stenosis caused by contracting scar tissue, which results in increasing obstruction weeks or months after extubation. Benjamin found that fiberoptic evaluation or laryngoscopy with the tube in situ was of limited value. The endotracheal tube obscured the view of the posterior glottis and subglottis. These lesions were best identified by rigid telescopes with image magnification during general anesthesia. This permitted the anticipation of problems and the development of a management strategy. His recommendations are based on the experience gained from performing approximately 400 endoscopic procedures in infants and children and 300 in adults each year. Although these observations are vast and impressive, they are uncontrolled.

Tracheomalacia may result from longstanding compression by intrathoracic goiter (see below) or as a consequence of prolonged intubation, presumably related to cuff-induced erosion of the tracheal cartilage with or without extension to the membranous portion. Tracheomalacia has been observed in 29% of 81 patients with long-term tracheostomies examined by fiberoptic bronchoscopy before decannulation. Diagnosis is made by visualization of tracheal collapse on spontaneous ventilation. Management may be conservative or may result in segmental resection, Marlex suspension, use of lyophilized dura mater with fibrin glue,[47] or repaired with ceramic rings.[48]

Laryngospasm is a common cause of upper-airway obstruction, particularly in children. Even in adults, Rose et al.[8] found that it accounted for 23.3% of critical postoperative respiratory events. Its occurrence at emergence from anesthesia was associated with an extremely high risk of such an event in the PACU (relative risk = 17.70).[8] (Critical respiratory events were defined as unanticipated arterial saturation of less than 90%, respiratory rate less than 8 breaths/min, $Paco_2 > 50$ mm Hg, or upper-airway obstruction requiring active intervention.) A variety of triggers are recognized, including cervical flexion or extension with an indwelling endotracheal tube; pain; pelvic or abdominal visceral stimulation; or vocal cord irritation from blood, vomitus, or oral secretions. These result in contraction of the lateral cricoarytenoids, the thyroarytenoid and the cricothyroid muscles mediated by the superior laryngeal nerve (supplying the cricothyroid muscle), and the recurrent laryngeal nerve (supplying the thyroarytenoid and the cricothyroid).[49] Management consists of elimination of the offending agent, administration of oxygen by sustained positive pressure, or the use of a short-acting neuromuscular blocker with or without reintubation if other measures are unsuccessful.[49]

E. VOCAL CORD PARALYSIS

Vocal cord paralysis results from injury to the vagus nerve or one of its branches and is a relatively rare complication associated mostly with head and neck, thyroid (see below), or thoracic surgery. However, Cavo[50] identified 30 cases in the literature of laryngeal nerve paralysis that could not be accounted for by the surgical site. Anatomic dissections identified a "zone of vulnerability," where the anterior division of the recurrent laryngeal nerve, supplying the adductors to the vocal cords, was in close proximity to the cuff of the endotracheal tube. This region was 6 to 10 mm below the posterior end of the free edge of the vocal cords. He recommended cuff placement at least 15 mm below the vocal cords. Presumably, this effect is more likely to occur with cuff overinflation.[51] *Unilateral* vocal cord paralysis generally produces little other than hoarseness, which usually improves without treatment.[51] *Bilateral* vocal cord paralysis, on the other hand, results in vocal cord adduction and airway obstruction apparent on extubation. The diagnosis is confirmed by laryngoscopy, and management generally requires reintubation and subsequent tracheostomy.[53] The same is true for bilateral recurrent laryngeal nerve (RLN) injury because the RLN provides motor innervation to all but the cricothyroid muscle, a weak vocal cord tensor supplied by the superior laryngeal nerve. *Bilateral recurrent laryngeal nerve paralysis* results in unopposed cricothyroid muscle contraction. This causes airway compromise despite adequate vocalization (see discussion of thyroid and carotid surgery below).

F. NEGATIVE-PRESSURE PULMONARY EDEMA

Acute pulmonary edema may complicate tracheal extubation when significant airway obstruction occurs.[54-60] In adults this generally occurs in patients with upper-airway tumors, severe laryngospasm, or rarely bilateral vocal cord palsy,[59] whereas in children it occurs most commonly as a complication of croup or epiglottitis.[57] Onset may be within minutes of the development of airway obstruction and generally resolves with relief of obstruction and supportive treatment for pulmonary edema.

G. LARYNGEAL INCOMPETENCE AND ASPIRATION

In a French, multicenter, prospective study looking at major complications associated with anesthesia, respiratory problems accounted for 52% of events. Of 198,103 anesthetic inductions, aspiration was identified in 27 cases, resulting in four deaths and two cases of anoxic encephalopathy.[61] Laryngeal function may be disturbed for at least 4 hours after tracheal extubation. This was demonstrated by detection of swallowed radiopaque dye on chest x-ray examination.[62] In this study, patients had been intubated for 8 to 28 hours during and after cardiac surgery. The mechanism of laryngeal incompetence was postulated to be primarily sensory because patients who aspirated dye did not cough. Aspiration may also result from obtundation or such conditions that impair vocal cord apposition (e.g., vocal cord paralysis and granulomata). Laryngeal dysfunction will be further discussed in the following section.

IV. HIGH-RISK EXTUBATIONS

At the time of extubation, some patients may be at greater risk because of preexisting medical conditions leaving them physiologically susceptible or as a result of surgical or anesthetic interventions. Prior identification of such patients permits consultation among involved physicians and surgeons and the development of an extubation strategy that one hopes will enhance patient safety. Patients may be at "high risk" at the time of extubation because they are more likely not to tolerate extubation or, alternatively, because of a greater risk of being unable to reestablish an airway. The former group includes patients who lose airway patency, experience a failure of ventilation or oxygenation, or lose the ability to clear pulmonary secretions or protect their airway. The latter group includes patients who had previously been difficult to intubate, those with restricted airway access, situations where available personnel may lack the required experience, or situations where airway injury has occurred. Postoperative patients may also be at risk for bleeding in and around the airway and may require reoperation (Box 39-2).

A. INABILITY TO TOLERATE EXTUBATION

1. Airway obstruction
a. PARADOXIC VOCAL CORD MOTION
The complications described above can complicate any extubation, and prediction of the patient at risk may be difficult. There are, however, numerous situations where complications are more likely to occur and anticipation of these situations may reduce complications. An interesting example is that of paradoxic vocal

---

BOX 39-2   High-risk extubations

I. Inability to tolerate extubation
  A. Airway obstruction
     1. Paradoxical vocal cord motion
     2. After thyroidectomy
     3. Recurrent laryngeal nerve palsy
     4. Neck hematoma
     5. Tracheomalacia
     6. After panendoscopy or laryngoscopy with biopsy
     7. After uvulopalatopharyngoplasty
     8. After carotid endarterectomy
        a. Wound hematoma
        b. Vocal cord palsy
        c. Hypoglossal nerve palsy
     9. Maxillofacial trauma
     10. Anterior cervical-spinal cord decompression
     11. Special preexisting medical conditions (Parkinson's syndrome, rheumatoid arthritis, epidermolysis bullosa, pemphigus)
     12. Obstructive sleep apnea
     13. No cuff leak
  B. Hypoventilation syndromes
     1. Central sleep apnea
     2. Severe chronic obstructive pulmonary disease
     3. Residual volatile anesthesia
     4. Residual neuromuscular blockade
     5. Preexisting neuromuscular disorders
     6. Diaphragmatic splinting
     7. Relative hypoventilation (excess carbon dioxide production)
  C. Hypoxemic respiratory failure
     1. Inadequate inspired oxygen concentration
     2. Ventilation-perfusion mismatch
     3. Right-to-left shunt
     4. Increased oxygen consumption
     5. Decreased oxygen delivery
     6. Impaired pulmonary diffusion
  D. Failure of pulmonary toilet
     1. Obtundation
     2. Pulmonary secretions
        a. Increased quantity
        b. Tenacious secretions
        c. Impaired mucociliary clearance
     3. Neuromuscular impairment
  E. Inability to protect airway
     1. Depressed level of consciousness
     2. Neuromuscular weakness
II. Difficulty reestablishing airway
  A. Previous airway difficulty
  B. Limited airway access
     1. Maxillomandibular fixation
     2. Cervical immobilization or instability
     3. Tracheal resection
     4. Major head or neck surgery
  C. Inexperienced personnel
  D. Airway injury
     1. Burns or smoke inhalation

From Cooper RM: *Anesthesiol Clinics North Am* 13(3):1995.

---

cord motion (PVCM), an uncommon and poorly understood condition that may be mistaken for asthma. Endoscopy reveals the cause of upper-airway obstruction to be vocal cord adduction on inspiration.[63-66]

Hammer et al.[65] described a 32-year-old woman with recurrent episodes of stridor, sometimes associated with cyanosis, despite normal flow volume loops and pulmonary function testing. The diagnosis of PVCM was made endoscopically and managed with "relaxation techniques." She was operated for a lumbar laminectomy. The anesthetic management included preoperative sedation, the topical application of lidocaine to the airway, bilateral superior laryngeal nerve blocks, and awake intubation over a fiberoptic bronchoscope. Extubation was performed once the patient became responsive; however, sustained inspiratory stridor developed, necessitating reintubation. A second attempt at extubation the next day was similarly complicated by obstruction, and inspiratory vocal cord adduction was documented. A tracheostomy was required for more than 58 days. Michelsen and Vanderspek[64] described a previously healthy 26-year-old woman who underwent general anesthesia and cesarean section for fetal distress. She was extubated once fully awake but stridor developed, leading to cyanosis. Conservative management failed and reintubation was required. Subsequent extubation was again complicated by stridor. Fiberoptic laryngoscopy revealed intermittent PVCM and a second reintubation was required. The third extubation attempt followed repeat laryngoscopy and bronchoscopy with the patient under general anesthesia. The patient breathed well while sedated but mild stridor developed when consciousness returned.

Most authors have advised that speech therapy, psychotherapy, hypnosis, and calm reassurance are helpful, but this is not always the case.[66] Some recent reports have recommended electromyographic-guided botulinum toxin injection into the thyroarytenoid muscle for recalcitrant cases. The optimal anesthetic management of these patients is not known. One report[64] recommended regional anesthesia, but presumably the potential for airway obstruction exists here as well, particularly if there is pain or the patient is under stress. Recognition of and familiarity with this condition, calm reassurance when there is prior suspicion, and extubation while the patient is under deep anesthesia would seem prudent. Recently, the author cared for a patient with recurrent stridor after extubation. The trachea was extubated during spontaneous ventilation under heavy propofol sedation. The airway was widely patent and anatomically and functionally normal. As the sedation was reduced and consciousness was regained, the false and true vocal cords increasingly constricted, obstructing the laryngeal inlet and producing stridor. Tracheal extubation with a continuous propofol infusion was accomplished by gradually weaning the sedation over 36 hours. Interestingly, this patient was a young, female nurse with coexistent asthma, fitting the description of the typical patient of Hayes et al.[66]

b. THYROID SURGERY

A variety of injuries have been described after thyroidectomies. Lacoste et al.[9] reviewed the records of 3008 patients who underwent thyroidectomies between 1968 and 1988. All patients had indirect laryngoscopy on the third or fifth postoperative day. Although the RLN had been identified intraoperatively in 2427 patients, unilateral RLN palsy occurred temporarily in 4.3% and permanently in 1.1% of patients. Three patients had bilateral RLN palsy and required tracheostomy. Eight other patients required a tracheostomy because of extensive thyroid cancer. Six of a total of 16 deaths during the first 30 postoperative days were attributed to respiratory complications. One death occurred after failed intubation caused by a deviated, constricted trachea. A second death occurred because of difficulties performing a tracheostomy. Two deaths resulted from aspiration or pneumonia, possibly related to RLN dysfunction.

Reviewing published reports with at least 1000 patients in which postoperative laryngoscopy was performed, the incidence of permanent nerve palsies with benign goiters was 0.5/100 operations. This was more common in substernal goiters (4%) and thyroid cancer (9%). In the latter group, it is sometimes necessary to sacrifice the nerve to achieve an adequate resection. Although bilateral RLN palsy is rare, thyroidectomy represents the leading cause of this injury. The external branch of the superior laryngeal nerve (ESLN) supplying the cricothyroid muscle, which tenses the vocal cords, is believed to be vulnerable during thyroid dissection; however, the frequency of this injury is unknown.[9]

In a literature review by Lacoste et al.[9] local hemorrhage or *hematoma* occurred postoperatively in 0.1% to 1.1% of the patients and in 0.36% in their series. These occurred from 5 minutes to 3 days postoperatively but required reexploration within the first day, only twice. Airway obstruction may result from significant laryngeal and pharyngeal edema, and wound evacuation may be of limited value in the relief of airway obstruction.[67] The prophylactic placement of surgical drains likely reduces the incidence of this complication.

Tracheal compression or displacement by a goiter was identified by preoperative x-ray films of the chest or neck in 26% and compressive symptoms were noted in 11% of 3008 patients scheduled for thyroid surgery.[9] Only 2.7% of patients in this series had dyspnea. Other studies observed preoperative tracheal compression in as many as 45% of patients, but this did not seem to be of clinical consequence. Tracheomalacia may result from long-standing compression by a goiter. This has been de-scribed after removal of giant goiters in Nigeria and has been suspected in some cases of postoperative airway obstruction. Although uncommon, it is theoretically more likely to become manifest when the tracheal support from the surrounding goiter is removed, although Wade[68] described a case in which airway obstruction occurred with the onset of muscle relaxation, necessitating urgent skin incision and mobilization of the strap muscles.

c. LARYNGOSCOPY AND PANENDOSCOPY

As mentioned above, patients undergoing laryngoscopy and panendoscopy are at increased postoperative risk of airway obstruction and are approximately 20 times as likely to require reintubation compared with a wide variety of other surgical procedures.[6] Hill et al.[6] retrospectively reviewed the records of 324 diagnostic laryngoscopies and 302 panendoscopies. They found that patients who had undergone laryngeal biopsy were at highest postoperative airway risk. Thirteen of 252 (5%) patients required reintubation, all within 1 hour of extubation. Twelve of these had undergone laryngeal biopsy. They did not state whether their patients had received topical anesthesia or vasoconstrictors. They had not received prophylactic steroids, although the value of this adjunct is not well established.[43]

Robinson[69] prospectively studied 183 patients having 204 endoscopic laryngeal procedures. Five of these patients had a tracheostomy before endoscopy and 2 of 12 patients, deemed to be at "high risk"—the criteria for which were not specified—underwent elective tracheostomy after endoscopy. Only one patient required reintubation. Indirect laryngoscopy, carried out between 4 and 6 hours after surgery, revealed mucosal hemorrhage or laryngopharyngeal swelling in 31% of cases. Because the patients undergoing tracheostomy were not described, it is possible that the low incidence of reintubation resulted from an aggressive approach to elective tracheostomy.

d. UVULOPALATOPHARYNGOPLASTY (UPPP)

Patients with obstructive sleep apnea are at risk of intermittent postoperative airway occlusion. The surgical removal of redundant oropharyngeal tissue, UPPP, has enjoyed clinical success. There is an expectation, however, that the procedure eliminates the risk of postoperative airway obstruction. Gabrielczyk[70] described one such patient, who after regaining spontaneous ventilation, experienced emergence delirium and after extubation had obstructive breathing at a slow respiratory rate develop. Bag-and-mask ventilation proved to be ineffective, despite the presence of nasopharyngeal airway. Needle cricothyroidotomy and manual ventilation (using a reservoir bag) were ineffective, and a tracheostomy was performed. Laryngoscopy was then performed with the patient under general anesthesia and revealed a moderately edematous palate and oropharynx. This assessment, however, was made after a period of considerable agitation. As well, the subsequent emergence with a tracheostomy in place was also stormy, despite the presence of an unobstructed airway. Thus the edematous airway may have been the result of a stormy emergence rather than its cause. No other cases of post-UPPP obstruction could be found in the literature, despite the popularity of this procedure. It should be noted that the sleep apnea syndrome may have a combination of central and obstructive components as this patient seemed to exhibit.

e. CAROTID ENDARTERECTOMY

Kunkel et al.[71] described 15 patients who had *wound hematomas* develop after carotid endarterectomy. Eight of these were evacuated with the patient under local anesthesia. In six of the seven cases in which general anesthesia was used, difficulties were encountered in airway management, resulting in two deaths and one patient with severe neurologic impairment. O'Sullivan et al.[72] described six patients with airway obstruction after carotid endarterectomy. Five of these patients had been taking antiplatelet medication preoperatively. They found that stridor was not relieved by wound evacuation. Of particular importance, the administration of muscle relaxants made manual ventilation by mask virtually impossible, whereas intubation was complicated by marked glottic or supraglottic edema. Cyanosis and extreme bradydysrhythmias or asystole occurred in four patients. Although the authors endorsed Kunkel's recommendation of the use of local anesthetic infiltration for wound evacuation, they believed that much of the airway compromise related to edema from venous or lymphatic congestion. They emphasized that the degree of external swelling may lead to an underestimate of the internal oropharyngeal edema. O'Sullivan et al. recommended wound evacuation with the patient under local anesthesia; if general anesthesia was required, an inhalation induction should be performed until the depth is sufficient to permit laryngoscopy or, alternatively, fiberoptic laryngoscopy with spontaneous ventilation until the airway is secured.

Accelerated carotid atherosclerosis may occur after *cervical irradiation*. Airway obstruction after carotid surgery occurred in two of five such patients described by Francfort et al.[73] The mechanisms of obstruction included supraglottic and glottic edema in one patient and periglottic trauma in the other patient.

Bilateral vocal cord[12] and bilateral *hypoglossal nerve palsies*[11] have been described after staged bilateral endarterectomies. In the latter case, the first procedure, done with the patient under regional anesthesia, had been complicated by a wound hematoma that resulted in numbness over the anterior neck and diminished sensation in the C2 and C3 distribution. The subsequent endarterectomy, done 4 weeks later with the patient

under deep cervical plexus block with subcutaneous infiltration resulted in intraoperative airway obstruction and asystole. The airway was secured but attempts at extubation resulted in obstruction caused by bilateral hypoglossal nerve palsy, which eventually improved.

f. MAXILLOFACIAL TRAUMA

Maxillofacial injuries are generally the result of unrestrained occupants of motor vehicles encountering an unyielding dashboard, windshield, or steering wheel. Gunshot wounds or physical altercations also cause maxillofacial injury. Airway obstruction is a primary cause of morbidity and mortality in these patients.[74] Most will present with a full stomach, and many will have associated head and neck injuries such as lacerations; loose or avulsed teeth; intraoral fractures; fractures extending into the paranasal sinuses, the orbit, or through the cribriform plate; and the potential for cervical-spine instability. Injury to the lower face raises the additional possibility of a laryngeal fracture. Intermaxillary fixation may be part of the surgical plan, necessitating nasal intubation or a surgical airway. Timing of endotracheal extubation is complex and based on consideration of factors such as the patient's level of consciousness, his/her ability to maintain satisfactory gas exchange, the integrity of protective airway reflexes, the difficulty encountered in establishing the airway, and the likelihood that reintubation would be more or less easy as a result of the surgery and passage of time. The lack of guidance provided by the literature makes communication between the anesthesiologist and the surgeon essential. Intermaxillary fixation requires that wire cutters be immediately available and that personnel know which wires to cut should this be necessary. If the expertise exists, a fiberoptic bronchoscope should be available at the time of extubation. Many would advocate that it be used to assess the airway if there is any suspicion of glottic or periglottic involvement. Fiberoptic bronchoscopy may also be helpful to exclude endotracheal tube entrapment. The ability to establish an emergency percutaneous airway (by needle or surgical cricothyrotomy) must exist. Ideally, extubation should be accomplished in a staged or "reversible" manner, permitting reintubation—blindly if necessary—while allowing oxygen administration by insufflation or jet ventilation as the airway is being secured[75-79] (see "Extubation Strategies").

g. ANTERIOR CERVICAL DECOMPRESSION

Emery et al.[10] retrospectively identified 7 of 133 (5.3%) patients undergoing cervical corpectomies who required postoperative reintubation. Three had been difficult intubations because of limited access or cervical immobility. The patients had undergone an anterior approach to achieve a three-level vertebral body and disk resection with bone grafting. Drains were placed and all patients were immobilized by halo-vest or a rigid head-cervical-thoracic orthosis. Three of the patients were extubated in the operating room and four were extubated at 12 to 91 hours postoperatively. Reintubation was necessary immediately in one case, within 30 minutes in two cases, and within 2 to 23 hours in four cases. Reintubation was required because of severe hypopharyngeal and supraglottic edema in four patients, but the indication was not specified in the other three. Five of the reintubations had no serious sequelae; these patients were extubated within 2 to 8 days. One patient required a cricothyrotomy, but delay resulted in hypoxic encephalopathy and death. The other patient was reintubated but died from severe adult respiratory distress syndrome.

The risk factors, identified by Emery et al.[10] included a smoking history, moderate or severe preoperative myelopathy, extensive multilevel decompression with prolonged surgery, and tissue retraction. The authors recommend 1 to 3 days of elective intubation postoperatively, determination of the presence of a "cuff leak" (see below), and direct laryngoscopy at extubation.

h. SPECIAL PREEXISTING MEDICAL CONDITIONS

i. Parkinson's syndrome. Parkinson's syndrome affects 2.5% of the population older than 65 years of age. Gastrointestinal dysmotility is common with excessive salivation and esophageal reflux. Aspiration is a common cause of death for patients with this condition, yet there are few reports of postoperative complications. Backus et al.[49] described a patient who shortly after taking cough medication became aphonic, had stridor, and had a respiratory arrest. Approximately 12 hours later, having been weaned from mechanical ventilation, she was extubated, and upper-airway obstruction recurred with vocal cord apposition. The patient subsequently extubated herself 4 days later with no further complications. The authors interpreted this laryngeal spasm as a "spontaneous" manifestation of Parkinson's syndrome. Others have noted upper-airway dysfunction, airflow limitation, and bilateral abductor vocal cord paralysis in association with Parkinson's syndrome. It is unclear whether the first episode occurred as a result of aspiration of the cough medicine. Nonetheless, there remains a possibility that such patients are more prone to laryngospasm, whether spontaneous or induced by glottic stimulation.

ii. Rheumatoid arthritis. This common collagen vascular disease is associated with numerous airway problems, including temporomandibular and cricoarytenoid arthritis and ankylosis, micrognathia, and cervical-spine instability. The specific indications for awake fiberoptic intubation in patients with this disorder are not known. Whether such an approach confers benefits beyond securing the airway were recently addressed in a retrospective review of 128 consecutive patients with this disorder, who had undergone posterior cervical-spine procedures.[80] Upper-airway obstruction after extubation occurred in 1 of 70 patients intubated fiberoptically but in 8 of 58 patients intubated by direct laryngoscopy. In the latter group, five of eight patients required reintubation with two near fatalities and one death. The two groups were apparently similar with respect to age, sex, American Rheumatology Association classification, ASA physical status, the duration of surgery and anesthesia, fluid balance, and postoperative immobilization. The time to extubation was significantly longer for the fiberoptic group (17.9 vs. 10.6 hr. P = .02), but this could bias the need for reintubation in either direction because of increased or resolved glottic edema. Using logistic regression, the authors concluded that patients with rheumatoid arthritis are less likely to experience postextubation airway obstruction if intubated by fiberoptic bronchoscopy. It is important to note that all patients, regardless of the group, were intubated awake. Furthermore, of the 58 patients intubated without the aid of a bronchoscope, 49 were intubated without visualization of the airway. It is not stated whether this was an a priori decision or done because the glottis could not be visualized without risking damage to the cervical spine. The authors did not describe their intubation techniques in detail; however, if conventional fiberoptic techniques were used, the bronchoscope was likely introduced through the glottis and the endotracheal tube was advanced "blindly" over the bronchoscope. This usually results in some coughing, a certain degree of tube rotation, and may be more traumatic to the airway—although perhaps less so to the cervical spine—than the insertion of an endotracheal tube with direct visualization of the glottis.

Unfortunately, this study, which was carried out over a 12-year period, was retrospective, and despite the apparent similarity in demographics, the absence of randomization leaves open the possiblity that there were unspecified differences between the groups. We do not know the basis for the decision to intubate fiberoptically or the skills of the anesthetists involved. Also, as previously mentioned, all patients intubated were intubated awake, and this may be more traumatic than when facilitated by muscle relaxation. Before accepting the authors' conclusions, it would be useful to randomize patients with the intention of visualizing the glottis and intubating under direct vision or fiberoptic intubation. These comments notwithstanding, the incidence of postextubation airway obstruction was high in patients with rheumatoid arthritis, and special precautions might be warranted.[81]

iii. Epidermolysis bullosa. This rare condition, with more than 25 described variations, results in the separation of layers of skin and mucous membranes with fluid accumulation caused by a deficiency in intercellular bridges. Shearing forces are particularly damaging and may result in separation, bullous formation, hemorrhage, and healing by scar formation and subsequent tissue contraction. Laryngeal involvement is extremely rare, and tracheal bullae have never been reported.[82] A retrospective report involving 33 patients undergoing 329 surgical procedures identified no postoperative airway problems, although microstomia was noted in 13 of the patients.[83] Giant oropharyngeal bullae and profuse bleeding from a ruptured oral bullus and a large fibrosing supraglottic bullus have, however, been reported to cause airway obstruction.[84]

iv. Pemphigus. Pemphigus embraces a group of rare immunologically mediated vesiculobullous diseases (vulgaris, foliaceus, pemphigoid, and others) that frequently involve mucous membranes. Ninety percent of patients with vulgaris have oromucosal involvement at some point.[85] Most lesions heal without scarring unless they become secondarily infected. Microstomia is not a feature. Management of such patients is similar to epidermolysis bullosa. Despite laryngeal and tracheal involvement, a literature search failed to identify reports of anesthetic complications.

i. NO CUFF LEAK

A variety of clinical conditions may lead to airway edema sufficient to encroach on the endotracheal tube, preventing leakage of gas around the deflated cuff. These include generalized edema, angioneurotic edema, anaphylaxis, hypopharyngeal infections, pemphigus, and epidermolysis bullosa. The most common situation likely occurs in the intensive care unit after prolonged intubation. Potgieter and Hammond[86] described a "cuff test" performed by deflation of the endotracheal tube cuff, digital occlusion of the tube, and an assessment of air movement around the tube. They evaluated this in 10 patients who required intubation for upper-airway obstruction caused by edema. They did not describe the extubation of patients without a cuff leak or the implications of leaving the tube in until a cuff leak develops. Kemper et al.[87] confirmed Potgieter's observation in a pediatric burn and trauma unit, concluding that the absence of a cuff leak was the best predictor of the need for reintubation or tracheostomy.

Fisher and Raper[88] observed that all of 60 patients with a cuff leak were successfully extubated, but two patients extubated without a cuff leak required reintubation, and five patients who repeatedly failed the test required tracheostomy. They subsequently studied 10 patients without a cuff leak, three of whom required reintubation or tracheostomy. It is significant that most tolerated extubation. This raises the question of how such patients should be best managed. Maintaining the presence of the endotracheal tube may contribute to airway injury and clearly increases patient discomfort and the cost of care. If the results of this very small series

can be generalized, most patients without a cuff leak remain intubated longer than necessary and some may unnecessarily be consigned to a tracheostomy.

The optimal management of this common clinical problem is not known. Traditional management has involved either continuing with tracheal intubation until a cuff leak develops or performing of a tracheostomy. A more "aggressive" approach has been to undertake tracheal extubation despite the absence of a cuff leak. A third option, namely extubation over a "jet stylet," will be presented below.

2. Hypoventilation syndromes

A wide variety of clinical conditions may give rise to postoperative ventilatory failure. In a large multicenter trial involving nearly 200,000 patients undergoing all forms of anesthesia, postoperative respiratory depression accounted for 27 of 85 respiratory complications that were life-threatening or resulted in serious sequelae. Such complications were responsible for seven deaths and five cases of hypoxic encephalopathy.[61] On the basis of a respiratory rate less than 8 breaths/min, Rose et al.[8] identified hypoventilation in .2% of patients in the PACU. Hypoventilation may be mediated centrally at the level of the upper motor neuron, the anterior horn cell, the lower motor neuron, the neuromuscular junction, or the respiratory muscles.[89] Clinical correlates include central sleep apnea, carotid endarterectomy,[90] medullary injuries, demyelinating disorders, direct injury to peripheral nerves, poliomyelitis, Guillain-Barré syndrome, motor neuron disease, myasthenia gravis, and botulism. As well, hypoventilation may result from the loss of lung or pleural elasticity, diaphragmatic splinting caused by abdominal distention or pain, thoracic deformities like kyphoscoliosis, or multifactorial entities such as morbid obesity and severe chronic obstructive pulmonary disease. Rarely, ventilatory failure will result from an excess of carbon dioxide production or a marked increase in physiologic dead space.

The residual effects of anesthetic drugs contribute to inadequate postoperative ventilation.[91-93] This may be aggravated by incomplete reversal of neuromuscular blockers; hypocalcemia or hypermagnesemia; or the administration of other drugs, including antibiotics, local anesthetics, diuretics, and calcium channel blockers, which may potentiate neuromuscular blockade.

3. Hypoxemic respiratory failure

There are many causes of postoperative hypoxemia, and a review of these is beyond the scope of this discussion. Generally, these might occur as a result of hypoventilation, a low inspired oxygen concentration, ventilation-perfusion mismatch, right-to-left shunting, increased oxygen consumption, diminished oxygen transport, or rarely an impairment of oxygen diffusion. Clearly there are clinical situations when such events are more likely, because of a preexisting medical condition or surgical and anesthetic interventions. If sufficiently severe, there may be a requirement for CPAP or reintubation and mechanical ventilation.

4. Failure of pulmonary toilet

Inadequate clearance of pulmonary secretions may be due to a depressed level of consciousness with impaired airway reflexes, an overproduction of secretions, an alteration in their consistency leading to inspissation and bronchial plugging, impaired mucociliary clearance or inadequate neuromuscular reserve. These may result in atelectasis or pneumonia with attendant hypoxemic respiratory failure. Alteration in pulmonary mechanics may also lead to hypercapnia, necessitating reintubation.

5. Inability to protect airway

ICU or postoperative patients may be unable to protect their airway because of preexisting obtundation, neurologic injury, or residual anesthetic effects. In the latter case, it may be possible to temporize by turning patients on their side, placing patients head down (or head up), or passing an oropharyngeal or nasopharyngeal airway. Clearly, these measures do nothing to restore airway reflexes; however, they may reestablish patency or diminish the risk of aspiration. If these measures are insufficient or the condition fails to improve, reintubation may be required.

B. DIFFICULTY REESTABLISHING THE AIRWAY

Reintubation under emergency conditions is an entirely different proposition from the controlled circumstances of an elective induction. In the latter case, the conditions have been optimized (e.g., putting the patient's head in a sniff position). In an emergency reintubation, there may be uncertainty about the ability to establish an airway, resulting in a reluctance to use muscle relaxants. This in turn may make the oropharynx inaccessible because of clenched teeth. Breath holding, vigorous coughing, blood, vomitus, or stomach contents may also complicate efforts. Bag-and-mask ventilation may be ineffective or increase the risk of contaminating an unsecured airway. This may also result in gastric distention, further increasing the risk of aspiration. Topical anesthesia may be less effective because of the presence of the above fluids[94,95] or the need to proceed before the medications have achieved their effects. Lastly, reintubation may be required because the patient is already hypoxemic, hypercapnic, agitated, or showing evidence of myocardial ischemia, dysrhythmias, or hemodynamic instability.

1. Previous difficulty

Although studies previously referred to indicate that only the occasional ICU patient and considerably fewer postoperative patients are likely to require reintubation, those who had been difficult to intubate under controlled conditions are likely to be particularly difficult in the emergency setting. Patients who had required multiple efforts by experienced individuals or who had undergone an awake, fiberoptic, or retrograde intubation should be treated differently at extubation. At the very least, extubation should be deferred until strict criteria are met. Additional precautions will be discussed below.

2. Limited access

Limited access to the airway is typified by the case of intermaxillary fixation. Similar situations exist in which airway access is restricted by a halo-vest, other cervical fixation methods, an unstable cervical spine, or recent tracheal resection. In the latter case, it is common practice to suture the chin to the chest so as not to allow distraction of the anastomosed trachea. Despite the airway edema and coexistent lung disease these patients may have, there is often pressure to extubate them early to minimize the risks of barotrauma and bacterial colonization. Access may also be limited by radical head and neck dissection, extensive head and neck irradiation, major facial reconstruction, and angioneurotic edema.

3. Inexperienced personnel

Many PACUs and ICUs do not enjoy the continuous presence of highly skilled airway practitioners. Thus complicated airway management problems may be left to trainees, delegated individuals, or on-call personnel who may not be immediately available and may have limited familiarity with the patient.

4. Airway injury

Burn patients with circumferential neck involvement or smoke inhalation are at particular risk of requiring reintubation.[2] Demling et al.[2] has suggested that the presence of the endotracheal tube may contribute to upper-airway damage and therefore should be removed as soon as standard criteria are met. These patients, however, are known to exhibit bronchorrhea, impaired mucociliary clearance and local defenses, laryngeal and supraglottic edema, increased carbon dioxide production, and progressive adult respiratory distress syndrome. Kemper et al.[96] reported on the management of 13 burn patients less than 15 years of age, 7 of whom exhibited postextubation stridor. Treatments with helium and oxygen resulted in lower stridor scores than patients treated with an air-oxygen mixture. In another report,[87] the authors found that 11 of 30 extubated burn victims required treatment for stridor after extubation, consisting of racemic epinephrine, helium-oxygen, reintubation (n = 5), or tracheostomy (n = 1). The absence of a cuff leak was considered to be the best predictor of failure with a sensitivity of 100% and a positive predictive value of 79%.

V. EXTUBATION STRATEGIES

To the extent that any of the "high-risk" conditions exist or are anticipated, it behooves the clinician to consider a strategy that does not cut off access to the airway. Ideally such a strategy should permit the continued administration of oxygen or the ability to ventilate a failing patient even while the airway is being reestablished. Such objectives are consistent with the ASA Task Force recommendations.[1]

These points have never been subjected to a controlled trial. The identification of patients at high risk for complications after extubation is largely anecdotal and influenced by the author's own clinical experience. This list will be enlarged or contracted by the reader's own experience. Most patients (even those in high risk categories) will not experience complications after extubation. As such, any proposed management strategy must carry low-risk; minimal patient discomfort; acceptable cost; and optimization of the objectives of airway access, oxygenation, and ventilation.

A. ROUTINE EXTUBATION

Extubation after the resumption of spontaneous respiration but while still in a surgical plane of anesthesia may be considered for patients in whom coughing or straining on emergence from anesthesia is particularly hazardous. This strategy may also be useful in patients with severe reactive airways disease or PVCM, although the latter situation has not been adequately evaluated. The disadvantage of such an approach is the increased risk of aspiration. The adult patient is commonly allowed to recover fully from neuromuscular blockade, reestablish adequate spontaneous respiration with acceptable oxygen saturation, and demonstrate recovery of consciousness. While breathing oxygen ($Fio_2 = 1.0$) sufficiently long to have eliminated nitrous oxide and the effects of diffusion hypoxia, the patient is instructed to open the mouth and the oropharynx is suctioned. The airway pressure can be allowed to rise to 5 to 15 cm H_2O[1,97] creating a "passive cough," the cuff is deflated, and the endotracheal tube is withdrawn, generally at peak inspiration so that secretions may be expelled on the subsequent exhalation.

B. POTENTIALLY DIFFICULT EXTUBATIONS OR REINTUBATIONS

Any extubation is potentially also a reintubation. However, there are situations where there is clear intention to exchange an existing endotracheal tube.

Although these may involve different problems and solutions, there is sufficient similarity that they warrant discussion together. This becomes problematic in the patient in whom securing the airway (1) had been difficult, (2) would now be difficult because of limited access or anatomic derangement, and/or (3) in whom physiologic instability makes the interruption of ventilation or oxygenation hazardous. A variety of options exist, many of which are safer than simply removing and attempting to reinsert the endotracheal tube.

1. Trial of extubation

Probably the most commonly practiced method of reintubation is to extubate the trachea and hope for the best. The justification for this approach stems from odds that generally favor the idea that reintubation will be unnecessary. In a similar way, advocates of the "trial by extubation" may argue that if reintubation is required, the likelihood of reintubation success is enhanced by the knowledge of the previous intubation difficulties and how they were overcome. An assumption of superior skill is occasionally invoked as well. Even if such assumptions are correct, the stakes are very high, particularly when dealing with a situation that is inherently unstable and where alternative methods exist that may be less hazardous.

2. Extubation or reintubation over a bronchoscope

In situations with the possibility of tube entrapment, extubation over a bronchoscope can detect and potentially avert disastrous outcomes. With a spontaneously breathing patient, extubation over a bronchoscope provides the opportunity of visually assessing vocal cord function. This can be very helpful in the patient suspected of having a vocal cord palsy or PVCM. It also permits an assessment of anatomic injury to the trachea, glottis, or supraglottic structures.[98] In the author's experience, such opportunities are maximized by reassurance and judicious sedation, administration of an antisialagogue, an auxiliary Yankauer sucker for oral secretions, placement of the bronchoscope above the carina, slow cuff deflation to minimize coughing, gradual withdrawal of the endotracheal tube into the oropharynx, very gradual withdrawal of the bronchoscope to the subglottic region, and, once the patient is comfortable, further withdrawal to a position just above the vocal cords. Even with such a deliberate technique, the exercise is frequently frustrated by excessive secretions, coughing, swallowing, or poor tolerance with insufficient opportunity of visualizing the anatomy or function.

If the technique is successful, it may enable the anticipation of complications. When significant abnormalities are noted, a decision must be made whether to immediately reinsert the tracheal tube or withdraw the bronchoscope and manage the patient with agents such as racemic epinephrine and helium/oxygen.[96,99] Bronchoscopic extubation does not provide a practical way of performing a "trial of extubation."

Hudes et al.[100] described two patients who had difficult intubations and required endotracheal tube changes. This was accomplished by the prior removal of the plastic connector on the original tube, mounting the new tube over a bronchoscope, advancement of the fiberoptic scope, and withdrawal of the original tube. The original tube was then filleted with a scalpel blade and peeled off to allow the replacement tube to be advanced. They claimed to have achieved this in 20 and 30 seconds. In this writer's limited experience, the technique is awkward and places the fiberoptic scope and the operator's fingers in jeopardy.

Others have used the bronchoscope to change endotracheal tubes. Rosenbaum and colleagues[101] placed a bronchoscope through the opposite nostril of a patient with an existing but inadequate nasotracheal tube. Watson[102] endorsed the use of a bronchoscope to exchange endotracheal tubes with the apparent advantages of minimizing sedation, the risk of aspiration, hemodynamic embarrassment and uncertainty about tube placement. His technique involved passing the "loaded" bronchoscope alongside the existing endotracheal tube. Such a technique had been successful in 13 of 15 attempts. Dellinger[98] considered the bronchoscope to offer the least likelihood of failure to reintubate, suggesting an admittedly "cumbersome" technique that places the bronchoscope alongside the tube to be replaced. A bronchoscope, preloaded with the new endotracheal tube, is introduced into and advanced within the trachea. The existing tube is removed and the new tube is advanced. He suggested that if the bronchoscope could not be advanced, it should be positioned just above the vocal cords and the existing tube withdrawn from the trachea followed by reintubation. Admittedly, this risks loss of the airway.

3. Extubation with a "string"

This technique is a variation on retrograde intubation.[5] Extubation with a string can be done if the original intubation used a retrograde intubation technique and is performed as follows: an epidural catheter is advanced through the cricothyroid membrane and retrieved from the oropharynx. A 30-inch length of silk is sutured to that end of the catheter. The other end of the silk is secured to the Murphy eye of the endotracheal tube. While the tongue is pulled forward, the epidural catheter is withdrawn through the cricothyroid membrane until the silk is retrieved. As tension on the silk is maintained, the endotracheal tube is advanced through the glottis. After ensuring placement of the endotracheal tube below the vocal cords, the silk is relaxed and the tube is advanced to the appropriate depth. The residual silk is taped to the

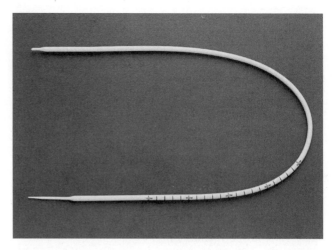

Fig. 39-1. Mettro (Mizus endotracheal tube replacement obturator). This device is available in 7.0 and 19 French sizes. It is solid but flexible, with tapered ends and designed to pass through endotracheal tubes larger than 3 and 7 mm inner diameter, respectively. It is well suited as a tube exchanger but does not permit oxygenation, ventilation, or capnography. (From Cooper RM: *Anesthesiology clinics of North America, The Difficult Airway—II* 13(3):1995.)

skin to be used for extubation. When extubation is performed, the proximal end of the silk is drawn out the mouth and the distal end is still secured to the neck and cheek with tape. If reintubation is required, the proximal end is once again tied to the Murphy eye and the tube is drawn into the trachea. There are no published reports of this technique and its success rate is not presently known.

4. Extubation over a bougie

A number of devices have been used to facilitate endotracheal tube exchange, including the protective plastic sleeve of a brachial CVP catheter,[103] Eschmann introducers,[104] and gum-elastic bougies.[105-107] Tomlinson described the use of a gum-elastic bougie to facilitate intubation when the glottis cannot be visualized but mentioned that "these introducers can be very useful for changing tracheal tubes in patients who had proved to be difficult to intubate on the first occasion."[106] Baraka[107] described the use of an esophageal bougie to change oral and nasal tubes but provided no details on the number of patients, success rate, or complications. Desai[104] described the use of an Eschmann introducer as a tube exchanger in more than 50 patients without difficulty. This device has an outer diameter of 15 French, is 65 cm long, and has a flexible tip.

5. Mettro (Mizus endotracheal tube replacement obturator)

This device (Fig. 39-1) manufactured by Cook Critical Care, (Bloomington, Indiana) was designed specifically for the replacement of endotracheal and tracheostomy tubes. It is available in two sizes, 70 cm, (7.0 French OD) for replacement of endotracheal tubes as small as 3 mm, and 80 cm long (19 French OD) that will pass through tubes 7 mm or larger. It is a flexible, solid device with a tapered tip. Recently, the manufacturer has modified the markings, replacing a single black band with specific distance indicators. There are also plans to alter the recommendations for use, although as of this writing, the user is directed to introduce the obturator through the existing endotracheal tube to a depth indicated by a black mark. This may result in carinal or endobronchial placement, which most awake patients do not tolerate, with the potential for coughing, discomfort, hypertension, and tachycardia. Tracheal perforation has been reported using different devices but following similar recommendations of advancing until resistance from the carina was encountered.[108,109]

Audenaert and colleagues[79] described the use of the smaller obturator as a tube exchanger to maintain airway access during 22 tracheostomies and for "tentative extubations" in seven patients. They stated that they preferred the smaller caliber device because there was minimal interference with spontaneous respiration, it was unobtrusive during the surgical tracheostomies, and it was well tolerated by their patients. The obturators were removed when it was apparent that reintubation was not required. In their experience, the 19 French obturator was not conducive to spontaneous breathing. Chipley et al.,[110] on the other hand, extubated the trachea of a obese 14-year-old with a fractured occipital condyle, recovering from respiratory failure using a Mettro obturator.[111] The authors did not indicate the size of the obturator used but it was left in place for 48 hours and removed once reintubation seemed unlikely.[110] As well, they used the obturator to stimulate coughing, a procedure that seems ill-advised in view of the potential for tracheal perforation mentioned above.

6. Nasogastric tube

Steinberg et al.[77] have described the use of a nasogastric tube as a means of maintaining airway access in the patient with intermaxillary fixation. Unfortunately, the authors provided no details as to the number of times this had been attempted, complications encountered, or whether any patients had been successfully reintubated. It is this author's experience and others[101] that a nasogastric tube is too pliable, and in fact softens further at body temperature, to serve as a reliable tube exchanger.

7. Bedger's "jet stylet"

Bedger and Chang[75] coined the term "jet stylet" to refer to a long (65-cm) plastic catheter with a removable 15-mm adapter for connection to an anesthesia circuit or jet injector. They created three side ports cut into the

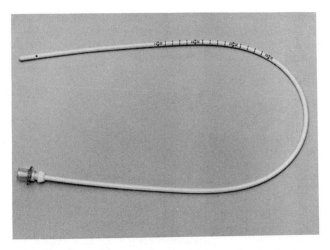

Fig. 39-2. Cook airway exchange catheters. The Cook airway exchange catheters are available in four outer diameters ranging from 2.7 to 6.33 mm. The smallest caliber is 45 cm long but all others are 83 cm long. They will pass through endotracheal tubes with inner diameters ranging from greater than 3.0 to 7.0 mm. Note the two distal side holes and the patented Rapi-Fit. 15-mm connector for connection to an anesthesia circuit or resuscitation bag. There is also a Rapi-Fit adapter for jet ventilation (see Fig. 39-3). These are designed for quick removal and replacement when off-loading or reloading an endotracheal tube. (From Cooper RM: *Anesthesiology clinics of North America, The Difficult Airway—II* 13(3):1995.)

distal 5 cm to minimize catheter whip. Their paper stated that the stylet had been for the intubation or reintubation of 59 patients. It functioned "adequately" in the patients in whom it was used for jet ventilation and oxygen insufflation. Although no complications were encountered in this series, the same authors, in an earlier report, described tension pneumothoraces in 3 patients of 600 ventilated through a 3.5-mm (OD) pediatric chest tube (at 15 pounds psi).[112] This "stylet" had been used to provide airway access and ventilation during direct laryngoscopy. They speculated that the pneumothoraces may have resulted from endobronchial migration of the catheter. They did not consider the possibility that barotrauma occurred as a result of jet ventilation against apposed vocal cords as their patients recovered from neuromuscular blockade. Nonetheless, their brief paper[75] discussed all the essential concepts of a reversible extubation.

8. Cook airway exchange catheters

Cook Critical Care (Bloomington, Indiana) has developed a family of hollow stylets, known as Airway Exchange Catheters (Fig. 39-2). According to information provided by the manufacturer, these have outer diameters of 2.7, 3.7, 4.7, and 6.33 mm (or 8, 11, 14, and 19 French, respectively) for use with endotracheal tubes greater that 3.0, 4.0, 5.0, and 7.0 mm inner diameter,

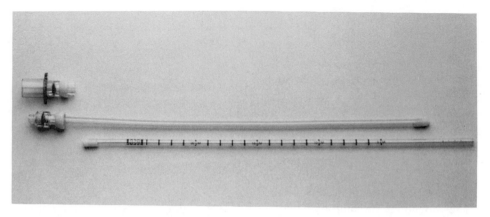

Fig. 39-3. Patil two-part intubation catheter. Shown here is the disassembled two-part intubation catheter. The first part is attached to the second by an integrated threaded connector. Note the two Rapi-Fit connectors, which are easily attached and removed by sliding the plastic collar up to disengage or down to secure the adapter. The jet adapter is shown attached to the "second part." There are eight distal side holes in addition to an end hole. A malleable stylet inserted through the "first part" can facilitate intubation (see text), whereas the extended device can be used as a tube exchanger or to accomplish reversible extubation. (From Cooper RM: *Anesthesiology clinics of North America, The Difficult Airway—II* 13(3):1995.)

respectively. The smallest diameter catheter is 45 cm long but all others are 83 cm. The catheters are radiopaque, have distance markings every centimeter and are blunt-ended. They are provided with a patented Rapi-Fit 15-mm connector for connection to an anesthesia circuit or resuscitation bag and a Luer lock adapter to permit jet ventilation. The Rapi-Fit was designed for easy adapter removal as the endotracheal tube is being off-loaded and subsequent reattachment for ventilation while the new tube is being introduced. All but one tube (C-CAE-11.0-83) has one end hole and two distal side holes. This 11Fr catheter has six side ports.

The length and inner diameters (1.6 to 3.4 mm) make manual ventilation with a resuscitation bag impractical because resistance is so high. Thus the 15-mm Rapi-Fit connector serves primarily as a means of connecting an exchange catheter to an oxygen insufflation source. During jet ventilation, the paucity of distal side holes potentially increases catheter whip and the risk of barotrauma.[113] However, the rigidity of the Cook catheter and the outer diameter, particularly of the largest model (C-CAE-19.0-83), make it especially suitable when a tube exchange, rather than a "reversible extubation," is intended. Neither the manufacturer nor the author has been able to identify any clinical reports of this catheter's performance.

9. Patil two-part intubation catheter

This device (Fig. 39-3) is also manufactured by Cook Critical Care. Patil has used this, or a similar device, for approximately 10 years (personal communication), but there are no clinical reports of its use for extubation or reintubation, although success is alluded to in another

paper by the inventor.[114] Its total length is 63 cm with an outer and inner diameter of 6.0 and 3.4 mm, respectively. It is manufactured of polyvinyl chloride and has a radiopaque stripe. The catheter is said to be suitable for endotracheal tubes with an inner diameter of greater than 7 mm. There are a total of eight side ports.

The *"first part"* can be used to facilitate intubation if a malleable stylet is inserted. A novel application is that of "magnetic intubation," whereby a strong magnet is placed over the thyroid cartilage drawing a ferrous stylet anteriorly into the larynx.[114] As well, the device can apparently be passed through a laryngeal mask airway (LMA), thereby permitting the removal of the LMA and replacement with an endotracheal tube of adequate size. Although a success rate of 84% has been reported using a gum-elastic bougie through a LMA and subsequently introducing an endotracheal tube of a desired size,[115] a recent report using the Cook Airway Exchange Catheter (C-CAE 19-83) through a properly positioned LMA was successful in only 6 of 20 efforts.[116] Given the lack of success with the CAEC, the superior performance of the Patil catheter requires documentation.

If tracheal tube exchange is anticipated, the *"second part"* is connected to the first, thereby extending its length to 63 cm. The endotracheal tube may then be removed and a replacement endotracheal tube advanced over the Patil catheter. The Rapi-Fit connector or Luer-Lok adapter is then attached, permitting either manual or jet ventilation.

10. Sheridan tracheal tube exchanger (TTX)

The Sheridan Catheter Corporation (Argyle, New York) manufactures the TTX in four sizes, with outer diameters of 2.0, 3.3, 4.8, and 5.8 mm (Fig. 39-4). The

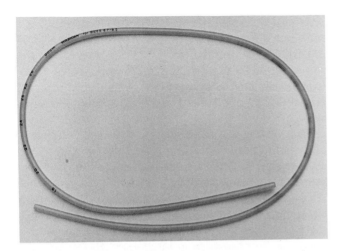

Fig. 39-4. Sheridan tracheal tube exchanger (TTX). The TTX is available in four sizes (2.0 to 5.8 mm OD). The smallest is 56 cm long whereas the others are 81.25 cm. Both ends are identical and distance markings, which only extend to 28 cm, begin at each end. There is only one distal end hole and no connector for it is provided, although the user can adapt the TTX for jet ventilation by one of two methods described in the text. The absence of distal side holes may create excessive catheter whip and high distal pressures during jet ventilation. (From Cooper RM: *Anesthesiology clinics of North America, The Difficult Airway—II* 13(3):1995.)

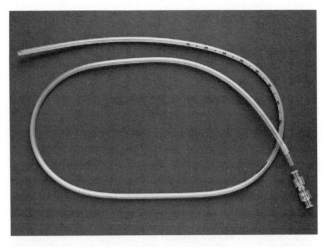

Fig. 39-5. JETTX (jet ventilation tracheal tube exchanger). This catheter overcomes the connector problem associated with the TTX. It is 4.8 mm external diameter, 100 cm long, and has a single distal end hole. It incorporates a Luer-Lok adapter with a jam fitting for easy removal and attachment. The jam fitting has a smaller external diameter than the catheter so that there is no problem off-loading or on-loading an endotracheal tube.

smallest (pediatric) is 56-cm long, whereas the others (small, medium, and large) are 81.25-cm long. This catheter has a single distal end-hole and no connectors. There is a radiopaque marker and distance markings every 5 cm. With the exception of the pediatric model, the catheters have a durometry of 85 Shore. According to the manufacturer, the device is thermolabile and softens to some extent at body temperature. Although less likely to cause injury, a softer catheter is possibly less reliable as a stylet.

Benumof[117] has described the combined use of a TTX and fiberoptic bronchoscope in replacing a 7.0-mm nasotracheal tube with a 8.0-mm orotracheal tube in a patient in halo fixation. The patient's epiglottis could not be visualized by direct laryngoscopy. An endotracheal tube loaded on a fiberoptic bronchoscope was passed alongside the existing tube and through the glottis anterior to the existing tube. The nasotracheal tube was withdrawn over the TTX and the orotracheal tube was advanced over the fiberoptic bronchoscope.

This catheter has been modified and described in the literature, notably by Benumof. Benumof's original connection of a Sheridan TTX to a jet ventilator involved wedging the hub of an intravenous catheter into the tube exchanger, using 18-, 16-, and 14-gauge IVs for small, medium, and large TTX's, respectively.[118] Because of the time and force required for assembly, the authors have refined the connection. Prior assembly is required and involves a metal or plastic female Luer Lok–barbed cone adapter inserted into a segment of 3.0, 4.0, or 5.0

inner diameter endotracheal tube, which in turn, fits over the proximal end of a small, medium, or large TTX.[119] This creates a very snug fit and allows secure attachment to a jet ventilator. It may present difficulties in removing the adapter when the original endotracheal tube is off-loaded.

11. JETTX

Based on the Benumof modifications, Sheridan Catheter Corporation has recently introduced the JETTX (Jet Ventilation/Tracheal Tube Exchanger) (Fig. 39-5). It is a longer (100 cm) modification of the 4.8-mm TTX, with a single distal end hole. It incorporates a Luer-Lok adapter with a jam fitting, allowing for easy attachment and removal. The manufacturer recommends that it be introduced into the existing endotracheal tube until its markings coincide with the distance markings on the tracheal tube. As yet, there are no clinical reports of its use for tube exchange, jet ventilation, or oxygen insufflation.

12. CardioMed endotracheal ventilation catheter (ETVC)

This device is manufactured by CardioMed Supplies (Gormley, Ontario, Canada) and was designed by the author* (Fig. 39-6). It is a 65-cm long hybrid plastic catheter with an outer and inner diameter of approximately 4 and 3 mm, respectively. It has distance markings at 4-cm intervals and a radiopaque stripe along its entire length. Proximally, it has a male hose barb with a

---

*The author has no financial interest in CardioMed Supplies Inc. but receives limited royalties from the sales of the ETVC.

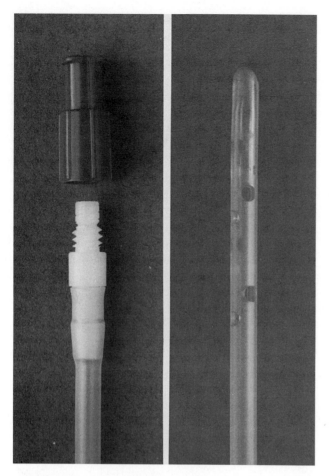

Fig. 39-6. CardioMed Endotracheal Ventilation Catheter (ETVC). The ETVC is currently available in only one size (4 mm OD, 65 cm long), although different configurations are planned by the manufacturer. This photograph shows closeups of the proximal (*left*) and the distal (*right*) ends of the ETVC. The adapter is removed for off-loading and reloading the endotracheal tube. It can be quickly reattached to permit jet ventilation or capnography with its Luer-Lok fitting. The distal end is blunt, with eight side holes and an end hole to minimize catheter whip and pressures during jet ventilation. (Cooper RM, Cohen DR: *Can J Anaesth* 41:1198, 1994.)

threaded adapter welded into the catheter. These attachments have been constructed so as not to restrict the catheter's inner diameter. The threaded adapter connects to an easily removed Luer-Lok adapter. Distally, it is blunt-ended with one end hole and eight helically arranged side holes to minimize catheter whip and jet ventilation pressure. Studies by the manufacturer indicate no significant softening over time at body temperature. This is desirable if the catheter is to remain in situ and is subsequently required to serve as a stylet.

The ETVC was designed to facilitate reversible extubation.[76] It has been used in more than 300 patients at the author's institution.[120] Data collected on the clinical application of the device in the first 202 consecutive cases revealed the following: for postoperative

or intensive care airway access (n = 120 patients), as a tube exchanger (n = 10), for tracheal reintubation (n = 22), for oxygen insufflation (n = 31), for jet ventilation (n = 45), and for capnography after extubation (n = 54). In most circumstances, the ETVC was placed to facilitate reintubation, although this was infrequently required.

Reintubation was successful in 20 of the 22 attempts. One failure occurred with a softer prototype catheter. The second failure resulted when an unsupervised operator with no previous instruction or experience attempted a tube exchange. Difficulty was occasionally encountered advancing the endotracheal tube through the glottis, similar to that experienced when using a fiberoptic bronchoscope to intubate.[121] Rotation of the endotracheal tube usually remedied this situation. Most of the patients in whom the ETVC was used had undergone orthognathic surgery (n = 44), had been difficult to intubate (n = 52), had sustained airway burns, had undergone prolonged intubation (n = 22), or concern existed about airway encroachment from soft tissue swelling (n = 15). Tube exchanges were required because of cuff damage or need for a longer endotracheal tube. Even if reintubation over the ETVC was unsuccessful, maintaining airway access with the ability to oxygenate or ventilate allows for alternative strategies to be considered in a more controlled manner.

Oxygen *insufflation* was achieved by connecting the male component of the ETVC to an oxygen flow meter with 2 to 4 L/min flow, titrated to the arterial saturation required. *Jet ventilation* will be discussed below. The ETVC has also been used to facilitate *intubation* when the glottis could only be seen through a rigid bronchoscope, in a limited number of patients to introduce an endotracheal tube through a LMA, and for *capnography* after extubation.[122,123]

Complications included barotrauma, intolerance, unintended dislodgment, and tracheal penetration. Barotrauma will be discussed along with jet ventilation. *Intolerance* occurred in 5 of 202 patients (generally because of carinal irritation) and in 1 patient recently recovered from status asthmaticus. Most patients with reactive airways have tolerated the ETVC without difficulty. *Dislodgment* occurred when the ETVC was inadequately secured or the patient "tongued" the catheter out. Tracheal or bronchial *perforation*, with different instrumentation, has been described previously.[108,109] In our case, it occurred in a patient with obstructing proliferative tracheal papillomatosis and a chronic tracheostomy. A rigid prototype catheter was inserted alongside the tracheostomy, penetrating the posterior tracheal wall. Jet ventilation resulted in fatal barotrauma. *Aspiration* and *laryngospasm* have not been observed.

VI. EXCHANGE OF DOUBLE-LUMEN TUBES

A double-lumen endobronchial tube (DLT) required for thoracic surgery is not well suited for postoperative ventilation should this be necessary. As well, the cuff of a DLT may have been damaged or it may become apparent that a different size DLT is required. If the patient was difficult to intubate or is considered a "high-risk extubation" the replacement of a DLT with a single-lumen endotracheal tube or a new DLT could be hazardous. Hannallah[124] and Cooper and Cohen[125] have observed that the length of the TTX and ETVC respectively are inadequate to function as exchange catheters for DLTs.

A. SHERIDAN E.T.X.

The E.T.X. has recently been introduced by Sheridan Catheter Corporation in collaboration with Hannallah. It is 100-cm long, with an outer diameter of 4.8 mm and was designed for use with 35 to 41 French Sheri-I-Bronch endobronchial tubes. It has one distal end hole. There are distance markings and "tracheal" and "bronchial" markings to indicate when the distal tip of the E.T.X. is at the opening of the distal lumen. The manufacturer discourages advancement beyond that point. Also, there is no attachment for jet ventilation, and Sheridan discourages jet ventilation with this device.

B. COOK AIRWAY EXCHANGE CATHETERS — DLT

Cook has recently introduced two sizes of double-lumen airway exchange catheters with outer diameters of 11 (OD, 3.7 mm) and 14 French (OD, 6.3 mm). These models (designated C-CAE-11.0-83-DLT and C-CAE-14.0-83-DLT, respectively) are intended for exchange of tubes with an inner diameter of 4 mm and 5 mm or larger. Both are 83-cm long and are provided with 15-mm and Luer-Lok Rapi-Fit adapters. Although the length will only allow for passage through the tracheal lumen, Cook will provide these at any length specified by a user (personal communication, Cook Critical, September, 1994). There are no clinical reports of this product's use.

C. CARDIOMED SUPPLIES

CardioMed has a DLT exchanger under development but specifications are not yet available.

VII. JET VENTILATION THROUGH STYLETS
A. IN VITRO STUDIES

Transtracheal jet ventilation, using an intravenous catheter, has been advocated in the management of the difficult airway, particularly when the trachea cannot be intubated nor the lungs ventilated.[1,78,118] In general, the inspiratory volume depends on gas flow rate, injection time, compliance of the respiratory system, and airway resistance. The expiratory volume will depend on the exhalation time, elastic recoil of the lungs, and resistance of the airway.[126] In vitro studies using jet stylets have been conducted to determine flow, pressure, and entrainment characteristics. Using an in vitro model, with three sizes of Sheridan TTX catheters, Dworkin et al.[126] measured inspiratory and expiratory flow resulting from 50 psi injection as these parameters were manipulated. Gas flows of 63, 33, and 12 L/min were achieved with the large, medium, and small diameter TTX catheters, respectively. The effective tracheal diameter was the difference between the tracheal and TTX diameters, varying according to TTX size. They also varied expiratory resistance by simulating a partial upper-airway obstruction. In their model, if the difference between the tracheal and TTX diameters resulted in an effective tracheal diameter that was greater than 4 to 4.5 mm, air trapping did not occur. Because increased upper-airway resistance and reduced effective tracheal diameter resulted in larger tidal volumes, they concluded that jet ventilation through a long catheter, positioned close to the carina, caused little Venturi effect. Such ventilation was not greatly dependent on air entrainment.

In another in vitro model, calculations based on oxygen dilution and direct measurement using a pneumotachograph revealed that air entrainment accounted for 0% to 31% of the inspired volume. The largest TTX and "lung compliance" resulted in the greatest entrainment.[127] Similarly, this combination resulted in the largest end expiratory volume with a fixed I/E ratio of 1:1 within a compliant system (50 ml/cm H_2O) all three sizes of TTX (5.8-to-3.3 mm OD) resulted in satisfactory tidal volumes. Indeed, with the large size TTX, even in a low-compliance setting, the tidal volume was 1680 ml, prompting the authors to suggest that expiratory times be increased and inspiratory times decreased when using the medium or large TTX.

Prolonging expiratory time reduces the minute ventilation by reducing the respiratory rate while still subjecting the lungs to potentially injurious tidal volumes. An alternative approach would be to reduce the driving pressure. Gaughan et al.[128] assessed the tidal volumes and air entrainment in a model lung, with a range of compliance sets, ventilated by high and low flow regulators through 14-gauge and 20-gauge intravenous catheters. Their high flow regulator, at steady state, produced flow rates of 320 L/min at 100 psi, whereas the low flow regulator produced flows up to 15 L/min at 0 to 5 psi. Intravenous catheters, because of their short length, offer considerably less resistance to flow. They also resulted in significantly greater air entrainment (15% to 74%). Both high and low flow regulators allowed adequate minute ventilation in the setting of normal tracheal and bronchial diameters and normal compliance. Gaughan et al. recommended that during

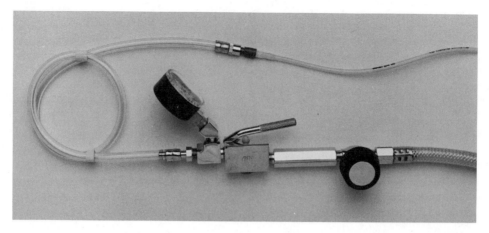

Fig. 39-7. ETVC connected to jet injector. This photograph shows the ETVC attached to a hand-held, jet injector. The ETVC is securely attached by its Luer-Lok adapter (see Fig. 39-6). Only the proximal end of the ETVC is visible in the photograph. The jet injector shown is a pressure-regulator and a gauge, allowing the selection of the lowest ventilation pressure resulting in adequate chest expansion. (Cooper RM, Cohen DR: *Can J Anaesth* 41:1197, 1994.)

transtracheal jet ventilation, when low flow regulators were used, an I/E ratio of 1:1 should be used because it yields the greatest minute ventilation. Although this observation is undoubtedly true, it remains to be determined whether such minute volumes are either clinically necessary or safe.[125,129]

Egol[113] has compared a variety of delivery devices and demonstrated that the pressure at the distal end was inversely related to the number of side holes. Others[75,130] have noted the advantage of multiple distal side holes to minimize catheter whip and center the catheter within the trachea during jet ventilation.

B. IN VIVO STUDIES

Chang et al.[112] provided intraoperative jet ventilation using a 3.5-mm pediatric chest tube as a jet catheter. Ventilating with 15 psi at 10 to 16 breaths/min, they continued until spontaneous ventilation was deemed adequate. The patient recovered and was noted to have a left pneumothorax that the authors attributed to catheter migration and unilateral ventilation. They mentioned that they had encountered three cases of pneumothoraces and one pneumoperitoneum in about 600 such procedures. The authors draw attention to the importance of catheter placement and advise that even brief airway obstruction can result in barotrauma. However, they failed to mention that vocal cord apposition, as recovery occurs, may promote such a complication. In a subsequent paper (see Bedger's Jet Stylet), the authors stated that the "jet stylet" had been used for the ventilation of six patients resulting in normocarbia and adequate oxygenation.[74]

Egol et al. described barotrauma in three patients using a variety of delivery devices and ventilating pressures: a hollow stylet at 50 psi, a nasogastric sump

tube at 20 psi, (I/E = 1:3), and a fiberoptic laryngoscope at 40 psi. They attributed the pneumoperitoneum and pneumothorax they saw in three patients to incorrect catheter placement, ventilation during phonation, and possible direct tissue injury from jet injection. They recommended minimizing airway pressure, providing an adequate expiratory time and using jet catheters with side holes.

The ETVC has been used to provide jet ventilation during general anesthesia, with muscle relaxation on 45 occasions in 40 patients, including 30 tracheostomies[32,130] and endoscopies. The attachment to a hand-held jet injector is illustrated in Fig. 39-7. Irish et al.[32] have described the use of the ETVC in the airway management of 25 patients undergoing percutaneous dilational tracheostomies. They had routinely used driving pressures of 50 psi in anesthetized, paralyzed patients, one of whom had a pneumothorax develop. Arterial blood gas analysis in 12 consecutive patients revealed (mean ± SD) a pH of 7.37 ± 0.09, $PaCO_2$ 45.5 ± 10.8, and PaO_2 256 ± 126. In a subsequent report, a patient ventilated for 90 minutes at only 20 psi, had a pneumothorax develop.[125] Although this may have been a consequence of catheter migration, gas penetration through tissue planes, tracheal instrumentation, or a ball-valve effect from a polypoid bronchial lesion, the authors and others[129] have strongly advised the use of a ventilating pressure adequate to provide chest expansion, muscle relaxation, short inspiratory and long expiratory times, and optimal positioning.

The risks of barotrauma should be carefully weighed against the need for jet ventilation, bearing in mind the possibility of oxygen insufflation. In the author's hands, using the ETVC for jet ventilation, barotrauma complicated 5 of 45 (11%) instances of jet ventilation. Although jet ventilation with the ETVC had in some cases been used in life-threatening circumstances, this complication rate is higher than that which has been previously reported for jet ventilation by stylet.[75,112] Barotrauma will depend on patient selection and techniques that minimize airway pressures or direct tissue injection.[113,125,129]

VIII. CONCLUSION

Successful airway management does not end with tracheal intubation. The ASA Task Force on Management of the Difficult Airway has recommended that each anesthesiologist have a preformulated strategy for extubating the difficult airway. The concept of a "reversible extubation" has been proposed, which allows maintenance of airway access after extubation and facilitates oxygenation, ventilation, and reinsertion of an endotracheal tube should this become necessary. The complications that may accompany routine endotracheal extubations were reviewed. As well, an attempt was made to identify those patients who may be at higher risk after extubation. Very few clinical studies have addressed this issue. Because even high-risk patients are statistically unlikely to require reintubation, any extubation strategy must provide benefits that clearly exceed the risks. Potential benefits include the opportunity of maintaining airway access even after extubation, maintaining oxygenation by insufflation or positive-pressure ventilation, and the possibility of reintubation even when the glottis cannot be seen. Potential risks include discomfort, dislodgment, tracheal aspiration, and trauma. A variety of strategies were reviewed. As yet, there have been no clinical trials or comparisons of these extubation strategies.

REFERENCES

1. Caplan RA, Benumof JL, Berry FA et al: Practice guidelines for management of the difficult airway: a report by the American Society of Anesthesiologists Task Force on Management of the Difficult Airway, *Anesthesiology* 78:597, 1993.
2. Demling RH, Read T, Lind LJ et al: Incidence and morbidity of extubation failure in surgical intensive care patients, *Crit Care Med* 16:573, 1988.
3. Gandia F, Blanco J: Evaluation of indexes predicting the outcome of ventilator weaning and the value of adding supplemental inspiratory load, *Intensive Care Med* 18:327, 1992.
4. Tahvanainen J, Salmenpera M, Nikki P: Extubation criteria after weaning from intermittent mandatory ventilation and continuous positive airway pressure, *Crit Care Med* 11:702, 1983.
5. Sanchez TF: Retrograde intubation, *Anesthesiology clinics of North America,* 13:2, 1995.
6. Hill RS, Koltai PJ, Parnes SM: Airway complications from laryngoscopy and pandenoscopy, *Ann Oto Rhinol Laryngol* 96:691, 1987.
7. Mathew JP, Rosenbaum SH, O'Connor T et al: Emergency tracheal intubation in the postanesthesia care unit: physician error or patient disease: *Anesth Anal* 71:691, 1990.
8. Rose DK, Cohen MM, Wigglesworth DF et al: Critical respiratory events in the postanesthesia care unit, *Anesthesiology* 81:410, 1994.
9. Lacoste L, Gineste D, Karayan J et al: Airway complications in thyroid surgery, *Ann Otol Rhinol Laryngol* 102:441, 1993.
10. Emery SE, Smith MD, Bohlman HH: Upper-airway obstruction after multilevel cervical corpectomy for myelopathy, *Bone Joint Surg* 73:544, 1991.
11. Levelle JP, Martinezx OA: Airway obstruction after bilateral carotid endarterectomy, *Anesthesiology* 63:220, 1985.
12. Tyers MR, Cronin K: Airway obstruction following second operation for carotid endarterectomy, *Anaesth Intensive Care* 14:314, 1986.
13. Miller KA, Harkin CP, Bailey PL: Postoperative tracheal extubation, *Anesth Analg* 80:149-172, 1995.
14. Hartley M, Vaughan RS: Problems associated with tracheal extubation, *Br Anaesth* 71:561, 1993 (review).
15. Coppolo DP, Maty JJ: Self-extubations: a 12-month experience, *Chest* 98:165, 1990, (see comments).
16. Vassal T, Anh NG, Gabillet JM et al: Prospective evaluation of self-extubations in a medical intensive care unit, *Intensive Care Med* 19:340, 1993.
17. Levy H, Griego L: A comparative study of oral endotracheal tube securing methods, *Chest* 104:1537, 1993.
18. Lall NG: Difficult extubation: a fold in the endotracheal cuff, *Anaesthesia* 35:500, 1980.
19. Khan RM, Kahn TZ, Ali M et al: Difficult extubation, *Anaesthesia* 43:515, 1988.
20. Tanski J, James RH: Difficult extubation due to a kinked pilot tube, *Anaesthesia* 41:1060, 1986.
21. Gillespie JA: Difficulty in extubation, *Anaesthesia* 47:715, 1992, (letter; comment).
22. Brock-Utne JG, Jaffe RA, Robins B et al: Difficulty in extubation: a cause for concern, *Anaesthesia* 47:229, 1992 (see comments).
23. Sprung J, Conley SF, Brown M: Unusual cause of difficult extubation, *Anesthesiology* 74:796, 1991, (letter).
24. Heyman DM, Greenfeld AL, Roger JS et al: Inability to deflate the distal cuff of the Laser-Flex tracheal tube preventing extubation after laser surgery of the larynx, *Anesthesiology* 80:236, 1994, (letter).
25. Lee C, Schwartz S, Mik MS: Difficult extubation due to transfixation of a nasotracheal tube by a Kirschner wire, *Anesthesiology* 46:427, 1977.
26. Lang S, Johnson DH, Lanigan DT et al: Difficult tracheal extubation, *Can J Anaesth* 36:340, 1989.
27. Akers JA, Riley RH: Failed extubation due to "sutured" double-lumen tube, *Anaesth Intensive Care* 18:577, 1990 (letter).
28. Dryden GE: Circulatory collapse after pneumonectomy (an unusual complication from the use of a Carlens catheter): case report, *Anesth Anal* 56:451, 1977.
29. Fagraeus L: Difficult extubation following nasotracheal intubation, *Anesthesiology* 49:43, 1978.
30. Hilley MD, Henderson RB, Giesecke AH: Difficult extubation of the trachea, *Anesthesiology* 59:149, 1983.
31. Ciaglia P, Firsching R, Syniec C: Elective percutaneous dilatational tracheostomy: a new simple bedside procedure; preliminary report, *Chest* 87:715, 1985.
32. Irish JC, Brown DH, Cooper RM: How I do it: airway control during percutaneous tracheotomy, *Laryngoscope* 104:1178, 1994.
33. Schwartz LB, Sordill WC, Liebers RM et al: Difficulty in removal of accidentally cut endotracheal tube, *J Oral Maxillofac Surg* 40:518, 1982.
34. Dyson A, Isaac PA, Pennant JH et al: Esmolol attenuates cardiovascular responses to extubation, *Anesth Analg* 71:675, 1990.
35. Muzzi DA, Black S, Lasasso TJ et al: Labetalol and esmolol in the control of hypertension after intracranial surgery, *Anesth Analg* 70:68, 1990.
36. O'Dwyer JP, Yorukoglu D, Harris MN: The use of esmolol to

attenuate the haemodynamic response when extubating patients following cardiac surgery: a double-blind controlled study, *Eur Heart J* 14:701, 1993.

37. Paulissian R, Salem MR, Joseph NJ et al: Hemodynamic responses to endotracheal extubation after coronary artery bypass grafting, *Anesth Analg* 73:10, 1991.

38. Wellwood M et al: Extubation and myocardial ischemia, *Anesthesiology* 61:a132, 1984.

39. Rocke DA, Scoones GP: Rapidly progressive laryngeal oedema associated with pregnancy-aggravated hypertension, *Anaesthesia* 47:141, 1992.

40. Tolley NS, Cheesman TD, Morgan D et al: Dislocated arytenoid: an intubation-induced injury, *Ann R Coll Surg Eng* 72:353, 1990.

41. Blanc VF, Tremblay NAG: The complications of tracheal intubation: a new classification with a review of the literature, *Anesth Analg* 53:202, 1974.

42. Koka BV, Jean IS, Andre JM et al: Postintubation croup in children, *Anesth Analg* 56:501, 1977.

43. Darmon JY, Rauss A, Dreyfuss D et al: Evaluation of risk factors for laryngeal edema after tracheal extubation in adults and its prevention by dexamethasone: a placebo-controlled, double-blind, multicenter study, *Anesthesiology* 77:245, 1992.

44. Gaussorgues P, Boyer F, Piperno D et al: Laryngeal edema after extubation. Do corticosteroids play a role in its prevention? *Presse-Med* 16:1531, 1987.

45. Lewis IH: Required sample size for randomized clinical trials, *Anesthesiology* 78:609, 1993.

46. Benjamin B: Prolonged intubation injuries of the larynx: endoscopic diagnosis, classification, and treatment, *Ann Otol Rhinol Laryngol* 160(suppl):1, 1993 (review).

47. Ikeda S, Hanawa T, Konishi T et al: [Diagnosis, incidence, clinicopathology and surgical treatment of acquired tracheobronchomalacia]. [Japanese], *Nippon Kyobu Shikkan Gakkai Zasshi [Japanese Journal of Thoracic Diseases]* 30:1028, 1992.

48. Amedee RG, Mann WJ, Lyons GD: Tracheomalacia repair using ceramic rings, *Otolaryngology Head Neck Surg* 106:270, 1992.

49. Backus WW, Ward RR, Vitkun SA et al: Postextubation laryngeal spasm in an unanesthetized patient with Parkinson's disease, *J Clin Anesth* 3:314, 1991 (review).

50. Cavo JW, Jr: True vocal cord paralysis following intubation, *Laryngoscope* 95:1352, 1985.

51. Minuck M: Unilateral vocal cord paralysis following endotracheal intubation, *Anesthesiology* 45:448, 1976.

52. Ellis PDM, Pallister WK: Recurrent laryngeal nerve palsy and endotracheal intubation, *J Laryngol Otol* 89:823, 1975.

53. Gibbin KP, Egginton MJ: Bilateral vocal cord paralysis following endotracheal intubation, *Br J Anesth* 53:1091, 1981.

54. Frank LP, Schreiber GC: Pulmonary edema following acute upper airway obstruction, *Anesthesiology* 65:106, 1986.

55. Oswalt CE, Gates GA, Holmstrom FMG: Pulmonary edema as a complication of acute airway obstruction, *JAMA* 238:1833, 1977.

56. Jenkins JG: Pulmonary edema following laryngospasm, *Anesthesiology* 60:611, 1984.

57. Lang SA, Duncan PG, Shephard DAE et al: Pulmonary oedema associated with airway obstruction, *Can J Anaesth* 37:210, 1990.

58. Halow KD, Ford EG: Pulmonary edema following post-operative laryngospasm: a case report and review of the literature, *Am Surg* 59:443, 1993 (review).

59. Dohi S, Okubo N, Kondo Y: Pulmonary oedema after airway obstruction due to bilateral vocal cord paralysis, *Can J Anaesth* 38:492, 1991.

60. Holmes JR, Hensinger RM, Wojtys EW: Postoperative pulmonary edema in young, athletic adults, *Am J Sports Med* 19:365, 1991.

61. Tiret L, Desmonts J, Hatton F et al: Complications associated with anaesthesia: a prospective survey in France, *Can J Anaesth* 33:336, 1986.

62. Burgess GE, Cooper JR, Marino RJ et al: Laryngeal competence after tracheal extubation, *Anesthesiology* 51:73, 1979.

63. Christopher KL, Wood RP, Eckert C et al: Vocal-cord dysfunction presenting as asthma, *New Engl J Med* 308:1566, 1983.

64. Michelsen LG, Vanderspek AFL: An unexpected functional cause of upper airway obstruction, *Anaesthesia* 43:1028, 1988.

65. Hammer G, Schwinn D, Wollman H: Postoperative complications due to paradoxical vocal cord motion, *Anesthesiology* 66:686, 1987.

66. Hayes JP, Nolan MT, Brennan N et al: Three cases of paradoxical vocal cord adduction followed up over a 10-year period, *Chest* 104:678, 1993.

67. Bexton MDR, Radford R: An unsual cause of respiratory obstruction after thyroidectomy, *Anaesthesia* 37:596, 1982.

68. Wade H: Respiratory obstruction in thyroid surgery, *Ann R Coll Surg Eng* 62:15, 1980.

69. Robinson PM: Prospective study of the complications of endoscopic laryngeal surgery, *J Laryngol Otol* 105:356, 1991.

70. Gabrielczyk MR: Acute airway obstruction after uvulo-palatopharyngoplasty for obstructive sleep apnea syndrome, *Anesthesiology* 69:941, 1988.

71. Kunkel JM, Gomez ER, Sebar MJ et al: Wound hematomas after carotid endarterectomy, *Am J Surg* 148:844, 1984.

72. O'Sullivan JC, Wells DG, Wells GR: Difficult airway management with neck swelling after carotid endarterectomy, *Anaesth Intensive Care* 14:460, 1986.

73. Francfort JW, Smullens SN, Gallagher JF et al: Airway compromise after carotid surgery in patients with cervical irradiation, *J Cardiovasc Surg* 30:877, 1989.

74. Phero JC, Weaver JM, Peskin RM: Anesthesia for maxillofacial/mandibular trauma. In Sosis MB: *Anesthesiology clinics of North America,* Philadelphia, 1993, W.B. Saunders.

75. Bedger RC, Chang JL: A jet stylet endotracheal catheter for difficult airway management, *Anesthesiology* 66:221, 1987.

76. Cooper RM, Levytam S: Use of an endotracheal ventilation catheter for difficult extubations, *Anesthesiology* 77:A1110, 1992.

77. Steinberg MJ, Chmiel RA: Use of a nasogastric tube as a guide for endotracheal reintubation, *J Oral Maxillofac Surg* 47:1232, 1989.

78. Benumof JL: Management of the difficult adult airway: with special emphasis on awake tracheal intubation, *Anesthesiology* 75:1087, 1991.

79. Audenaert SM, Montgomery CL, Slayton D et al: Application of the Mizus endotracheal obturator in tracheostomy and tentative extubation, *J Clin Anesth* 3:418, 1991.

80. Wattenmaker I, Concepcion M, Hibberd P et al: Upper-airway obstruction and perioperative management of the airway in patients managed with posterior operations on the cervical spine for rheumatoid arthritis, *J Bone Joint Surg Am* 76:360, 1994.

81. Cooper RM: Upper-airway obstruction after multilevel cervical corpectomy for myelopathy, *J Bone Joint Surg Am* (in press).

82. Broster T, Placek R, Eggers GWN: Epidermolysis bullosa: anesthetic management for cesarean section, *Anesth Analg* 66:341, 1987.

83. James I, Wark H: Airway management during anesthesia in patients with epidermolysis bullosa dystrophica, *Anesthesiology* 56:323, 1982.

84. Fisher GC, Ray DAA: Airway obstruction in epidermolysis bullosa, *Anaesthesia* 44:449, 1989.

85. Yancey KB, Lawley TJ: Immunologically mediated skin diseases. In Wilson JD, Braunwald E, Isselbacher KJ et al: *Harrison's principles of internal medicine,* New York, 1991, McGraw-Hill.

86. Potgieter PD, Hammond JMJ: "Cuff" test for safe extubation following laryngeal edema, *Crit Care Med* 16:818, 1988.

87. Kemper KJ, Benson MS, Bishop MJ: Predictors of postextubation stridor in pediatric trauma patients, *Crit Care Med* 19:352, 1991.

88. Fisher MM, Raper RF: The "cuff-leak" test for extubation, *Anaesthesia* 47:10, 1992.

89. Nunn JF: Ventilatory failure. In Anonymous: *Applied respiratory physiology*, London, 1987, Butterworths.

90. Wade JG, Larson CPJ, Hickey RF: Effect of carotid endarterectomy on carotid chemoreceptor and baroreceptor function in man, *N Engl J Med* 282:823, 1970.

91. Knill RL, Gelb AW: Ventilatory responses to hypoxia and hypercarbia during halothane sedation and anaesthesia in man, *Anesthesiology* 49:244, 1978.

92. Goodman NW: Volatile agents and the ventilatory response to hypoxia, *Br J Anaesth* 72:503, 1994.

93. Nagyova B, Dorrington KL, Robbins PA: Effect of low-dose enflurane on the ventilatory response to hypoxia in humans, *Br J Anaesth* 72:509, 1994.

94. Kopriva CJ, Eltringham RJ, Siebert PE: A comparison of the effects of intravenous innovar and topical spray on the laryngeal closure reflex, *Anesthesiology* 40:596, 1974.

95. Mlinek EJ, Clinton JE, Plummer D et al: Fiberoptic intubation in the emergency department, *Ann Emerg Med* 19:359, 1990.

96. Kemper KJ, Ritz RH, Benson MS et al: Helium-oxygen mixture in the treatment of postextubation stridor in pediatric trauma patients, *Crit Care Med* 19:356, 1991.

97. Garla PG, Skaredoff M: Tracheal extubation, *Anesthesiology* 76:1058, 1992.

98. Dellinger RP: Fiberoptic bronchoscopy in adult airway management, *Crit Care Med* 18:882, 1990.

99. Kemper KJ, Izenberg S, Marvin JA et al: Treatment of postextubation stridor in a pediatric patient with burns: the role of heliox, *J Burn Care Rehabil* 11:337, 1990.

100. Hudes ET, Fisher JA, Guslitz B: Difficult endotracheal reintubations: a simple technique, *Anesthesiology* 64:515, 1986.

101. Rosenbaum SH, Rosenbaum LM, Cole RP et al: Use of the flexible fiberoptic bronchoscope to change endotracheal tubes in critically ill patients, *Anesthesiology* 54:169, 1981.

102. Watson CB: Use of a fiberoptic bronchoscope to change endotracheal tube endorsed, *Anesthesiology* 55:476, 1981.

103. Finucane BT, Kupshik HL: A flexible stilette for replacing damaged tracheal tubes, *Can Anaesthetists' Soc J* 25:153, 1978.

104. Desai SP, Fenci V: A safe technique for changing endotracheal tubes, *Anesthesiology* 53:267, 1980.

105. Robles B, Hester J, Brock-Utne JG: Remember the gum-elastic bougie at extubation, *J Clin Anesth* 5:329, 1993.

106. Tomlinson AA. Difficult tracheal intubation, *Anaesthesia* 40:496, 1985.

107. Baraka A: A simple manoeuver for changing the tracheal tube, *Intensive Care Med* 13:216, 1987.

108. deLima L, Bishop M: Lung laceration after tracheal extubation over a plastic tube changer, *Anesth Analg* 73:350, 1991.

109. Seitz PA, Gravenstein N: Endobronchial rupture from endotracheal reintubation with an endotracheal tube guide, *J Clin Anesth* 1:214, 1989.

110. Chipley PS, Castresana M, Bridges MT et al: Prolonged use of an endotracheal tube changer in a pediatric patient with a potentially compromised airway, *Chest* 105:961, 1994.

111. Cooper RM: Prolonged use of an endotracheal tube changer in a pediatric patient with a potentially compromised airway, *Chest* (in press).

112. Chang JL, Bleyaert A, Bedger RC: Unilateral pneumothorax following jet ventilation during general anesthesia, *Anesthesiology* 53:244, 1980.

113. Egol A, Culpepper JA, Snyder JV: Barotrauma and hypotension resulting from jet ventilation in critically ill patients, *Chest* 88:98, 1985.

114. Patil VU, Buckingham T, Willoughby P et al: Magnetic orotracheal intubation: a new technique, *Anesth Analg* 78:749, 1994.

115. Allison A, McCrory J: Tracheal placement of a gum-elastic bougie using the laryngeal mask airway, *Anaesthesia* 45:419, 1990.

116. Brimacombe J, Berry A: Placement of a Cook airway exchange catheter via the laryngeal mask airway, *Anaesthesia* 48:351, 1993.

117. Benumof JL: Additional safety measures when changing endotracheal tubes, *Anesthesiology* 75:921, 1991.

118. Benumof JL, Scheller MS: The importance of transtracheal jet ventilation in the management of the difficult airway, *Anesthesiology* 71:769, 1989.

119. Benumof JL, Gaughan SD, Ozaki GT et al: Connecting a jet stylet to a jet injector, *Anesthesiology* 74:963, 1991.

120. Cooper RM: Clinical use of an endotracheal ventilation catheter for airway management, *Can J Anaesth* (in press).

121. Katsnelson T, Frost EAM, Farcon E et al: When the endotracheal tube will not pass over the flexible fiberoptic bronchoscope, *Anesthesiology* 76:151, 1992.

122. Levytam S et al: Distal tracheal capnography following general anesthesia, *Anesth Analg* 76:S223, 1993.

123. Athayde JT, Cooper RM, Sandler AN: Use of endotracheal ventilation catheter in monitoring end-tidal CO$_2$ in postoperative cardiac patients after "early extubation," *Anesth Analg* 78:S13, 1994.

124. Hannallah M: Evaluation of tracheal tube exchangers for replacement of double-lumen endotracheal tubes, *Anesthesiology* 77:609, 1992.

125. Cooper RM, Cohen DR: The use of an endotracheal ventilation catheter for jet ventilation during a difficult intubation, *Can J Anaesth* 41:1196, 1994.

126. Dworkin R, Benumof JL, Benumof R et al: The effective tracheal diameter that causes air trapping during jet ventilation, *J Cardiothorac Anesth* 4:731, 1990.

127. Gaughan SD, Benumof JL, Ozaki GT: Quantification of the jet function of a jet stylet, *Anesth Analg* 74:580, 1992.

128. Gaughan SD, Ozaki GT, Benumof JL: A comparison in a lung model of low- and high-flow regulators for transtracheal jet ventilation, *Anesthesiology* 77:189, 1992.

129. Benumof JL, Gaughan SD: Concerns regarding barotrauma during jet ventilation, *Anesthesiology* 76:1072, 1992.

130. Cooper RM, Irish JC, Brown DH: A new technique for percutaneous dilatational tracheostomies using an endotracheal ventilation catheter, *Can J Anaesth* 40:A71, 1993.

Chapter 40

COMPLICATIONS OF MANAGING THE AIRWAY

Cedric R. Bainton

I. INTRODUCTION

Closed claims analysis[1] reveals that adverse outcomes associated with respiratory events constitute the single largest injury to patients. Three mechanisms, failure to ventilate (38%), failure to recognize esophageal intubation (18%), and difficult or failed intubation (17%), accounted for 75% of the adverse events. Death or brain damage occurred in 85% of these cases. In most cases these were errors of omission (i.e., failure to recognize the magnitude of a problem, failure to make appropriate observations, or failure to act in a timely manner).

Other injuries are those of commission with a spectrum from trivial to life-threatening. Injury to the lips and to the nasal, oral, pharyngeal, laryngeal, and tracheal passages is an unavoidable fact of anesthetic practice. As we force entry into the pharynx for a view of the glottis or blindly probe to find this structure, we introduce sharply pointed metal and hard plastic objects to achieve our goal. For the most part we are successful and do not violate the delicate mucosal surfaces of these structures as long as we obey the rules to be gentle; never force; lift, do not pry; be conservative; opt if possible for a direct view; and avoid forceful, blind probing.

To minimize injury we must examine the airway carefully, identify the hurdles that must be overcome, devise a plan with minimal risk for injury, have practiced our skills ahead of time, and have sufficient time to follow out our plan. If time is short, some of these cautions may be pushed aside. For example, in the "no ventilate — difficult intubate" situation, to lose a tooth in the process of intubation is insignificant when survival is in the balance. Common sense should prevail. Quality assurance bodies assume that when injury occurs a mistake has been made. The suggestion of guilt for each injury implies that full knowledge is possible. Rather medical knowledge is incomplete and continues to evolve. Complications are to be evaluated for the new insights and revelations they bring and not simply the rules we may have trespassed. Mistakes can be both logical and technical and can happen at any point in our management, our knowledge base, problem evaluation, conception of a plan, execution of the plan, thinking on our feet and evaluation of what went wrong. Problems also come in the use of new devices and techniques. We must explore these new possibilities but accept the fact that as we gain experience we will discover defects and difficulties we could not possibly have anticipated. This chapter will review the long list of potential pitfalls we can fall into in management of the airway with the hope that the collective experience of our colleagues can reduce the need for each of us, individually, to experience all problems before our education is complete.

II. USE OF THE MASK (SEE CHAPTER 12)

As innocuous as the anesthetic mask may seem, it can be the source of several problems as can mask ventilation.

A. CHEMICAL BURNS

If a reusable mask is used it should be checked for any pinhole defects in the air-filled bladder before it is applied to a patient. If air or fluid is expressed when pressure is applied to the air bladder, the mask must be discarded. Durkan and Fleming[2] reported on how sterilizing solutions found access to the air bladder of such a mask in the process of cleaning. During anesthetic induction, the solution leaked onto the patient's face causing burning and irritation of the patient's eye. Parenthetically such precautions apply to any reusable item. Grigsby et al.[3] incriminate residual gluteraldehyde

on an improperly rinsed laryngoscope blade as the cause of life-threatening allergic glossitis. Cold sterilizing solutions must be thoroughly washed from all surfaces. This is particularly pertinent to a fiberoptic laryngobronchoscope (fiberscope); it is easy to forget the suction channel as a source of caustic gluteraldehyde. The channel must be thoroughly rinsed with water after the cold sterilizing process or gluteraldehyde will drip on the larynx and trachea during laryngoscopy and burns will result. Similarly, the strict rules for ethylene oxide shelf time must be adhered to so that ethylene oxide does not have contact with mucosal surfaces of the patient.

B. DIFFICULTIES WITH MASK FIT AND MAINTENANCE OF AIRWAY

During anesthetic induction, the mask is gently placed on the face for preoxygenation. It is important to note whether the compliant air-filled portion of the mask is properly inflated so that the rigid parts of the mask do not make contact with the bridge of the nose or mandible. Otherwise, bruising will occur at these contact points as pressure is more firmly applied. As induction proceeds, firmer mask pressure will be necessary to provide positive airway pressure to distend pharyngeal structures, maintain pharyngeal air space, and provide ventilation. It will be necessary to apply pressure with fingers to the angle of mandible to maintain a tight mask fit. It is important not to depress the soft submandibular tissues, particularly in the child, or airway obstruction can occur. As greater pressure is applied to the mandible, it may be hard to avoid the mandibular branch of the facial nerve as it crosses over the mandible. Glauber[4] describes how he managed to injure this nerve in a physician colleague who he hoped to avoid intubating for risk of a sore throat. Instead the physician had facial nerve paresis for 3 weeks. Azar and Lear[5] report numbness of the lower lip in two patients. They attribute the injury to excessive pressure exerted by the rim of the mask on the mental nerves where they emerge from the mental foramina in the mandible. Positive airway pressure does not always distend and lift pharyngeal structures. Andersen et al.[6] describe how a large lax epiglottis was pushed caudally to impact in the glottic opening and cause airway obstruction with continuous positive pressure breathing. As induction proceeds, the tongue may fall to the back of the pharynx and obstruct the airway. Oral airways need to be inserted gently to avoid scratching the mucosal surfaces, breaking teeth, or impacting the epiglottis into the glottic opening. Equal care should be given to inserting a nasal airway to avoid a troublesome nosebleed. At some point it may be necessary to apply firm lifting pressure on the angle of the mandible and even sublux the temporomandibular joint (TMJ). Patients may later complain of bruising and pain over these points, and some may have persistent dislocation of the jaw. With airway obstruction, positive pressure may force air quite easily into the stomach instead of the trachea. The stomach may distend, making the patient more prone to regurgitation with increased risk for aspiration. Cricoid pressure can help reduce the possibility of gastric ventilation during this difficult time. Edentulous patients are difficult to mask ventilate. Other patients are those with full beards, large tongues, heavy jaw muscles that resist subluxation of the mandible, poor atlanto-occipital extension, uncertain pharyngeal pathologic lesions, and burns to the face or facial deformities. In such cases it may be best to avoid mask ventilation and opt instead for direct laryngoscopy, if judged to be easy, or awake fiberoptic laryngoscopy. Patients with traumatic rents in pharyngeal mucosa are at risk for pharyngeal emphysema. Playing wind instruments produces intrapharyngeal pressure sufficient to cause diverticula and laryngoceles in the lateral pharynx.[7] These might be at risk for distention during mask ventilation.

C. PROLONGED MASK USE

When a mask is used for a prolonged period, it is important to examine pressure points frequently to make sure blood supply is not being compromised. The bridge of the nose and skin over the mandible are most vulnerable.[8] These areas can be massaged and the mask replaced or it may be necessary to abandon mask ventilation if there is concern. Mask ventilation does not isolate the trachea, thus the patient is at risk for aspiration from silent regurgitation. The anesthetist must be alert to any sign of unexpected coughing or airway noise. Transparent masks are superior to opaque in that they permit a good view of the lips while the mask is in place and more prompt recognition of vomitus. Corneal abrasion is a real possibility. It is important to keep lids closed and avoid undo mask pressure, particularly where there is an open globe injury. Patients with basilar skull fractures are at risk for pneumoencephalus[9,10] with continuous pressure mask ventilation. Rarely otorrhagia can occur.[11]

III. INTUBATION: NASAL
A. CRANIAL INTUBATIONS

Nasal intubation can be hazardous. The classic picture of a nasogastric tube sitting inside the cranium passing through a basilar skull fracture[12] is now surpassed by the frightening picture of an endotracheal tube sitting in that same location.[13] Patients with major facial trauma and basilar skull fractures are not candidates for this approach. Bähr and Stoll[14] challenge this cautious approach. They report that the complication rate in 160 patients with frontobasal skull fractures was not different whether intubation was oral or nasal. They believe that a careful intubation with the help of fiberoptic instrumentation can avoid any problem.

B. NASAL INJURY AND FOREIGN BODIES

All too common and particularly troublesome are nosebleeds. It is so much easier to prevent than to treat one. Thus every consideration must be made for prevention. Nosebleeds can be minimized by using a small endotracheal tube (ET); constricting the nasal mucosa, inserting a soft stint over which the tube can slide, and never using extreme force. An adult male can actually breathe adequately through a 5-mm tube, thus *think small.* A vasoconstrictor must be applied to the nasal mucosa; 0.5% neosynephrine in 4% lidocaine works well, as does 4% cocaine. One approach is to dilate the nasal passage with nasal airways of progressively increasing size before ET insertion. I prefer to gently pass a well-lubricated pediatric esophageal stethoscope through the nose to establish that a channel a priori exists and to gain entrance to the pharynx. The ET can then be passed over this stethoscope as a stent. This prevents the sharp tip of the ET from cutting into the nasal and pharyngeal mucosa to cause bleeding or even a false submucosal passage. Such rents can progress to a retropharyngeal abscess.[15] It also protects the turbinates,[16,17] adenoids, and tonsils from partial excision and minimizes the chance to penetrate a pointing abscess. Foreign bodies in the nares are legion. Smith et al.[18] describe a rhinolith formed around a rubber tire of a toy car that was dislodged during nasal intubation 30 years later. The rhinolith had caused no symptoms. These bodies can be pushed from the nose and into the pharynx without lodging in the tip of the ET by the described method. The esophageal stethoscope can then be removed and the tube suctioned for any blood, saliva, or debris. A similar technique can be used to insert a "split" tube when nasogastric (NG) tube placement is troublesome and a rigid split channel is necessary to guide the NG tube into the esophagus. If a nosebleed does occur, it is important to leave the ET in place in an attempt to tamponade the bleeding. The cuff of the ET can be inflated and the ET retracted to impact into the nasopharynx until bleeding stops. Once the trachea is intubated, it is important to position the ET centrally as it enters the naris. Distortion of the naris can lead to ischemia and necrosis and nasal adhesion. Postintubation sequelae can occur. Sherry and Murday[19] describe an obstructing adhesion extending from the septum to the inferior turbinate occurring 4 months after nasal intubation. Although paranasal sinusitis tends to occur some days after nasal intubation,[20,21] nasal septal abscess and retropharyngeal abscess can occur after short-term intubation.[15]

IV. INTUBATION: ORAL
A. ANATOMIC REQUIREMENTS

There are four anatomic requirements for successful oral laryngoscopy. If any of these is lacking, oral laryngoscopy will be difficult to impossible. Unless thought through carefully, the anesthetist may choose an approach that will increase the chance for injury and complications or leave the anesthetist in the difficult position of "failed intubation." These requirements are adequate oral entry, sufficient pharyngeal space, compliant submandibular tissue, and adequate atlanto-occipital extension.

1. Adequate oral entry

Oral entry may be limited by facial scars, TMJ disease, a large tongue, and, most important, dental disease. Blind nasal or fiberoptic techniques can obviate these problems.

2. Sufficient pharyngeal space

Pharyngeal space can be restricted by tumors, infection, traumatic or surgical disruption, and edema. Whenever the anatomy is distorted, it is important to create the best possible view. There is great merit in intubating while the patient is awake because wakefulness imparts greater pharyngeal space. A tubular blade[22] may be necessary (see Chapter 2c). It is imperative to identify structures properly. If an ET is unwittingly passed through rents in the mucosa of the pharynx, the results can be disastrous.

3. Compliant submandibular tissue

Compliance of submandibular tissue is essential in direct laryngoscopy if the tongue is to be displaced from the pharynx to view the glottis. Compliance is decreased by scarring, after radiation, and by submandibular infection. Direct laryngoscopy will be very difficult in such circumstances, increasing the risk for injury if one persists. It is prudent to start with blind nasal or fiberoptic techniques as they are safer, quicker, and less injury prone.

4. Adequate atlanto-occipital extension

Atlanto-occipital extension is essential to lift the epiglottis off the posterior wall of the pharynx during direct laryngoscopy. If the epiglottis cannot be elevated, glottic structures will not be seen. The fused, fixed, or unstable spine will thus be a problem. Blind nasal or fiberoptic techniques should be used to minimize injury.

B. DENTAL INJURY

Dental injury from the administration of general anesthesia is one of the most common anesthesia-related malpractice claims.[23] Injury is variously reported to range from 1:150 to 1:1000.[24] In New Zealand damage to teeth is viewed as an accepted risk of general anesthesia and not therefore compensatable.[25] Thus anesthesiologists may be personally liable for these expensive repairs. Teeth are dislodged because of poor bony support

structure. Children's primary dentition is poorly supported. Children should be asked to identify teeth that are mobile and be notified that it would be to their advantage to have these removed before or at the time of general anesthesia. When orthodontic braces are removed, the teeth are quite mobile with poor structural support for many months. Periodontal disease destroys structural support for teeth. Minimal pressures applied to these teeth can extract them. If extraction occurs, the tooth should be retrieved and saved in moist gauze without cleansing. The oral surgeon or dentist should be notified. Some teeth, reimplanted and braced, will survive. Carious teeth, capped teeth, and bridges are fragile and easily broken if not removed. Thus teeth can be injured easily in what might otherwise be considered easy intubation circumstances. If other anatomic difficulties for intubation are present, the risk for dental injury goes up exponentially. The prudent choice where risk is high and time permits, is to do an awake blind nasal or fiberoptic intubation to avoid this hazard.

It is extremely important to make a careful dental examination before intubation. All diseased, loose, chipped, and capped teeth are identified, a note made in the chart, and the patient advised as to the risk of damage. Teeth protectors can be used but may be awkward and can obstruct vision.[26]

C. CERVICAL NECK PROBLEMS

If the neck is fused because of ankylosing spondylitis, attempts at direct laryngoscopy have limited chance for success and may create cervical fractures and quadriplegia.[27] The head fixed in a halo-jacket does not permit atlanto-occipital extension and has limited chance to succeed at direct laryngoscopy. These problems lend themselves to blind nasal or fiberoptic intubation as the greatest chance for success. The neck that is unstable because of acute cervical fracture can be supported by axial traction if intubation must proceed promptly. Special concern should be noted for C1 and C2 injuries where any degree of extension might be disastrous for spinal cord survival. A recent report by Hastings and Kelly[28] documents neurologic deterioration associated with direct laryngoscopy in a cervical-spine–injured patient. If time permits, blind nasal and fiberoptic techniques are preferable. Down syndrome and other congenital anomalies are associated with atlanto-axial subluxation.[29] Williams et al[30] describe a child with Down syndrome who complained of severe neck pain on attempted motion 1 month after anesthesia. The child had rotary subluxation of the atlanto-axial joint but no other neurologic symptoms. The child was successfully treated with C-1–C-2 fusion. In these patients a test of full range of motion and degree of atlanto-occipital extension should be established while the patient is awake. If any question exists, neurosurgeons should be consulted. Again, blind nasal fiberoptic techniques should be used to minimize potential injury.

Dong[31] points up the hazard of intubation in undiagnosed Arnold-Chiari malformations. Cerebellar tonsil herniation occurred during intubation for tonsillectomy. The child was seen 1 week after intubation with acquired torticollis, clonus, and hyperactive deep tendon reflexes. Surgical correction was successful and symptoms were resolved.

D. PREEXISTING LARYNGOTRACHEAL TRAUMA

If injury is suspected in larynx or trachea, it is imperative that the lesion be visualized directly or with a fiberscope. The fiberscope can be passed distal to the lesion and the ET passed over the fiberscope as a stent without further injury. If this approach is not used, the results can be disastrous. If time does not permit fiberscope use, the smallest possible tube must be passed gently through the glottic opening. If the tube meets any resistance, the tube must be removed and a tracheostomy performed.

E. CORNEAL ABRASION

Corneal abrasion is possible during the act of intubation. Loosely fitting watch bands, ID tags, and jewelry can scrape the cornea.[32] The ubiquitous stethoscope slung around the neck can fall forward to strike the forehead and eyes.

F. DAMAGE TO THE UVULA

Uvular edema and necrosis can occur in association with intubation.[33,34] It is postulated that direct pressure to the ET or overzealous suctioning may be the cause.

G. VOCAL CORD PARALYSIS

Several authors[35-38] report vocal cord paralysis after endotracheal intubation and difficult gastric tube insertion[39] with no other obvious cause for paralysis. Cavo[36] and Brandwein et al.[35] believe the likely site of injury is pressure of the cuff on the recurrent laryngeal nerve close to or slightly caudad to the vocal process of the arytenoid cartilage. Inflating the cuff below this area would seem an obvious solution. The paralysis is usually temporary.

Mayhew et al.[40] remind us that vocal cord paralysis can have a central origin as well and report paralysis of the left vocal cord in an infant with a Dandy-Walker cyst after insertion of a cyst-to-peritoneal shunt.

H. OTHER NERVE INJURIES

Teichner[41] reports a compression injury to the lingual nerve during a difficult intubation with loss of tongue sensation for 1 month. Aucott et al.[42] identify two patients who had signs of aspiration resulting from supraglottic anesthesia. The authors postulate that the internal branch of the superior laryngeal nerve was damaged during difficult intubation.

I. MACROGLOSSIA

Macroglossia developed 20 minutes after extubation in a 16-month-old child after craniotomy in the sitting position.[43] The case was long (5 hours) and the head was in an extreme flexed position. There was no oral airway or bite block present. The cause is not clear. Teeple et al.[44] describe a similar problem in a 56-year-old woman, despite the fact that they followed the suggestions to avoid an oral airway, bite block, soft tissue compression of chin, and extreme flexion of the head. They suggest that the ET may have severely compressed circulation to the right side of the tongue. They recommend hourly checks of the tongue intraoperatively to identify the problem. Macroglossia was accompanied by marked swelling of the head and neck in a procedure with the head in severe flexion. The authors[45] suggest that major venous compression was the cause. These three cases point to the hazards of severe neck flexion during prolonged surgery. Pressure from the ET on the tongue may play a role, although cause is not clear at this time.

Patane and White[46] point to the insidious development of macroglossia after prolonged cleft palate repair. They caution careful postoperative observation in cases in which the tongue is severely retracted and the procedure lasts longer than 3 hours. Although anesthetic maneuvers may have played no role in producing these cases of macroglossia, the postoperative sequelae of life-threatening airway obstruction is very much our concern.

Massive tongue swelling can occur when the oral ET obstructs the submandibular duct.[47] Patients with airway hemangiomas are at risk for sudden engorgement causing airway obstruction. A child with a diffuse orofacial cavernous hemangioma had severe airway obstruction develop quite unexpectedly after an intramuscular ketamine injection.[48] Hemangiomas are deficient in normal anatomic control. The authors postulate that ketamine, by directly dilating vessels of the hemangioma and increasing systemic pressure, caused the hemangioma to engorge. They conclude that ketamine should be avoided in such circumstances. Exciting new therapy for airway hemangiomas has been identified in recombinant interferon alfa-2a.[49] Interferon alfa-2a is presumed to act as an antiangiogenesis agent.

Macroglossia and angioedema is associated with ACE inhibitors. The edema demonstrates an unusual predilection for the head and neck. Edema of the tongue is commonly the presenting symptom, but involvement of the face, lips, floor of mouth, pharynx, glottis, or larynx is frequently seen. Kharasch[50] describes a case associated with endotracheal intubation. This case reminds us that angioedema can be expected to be an increasing problem now that ACE inhibitors are in such wide use for hypertension control.

J. ASPIRATION

Aspiration of gastric contents is a constant concern when intubating the patient with a full stomach. The use of cricoid pressure has taken a great deal of worry out of the "crash induction." Cricoid pressure is effective even in the presence of an NG tube.[51] It is imperative to make a careful assessment of "ease of intubation" when considering a crash intubation because it is very troublesome to be caught unable to intubate after giving paralyzing drugs. Clearly any patient with limited oral entry, restricted pharyngeal space, diminished submandibular tissue compliance, and limited atlanto-occipital extension will be a poor candidate for a "crash" induction. If ease of intubation is uncertain, it is advisable to secure additional information while the patient is awake. Using oral analgesia it is possible to perform limited pharyngoscopy to determine whether there will be adequate pharyngeal space. If uncertainty persists, awake blind or fiberoptic techniques should be used.

The application of cricoid pressure can sometimes cause complete airway obstruction. This can occur with a lingual tonsil and lingual thyroid gland.[52] It can be a warning of undiagnosed laryngeal trauma.[53] It can occur associated with the use of the LMA.[54]

Harris et al.[55] report an unusual case with the potential for aspiration. The patient had percutaneous lithotripsy for intrahepatic cholelithiasis. At the conclusion of the procedure, 7 liters of 0.9% saline was infused into the common duct for irrigation. Saline refluxed through an "incompetent" pyloric sphincter. During emergence, the patient vomited 1 liter of thin watery gastric contents to the surprise of anesthetists. Vomiting was repeated in the recovery room.

K. ESOPHAGEAL INTUBATION

Esophageal intubation must be recognized promptly (see Chapter 27). A direct view of the ET passing through the glottic opening is very reassuring but not always achieved. It is important to see that the arytenoids are inferior to the ET. Ford[56] describes how posterior displacement of the tube toward the palate assists in providing this view. End-tidal CO_2 confirms proper intratracheal tube placement. The sharp upslope and downslope of breath-by-breath CO_2 tracing marching across the oscilloscope ends all doubt. All other signs can be misleading (good breath sounds, axillary breath sounds, absence of gastric breath sounds, etc.)

Esophageal intubation can briefly produce an end-tidal CO_2[57] tracing, but the concentration decreases rapidly after 5 breaths.

Tracheal intubation is not invariably confirmed by capnography if there is profound bronchospasm[58] or there is no CO_2 delivery to the lung because of absent cardiac output.

L. LESIONS OF THE LARYNX

Kambic and Radsel[59] examined 1000 patients for laryngeal lesions after intubation; 6.2% had severe lesions, 4.5% had hematoma of the vocal cord. Hematoma of the supraglottic region and laceration of vocal cord mucosa were approximately 1% each. They suggest that because intubation almost always has some degree of trauma, the anesthetists should examine the larynx before and after intubation so that lesions can be recognized and proper therapy implemented.

Peppard and Dickens[60] found a small but significant number of patients with laryngeal injury after short-term intubation. Recovery was generally prompt.

Arytenoid displacement is a rare event. Frink and Pattison[61] report a case that followed a traumatic endotracheal intubation. They suggest the natural curve of the ET from mouth to larynx places a force against the arytenoid sufficient to cause dislocation. In other cases it is likely that the forceful technique necessary in a difficult intubation is the cause.[62] Debo et al.[63] report arytenoid subluxation after blind intubation with a lighted wand.

Repeated intubations may result in laryngeal trauma. Wackym et al.[64] report recrudescence of herpes zoster of the larynx under such circumstances.

The vocal process of the arytenoid is the most likely site of damage from the ET as it sits between the cords. Bishop et al.[65] show clearly that the degree of injury increases with increasing size of the ET. It is this point that is the most common site for later granulation formation. Granulations are usually a late complication after long-term intubation but can occur after short-term intubation as well.[66] Longer term intubation results in varying degrees of laryngeal edema and vocal fold ulceration.[67,68]

M. BRONCHIAL INTUBATION

Bronchial intubation occurs frequently and is sometimes hard to identify. Undetected, it leads to atelectasis and hypoxemia. Kramer et al.[69] describe three cases of pulmonary edema after intubation of the right mainstem bronchus. Measurement of tube length can be estimated by placing the tube alongside the face and neck with bifurcation of the trachea taken at the angle of Louis. Transmitted light from a lightwand can identify the tip of the ET in the neck[70] as can a fiberoptic bronchoscope. Palpation of the sharply inflated cuff in the neck above the sternal notch is useful. The tube can be deliberately passed into a mainstem bronchus and then removed until bilateral breath sounds are equal. If there is any question, a fiberscope can give the definitive answer. The tube can advance into a mainstem bronchus with flexion of the head and/or steep Trendelenburg positioning. Thus tube position should be checked after repositioning the patient.

N. TRACHEAL TRAUMA

Tracheal trauma can occur from the use of oversized ETs, overzealous inflation of ET cuffs, and sharp stylets that protrude from the ET. These injuries can produce mucosal tears, hemorrhage, and rupture of the trachea, progressing to mediastinal emphysema and pneumothorax. Seitz and Gravenstein[71] report endobronchial rupture from use of an ET guide or tube changer. They recommend special caution in use of these guides.

ET cuffs inflated to a pressure greater than 30 torr (capillary perfusion pressure) run the risk of devitalizing the mucosa, which progresses to ulceration, necrosis, and loss of structural integrity of the trachea. If the patient is hypotensive, this problem will occur at progressively lower pressures. The need for larger cuff volumes to sustain a positive tracheal seal is an ominous sign that may herald tracheomalacia. The patient with Mounier-Kuhn syndrome (tracheobronchomegaly) is particularly vulnerable to this problem even at very low pressures.[72] It may be necessary to manage these patients with an uncuffed ET and pack the throat with gauze to maintain an airway seal. Massive gastric distention in the intubated patient may herald the presence of a tracheoesophageal fistula as the cuff continues to erode into the esophagus.[73] Patients bleeding more than 10 ml from the ET without cause are suspect for tracheocarotid artery fistula.[74]

O. DOUBLE-LUMEN TUBES

Benumof et al.[75] have defined the limits for safe placement of modern double-lumen ETs. In large part fiberoptic bronchoscopes have taken the mystery out of proper tube placement. The tube can be placed blindly with fiberscope confirmation and readjustment. Alternatively, the fiberscope can be passed through right or left channel into the appropriate mainstem bronchus and the double-lumen tube inserted over the fiberscope as a stent. Problems intraoperatively are again best confirmed and resolved by direct fiberscope observation. Tracheobronchial tree injuries can occur. Bronchial rupture is a serious complication that must be attended to immediately. Precautions are listed: remove the stylet after the tip of the tube is passed through the cords, deflate cuffs when repositioning the patient, and never overinflate cuffs. Wagner et al.[76] were unable to explain the cause of the rupture of the membranous trachea in their patient. Hannallah and Gomes[77] believed the ET was too large for their small patient, resulting in rupture of the left mainstem bronchus.

Benumof[78] provides a technique to prevent overinflation of the left bronchial cuff. With the tracheal cuff inflated and the right (tracheal) lumen open to air, the left lung is inflated. The left cuff is then inflated until the leak disappears.

P. BAROTRAUMA

Barotrauma occurs with high-pressure distention or normal pulmonary structures or at much lower intrapulmonary pressures where disease has weakened tissue. Most notable are high-flow insufflation techniques with a small catheter distal to the larynx. If laryngospasm or some other form of expiratory obstruction develops, there is suddenly no egress for oxygen, and before the anesthesiologist recognizes the problem, the lungs may become overdistended and rupture. These problems are not uncommon in microlaryngeal surgery where jet ventilation is used.[79-83] Egol et al.[81] suggest that direct impingement of the catheter tip on the mucosal surface is a possible cause. They report the problem using the suction part of a fiberoptic laryngoscope for jet delivery of oxygen. Safety mechanisms must be in place to stop oxygen flow if intrapulmonary pressure increases to a dangerous level. For diseased pulmonary tissue, as seen in pneumocystic pneumonia, it is important to devise ways to ventilate at minimal intrapulmonary pressure to avoid a parenchymal blowout. This holds true for the trauma victim with blunt trauma to the chest and subcutaneous emphysema. The patient has an intrapulmonary bronchial leak until proven otherwise, and low-pressure ventilation must be sustained if possible until the lesion is located. Chest tubes obviously help relieve the problem until definitive surgery can be performed.

Q. ESOPHAGEAL PERFORATION AND RETROPHARYNGEAL ABSCESS

Perforation of the esophagus can occur with nasogastric and endotracheal intubation.[84-91] Perforation occurs most often over the cricopharyngeus muscle on the posterior wall of the esophagus. The esophagus is markedly thin and narrowed in this location. Bacterial contamination leads to diffuse cellulitis. Early diagnosis and treatment is extremely important. If mediastinitis results, the mortality rate is more than 50%. Life-threatening airway emergency, subcutaneous emphysema, and pneumothorax can result. Esophageal perforation can also occur in the delivery suite during aggressive airway management of meconium aspiration.[92] Esophageal perforation should be suspected in a patient with subcutaneous emphysema, fever, dysphagia, and a history of difficult intubation.

Traumatic tracheal perforation is reported by way of the esophagus.[93] Intubation was complicated by contractures and poor cervical neck extension. After several attempts, it was believed that the trachea had been intubated and apparently confirmed by a return to 100% oxygen saturation. A postintubation x-ray film revealed that the ET was indeed intratracheal but had taken a unique path by perforating, in turn, the esophagus and membranous trachea.

R. NASOGASTRIC TUBES AND ESOPHAGEAL STETHOSCOPES

Placement of NG tubes can cause many of the same problems of placement caused by ETs: nosebleed, retropharyngeal dissection, perforation of the esophagus, and intracranial intubation.[12] The not uncommon occurrence of finding that the NG tube has passed into the trachea is repeated by Wood et al.[94] In this case the peculiar circumstance of changing head position unkinked the NG tube, which was coiled up in the mouth. The NG tube, not functioning up to that time, suddenly began to evacuate the lung and activated the low-pressure airway alarm.

The esophageal stethoscope can also find its way into the trachea. Pickard and Reid[95] report that a stethoscope found its way into the right lower lobe bronchus, causing collapse of that lobe and significant hypoxemia until it was recognized.

S. LARYNGOSPASM

Reflex responses to intubation can be troublesome. Laryngospasm as described by Fink[96] is more than spastic closure of vocal cords. Rather it constitutes an infolding of arytenoids and aryepiglottic folds, which, in turn, are finally covered by the epiglottis. This explains why vigorous pressure on the angle of the jaw, which elevates the hyoid, in turn puts stretch on the epiglottis and aryepiglottic folds to open the forced closure and help break the spasm. Positive mask airway pressure may be helpful but not necessarily sufficient to break laryngospasm. Thus, succinylcholine may be necessary if hypoxia is to be avoided. Prevention of laryngospasm is the real objective. It is extremely important that no saliva, blood, or gastric contents touch the glottic structures to incite spasm. In situations where every measure must be taken to ensure a laryngospasm-free awakening from anesthesia, it is wise to perform direct laryngoscopy while the patient is deeply anesthetized and suction any suspicious material away from the glottis. Traditional wisdom suggests that the patient should then be extubated while a "deep" level of anesthesia exists or conversely when the patient is responding appropriately to verbal commands. The "danger" period between these two states should be avoided. The patient with a full stomach must have intact pharyngolaryngeal reflexes if aspiration and laryngospasm are to be avoided. These patients fall into the group that must be responding to verbal commands before extubation is contemplated.

T. BRONCHOSPASM

Bronchospasm occurs in response to tracheal irritation of the ET and can be quite intense. It can be broken with administration of inhaled β_2-agonist, deepening inhalant anesthetic, or epinephrine. The best plan is to avoid the problem entirely. In patients with reactive airways, ketamine and inhalant drugs are ideal. A "deep" level of anesthesia should be achieved before the trachea is instrumented. Tracheal lidocaine can be administered as a spray before actual intubation. Sometimes the bronchospasm from this alone is alarming, but usually short-lived. Intravenous lidocaine can also be given before instrumentation.

U. COUGHING AND BUCKING

Coughing and bucking are responses to tracheal intubation and are to be avoided when there is increased intracranial pressure; blood pressure must not be elevated or increased abdominal pressure could rupture an abdominal incision. While the patient is well anesthetized, the trachea can be sprayed with lidocaine particularly at the level of the irritating ET cuff. Intravenous lidocaine can be given just before extubation and again the tube can be removed while a "deep" level of anesthesia persists. It is extremely important to clean the pharynx of any irritating material before extubation as described.

V. APNEA

Apnea is occasionally seen as a reflex tracheal response to irritation of the ET. If the patient has not had narcotics, has a light level of anesthesia, and no other central explanation for apnea exists, the ET may be removed (if it was easy to insert in the first place), to see whether breathing will begin. Reintubation can always be done if necessary.

W. VOMITING

Vomiting as a response to tracheal irritation is not unexpected with a full stomach. However, it need not be a problem. If the airway is secure, the ET must simply be kept in place until the patient clearly responds to verbal commands in a comprehensible fashion. At that point it is safe to remove the ET, but only then.

V. PROBLEMS WHILE THE PATIENT IS INTUBATED
A. AIRWAY OBSTRUCTION

Airway obstruction can occur in every imaginable form. Tubes can kink; be bitten to closure; or become obstructed with blood, mucous casts, foreign bodies, and lubricant. The "saber-sheath" trachea with its narrow elliptical shape can obstruct the tracheal lumen of the double-lumen tube.[97] The plastic coating sheared from a stylet has been described.[98,99] Obstruction of an ET by a prominent aortic knuckle is reported.[100] Gas bubbles trapped in the walls of an ET expanded in the presence of N_2O to obstruct the ET.[101] The anode wire tube is not immune to problems. It can kink at a point between the end of the ET adapter and before the support wire begins. The soft distal tip can fold into the tube and obstruct. Despite its added strength, a patient can bite through the tube.[102] If an anode tube is placed through a tracheostomy site no further than the proximal edge of the cuff, the inflated cuff can alter tube position and abut the tube bevel against the tracheal wall and obstruct the tube.[103] The inflated cuff may compress the ET inward.[104] The cuff may herniate over the tip.[105] The practical solution when confronted by these problems is to pass a suction catheter or fiberoptic bronchoscope down the lumen if time permits. If time does not permit, the tube should be removed and the patient reintubated.

Airway obstruction can also occur by unusual pathologic processes. Two papers report complete airway obstruction caused by achalasia and massive esophageal dilation. One was treated successfully by nitroglycerin,[106] the other by esophageal aspiration.[107]

The widespread use of laparoscopy is revealing unique forms of pathophysiology tension hydrothorax and circulatory compromise in patients with ascites[108] and during operative hysteroscopy.[109]

B. LASER FIRES (SEE CHAPTER 33)

The risk of ET contact with a laser beam is 1:2.[110] Laser fires are commonplace. The laser penetrates the plastic ET. If high concentrations of oxygen are present, the laser creates a fire that propagates in both directions. A "blowtorch" is created, fed by the combustible fuel of pyrolysis, and intensified by high oxygen flow rates. To quench the fire, oxygen and all anesthetics should be turned off and the tube removed. Fire should be extinguished with saline. The airway should be examined for damage and the need for reintubation assessed. Pashayan et al.[111] offer a "helium protocol" to reduce fires. It consists of helium in a concentration of 60% to 80%, the use of unmarked polyvinyl chloride tubes, a limit to laser power, and surgical technique characterized by short repeated bursts of power. Nitrogen works equally well to retard combustion at 80% concentration, but obviously prevents an enriched oxygen environment. N_2O must not be used[112] because N_2O supports combustion. Barium sulfate strip and markings make polyvinyl chloride more flammable.[113-115] Sosis and Dillon[116] have identified the best protective tapes. The new Xomed Laser-Shield is not effective.[117] Intermittent apneic techniques and metal LaserFlex tubes work well.[118] A rigid bronchoscope can also be used effectively.

VI. PROBLEMS OF EXTUBATION (SEE CHAPTER 40)

Sometimes the ET cannot be removed. Surgeons may inadvertently include the ET in their suturing process. Care must be taken to observe the proximity of surgical sutures. Lang et al.[119] advise the frequent inward-outward movement of the tube to identify fixation if the possibility is suspect, as well as routine fiberoptic bronchoscopy through the tube to check for surgical proximity to the ET. When ET cuffs cannot be deflated, it is recommended that the cuff be pierced with transtracheal needle puncture.

VII. EARLY POSTEXTUBATION PROBLEMS
A. HOARSENESS

Lesser and Williams[120] believe that hoarseness, although transient, is due to laryngeal damage because subjective change correlates well with objective changes in voice frequency histogram. Beckford et al.,[121] on the other hand, found little evidence of intrinsic vocal fold trauma. They postulate that extralaryngeal factors may be equally important. Several investigators suggest that acoustic measures may be very useful in identifying and monitoring minor intubation-related trauma.[122,123]

B. POSTOBSTRUCTIVE PULMONARY EDEMA

Postobstructive pulmonary edema has been described in a variety of circumstances.[124-128] The cause is not clear. A common denominator is hypoxia in association with airway obstruction, even for brief periods of time. Other theories suggest a role for negative intrathoracic pressure that develops against a closed glottis and catecholamine activation.[126] The onset can be delayed for some time after the episode of obstruction.[129] It is uncertain how to avoid the problem other than by preventing hypoxia. Any period of airway obstruction with hypoxia is suspect. The condition should be recognized promptly. Reintubation, oxygen, and positive end-expiratory pressure (PEEP) are curative. The condition is usually self-limited when promptly treated.

Naloxone-induced pulmonary edema is a rare but potentially fatal drug reaction. Its cause is uncertain but sympathetic overactivity may play a role. On the basis of this concept, Brimacombe et al.[130] treated one patient with phentolamine with dramatic success.

C. SORE THROATS

Sore throat is a common finding in patients after intubation. Monroe et al.[131] could find no difference in incidence if plastic oropharyngeal airways or gauze bite blocks were used. The incidence was in the range of 40% for both. The incidence was increased to 65% when blood was found on airway instruments. They incriminate aggressive oral suctioning as the likely cause.

Klemola et al.[132] suggest that lidocaine jelly not be used. The incidence of sore throat was greatest when it was used in combination with lidocaine spray.

VIII. PROBLEMS WITH SPECIAL TECHNIQUES

A. LIGHTED STYLET (SEE CHAPTER 18)

The lighted stylet is a recent innovation in which a light at the tip of a flexible stylet transilluminates light through soft tissues so that the position of the stylet can be identified as it is passed through the pharynx, larynx, and trachea. The device can be quite effective in probing for the glottic opening blindly without laryngoscopy[133-135] or as an aid where direct laryngoscopy provides only partial vision. It is also a precise method to locate the tip of an ET placed in the cervical trachea and thus establish that the tube is not inserted too far.[136,137] The use of the lighted stylet suffers from being a blind procedure, thus unsuspected pharyngeal pathologic process will be missed. Likewise if placement of the stylet is not straightforward, one may be reluctant to proceed not knowing whether the problem is a lack of technical skill or a pathologic process that might be made worse with probing.

Complications, real and potential, have been reported; detachment of the bulb,[138] failure to remove a protective tubing that might have become dislodged in the trachea,[139] and arytenoid subluxation[64] have all been reported.

B. RETROGRADE WIRE INTUBATION (SEE CHAPTER 17)

Retrograde wire intubation is an ingenious way to secure a difficult airway. The technique can be used where anatomic limitations prevent a view of glottic structures, including blood, saliva, and traumatic disruption. The blind nature of the technique demands caution such that existing pathologic conditions or traumatic damage is not made worse. A wire is passed cephalad through the cricothyroid or subcricoid region[140] until it is observed protruding from the nose or mouth. An ET is then slipped over the wire and introduced through the pharyngeal and glottic opening until it reaches the point where the wire enters the trachea. The wire is then removed and the ET is advanced into the trachea.

The technique is easy in principle, but there can be problems. The procedure takes time. Often the tip of the endotracheal will "hang up" on glottic structures and not enter the laryngeal opening. A tapered dilator inside the ET can lessen this problem. Alternatively, an epidural catheter can be used as "the wire" that can be looped[141] or tied through the Murphy eye and the tip of the ET. The tip of the ET can now be pulled into the glottic opening avoiding "hang up" on the epiglottis or arytenoids.

There are additional problems. Bleeding can occur at the needle puncture site enough to cause a tracheal clot and potential obstruction. Laryngospasm can occur with irritation of the "wire" unless the laryngeal cords are anesthetized or paralyzed. Thus the technique is not appropriate for the patient with full stomach because the airway cannot be protected.

Faithfull[142] reports injury to the terminal branches of the trigeminal nerve with this technique.

C. FIBEROPTIC NASAL-ORAL ENDOTRACHEAL INTUBATIONS (SEE CHAPTER 16)

The flexible fiberoptic intubating bronchoscope has proved its worth. It combines direct vision with the flexibility to probe the pharynx when oral laryngoscopy is difficult or impossible. It takes time to perform and requires patience, but the rewards are well worth the effort. There is a temptation to believe that this elegant technology can solve all airway problems, and this is simply not so. Fiberoptic intubation should not be attempted when the pharynx is filled with saliva and blood, when there is no pharyngeal space to look around and identify pharyngeal structures, or when time has run out and a surgical cricothyrotomy is the immediate priority. The corollary to these warnings is that every effort must be made to provide a dry field and prevent a nosebleed while performing fiberoptic laryngoscopy. Another potential hazard to the patient is the practice of insufflating oxygen through the suction channel. This technique has the advantage to help keep the fiber tip clean by blowing saliva and blood from the fiber tip and by providing high inspired oxygen. I have had the unfortunate experience to have the sharp fiber tip cut the pharyngeal mucosa. Insufflation oxygen then dissected under the mucosa to cause significant emphysema of pharynx, face, and periorbital areas. This can happen intratracheally if the fiber tip becomes submucosal,[82] with potentially disastrous results.

D. TRANSTRACHEAL VENTILATION (SEE CHAPTER 23)

Transtracheal ventilation is an elegant method to salvage a "can't ventilate—can't intubate" situation.[143,144] Yealy et al.[145] demonstrate that the technique can effectively prevent aspiration in a canine model at specific frequencies and head elevation. It can be an aid to fiberoptic intubation.[146] But there are life-threatening problems associated with this technique. It is often recommended that a 3 to 4-inch catheter be used to deliver oxygen to the trachea through the cricothyroid membrane. If this catheter should be displaced to a subcutaneous position, oxygen delivered could produce subcutaneous emphysema progressing quickly to mediastinal emphysema, pneumothorax, and death. The natural movement of compliant skin in the neck can be 3 to 4 inches. Thus a catheter of this length, sutured to the skin, can be displaced to the subcutaneous position if tension occurs inadvertently at the skin suture site, for example, if someone should stumble over the oxygen source hose attached to this transtracheal catheter. This problem can be solved by using an 8-inch catheter, which can more than accommodate to any accidental skin displacement. Barotrauma is equally serious.[147,148] Oxygen delivered through a transtracheal catheter must have free egress through the larynx or overdistention can lead to lung rupture. Laryngospasm can obstruct oxygen egress. It must be prevented by either local analgesia of the laryngeal structures or by muscle paralysis if jet ventilation is planned.[148] If the larynx is totally obstructed because of a foreign body, only low-flow oxygen can be given through the catheter in an amount equal to metabolic oxygen consumption. If jet ventilation is being supplied by an intratracheal route, these same admonitions apply. If the delivery line is inadvertently introduced into the stomach, gastric rupture can occur.[149]

Slow intratracheal bleeding can be a final problem of this technique. This has been a problem for internists who may leave transtracheal catheters in for many days to aspirate repeated sputum samples. For anesthesiologists who use the technique acutely, this has not been a reported problem.

E. THE LARYNGEAL MASK AIRWAY (SEE CHAPTER 19)

The LMA is composed of a conventional tracheal tube that has been cut diagonally at approximately 20 cm from the proximal end. An elliptical mask is attached to the distal end of the tracheal tube, the rim of which can be inflated or deflated by means of an attached pilot tube. The mask is inserted into the posterior pharynx, and when inflated forms a snug fit directly over the glottic opening. The attached tracheal tube projecting from the mouth is attached to the gas delivery system. There can be difficulties in placement of the mask. The mask can fold over on itself. The epiglottis can be impacted into the glottic opening or entrapped into the laryngeal inlet of the mask. Despite these imperfect applications, it is remarkable that airway patency is maintained in most cases.

In the few years since its introduction, the LMA has achieved broad acceptance and wide use. A recent review by Pennant and White[150] thoroughly discusses all aspects of LMA use. The LMA would seem to have a clear advantage when laryngeal trauma must be minimized (singers); standard mask fit is impossible or undesirable because of facial burns, delicate skin, or full beard; light planes of anesthesia are desired; and/or

patients are returning for frequent repeated procedures. It has also saved many difficult situations where mask ventilation was ineffective and direct laryngoscopy impossible.

There are also contraindications to its use. Because the LMA does not isolate the trachea from the esophagus, its use will be risky when the patient has a full stomach or when high airway pressures are necessary to ventilate the patient. This problem is compounded by the fact that cricoid pressure may prevent insertion of the LMA[151] and the LMA relaxes the lower esophageal sphincter.[152] Complications are thoroughly discussed in the Pennant and White review.[150] These include aspiration pneumonitis, inflation of the stomach, impacting a floppy epiglottis into the glottic opening, laryngospasm, epiglottic edema, dysarthria, mask overinflation causing airway obstruction, uvular bruising, and posterior pharyngeal wall edema.

Since this review, hypoglossal nerve paralysis has been identified[153,154] presumably caused by an overinflated laryngeal mask compressing the nerve against the hyoid bone. Postobstructive pulmonary edema[155] and tongue cyanosis[156] are reported.

F. COMBITUBE (SEE CHAPTER 22)

The Combitube (Sheridan Catheter Corporation, Argyle, New York) is an esophagotracheal double-lumen airway. It is designed for emergency use when standard measures of airway management have failed. The Combitube is inserted blindly into the mouth and advanced to preset markings. The distal tube will usually be positioned in the esophagus at this point. A distal cuff on the esophageal tube is inflated (15 cc). The pharyngeal cuff (100 cc) is also inflated. Ventilation is then attempted through the esophageal tube. If ventilation through the esophageal tube does not occur after repositioning the device, cautious ventilation of the ET should establish whether it is positioned in the trachea.

This device is new. Most reports are enthusiastic discriptions of its success in difficult situations. One paper[157] describes how too deep an insertion of the Combitube will cause the large pharyngeal cuff to lie directly over the glottic opening and obstruct the glottis when inflated. Withdrawing the Combitube a few centimeters from the mouth can solve the problem.

IX. CONCLUSION

I have dealt with the complications anesthesiologists may encounter in management of the airway. Errors can be both technical and judgmental. We need to study these events for the lessons we can learn. To minimize problems, it is important to think out problems ahead of time, devise safe plans, instrument under direct vision, be gentle, avoid sharp objects, be conservative, and use common sense.

REFERENCES

1. Caplan RA et al: Adverse respiratory events in anesthesia: a closed claims analysis, *Anesthesiology* 72:828, 1990.
2. Durkan W, Fleming N: Potential eye damage from reusable masks, *Anesthesiology* 67:444, 1987.
3. Grigsby EJ et al: Massive tongue swelling after uncomplicated general anaesthesia, *Can J Anaesth* 37:825, 1990.
4. Glauber DT: Facial paralysis after general anesthesia, *Anesthesiology* 65:516, 1986.
5. Azar I, Lear E: Lower lip numbness following general anesthesia, *Anesthesiology* 65:450, 1986.
6. Andersen APD et al: Obstructive sleep apnea initiated by lax epiglottis: a contraindication for continuous positive airway pressure, *Chest* 91:621, 1987.
7. Langley JM, Salisbury SR: Trombonist's Torment, *N Engl J Med* 327:1533, 1992.
8. Smurthwaite GJ, Ford P: Skin necrosis following continuous positive airway pressure with a face mask, *Anaesthesia* 48:147, 1993.
9. Jarjour NN, Wilson P: Pneumocephalus associated with nasal continuous positive airway pressure in a patient with sleep apnea syndrome, *Chest* 96:1425, 1989.
10. Klopfenstein CE, Forster A, Suter PM: Pneumocephalus: a complication of continuous positive airway pressure after trauma, *Chest* 78:656, 1980.
11. Weaver LK, Fairfax WR, Greenway L: Bilateral otorrhagia associated with continuous positive airway pressure, *Chest* 93:878, 1988.
12. Seebacher J, Nozik D, Mathieu A: Inadvertent intracranial introduction of a nasogastric tube: a complication of severe maxillofacial trauma, *Anesthesiology* 42:100, 1975.
13. Horellou MF, Mathe D, Feiss P: A hazard of naso-tracheal intubation, *Anaesthesia* 33:73, 1978.
14. Bähr W, Stoll P: Nasal intubation in the presence of frontobasal fractures: a retrospective study, *J Oral Maxillofac Surg* 50:445, 1992.
15. Hariri MA, Duncan PW: Infective complications of brief nasotracheal intubation, *J Laryngol Otol* 103:1217, 1989.
16. Cooper R: Bloodless turbinectomy following blind nasal intubation, *Anesthesiology* 71:469, 1989.
17. Wilkinson JA, Mathis RD, Dire DJ: Turbinate destruction: a rare complication of nasotracheal intubation, *J Emerg Med* 4:209, 1986.
18. Smith WD, Timms MS, Sutcliffe H: Unusual complication of nasopharyngeal intubation, *Anaesthesia* 44:615, 1989.
19. Sherry KM, Murday A: A nasal adhesion following prolonged nasotracheal intubation, *Anaesthesia* 42:651, 1987.
20. Arens JF, LeJeune FE Jr, Webre DR: Maxillary sinusitis, a complication of nasotracheal intubation, *Anesthesiology* 40:415, 1974.
21. Fassoulaki A, Pamouktsoglou P: Prolonged nasotracheal intubation and its association with inflammation of paranasal sinuses, *Anesth Analog* 69:50, 1989.
22. Bainton CR: A new laryngoscope blade to overcome pharyngeal obstruction, *Anesthesiology* 67:767, 1987.
23. Rosenberg MB: Anesthesia-induced dental injury, *Int Anesthesiol Clin* 27:120, 1989.
24. Lockhart PB et al: Dental complications during and after tracheal intubation, *J Am Dent Assoc* 112:480, 1986.
25. Burton JF, Baker AB: Dental damage during anaesthesia and surgery, *Anaesth Intensive Care* 15:262, 1987.
26. Aromaa U et al: Difficulties with tooth protectors in endotracheal intubation, *Acta Anaesthesiol Scand* 32:304, 1988.
27. Salathé M, Jöhr M: Unsuspected cervical fractures: a common problem in ankylosing spondylitis, *Anesthesiology* 70:869, 1989.
28. Hastings RH, Kelly SD: Neurologic deterioration associated with airway management in a cervical spine-injured patient, *Anesthesiology* 78:580, 1993.
29. Crosby ET, Lui A: The adult cervical spine: implications for airway management, *Can J Anaesth* 37:77, 1990.
30. Williams JP et al: Atlanto-axial subluxation and trisomy-21: another perioperative complication, *Anesthesiology* 67:253, 1987.
31. Dong ML: Arnold-Chiari malformation type I appearing after tonsillectomy, *Anesthesiology* 67:120, 1987.
32. Watson WJ, Moran RL: Corneal abrasion during induction, *Anesthesiology* 66:440, 1987.
33. Krantz MA, Solomon DL, Poulos JC: Uvular necrosis following endotracheal intubation, *J Clin Anesth* 6:139, 1994.
34. Diaz J: Is uvular edema a complication of endotracheal intubation? *Anesth Analg* 76:1139, 1993.
35. Brandwein M, Abramson AL, Shikowitz MJ: Bilateral vocal cord paralysis following endotracheal intubation, *Arch Otolaryngol Head Neck Surg* 112:877, 1986.
36. Cavo JW Jr: True vocal paralysis following intubation, *Laryngoscope* 95:1352, 1985.
37. Lim EK, Chia KS, Ng BK: Recurrent laryngeal nerve palsy following endotracheal intubation, *Anaesth Intensive Care* 15:342, 1987.
38. Nuutinen J, Kärjä J: Bilateral vocal cord paralysis following general anesthesia, *Laryngoscope* 91:83, 1981.
39. Ibuki T, Ando N, Tanako Y: Vocal cord paralysis associated with difficult gastric tube insertion, *Can J Anaesth* 41:431, 1994.
40. Mayhew JF, Miner ME, Denneny J: Upper airway obstruction following cyst-to-peritoneal shunt in a child with a Dandy-Walker cyst, *Anesthesiology* 62:183, 1985.
41. Teichner RL: Lingual nerve injury: a complication of orotracheal intubation, *Br J Anaesth* 43:413, 1971.
42. Aucott W, Prinsley P, Madden G: Laryngeal anaesthesia with aspiration following intubation, *Anaesthesia* 44:230, 1989.
43. Mayhew JF, Miner M, Katz J: Macroglossia in a 16-month-old child after a craniotomy, *Anesthesiology* 62:683, 1985.
44. Teeple E, Maroon J, Rueger R: Hemimacroglossia and unilateral ischemic necrosis of the tongue in a long-duration neurosurgical procedure, *Anesthesiology* 64:845, 1986.
45. Ellis SC, Bryan-Brown CW, Hyderally H: Massive swelling of the head and neck, *Anesthesiology* 42:102, 1975.
46. Patane PS, White SE: Macroglossia causing airway obstruction following cleft palate repair, *Anesthesiology* 71:995, 1989.
47. Huehns TY, Yentis SM, Cumberworth V: Apparent massive tongue swelling, *Anaesthesia* 49:414, 1994.
48. Baronia AK, Pandey CK, Kaushik S: Diffuse oral facial cavernous hemangioma causing severe airway obstruction after intramuscular ketamine, *Anesthesiology* 79:142, 1993.
49. Ohlms LA et al: Interferon alfa-2a therapy for airway hemangiomas, *Ann Otol Rhinol Laryngol* 103:1, 1994.
50. Kharasch ED: Angiotensin-converting enzyme inhibitor-induced angioedema associated with endotracheal intubation, *Anesth Analg* 74:602, 1992.
51. Salem MR et al: Cricoid compression is effective in obliterating the esophageal lumen in the presence of a nasogastric tube, *Anesthesiology* 63:443, 1985.
52. Georgescu A, Miller JN, Lecklitner ML: The Selleck maneuver causing complete airway obstruction, *Anesth Analg* 74:457, 1992.
53. Shorten GD, Alfille PH, Gliklich R: Airway obstruction following application of cricoid pressure, *J Clin Anesth* 3:403, 1991.
54. Brimacombe JR, Berry A: Mechanical airway obstruction after cricoid pressure with the laryngeal mask airway, *Anesth Analg* 78:601, 1994.
55. Harris M et al: Gastroduodenal reflux of irrigating solution during percutaneous lithotripsy for intrahepatic cholelithiasis, *Anesthesiology* 62:182, 1985.

56. Ford RWJ: Confirming tracheal intubation: a simple manoeuvre, *Can Anaesth Soc J* 30:191, 1983.

57. Sum Ping ST: Esophageal intubation, *Anesth Analg* 66:483, 1987.

58. Dunn SM et al: Tracheal intubation is not invariably confirmed by capnography, *Anesthesiology* 73:1285, 1990.

59. Kambic V, Radsel Z: Intubation lesions of the larynx, *Br J Anaesth* 50:587, 1978.

60. Peppard SB, Dickens JH: Laryngeal injury following short-term intubation, *Ann Otol Rhinol Laryngol* 92(4 pt 1):327, 1983.

61. Frink EJ, Pattison BD: Posterior arytenoid dislocation following uneventful endotracheal intubation and anesthesia, *Anesthesiology* 70:358, 1989.

62. Gray B, Huggins NJ, Hirsch N: An unusual complication of tracheal intubation, *Anaesthesia* 45:558, 1990.

63. Debo RF et al: Cricoarytenoid subluxation: complication of blind intubation with a lighted stylet, *Ear Nose Throat J* 68:517, 1989.

64. Wackym PA, Gray GF Jr, Avant GR: Herpes zoster of the larynx after intubational trauma, *J Laryngol Otol* 100:839, 1986.

65. Bishop MJ, Weymuller EA Jr, Fink BR: Laryngeal effects of prolonged intubation, *Anesth Analg* 63:335, 1984.

66. Drosnes DL, Zwillenberg DA: Laryngeal granulomatous polyp after short-term intubation of a child, *Ann Otol Rhinol Laryngol* 99:183, 1990.

67. Alessi DM, Hanson DG, Berci G: Bedside videolaryngoscopic assessment of intubation trauma, *Ann Otol Rhinol Laryngol* 98:586, 1989.

68. Colice GL, Stukel TA, Dain B: Laryngeal complications of prolonged intubation, *Chest* 96:877, 1989.

69. Kramer MR, Melzer E, Sprung CL: Unilateral pulmonary edema after intubation of the right mainstem bronchus, *Crit Care Med* 17:472, 1989.

70. Mehta S: Guided orotracheal intubation in the operating room using a lighted stylet, *Anesthesiology* 66:105, 1987.

71. Seitz PA, Gravenstein N: Endobronchial rupture from endotracheal reintubation with an endotracheal tube guide, *J Clin Anesth* 1:214, 1989.

72. Messahel FM: Tracheal dilatation followed by stenosis in Mounier-Kuhn syndrome, *Anaesthesia,* 44:227, 1989.

73. Tessler S et al: Massive gastric distention in the intubated patient, *Arch Intern Med* 150:318, 1990.

74. LoCicero J III: Tracheo-carotid artery erosion following endotracheal intubation, *J Trauma* 24:907, 1984.

75. Benumof JL et al: Margin of safety in positioning modern double-lumen endotracheal tubes, *Anesthesiology* 67:729, 1987.

76. Wagner DL, Gammage GW, Wong ML: Tracheal rupture following the insertion of a disposable double-lumen endotracheal tube, *Anesthesiology* 63:698, 1985.

77. Hannallah M, Gomes M: Bronchial rupture associated with the use of double-lumen tube in a small adult, *Anesthesiology* 71:457, 1989.

78. Benumof JL: Physiology of the open chest and one lung ventilation. In Benumof JL, editor: *Anesthesia for Thoracic Surgery,* ed 2, Philadelphia, 1994, Saunders.

79. Badran I, Jamal M: Pneumomediastinum due to Venturi system during microlaryngoscopy, *Middle East J Anesthesiol* 9:561, 1988.

80. Chang JL, Bleyaert A, Bedger R: Unilateral pneumothorax following jet ventilation during general anesthesia, *Anesthesiology* 53:244, 1980.

81. Egol A, Culpepper JA, Snyder JV: Barotrauma and hypotension resulting from jet ventilation in critically ill patients, *Chest* 88:98, 1985.

82. O'Sullivan TJ, Healy GB: Complications of Venturi jet ventilation during microlaryngeal surgery, *Arch Otolaryngol* 111:127, 1985.

83. Wetmore SJ, Key JM, Suen JY: Complications of laser surgery for laryngeal papillomatosis, *Laryngoscope* 95(7 pt 1):798, 1985.

84. Eldor J, Ofek B, Abramowitz HB: Perforation of oesophagus by tracheal tube during resuscitation, *Anaesthesia* 45:70, 1990.

85. Johnson KG, Hood DD: Esophageal perforation associated with endotracheal intubation, *Anesthesiology* 64:281, 1986.

86. Kras JF, Marchmont-Robinson H: Pharyngeal perforation during intubation in a patient with Crohn's disease, *J Oral Maxillofac Surg* 47:405, 1989.

87. Levine PA: Hypopharyngeal perforation: an untoward complication of endotracheal intubation, *Arch Otolaryngol* 106:578, 1980.

88. Majumdar B, Stevens RW, Obara LG: Retropharyngeal abscess following tracheal intubation, *Anaesthesia* 37:67, 1982.

89. Norman EA, Sosis M: Iatrogenic oesophageal perforation due to tracheal or nasogastric intubation, *Can Anaesth Soc J* 33:222, 1986.

90. Wengen DF: Piriform fossa perforation during attempted tracheal intubation, *Anaesthesia* 42:519, 1987.

91. Young PN, Robinson JM: Cellulitis as a complication of difficult tracheal intubation, *Anesthesia* 42:569, 1987 (letter).

92. Topsis J, Kinas HY, Kandall SR: Esophageal perforation: a complication of neonatal resuscitation, *Anesth Analg* 69:532, 1989.

93. Reyes G, Galvis AG, Thompson JW: Esophagotracheal perforation during emergency intubation, *Am J Emerg Med* 10:223, 1992.

94. Wood G et al: Ventilatory failure due to an improperly placed nasogastric tube, *Can J Anaesth* 37:587, 1990.

95. Pickard WA, Reid L: Hypoxia caused by an esophageal stethoscope, *Anesthesiology* 65:534, 1986.

96. Fink BR: Laryngeal complications of general anesthesia. In: Orkin FK, Cooperman LH, editors: *Complications in anesthesiology,* Philadelphia, 1983, JB Lippincott.

97. Bayes J et al: Obstruction of a double-lumen tube by a saber-sheath trachea, *Anesth Analg* 79:186, 1994.

98. Cook WP, Schultetus RR: Obstruction of an endotracheal tube by the plastic coating sheared from a stylet, *Anesthesiology* 62:803, 1985.

99. Zmyslowski WP, Kam D, Simpson GT: An unusual cause of endotracheal tube obstruction, *Anesthesiology* 70:883, 1989.

100. Sapsford DJ, Snowdon SL: If in doubt, take it out: obstruction of tracheal tube by prominent aortic knuckle, *Anaesthesia* 40:552, 1985.

101. Populaire C, Robard S, Souron R: An armoured endotracheal tube obstruction in a child, *Can J Anaesth* 36(3 pt 1):331, 1989.

102. Gemma M, Ferrazza C: "Dental trauma" to oral airways, *Can J Anaesth* 37:951, 1990.

103. Riley RH, Mason SA, Barber CD: Obstruction of a preformed armoured tracheostomy tube, *Can J Anaesth* 37:824, 1990.

104. Wright PJ, Mundy JVB, Mansfield CJ: Obstruction of armoured tracheal tubes: cause report and discussion, *Can J Anaesth* 35:195, 1988.

105. Treffers R, de Lange JJ: An unusual case of cuff herniation, *Acta Anaesthesiol Belg* 40:87, 1989.

106. Westbrook JL: Oesophageal achalasia causing respiratory obstruction, *Anaesthesia* 47:38, 1992.

107. Kendall AP, Lin E: Respiratory failure as presentation of achalasia of the esophagus, *Anaesthesia* 46:1039, 1991.

108. McConnel MS, Finn JC, Feeley TW: Tension hydrothorax during laparoscopy in a patient with ascites, *Anesthesiology* 80:1390, 1994.

109. Gallagher M, Roberts-Fox M: Respiratory and circulatory compromise associated with acute hydrothorax during operative hysteroscopy, *Anesthesiology* 79:1129, 1993.

110. Pashayan AG, Gravenstein N: High incidence of CO_2 laser beam contact with the tracheal tube during operations on the upper airway, *J Clin Anesth* 1:354, 1989.

111. Pashayan AG et al: The helium protocol for laryngotracheal

operations with CO_2 laser: a retrospective review of 523 cases, *Anesthesiology* 68:801, 1988.

112. Wolf GL, Simpson JI: Flammability of endotracheal tubes in oxygen and nitrous oxide enriched atmosphere, *Anesthesiology* 67:236, 1987.

113. Geffin B et al: Flammability of endotracheal tubes during Nd-YAG laser application in the airway, *Anesthesiology* 65:511, 1986.

114. Pashayan AG, Gravenstein JS: Helium retards endotracheal tube fires from carbon dioxide lasers, *Anesthesiology* 62:274, 1985.

115. Pashayan AG, Gravenstein JS: On reducing the flammability of PVC, *Anesthesiology* 68:173, 1988.

116. Sosis MB, Dillon F: What is the safest foil tape for endotracheal tube protection during Nd-YAG laser surgery? A comparative report, *Anesthesiology* 72:553, 1990.

117. Sosis MB: Airway fire during CO_2 laser surgery using a Xomed laser endotracheal tube, *Anesthesiology* 72:747, 1990.

118. Hawkins DB, Joseph MM: Avoiding a wrapped endotracheal tube in laser laryngeal surgery: experiences with apneic anesthesia and metal Laser-Flex endotracheal tubes, *Laryngoscope* 100:1283, 1990.

119. Lang S et al: Difficult tracheal extubation, *Can J Anaesth* 36(3 pt 1):340, 1989.

120. Lesser T, Williams G: Laryngographic investigation of postoperative hoarseness, *Clin Otolaryngol* 13:37, 1988.

121. Beckford NS et al: Effects of short-term endotracheal intubation on vocal function, *Laryngoscope* 100:331, 1990.

122. Priebe H-J, Henke W, Hedley-Whyte J: Effects of tracheal intubation on laryngeal acoustic waveforms, *Anesth Analg* 67:219, 1988.

123. Yonick TA et al: Acoustical effects of endotracheal intubation, *J Speech Hearing Disord* 55:427, 1990.

124. Frank LP, Schreiber GC: Pulmonary edema following acute upper airway obstruction, *Anesthesiology* 65:106, 1986.

125. Herrick IA, Mahendran B, Penny FJ: Postobstructive pulmonary edema following anesthesia, *J Clin Anesth* 2:116, 1990.

126. Lang SA et al: Pulmonary oedema associated with airway obstruction, *Can J Anaesth* 37:210, 1990.

127. Warner LO, Beach TP, Martino JD: Negative pressure pulmonary oedema secondary to airway obstruction in an intubated infant, *Can J Anaesth* 35:507, 1988.

128. Wilder RT, Belani KG: Fiberoptic intubation complicated by pulmonary edema in a 12-year old child with Hurler syndrome, *Anesthesiology* 72:205, 1990.

129. Glasser SA, Siler JN: Delayed onset of laryngospasm-induced pulmonary edema in an adult outpatient, *Anesthesiology* 62:370, 1985.

130. Brimacombe J et al: Two cases of naxolone-induced pulmonary oedema: the possible use of phentolamine in management, *Anaesth Intensive Care* 19:578, 1991.

131. Monroe MC, Gravenstein N, Saga-Rumley S: Postoperative sore throat: effect of oropharyngeal airway in orotracheally intubated patients, *Anesth Analg* 70:512, 1990.

132. Klemola U-M, Saarnivaara L, Yrjölä H: Post-operative sore throat: effect of lignocaine jelly and spray with endotracheal intubation, *Eur J Anesthesiol* 5:391, 1988.

133. Ellis DG et al: Guided orotracheal intubation in the operating room using a lighted stylet: a comparison with direct laryngoscopic technique, *Anesthesiology* 64:823, 1986.

134. Hartman et al: Rapid orotracheal intubation in the clenched-jaw patient: a modification of the light wand technique, *J Clin Anesthesia* 4:245, 1992.

135. Fox DJ, Matson MD: Management of the difficult pediatric airway in an austere environment using the light wand, *J Clin Anesthesia* 2:123, 1990.

136. Stewart RD et al: Correct positioning of an endotracheal tube using a flexible lighted stylet, *Crit Care Med* 18:97, 1990.

137. Mehta S: Transtracheal illumination for optimal tracheal tube placement, *Anaesthesia* 44:970, 1989.

138. Dowson S, Greenwald KM: A potential complication of lightwand-guided intubation, *Anesth Analg* 74:169, 1992 (letter).

139. Monkabary K, Peterson CJ, Kingsley CP: A potential complication of the lightwand, *Anesthesiology* 81:523, 1994 (letter).

140. Shantha TR: Retrograde intubation using the subcricoid region, *Br J Anaesthesia* 68:109, 1992.

141. Abou-Madi MN: Pulling versus guiding: a modification of retrograde guided intubation, *Can J Anaesthesia* 36:336, 1989.

142. Faithfull NS: Injury to terminal branches of the trigeminal nerve following tracheal intubation, *Br J Anaesth* 57:535, 1985.

143. Benumof JL, Scheller MS: The importance of transtracheal jet ventilation in the management of the difficult airway, *Anesthesiology* 71:769, 1989.

144. Weymuller EF Jr et al: Management of difficult airway problems with percutaneous transtracheal ventilation, *Ann Otol Rhinol Laryngol* 96(1 pt 1):34, 1987.

145. Yealy DM et al: Manual translaryngeal jet ventilation and the risk of aspiration in a canine model, *Ann Emerg Med* 19:1238, 1990.

146. Boucek CD, Gunnerson HB, Tullock WC: Percutaneous transtracheal high-frequency jet ventilation as an aid to fiberoptic intubation, *Anesthesiology* 67:247, 1987.

147. Craft TM et al: Two cases of barotrauma associated with transtracheal jet ventilation, *Br J Anaesth* 64:524, 1990.

148. Schumacher P et al: Laryngospasm during transtracheal high frequency jet ventilation, *Anaesthesia* 47:855, 1992.

149. Sichel et al: Complications of jet ventilation during microlaryngeal surgery, *Ann Otol Rhinol Laryngol* 103:624, 1994.

150. Pennant JH, White PF: The laryngeal mask airway: its use in anesthesiology, *Anesthesiology* 79:144, 1993.

151. Ansermino JM, Blogg CE: Cricoid pressure may prevent insertion of the laryngeal mask airway, *Br J Anaesthesia* 69:465, 1992.

152. Rabey PG et al: Effect of the laryngeal mask airway on lower oesophageal sphincter pressure in patients during general anesthesia, *Br J Anaesthesia* 69:346, 1992.

153. King G, Street MK: Twelfth cranial nerve paralysis following use of a laryngeal mask airway, *Anaesthesia* 49:786, 1994.

154. Nagai K, Sakuramoto C, Goto F: Unilateral hypoglossal nerve paralysis following the use of the laryngeal mask airway, *Anaesthesia* 49:603, 1994.

155. Ezri T et al: Laryngeal mask and pulmonary edema, *Anesthesiology* 78:219, 1993.

156. Wynn JM, Jones KL: Tongue cyanosis after laryngeal mask airway insertion, *Anesthesiology* 80:1403, 1994.

157. Green KS, Berger TH: Proper use of the Combitube, *Anesthesiology* 81:513, 1994.

Part VII

SOCIETAL CONSIDERATIONS

Chapter 41

TEACHING MANAGEMENT OF THE AIRWAY: THE UCSD AIRWAY ROTATION

Sheila D. Cooper
Jonathan L. Benumof

I. BASIC PRINCIPLES

A. HISTORY OF THE DIFFICULT AIRWAY ALGORITHM

The fundamental responsibility of an anesthesiologist is to maintain adequate gas exchange. To do this, the airway must be managed in such a way that it is almost continuously patent. Failure to maintain a patent airway can result in brain damage or death, therefore, it is not surprising that 85% of all respiratory-related closed malpractice claims involve a brain-damaged or dead patient.[1] In fact, it has been estimated that the inability to successfully manage a difficult airway has been responsible for as many as 30% of deaths that are totally attributable to anesthesia.[2,3] In response to these statistics, an American Society of Anesthesiologists (ASA) Task Force developed a difficult airway (DA) algorithm. The primary focus of this algorithm is the maintenance of airway patency at all times with a series of management options for a specific clinical scenario (preconceived plans A and B and so forth). It is thought that adherence to the principles presented in this algorithm should both reduce respiratory catastrophes and decrease anesthesia-related morbidity and mortality rates. Conceptually this is an admirable goal, but realistically many anesthesia care providers lack the fundamental clinical skills necessary to implement many of the options presented in the DA algorithm.

B. LEARNING THE MANAGEMENT OPTIONS

Theoretically, every anesthesiologist should be familiar with and well practiced in a variety of the intubation techniques that are presented in the DA algorithm so that when an airway problem occurs, it can be managed with a solid armamentarium of information and experience. However, with the rapid advancements in airway management technology, many of the newer airway devices are foreign to most anesthesiologists. Acquiring the equipment is not the problem: learning to use it is. Self-teaching, learning from clinical material as it presents itself, and attending specialized airway workshops are a beginning, but each of these solutions has major limitations or deficiencies.

Self-teaching through reading product information literature and clinical studies that critically evaluate the equipment, viewing instructional videotapes, and attending specialized lectures are a beginning in understanding the concepts behind the development of a particular technique or device, but they do not substitute for hands-on experience. Learning to use the equipment when an airway management problem presents itself is an extremely common occurrence, but it is usually an unrewarding situation that impacts negatively on the practitioner and the patient. Participating in specialized airway courses and workshops is an excellent means of introducing the manual skills required to implement airway devices, but practice in mannequins does not accurately simulate "real" patients and therefore is often not directly applicable. Mannequins have wide open, patent channels with immobile airway structures, which is markedly different from an actual airway. Therefore, although these options are a beginning to learning about various airway management techniques and devices, they all have limitations. At the University of California at San Diego Medical Center we have recognized these limitations and have developed a difficult airway residency rotation with the goal of creating nonurgent, nonstressful learning situations in which a multitude of airway management techniques can be mastered in actual patients.[4] This chapter details this rotation.

II. SETTING UP AN AIRWAY ROTATION
A. ADMINISTRATION

The administrative aspects of setting up a successful airway rotation involve the following: (1) approval by the residency education director or committee, or both, (2) selecting faculty to serve as instructors, (3) careful scheduling, (4) formulating a didactic program, and (5) having the appropriate equipment. Each of these issues is discussed separately in the following sections.

1. Approval by residency education director or committee

The initial step in setting up a successful airway rotation is gaining approval by the residency education director or committee, or both. We petitioned the committee to adopt this rotation as a mandatory part of every resident's training and education, stressing the ASA's goal of reducing respiratory catastrophes with the introduction of the DA algorithm. After obtaining the

commitment of the committee to incorporate this rotation as an essential component of the residency program, we integrated it as part of the subspecialty cascade rotation series. Eligible residents include those who have been through a minimum of 9 months of basic anesthesia training; to date we have had, exclusively, second or third year clinical anesthesia "airway" residents.

2. Faculty instructors

Two criteria are essential for the faculty chosen to serve as instructors. Above all, they should have an interest in advanced airway management and a broad depth of experience with current airway management devices and techniques. It is impossible to teach something if unfamiliar with it and, as previously stated, this approach is not only doomed to failure but it is extremely unrewarding. The second important consideration is that it is helpful if the faculty is actively involved in clinical research using airway management devices. This is beneficial in several ways: (1) the faculty are more likely to keep current on the literature, (2) companies promoting new airway devices and techniques may ask for their evaluation, and most important, (3) the clinical research interests of the faculty may stimulate resident involvement, resulting in an active clinical research program. We have two dedicated faculty members who teach advanced airway management.

3. Scheduling considerations

Careful scheduling, of both the monthly and the daily schedules, is of the utmost importance. Two features of our schedule that we pay particular attention to are that both members of the faculty are not absent at the same time during the month-long rotation and that one of the faculty is assigned daily clinical duties concurrent with the airway resident's clinical duties. This requires that the faculty schedule maker and the chief resident, who writes the resident schedule, coordinate the faculty and airway resident's schedules to ensure daily supervision, which optimizes the learning experience during the month-long rotation.

At our institution the clinical director is responsible for the daily assignment of cases for the faculty and residents. Selecting appropriate patients for learning airway management techniques is crucial to a good learning experience; the patient should require general anesthesia for a procedure in which there is no competing anesthesia and surgical interest for the airway and in which patient positioning is suitable (i.e., supine with the patient's head near the anesthesiologist and readily accessible). For example, many orthopedic, pelvic, lower to midabdominal, and plastic surgery procedures are very suitable because of no competition for access to the airway or major early patient position changes. The airway rotation resident also has a high priority on patients who require awake intubation. We find it helpful for the airway resident or faculty, or both, to consult with the clinical director on daily case assignment when the finalized daily schedule is available to ensure the best learning situation.

4. Didactics

Prior to the rotation the airway resident receives a syllabus that contains the classic and current articles on airway management devices and techniques. This syllabus serves as the foundation for formal didactic teaching sessions and serves as the nidus for informal teaching in the operating room.

Before any new or unfamiliar airway device is used in a patient, a thorough and complete discussion takes place with regard to theory, description, technique, and current clinical experience. Once the resident is familiarized with the device, the technique is practiced in models or mannequins, or both, so that the essential mechanical aspects are mastered. For example, when the airway resident is introduced to fiberoptic bronchoscopy, special models that teach maneuvering skills[5] and lung casts are used extensively until the resident can successfully manipulate the bronchoscope. When more invasive techniques are introduced, such as retrograde intubations and percutaneous cricothyrotomy, special workshops are held at the medical school anatomy laboratory where cadavers are used as "models" to teach the residents the necessary mechanical skills.

Recently, we acquired the Medical Plastics Laboratory, Inc., DA management trainer mannequin (model no. DA-1100). The head of the mannequin is a realistic, life-size intubation trainer with a flexible tongue, arytenoid cartilage, epiglottis, vallecula, vocal cords, trachea, and esophagus. The head can be tilted forward or backward or rotated 90 degrees to either side. The head has a neck opening and replaceable skin for practicing cricothyrotomy techniques. Since the larynx is replaceable, the mannequin allows repeated practice of retrograde intubation, transtracheal jet ventilation (the mannequin contains a chest with expandable lungs), needle and surgical cricothyrotomy, and lightwand intubation, as well as oral and nasal fiberoptic and standard conventional intubation. The cost of the mannequin is approximately $1200. The benefit of each airway resident being able to "go through the motions" ad infinitum seems to be immense.

5. Equipment

Access to the proper equipment is paramount to a successful airway rotation. We have organized a self-contained dedicated anesthesia "airway" cart that contains a multitude of airway devices. The actual cart we use is pictured in Fig. 41-1. Each drawer in the cart has been organized to contain the necessary equipment for

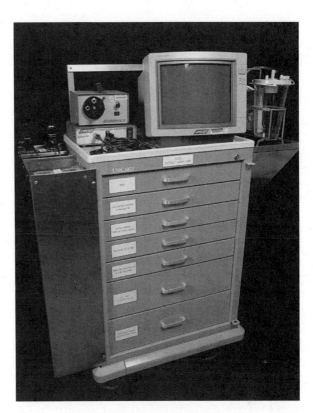

Fig. 41-1. The dedicated airway cart containing all the equipment necessary to master a number of different airway management techniques. The contents of this cart, drawer by drawer, are listed in Box 41-1.

a particular airway technique, and most of the available, currently used airway devices on the market are contained in one of these drawers. A complete listing, drawer by drawer, of the contents is found in Box 41-1. Adult and pediatric bronchoscopes are in a side compartment for easy access. A surgical video camera with a universal adapter that can couple with different viewing lenses (e.g., a fiberoptic bronchoscope or the Bullard laryngoscope), along with a video monitor and an external light source, is mounted on top of the cart. The video monitor greatly facilitates on-the-spot teaching. We also have a video cassette recorder to provide material for future teaching and review.

III. DAILY APPLICATION

A. PATIENT SELECTION

Proper patient selection is crucial to a good learning experience. When the daily operating room schedule is completed, the clinical director assigns cases to the faculty and residents. Since the inception of this rotation 3 years ago, we have familiarized our clinical director with the patient population we think is best suited for the residents to practice and learn airway management techniques. Before gaining this familiarity, we found it helpful for the airway resident or faculty, or both, to

BOX 41-1   University of California at San Diego Medical Center difficult airway cart

Drawer 1: Preps

Alcohol prep
Atomizer sprayer
Catheter, 22-gauge angio × 1 inch
Cetacaine topical spray
Gauze, 3 × 3 inch
Glycopyrrolate, 0.2 mg/ml
Lidocaine, 1%, 50 ml
Lidocaine, 2%, 50 ml
Needle, 25-gauge × 3.5 inch spinal
Needles, 19-gauge × 1.5 inch

Oxymetazoline hydrochloride spray (Afrin)
Silicone lubricant
Stopcocks, three-way
Syringes, 3 cc
Tetracaine, .45%, 49 ml
Tongue depressor
Xylocaine 2%, jelly
Xylocaine 5%, ointment
Xylocaine prep 4%, for topical spray

Drawer 2: Laryngeal mask airway, suction catheter, and Yankauer tip

No. 1 laryngeal mask (neonate/infants)
No. 2 laryngeal mask (babies/children)
No. 2.5 laryngeal mask (babies/children)
No. 3 laryngeal mask (children/small adults)
No. 4 laryngeal mask (normal/large adults)

Laryngeal mask tube extensions
Catheter, suction, 14 F, adult
Catheter, suction, 8 F, pediatric
Yankauer suction tips

Drawer 3: Blades, handles, and Combitube

Combitube
Laryngoscope handle (regular)
Laryngoscope handle (short)
Macintosh blade no. 2 (child)
Macintosh blade no. 3 (adult, medium)
Macintosh blade no. 4 (adult, large)

Magill forceps (small)
Magill forceps (large)
Miller blade no. 1 (infant)
Miller blade no. 2 (child)
Miller blade no. 3 (adult, medium)

Drawer 4: Retrograde set and transtracheal jet ventilation (TTJV)

0.035 × 145 cm guidewire
Catheter, 14-gauge intravenous (IV) (TTJV)
Catheter, red rubber, Robinson urethral
Clamps, Kelly
Needle, 18-gauge thin-wall

Needle, epidural with catheter
Nerve hooks
Retrograde set (Cook)
Sutures, silk

Drawer 5: Airways and tube exchangers

Airway, Berman oral, 100 mm
Airway, Berman oral, 80 mm
Airway, Berman oral, 90 mm
Catheter, 14-gauge × 2 inch
Catheter, 16-gauge × 2 inch
Catheter, 18-gauge × 2 inch
Melker emergency cricothyrotomy set
Nasopharyngeal airway, 26F
Nasopharyngeal airway, 28F

Nasopharyngeal airway, 30F
Nasopharyngeal airway, 32F
Nasopharyngeal airway, 34F
Needle, Benumof transtracheal (Cook)
Syringe, 20 cc
Tube exchanger, large with adapter (Sheridan)
Tube exchanger, medium with adapter (Sheridan)
Tube exchanger, small with adapter (Sheridan)

Drawer 6: Endotracheal tubes and lighted stylets

2.5 mm, uncuffed
3.0 mm, cuffed
3.0 mm, uncuffed
3.5 mm, uncuffed
4.0 mm, cuffed
4.0 mm, uncuffed
4.5 mm, cuffed
4.5 mm, uncuffed
5.0 mm, cuffed
5.0 mm, uncuffed
5.5 mm, uncuffed

6.0 mm, cuffed
7.0 mm, cuffed
7.0 mm, armoured
8.0 mm, armoured
Stylet, adult
Stylet, pediatric
Lighted stylet, Anesthesia Medical Specialties
Lighted stylet, Imagica
Lighted stylet, Imagica sheaths
Lighted stylet, Laerdal, handle
Lighted stylet, Laerdal, disposable stylets

Continued.

BOX 41-1 **University of California at San Diego Medical Center difficult airway cart—cont'd**

Drawer 7: Mask, specialty blades, and miscellaneous

No. 2 Patil-Syracuse mask fiberoptic bronchoscope (FOB)
No. 3 Patil-Syracuse mask fiberoptic bronchoscope (FOB)
No. 4 Patil-Syracuse mask fiberoptic bronchoscope (FOB)
No. 5 Patil-Syracuse mask fiberoptic bronchoscope (FOB)
No. 6 Patil-Syracuse mask fiberoptic bronchoscope (FOB)
Airway, Ovassapian
Airway, Williams, 10 cm
Airway, Williams, 9 cm
Augustine guide
Belscope, adult

Belscope, small
Bronch swivel elbow
Bullard blade, adult
Bullard blade, small
CO_2 analyzer, Easy Cap, disposable
Scissors
Tubing, O_2 supply
Tubing, suction connection
WuScope, adult
WuScope, small

---

consult with the clinical director when the cases are being assigned for the next day. The patient population that is best suited to practice airway management skills on is relatively straightforward. They are patients in ASA class I or II who require a general anesthetic without the need for extensive or invasive monitoring or setup. The patient must be operated on in the supine position with easy access to the airway, and the surgical procedure cannot involve the head or neck, which would obviously create competition for the airway. If a patient scheduled for surgery requires specialized airway management (i.e., an awake intubation), the case is prioritized to the airway resident. We try to avoid having the resident move from room to room to gather experience; rather, the airway resident is assigned to specific cases in a single operating room. With this type of scheduling the resident gains experience on two to four patients each day, practicing intubation techniques on approximately 40 to 50 patients over the 1-month rotation.

B. PREOPERATIVE CONSIDERATIONS

1. Airway evaluation (see Chapter 7)

The patient's airway is evaluated by the airway resident, and the findings discussed with the faculty. The evaluation includes oropharyngeal classification, measurement of the mandibular space, range of motion of the head and neck, length and thickness of the neck, length and looseness of teeth, override of the maxillary teeth on the mandibular teeth, configuration of the palate and other remarkable findings such as beards or large breasts, and, very important, of course, preexisting disease. With many cases (e.g., thoracic-lung separation) radiologic findings are also discussed.

2. Proper preparation for awake intubation (see Chapter 9)

If awake intubation is indicated, the airway resident with the faculty physiologically and pharmacologically

prepares the patient and administers topical anesthetic and nerve block to the upper airway.

C. TYPICAL GENERAL ANESTHESIA AND AIRWAY PROCEDURE SEQUENCES

Before induction of anesthesia all patients are premedicated with an antisialagogue to help decrease secretions, which can interfere with visualization through fiberoptic instruments, and an anxiolytic (unless contraindicated). Baseline measurements of heart rate, blood pressure, oxygen saturation, and end-tidal carbon dioxide (CO_2) are recorded during preoxygenation. Anesthesia can be induced with any of a number of appropriate agents, and the patient is paralyzed with an intermediate-acting neuromuscular blocking agent. Anesthesia is maintained with inhalational or intravenous agents, or both. As soon as mask ventilation is established, the surgeons are encouraged to ready the patient for the operative procedure and a drape is placed between the anesthesiologist and the surgical field; mask ventilation is continued. Once complete paralysis has been established (train-of-four = 0/4), a number of intubation techniques can be practiced in a controlled, unrushed manner while surgery proceeds under mask general anesthesia. Typical intubating sequences are depicted in Fig. 41-2.

A laryngeal mask airway (LMA), for example, may be initially inserted, and ventilation continued through the LMA (Fig. 41-2). A fiberoptic elbow adapter with a self-sealing diaphragm is then interposed between the proximal end of the LMA and the breathing circuit. A fiberoptic bronchoscope can then be introduced through this adapter and through the LMA channel with or without a preloaded, appropriately sized endotracheal tube (ET) (i.e., a cuffed 6.0-mm internal diameter [ID] ET with a size 4 LMA). If the fiberoptic bronchoscope is used strictly as a learning device, to show how the LMA seats itself around the larynx (and therefore to

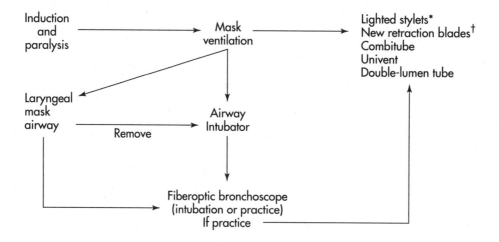

Fig. 41-2. A schematic of typical intubating sequences. After induction of general anesthesia and establishment of adequate mask ventilation, the patient is paralyzed with an intermediate-acting neuromuscular blocking agent. A number of different intubating techniques can be employed at this point, as illustrated.

demonstrate the ease of intubation through the LMA), it is maneuvered through the grids on the LMA and the vocal cords are identified. The vocal cords are not entered unless the fiberoptic bronchoscope is used as an aid to intubation. Once the vocal cords are identified, the fiberoptic bronchoscope is removed and the diaphragm on the elbow adapter is resealed. Mask ventilation continues uninterrupted throughout this sequence. Ventilation and oxygenation can continue through the LMA, but usually the LMA is removed and mask ventilation reestablished with an airway intubator as an oropharyngeal airway (instead of conventional Guedel oropharyngeal airway) and an anesthesia mask with a self-sealing fiberoptic port (instead of a conventional anesthesia mask). Fiberoptic visualization of the larynx can then be practiced while the faculty ventilates the lungs, or the trachea may be fiberoptically intubated through the anesthesia mask with fiberoptic port and airway intubator at this time. As an alternative, removal of the LMA can be followed by other definitive airway techniques such as use of lighted stylets, new retraction blades, or a Combitube, or if indicated, a Univent Bronchial Blocker or double-lumen tube can be used to facilitate intubation of the patient's trachea. Once the patient's trachea has been intubated, no other devices or techniques are employed. At all times, gentleness is mandatory, all manuevers are strictly supervised by the faculty (most are visualized on the television screen), and absolutely no trauma to the patient is permitted. Under these circumstances, we have never had a patient complication or injury occur in the 3 years of the airway rotation. Since there is no competition for the airway, the surgeons can begin working as soon as mask ventilation is established, enabling the airway resident to learn these skills in an unhurried, unpressured fashion. In a number of cases, and while the lungs are being continuously ventilated, a fiberoptic bronchoscope is inserted through a bronchoscopy elbow and the resident is asked to identify for the faculty all the lobar bronchial orifices (as viewed on the television screen).

IV. EVALUATION

Experience with various airway management techniques before participating in the airway rotation is extremely variable. During the DA rotation the resident typically participates in three cases per day, 4 days per week (the day after an in-house call is nonclinical), for 4 weeks, or 48 cases. These cases include at least 15 fiberoptic intubations, multiple LMA insertions, use of a Combitube, intubations with a variety of lighted stylets and new retraction blades, and experience with double-lumen and Univent Bronchial Blocker tubes. Retrograde intubation, insertion of transtracheal jet ventilation catheters, and percutaneous cricothyrotomy are taught and practiced on cadavers in a separate dedicated workshop, as well as on our newly acquired DA trainer mannequin, unless a clinical opportunity arises during the rotation.

We think the airway rotation as outlined in this chapter is a good one for several reasons. First, the residents greatly enjoy learning many new skills and acquiring a great deal of knowledge in a short time. Second, the stress-free learning environment is unique and greatly facilitates learning and interest. Third, the one-on-one intense relationship with a knowledgeable faculty person also greatly promotes learning. Fourth, the residents go on with much confidence to use their acquired skill and knowledge at a much greater frequency during the rest of their residency.

V. PLANNING AHEAD: A FUTURE REQUIREMENT IN ANESTHESIA TRAINING?

If every anesthesiologist is to become competent at managing airway difficulties, teaching and training of the necessary skills must be intensified. The question is how to best achieve this goal. With fiberoptic intubation, for example, there has been slow dissemination of the technique within the anesthesia community, particularly in the United Kingdom[6] despite the formal establishment of various training programs and workshops.[7,8] Reasons for the slow acceptance of fiberoptic or for that matter any new airway technology have included the high initial cost and subsequent repair or replacement of equipment, lengthy cleaning and disinfecting routines, and difficulty in learning and mastering the techniques.[9] In Europe surveys have shown that a lack of training and teaching is more of a problem than purchasing the equipment.[10] Several training programs for teaching fiberoptic intubation have been implemented, and studies have shown that although intubation takes significantly longer with trainees than does a conventional direct laryngoscopic technique,[11,12] none of the potential problems associated with prolonged intubation time[13] have been reported. In fact, one study emphasized, just as we do, the importance of careful patient selection,[14,15] which may directly affect the low complication rate.

In addition to teaching fiberoptic intubation, we teach our residents how to use most of the airway devices available to the anesthesia community (and some that are not) in a concentrated 1-month rotation. To learn how to use these various devices and perform different management techniques obviously requires the acquisition of the devices and equipment. This can translate into a significant financial outlay, which may be prohibitive to many institutions and individuals who want to develop a teaching program similar to ours. We have managed to finance our rotation through institutional hospital support and individual company support.

With the endorsement of this educational endeavor by the entire anesthesia department, we approached the hospital administration for financial support in purchasing the most expensive items, the three fiberoptic bronchoscopes. Our proposal was strengthened by our department's commitment to finance the purchase of the surgical video camera, video monitor, light source, and video cassette recorder. The bulk purchase of all of these items greatly reduced the cost as quoted by every company we approached. In addition, the pulmonary and cardiothoracic departments endorsed the purchase, which helped emphasize the necessity of obtaining the requested equipment.

The second source of support we sought was individual companies. We have been successful in soliciting companies to loan us their devices or equipment on a trial basis, which in some situations has extended into an indefinite loan period. In turn, the companies have reaped the benefit of several published clinical studies and exposure of their devices to all of our residents, who often purchase the equipment upon graduation or convince the group they join to purchase it, which means additional exposure to multiple anesthesiologists. This symbiotic relationship has extended to involve multiple companies who regularly donate supplies and devices.

With some persistence and ingenuity the entire realm of equipment necessary to simulate what we have assimilated for our airway rotation can be attained with minimal out-of-pocket expense. The experience our residents gain during this rotation is extrapolated to numerous clinical situations throughout the remainder of their training, so every graduating anesthesia resident has gained the skills necessary to approach a difficult airway with confidence in a well-planned, precise, and logical manner. It is our hope that other teaching institutions recognize the value and necessity of the rotation that we have described and will adopt, foster, and incorporate a similar program into their residency training curriculum so that all anesthesia resident graduates gain proficiency in the most basic skill: effective airway management.

REFERENCES

1. Caplan RA, Posner KL, Ward RJ et al: Adverse respiratory events in anesthesia: a closed claims analysis, *Anesthesiology* 72:828, 1990.
2. Benumof JL, Scheller MS: The importance of transtracheal ventilation in the management of the difficult airway, *Anesthesiology* 71:769, 1989.
3. Bellhouse CP, Dore C: Criteria for estimating the likelihood of difficulty of endotracheal intubation with Macintosh laryngoscope, *Anaesth Intensive Care* 16:329, 1988.
4. Cooper SD, Benumof JL: Teaching the management of the difficult airway: the UCSD airway rotation, *Anesthesiology* 81: A1241, 1994.
5. Bainton CR: personal communication.
6. King TA, Adams AP: Failed tracheal intubation, *Br J Anaesth* 65:400, 1990.
7. Vaughan RS: Training in fibreoptic laryngoscopy, *Br J Anaesth* 66:538, 1992.
8. Dykes MHM, Ovassapian A: Dissemination of fibreoptic airway endoscopy skills by means of a workshop utilizing models, *Br J Anaesth* 63:595, 1989.

9. Coe PA, King TA, Towey RM: Teaching guided fibreoptic nasotracheal intubation: an assessment of an anaesthetic technique to aid in training, *Anaesthesia* 43:410, 1988.

10. Mason RA: Learning fibreoptic intubation: fundamental problems, *Anaesthesia* 47:729, 1992.

11. Wood PR, Dresner M, Lawler PGP: Training in fibreoptic tracheal intubation in the North of England, *Br J Anaesth* 69:202, 1992.

12. Smith JE, MacKenzie AA, Scott-Knight VCE: Comparison of two methods of fibreoptic-guided tracheal intubation, *Br J Anaesth* 66:546, 1991.

13. Finfer SR, MacKenzie SIP, Saddler JM et al: Cardiovascular responses to tracheal intubation: a comparison of direct laryngoscopy and fibreoptic intubation, *Anaesth Intensive Care* 17:44, 1989.

14. Hartley M, Morris S, Vaughan RS: Teaching fibreoptic intubation: effect of alfentanyl on the haemodynamic response, *Anaesthesia* 49:335, 1994.

15. Schaefer HG, Marsch SCU, Keller HL et al: Teaching fibreoptic intubation in anaesthetised patients, *Anaesthesia* 49:331, 1994.

Chapter 42

TEACHING AND LEARNING AIRWAY MANAGEMENT OUTSIDE THE OPERATING ROOM: GENERAL AND BASIC USE OF COMPUTERS

Phil Liu
Marc D. Posner
Letty M. P. Liu

I. BACKGROUND

With all the exhilarating new material and concepts in the field of airway management that have been presented in the previous chapters in this textbook, high-quality, efficient instructional methods are needed to educate all medical and health-care workers in need of airway management skills. As wonderful as textbooks are, reading textbooks is only part of the traditional approach to education.

For some time, anesthesia educators have been in the forefront of medical education. In 1980, anesthesiologists were among the first medical specialists to form a society devoted to education (Society for Education in Anesthesia). Anesthesiology was the first medical specialty to innovate a successful "problem-based learning" continuing education program at the ASA's annual meeting. Anesthesiology is also the only medical specialty that is embarking on the extensive use of simulators for medical skills training. Thus it is a natural progression that anesthesiologists develop the cutting-edge technology of computer-aided instruction to educate personnel in areas of expertise of anesthesiologists, such as airway management.

The use of computers as an educational tool has increased exponentially in recent years. Computer programs have been developed to teach students of all ages, from preschool children to adults interested in continuing education. Computer-aided instruction and learning of concepts of airway management is one of the more exciting developments in anesthesia. Computer programs that efficiently teach airway management can be educational and also entertaining for the learner.

This chapter describes our approach to the use of the computers in the teaching and learning of airway

911

management. The advantages and disadvantages of this educational format are presented, and the rapidly changing software and programming options are discussed for those interested in embarking on creating computer-based educational material.

II. PRINCIPLES OF DESIGNING AN INSTRUCTIONAL PROGRAM

The principles of designing an instructional program for airway management is identical to the process of designing any medical instructional program. The process involves the following steps: (1) defining the students, (2) defining the objectives, (3) designing the instructional activity, and (4) evaluation.[1]

Defining the students for which the educational activity is intended is the initial step in systematic course design. One must define the professional responsibility of the intended learners. The skills, knowledge, values, and attitudes that these students will need in order to fulfill their professional responsibilities vis-à-vis the educational topic need to be stated. The knowledge base of the learners must also be considered. What is the educational background of the learners? Is the extent of their medical knowledge similar, or does the instructional program have to address the needs of learners with different training, for example, lay persons as well as trained health-care professionals. The proficient instructor takes the time to address these key issues and sort them out before embarking on designing the instructional program.

Objectives are statements of the goals of the instruction. By defining the needs of the students in terms of the knowledge, skills, values, and attitudes that they require to fulfill their professional responsibilities, the instructor next states the objectives of the instructional program. Objectives are statements that define the instructor's expectations when the student encounters a situation or circumstance after the course of instruction. For example, in airway management a reasonable objective would be the following: After the course of instruction the student will be able to establish a patent airway in a comatose but spontaneously breathing patient without equipment by neck extension and/or mandibular jaw thrust. The objectives define the intent of the instructional program.

Once the educational objectives have been delineated, the creative aspect of designing instructional activities to accomplish the learning expressed in the objective can be undertaken. For example, neck extension and jaw-thrust maneuver for opening an obstructed airway can be taught by presenting a problem case with instructional material on a computer. On the other hand, medical students can be taught head extension and jaw thrust on mannequins or anesthetized patients in the operating room. There are almost limitless options confronting the inventive teacher. However, efficiency and realistic use of resources are factors in choosing instructional activities. For example, crisis scenarios that should never be allowed to happen during training on real patients are possible in simulators.

The final step in systematic course design is evaluation. All complete instructional designs contain evaluation. Only by assessment is the instructor certain that the students have achieved the educational objectives that the instructor has defined. As in instructional activities, compromises may have to be made in the evaluation format for the sake of efficiency and practicality.

The application of the four previously identified principles before embarking on teaching requires a significant amount of initial effort. Nevertheless, the time spent in designing rational, systematic educational endeavors is amply rewarded in student learning. There are too many examples of poor educational outcomes due to haphazard design.

III. COMPUTER-AIDED INSTRUCTIONAL PROGRAMS

Why are we so excited about computer-aided instruction? An inescapable aspect of a learner in front of a computer is the *interactive* nature of the encounter. Almost inevitably, computer-aided instruction is a form of *active learning* contrasted with *passive learning*.[2] To simply get the computer software to advance, the learner must be active. Unlike sitting in a lecture, computer-aided instruction can force the learner to think, to react, and to act! Immediate feedback can be given to the learner as fast as the next screen appears. Objectives can be presented directly to the learner. Video and animated illustrated instruction with audio is possible. The learner can control the speed of the instruction to his or her individual pace. The learner can choose from a variety of instructional options. Some learners may prefer problem-based case scenarios, others may choose to review instructional material, and others may opt for the pretest and posttest evaluation.

Although significant effort by the instructor is invested initially in developing and field testing high-quality educational software, a computer-aided instructional program can free the faculty for other activities and large numbers of learners can be instructed once the hardware and the software are in place. In addition, evaluation can be directly incorporated into the program. Remediation can also be built into the program, so that if learner deficiencies are discovered, remediation can be offered immediately.

What are the disadvantages of computer-aided instruction? Despite our enthusiasm for this educational format, there are some drawbacks. For some learners,

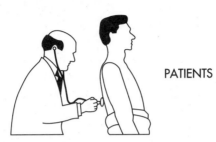

**Who Can Benefit from Airway
Management Preceptor?**

PATIENTS

- Anesthesiologists
- Anesthesia Residents
- Nonanesthesiologist M.D.s
- Medical Students

- Nurses
- Dentists
- Paramedics
- * Firefighters

Specific curriculum can be designed for each category of
learner by selecting relevant cases and teaching material

Fig. 42-1. Classes of individuals who can benefit from using the *Airway Management Preceptor
Computer Educational Program.*

**Airway Management Preceptor
Case: The Impudent Oyster**

You are at a societal sherry party when you see
someone in distress. He seems to be struggling
to say something, but cannot. As you watch, his
face turns dark red, and he collapses onto the
plush carpet with his **hands at his throat.**

What will you do now?   Related Stacks

|

Restart   Explain   Continue

Fig. 42-2. An opening page of a case in the *Airway Management Preceptor Educational Program.*

BOX 42-1   Steps in laryngoscopy

- Opening the mouth
    Intraoral or "scissor" technique
    Extraoral technique (preferred method)
- Placement of laryngoscope blade to right of tongue
- Advancement of blade to vallecula
- Visualize epiglottis
- Direction of force applied to blade
- Visualize larynx
    Identify structures of larynx (e.g., vocal cords)
- View of correct placement of Mac #3 for intubation
- Difference between straight blade and a Mac #3

From Benumof JL: Conventional (laryngoscopic) orotracheal and nasotracheal intubation (single-lumen tube). In Benumof JL: *Clinical procedures in anesthesia and intensive care,* Philadelphia, 1992, JB Lippincott.
NOTE: Each step on this page in the *Airway Management Preceptor* educational program is followed by an illustration of the step (see Fig. 42-3 A and B).

computers are not friendly. Some individuals simply have *computer phobia.* In addition, one can argue cogently that traditional educational methods have a track record of success. Inevitably, everyone who has worked with computers realizes that eventually one encounters *software and hardware glitches* that are extraordinarily frustrating. Another consideration is the expense of both software and hardware for this type of education. It is hoped that the educational software you purchase will be worth the expense, and not merely a book page on a screen. We cannot overemphasize the tremendous amount of time and effort necessary to create high-quality educational software. We have been working on a computer-aided teaching and learning program in airway management for several years. At the American Society of Anesthesiologists annual meeting in 1993 we presented a prototype of our program, *Airway Management Preceptor.*

IV. CHANGING DOMAIN OF SOFTWARE PLATFORMS FOR DEVELOPMENT OF EDUCATIONAL SOFTWARE

In our development of *Airway Management Preceptor* we have chosen to concentrate our programing efforts on the Macintosh family of computers for several reasons. First, the Macintosh is an easily accessible machine by its nature and graphic interface; most new computer users can easily understand how to operate the machine. As a result, we can at least partially overcome the computer phobia mentioned earlier. Second, the Macintosh has complete integration of graphic material with text and sound. Third, the convenience of ready-made platforms for development of educational material, specifically, *SuperCard,* gave us a foundation on which to build.

BOX 42-2   Checklist for novices (review after esophageal intubation)

- Incorrect head and neck position (lack of "sniff" position)
- Inadequate mouth opening
- Unsatisfactory displacement of the tongue to the left as the blade is positioned in the midline
- Rotating or pivoting the wrist when the epiglottis comes into view instead of lifting up and forward (laryngoscope blade traumatizing upper incisors)
- Failure to overcome parallax by not dropping your head in order to look beyond the tip of the laryngoscope
- Rushing, being inappropriately overconfident
- Being overcautious and timid
- Taking your eyes off the tube as it passes through the vocal cords
- Vocal cords can be observed while passing the tube because tube not passed directly down the laryngoscope view channel
- Unable to maneuver tube to clearly visible vocal cords

From Benumof JL: Conventional (laryngoscopic) orotracheal and nasotracheal intubation (single-lumen tube). In Benumof JL: *Clinical procedures in anesthesia and intensive care,* Philadelphia, 1992, JB Lippincott.

BOX 42-3   After an esophageal intubation

1. Remove the esophageal tube.
2. Immediately establish the ability to ventilate with a face mask. This is critical and must be assessed prior to any other attempt at intubation.
    After mask ventilation is established, further intubation strategies can progress in an orderly nonemergent manner.
3. Check vital signs, end-tidal CO_2, and O_2 saturation before proceeding. Ventilate by mask or administer drugs or fluid to correct abnormal values.

From Benumof JL: Conventional (laryngoscopic) orotracheal and nasotracheal intubation (single-lumen tube). In Benumof JL: *Clinical procedures in anesthesia and intensive care,* Philadelphia, 1992, JB Lippincott.

Fourth, Macintosh was the most available hardware platform for us to use.

Before *SuperCard* there was *HyperCard.* This development environment was originally bundled with all new Macintosh units when it was first developed. It was a simple, straightforward platform designed to let the average user dabble in programing. The resulting "stacks" could be made quite elegant, but the program lacked the power of a true language. In addition, the stacks depended on the presence of the original program to run. In addition, *HyperCard* did not allow the use of

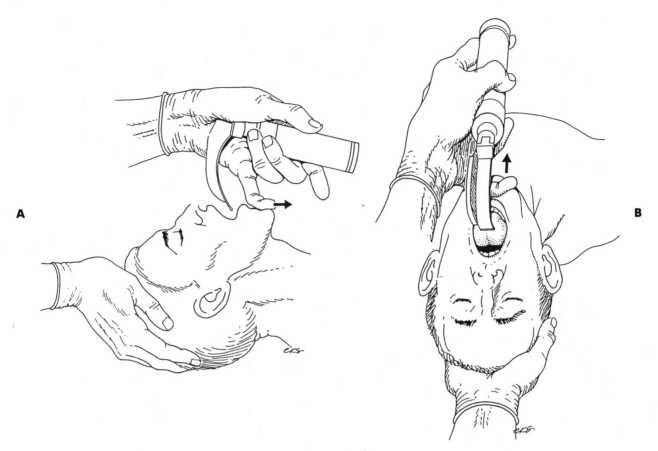

Fig. 42-3. Illustration of one of the steps listed in Box 42-1, the extraoral technique for opening the mouth. **A,** Lateral view. **B,** Frontal view. (From Benumof JL: Conventional [laryngoscopic] orotracheal and nasotracheal intubation [single-lumen tube]. In Benumof JL: *Clinical procedures in anesthesia and intensive care,* Philadelphia, 1992, JB Lippincott.)

color, could only support one open window, and was limited in its capabilities.

To answer all of these weaknesses, *SuperCard* was written. This program attempted to address many of the shortcomings of *HyperCard:* color was now fully supported, as were multiple windows. The programing language, *SuperTalk,* was more powerful than its predecessor, *HyperTalk,* yet still maintained its accessibility. Stacks could be converted into stand-alone programs, although they were still interpreted by a run-time package, limiting their speed. We began our work in *SuperCard,* hoping that it would provide for the needs of our project.

As we progressed, carefully and tediously entering each "card" of every case and placing every graphic, it became clear that *SuperCard* was not powerful enough for our needs. Our program quickly increased in size, and as a result ran very slowly. While we were generally able to accomplish what we needed with *SuperTalk,* we found, after several years, that this platform would not be sufficient to fully encompass all that we had set out to do.

As a result, we decided to write a new platform specifically designed for the task we had chosen. The language *FutureBasic* was chosen, since it is accessible, yet powerful. As an interpreted language, the project would be compiled into a real program, running at the same speed as any other commercially available program, rather than as an interpreted "stack" like *Super-Card.* In addition, we could easily add all the capabilities we wanted and make the interface look exactly as we desired, since we were developing the new environment from scratch. Early prototypes of the new project look and feel much like the successful *SuperCard* prototype displayed at the American Society of Anesthesiologists meeting, with few important differences. The program is now much smaller and faster, and development of new cases and review materials will take a fraction of the time it took previously. This new platform will permit a much more effective and usable product.

Every week, it seems, new platforms are announced for multimedia production development. While they differ in their strengths and weaknesses, they all offer the user a chance to develop educational material on his or her own. Microsoft and IBM have recently announced platforms, and more are sure to follow. It is hoped that software designers will develop more usable platforms for development of educational material so that computer-aided instruction will be easier to develop. In this way computer-aided instruction will be able to fulfill the potential that we envision.

V. AIRWAY MANAGEMENT COMPUTER PROGRAM

Airway Management Preceptor is just one example of a computer software program for teaching airway management. The program was designed for students who need to learn airway management skills (Fig. 42-1 on p. 913).

A learner can use this computer-aided instructional program by starting in the case-based teaching stack, in the instructional stacks, or in the stacks relating to the evaluation of knowledge and skills in airway management. The choice of where to begin is the option of the learner. As the learner progresses through any of these choices, he or she has the option to digress into the other two domains at any time. Many learners prefer the case-based problems because these are clinical scenarios that are relevant to their professional clinical activities. However, as learners progress in a scenario, they may realize that they need instruction on the topic. In this case, a learner may choose to select the button "related stacks," which will lead him or her into the instructional material related to the topic of the clinical scenario.

Figure 42-2 on p. 913 shows an opening case and the screen that the learner will be confronted with. The computer asks the learner, "What will you do now?" The learner responds by typing his response in the response box. The computer then provides immediate feedback to the learner's typed response. The student may also select the "explain" button instead of typing a response. When this option is chosen, a clue will be provided. The learner progresses through a series of screens until the clinical scenario is resolved.

Much of the material in the teaching stacks of *Airway Management Preceptor* are illustrations of airway management skills. The steps in laryngoscopy are listed in Box 42-1 on p. 914. Each of the items listed is followed by a series of illustrations that demonstrate steps in the skill described. For example, the extraoral technique of opening the mouth during laryngoscopy is illustrated in Fig. 42-3 on p. 915.

In other portions of the teaching stacks the focus of the educational material is more conceptual. A checklist for novices to review after they have intubated the esophagus instead of the trachea is presented in Box 42-2 on p. 914. A second conceptual teaching stack is given in Box 42-3 on p. 914. This screen describes the immediate actions the learner should perform after an esophageal intubation.

The preceding examples are provided to give the reader an overview of the type of material provided in the *Airway Management Preceptor* computer program.

VI. CONCLUSION

In this chapter we have attempted to describe the awesome potential that we envision for computer-aided instruction. We have described the process of development of logical, systematic educational programs. Advantages and disadvantages of computer-aided instruction have been presented. A discussion of the evolving domain of software platforms in the development of educational software was rendered, and an overview of one instructional computer program on airway management has been presented.

REFERENCES
1. Segall AJ, Vanderschmidt H, Burglass R et al: *Systematic course design for the health fields,* New York, 1975, John Wiley & Sons.
2. Physicians for the Twenty-first Century: *The GPEP report: report of the panel on the general professional education of the physician and college preparation for medicine,* Washington, DC, 1984, Association of American Medical Colleges.

Chapter 43

TEACHING AIRWAY MANAGEMENT OUTSIDE THE OPERATING ROOM: USE OF COMPUTERS WITH SPECIAL EMPHASIS ON CLINICAL CONCERNS AND THE ASA ALGORITHM

George J. Sheplock
Stephen F. Dierdorf

I. BACKGROUND

In 1985 the American Society of Anesthesiologists' Committee on Professional Liability began to analyze closed claim malpractice cases in order to objectively assess adverse outcomes from anesthesia. Respiratory events accounted for 37% of the claims (762 of 2046 cases). Eighty-five percent of the respiratory events resulted in permanent neurologic injury or death.[1] Three common mechanisms of adverse outcome from respiratory events accounted for 75% of the adverse respiratory events: inadequate ventilation (38%), esophageal intubation (18%), and difficult endotracheal intubation (17%).[2] The reviewers concluded that 90% of the cases of inadequate ventilation and esophageal intubation were preventable if monitoring with capnography and pulse oximetry had been employed. It was also concluded that only 36% of the cases of difficult endotracheal intubation were preventable.

Because of the disproportionately high incidence of adverse outcome from respiratory events and the finding that most cases of difficult endotracheal intubation were not easily preventable, the Task Force on Guidelines for Management of the Difficult Airway was convened. After an exhaustive search and evaluation of the available medical literature concerning airway management published between 1973 and 1991, the task force

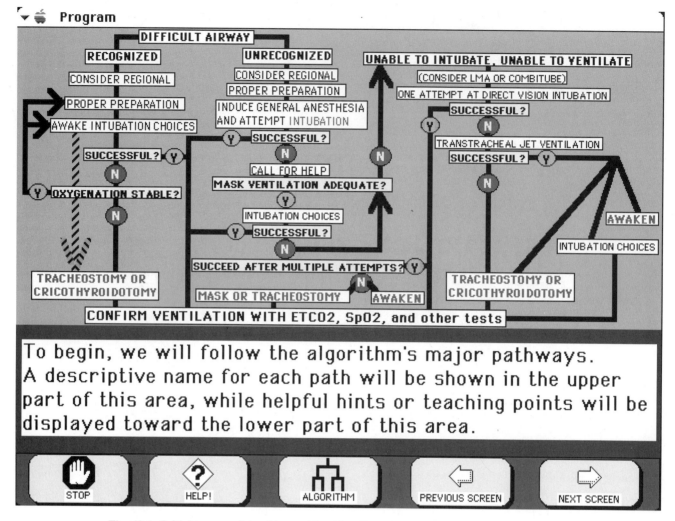

Fig. 43-1. Initial screen of the Airway Algorithm Program demonstrating the entire airway algorithm.

published "Practice Guidelines for Management of the Difficult Airway" in March 1993.[3] These guidelines included recommendations for evaluation of the airway, basic preparation for difficult airway management, strategy for intubation of the difficult airway, strategy for extubation of the difficult airway, and follow-up care. The task force also developed an algorithm for management of the difficult airway.[3] The purpose of these guidelines is to reduce the likelihood of adverse outcomes from untoward respiratory events. Most notably, the algorithm focuses on important decision points in management of the difficult airway and does not recommend specific airway management techniques. Although the published guidelines provide a list of different methods of ventilation and endotracheal intubation techniques for the difficult airway, there are no endorsements of particular techniques. The specific management technique must be determined by the anesthesiologist and depends on the airway problem and

the expertise of the anesthesiologist with different management techniques.

Although respiratory events are more likely to result in an adverse outcome, the incidence of patients with a difficult airway in clinical practice is, in actuality, very low. The incidence of failure to intubate the trachea in a large series of surgical patients was only 0.3%.[4] Since the incidence of patients with a difficult airway is so low, how can an anesthesiologist in clinical practice learn and practice new airway management techniques? How can the ramifications of the critical decision points in airway management be learned? There is evidence that performance during infrequent critical clinical events is improved by regular simulated practice.[5] New developments in computers and software have provided the necessary tools for producing interactive programs directed at learning the algorithm and evaluating the merits of different airway management techniques. The interactive pro-

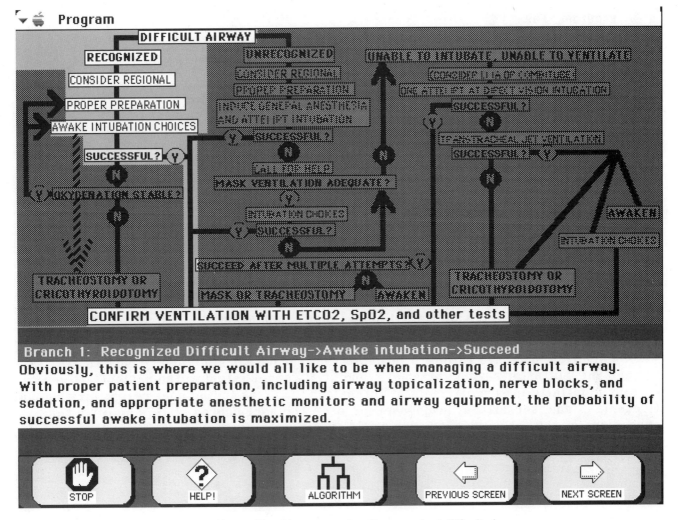

Program

Branch 1: Recognized Difficult Airway->Awake intubation->Succeed
Obviously, this is where we would all like to be when managing a difficult airway. With proper patient preparation, including airway topicalization, nerve blocks, and sedation, and appropriate anesthetic monitors and airway equipment, the probability of successful awake intubation is maximized.

STOP HELP! ALGORITHM PREVIOUS SCREEN NEXT SCREEN

Fig. 43-2. Airway Algorithm concerning the recognized difficult airway.

grams can be used frequently and repeatedly at relatively little cost.

II. LEARNING SKILLS FOR MANAGEMENT OF THE DIFFICULT AIRWAY

After presentation of didactic material that details the theory and use of different ventilation and endotracheal intubation techniques, these skills can be practiced with the aid of specially designed mannequins. These techniques are designed to teach the correct procedures for insertion and use of airway devices. The mannequins can be specially designed to demonstrate a single device or can be designed to accommodate a number of different airway devices. Most clinical anesthesiologists, with proper instruction and practice, develop the skill to use these devices in mannequins quickly and without difficulty. There may, however, be considerable reticence to transfer these newly learned skills to use in patients. Clearly, insertion of airway devices in mannequins may be considerably different from insertion and use in patients for a variety of reasons.

The other aspect of learning techniques for management of the difficult airway is the development of an understanding of the critical decision points in the course of airway management. There are times when the clinical situation demands a rapid decision about airway management. The consequences of that decision may result in successful resolution of the airway problem or may produce severe hypoventilation, hypoxemia, neurologic injury, or death. The recognition and resolution of these decision points cannot be effectively taught in a lecture format or with mannequins. These traditional teaching techniques cannot convey the sense of time limitation that occurs during a true airway emergency.

III. COMPUTER-ASSISTED INSTRUCTION

The use of computer-assisted instruction in education has increased dramatically in recent years. Early computer-assisted instruction consisted of little more than placing text into a file of a word processor for the user to read. These computer presentations consisted of

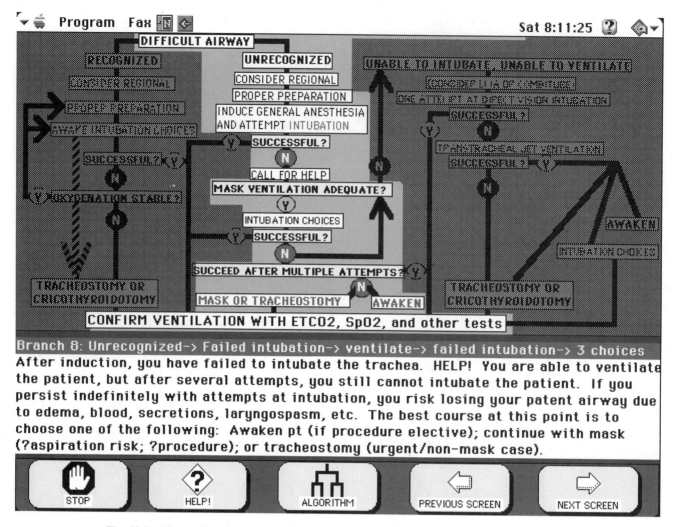

Fig. 43-3. Airway Algorithm concerning the initial part of the unrecognized difficult airway.

drills and tutorials and offered little more to the user than a textbook. Consequently, the results of this type of instruction could not be demonstrated to be any more effective than reading printed material. However, by the 1970s it could be demonstrated that computer-assisted instruction did have positive and lasting educational benefits for secondary education students.[6] In addition to proving that computer-assisted instruction produced a positive effect on learning, the time to learn was markedly reduced. As a result, the efficiency of learning was increased. Despite recommendations in 1984 that medical schools rely less on lecture-based instruction and more on independent learning, it was evident in 1993 that most medical schools had made only negligible progress in developing and implementing self-paced computer-assisted learning programs.[7] Assessment of the value of computer-assisted instruction has been difficult because of the inability to establish effective control and experimental groups. This difficulty may result because successful parts of a hypermedia

computer-assisted instruction program may inadvertently be transferred to the control group in a different format. This transfer problem may eliminate the detection of learning differences between the control and experimental groups, but in fact enhances learning in both groups. Despite this controversy, it seems evident that hypermedia computer-assisted instruction is extremely popular with students at all educational levels and is an extremely efficient means of disseminating new information and clinical techniques.

Multimedia devices such as slides, video, audio, and overhead projectors have been used for educational purposes for many years. These devices certainly enhanced learning but in the past could not be linked to each other. However, recent technologic developments have dramatically expanded the capabilities of personal computers and now permit the linkage of multiple media. The technology to link multimedia in an organized manner that permits the user to acquire data conveniently in different formats is the cornerstone of

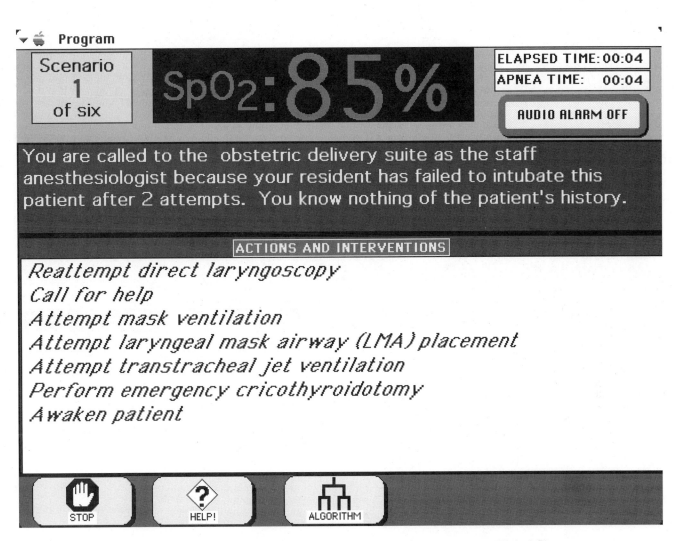

Fig. 43-4. Initial screen of a clinical scenario from the Airway Program. Clinical history, elapsed time, pulse oximetry data, and interventional options are apparent.

modern computer-assisted instruction. This linkage of multiple types of media into a single system is called hypermedia.[8] Hypermedia permits the acquisition of information from many sources and can be modeled to mimic normal thought and learning processes. The patterns of learning may vary between individuals, and hypermedia allows the pattern of data acquisition to be varied by the user. This versatility defines the true value and power of application of computer-assisted instruction.

New developments in software also permit the assembly of interactive programs by anesthesiologists with expertise in airway management based on real situations from clinical practice. The combination of text material with imported photographs and diagrams can be used to explain concepts and techniques in considerable detail. After these aspects of the material have been learned, imported videos and internal algorithms can be used to present a true clinical situation with

different management options in real time. This allows the student to explore different management options with accurate clinical information and time constraints as they would occur in clinical practice. The design of the teaching program permits rapid feedback of the results of the learner's decision. After evaluating the clinical scenario, making a management decision, and seeing the consequences of that decision, the learner can review didactic material germane to that clinical scenario. It is hoped that practicing these clinical decision processes in real time will reduce the reaction time and sense of panic that may accompany the true airway emergency.

The capabilities of current personal computers allow the storage of large amounts of information in different formats in a self-contained medium. The student can progress at his or her own pace but have the advantage of mimicking real situations. Considerable effort has been devoted to the design of all-purpose anesthesia simulators. These are very expensive and require per-

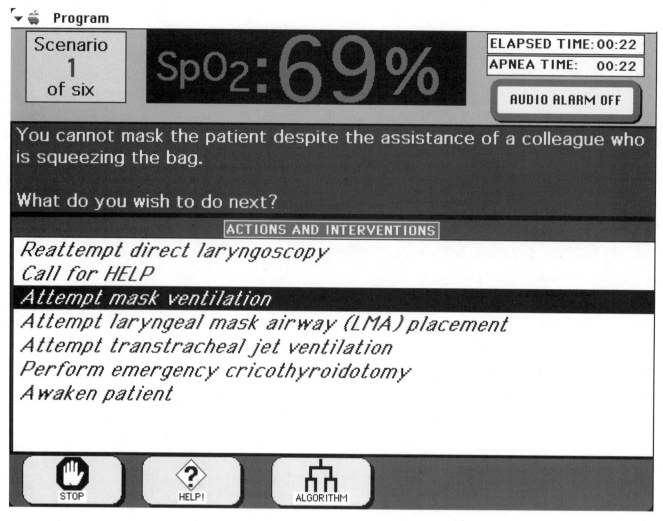

Fig. 43-5. Second screen of the clinical scenario in which the initial intervention of mask ventilation has not been successful. The arterial oxygen saturation level has decreased.

sonnel for operation. Interactive programs are relatively inexpensive to develop and require only a personal computer for operation. In addition, interactive computers can be used at any time that is convenient for the user.

In general, the technologic advances that have provided these tools are faster and more powerful microprocessors, increased storage capacity, and high-resolution graphics.[9] It is also financially feasible to produce CD-ROMs for computer-assisted instruction. The CD-ROM stores extremely large quantities of information (680 megabytes) on a small optical disk. These components are now readily available in affordable personal computers. In addition, new authoring languages permit nontechnical anesthesia educators to produce high-quality, interactive multimedia teaching programs.[10,11] Interactive computer-assisted instructional programs are well established for regional anesthesia.[12-14] It is well recognized that learning

anatomy for regional anesthesia is enhanced by cadaver dissection. However, cadaver dissection is not readily available to all anesthesiologists. Anatomic cadaver photographs at different dissection levels can be scanned, digitized, and imported into the personal computer. Once imported into the computer, the image can be enhanced, sharpened, and resized. The same format can be used for developing an interactive airway management program.

IV. THE INTERACTIVE AIRWAY MANAGEMENT INSTRUCTIONAL PROGRAM

There are several aspects of the Interactive Airway Management Instructional Program. The first part of the program is devoted to the ASA difficult airway algorithm.[15] Initially the entire algorithm is reviewed, and the user can explore the different branches of the algorithm (Fig. 43-1 on p. 918). The primary goal of this section is to focus the user's attention on making critical

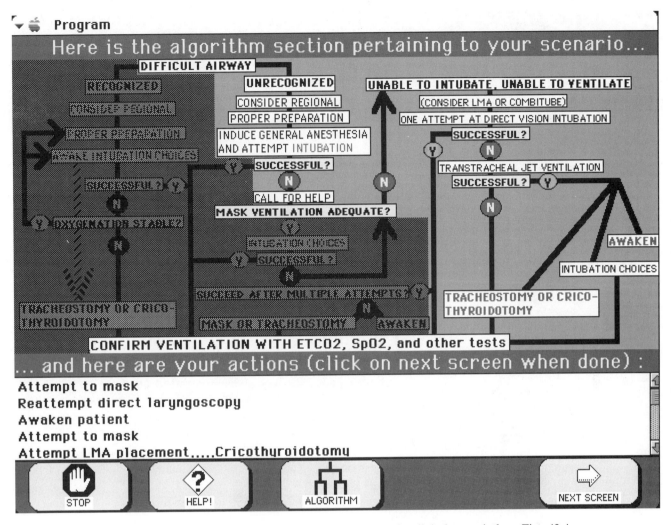

Fig. 43-6. Section of the Airway Algorithm pertaining to the clinical scenario from Figs. 43-4 and 43-5. This branch can be reviewed after completion of the clinical scenario.

airway management decisions in real time. The first critical decision point in the algorithm occurs after the initial evaluation of the patient's airway. If the evaluation indicates that the airway is abnormal and difficult ventilation is anticipated, an awake intubation is mandated[16] (Fig. 43-2 on p. 919). If an awake intubation cannot be achieved, the next decision to make is whether an airway by surgical access must be established.

The next branch of the algorithm concerns the unrecognized difficult airway (Fig. 43-3 on p. 920). If the preoperative airway evaluation indicates that the airway is normal, induction of general anesthesia may proceed. If, after induction of general anesthesia, it is discovered that endotracheal intubation is difficult but positive pressure ventilation can be administered, alternative intubation techniques may be employed. Should ventilation also become difficult, a rapid decision must be made as to how ventilation can be achieved. This decision point must be appreciated because the inability

to provide adequate ventilation will very quickly lead to hypoxemia and neurologic injury or death.

The interactive program emphasizes the preceeding critical decision points. Each branch of the algorithm may be isolated and displayed. Accompanying the display of each branch is text material that provides the user with an explanation of the purpose of the branch and the likelihood that the intervention will be successful. The user is also instructed in how confirmation of successful ventilation should be confirmed. The text information can also provide the consequences of inappropriate intervention techniques. Each branch may be reviewed until the critical decision points in difficult airway management are thoroughly understood.

After an understanding of the algorithm is achieved, the user is presented with a clinical scenario mimicking some airway situation. Pulse oximetry data and audio signals are provided, and a clock is set into motion so that the user must respond within an appropriate interval.

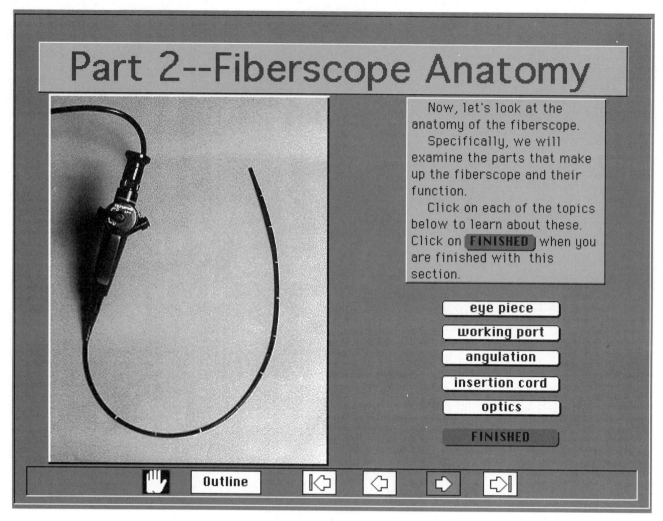

Fig. 43-7. Initial screen of the fiberoptic intubation section of the Airway Program demonstrating the function of the fiberoptic laryngoscope.

Total elapsed time and apnea time are continually displayed (Fig. 43-4 on p. 921). As the user selects a management option, he or she receives information that describes the patient's response to the intervention. If the intervention is successful, the problem is resolved. If, however, the intervention is unsuccessful or inappropriate, the patient's condition may deteriorate and another intervention technique must be selected (Fig. 43-5 on p. 922). After completion of the interactive clinical scenario, it is displayed for further study (Fig. 43-6 on p. 923). Intervention techniques may also introduce other complicating factors into the clinical scenario. The designer of the program can feature or highlight any clinical situation or response that he or she feels needs to be emphasized. For example, if the educator would like to emphasize use of the laryngeal mask airway (LMA), the clinical scenarios can be designed to direct the student to that conclusion.

The second part of the program is directed at presenting fiberoptically assisted endotracheal intubation.[17] The fiberoptic laryngoscope or bronchoscope is the most versatile of difficult airway management techniques. Consequently, fiberoptically assisted intubation has become an integral part of difficult airway management protocols. The program initially presents the structure and mechanics of the fiberscope (Fig. 43-7). A thorough knowledge of the operational aspects of the fiberoptic laryngoscope increases the rapidity with which the user masters fiberscope manipulation skills. After the beginning endoscopist learns how to manipulate the fiberscope, navigation of the fiberscope through an abnormal airway becomes relatively easy. Imported photographs of the fiberscope in conjunction with text material are used to identify the different parts of the fiberscope and explain each part's function. Short videos demonstrate the function of each part. Adjuncts to fiberoptically directed endotracheal intubation, such as intubating airways, are also shown and described.

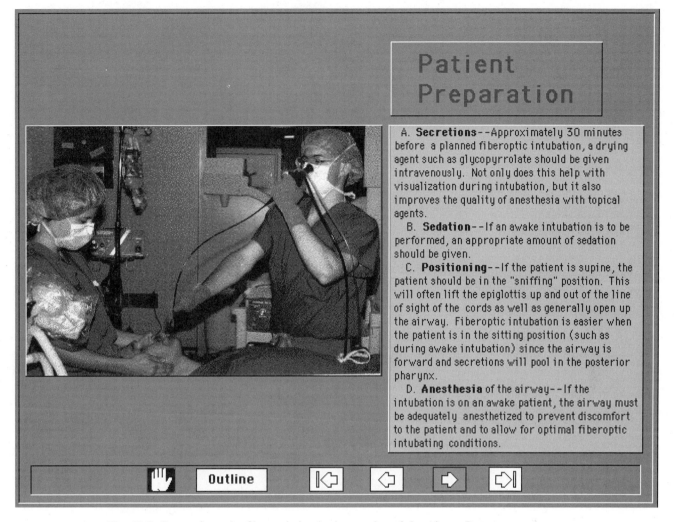

Patient Preparation

A. **Secretions**--Approximately 30 minutes before a planned fiberoptic intubation, a drying agent such as glycopyrrolate should be given intravenously. Not only does this help with visualization during intubation, but it also improves the quality of anesthesia with topical agents.
  B. **Sedation**--If an awake intubation is to be performed, an appropriate amount of sedation should be given.
  C. **Positioning**--If the patient is supine, the patient should be in the "sniffing" position. This will often lift the epiglottis up and out of the line of sight of the cords as well as generally open up the airway. Fiberoptic intubation is easier when the patient is in the sitting position (such as during awake intubation) since the airway is forward and secretions will pool in the posterior pharynx.
  D. **Anesthesia** of the airway--If the intubation is on an awake patient, the airway must be adequately anesthetized to prevent discomfort to the patient and to allow for optimal fiberoptic intubating conditions.

Outline

Fig. 43-8. Screen from the fiberoptic intubation section of the Airway Program.

After the fiberscope has been described and its function explained, patient preparation, including management of secretions, sedation, positioning, and anesthesia, are presented (Fig. 43-8). A video sequence is then shown that demonstrates fiberoptic intubation (Fig. 43-9).

The next part of the interactive program is designed to display upper airway anatomy with special reference to sensory innervation of the upper airway in preparation for establishing adequate topical anesthesia. The importance of learning techniques for producing anesthesia of the airway in the awake patient cannot be overestimated.[18] When the patient is well anesthetized and cooperative, fiberoptic laryngoscopy is almost always successful. Fiberoptic laryngoscopy becomes extremely difficult when the patient is poorly anesthetized, gagging, and coughing. The program displays the anatomy of the upper airway and displays areas innervated by different sensory nerves. The different sensory zones are color coded and the user quickly appreciates the fact that

multiple sensory nerves supply the upper airway. The viewer can access this information in two ways. When the cursor is placed on a colored area, the program will reveal the nerve supplying sensation to that area. Conversely, when the cursor is placed on the name of the nerve, the area that nerve supplies will be highlighted in color. The fiberscope and its components are also demonstrated to the user in a similar fashion. Devices that may assist fiberoptic intubation, such as intubating airways, are also displayed. The purpose of this phase of the program is to teach how the fiberscope operates and its advantages and limitations.

The next section of the second part of the tutorial contains video clips that demonstrate the use of the fiberoptic laryngoscope in patients (Fig. 43-10). Real-time video clips are powerful educational additions to any computer-assisted educational program. Students at all levels quickly focus their attention on real-time video sequences. The user can halt most of the video clips at any time for further inspection of the still picture.

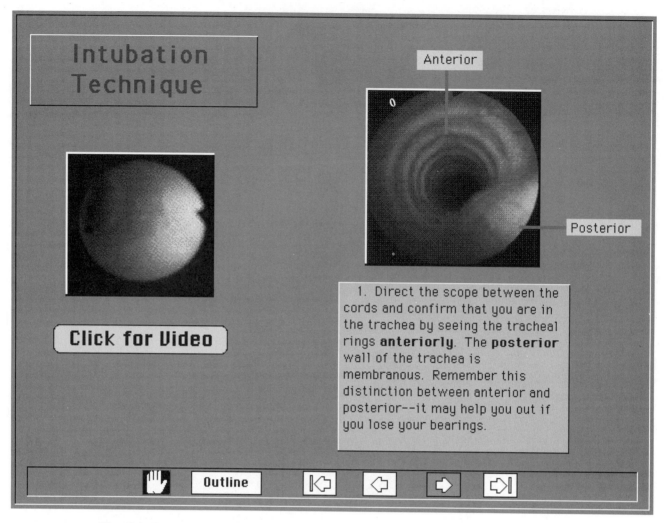

Fig. 43-9. Screen from the fiberoptic intubation section of the Airway Program. A video sequence demonstrating a normal fiberoptic view of anatomy is included.

The third section of the tutorial is a series of video clips that were taped in the clinical practice of fiberoptic examination of the airway or fiberoptically assisted endotracheal intubation, or both. These videos demonstrate normal upper airway anatomy and upper airway disease. Pathologic conditions include laryngeal tumors, rheumatoid arthritis, vocal cord polyps, superior vena cava syndrome. Many of these videos were produced with the new Olympus BF-200 videobronchoscope, which produces wide-angle upper airway images with outstanding resolution (Fig. 43-11). This videobronchoscope has a charge-coupled device (CCD) chip at the distal end of the fiberscope. The CCD chip converts light signals to electrical signals, which are relayed to the fiberscope's microprocessor, and the image is constructed and displayed on a video monitor. There are no fiberoptic imaging bundles in this fiberscope. This imaging technology provides excellent resolution and eliminates the optical distortion introduced by long fiberoptic imaging bundles.

These video sequences show many different types of airway abnormalities and pathologic conditions. The videos can be directly imported into the computer from a tape deck and edited via the computer. Text material can also be added to the program for explanation of the video. The imported video material can be tailored by the developer to selected, specific clinical situations to emphasize features that the educator considers important.

V. THE ANESTHESIOLOGY ACADEMIC COMPUTER LABORATORY

The primary purpose of an academic computer laboratory is to develop computer-assisted multimedia presentations and interactive educational software using input from multiple media sources including digitized sound, digitized color images from a flatbed scanner and 35 mm slide scanner, and digitized video from camcorders or video cassette recorders (VCRs) (Fig. 43-12; Box

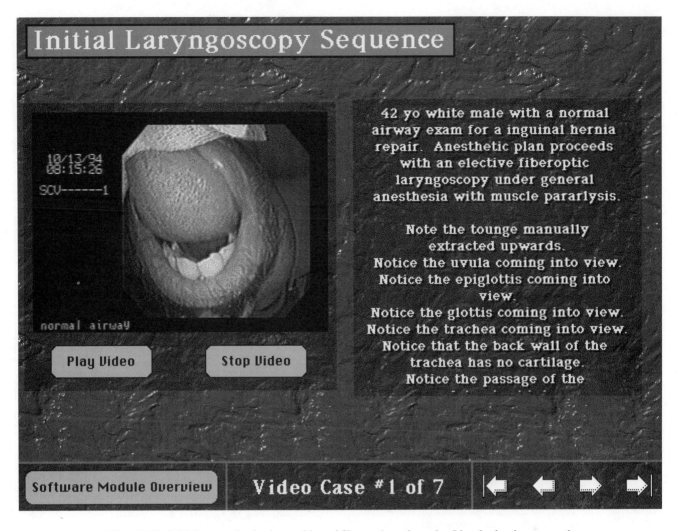

Fig. 43-10. Initial screen beginning a video of fiberoptic endotracheal intubation in a normal patient.

43-1). Animation and three-dimensional modeling can also be included. Once the format is developed, this instructional software can be used to teach any facet of anesthesiology. Educators preparing these programs use basic computer literacy skills developed from using software for word processing, spreadsheets, animation, painting and drawing, slide-making, scanning, digitizing audio and video inputs, and other presentation programs (Box 43-2). It is not, however, necessary that all anesthesiologists participating in the development process be facile with all aspects of the techniques. If an anesthesiology department has one or two faculty members with these skills, the other contributors can gain the necessary expertise as the project progresses. In fact, another primary purpose of the academic computing laboratory is to increase computer literacy skills among the residents and faculty.

After selection of the subject to be presented and establishment of the instructional goals, a database must be established that contains material to be imported into the program and all necessary reference information. The database should be dynamic and allow for updates and revisions. Interactive basic science software models that demonstrate the application of physiology and pharmacology to the understanding and management of pathologic processes in the clinical setting are extremely valuable for the learner. Computer-assisted instruction can demonstrate many of these basic principles in new formats that enhance learning.

Functional models of anesthesia equipment, both anesthesia delivery systems and monitoring devices, can be introduced. These models, with the aid of animation, can be used to effectively teach operational principles, limitations, and diagnosis of malfunctions. Computer-derived equipment models are extremely important and will occupy a pivotal role in future educational projects. Past generations of anesthesiology residents were able to disassemble, examine, and reassemble anesthesia ma-

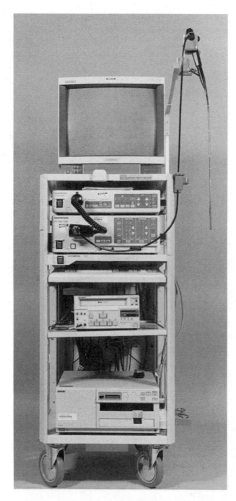

Fig. 43-11. The Olympus BF-200 videobronchoscope. This bronchoscope produces extremely high-resolution images. These images can be imported into interactive instructional programs.

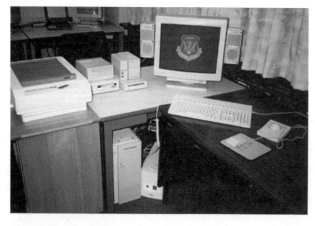

Fig. 43-12. The multimedia computer production station used to produce the Interactive Airway Program.

BOX 43-1   Computer hardware for the production station of an anesthesia interactive computer-assisted learning laboratory (Macintosh based)

Central processing unit with audiovisual capabilities
    Apple PowerMac 8100/100 AV
        64-megabyte RAM
        2-gigabyte hard disk drive
        CD-ROM
        Modem, networking hardware
        AV digitizing card
    Optional advanced components
        High-performance AV digitizing boards (permit faster frame rates and window size with improved quality)
        Hard drive disk array (2 to 10 gigabytes)
            High-capacity, high-speed drive that operates in conjunction with AV board and improves overall system performance
Accessory hardware
    External hard disk drive for mass data storage
    Storage media
        Removable cartridge drives (45 to 270 megabytes)
        Optical cartridge drive (120 to 1300 megabytes)
        Digital tape
    Scanners (flatbed scanner, slide scanner)
    Digitizing and drawing tablet
    Printers (laser printer, color printer)

---

chines. These exercises resulted in an exceptional understanding of how the devices functioned. As anesthesia equipment became more complex, the process of disassembly and reassembly was no longer practical or safe. The computer model, however, is a perfect substitute and may be superior to more traditional methods of demonstrating equipment function. Animation can be used to demonstrate gas flows through delivery systems, vaporizers, valves, and breathing circuits. Interactive features permit the user to see how changing position of the valves, components, or gas inlet lines may affect function of the system.

Once the basic format of the instructional program has been established, specific "specialty modules" such as regional anesthesia, fiberoptic laryngoscopy, transesophageal echocardiography, and equipment function can be developed. Faculty, organized into small groups, can develop a comprehensive departmental educational program with a series of instructional modules. Once the necessary programs have been developed, most of the lectures and formal didactic presentations can be delivered with a portable computer and a color LCD projection panel.

There is considerable benefit to a teaching program to be able to develop computer-assisted instructional

---

BOX 43-2   Production software for computer-assisted learning laboratory

Image processing

Photo processing-editing (Adobe Photoshop)
Video processing (Adobe Premiere)

Development software: interactive use of digital video, audio, video, and text

SuperCard (Alegiant Technologies)
HyperCard (Claris)
Director (MacroMind)
Authorware (MacroMind)
Script X (Klieda)

Painting and drawing

Canvas (Deneba)
Illustrator (Adobe)
Freehand (Aldus)

Three-dimensional modeling

Swivel 3D Pro (Swivel)
Showplace, MacRenderman (Pixar)
3D, Macromodel Bundel (MacroMind)
Studio Pro (Strata)
Sketch (Alias)

Data acquisition and modeling

LabView (National Instruments)

Database

4th Dimension
Filemaker Pro (Claris)

Supporting software

Word processing: Microsoft Word, Excel, PowerPoint
Page layout (Adobe Pagemaker)
Slide making (Aldus Persuasion)

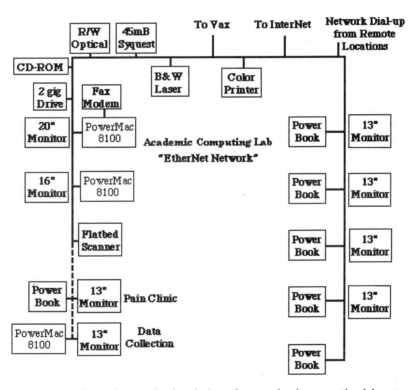

Fig. 43-13. A schematic organizational plan of an academic computing laboratory.

presentations by incorporating images and videos from their own department's clinical practice. Anesthesiology residents are then able to learn procedures and techniques exactly as they will be taught by the faculty of that department. These programs can be completed by the resident prior to actual performance of the procedure. This capability to specifically design the instructional material is superior to commercially prepared programs, which may present different techniques that may introduce confusion into the teaching process. To further enhance the educational opportunities and computer literacy of the anesthesiology residents, electives can be developed during the CA-3 year that permit the resident to construct an interactive program.

To facilitate development of an educational computer laboratory, resources and personnel from outside the department may prove invaluable. Networking personnel from the hospital or university, if the department is university affiliated, can assist with the local area network, access to the institution's network, and access to Internet. These personnel can also help with hardware and software compatibility within the institution. However, the department must select hardware and software that best suits its needs and is the easiest to use. Once the necessary computers have been obtained, they can be networked for educational purposes (Fig. 43-13 on p. 929). Internet access permits the communication and transfer of information with other educational institutions throughout the world.

The computer laboratory can also provide other services for the anesthesiology department. Functions such as data collection for quality assurance information, data collection for clinical research, and statistical analysis can all be performed with the network.

VI. CONCLUSION

The development of powerful personal computers and the introduction of software that permits construction of interactive programs with little expertise in software use will revolutionize medical education for medical students, residents, and practitioners. The ability to import and integrate images and video sequences into an interactive instructional program markedly enhances presentation. These presentations can be specifically designed to demonstrate actual clinical scenarios encountered in the programer's practice. For the user there are multiple ways to access the information and the interactive sequences. Consequently, the user can employ the program in a manner that is most suitable for the learning techniques of that individual. Critical clinical events can be learned and practiced repeatedly at the user's pace until the concepts are thoroughly understood. Future improvements in computer technology and software capability will further increase our instructional effectiveness.

REFERENCES

1. Caplan RA, Posner KL, Ward RJ et al: Adverse respiratory events in anesthesia: a closed claims analysis, *Anesthesiology* 72:828, 1990.
2. Cheney FW, Posner KL, Caplan RA: Adverse respiratory events infrequently leading to malpractice suits, *Anesthesiology* 75:932, 1991.
3. American Society of Anesthesiologists Task Force on Management of the Difficult Airway: Practice guidelines for management of the difficult airway, *Anesthesiology* 78:597, 1993.
4. Rose DK, Cohen MM: The airway: problems and predictions in 18,500 patients, *Can J Anaesth* 41:372, 1994.
5. Schwid HA, O'Donnell DO: Anesthesiologists' management of simulated critical events, *Anesthesiology* 76:495, 1992.
6. Kulik JA, Bangert RL, Williams GW: Effects of computer-based teaching on secondary school students, *J Educational Psychology* 75:19, 1983.
7. Jelovsek FR, Adebonojo L: Learning principles as applied to computer-assisted instruction, *MD Comput* 10:170, 1993.
8. Wishnietsky DH: *Hypermedia: the integrated learning environment*, Bloomington, Ind., 1992, Phi Kappa Delta Educational Foundation.
9. Dean JM: *Heartlab, MD Comput* 4:46, 1987.
10. Brahmi FA: The Macintosh in medicine, *MD Comput* 6:44, 1989.
11. Eberts RE: Computer-aided education, *MD Comput* 3:20, 1986.
12. Sheplock GJ, Thomas PS and Camporesi EM: An interactive computer program for teaching regional anesthesia, *Anesthesiol Rev* 20:53, 1993.
13. Hahn MB, McQuillan PM, Sheplock GJ: *Regional anesthesia*, St Louis, 1995, Mosby.
14. Fernandez O, Galindo A, Galindo P: *Interactive regional anesthesia*, New York, 1995, Churchill Livingstone.
15. Jones R, Sheplock G, Goldstoff M: Airway algorithm program: scientific exhibit. Presented at the annual meeting of the American Society of Anesthesiologists, San Francisco, Oct 1994.
16. Benumof JL: Management of the difficult adult airway, *Anesthesiology* 75:1087, 1991.
17. Start R, Sheplock G, Goldstoff M et al: Fiberscope training program: scientific exhibit. Presented at the annual meeting of the American Society of Anesthesiologists, Washington DC, Oct 1993.
18. Reed AP: Preparation of the patient for awake flexible fiberoptic bronchoscopy, *Chest* 101:844, 1992.

Chapter 44

EFFECTIVE DISSEMINATION OF CRITICAL AIRWAY INFORMATION: THE MEDIC ALERT* NATIONAL DIFFICULT AIRWAY/ INTUBATION REGISTRY

Lynette Mark
James Schauble
Gordon Gibby
Joyce Drake
Susan Turley

*Medic Alert is a federally registered trademark and servicemark of the nonprofit, tax-exempt Medic Alert Foundation.

I. OVERVIEW

Communication of critical airway information traditionally has been accomplished by brief notes in the medical record, by letter, or by verbal communication to patients and physicians, or by a combination of these. Significant shortcomings of these types of communication include questionable patient or future provider understanding of the significance of the airway difficulty and potential implications to future airway management, nonuniformity in documentation, and an inability to reaccess legible hard copy of these communications in a timely way. The Medic Alert National Difficult Airway/Intubation Registry was established in 1992 to facilitate uniform documentation and effective dissemination of standardized critical information related to complex airway management. The Registry was created by the Anesthesia Advisory Council, a volunteer multidisciplinary team of anesthesiologists, otolaryngologists, and experts in quality assurance and risk management. The Registry is expected, through dissemination of critical airway information and maintenance of a research database, to accomplish the goals of improving patient safety and practitioner security and to facilitate long-term tracking and outcome studies of patients. Such outcome studies may allow refinement of airway techniques, allow better anticipation of complex airway problems, and reduce future adverse outcomes.

The core of the Registry is the nonprofit Medic Alert Foundation, the oldest and foremost international personal emergency medical information system. To create the Registry, the Medic Alert Foundation system, which includes a 24-hour computerized emergency response center (with telephone access nationally and internationally without charge to the caller), wallet card, and identification emblem, was expanded to accommodate a more extensive database and a fax service for hard copy. Medic Alert Foundation has been endorsed by more than 50 organizations including the American Society of Anesthesiologists (ASA) in 1979, the World Federation of Societies of Anaesthesiologists in 1992, and the American Academy of Otolaryngology–Head and Neck Surgery Foundation in 1993. Medic Alert Foundation International currently is organized in more than 35 countries worldwide. International expansion of the Registry can be encouraged and promoted by Medic Alert Foundation and facilitated by the World Federation of Societies of Anaesthesiologists.

This chapter discusses the Medic Alert Foundation and the Registry, specifically addressing issues of documentation and dissemination of critical, standardized, clinically appropriate airway information. Objectives, components, and benefits of the Registry are presented, as well as future plans for a comprehensive and integrated system on national and international levels. Strategies for implementation of the Registry into clinical practice, including patient enrollment and subsequent practitioner access to the Registry, are discussed. Information on how to contact Medic Alert Foundation, receive Difficult Airway/Intubation Registry enrollment forms, or query the Registry appears in Appendix B.

II. DIFFICULT AIRWAY/INTUBATION: A MULTIFACETED PROBLEM

Complex airway management is a multifaceted problem involving health-care providers in a variety of clinical settings. The consequences of failed airway maintenance or endotracheal intubation, or both, can be devastating to the patient, the practitioner, and the health-care system. Critical issues include identification of difficult airway/intubation patients, documentation of airway management techniques, dissemination of critical airway information to future health-care providers, and medicolegal considerations.

A. PATIENT IDENTIFICATION

Controversies regarding predictors and definitions of "difficult" exist, both intraspecialty and interspecialty and dependent and independent of practitioner skill, related to specific techniques and complicated by changing patient pathophysiology.[1] Historically, anesthesiology literature cites an incidence of 1% to 3% of unanticipated difficult airway/intubation in patients undergoing general endotracheal anesthesia.[2-5] The airway management technique used to define "difficult" in this literature was conventional rigid laryngoscopy (Macintosh or Miller blades). Despite advances in airway management techniques and refinement of difficulty predictors, the 1% to 3% incidence of unanticipated difficulty cited has not changed and is still defined by conventional laryngoscopy.[5-7]

In an institution with approximately 25,000 general endotracheal anesthetic procedures annually, there are potentially 250 to 750 unanticipated difficult airway/intubations per year. Based on an ASA membership, which represents 90% of practicing anesthesiologists, and assuming that a full-time practicing anesthesiologist would encounter one unanticipated difficult intubation per year, there are potentially 30,000 to 90,000 unanticipated difficult airway/intubations annually in the United States. However, these numbers may underestimate the true incidence, since anesthesiologists may not recall many near misses as vividly as a smaller number of difficult intubations in which, despite the effort, the result was suboptimal. On a national and international level the scope of this problem and its impact on patients, practitioners, and the health-care system is sufficient to warrant vigorous efforts to identify solutions.

In addition to patients who have unanticipated difficult airways on initial presentation, cohorts of patients have anticipated complex airway management, which can be successfully managed by a variety of innovative and specialty-specific techniques employed by other airway specialists (otolaryngology–head and neck surgeons, pulmonologists, emergency department physicians, and the like). Some of these techniques (laryngeal mask airway and Combitube) are readily available, require minimal practitioner education or training, and are inexpensive, whereas others may be available primarily in specialty centers, may require extensive practitioner skill, and may be relatively expensive (fiberoptic bronchoscope, surgical airway, specialized rigid laryngoscopes, and fluoroscopic-assisted intubation).

Some patients may have undergone head and neck surgery and have visible or hidden implants (laryngeal stents, thyroplasties, and so forth). For these patients, specific considerations for airway management may be unknown to future providers (e.g., thyroplasty patients might require smaller endotracheal tubes than anticipated), compromising patient safety and increasing practitioner risk for preventable adverse events.

Successful future management of previously unanticipated difficult airway/intubations may be facilitated by identification of patients and by documentation and dissemination of information detailing successful and unsuccessful airway management techniques and primary difficulty encountered. For anticipated difficult airway patients, availability of this same information promotes quality of care.

B. DOCUMENTATION AND DISSEMINATION OF CRITICAL INFORMATION

Written documentation of airway events is institution specific and specialty variable. No standardized, uniform, readily available document exists to precisely record airway events and summarize salient issues.

When complex airway management patients are discharged, information about critical airway events may be inadvertently not communicated or miscommunicated. Verbal communication of difficult airway information by the provider to the patient is unreliable. Communication may be hindered by patient intubation or sedation, or both. The patient may be expeditiously discharged from the health-care facility or discharged by personnel other than primary health care provider before airway events have been fully communicated. Miscommunication may arise because of patients' lack of medical knowledge or overriding anxiety related to their primary medical condition. In addition, providers may underrepresent the severity of difficulty, attempting to allay patients' anxiety or fearing liability exposure. Written communication of difficult airway information by the provider to the patient may be a more effective strategy, but the patient may fail to accurately and comprehensively convey this information to future health-care providers. Patients may lose the anesthesiologist's letter or memo or fail to give a copy of it to their primary care provider, and in an emergency the information will most likely be inaccessible.

When difficult airway/intubation patients reenter the health-care system electively or emergently, they may relate vague verbal histories, deny any difficult airway history, or be physically unable to communicate. Attempts to retrieve prior anesthesia records and documentation should be initiated but may be unsuccessful because of constraints of time or availability. When available, written documentation may be incomplete and difficult for other health-care providers to decipher. Both of these situations create confusion as to the exact nature of the airway difficulty encountered and airway management employed, potentially delaying or compromising patient care.

Even when written documentation is adequate, dissemination of critical information is usually limited to the patient's medical record. Subsequent elective or emergent retrieval of records by future health-care providers, separated by geography or time, may be untimely or impossible.

C. CONSEQUENCES OF DIFFICULT AIRWAY MANAGEMENT

The consequences of a difficult airway/intubation with or without adverse outcomes may be as unsettling as the event itself. There may be patient-perceived threat to future anesthetic safety or lack of understanding as to the significance of the difficulty. There may be practitioner-perceived threat to professional security. The impact in direct and indirect costs to the health-care system for complex airway management–related events is far-reaching.

Three studies specifically demonstrated the consequences of difficult airway management on liability exposure.[8-10] In an analysis of approximately 5000 claims filed in the Maryland legal system over a 15 year period that named one or more anesthesiologists as a defendant, insertion of an endotracheal tube was the sixth most common medical procedure leading to a liability claim. The great majority of these claims also included as defendants other members of the operating room team (e.g., general surgeons, nurse anesthetists, orthopedic surgeons, otolaryngologists, plastic surgeons, cardiac surgeons, dentists, and nurses). Forty-five claims have been resolved as of 1994; one resulted in a jury award of $5 million.[8]

In a 1992 loss analysis study conducted by the Physicians Insurers Association of America (PIAA), files retrieved from an aggregate of 43 physician-owned malpractice insurance companies (representing approximately 2000 anesthesiologists nationally) ranked "intubation problems" as the third most prevalent misadventure (behind "tooth injury" and "no medical misadventures"). The average paid indemnity for 175 of 339 files was $196,958.[9]

The ASA Committee on Professional Liability closed claims study found that respiratory events were the most common cause of brain damage and death during anesthesia, with difficult intubation being the likeliest category for risk reduction. The median payment for respiratory claims was $200,000.[10]

To put these statistics in perspective, the following must be considered: (1) The number of malpractice claims reported represent only a small fraction (one eighth) of all adverse outcomes,[11] with one malpractice claim filed for every 7.5 patient injuries from difficult airway events and adverse outcomes that are not the subject of a claim;[12] (2) claims may often be aborted by good physician-patient communication; (3) claims are often initiated against physicians because of poor communication and inadequate records.[13]

III. DIFFICULT AIRWAY/INTUBATION: RESPONSES TO THE PROBLEM

A. AMERICAN SOCIETY OF ANESTHESIOLOGISTS GUIDELINES

In response to the previously mentioned issues the ASA developed and published *Practice Guidelines for Management of the Difficult Airway*. These guidelines heightened practitioners' awareness of the scope and magnitude of problems related to complex airway management. They encouraged familiarity with a standardized clinical airway algorithm and stressed availability of technologies in addition to conventional rigid laryngoscopy for difficult airway management. The guidelines recommended that the anesthesiologist document in the medical record the presence and nature of airway difficulties, the various airway management techniques employed, and whether they were beneficial or detrimental in managing the difficult airway. Recommendations for dissemination of critical information included informing the patient (or responsible person) of the presence of a difficult airway, apparent reasons for difficulty, and implications for future care.[5]

B. ANESTHESIA ADVISORY COUNCIL

Coincident with the development of these guidelines, an Anesthesia Advisory Council (Appendix A) representing anesthesiologists, otolaryngologists, and experts in risk management joined together to create a comprehensive system for uniform documentation and effective dissemination of critical airway information. Specifically, they addressed the following questions: (1) Once an airway event happens, is there a consistency in documentation and easy access to a central internationally accessible database? (2) Is there a uniform way that patients and health-care personnel can be informed of critical airway information? The Council identified and investigated two existing systems that were successful in documentation and dissemination of critical airway information: The University of Michigan Airway Clinic and the Medic Alert Foundation.

C. THE UNIVERSITY OF MICHIGAN AIRWAY CLINIC[14]

Martin L. Norton and colleagues at the University of Michigan pioneered efforts to more fully evaluate patients with complex airway management problems and to effectively disseminate critical information to patients and future health-care providers. The University of Michigan Airway Clinic was established in 1987 as a multidisciplinary, national and international referral center. The core of its clinical documentation consisted of a handwritten airway consultation record, photodocumentation, and an information response center. As the Clinic grew in size, it became increasingly apparent to house staff that the existing Medic Alert Foundation could more readily accommodate 24-hour emergency requests for information, and selected Clinic patients were enrolled.

D. MEDIC ALERT FOUNDATION

Medic Alert Foundation is a 501(c)3 nonprofit organization that has 40 years of experience with information exchange. Its stated mission is to protect and save lives by disseminating critical patient information immediately and accurately while maintaining patient confidentiality and privacy. This service comprises a three-part system: a 24-hour emergency response center, a visible alert emblem worn by the patient (Fig. 44-1), and a wallet card (Fig. 44-2). Medic Alert reliably tracks patients and updates their medical information. An initial enrollment fee of $35 to $75 (depending on the type of metal selected for the emblem) is waived for patients who are unable to pay, if enrollment is accompanied by a letter from the health-care provider. Patients are contacted yearly to update medical information, and a $15 annual fee is requested. In 1979, Medic Alert Foundation was endorsed by the ASA House of Delegates. In 1992 the Anesthesia Advisory

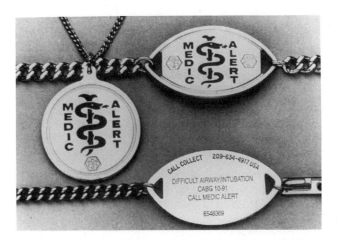

Fig. 44-1. *Clockwise from left,* The Medic Alert emblem as a necklace, the Medic Alert emblem as a bracelet, and the reverse side of the Medic Alert emblem, which shows the Medic Alert collect phone number (accessible nationally and internationally without charge to the caller), the Difficult Airway/Intubation Registry designation, and the patient's unique identification number for the Medic Alert system.

Council recommended the creation of the National Difficult Airway/Intubation Registry within the Medic Alert Foundation.

For years anesthesiologists have recognized the value of the Medic Alert emergency response system for patients with malignant hyperthermia (INDEX ZERO hotline) and have enrolled patients with difficult airways in a nonuniform way. The establishment of the National Difficult Airway/Intubation Registry within Medic Alert has promoted a standardization of terminology and an expanded database specifically for airway patients.

IV. THE MEDIC ALERT NATIONAL DIFFICULT AIRWAY/INTUBATION REGISTRY
A. OBJECTIVES OF THE REGISTRY

The major objectives of the Medic Alert Anesthesia Advisory Council for this Registry are (1) to develop and implement mechanisms for uniform documentation and dissemination of critical information, (2) to establish a central databank of airway management information for research purposes, (3) to analyze and refine predictors of difficulty, (4) to develop innovative airway management technologies based on analysis of successful and unsuccessful techniques employed, (5) to analyze and refine difficult airway management based on clinical practices, (6) to conduct long-term tracking of patients to assess implications of adverse outcomes on future management, (7) to create a multidisciplinary concept of "difficult airway/intubation," and (8) to determine whether rapid and economical dissemination of currently unavailable critical airway information will have a positive impact on future patient care and overall cost to the health-care system.

B. "DIFFICULT AIRWAY/INTUBATION" CATEGORY AND PATIENT IDENTIFICATION

The Council established the uniform category "difficult airway/intubation" to provide standard nomenclature on the Medic Alert identification emblem. Patients are identified for enrollment in the Registry after their surgery and medical management or via documented airway difficulty on their medical record, or both. They can be divided into at least three distinct groups: (1) anticipated difficult airway based on accepted predictors (genetic, disease specific, anatomic or physiologic, and patient experience), (2) previously unanticipated difficult airway, and (3) otolaryngology–head and neck surgery patients (with or without airway implants).

In an effort to circumvent controversies regarding the definition of "difficult," patients are enrolled by providers who have medicolegal responsibility for them, enabling primary providers to use their own definition of "difficult." To facilitate a common orientation for difficult airway management by various specialists, the following concept, adopted by the Council, is useful:

Knowing what you now know about this patient's airway and successful/unsuccessful airway management techniques employed, if this patient required emergency surgery and endotracheal intubation, would you do a 'rapid sequence induction'? IF your answer is NO!—and you documented on the patient's medical record "difficult airway/intubation"—that's a difficult airway/intubation!

C. COMPONENTS OF THE REGISTRY

The core of the Registry is the Medic Alert emergency response service: 24-hour emergency response center with phone and facsimile (fax) capability, identification (ID) emblem, and wallet card. The Medic Alert phone number (209-634-4917) is imprinted on the emblem. Callers are instructed to call collect. The number is accessible nationally and internationally, unlike an 800 number, which cannot be accessed outside the United States.

The basic Medic Alert service was expanded to include the following components:

1. Specialized enrollment brochure
Enrollment in the Registry is facilitated by a brochure specifically designed to address the concerns of health-care providers and patients (Fig. 44-3). It consists of the following:
a. HEALTH-CARE PROVIDER INFORMATION PANEL
Questions frequently asked by providers are addressed, such as the following:
Why the Medic Alert National Difficult Airway/Intubation Registry? Up to 3% of all patients undergoing anesthetics have unanticipated difficult air-

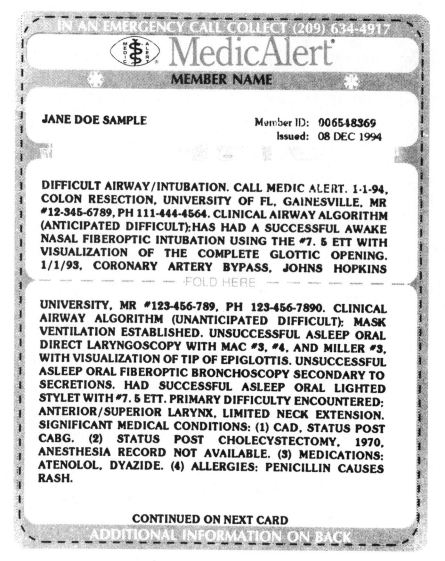

Fig. 44-2. The Medic Alert wallet card.

way/intubations. Knowledge of your experiences with these patients may facilitate future uncomplicated airway management. Medic Alert provides immediate access to this critical information with an alerting emblem, 24-hour emergency response center and database, and wallet card.

What is a difficult airway/intubation? Most practitioners use an "intuitive definition" to qualify a difficult airway/intubation. If your response to the question, "If this patient returned for emergency surgery requiring general endotracheal anesthesia in the middle of the night, would you do a rapid sequence induction?" is NO!—that's a difficult intubation!

I've never had an airway that I could not ultimately manage. In urgent and emergency situations, medical personnel with less daily airway experience than you may be the first to manage this patient's airway. Give them the benefit of your experiences.

I already provide letters of explanation for patients with

difficult airway/intubations. Medic Alert provides a uniform document to disseminate critical information. Incorporating Medic Alert into your practice for select patients may save you time and money, and will protect them.

Should I enroll patients with airways that are anticipated to be difficult—either by examination or by history, or both? Any patient who requires special techniques for airway management may benefit from enrollment in the Registry.

I just encountered a Registry patient and had no difficulty with airway management. Now what? The Registry provides a chronology of patient events. Medic Alert invites review by members and their physicians and regularly updates patients' files and wallet cards.

How detailed should I be in completing this application? Please complete and sign the airway databank section, especially the medical record number, and

Medic Alert
National Registry
for Difficult
Airway/Intubation

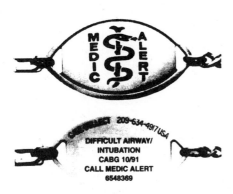

Protect Your Patients,
Inform Your Colleagues.

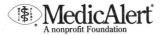
A nonprofit Foundation

Endorsed by the American Society of Anesthesiologists,
World Federation of Societies of Anaesthesiologists,
American Academy of Otolaryngology
Head and Neck Surgery

Fig. 44-3. The cover of the Medic Alert National Difficult Airway/Intubation Registry enrollment brochure.

obtain the patient's signature. Give the form to a patient or family member to mail with the enrollment fee.

How do I enroll patients who are unable to pay for membership? Medic Alert is a nonprofit foundation and will provide membership without charge for an indigent patient if the completed enrollment form is accompanied by a statement of the financial need, written on official letterhead, and signed by the practitioner.

b. PATIENT INFORMATION PANEL

Many health-care providers use candid questions and responses to facilitate perioperative discussion with patients. Questions most often asked by patients include the following:

What is difficult airway/intubation? During general anesthesia a specially trained professional assists your breathing. For the majority of patients, this is easily done by placing a mask over your nose and mouth or inserting a breathing tube into your windpipe, or both. Individual differences in jaw structure, mouth opening and dentition, and neck

movement might make some patients more difficult to manage than others. If the physician can anticipate or is alerted to previous airway difficulty, he or she can implement special techniques that are safe and comfortable.

How can Medic Alert help? Medic Alert can provide readily available information regarding your history of difficult airway/intubation for future elective and emergency medical situations. This is important, particularly in emergency situations, when someone other than your primary physician may provide you with emergency health care. The Medic Alert emblem will immediately alert the health-care provider to vital information that is critical to your safety.

How can I enroll in Medic Alert? If your physician noted airway difficulty and thinks you should be enrolled in the Medic Alert program, he or she will provide information about your airway management on this form. You must provide personal data and other significant medical conditions. When completed, please sign the form and mail with the enrollment fee.

c. MEDIC ALERT SERVICE

A visual and written description of the Medic Alert service is included for practitioner and patient education, including information on updating patient information and Medic Alert's 24-hour emergency response number (209-634-4917), a collect number for access nationally and internationally without charge to the caller).

d. MEDIC ALERT ANESTHESIA ADVISORY COUNCIL

A list of names and affiliations of members of this voluntary Council serves as a resource for questions, comments, or concerns that may arise regarding the Registry (Appendix A).

e. LEGAL STATEMENT

A legal statement, designed to address practitioner and institutional liability exposure and facilitate research, must be signed by all patients prior to enrollment in the Registry. The statement is as follows:

The member agrees not to wear the emblem or carry the wallet card until the emergency record has been carefully checked by the member for correctness, and agrees to inform Medic Alert in writing of any error found. The member authorizes Medic Alert to relay information in response to emergency telephone calls. The member agrees to immediately notify Medic Alert whenever his/her medical condition or address changes.

Enrolling hospital/physician's sole responsibility is to provide information to Medic Alert. How information is used is the sole responsibility of provider and therefore member hereby holds harmless the enrolling institution, physician and Medic Alert for actions taken based on information provided.

CLINICAL SETTING

○ ANESTHESIOLOGIST ○ CRNA ○ ENT ○ ED-MD ○ Other

ASA Class ○ 1 ○ 2 ○ 3 ○ 4 ○ 5 ○ E

HEIGHT ○ CM ○ IN [ ][ ] WEIGHT ○ KG ○ LBS [ ][ ]

SITE ○ OR ○ PACU ○ ICU ○ WARD ○ ED ○ Other

MONITORS ○ Capnograph ○ Oximetry ○ Auscult ○ None ○ Other

The difficult airway was ○ unanticipated ○ anticipated

Type of difficult airway encountered:
○ mask/ventilation
○ intubation
○ extubation
○ other

Why was it anticipated?
○ pt/family interview ○ prior paralysis
○ medical record ○ prior teflon inj
○ physical exam ○ prior thyroplasty
○ diagnostic tests ○ prior trach. stent
○ consults ○ existing trach
○ prior stenosis ○ other

Cause of difficulty (check all applicable):
○ redundant/swollen tiss
○ small mouth
○ tongue
○ dentition
○ ant/sup larynx
○ limited jaw op/mob
○ limited neck ext
○ c-spine instab
○ distorted anat
○ stricture
○ infection
○ other [ ]

Overall clinical assessment:
○ no difficulty
○ mildly difficult
○ moderately
○ severely

Airway management time:
○ <10 mins
○ 10-20 mins
○ >20 mins

Clinical outcome -- CONFIDENTIAL, for research purposes only
○ Not adverse ○ Minimal ○ Major

○ dental trauma ○ aspiration
○ desaturation ○ CV compromise
○ soft tissue/nasal ○ Tracheostomy
○ esoph trauma ○ No airway mngmnt.
○ laryng trauma   req. for this proc.
○ vocal cord trauma ○ Other
○ procedure cancelled [ ]

Clinically applied algorithm and comments

Signature of Anesthesiologist _____
Print Name/Phone _____

Check the details of each technique used in sequence:

TECHNIQUE #	1	2	3	4	5	6
Successful	○	○	○	○	○	○
Unsuccessful	○	○	○	○	○	○
# of Attempts	[ ]	[ ]	[ ]	[ ]	[ ]	
Awake	○	○	○	○	○	○
Asleep	○	○	○	○	○	○
Rapid sequence	○	○	○	○	○	○
Paralysis	○	○	○	○	○	○
Mask vent OK	○	○	○	○	○	
Nasal	○	○	○	○	○	○
Oral	○	○	○	○	○	○
Blind Nasal	○	○	○	○	○	○
Mac blade	○	○	○	○	○	○
Miller blade	○	○	○	○	○	○
Special blade	○	○	○	○	○	○
Blade size (if half size, enter next smaller size)	[ ]	[ ]	[ ]	[ ]	[ ]	
Tube size (or next smaller size)	[ ]	[ ]	[ ]	[ ]	[ ]	
Rigid Scope	○	○	○	○	○	○
Bougie/guide	○	○	○	○	○	○
Fiberoptic	○	○	○	○	○	○
Retrograde	○	○	○	○	○	○
Light wand	○	○	○	○	○	○
Laryngeal mask	○	○	○	○	○	○
Combitube	○	○	○	○	○	○
Transtrach	○	○	○	○	○	○
Cricothyroidotomy	○	○	○	○	○	○
Tracheostomy	○	○	○	○	○	○
Other	○	○	○	○	○	○
Only tip epigl. seen	○	○	○	○	○	
Only arytenoids seen	○	○	○	○	○	
Partial glottis seen	○	○	○	○	○	
All glottis seen	○	○	○	○	○	

Hospital _____

Medical Record Number _____

Procedure/Date _____

Patient or Guardian Signature _____

I understand and accept legal statement below. | 1844

Fig. 44-4. Airway management database section of the Medic Alert National Airway/ Intubation Registry enrollment form. It can be scanned and faxed to facilitate rapid dissemination of critical airway information.

Member agrees to permit any information on this form to be collected and used anonymously for scientific and educational research.

f. ENROLLMENT SECTION

Information requested for enrollment in Medic Alert includes patient demographics, emergency contacts, medical information to be engraved on the emblem, and other emergency medical information. Specific Registry information that is supplied by the practitioner includes hospital name, medical record number, surgical procedure, date of procedure, clinical anesthesia profile, nature of difficulty encountered, reason(s) for difficulty, successful and unsuccessful techniques, best visualization of airway anatomy, clinically applied algorithm, and clinical outcome. This section of the brochure is scannable and faxable (Fig. 44-4). The enrolling health-care provider's signature facilitates verification, and anonymity is honored, if requested. Select information from this database is compiled in paragraph form, printed on the patient's wallet card, and sent by fax when requested. With the exception of specific airway requirements (due to tracheal surgery, stenosis, or other conditions requiring specific size of endotracheal tubes), recommendations for future airway management are *not* made, thereby avoiding conflicts with other practitioners' choices for future airway management techniques. Clinical outcome information is confidential, collected for research purposes only, and not disseminated to the patient or future health-care providers.

g. PATIENT SIGNATURE

Informed consent must be obtained for enrollment.

2. Patient confidentiality

For more than 40 years there have been no claims against Medic Alert for breach of confidentiality or dissemination of incorrect medical information. Information contained in the Registry is available from the patient's medical record. When patients sign the informed consent for enrollment in Medic Alert, they are agreeing to confidential exchange of physician-verified medical information.

3. Physician education service

Primary or specialty physicians, or both, who are identified by the patient on the Registry enrollment form are notified of the patient's difficult airway/intubation by first-class mail. The notification is intended to be placed in the patient's file for future reference.

4. Long-term tracking

In addition to the initial enrollment fee, a nominal annual fee enables Medic Alert to maintain current medical information and track patients on a long-term basis. Medic Alert sends updating forms (via first-class mail) to all members and encourages them to review and update their medical information. Unopened returned envelopes are address-searched through the U.S. Postal Service and Social Security Administration. In this way, a current accounting of active members is maintained. In addition to this annual updating initiated by Medic Alert, patients are encouraged to update their medical information as often as necessary. Long-term tracking by Medic Alert will allow the Registry to compile a chronology of patient airway events. This reflects changing patient pathophysiology, which may have presented as complex airway management on one occasion and uncomplicated airway management on another (different techniques and algorithms used). By providing a chronology of events, any concerns of permanently labeling a patient as "difficult" are negated.

5. Research database

When patients sign the informed consent for enrollment, they agree to allow information in the Registry database to be used anonymously for educational and research purposes. Patient information updates are automatically reflected in the Registry database. Inquiries to the Registry database by researchers are reviewed by the Anesthesia Advisory Council and granted by the Medic Alert Foundation board.

D. BENEFITS OF THE REGISTRY

1. Patient safety

Knowledge of prior airway events, as provided by the Registry emergency response system, may significantly improve patient safety by detailing for future care providers unsuccessful and successful airway techniques used in the past.

Lack of definitive predictors of airway difficulty,[15-17] changing patient pathophysiology, and the use of conventional laryngoscopy as the first choice for airway management contribute to an unchanged incidence of 1% to 3% for unanticipated difficult airway/intubation. Until more accurate and comprehensive predictors of airway difficulty are identified, relatively healthy patients are at continued risk during anesthetic events—risk that cannot be completely addressed by improved monitoring techniques or through increased practitioner vigilance.

Identification of various combinations of anatomic abnormalities (as noted on the Registry enrollment form) may contribute to the development of a difficult airway/intubation profile that is more accurate than any single predictor.

With enrollment in the Registry, the patient's primary physician and specialist (as noted on the enrollment form) are notified of the patient's difficult airway/intubation status, thus providing for continuity of care.

2. Practitioner security

Practitioner security could be increased by the Registry in two ways: (1) by improving provider-patient communication and (2) by documenting and disseminating critical airway information for future health-care providers.

Malpractice claims are often initiated because of poor communication.[13] Enrollment in the Registry gives providers an opportunity to inform patients of their airway difficulties and adverse events while offering a way to protect them in the future. A survey of Registry patients showed that, despite experiencing adverse outcomes (cancellation of surgery, dental trauma, soft tissue trauma, desaturation, cardiovascular compromise, and cricothyrotomy or tracheostomy), 100% were satisfied with enrollment in the Registry and had a sense of comfort that future health-care providers would understand the significance of their difficult airway/intubation and the concept of Medic Alert.[18]

Patients may also favorably respond, after a difficult experience, to their anesthesiologists' knowledgeable presentation of organized efforts to register their problem and reduce the risk of recurrence.

Malpractice claims are often initiated because of poor documentation.[19] For future events, the intraoperative anesthesia record does not provide information in a standardized, easily readable form and is not readily accessible. Information from the Registry is standardized and detailed, and can be obtained via telephone or fax within 5 minutes of the request.

Enrollment in the Registry, as documented in patients' charts, is a positive reflection on the providers' concern for future patient safety.

3. Cost savings

The cost of initial enrollment in the Registry may be justified by future savings realized by the patient and provider or institution. A preliminary study of selective patient charges for anesthesia preparation time (i.e., anesthesiologist's professional fee, anesthesia resident's charge, drug and supply charges, and operating room time charges) was done for all 690 patients undergoing coronary artery bypass graft (CABG) surgery as the first procedure of the day at the Johns Hopkins Hospital during a 10-month period. Of these patients, 684 had no airway difficulty (control group); 6 had difficult airway/intubation and were subsequently enrolled in the Medic Alert National Difficult Airway/Intubation Registry. The results showed that the mean selective patient charge for anesthesia preparation time for the Registry group was $1578.24; this represented a 59% increase over the control group mean selective patient charge of $990.71.[20] Knowledge of difficulties previously encoun-

Table 44-1. Characteristics of patients enrolled in the Medic Alert National Difficult Airway/Intubation Registry (n = 111)

Characteristic	Cases (%)
Adult (age >18 years)	99
Emergency	1
ASA classes I and II	54
ASA classes III and IV	46
ASA class V	0
Anticipated difficult	44
Unanticipated difficult	56
Difficult mask airway	10
Difficult intubation	97

ASA, American Society of Anesthesiologists.

Table 44-2. Airway management techniques used for patients in the Medic Alert National Difficult Airway/Intubation Registry

Technique	Outcome	
	Successful (n = 110)	Unsuccessful (n = 200)
Conventional laryngoscopy	20	170
Fiberoptic bronchoscopy	66	13
Lighted stylet	1	1
Surgical airway	11	3
Specialized others	12	13

Table 44-3. Adverse outcomes for patients in the Medic Alert National Difficult Airway/Intubation Registry

Type	Frequency (n = 31)
Cancellation	9
Dental trauma	3
Desaturation	7
Soft tissue or nasal trauma	8
Tracheal trauma	3
Cardiovascular compromise	2
Other	7

tered and techniques used could promote cost-effective use of equipment and operating room time.

Anticipation and preparation for a difficult airway/intubation patient, as identified by the Registry, may decrease the incidence of cancellations, adverse outcomes, and malpractice claims. Even one settlement can cost the provider or institution significantly more than the time, effort, and cost of enrolling many patients in the Registry.

4. Outcomes studies

The database of the Registry is accessible for educational and research purposes via request to the Anesthesia Advisory Council. It is anticipated that this data will be used to improve anesthetic practice by refining airway techniques, identifying difficult airway/intubation patients more accurately, and decreasing the incidence of adverse outcomes.

E. CHARACTERISTICS OF REGISTRY PATIENTS

Between 1992 and 1994, more than 250 adult and pediatric patients throughout the United States were enrolled in the Medic Alert National Difficult Airway/Intubation Registry. Approximately 50% were in ASA classes I to II, and 50% were in ASA classes III to IV. Enrolled patients required general anesthesia, had difficulty, and/or did not require airway management at the time of enrollment but had a documented history of prior airway management. Patients were enrolled from private and academic institutions, outpatient surgical centers, and by self-referral. In a preliminary report of 111 of these patients, a variety of airway techniques were used and adverse outcomes were reported[21] (Tables 44-1 to 44-3). To ensure patient safety, providers encouraged these patients to enroll when there were minor or major adverse outcomes, despite concerns of liability exposure.

F. CLINICAL PRACTICES: IMPLEMENTATION OF THE MEDIC ALERT REGISTRY

1. Institutional level

Patients presenting themselves for surgery may have a history or physical features that suggest difficult airway management with conventional laryngoscopy, as identified by the provider. For these patients the provider may suggest enrollment in the Registry during the preoperative interview. For all patients a simple, direct statement included as part of the anesthesia consent, mentioning the potential for unanticipated airway difficulty and the Registry, may be appropriate. An institutional team approach has been instrumental in successful identification and enrollment of patients in the Registry.

At the Johns Hopkins Medical Institutions the following system has been implemented. The anesthesiologist identifies the difficult airway/intubation patient based on clinical experiences and completes an in-hospital quality assurance scan form similar to the Medic Alert Registry scan form, or simply uses the Medic Alert form. Medic Alert is the first registry to use a scan form system, which will allow reductions in costs of registry data entry.[22] The form can be submitted by fax to the Registry within minutes, or mailed. The nursing critical pathway, a key element in the successful education and enrollment of difficult airway/intubation patients,

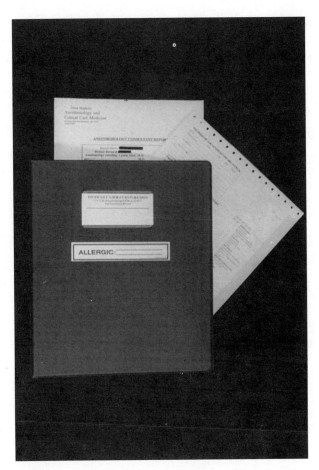

Fig. 44-5. Institutional difficult airway/intubation alert label for patient's record.

prompts nursing personnel to specifically query difficult airway preoperatively and on arrival in the recovery room. If the condition is present, the critical pathway initiates implementation of a specific protocol that includes in-hospital identification, patient-family teaching, and enrollment in the Registry.[23] Difficult airway/intubation patient identification also includes a green identification wristband and a patient chart airway alert label (Fig. 44-5). The wristband contains the Medic Alert insignia with the word "Temporary." This facilitates physician-patient communication and transition from a temporary in-hospital registry to the permanent Medic Alert Registry. Like an allergy alert band, the green difficult airway/intubation band provides continued patient identification and safety during hospitalization. The Joint Committee on Clinical Investigations at Johns Hopkins Medical Institution issued a waiver to written informed consent to place wristbands on identified difficult airway/intubation patients. Health-care personnel and patients recognize the tremendous implications to patient safety (vs. breach of confidentiality) as modeled in existing in-hospital "allergy alert" temporary

wristbands and out-of-hospital permanent medical alert bracelets.[24]

The Registry database information in the Medic Alert enrollment brochure is filled out by the anesthesiologist, and patient informed consent and signature are obtained to initiate Medic Alert Foundation personnel completing Registry enrollment. Issues of payment are discussed at this time. (See Notes to Practitioner in brochure description IV.C.1.a.)

Implementation at the institutional level should include physicians, nurses, and other health-care providers from all areas that identify and treat difficult airway/intubation patients (anesthesiology, otolaryngology–head and neck surgery, pulmonology, emergency department, and so forth).

2. National level

National implementation of a comprehensive and integrated system for Registry enrollment will involve identification of difficult airway/intubation patients at the point of entry into the health-care system—physician's office, clinic, ambulatory surgery center, emergency department, or hospital—or during the episode of care (intraoperatively). All enrolled patients will then be readily identified upon reentry into the health-care system, independent of time or place.

National availability of Registry enrollment forms will be accomplished through distribution by airway equipment manufacturers (Laerdal and others) who have agreed to include Registry forms in each box of equipment they ship, and through printing the Medic Alert collect phone number on the malignant hyperthermia posters distributed to all anesthesia departments. (Medic Alert is the Malignant Hyperthermia INDEX ZERO hotline.)

Interest has been high for several years in the concept of a national computerized patient record. In 1991 the Institute of Medicine set a goal of 10 years for widespread use of the computerized patient record. In January 1994 the Computer-Based Patient Record Institute, Inc., announced that it would seek major funding to finalize the development of standards for health care informatics. It seems inevitable, given the current interest and effort by government and private sectors, that a national computerized patient record will become a reality. However, because of the complexity and scope of issues involved, the time frame for accomplishing this goal remains far from certain. The objectives of the Registry are in agreement with those organizations supporting development of the computerized patient record. The Medic Alert system (with its centralized and computerized database of medical information accessible via telephone or fax within 5 minutes and with Internet access in development), already embodies many of the concepts of the computerized patient record. Proposals are being developed to allow electronic data transfers while accommodating patient confidentiality and medical records security through appropriate documentation and encryption techniques. Once these safety mechanisms are in place, automated queries of the Registry will become possible, obviating the need for telephone calls which interrupt the flow of patient evaluation in busy outpatient practices. As computerized medical records become more common in preanesthetic evaluation,[25] such automated queries of the Registry will become commonplace. Future developments could include supplementary photodocumentation. As development of the computerized patient record continues, Medic Alert's goals and information format will easily mesh with the infrastructure of an emerging computerized patient record.

3. International level

The technologic development of an internationally accessible Registry is now quite feasible and can be realized through the cooperative efforts of the Medic Alert Foundation, the World Federation of Societies of Anaesthesiologists, and the Society for Technology in Anesthesia. Encryption techniques now easily allow the Internet or alternative commercial packet-switched networks to be used for extremely fast data transmission throughout most of the world. The prodigious advance of technology now makes the required equipment both inexpensive and plentiful. Even where computer technology is lacking, however, enrollment can be accomplished using only a telephone, mail, or the ubiquitous fax machine, and queries can be accomplished by using the telephone. By 1994, Medic Alert Foundation International existed in more than 35 countries worldwide. Attention must be given to disparities in availability of technology. Many countries will be able to technically implement and support a comprehensive system as described earlier; other countries may not. Enrollment can be facilitated with only a pencil and the Registry enrollment form (or regular Medic Alert enrollment form).

V. CONCLUSION

The Medic Alert National Difficult Airway/Intubation Registry documents and disseminates critical airway information about difficult airway/intubation patients in a timely and standardized way to future health-care providers. Implementation of the Registry on a national and international scale may improve patient safety, increase practitioner security, and facilitate refinement of airway predictors and techniques.

ACKNOWLEDGMENTS

We wish to acknowledge Martha Chalmers, Sharon Buie, Margaret Leonard, Geneva Keaton, and Suzette Johnson for their continuing support of this project.

APPENDIX A: THE ANESTHESIA ADVISORY COUNCIL OF THE MEDIC ALERT FOUNDATION

Lynette Mark, MD,
The Johns Hopkins University
Chairman

Charles Beattie, PhD, MD,
Vanderbilt University

Charles W. Cummings, MD,
The Johns Hopkins University

Paul W. Flint, MD,
The Johns Hopkins University

Robert Forbes, MD,
University of Iowa College of Medicine

Gordon Gibby, MD,
University of Florida School of Medicine

Paul Goldiner, MD,
The Mount Sinai Medical Center

J.S. Gravenstein, Sr., MD,
University of Florida School of Medicine

Martin L. Norton, MD, JD,
University of Michigan Medical Center

Andranik Ovassapian, MD, FACP,
Northwestern University Medical School
Veterans Administration Lakeside Medical Center

A. Thomas Pedroni, Jr., Esq.,
Alexander & Alexander

Ellison C. Pierce, Jr., MD,
New England Deaconess Hospital

J.G. Reves, MD,
Duke University Medical Center

James Roberts, MD,
Massachusetts General Hospital

Mark C. Rogers, MD,
Duke University Medical Center

Henry Rosenberg, MD,
Hahnemann University and Hospital

James F. Schauble, MD,
The Johns Hopkins University

Alan Jay Schwartz, MD, MS Ed,
Medical College of Pennsylvania

Richard S. Wilbur, MD, JD,
Medic Alert Foundation

John F. Williams, Jr, MD,
George Washington University Medical Center

APPENDIX B: ADDRESSES

Completed Registry enrollment forms should be mailed to the Medic Alert Foundation, 2323 Colorado Ave., Turlock, CA 95382.

Requests for additional Registry enrollment forms should be directed to the Medic Alert Foundation, 2323 Colorado Ave., Turlock, CA 95382.

Phone: 1-800-432-5378

Fax: 1-209-669-2450

Internet: medcalrt@koko.csustan.edu

Requests to query the Registry database should be directed to Lynette Mark, MD, Chairman, Anesthesia Advisory Council, c/o Department of Anesthesiology and Critical Care Medicine, The Johns Hopkins Medical Institutions, 600 N Wolfe St., Tower 711, Baltimore, MD 21205.

Phone: 410-955-0631

Fax: 410-955-0994

Internet: lm@welchlink.welch.jhu.edu

REFERENCES

1. Benumof JL: Management of the difficult adult airway, *Anesthesiology* 75:1087, 1991.
2. Wilson ME, Spiegelhalter D, Robertson JA et al: Predicting difficult intubation, *Br J Anaesth* 61:211, 1988.
3. Mallampati SR, Gatt SP, Gugino LD et al: A clinical sign to predict difficult intubation: a prospective study, *Can Anaesth Soc J* 32:429, 1985.
4. Caplan RA, Posner K, Ward RJ et al: Adverse respiratory events in anesthesia: a closed claims analysis, *Anesthesiology* 72:828, 1990.
5. American Society of Anesthesiologists Task Force on Guidelines for Management of the Difficult Airway: Practice guidelines for management of the difficult airway, *Anesthesiology* 78:597, 1993.
6. Williamson JA, Webb RK, Szekely S et al: Difficult intubation: an analysis of 2000 incident reports, *Anaesth Intensive Care* 21:602, 1993.
7. Rose DK, Cohen MM: The airway problem and predictors in 18,500 patients, *Can J Anaesth* 41(5):372, 1994.
8. Morlock L: Personal communication to Lynette Mark, July 17, 1994.
9. Mark L, Drake J: Professional liability and patient safety: the Medic Alert national difficult airway/intubation registry, *Anesthesiology Alert* 3(4):1, 1994.
10. American Society of Anesthesiologists Committee on Professional Liability: Preliminary study of closed claims, *ASA Newsletter* 52:8, 1988.
11. Caplan RA: Anesthetic liability: what it is and what it isn't. In *1992 Review Course Lectures,* Cleveland, 1994, International Anesthesia Research Society.
12. Morlock L: Personal communication to Lynette Mark, July 17, 1994.
13. Kidwell R: Personal communication to Lynette Mark, July 17, 1994.
14. Norton ML, editors: *Atlas of the Difficult Airway,* St Louis, 1991, Mosby.
15. Ovassapian A, Krejcie TC, Yelch SJ et al: Awake fiberoptic intubation in the patient at high risk of aspiration, *Br J Anaesth* 62:13, 1989.
16. Wilson ME, John R: Problems with the Mallampati sign, *Anaesthesia* 45:486, 1990.
17. Vaughan RS: Airways revisited, *Br J Anaesth* 62:1, 1989.
18. Cherian M, Mark L, Schauble J et al: The national Medic Alert difficult airway/intubation registry: patient safety and patient satisfaction. Presented at the annual meeting of the American Society of Anesthesiologists, San Francisco, October 1994 (abstract).
19. How to avoid small complaints about quality of care, *Maryland BPQA (Maryland Board of Physician Quality Assurance) Newsletter* 1(4):1, 1993 (editorial).
20. Mark L, Schauble J, Turley S et al: The Medic Alert national difficult airway/intubation registry: technology that pays for itself. Presented at the annual meeting of the Society for Technology in Anesthesia, 1995 (abstract).
21. Mark L, Gibby G, Fleisher L et al: Practice guidelines to clinical practices: Medic Alert difficult airway/intubation registry. Presented at the annual meeting of the American Society of Anesthesiologists, 1994 (abstract).
22. Gibby GL, Mark L, Drake J: Effectiveness of Teleforms scan-based input tool for difficult airway registry: preliminary results. Presented at the annual meeting of the Society for Technology in Anesthesia, 1995 (abstract).
23. Krenzischek E: Personal communication to Lynette Mark, November 1, 1994.
24. Mark L, Beattie C, Ferrell C et al: The difficult airway: mechanisms for effective dissemination of critical information, *J Clin Anesth* 4:247, 1992.
25. Gibby GL, Jackson KI, Gravenstein JS et al: Development of problem categories for computerized preanesthesia evaluation of outpatients, *J Clin Monit* 8:156, 1992 (abstract).

Chapter 45

MEDICAL-LEGAL CONSIDERATIONS: THE ASA CLOSED CLAIMS PROJECT

Robert A. Caplan
Karen L. Posner

The opinions expressed herein are those of the authors and do not represent the policy of the American Society of Anesthesiologists.

I. HISTORICAL PERSPECTIVE

Anesthesiologists have a long-standing appreciation for risks associated with airway management. During the past five decades, a variety of studies have demonstrated that events involving the respiratory system are a prominent cause of adverse outcomes in anesthesia practice.[1-9] A few examples help illustrate this point. The Anesthesia Study Commission, which investigated anesthesia-related fatalities in metropolitan Philadelphia between 1935 and 1944, identified respiratory factors such as airway obstruction, hypoxia, and aspiration as the probable cause of death in approximately 19% of cases.[1] A large, multicenter study by Beecher and Todd, conducted about a decade later when curare and other muscle relaxants were first entering clinical practice, led to the recognition of excess mortality associated with perioperative respiratory depression.[2] In the 1970s, Utting and colleagues analyzed a seven-year series of anesthesia accidents reported to the Medical Defence Union of the United Kingdom.[3] Of 227 cases resulting in death or brain damage, 36% involved adverse respiratory events such as esophageal intubation, ventilator misuse, and aspiration.

Critical-incident studies have offered a similar picture. Cooper's landmark study of the late 1970s, revealed that 29% of reported incidents were related to respiratory events such as airway mismanagement or failure and misuse of ventilators and breathing circuits.[4] Most recently, the Australian Incident Monitoring Study has provided a detailed analysis of the first 2000 cases that have been voluntarily submitted since the late 1980s.[5] In this collection of critical incidents, problems with ventilation accounted for 16% of reports from practitioners in Australia and New Zealand.

II. THE CLOSED-CLAIMS PERSPECTIVE

Closed medical malpractice claims represent an important resource for the study of professional liability associated with airway management. To better appreciate this resource, it is helpful to describe some basic features of claims data.

A medical malpractice claim is a demand for financial compensation by an individual who has sustained injury in connection with medical care. Resolution of a claim usually occurs by either an out-of-court process or litigation. Once a claim is resolved, its file is *closed*. A closed claim file typically contains a broad assortment of documents relating to the adverse outcome. These documents may include medical records, narrative statements of the involved health-care personnel, expert and peer reviews, deposition summaries, outcome and follow-up reports, and the cost of settlement or jury award.

Claims represent only a small fraction of all adverse outcomes arising from medical care. The Harvard Medical Practice Study of patients in New York State in 1984 reported that approximately 4% of patients sustained an iatrogenic injury during hospitalization.[10] Malpractice claims, however, were filed by only one eighth of all injured patients. Similar findings were described 10 years earlier by the Medical Insurance Feasibility Study in California.[11] These small fractions make it unlikely that claims can be regarded as a representative cross section of all adverse outcomes.

Although claims may not serve as a representative sample of the entire population of adverse outcomes, these cases have a direct and important implication for the study of professional liability: the cost of claims plays an important role in determining the cost of medical malpractice premiums. By studying a large collection of claims, it may be possible to identify types of adverse events that consistently make a large contribution to insurance costs. This information helps focus research and risk-management strategies on areas of clinical practice associated with the greatest losses. Successfully reducing losses may lead to lower premiums, with accompanying savings for physicians, patients, and associated third-party participants. Since many types of adverse outcomes are relatively rare, claims files also represent an enriched environment for collecting information about infrequent but catastrophic events. Examining a large set of rare or unusual adverse outcomes with a common theme provides an opportunity to generate hypotheses of causation and remedy that may not be evident to practitioners who experience such cases as isolated events.

Since 1985, the Committee on Professional Liability of the American Society of Anesthesiologists (ASA) has

Table 45-1. Most common damaging events

Respiratory system	34%
Equipment problem	6%
Cardiovascular system	4%
Wrong drug/dose	4%
Convulsion	2%

n = 1541. ASA Closed Claims Database 1990.
Adapted from Caplan RA, Posner KL, Cheney FW et al: *Anesthesiology* 72:828, 1990.

engaged in a structured analysis of closed anesthesia claims in the United States. This undertaking is designated as the ASA Closed Claims Project. Cases involving adverse anesthetic outcomes are retrieved from the closed claims files of 34 U.S. medical-liability insurance carriers who voluntarily participate in this project. Claims for dental injury are not included in this project. In aggregate, the 34 participating carriers provide coverage for approximately 50% of U.S. anesthesiologists. Since several years often elapse between the occurrence of an adverse event and the closure of its associated claim, the majority of cases span an interval from the late 1970s to the mid-1980s. The database now contains more than 3000 cases.

A detailed description of data-collection procedures for the Closed Claims Project has been reported previously.[12] In brief, each claim file is reviewed by a practicing anesthesiologist, and a standardized form is used to record detailed information on patient characteristics, surgical procedures, anesthetic agents and techniques, involved personnel, sequence of events, standard of care, critical incidents, clinical manifestations, types of error, responsibility, and outcome. Standard of care is rated as appropriate (standard), less than appropriate (substandard), or impossible to judge, based upon reasonable and prudent practices at the time of the event. Practice patterns that may have evolved at a later date are not retrospectively applied when the standard of care is rated. An adverse outcome is deemed preventable with better monitoring if the reviewer finds that the use—or better use—of any monitor would probably have prevented the outcome, whether or not such monitor was available at the time of the event. An acceptable level of interrater reliability has been established for reviewer judgments on the standard of care and preventability of adverse outcomes with better monitoring.[13]

A. PRINCIPAL FEATURES OF ADVERSE RESPIRATORY OUTCOMES AND HIGH-FREQUENCY ADVERSE RESPIRATORY EVENTS

1. Basic features

Adverse respiratory events constitute the single largest source of injury in the closed-claims project

Table 45-2. Comparison of respiratory and nonrespiratory events

	Respiratory	All others
Incidence	34%	66%
Death or brain damage	85%	30%
Preventable	72%	11%
Substandard care	76%	30%
Payment frequency	72%	51%
Median payment	$200,000	$35,000

n = 1541. ASA Closed Claims Database 1990.
Adapted from Caplan RA, Posner KL, Cheney FW et al: *Anesthesiology* 72:828, 1990.

Table 45-3. Most common claims for adverse respiratory events

Event	Number of cases	% of 522 respiratory claims	% of 1541 total claims
Inadequate ventilation	196	38	13
Esophageal intubation	94	18	6
Difficult endotracheal intubation	87	17	6
Total	377	73%	25%

Other adverse respiratory events (e.g., aspiration, airway obstruction, bronchospasm, premature extubation, unintended extubation, endobronchial intubation) exhibited an overall incidence ≤5%. n = 1541. ASA Closed Claims Database 1990. Adapted from Caplan RA, Posner KL, Cheney FW et al: *Anesthesiology* 72:828, 1990.

(Table 45-1). A detailed analysis of these events was initiated when the database reached a total of 1541 claims.[14] The contrast between adverse respiratory events and other claims was particularly unfavorable. In particular, respiratory-related claims were characterized by a high frequency of devastating outcomes and costly payments (Table 45-2).

Just three mechanisms of injury accounted for nearly three fourths of all claims for adverse respiratory events (Table 45-3). These mechanisms were inadequate ventilation (38% of cases), esophageal intubation (18%), and difficult intubation (17%). The remaining adverse respiratory events were produced by a variety of low-frequency mechanisms including aspiration, airway obstruction, bronchospasm, premature and unintentional extubation, endobronchial intubation, inadequate inspired oxygen delivery, and equipment failure. Each low-frequency mechanism represented no more than 5% of the overall database. Special features of low-frequency events are discussed later in this chapter.

A detailed display of outcome and payment data for the three most common types of adverse respiratory events is shown in Table 45-4. Death and permanent brain damage were more frequent in claims for inadequate ventilation and esophageal intubation (>90%) than in claims for difficult tracheal intubation (56%; $P < .05$). Overall, payment for respiratory-related claims ranged from $1000 to $6 million. Nearly three fourths (72%) of claims resulted in payment. Median payment was highest for inadequate ventilation ($240,000) and lowest for difficult tracheal intubation ($76,000). Claims for adverse respiratory events generally involved healthy adults undergoing nonemergency surgery with general anesthesia (Table 45-5).

The reviewers judged that better monitoring would have prevented the adverse outcome in 376 (72%) of the 522 claims for adverse respiratory events (Fig. 45-1). This differs from nonrespiratory claims, in which only 11% of cases were judged preventable with better monitoring ($P < .05$). Almost all (>90%) claims for inadequate ventilation and esophageal intubation were considered preventable with better monitoring, as opposed to 36% of claims for difficult endotracheal intubation. For the 376 claims considered preventable with better monitoring, the reviewers chose pulse oximetry, capnometry, or both of these devices in 98% of cases. The combination of pulse oximetry and capnometry was the most common choice for prevention of esophageal intubation (84%) and inadequate ventilation (50%), but pulse oximetry alone was chosen most often for prevention of adverse outcomes associated with difficult endotracheal intubation (74%). Data on the role of better monitoring in the prevention of adverse outcomes must be interpreted with particular care, as the reviewers were not asked to consider confounding factors such as equipment malfunction, diversion of attention, misinterpretation and misuse of data, or the impact of false-positive and false-negative results. Thus the reviewers' judgments should be regarded as a near-maximum (and probably unattainable) estimate of the efficacy of better monitoring.

2. Inadequate ventilation

The largest class of adverse respiratory events was inadequate ventilation. The distinguishing feature in this group of claims was the reviewer's inability to identify a specific mechanism of injury. In part, the inability to assign a mechanism of injury may reflect uncertainty on the part of the original health-care providers. Since most adverse events occurred before the widespread use of pulse oximetry and capnometry, the uncertainty may be due to the limitations of traditional clinical signs such as chest excursion, reservoir-bag motion, and breath sounds. With increasing use of quantitative measures of ventilation, fewer cases may be assigned to the category of inadequate ventilation. It is also possible that a delayed rather than contemporaneous approach to the inves-

Table 45-4. Outcome, payment, and payment frequency for the most common adverse respiratory events

	Inadequate ventilation n = 196	Esophageal intubation n = 94	Difficult endotracheal intubation n = 87	All nonrespiratory events n = 1019
Outcome		(% of cases)		
Death	71*	81*	46*	22
Permanent brain damage	23*	17*	10	8
Other permanent injury	1*	1*	18	25
Temporary injury	4*	1*	24*	39
No injury	1*	0*	1*	6
Payment		(in $1000s)		
Range	1.5-6000	30-3400	1-4700	<1-5400
Median	240*	217*	76*	35
Payment frequency		(% of claims paid)		
	73*	82*	67*	51

Percentages do not always sum to 100 because of rounding error. *$P < .05$ compared to nonrespiratory events. n = 1541. ASA Closed Claims Database 1990. Adapted from Caplan RA, Posner KL, Cheney FW et al: *Anesthesiology* 72:828, 1990.

Table 45-5. Basic clinical features of cases involving adverse respiratory events

	All respiratory events n = 522	All nonrespiratory events n = 1019
Age in years (mean ± SD)	37 ± 21	41 ± 20
ASA physical class (median)	2	2
Emergency (%)	25	17
Male/female (%)	40/58	40/59
Primary anesthetic (%)		
General	85	63
Regional	11	32
Other*	4	5

Percentages do not always sum to 100 because of missing data and/or rounding.
*Includes combined regional and general techniques, anesthesia standby, monitored anesthesia care, and nonoperative events involving an anesthesiologist. n = 1541. ASA Closed Claims Database 1990. Adapted from Caplan RA, Posner KL, Cheney FW et al: *Anesthesiology* 72:828, 1990.

tigation of adverse outcomes is not powerful enough to provide an understanding of many events.

3. Esophageal intubation

Prompt detection of esophageal intubation is a primary concern in anesthesia practice. A disturbing feature in this series of claims is that the detection of esophageal intubation required five or more minutes in the majority of cases (97%). Incompetence and negligence (e.g., intubation performed by a legally blind practitioner or minimal attention to the patient during the first half hour of the case) provide straightforward explanations for delayed detection. However, we found only eight claims (9%) in which this type of obviously inadequate behavior played a primary role.

Why, then, was delayed recognition such a prominent feature in these claims for esophageal intubation? We speculate that reliance on indirect tests of ventilation may have been an important factor contributing to delay. For example, cyanosis is an indirect test of ventilation that might be used as a clue of esophageal intubation. This approach, however, is limited by the insensitivity of the human eye to the changes in skin color that occur during arterial desaturation.[15,16] Furthermore, effective preoxygenation before intubation may extend the time before significant arterial desaturation develops.[17] In this context, it is not surprising that cyanosis preceded the recognition of esophageal intubation in only 34% of cases.

One might also expect cardiovascular clues to accompany hypoxemia or hypercarbia. Indeed, one or more major hemodynamic derangements were recorded in 79 of the 94 claims (84%) for esophageal intubation. In order of frequency, these derangements included bradycardia, asystole, hypotension, unspecified arrhythmia, tachycardia, and ventricular fibrillation (Table 45-6). It is particularly noteworthy that hemodynamic derangements preceded the recognition of esophageal intubation in 60 claims (65%). One can readily appreciate how the life-threatening nature of such derangements could have drawn effort away from detection of the underlying problem. The severity of the hemodynamic changes also suggests that the respiratory and metabolic consequences of esophageal intubation were so far advanced that some degree of irreversible damage had already

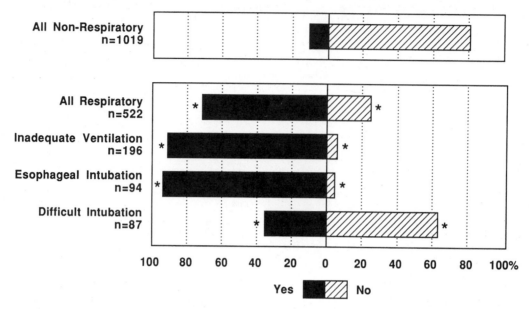

Fig. 45-1. Percentage of adverse respiratory outcomes considered preventable or not preventable with better monitoring. Incidence of claims considered impossible to judge was 1%-3% in respiratory groups and 9% in nonrespiratory group. *$P < .05$ compared with nonrespiratory claims. n = P1541. ASA Closed Claims Database 1990. (Reproduced from Caplan RA, Posner KL, Cheney FW et al: *Anesthesiology* 72:828, 1990.)

Table 45-6. Major hemodynamic derangements accompanying esophageal intubation claims

Hemodynamic derangement	% of claims (n = 94)
Bradycardia	57
Asystole	55
Hypotension	49
Unspecified arrhythmia	10
Tachycardia	5
Ventricular fibrillation	1

Percentages sum to more than 100 because of multiple derangements. n = 1541. ASA Closed Claims Database 1990.
Adapted from Caplan RA, Posner KL, Cheney FW et al: *Anesthesiology* 72:828, 1990.

occurred. Thus, from the standpoint of timely detection and intervention, skin color and routine hemodynamic measurements do not seem to provide useful clues of esophageal intubation.

Auscultation of breath sounds is another widely used test of ventilation. In this series of claims, breath-sound auscultation was documented in 62 of the 94 claims for esophageal intubation (63%). In three of these cases (5%), breath-sound auscultation led to a correct diagnosis of esophageal intubation. In 30 cases (48%),

auscultation led to the erroneous conclusion that the endotracheal tube was located in the trachea when it was actually in the esophagus. This result was termed a *misdiagnosis of tracheal intubation*. The diagnostic error in such cases was recognized in a variety of ways, including later reexamination with direct laryngoscopy, absence of any object in the trachea at the time of an emergency tracheostomy (despite ongoing "ventilation" through an endotracheal tube), resolution of cyanosis following reintubation (often by a second participant), and discovery of esophageal intubation at autopsy. In 29 of the 62 claims (47%) in which auscultation was documented, the records did not contain sufficient information to determine how the auscultatory findings were interpreted.

The preceding paragraph presents the grim finding that breath-sound auscultation was associated with a misdiagnosis of endotracheal intubation in nearly half of cases (48%). Let us try to place these data in a more favorable context by devising an analysis based upon a best-case scenario in which we assume that auscultation led to a correct diagnosis in (1) the 3 cases in which it actually did so, (2) the 29 cases in which the role of auscultation was unclear, and (3) the 32 cases in which there was no information about the use of auscultation. With this approach, the results are still unsettling:

misdiagnosis occurred at a rate of 32% (30 out of 94 cases).

Although the limitations of auscultation have been well described previously,[18] this set of claims provides the first evidence for a recurring pattern of risk: *if esophageal intubation has occurred, the use of auscultation to distinguish between endotracheal and esophageal location may delay the restoration of effective ventilation by producing a false impression of correct endotracheal placement.* We do not wish to imply that the risk of auscultation is related primarily to the mechanical act of listening to breath sounds (which is innocuous by itself) or the simple existence of false-positive and false-negative results (which can occur with any test). We speculate that the risk develops when auscultatory findings are obtained in a clinical environment that promotes misinterpretation. The risk of misinterpretation may be greatest when quantitative data from capnometry and oximetry are unavailable and other indirect clues of esophageal intubation (e.g., gastric distention, cyanosis, hemodynamic changes) are not readily evident or not yet manifest.

The most likely setting for misinterpretation of breath sounds is probably the first few minutes following esophageal intubation in the patient who has been adequately preoxygenated during an otherwise uncomplicated induction of general anesthesia. In the context of this transiently benign-appearing state, there may be a tendency to interpret equivocal or ambiguous auscultatory findings as normal. The reasoning process leading to this error might take a course similar to the following: "The breath sounds are somewhat distant, but everything else seems fine. Therefore, the abnormal quality of breath sounds is more likely due to obesity (or has some other underlying condition that can hamper auscultation), rather than esophageal intubation." Since quantitative data from capnometry and oximetry are also subject to misinterpretation, these monitors cannot be regarded as definitive remedies. The fundamental problem is the potential for error that arises from the interaction between preconceived notions of likelihood, reflex clinical behaviors, conflicting environmental data, the potential for a rapid and poorly reversible cascade of critical events, and the inherent limitations of all diagnostic tests (see Chapter 7). The theoretical background for exploring this type of interaction and developing more-effective clinical algorithms has been reviewed by Gaba and colleagues.[19,20]

4. Difficult intubation

Claims for difficult intubation were distinguished by a relatively small percentage of cases in which care was considered less than appropriate (38% vs. >80% for inadequate ventilation and esophageal intubation), and a similarly small percentage of cases in which better

monitoring would have prevented the complication (36% vs. >90% for inadequate ventilation and esophageal intubation). Although these findings seem outwardly favorable, the comparisons are not so attractive from the perspective of risk reduction. If the majority of cases of difficult intubation cannot be linked to obvious inadequacies in care or deficiencies in monitoring, then it is unlikely that claims analysis alone can point to effective or broad-based remedies. Simulators, algorithms, and drill routines have generated considerable interest in recent years. These newer educational tools and management strategies may provide an important opportunity for clinicians to gain concentrated exposure to relatively infrequent events. An evidence-based guideline for management of the difficult airway has recently been developed by the American Society of Anesthesiologists.[21] Key features of this guideline are discussed in Chapter 8.

B. LOW-FREQUENCY ADVERSE RESPIRATORY EVENTS

1. Basic features

The foregoing discussion has focused on the most common mechanisms of respiratory injury in the closed-claims database. A formal study of low-frequency adverse respiratory events was conducted in 1991 when the closed-claims database had reached 2046 cases.[22] Although these events are much less common—each category representing no more than 5% of the overall database—sufficient claims have been collected to permit the identification of recurrent themes that may contribute to liability. Five categories of events have been studied in depth, each category containing at least 40 claims and together encompassing 300 claims, or about 15% of the overall database. These categories include airway trauma, pneumothorax, airway obstruction, aspiration, and bronchospasm. Death or brain damage occurred in nearly half (47%) of these cases, and the median payment was $60,000 (Table 45-7).

2. Airway trauma

Airway trauma was the most common type of low-frequency airway event, accounting for 97 claims or 5% of the overall database. Difficult intubation was associated with 41 of these claims (42%). The most frequent sites of injury were the larynx, pharynx, and esophagus (Table 45-8), together accounting for 70% of injuries associated with airway-trauma claims. The pharynx and esophagus were more likely to be the site of injury in claims associated with difficult intubation (39%) than claims in which intubation apparently proceeded in a routine manner (18%). In contrast, there was no statistically significant difference between these two groups for the incidence of laryngeal injury. Pharyngeal and esophageal injuries most commonly consisted of

Table 45-7. Low-frequency adverse respiratory events

Type of claim	n (% of total)	Death (%)	Brain damage (%)	Payment frequency (%)	Median payment ($)
Airway trauma	97 (4.7)	12	0	60	22,000
Pneumothorax	67 (3.3)	24	10	63	19,000
Airway obstruction	56 (2.7)	64	23	63	300,000
Aspiration	56 (2.7)	45	5	66	60,000
Bronchospasm	40 (1.9)	70	18	53	218,000
All infrequent respiratory*	300 (14.6)	37†‡	10†	60†‡	60,000†
Other respiratory	462 (22.6)	70	23	75	233,000
All nonrespiratory	1284 (63.7)	22	9	59	40,000

*More than one adverse respiratory event occurred in 16 claims, so the total number of claims for 316 events is 300. $P \leq .01$ compared to other respiratory claims (†) or nonrespiratory claims (‡). n = 2046. ASA Closed Claims Database 1991. Adapted from Cheney FW, Posner KL, Caplan RA et al: *Anesthesiology* 75:932, 1991.

Table 45-8. Sites of airway trauma

Location of injury	Difficult intubation present (n = 41)	Difficult intubation absent (n = 56)
	% associated with airway trauma	
Larynx	35	50
Pharynx or esophagus	39*	17
Nasopharynx, nose	4	8
Temporomandibular joint	0**	12
Mouth, gums, or lips	13	10
Trachea	11	3

Distribution of airway-trauma sites, based on the presence or absence of concomitant difficult intubation. * $P \leq .05$. ** $P \leq .01$. n = 2046. ASA Closed Claims Database 1991. Adapted from Cheney FW, Posner KL, Caplan RA et al: *Anesthesiology* 75:932, 1991.

lacerations or perforations leading to mediastinitis or mediastinal abscess. The most common laryngeal injuries in both groups included vocal-cord paralysis (14 cases), arytenoid dislocation (4 cases), and granuloma (2 cases). Of the 56 cases (58%) in which intubation was routine, the injury was believed to be due to endotracheal intubation in 43 cases. Of the 13 cases in the routine intubation group in which endotracheal intubation played no role, 8 were due to passage of a nasogastric tube and 2 to a nasal or oral airway. Three were not classified. None of the temporomandibular-joint injuries was associated with difficult intubation.

These claims provide several useful insights. Circumstances surrounding difficult intubation clearly put the tissues of the pharynx and esophagus at risk. The clinical implication is that patients in whom endotracheal intubation has been difficult should be observed for, or told to watch for, the development of signs and symptoms of pharyngeal abscess or mediastinitis. Since soft-tissue infections may develop slowly over a period of days, an apparent lack of complications in the first few hours after

surgery should not be regarded as a definitive outcome in patients who have experienced difficult intubation. This is especially important to remember in the ambulatory surgery setting.

Although it is easy to understand how difficult intubation may lead to trauma of the larynx, it is less apparent why laryngeal injuries appeared so frequently in the routine intubation group. The reason for vocal-cord paralysis, granuloma, and arytenoid dislocation in the routine intubation group was not apparent from the data available in the claim file. Similarly, it is curious that temporomandibular-joint injury was present only in the routine intubation group. One might expect that temporomandibular-joint injury would be more commonly associated with difficult intubation, in which forces applied to the jaw during airway manipulation and laryngoscopy might be more intense or prolonged than those encountered during routine intubation. These observations suggest that many injuries to the larynx and temporomandibular joint may be related to predisposing factors or underlying patient characteristics that we do not yet understand. Kroll et al. observed a similar phenomenon in a review of closed claims for peripheral nerve injuries.[23]

3. Pneumothorax

Pneumothorax was the second most common type of low-frequency airway event. Clinical activities that were not directly or clearly related to airway management were associated with 43 of the 67 claims for pneumothorax (64%; Table 45-9). In particular, five types of nerve blocks (supraclavicular, intercostal, stellate ganglion, interscalene, and suprascapular) were responsible for 40% of pneumothorax claims. Airway instrumentation was associated with pneumothorax in 19% of cases. The actual mechanism of pneumothorax was not anatomically proven in most cases, but was usually attributed to laryngoscopy, endotracheal-tube placement, or bronchoscopy on the basis of clinical events and reviewer

Table 45-9. Clinical factors associated with pneumothorax claims

Clinical factor	Claims	% of total
Airway related		
Airway instrumentation	13	19
Barotrauma	11	16
Non–airway related		
Regional block	27	40
Central line	5	7
Spontaneous/unknown	5	7
Other	6	9
Total	67	100

n = 2046. ASA Closed Claims Database 1991. Adapted from Cheney FW, Posner KL, Caplan RA et al: *Anesthesiology* 75:932, 1991.

judgments. Barotrauma was the cause of pneumothorax in 11 claims (16%), mostly arising from obstruction of the expiratory limb of a mechanical ventilator or the use of excessive tidal volumes (seven cases).

A notable feature of pneumothorax claims was the marked disparity in outcome between events associated with airway instrumentation and events arising from nerve blocks and central-line placement. In the subset of 24 claims involving airway instrumentation, the outcome in 16 cases (67%) was death or permanent brain damage. In contrast, there were no instances of death or brain damage in the 16 cases of pneumothorax that arose after nerve blocks or central-line placement. We speculate that this difference may be due at least in part to the more rapid compromise of respiratory and circulatory function that occurs under conditions of mechanical ventilation and positive-pressure gas delivery. Not surprisingly, the median payment for pneumothorax associated with nerve-block or central-line placement was only $6,000, while the median payment for cases associated with airway instrumentation was $75,000.

4. Airway obstruction

Airway obstruction accounted for 56 claims or approximately 3% of the database. Most cases (89%) occurred during general anesthesia. Obstruction was attributed to an upper-airway site in 39 claims (70%), although an exact cause or site was identifiable in only half of these claims. Laryngospasm was the most common cause of upper-airway obstruction, accounting for 11 (28%) of 39 cases. Other causes of upper-airway obstruction included foreign body (four cases), laryngeal polyps (two cases), laryngeal edema (one case), and pharyngeal hematoma (one case). In 10 cases of upper-airway obstruction, emergency tracheostomy was performed. Causes of lower-airway obstruction (21% of claims) included blood clots or mucous plugs in the tracheal lumen, or external compression due to medi-

astinal tumor masses or blood. Endotracheal-tube obstruction accounted for 9% of cases and was attributed to blood clots in the lumen of the endotracheal tube or kinking of the tube itself. Other factors associated with claims for airway obstruction included concurrent difficult intubation (17 cases, 30%), operation on the airway (13 cases, 23%), and pediatric age group (10 cases, 18%). The outcome in almost all claims for airway obstruction (87%) was death or brain damage.

5. Aspiration

Claims for aspiration accounted for 3% of the database (56 cases). Almost all cases (95%) occurred in patients who received general anesthesia. The aspirated material was gastric contents in 88% of cases; other cases involved aspiration of blood, pus, or teeth. Approximately one third (34%) of aspirations took place during anesthetic induction just prior to endotracheal intubation (34%). In six of these cases, aspiration occurred during a rapid-sequence induction; in another six, the aspiration occurred under circumstances in which the reviewer believed that a rapid-sequence induction was indicated but not used. Another one third of aspiration cases (36%) took place during the maintenance phase of mask general anesthetic. Of note, only two cases occurred (4%) during the maintenance phase of general endotracheal anesthesia. Aspiration occurred in one of these cases when the endotracheal tube was removed to facilitate the passage of a nasogastric tube. In the other case, aspiration occurred while an endotracheal tube with a leaking cuff was being replaced with a new tube. The remaining cases took place during emergence from anesthesia (18%).

Two clinical factors—pregnancy and emergency surgical status—were particularly prevalent in claims for aspiration. Obstetrical patients account for 12% of the overall database, but represent 29% of all aspiration claims ($P \le .05$). Emergency-surgery patients account for 19% of the database, but represent 45% of all aspiration claims ($P \le .01$). It is also noteworthy that 23% of aspiration claims involved a problem with airway management such as difficult intubation (nine cases) or esophageal intubation (four cases). This relationship was previously reported by Olsson and colleagues.[24]

Overall, aspiration accounted for only 3% of claims in the database. In terms of contemporary experience, this is consistent with the observation by Warner and colleagues[25] that the incidence of aspiration in more than 200,000 patients who underwent elective and emergency surgery between 1985 and 1991 was very low (1 in 3216). These observations suggest that current strategies to prevent aspiration in the United States are generally successful. It is interesting to contrast this picture with the findings of Tiret and colleagues' prospective survey[9] of anesthesia complications in

France between 1972 and 1982. This large study identified 163 complications that were totally attributable to anesthesia. Of these, aspiration accounted for 17% of all complications and 30% of complications that were specifically related to respiratory events. Moreover, almost 50% of cases in the Tiret series occurred in the postanesthetic period. This high incidence of aspiration in the Tiret study has been attributed to a lack of post-anesthetic care units in French hospitals during the years encompassed by the study.[9]

6. Bronchospasm

Adverse outcomes arising from bronchospasm accounted for 40 claims, or almost 2% of the database. Most of these claims (80%) occurred during the administration of general anesthesia as the primary anesthetic technique. Nearly half (48%) of the patients had a medical history that included at least one of the following; asthma, chronic obstructive pulmonary disease, or smoking. In cases involving the administration of general anesthesia, the first occurrence of bronchospasm was more often at the time of intubation (69%) than during maintenance (25%) or emergence (6%).

Twenty percent of claims for bronchospasm were associated with the conduct of regional anesthesia. In most of these cases, bronchospasm occurred during cesarian section when endotracheal intubation was required for management of a failed block or a high block in a patient with a history of asthma. These cases illustrate the concept that regional anesthesia does not in itself obviate the risk associated with intraoperative management of reactive airway disease. In particular, the risk of bronchospasm may be especially pronounced in this setting because relatively modest doses of intravenous agents are often employed in an effort to minimize anesthetic effects on the fetus.

Bronchospasm claims were also notable in cases that involved a difficult differential diagnosis. The claims files indicated that clinicians had difficulty distinguishing between bronchospasm and the presence of esophageal intubation (six cases) or pneumothorax (four cases). End-tidal carbon dioxide concentration was not used in any of the six cases in which the failure to make a correct and timely differential diagnosis between esophageal intubation and bronchospasm led to an adverse outcome. Since end-tidal carbon dioxide is now an ASA standard for verification of endotracheal-tube placement, it is possible that this pathway of injury will become less common. However, it is important to recognize that failure to differentiate between bronchospasm and esophageal intubation may still occur in cases in which bronchospasm is so severe that ventilation is impossible and carbon dioxide cannot reach the detector in clinically useful amounts. In this circumstance, fiberoptic bronchoscopy might prove helpful.

C. EMERGING TRENDS FROM THE ASA CLOSED CLAIMS PROJECT

The database of the closed claims project is now sufficiently large that it can be studied for evidence of changing trends in the overall distribution of adverse events and outcomes. In doing so, two key limitations must be emphasized. First, these data cannot be used to generate any general estimates of risk. This limitation arises from a lack of denominator data, a probable bias toward severe outcomes, and partial reliance on the observations of direct participants. Second, the resolution of a claim is a lengthy process. Typically, this leads to a delay of about five years between the occurrence of a claim and its entry into the database. Thus the most recent trends (which are usually of greatest interest) must be viewed as especially tentative because they may show considerable change as additional claims are resolved and processed.

In 1994 a preliminary examination of trends was conducted.[26] At that point the database consisted of more than 3000 claims drawn from 34 U.S. insurance organizations. Two major trends were evident. First, the overall incidence of adverse respiratory events was declining (Fig. 45-2). During the earliest interval between 1975 and 1979, 35% of claims arose from respiratory system events. This percentage decreased to 28% between 1980 and 1984, and further decreased to 17% in the group of claims occurring from 1990 onward. The second trend involved the severity of injury. This, too, showed a general decrease, and was specifically characterized by a declining incidence of claims for death and brain damage (Fig. 45-3). Between 1975 and 1979, for example, 56% of claims involved death or brain damage. In contrast, death or brain damage accounts for only 33% of claims that have thus far occurred in the decade of the 1990s. It is tempting to infer that the overall decline in adverse respiratory events is linked to the decline in death and brain damage, but the current limitations of the closed-claims database have yet to permit us to establish this relationship in a rigorous way.

Nonetheless, some tentative associations can be discerned. In recent years, there have been several changes in monitoring and clinical practice that may have had an impact on adverse respiratory events. Pulse oximetry and end-tidal capnometry have been widely available since the mid-1980s. Moreover, the ASA Standards for Basic Intra-Operative Monitoring specify the use of pulse oximetry for basic intraoperative monitoring (as of January 1, 1990) and end-tidal CO_2 for verification of endotracheal intubation (as of January 1, 1991).

Is the presence of these monitors reflected in the pattern of liability for closed claims? This question was explored in 1992 when the overall database contained

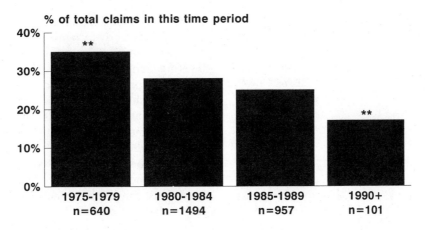

Fig. 45-2. Claims for respiratory system damaging events as proportion of all claims in 1994 ASA Closed Claims Database by five-year periods. Time periods n do not sum to N because some claims in database (prior to 1975) have no recorded occurrence date. (Adapted from Cheney FW: *American Society of Anesthesiologists Newsletter* 58(6):7, June 1994.)

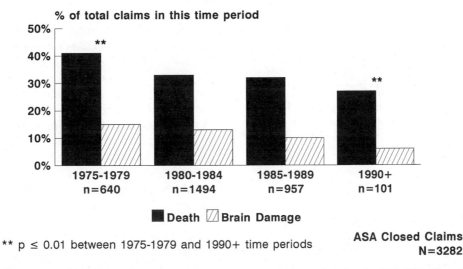

Fig. 45-3. Claims for death and brain damage as proportion of all claims in 1994 ASA Closed Claims Database by five-year periods. (Adapted from Cheney FW: *American Society of Anesthesiologists Newsletter* 58(6):7, June 1994.)

2500 cases.[27] Claims involving adverse events that arose intraoperatively during general anesthesia were studied (1237 cases). This type of case was selected to focus on the setting in which one might expect the greatest benefit from use of pulse oximetry and capnography. Overall, neither Sao_2 or $ETco_2$ were monitored in 1132 of 1237 claims (91%). Sao_2 alone was monitored in 60 claims, $ETco_2$ alone was monitored in 20 claims, and both Sao_2 and $ETco_2$ were monitored in 25 claims. As shown in Table 45-10, respiratory-system events constituted 44% of claims when neither monitor was used, as opposed to 28% to 35% of claims when one or both monitors was present.

A focused examination of the three most common adverse respiratory events (inadequate ventilation, esophageal intubation, and difficult intubation) revealed a further association. In aggregate, these outcomes constituted 536 cases, or 43% of the 1132 claims. All three adverse outcomes occurred with approximately equal frequency when neither Sao_2 or $ETco_2$ was present, and the three adverse outcomes were also represented when $ETco_2$ was used alone (Table 45-11). However, claims for inadequate ventilation were absent in cases where Sao_2 was used alone or in combination with $ETco_2$. This observation suggests that most claims attributed to inadequate *ventilation* probably have a

Table 45-10. Overview of respiratory system damaging events during general anesthesia

Monitors used	% respiratory system–damaging events
No SpO_2/no $ETCO_2$	44
SpO_2 only	35
$ETCO_2$ only	35
SpO_2 and $ETCO_2$	28

Table shows percent of claims in each monitoring group that involved respiratory system damaging events. Only intraoperative general-anesthesia claims (1237 cases) were studied. n = 2500. ASA Closed Claims Database 1992. Adapted from Cheney FW: *American Society of Anesthesiologists Newsletter* 56(6):6, June 1992.

Table 45-11. Most common respiratory system damaging events during general anesthesia

Monitors used	Inadequate ventilation (%)	Esophageal intubation (%)	Difficult intubation (%)
No SpO_2/no $ETCO_2$	28	23	22
SpO_2 only	0*	33	33
$ETCO_2$ only	14	29	14
SpO_2 and $ETCO_2$	0	57	14

Percent of claims in each monitoring group that involved inadequate ventilation, esophageal intubation, or difficult intubation. Only intraoperative general anesthesia claims (n = 1237) were studied. *$P \le .01$ compared to no SpO_2/no $ETCO_2$. n = 2518. ASA Closed Claims Database 1992. Adapted from Cheney FW: *American Society of Anesthesiologists Newsletter* 56(6):6, June 1992.

more specific cause—inadequate *oxygenation*. This group of cases also provides an important lesson about the limitations of monitoring. In most of the cases where pulse oximetry or capnography was available either alone or in combination, the adverse outcome was associated with human factors such as failure to use the monitor, misinterpretation of monitor data, or turning off the audible alarm signal.

As mentioned previously, evidence-based guidelines for management of the difficult airway have recently been developed by the American Society of Anesthesiologists.[21] The impact of this set of guidelines on claims involving difficult airway management is now under study in the closed-claims project. At present, it is too early to explore this data for any patterns.

Clinicians often worry that the recent proliferation of practice guidelines will lead to a general increase in liability. It is important to remember that modern-day, evidence-based guidelines have a relatively flexible place in medical practice that differs from standards. Standards are typically used for straightforward aspects of care that command high levels of agreement and acceptance. Noncompliance implies an action that is outside of a clearly recognized norm; in some instances, such actions may be accompanied by sanctions. Guidelines are employed for more complex aspects of care that cannot be precisely codified and accepted in a near-uniform fashion. Thus guidelines are intended as *recommendations* that can assist the practitioner and the patient in making decisions about health care. Guidelines may be accepted, modified, or even rejected according to specific clinical needs and constraints. This means that not following a guideline, under some clinical conditions, can still be a decision that is consistent with reasonable and prudent practice.

III. CONCLUSION

The database of the ASA Closed Claims Project indicates that adverse events involving the respiratory system constitute the single largest source of liability in anesthetic practice. These events represent a particularly urgent target for research and preventive strategies because they are characterized by a high frequency of severe outcomes and costly payments.

Inadequate ventilation, esophageal intubation, and difficult intubation account for nearly three fourths of all adverse respiratory events. Emerging trends suggest that inadequate oxygenation plays a major role in claims attributed to inadequate ventilation. The widespread use of pulse oximetry may minimize this source of liability. Claims for difficult intubation are characterized by a high rate of misdiagnosis of endotracheal intubation. Misdiagnosis seems to arise from reliance on indirect tests of endotracheal intubation, particularly breath sound auscultation. The use of capnography may facilitate the recognition of incorrect placement and reduce the severity of outcomes associated with delayed recognition of esophageal intubation.

The in-depth analysis of low-frequency respiratory events also provides valuable lessons. Complications associated with airway trauma may not manifest in the immediate postoperative period. This suggests that explicit follow-up plans and communication are particularly important for outpatients who have experienced airway-management difficulties. Severe bronchospasm is not a common cause of claims in the overall database, but the desire to minimize fetal exposure to anesthetic agents may be a factor leading to a relatively high incidence of bronchospasm claims in obstetrical patients receiving general anesthesia for cesarian section.

Overall, reviewers have found that most claims involving adverse respiratory events might have been prevented by the use of pulse oximetry and capnography (either alone or in combination). Since most claims took place before the widespread use of these two monitors, it is difficult to know if this perception is accurate in its own right, or a reflection of wishful hindsight and unrealistic expectations. Tentative support for a preventive role comes from the observation that adverse respiratory events constitute a decreasing proportion of database claims, particularly for claims occurring in the 1990s.

ACKNOWLEDGMENTS

The Closed Claims Project is supported by funds from the American Society of Anesthesiologists. The project committee gratefully acknowledges the contributions of insurance companies who have granted access to closed-claims files and the members of the American Society of Anesthesiologists who have served as reviewers of closed claims and participants in studies of peer review.

REFERENCES

1. Ruth HS, Haugen FP, Grove DD: Anesthesia Study Commission: findings of eleven years' activity, *JAMA* 135:881, 1947.
2. Beecher HK, Todd DP: A study of the deaths associated with anesthesia and surgery based on a study of 599,548 anesthesias in ten institutions, 1948-1952, inclusive, *Ann Surg* 140:2, 1954.
3. Utting JE, Gray TC, Shelly FC: Human misadventure in anaesthesia, *Can Anaesth Soc J* 26:472, 1979.
4. Cooper JB, Newbower RS, Long CH et al: Preventable anesthetic mishaps: a study of human factors, *Anesthesiology* 49:399, 1978.
5. Russell WJ, Webb RK, Van Der Walt JH et al: Problems with ventilation: an analysis of 2000 incident reports, *Anaesth Intensive Care* 21:617, 1993.
6. Harrison GC: Death attributable to anaesthesia: a ten-year survey, 1967-1976, *Br J Anaesth* 50:1041, 1978.
7. Holland R: Anaesthesia-related mortality in Australia, *Int Anesthesiol Clin* 22:61, 1984.
8. Keenan RL, Boyan CP: Cardiac arrest due to anesthesia: a study of incidence and causes, *JAMA* 253:2373, 1985.
9. Tiret L, Desmonts JM, Hatton F et al: Complications associated with anaesthesia: a prospective survey in France, *Can Anaesth Soc J* 33:336, 1986.
10. Brennan TA, Leape LL, Laird NM et al: Incidence of adverse events and negligence in hospitalized patients: results of the Harvard Medical Practice Study I, *N Engl J Med* 324:370, 1991.
11. Hiatt HH, Barnes BA, Brennan TA et al: A study of medical injury and medical malpractice: an overview, *N Engl J Med* 321:480, 1989.
12. Cheney FW, Posner K, Caplan RA et al: Standard of care and anesthesia liability, *JAMA* 261:1599, 1989.
13. Posner KL, Sampson PD, Caplan RA et al: Measuring interrater reliability among multiple raters: an example of methods for nominal data, *Stat Med* 9:1103, 1990.
14. Caplan RA, Posner KL, Ward RJ et al: Adverse respiratory events in anesthesia: a closed claims analysis, *Anesthesiology* 72:828, 1990.
15. Comroe JH Jr, Botelho S: The unreliability of cyanosis in the recognition of arterial anoxemia, *Am J Med Sci* 214:1, 1947.
16. Coté CJ, Goldstein EA, Coté MA et al: A single-blind study of pulse oximetry in children, *Anesthesiology* 68:184, 1988.
17. Heller ML, Watson TR Jr: Polarographic study of arterial oxygenation during apnea in man, *N Engl J Med* 264:326, 1961.
18. Birmingham PK, Cheney FW, Ward RJ: Esophageal intubation: a review of detection techniques, *Anesth Analg* 65:886, 1986.
19. Gaba DM, Maxwell M, DeAnda A: Anesthetic mishaps: breaking the chain of accident evolution, *Anesthesiology* 66:670, 1987.
20. Gaba DM: Human error in anesthetic mishaps, *Int Anesthesiol Clin* 27:137, 1989.
21. American Society of Anesthesiologists: Practice Guidelines for management of the difficult airway: a report by the American Society of Anesthesiologists Task Force on Management of the Difficult Airway, *Anesthesiology* 78:597, 1993.
22. Cheney FW, Posner KL, Caplan RA: Adverse respiratory events infrequently leading to malpractice suits: a closed claims analysis, *Anesthesiology* 75:932, 1991.
23. Kroll DA, Caplan RA, Posner K et al: Nerve injury associated with anesthesia, *Anesthesiology* 73:202, 1990.
24. Olsson GL, Hallen B, Hambraeus-Jonzon K: Aspiration during anaesthesia: a computer-aided study of 185,358 anaesthetics, *Acta Anaesthesiol Scand* 30:84, 1986.
25. Warner MA, Warner ME, Weber JG: Clinical significance of pulmonary aspiration during the perioperative period, *Anesthesiology* 78:56, 1993.
26. Cheney FW: Committee on Professional Liability: overview, *American Society of Anesthesiologists Newsletter* 58(6):7, June 1994.
27. Cheney FW: ASA Closed Claims Project progress report: the effect of pulse oximetry and end-tidal CO_2 monitoring on adverse respiratory events, *American Society of Anesthesiologists Newsletter* 56(6):6, June 1992.

INDEX

Page numbers in *italics* indicate illustrations; page numbers followed by a *t* indicate a table.